Essentials of Ear, Nose and Throat

Essentials of Ear, Nose and Throat

Mohan Bansal MS PhD FICS FACS
Guest Professor ENT, Clinical College of Dali University,
Dali Yunnan, PR China
Consultant Otolaryngologist Head and Neck Surgeon
Anand, Gujarat

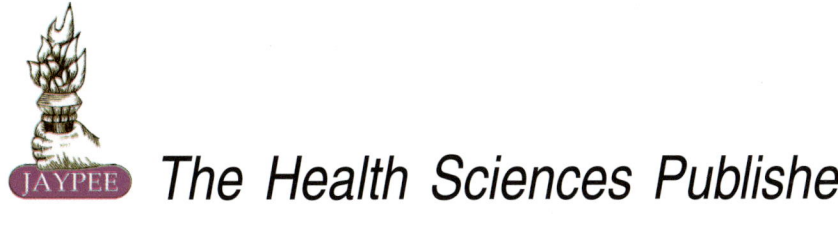

The Health Sciences Publisher
New Delhi | London | Philadelphia | Panama

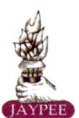
Jaypee Brothers Medical Publishers (P) Ltd

Headquarters
Jaypee Brothers Medical Publishers (P) Ltd
4838/24, Ansari Road, Daryaganj
New Delhi 110 002, India
Phone: +91-11-43574357
Fax: +91-11-43574314
Email: jaypee@jaypeebrothers.com

Overseas Offices

J.P. Medical Ltd
83 Victoria Street, London
SW1H 0HW (UK)
Phone: +44-2031708910
Fax: +02-03-0086180
Email: info@jpmedpub.com

Jaypee Medical Inc.
The Bourse
325 Chestnut Street, Suite 412
Philadelphia, PA 19106, USA
Phone: +1 267-519-9789
Email: joe.rusko@jaypeebrothers.com

Jaypee Brothers Medical Publishers (P) Ltd
Bhotahity, Kathmandu, Nepal
Phone: +977-9741283608
Email: kathmandu@jaypeebrothers.com

Jaypee-Highlights Medical Publishers Inc.
City of Knowledge, Bld. 237, Clayton
Panama City, Panama
Phone: +1 507-301-0496
Fax: +1 507-301-0499
Email: cservice@jphmedical.com

Jaypee Brothers Medical Publishers (P) Ltd
17/1-B Babar Road, Block-B, Shaymali
Mohammadpur, Dhaka-1207
Bangladesh
Mobile: +08801912003485
Email: jaypeedhaka@gmail.com

Website: www.jaypeebrothers.com
Website: www.jaypeedigital.com

© 2016, Jaypee Brothers Medical Publishers

The views and opinions expressed in this book are solely those of the original contributor(s)/author(s) and do not necessarily represent those of editor(s) of the book.

All rights reserved. No part of this publication may be reproduced, stored or transmitted in any form or by any means, electronic, mechanical, photocopying, recording or otherwise, without the prior permission in writing of the publishers.

All brand names and product names used in this book are trade names, service marks, trademarks or registered trademarks of their respective owners. The publisher is not associated with any product or vendor mentioned in this book.

Medical knowledge and practice change constantly. This book is designed to provide accurate, authoritative information about the subject matter in question. However, readers are advised to check the most current information available on procedures included and check information from the manufacturer of each product to be administered, to verify the recommended dose, formula, method and duration of administration, adverse effects and contraindications. It is the responsibility of the practitioner to take all appropriate safety precautions. Neither the publisher nor the author(s)/editor(s) assume any liability for any injury and/or damage to persons or property arising from or related to use of material in this book.

This book is sold on the understanding that the publisher is not engaged in providing professional medical services. If such advice or services are required, the services of a competent medical professional should be sought.

Every effort has been made where necessary to contact holders of copyright to obtain permission to reproduce copyright material. If any have been inadvertently overlooked, the publisher will be pleased to make the necessary arrangements at the first opportunity.

Inquiries for bulk sales may be solicited at: jaypee@jaypeebrothers.com

Essentials of Ear, Nose and Throat

First Edition: **2016**

ISBN: 978-93-5152-331-4

Printed at Sanat Printers

By always praising the all pervading being, who is without beginning and without end, who is the supreme Lord of all the worlds, and who is the eternal controller of the universe, one gets beyond all grief.

Om. From the unreal, lead me to the real. From darkness, lead me to light. From death, lead me to immortality.

Om. O God, may we hear with our ears what is auspicious. O Ye adorable ones, may we see with our eyes what is auspicious. May we sing praises to Ye and enjoy with strong limbs and body, the life allotted to us by the God. "Om Peace, Peace, Peace".

Om. May almighty God protect us both, the preceptor and the disciple. May he nourish us both. May we work together with great energy. May our study be vigorous and fruitful. May we not hate each other "Om Peace, Peace, Peace".

We offer our salutations to thee, the giver of happiness and well-being. We offer our salutations to thee, the promoter of good and auspiciousness. We offer our salutations to thee, the bestower of bliss and still greater bliss.

O Lord, thou art the embodiment of infinite energy; do thou fill me with energy. Thou art the embodiment of infinite virility; do thou endow me with virility. Thou art the embodiment of infinite strength; do thou bestow strength upon me. Thou art the embodiment of infinite power; do thou grant power unto me. Thou art the embodiment of infinite courage; do thou inspire me with courage. Thou art the embodiment of infinite fortitude; do thou steel me with fortitude.

May I be able to look upon all beings with the eye of a friend. May we look upon one another with the eye of a friend.

PREFACE

As long as I live I learn
Bhagwan Shri Ramakrishna Dev

"Essentials of Ear, Nose and Throat" is intended to serve medical students in the diagnosis and management of diseases of ear, nose, throat, head and neck region. This 'all in one' up-to-date textbook present the essential material in a clear, direct manner, anticipating questions that occur during examination and providing specific information to allow an individualized approach to diagnosis and treatment. The students will find boxes, tables, flow charts, line diagrams and photos that enhance learning. The book is comprehensive and of broader scope and would be useful for even residents and practitioners. The brevity, conciseness, readable format and easy accessibility of key information will facilitate students' learning and memorizing. The socratic approach of posing questions is followed throughout the book. Each chapter begins with the Specific Learning Objectives that consists of the questions which students are supposed to answer after going through the chapter. The chapters end with the Self-Evaluation Exercises that offers MCQs, filling the blanks, matching and true and false sentences. Each chapter has highlighted key points for the quick revision of the students. At the end of some of the chapters are given the additional Pearls and Nuggets and Problem-oriented Cases, which will be of immense use and interest to the students.

I would like to acknowledge my parents, the late Ramchandra Bansal and Kalawati Devi Bansal as I owe a lot to them. I appreciate the patience and understanding of my wife Sushma and kids Mohit, Tejal, Astha and Agastyaa, which are essential for the completion of such project. I wish to thank all the faculties who spared their valuable time in reviewing the chapters. The process of learning is truly life-long. Creating this textbook allowed me to continue to become invigorated and inspired by ENT. I hope that students will find my efforts useful and will inform me regarding further improvements that I can make in the next edition.

Mohan Bansal
mohanbansal@yahoo.com

ACKNOWLEDGMENTS

It has been a pleasure to work with Mr Jitendar P Vij (Group Chairman) and Mr Ankit Vij (Group President), who have provided excellent leadership and added tremendously to the production of this book. I would like to acknowledge the collaboration of all the reviewers for their excellent scientific input. I also thank the dedicated editorial and production team at Jaypee Brothers Medical Publishers especially Ms Sunita Katla and Ms Nitasha Arora. I would also like to acknowledge the support of my following colleagues: Alpesh Fefar (Rajkot), Amit Goyal (Jodhpur), Arvind Sangavi (Raichur), Chandrashekharayya (Bagalkot), Chetan Ghorpade (Kolhapur), Hiren Soni (Vadodara); L Sudarshan Reddy (Nizamabad), Manish Tyagi (Udaipur), Mayur Ingale (Pune), ND Zingade (Belgaum), Navneet Agarwal (Jodhpur), Parvinderjit Singh Kohli (Patiala), Pawan Singhal (Jaipur), Priyanka Singla (Bhatinda), Rahul Modi (Mumbai), Rakesh Srivastava (Lucknow), Sandeep Bansal (Chandigarh), Saurabh Agarwal (Mumbai), Saurav Sarkar (Bhubaneshwar), Shailendra Inamdar (Kenya), Shashidhar Suligavi (Bagalkot); Sudipta Chandra (Kolkata), Suhail Amin Patigaroo (Srinagar), Sunita Chapola Shukla (Mumbai), Vaibhav Kuchhal (Haldwani), Vinod Felix (Thiruvananthapuram) and Vishal Dave (Ahmedabad).

REVIEWERS

Following senior faculties mostly Professors ENT were contacted for emailing the chapters. Majority of them sent their valuable inputs. Their insightful suggestions for improvement helped me maintain book's accuracy and clarity. I am extremely grateful to them. The chapters were modified significantly after getting the feedbacks from them, other colleagues and students. To make the textbook 'All-in-one' and students' friendly, sections of Specific Learning Objectives, Self-evaluation Exercises, Problem-oriented Cases and additional Pearls and Nuggets were introduced in the chapters.

- AK Gupta, HOD, Geetanjali MC, Udaipur
- AS Harugop, JNMC, Belgaum
- Achal Gulati, HOD and Director, MAMC, New Delhi
- Ahilasamy, MMC, Chennai
- Aniece Chowdary, HOD, MC, Lucknow
- Anil Kumar Jain, HOD, Chirayu MC, Bhopal
- Arjun Dass, HOD, GMC, Chandigarh
- Arun Kumar Agarwal, Director-Professor and Ex-Dean, MAMC, New Delhi
- Arun Patel, JMC, Jhalawar
- Ashish Katarkar, HOD, GMERS, Gandhinagar
- Ashish Varghese, CMC, Ludhiana
- Atul Kansara, HOD, AMC MET MC, Ahmedabad
- Avadh Chouhan, Peoples MC, Bhopal
- B Viswanatha, Bangalore MC, Bangalore
- Bela Prajapati, BJMC, Ahmedabad
- Bikash Lal Shrestha, KUH, Kavre, Nepal
- CS Gohil, HOD, Shardaben MC, Ahmedabad
- Chandra Shekhar, HOD, NMC, Patna
- Chetana S Naik, SK Navale MC, Pune
- D Barman, HOD, Burdwan MC, Midnapore
- Dalbir Singh, PIMS, Jalandhar
- Deep Chand, HOD, SPMC, Bikaner
- Devendra M Mahore, HOD, GMC, Miraj
- Dharmendra Kumar, SN MC, Agra
- G Shankar, HOD, VIMS Cant, Bellary
- GS Renukananda, JJM MC, Davangere
- Gangadhara Somayaji, HOD, YMC, Mangalore
- Girish Mishra, HOD, PSMC, Anand
- HS Bhuie, HOD, RNT MC, Udaipur
- H Priyosakhi Devi, HOD, RIMS, Imphal

Acknowledgments

- Hardik Shah, Sola MC, Ahmedabad
- Hari Mohan Sharma, Dean, Jhalawar MC, Jhalawar
- Haritosh Velankar, DYP MC, Navi Mumbai
- HC Taneja, UCMS, New Delhi
- Hemant Chopra, HOD, DMC, Ludhiana
- Ishwar Singh, MAMC, New Delhi
- J Paul, ASCMS, Jammu
- JK Sharma, Dean, RD Gardi MC, Ujjain
- JC Passey, HOD, MAMC, New Delhi
- Jaymain Contractor, HOD, GMC, Surat
- Janakiraman TN, Trichy
- Jawahar Talsania, Ex HOD, VS NHLMC, Ahmedabad
- Jyoti Dabholkar, HOD, Seth GSMC, Mumbai
- KB Mothilal, HOD, KFMSR, Coimbatore
- K Srinivasan, Saveetha MC, Thandalam, Kanchipuram
- KS Gangadhar, HOD, SIMS, Shimoga
- KV Lokanath, HOD, JJMMC, Davangere
- Karan Sharma, HOD, GMC, Amritsar
- Kiran J Shinde, HOD, SKN MC, Pune
- Kiran Naik, ASRC, BG Nagar, Nagamangala, Mandya
- Kishore Chandra Prasad, Kasturba MC, Manipal
- Lathadevi, BM Patil MC, Bijapur
- Madhavi Raibagkar, HOD, VS NHL MC, Ahmedabad
- Mangal Singh, HOD, MLN MC, Allahabad
- Manish R Mehta, HOD, PDU MC, Rajkot
- Manish Munjal, DMC, Ludhiana
- Man Prakash Sharma, HOD, SMS MC, Jaipur
- Mohan V Jagade, HOD, Grant MC, Mumbai
- Muraleedharan A, Stanley GMC, Chennai,
- NH Kulkarni, BMP MC, Bijapur
- Nayanna Karodpati, DYP MC, Pune
- Neelima Gupta, UCMS, New Delhi
- Nirmal Kumar Soni, Ex HOD, SPMC, Bikaner
- Nitin Deosthale, NKPS IMSRC, Nagpur
- Nitin Nagarkar, Director, AIIMS, Raipur
- Nitish Baisakhiya, HOD, MMIMSR, Mullana, Ambala
- P Devan, AJIMS, Mangaluru
- P Karthikeyan, HOD, MGMC&RI, Pondicherry
- Pankaj Shah, HOD, CUS MC, Surendranagar
- Prakash Mishra, Ex HOD, SMSMC, Jaipur
- Pramod Jadhav, RIMS, Adilabad
- Pratibha Vyas, MGNIMS, Jaipur
- RK Mundra, MGMMC, Indore
- RS Mudhol, Vice-Principal, JNMC, Belgaum
- RA Patigaro, Era MC, Lucknow
- Rahul Kawatra, MC, Lucknow
- Rajesh Vishwakarma, HOD, BJMC, Ahmedabad
- Rajeshwary A, HOD, KSEMA, Mangaluru
- Rakesh Gupta, Hon Secretary AOI, Raipur, Chhattisgarh
- Raman Wadhera, PGIMS, Rohtak
- RC Deka, Ex Director, Dean of AIIMS, New Delhi
- Ranjan Aiyar, HOD, GMC, Vadodara
- Rashmi Goyal, HOD, MIMSR, Badwai, Bhopal
- Ravi D, MIMS, Mandya
- Ravinder Sharma, Subharti MC, Meerut
- Rohit Saxena, HOD, Sharda MC, Greater Noida
- Rupa Parikh, HOD, MMC, Surat
- SC Gupta, (Surg Cmde), Naval HQ
- SA Jagdish kumar, Dy VC Acad IMTU, Tanzania
- SF Hashmi, JNMC, AMU, Aligarh
- SP Srivastava, HOD, NIMS, Jaipur
- SS Bist, HIHT University, Dehradun
- Samir Joshi, BJMC, Pune
- Sandeep Kaushik, HOD, GMC, Kannauj, UP
- Sanjay Agarwal, President-Elect AOI, Indore
- Sanjeev Tadasadmath, HOD, KBNIMS, Gulbarga
- Sanjeev Mohanti, HOD, SRMC, Porur, Chennai
- Santosh UP, JJM MC, Davangere
- SP Dubey, Editor IJOHNS, AOI, Bhopal
- Saumindranath Bandyopadhyay, MC, Kolkata
- Saurabh Varshney, Sub Dean Acad, AIIMS, Rishikesh
- Sham Somani, Medical College, Latur
- Shenal Kothari, SAIMS MC, Indore
- Shreeya Kulkarni, VRP MC, Nasik
- Sivakumar, GMC, Vellore
- SK Pippal, Jt Dir Med Edu, Bhopal
- SP Aggarwal, HOD, CSMMU, Lucknow
- Sudhakar Vaidya, HOD, RD Gardi MC, Ujjain

- Surendra Gawarle, HOD, GMC, Nagpur
- Sushil Jha, HOD, GMC, Bhavnagar
- Suvamoy Chakraborty, HOD, SMIMS, Gangtok
- Swagata Khanna, Guwahati MC, Guwahati
- TS Chaudhary, People MC, Bhopal
- TS Anand, HOD and Director, LHMC, New Delhi
- UB Shah, Ex Dean, Sola GMERS, Ahmedabad
- V Phaniendra Kumar, Professor-Emeritus, Guntur
- VK Poorey, HOD, SS MC, Rewa, Madhya Pradesh
- VM Rao (Gp Capt), Mamata MC, Khammam
- VP Venkatachalam, HOD, VMMC, New Delhi
- Vadish Bhat, KS HMA, Mangaluru
- Venkataramanan R, SLN, Pondicherry
- Vijaya Ambulekar, HOD, GMC, Nanded, Maharashtra
- Vijayendra Honnurappa, JN MC, Bangaluru
- Viral A Chhaya, President AOI, Jamnagar
- Vishala Pandya, HOD, Gotri MC, Vadodara
- Vivek R Sinha (Col), Army Hospital, Delhi Cantt
- Yogesh Dabholkar, DYP MC, Nerul, Mumbai
- Yogesh Gajjar, HOD, GMERS, Patan, Gujarat
- Yojana Sharma, PSMC, Anand, Gujarat

CONTENTS

SECTION 1 — General

1. History and examination — 1
   - Introduction to otorhinolaryngology
   - History taking and Physical examination
   - General set-up

SECTION 2 — Ear

2. Anatomy of ear — 4
3. Physiology of hearing and vestibular system — 24
4. Otologic symptoms and examination — 30
   - Ear symptoms and examination
   - Otalgia (earache)
   - Otorrhea (ear discharge)
   - Ear polyp
   - Tinnitus
5. Hearing evaluation — 38
   - Audiology and acoustics
   - Types of hearing loss
   - Hearing evaluation
6. Conductive hearing loss and otosclerosis — 51
7. Sensorineural hearing loss — 59
8. Hearing impairment in infants and young children — 69
9. Hearing aids and cochlear implants — 76
10. Diseases of external ear and tympanic membrane — 85
11. Disorders of Eustachian tube — 95
12. Acute otitis media and otitis media with effusion — 101
13. Chronic suppurative otitis media and cholesteatoma — 109
14. Complications of suppurative otitis media — 117
15. Evaluation of vertigo — 130
16. Peripheral vestibular disorders — 136
    - Benign paroxysmal positional vertigo
    - Acute vestibular neuritis
    - Meniere's disease
    - Labyrinthitis
    - Perilymphatic fistula
17. Central vestibular disorders — 144
    - Migraine
    - Cerebrovascular strokes
    - Multiple sclerosis
    - Motion sickness
    - Psychophysiologic
    - Cervical vertigo
18. Facial nerve disorders — 148
19. Tumors of the ear and cerebellopontine angle — 160
    - Tumors of external ear
    - Tumors of middle ear and mastoid
    - Acoustic neuroma (Schwannoma)

SECTION 3 — Nose and Paranasal Sinuses

20. Anatomy and physiology of nose and paranasal sinuses — 169
21. Nasal symptoms and examination — 184
    - History taking and examination of nose
    - Smell
    - Nasal obstruction
    - Nasal valves disorders
    - Proptosis
    - Epistaxis (nosebleed)
22. Diseases of external nose and vestibule — 196

23. Infectious rhinosinusitis   200
    - Classification
    - Viral rhinosinusitis
    - Acute bacterial rhinosinusitis
    - Chronic rhinosinusitis
    - Complications of rhinosinusitis
    - Nasal polyps
24. Nasal manifestation of systemic diseases   213
    - Granulomatous conditions
    - Atrophic rhinitis
    - Rhinosporidiosis
    - Fungal sinusitis
25. Allergic and nonallergic (vasomotor) rhinitis   222
26. Nasal septum disorders   229
    - Diseases of nasal septum
    - Hypertrophied turbinates
    - Nasal synechia
    - Choanal atresia
27. Maxillofacial trauma   235
    - Maxillofacial injuries
    - Oroantral fistula
    - Cerebrospinal fluid rhinorrhea
    - Foreign body nose
    - Rhinolith
    - Nasal myiasis
28. Tumors of nose and paranasal sinuses   246

Section 4 Oral Cavity and Salivary Glands

29. Anatomy of oral cavity   255
30. Oral symptoms and examination   258
    - Oral cavity symptoms and examination
    - Evaluation of oral cancer patients
31. Oral mucosal lesions   262
    - Red/white lesions
    - Vesiculobullous/ulcerative lesions
    - Lesions of tongue
32. Disorders of salivary glands   271
    - Inflammatory disorders
    - Obstructive disorders (sialolithiasis)
    - Neoplasms
    - Xerostomia (Sjogren's syndrome)
    - Frey's syndrome (gustatory sweating)
33. Neoplasms of oral cavity   280
    - Benign tumors
    - Malignant tumors

Section 5 Pharynx and Esophagus

34. Anatomy and physiology of pharynx and esophagus   288
35. Pharyngeal symptoms and examination   297
    - Evaluation of pharynx
    - Evaluation of esophagus
    - Dysphagia
36. Pharyngitis and adenotonsillar disease   303
37. Obstructive sleep apnea   311
38. Tumors of nasopharynx   317
    - Juvenile nasopharyngeal angiofibroma
    - Nasopharyngeal carcinoma
    - Thornwaldt's disease
39. Tumors of oropharynx   325
    - Malignant tumors
    - Benign tumors
    - Parapharyngeal tumors
    - Stylalgia (Eagle's syndrome)
40. Tumors of hypopharynx   331
41. Disorders of esophagus   335

Section 6 Larynx, Trachea and Bronchus

42. Anatomy and physiology of larynx   346
43. Laryngeal symptoms and examination   355
    - Endoscopy examination and stroboscopy
    - Hoarseness of voice
    - Stridor

44. Infections of larynx 361
    - Acute infections of larynx
    - Chronic laryngitis
    - Edema of larynx
45. Benign tumors of larynx 368
    - Non-neoplastic
    - Neoplastic
    - Saccular swellings
46. Neurologic disorders of larynx 374
    - Laryngeal paralysis
    - Phonosurgery
47. Speech and voice disorders 379
48. Malignant tumors of larynx 382
49. Management of impaired airway 390
    - Tracheostomy
    - Cricothyrotomy
    - Percutaneous dilational tracheostomy
    - Congenital lesions of larynx
    - Foreign bodies of air passages
    - Laryngotracheal trauma

Section 7 Neck

50. Anatomy of neck 402
    - Lymph nodes of head and neck
    - Neck dissection
    - Thyroid and parathyroid glands
51. Cervical symptoms and examination 408
    - History and examination of neck and lymph nodes
    - History and examination of thyroid, hypothyroidism, hyperthyroidism and investigations
52. Neck masses 413
53. Neoplasms of thyroid 417
54. Deep neck infections 425
    - Pertinent anatomy
    - Head and neck space infections
    - Trismus

Section 8 Operative Procedures and Instruments

55. Middle ear and mastoid surgeries 432
    - Myringotomy and tympanostomy tubes
    - Simple cortical mastoidectomy
    - Radical mastoidectomy
    - Modified radical mastoidectomy
    - Tympanoplasty, myringoplasty and ossiculoplasty
56. Operations of nose and paranasal sinuses 441
    - Nasal endoscopy (sinuscopy)
    - Endoscopic sinus surgery
    - Antral puncture (lavage)
    - Inferior meatal antrostomy
    - Caldwell-Luc operation
    - Septoplasty
    - Submucous resection of nasal septum (SMR)
57. Adenotonsillectomy 450
58. Endoscopies 456
    - Direct laryngoscopy and microlaryngoscopy
    - Bronchoscopy rigid and flexible
    - Esophagoscopy rigid and flexible
59. Instruments 463
    - OPD instruments
    - Mastoid and earmicrosurgery
    - Operations of nose and paranasal sinuses
    - Mouth gags and retractors
    - Adenotonsillectomy and quinsy
    - Endoscopes
    - Tracheostomy and airway devices

Section 9: Related Disciplines

60. Diagnostic imaging — 475
    - Conventional radiology in ENT
    - CT anatomy of ear, nose, throat, head and neck
61. Radiotherapy and chemotherapy — 484
62. Laser surgery and cryosurgery — 492
    - Laser surgery
    - Photodynamic therapy
    - Radiofrequency surgery
    - Cryosurgery
    - Hyperbaric oxygen therapy
63. Human immunodeficiency virus infection — 498

Problem-oriented Cases — 168, 254, 354, 431
Pearls and Nuggets — 29, 58, 75, 129, 147, 221, 234, 261, 296, 324, 412, 424, 503

Index 505

Section 1: General

Chapter 1

History and Examination

⊙ Specific Learning Objectives
After going through the chapter, you should be able to answer the following questions:
- What do you mean by otorhinolaryngology?
- What are the subdivisions and subspecialization within the otorhinolaryngology?
- In which specific order would you like to perform the ear, nose, throat, head and neck examination so that you do not miss any component?
- How do you position the head mirror while performing the ENT examination?

OTORHINOLARYNGOLOGY

Otorhinolaryngology (oto: ear; rhino: nose; laryngo: larynx-throat), which is also called *otolaryngology*, is the specialty that deals with diseases of ear, nose, throat, head and neck region. Originally, the specialty was commonly called as **EENT** (eyes, ear, nose and throat) and included ophthalmology as well. But the two disciplines split many years ago because of the explosion of medical knowledge. In recent times, the specialty is usually called "otolaryngology–head and neck surgery". The doctor who deals with the specialty is called otolaryngologist/ear, nose, throat, head and neck surgeon.

Otolaryngology is both medical as well as surgical specialty. Approximately, only 10% of ENT patients require surgical interference. The otolaryngologist cares for all the age groups of patients such as children, adults and old.

The subdivisions which exist within the specialty are—otology, laryngology, rhinology and bronchoesophagology. The other subspecialties recognized in recent times because of information explosion are: pediatric otolaryngology, otolaryngologic allergy, rhinology and sinus surgery, facial plastic and reconstructive surgery and head and neck (oncology) surgery. Otology includes not only ear and temporal bone but also neurotology and skull base surgery. The recent developments have made some ENT surgeons to specialize in neurolaryngology, microvascular surgery, chemosensation (taste and smell disorders), audiology and speech disorders.

Evaluation of the patient with diseases of ENT requires patience and practice because the examiner will have to deal with the narrow and darker cavities of the ear, nose, pharynx and larynx, which have relatively complex anatomy and physiology.

HISTORY TAKING

On the basis of adequate history, many conditions can be accurately diagnosed. Table 1.1 shows the general scheme of case taking.
- ***Personal particulars:*** The name, age, sex, religion, social status, occupation and residential address of the patient are noted, as many a times they are quite relevant and associated with certain diseases.
- ***Chief complaints:*** The complaints, side of affection and their duration are recorded in a chronological order of their appearance. Table 1.2 shows the list of common complaints of ENT patients. It is very important to ask patient, "What made you to consult doctor?" The details of ear, nose and throat diseases are covered in the sections of ear, nose and paranasal sinuses, oral cavity and salivary glands, pharynx and esophagus, larynx, trachea and bronchus, and neck.

Table 1.1: General scheme of case taking

• **History taking**
  ▪ Personal particulars
  ▪ Chief complaints with duration
  ▪ History of present illness
  ▪ Past history
  ▪ Drug history
  ▪ History of allergy
  ▪ Personal history
  ▪ Family history
  ▪ History of immunization
• **Physical examination**
  ▪ General survey
  ▪ Local examination
  ▪ Systemic examination
	• **Provisional clinical diagnosis**
	• **Differential diagnosis**
	• **Investigations**
	  ▪ Laboratory
	  ▪ Radiological
	  ▪ Biopsy
	• **Final diagnosis**
	• **Treatment**
	  ▪ Medical
	  ▪ Surgical
	• **Progress and follow-up**
	• **Termination**

Table 1.2: Common complaints of ear, nose and throat

Ear	Nose/Sinuses	Oral cavity	Throat	Face	Neck
• Hearing loss • Discharge • Pain • Noises • Dizziness/vertigo • Itching • Deformities • Swelling • Facial palsy • Injury/foreign body	• Blocking • Sneezing • Disturbed sense of smell • Discharge • Nose bleed • Post-nasal drip • Headache • Facial pain • Swelling • Deformities • Injury/foreign body	• Ulcers • Swelling • Pain • Disturbed sense of taste/salivation • Trismus • Ankyloglossia • Cleft palate • Injury/foreign body • Halitosis	• Pain • Odynophagia • Stridor • Voice change • Nasal voice • Dysphagia • Snoring • Cough • Sputum • Injury/foreign body	• Pain • Cleft lip • Swelling • Injury • Parotid and submandibular swellings • Jaw swellings	• Pain • Swelling • Enlarge Nodes • Goiter • Injury • Cyst • Fistula • Sinus

General: Fever, headache, migraine, vomiting, convulsions, loss of weight and anorexia.
Personal: Chewing of *paan*, *sopari* and tobacco, smoking, alcohol, swimming, exposure to dust and noise.
Systemic: Anemia, asthma, bleeding tendencies, epilepsy, jaundice, tuberculosis, hernia, gastroesophageal reflux disease, peptic ulcer, diabetes, hypertension, chest pain, heart attack, diseases of kidneys and eyes and pregnancy.

- **History of present illness:** It includes the details of all the complaints mentioned in the chief complaints that begin with the appearance of first symptom and extend up to the time of consultation. It usually consists of the mode of onset (sudden/gradual), preceding events causing onset, course of symptoms (progressive/constant/fluctuant; and continuous/intermittent), factors aggravating/relieving, other accompanying complaints, and the treatment taken. The common causes of headache in women are migraine, tension and trigeminal. Diurnal headache is a feature of acute frontal sinusitis. Vacuum headache is also associated with frontal sinus. In cases of unilateral disorder, note the side and site of affliction. If both ears and/or both sides of nose are affected then it should be mentioned which is more affected. Many a times negative answers are equally important in arriving at a diagnosis. Inquiries are done for any systemic diseases, which a patient might be suffering from such as diabetes, hypertension, coronary artery disease, liver or kidney disease, tuberculosis, HIV/AIDS and any bleeding disorder.
- **History of past illness:** It includes history of similar complaints in the past and the treatment taken and history of surgeries, accidents, radiation exposure and any complications. All the diseases with which the patient has suffered in the past should be recorded in a chronological order, whether seemingly relevant or irrelevant.
- **Drug history:** All the drugs which patient was/is taking such as steroids, chemotherapy, insulin, antihypertensives, diuretics, monoamine oxidase (MAO) inhibitors, contraceptives and hormone replacement therapy should be recorded.
- **History of allergy:** It must not be missed as the consequences can be life-threatening. Patients can be allergic to certain drugs, diets, pollens, fungi, animals and dusts.
- **Personal history:** Patient's occupation, personal habits (smoking, alcohol and chewing of *paan*, *sopari* and tobacco), food habits (vegetarian/nonvegetarian, regular/irregular, spicy food), lifestyle (exercise or sedentary), and marital status are included in this. In women, menstrual history and number of pregnancies and miscarriages should be recorded.
- **Family history:** It is important as many ENT diseases run in families and have genetic basis such as otospongiosis, certain types of sensorineural hearing loss, malignancies and autoimmune disorders. Infectious diseases such as sexually transmitted diseases (STDs), tuberculosis, mumps, pediculosis, scabies and diphtheria can affect other family members.
- **History of immunization:** It should be asked in children.

PHYSICAL EXAMINATION

It consists of general survey, local examination and general examination.

General Survey

The general survey includes general assessment of illness, mental state, intelligence, build, nutrition, attitude, decubitus (patient's position in bed), skin color and eruptions, and vital parameters like pulse, blood pressure, respiration and temperature.

Cyanosis is not detectable in patients with severe anemia.

Local Examination

It includes inspection and palpation of the affected region. Percussion and auscultation are important in a few ENT conditions. Examination of the draining lymph nodes is the essential component of local examination. Detailed description of ENT examination is covered in the sections of ear, nose and paranasal sinuses, oral cavity and salivary glands, pharynx and esophagus, larynx, trachea and bronchus, and neck. The general set up of otorhinolaryngological head and neck examination will be discussed in this chapter. ENT head and neck examination also includes eyes and cranial nerves.

> Following a specific order facilitates complete examination without missing any region. It is always advisable to proceed from outside to inside. For example begin from external nose to nasal cavity.

The comprehensive examination of ear, nose, throat, head and neck include following components.
- *Ears:* See Chapter 'Otologic Symptoms and Examination'.
- *Nose:* See Chapter 'Nasal Symptoms and Examination'.
- *Oral cavity:* See Chapter 'Oral Symptoms and Examination'.
- *Pharynx:* For the details of oropharynx, nasopharynx, and laryngopharynx, see Chapter 'Pharyngeal Symptoms and Examination'.
- *Larynx:* See Chapter 'Laryngeal Symptoms and Examination'.
- *Head:* The examination of head includes face and scalp.
- *Neck:* Note movements, neck veins, lymph nodes, carotid pulsation and thyroid glands. For details, see Chapter 'Cervical Symptoms and Examination'.

Systemic Examination

It is especially required in chronic or systemic diseases, indoor patients and before surgery.

It consists of examination of all the systems such as gastrointestinal, respiratory, cardiovascular and neurological.

GENERAL SET-UP

Bull's Eye Lamp

The lamp house can be tilted and rotated and raised or lowered on the floor stand according to the need. It is a powerful source of light and provides an illumination of about 200 candlepower without any image of the filament. The patient is examined in a semi-dark room. The patient is seated erect on a stool or in a chair opposite the examiner. The head of the patient leans slightly forward towards the examiner. The child feels comfortable in mother's lap but should be held properly. Bull's eye lamp is placed on the left (some prefer right side) of the patient at the level of his shoulder. The examiner adjusts a head mirror on his/her right eye (some prefer left eye), which reflects light from the Bull's eye lamp onto the area of interest.

Head Mirror

It is a concave mirror with a central hole of 19 mm diameter. *The mirror has a focal length of about 25 cm and a diameter of 89 mm (3.5 inch).* It provides not only good illumination but also permits freedom to use both hands for other activities.

The perfect and comfortable use of Bull's lamp and head mirror needs some coordination, which requires practice and patience. However, some doctors prefer headlights. Both the electric bulb and fiber optic headlight of various types are available. Section 'Operative Procedures and Instruments' discusses some of the routinely used out patient department (OPD) instruments that are used for examining ENT patients.

Self-evaluation Exercises

1. Which of the following statements is not true?
   a. To ensure complete examination one should follow a specific order and it avoids missing of any component of examination
   b. During ENT examination, the hand that is holding the instrument should be stabilized against the patient and it prevents inadvertent injury upon sudden patient movement
   c. Before examination always assure and describe to the patient what you intend to do
   d. Adjust the patient's chair height in such a way that patient's head remain little lower than the examiner's head
   e. Transoral palpation is important because certain lesions such as submucosal mass/nodule of carcinoma tongue can be felt and not seen
2. The two most common causes of headache are _____ and _____.

True (T)/False (F)

3. Diurnal and vacuum headaches are features of frontal sinusitis.

Answers
1. d   2. tension, migraine   3. T

Section 2: Ear

Chapter 2

Anatomy of Ear

Specific Learning Objectives

After going through the chapter, you should be able to answer the following questions:
- What are the parts of external ear and their characteristic features and nerve supply?
- What are the contents and boundaries of middle ear?
- Name the different parts of all the three middle ear ossicles.
- Describe the intratympanic muscles and their functions.
- What are the different parts of the inner ear?
- Describe the anatomy of cochlea.
- What are the cochlear and vestibular aqueducts and their clinical significance?
- What do you know about the organ of Corti?
- Enumerate the structural and neural differences between the inner and outer hair cells.
- Trace the hearing pathway from the cochlea to the cerebrum.
- Name the vestibular reflexes and enumerate their importance.

The ear is a complex organ. Its functional components, the hearing apparatus and balancing organ are situated in the temporal bone of skull. Ear has intimate relationship to the brain occupying middle and posterior cranial fossa, jugular bulb, sigmoid sinus, internal carotid artery and cranial nerves V, VI, VII, VIII, IX, X, XI and XII. For the sake of description, the ear is divided into three parts (Fig. 2.1):
1. External ear
2. Middle ear
3. Internal ear

EXTERNAL EAR ANATOMY

The external ear is divided into auricle (pinna) and external acoustic or auditory canal (EAC). The tympanic membrane separates external ear from the middle ear.

AURICLE

The auricle (Figs 2.2A and B) is made up of a framework of a single piece of yellow elastic cartilage (except its lobule), which is covered with skin. The skin is adherent to the perichondrium on its lateral surface, while it is comparatively loose on the medial surface. Epithelium is squamous keratinizing. Sebaceous glands and hair follicles are found in the subcutaneous tissue. Adipose tissue is present only in the lobule. There are various elevations and depressions, which can be seen on the lateral surface of pinna. Incisura terminalis is devoid of cartilage and lies between the tragus and crus of the helix (Fig. 2.2B).

- **Endaural incision:** It is made in incisura terminalis for the surgery of external auditory canal (EAC) and middle ear. It does not cut through the auricular cartilage.
- **Frost bite:** The outer surface of pinna is more prone to frost bite because the skin is adherent to the underlying perichondrium. There is no subcutaneous tissue.

Contd...

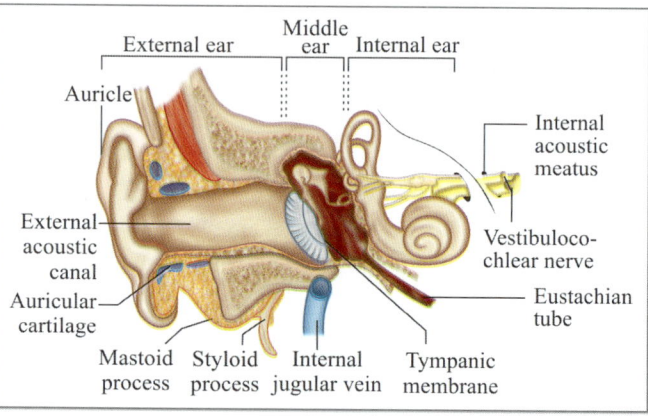

Fig. 2.1: Three parts of the ear: external, middle and internal

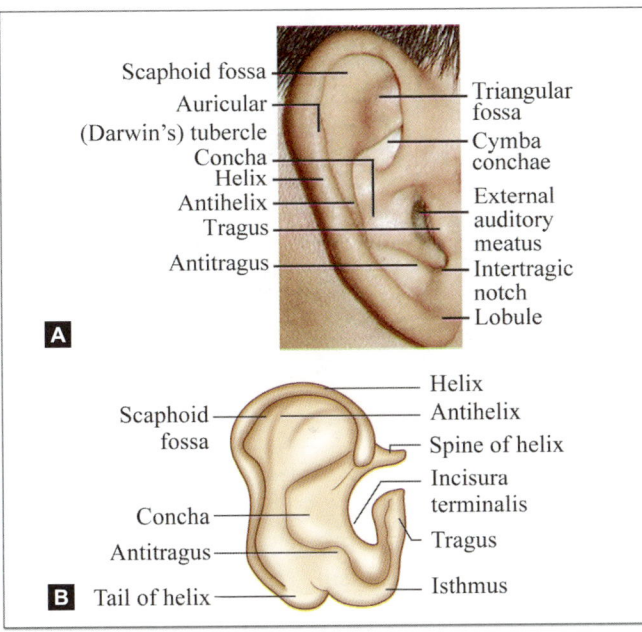

Figs 2.2A and B: External features of auricle. (A) Photographic; (B) Diagrammatic representation

Contd…

- **Sebaceous cysts:** They are more common on medial surface of pinna, especially lower part of retroauricular sulcus.
- **Grafts in rhinoplasty:** The conchal cartilage is frequently used to correct depressed nasal bridge. The composite grafts of the skin and cartilage can be used for repair of defects of ala of nose.
- **Grafts in tympanoplasty:** Tragal and conchal cartilage and perichondrium and fat from lobule are often used during tympanoplasty operations.

Nerve Supply (Figs 2.3A and B)

- **Auriculotemporal nerve (CN V_3):** It is a branch of mandibular division of trigeminal nerve and supplies anterosuperior part of lateral surface of pinna including tragus and crus of helix.
- **Facial nerve (CN VII):** It innervates the skin of concha and antihelix, lobule, and mastoid.
- **Vagus nerve (CN X):** Its auricular branch (Arnold's nerve) supplies to concha and postauricular skin.
- **Greater auricular nerve ($C_{2,3}$):** This nerve of cervical plexus supplies most of the medial surface of auricle and posterior part of lateral surface and the postauricular region.
- **Lesser occipital nerve (C_2):** This nerve of cervical plexus supplies upper part of medial surface of auricle and postauricular region.

EXTERNAL AUDITORY CANAL (EAC)

- **Dimensions:** It is 24 mm long and extends from the concha to the tympanic membrane. Its anterior wall is 6 mm longer than the posterior wall. EAC is usually divided into 2 parts: cartilaginous and bony. Its outer one-third (8 mm) is cartilaginous and inner two-third (16 mm) is bony.
- **Direction:** External auditory canal (EAC) is 'S' shaped and not straight. Its outer one-third cartilaginous part is directed upward, backward, and medially, while it's inner two-third bony part is directed downward, forward, and medially.

Examination of tympanic membrane: The pinna is pulled upward, backward, and laterally and this brings the two parts of EAC in alignment.

- **Cartilaginous EAC:** It is a continuation of the cartilage that forms the framework of the pinna.
    - **Skin glands:** The skin of the cartilaginous canal is thick and contains ceruminous and pilosebaceous glands that secrete wax. The hydrophobic, slightly acidic (pH 6.0–6.5) cerumen is formed in this part of EAC.

- **Fissures of Santorini:** Transverse slits in the floor of cartilaginous external auditory canal called **"fissures of Santorini"** provide passages for infections and neoplasms to and from the surrounding soft tissue (especially parotid gland). The parotid and mastoid infections can manifest in the EAC.
- **Hair follicles** are present only in the outer cartilaginous canal and therefore, furuncles (staphylococcal infection of hair follicles) are seen only in the cartilaginous EAC.

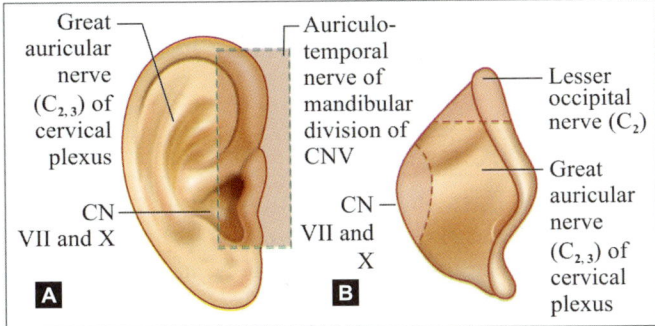

Figs 2.3A and B: Nerve supply of right pinna. (A) Lateral surface; (B) Medial surface

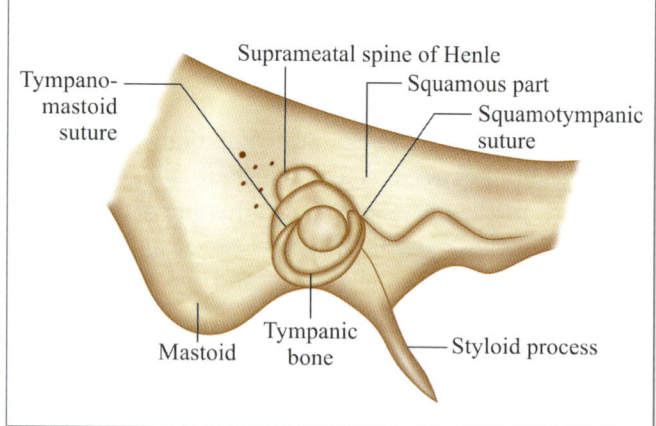

Fig. 2.4: Lateral view of temporal bone showing endomeatal spines and sutures

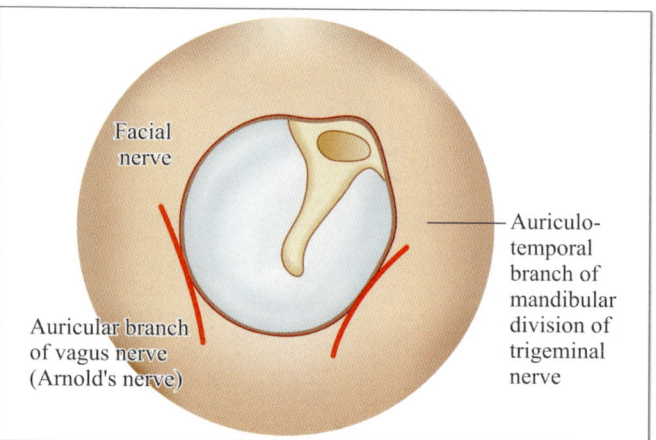

Fig. 2.5: Nerve supply of external auditory canal

- **Bony EAC:** It is mainly formed by the tympanic portion of temporal bone but roof is formed by the squamous part of the temporal bone (Fig. 2.4). In the anterosuperior region, squamous part articulates with tympanic bone (tympanosquamous suture). Inferiorly and medially squamous part joins with the lateral superior portion of the petrous bone (petrosquamous suture). Skin of the bony EAC is thin and continuous over the tympanic membrane. Here the skin is devoid of subcutaneous layer, hair follicles, and ceruminous glands.
  - *Isthmus:* Approximately, 6 mm lateral to tympanic membrane, bony EAC has a narrowing called the *isthmus*. Big solid foreign body impacted medial to bony isthmus of EAC are difficult to remove.
  - *Recess:* Anteroinferior part of the deep bony meatus, medial to the isthmus has a recess, which is called the *anterior recess*. The anterior recess of bony EAC acts as a cesspool for discharge and debris.
  - *Foramen of Huschke:* In children and occasionally in adults, anteroinferior bony EAC may have a deficiency that is called *foramen of Huschke*.

Foramen of Huschke permits spread of infections to and from external auditory canal and parotid.

  - **Relations of bony external auditory canal**
    - *Superior:* Middle cranial fossa
    - *Inferior:* Parotid gland
    - *Posterior:* Mastoid antrum and air cells and the facial nerve
    - *Anterior:* Temporomandibular joint (TMJ)
    - *Medial:* Tympanic membrane
    - *Lateral:* Cartilaginous EAC

Acute mastoiditis causes sagging of posterosuperior part of deeper bony external auditory canal because it is related with the mastoid antrum.

- *Epithelial migration:* The skin of EAC has a unique self-cleansing mechanism. This migratory process continues from the medial to lateral side. The sloughed epithelium is extruded out as a component of cerumen.

Nerve Supply (Fig. 2.5)
- *Auriculotemporal nerve (CN V_3):* It is a branch of mandibular division of trigeminal nerve and supplies anterosuperior wall of EAC.
- *Vagus nerve (CN X):* Its auricular branch (Arnold's nerve) supplies to inferoposterior EAC.
- *Facial nerve (CN VII):* It innervates the skin of the posterior part of EAC.

- **Hitzelberger's sign:** The hypoesthesia of posterior meatal wall occurs due to the pressure on facial nerve (sensory fibers are affected early) in patients with acoustic neuroma.
- **Vasovagal reflex:** While cleaning the EAC, patient may develop coughing, bradycardia, syncope, and even cardiac arrest. They occur because of Arnold's branch of vagus nerve.
- **Appetite:** Because of vagal innervation, instilling spirit in EAC before meal can stimulate appetite.
- **Ramsay Hunt syndrome:** Vesicles of herpes zoster oticus occur on mastoid and posterior meatal wall, which indicate that this part of external ear has facial nerve innervation.

TYMPANIC MEMBRANE
- *Dimensions:* Its dimensions are: 9–10 mm height, 8–9 mm width and 0.1 mm thickness.
- *Position:* Tympanic membrane is a partition wall between the EAC and the middle ear. It is positioned obliquely. It forms an angle of 55° with deep EAC. Its posterosuperior part is more lateral than its anteroinferior part.

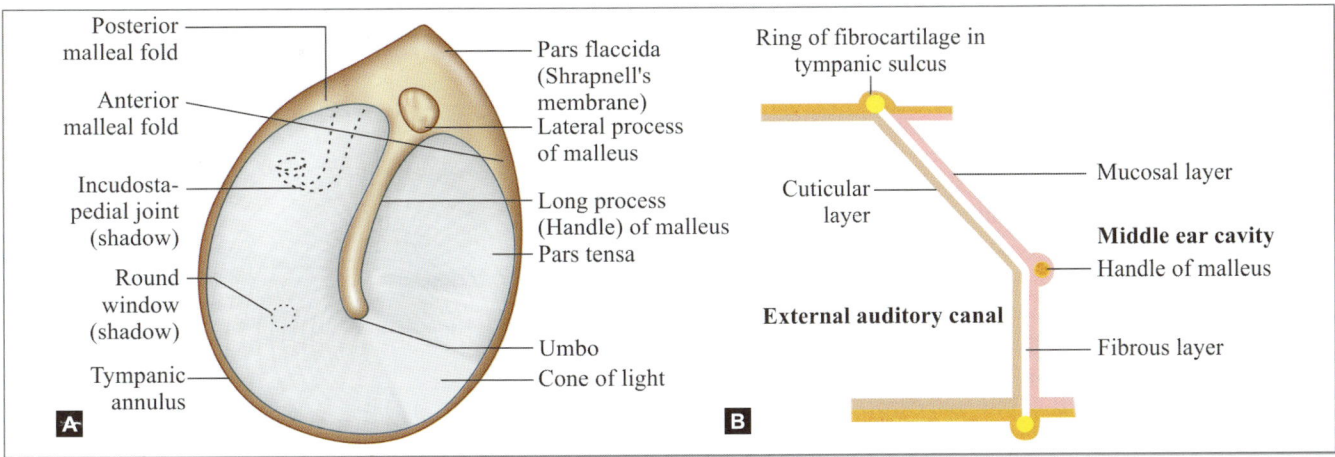

Figs 2.6A and B: (A) Tympanic membrane showing attic, malleus handle, umbo, cone of light and structures of middle ear seen through it on otoscopy; (B) Three layers of tympanic membrane

Parts

Tympanic membrane consists of two parts: Pars tensa and pars flaccida (Fig. 2.6A).
1. *Pars tensa:* It forms most of the tympanic membrane.
   - *Annulus tympanicus:* Tympanic membrane is thickened in the periphery and forms a fibrocartilaginous ring, called the **annulus tympanicus** that fits in the tympanic sulcus.
   - *Umbo:* The central part of tympanic membrane near the tip of malleus is tended inward and is called the **umbo**.
   - *Cone of light:* A bright cone of light radiating from the tip of malleus to the periphery in the anteroinferior quadrant is usually seen during otoscopy.
2. *Pars flaccida (Shrapnell's membrane):* It is situated above the lateral process of malleus between the notch of Rivinus and the anterior and posterior malleal folds. It is not as tense as pars tensa and may appear little pinkish.

Structure

Tympanic membrane consists of the following three layers (Fig. 2.6B):
1. *Outer epithelial layer:* It is continuous with the EAC skin.
2. *Middle fibrous layer:* It encloses the handle of malleus and consists of three types of fibers: radial, circular, and parabolic. In comparison to pars tensa, this layer is very thin in pars flaccida and not organized into various fibers.
3. *Inner mucosal layer:* It is continuous with the middle ear mucosa.
- *Otoscopy (Fig. 2.6A):* Normal tympanic membrane is shiny and pearly-gray in color. Its lateral surface is concave, which is more marked at the tip of malleus (umbo). Attic area lies above the lateral process of malleus and is slightly pinkish. Its transparency varies from person to person. Some middle ear structures can usually be seen through tympanic membrane, such as incudostapedial joint, round window and eustachian tube.
- *Mobility (seigalization):* A normal tympanic membrane is mobile and this can be tested with pneumatic otoscope or Siegel's speculum.

Nerve Supply

- *Auriculotemporal nerve (CN V_3):* It supplies anterior half of lateral surface of tympanic membrane.
- *Vagus nerve (CN X):* Its auricular branch (Arnold's nerve) supplies to posterior half of lateral surface of tympanic membrane TM.
- *Glossopharyngeal nerve (CN IX):* Its tympanic branch (Jacobson's nerve) supplies to medial surface of tympanic membrane.

MIDDLE EAR ANATOMY

The middle ear cleft (Fig. 2.7), which is lined by mucous membrane and filled with air, consists of the middle ear, eustachian tube, aditus ad antrum, mastoid antrum and mastoid air cells. Middle ear is a 1–2 cm³ air-filled cavity

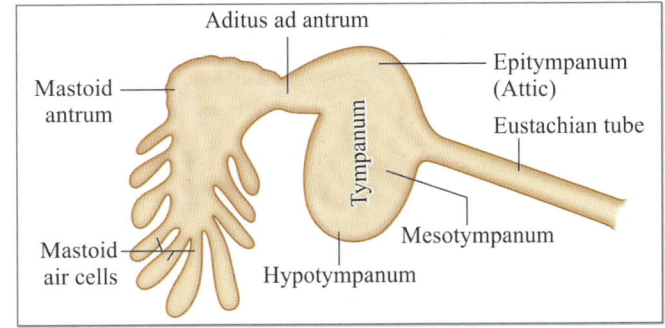

Fig. 2.7: Parts of middle ear cleft

that houses ossicles (malleus, incus, stapes), muscles (tensor tympani, stapedius) and nerves (chorda tympani, tympanic plexus).

Relations of Middle Ear Cleft

- *Roof:* Tegmen plate separates it from middle cranial fossa and its contents like meninges and temporal lobe of cerebrum.
- *Floor:* Jugular bulb.
- *Medial:* Labyrinth. Lateral semicircular canal lie posterosuperior to facial nerve.
- *Posterior:* Sigmoid intracranial venous sinus.
- *Anterior:* Petrous part of internal carotid artery lying in carotid canal.
- *Posteromedial:* Posteromedial to mastoid air cells is situated cerebellum in the posterior cranial fossa.
- *Cranial nerves:*
  - **CN V and CN VI:** They lie close to the apex of the petrous pyramid.
  - **CN VII:** The horizontal tympanic part is situated in the medial wall of middle ear, while vertical mastoid part runs between the middle ear and mastoid air cells system.

Parts of Middle Ear (Tympanum)

The dimensions of middle ear are shown in Figure 2.8. The tympanum is traditionally divided into three parts—mesotympanum, epitympanum, and hypotympanum (Fig. 2.9).

1. *Mesotympanum:* This is the portion of middle ear that lies at the level of pars tensa.
2. *Epitympanum (attic):* This is the portion of middle ear that lies above the level of pars tensa and medial to Shrapnell's membrane and the lateral bony attic wall.
3. *Hypotympanum:* This is the portion of middle ear that lies below the level of pars tensa.

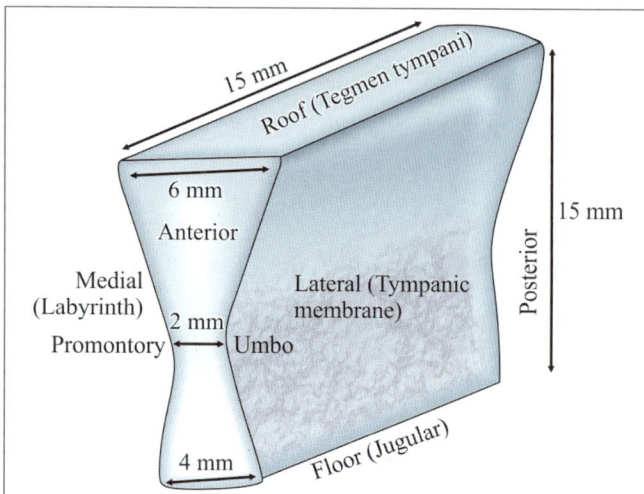

Fig. 2.8: Dimensions of tympanum

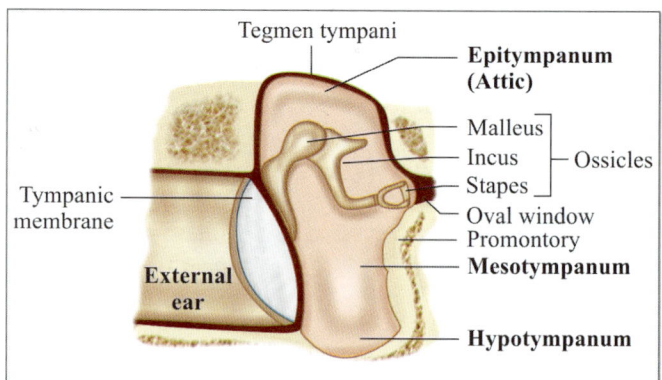

Fig. 2.9: Parts of middle ear seen on coronal section

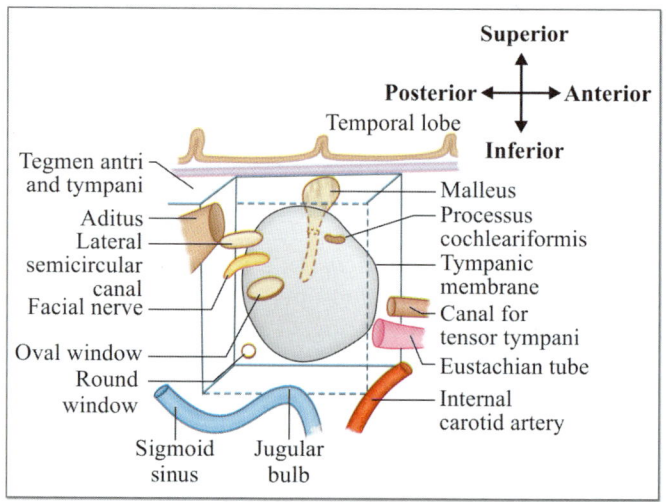

Fig. 2.10: Six boundaries of tympanum. Medial wall is seen through the tympanic membrane

- *Protympanum:* The portion of middle ear around the eustachian tube opening is termed as *protympanum*.

Boundaries of Middle Ear

Middle ear has six boundaries—roof, floor, and medial, lateral, anterior and posterior walls (Fig. 2.10).

1. *Roof (tegmental wall):* It is formed by tegmen tympani (a thin plate of bone), which extends posteriorly to form the roof of the aditus and antrum (tegmen antri). Tegmen tympani separates middle ear from the middle cranial fossa.
2. *Floor (jugular wall):* A thin plate of petrous temporal bone separates tympanic cavity from the jugular bulb.

> **Dehiscent roof of jugular fossa:** The floor of middle ear may be congenitally dehiscent. In such cases, jugular bulb projects into the middle ear and is at greater risk of injury during surgery because it is just covered by middle ear mucosa.

3. *Anterior (carotid wall):* A thin plate of petrous part of temporal bone separates the middle ear cavity from the internal carotid artery. The anterior wall has the following features:
   - *Eustachian tube:* It connects the middle ear with nasopharynx. It aerates and drains the middle ear. *See* Chapter on 'Disorders of Eustachian Tube'.

> *Otitis media:* Malfunctioning of Eustachian tube is the key cause of middle ear infections.

   - *Canal of tensor tympani muscle:* It is situated in the roof of eustachian tube.
   - Canal for chorda tympani nerve.
   - Attachment of anterior malleolar ligament.
4. *Posterior (mastoid wall):* It lies close to the mastoid air cells and presents following structures:
   - *Pyramid:* It is a bony projection through the summit of which appears the tendon of the stapedius muscle that is inserted to the neck of stapes.
   - *Aditus ad antrum:* It is an opening through which mastoid antrum opens into the attic. It lies above the pyramid. Its relations are following:
     * *Medial:* Bony prominence of the horizontal semicircular canal.
     * *Lateral:* Fossa incudis, to which is attached the short process of incus.
     * *Inferior:* Fallopian canal for facial nerve.
     * *Superior:* Tegmen antri.
   - *Facial nerve:* The vertical mastoid part of the fallopian canal for facial nerve runs in the posterior wall just behind and below the pyramid.
   - *Facial (suprapyramidal) recess (Fig. 2.11):* This recess is a depression in the posterior wall lateral to the pyramid. Its boundaries are following:
     * *Medial:* Vertical part of CN VII.
     * *Lateral:* Chorda tympani (branch of CN VII) and tympanic annulus.
     * *Superior:* Fossa incudis, in which lies short process of incus.

> *Intact canal wall mastoidectomy:* The middle ear is approached (posterior tympanotomy or facial recess approach) through the facial recess without disturbing posterior meatal wall (Fig. 2.12).

   - *Sinus (infrapyramidal) tympani:* This deep recess lies medial to the pyramid. It is bounded by the subiculum below and the ponticulus above.
5. *Medial (labyrinthine wall) (Figs 2.13 and 2.14):* It is formed by the lateral wall of labyrinth. It presents following structures:
   - *Promontory:* It is a bony bulge which is due to the basal coil of cochlea.
   - *Oval window (fenestra vestibuli):* The footplate of stapes is placed in this window.
   - *Round window (fenestra cochleae):* It is covered by the secondary tympanic membrane.
   - *Horizontal tympanic part of fallopian canal for facial nerve:* It lies above the oval window.

> *Facial palsy:* The tympanic segment of facial nerve canal may be congenitally dehiscent and the exposed facial nerve becomes vulnerable to injuries during middle ear surgeries and infection in cases of otitis media.

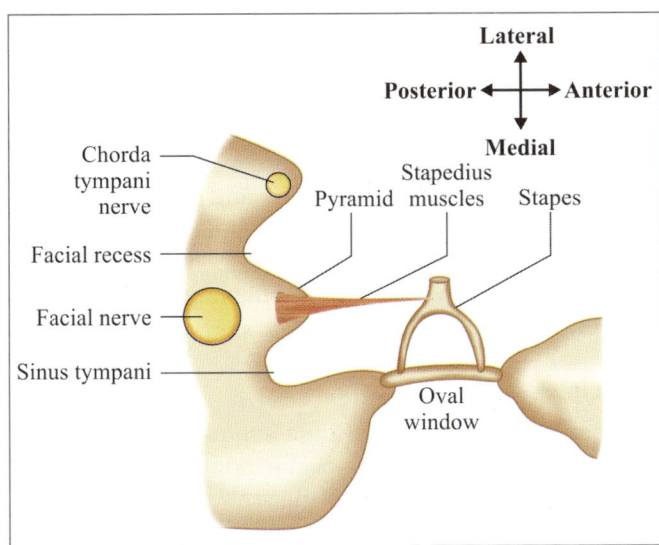

Fig. 2.11: Facial recess and sinus tympani relations with facial nerve and pyramidal eminence

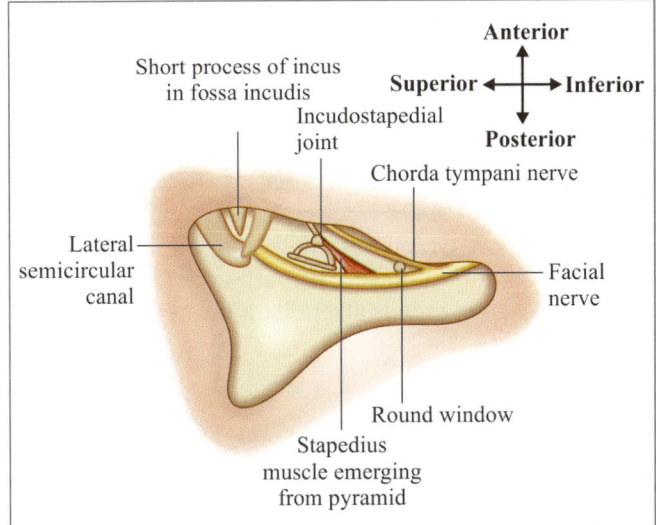

Fig. 2.12: Posterior tympanotomy. Structures of middle ear seen through the opening of facial recess

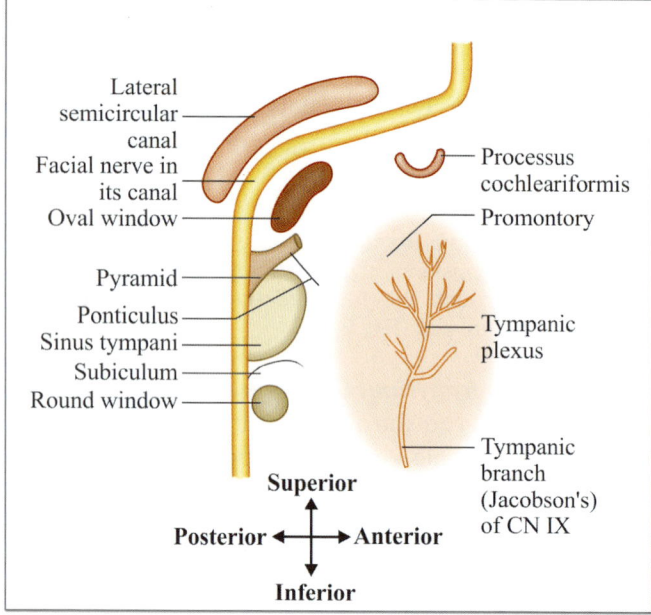

Fig. 2.13: Medial wall of middle ear

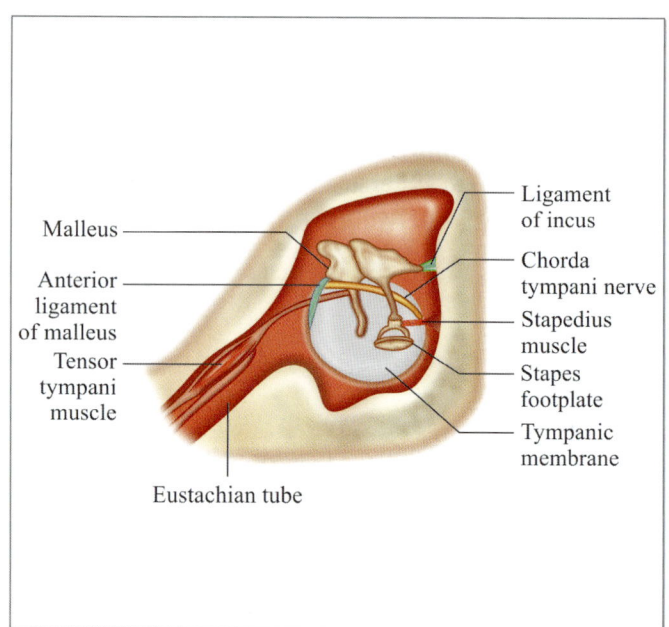

Fig. 2.15: Right tympanic membrane, ossicles, and eustachian tube seen from medial side

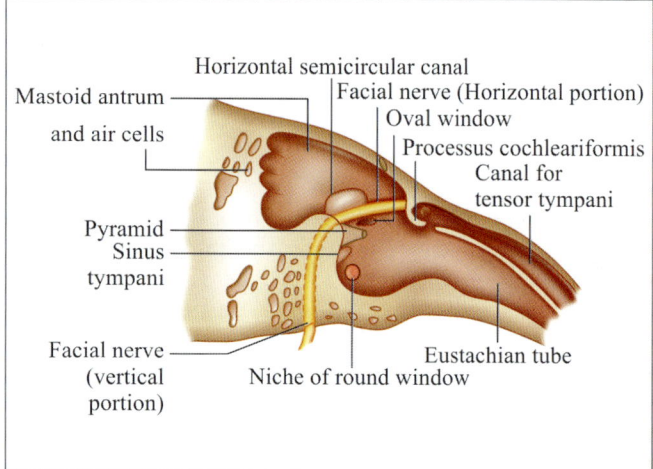

Fig. 2.14: Medial wall of middle ear cleft

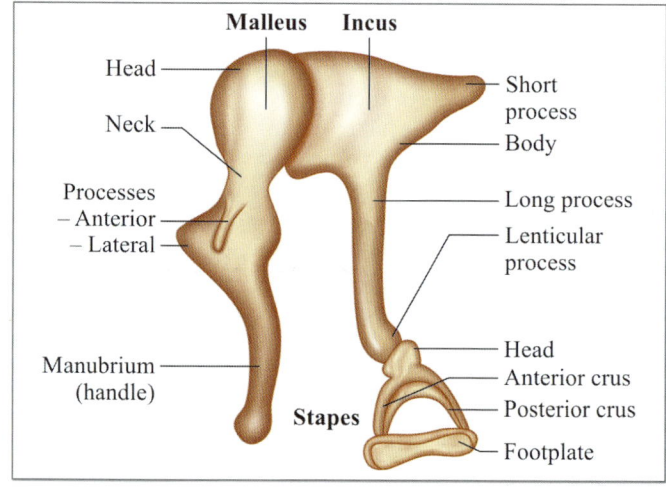

Fig. 2.16: Middle ear ossicles

- *Lateral semicircular canal:* It lies above the fallopian canal of facial nerve.
- *Processus cochleariformis:* It is a hook-like projection, which lies anterior to the oval window. The tendon of tensor tympani takes a turn on this process and then is inserted on the neck of malleus.

Processus cochleariformis is an important surgical landmark for the level of the genu of the facial nerve.

6. *Lateral (membranous wall) (Fig. 2.15):*
   - *Tympanic membrane:* Lateral wall is formed mainly by the tympanic membrane. Some structures of the middle ear (such as long process of incus, incudostapedial joint, round window, and eustachian tube) can be seen through the normal semitransparent tympanic membrane.
   - *Scutum:* An upper part of epitympanum is formed by outer bony attic wall called *scutum*.

Ossicles

The ossicles (Fig. 2.16) conduct sound energy from the tympanic membrane to the oval window. There are three middle ear ossicles—malleus, incus and stapes.

1. *Malleus (hammer):* It consists of a head, neck, handle (manubrium), and a lateral and an anterior process. It is the largest ossicle and measures 8 mm in length.

- *Head and neck:* They lie in the attic.
- *Manubrium:* It is embedded in the fibrous layer of the tympanic membrane.
- *Lateral process:* It appears as a knob-like projection on the outer surface of the tympanic membrane and provides attachments to the anterior and posterior malleal folds.

2. *Incus (anvil):* It consists of following parts:
   - *Body and short process:* They lie in the attic.
   - *Long process:* It hangs vertically and forms incudostapedial joint with the head of stapes.
3. *Stapes (stirrup):* This smallest bone of body measures about 3.5 mm. It consists of head, neck, anterior and posterior crura, and footplate. The footplate is positioned in the oval window by annular ligament.

Intratympanic Muscles

There are two middle ear muscles—tensor tympani and stapedius.

1. *Tensor tympani (Fig. 2.15):* It runs above the eustachian tube. Its tendon turns round the processus cochleariformis and passes laterally. It tenses the tympanic membrane.
   - *Origin:* Bony tunnel above the osseous part of eustachian tube.
   - *Insertion:* Just below the neck of malleus.
   - *Nerve supply:* It develops from the 1st branchial arch and is supplied by a branch of mandibular division of trigeminal nerve (CN V_3).
2. *Stapedius (Fig. 2.15):* On contraction, it dampens the loud sounds and prevents noise trauma to the inner ear.
   - *Origin:* Conical cavity and canal within pyramid.
   - *Insertion:* It inserts on the neck of stapes.
   - *Nerve supply:* It is developed from the second branchial arch and is supplied by a branch of CN VII (nerve to stapedius).
   - *Functions:* Acoustic reflex protects ear from loud sounds.
     * Dampening of middle ear mechanics: Loud sounds (80 dB and above) cause contraction of stapedius that limits stapes movement.
     * Gain control mechanism: Acoustic reflex keep cochlear input more constant and expand dynamic range.
     * Reduction in self generated noise: Stapedius muscle contracts with chewing and vocalization.

Intratympanic Nerves (Figs 2.11 to 2.15)

- *Tympanic plexus (nerve supply of middle ear):* The tympanic nerve plexus, which lies on the promontory, supplies to the medial surface of the tympanic membrane, tympanic cavity, mastoid air cells, and the bony eustachian tube. It is formed by following nerves:
  - *Tympanic branch (Jacobson) of glossopharyngeal:* It carries secretomotor fibers to the parotid gland. The pathway of secretomotor fibers to the parotid gland consists of inferior salivary nucleus → CN IX → Jacobson's tympanic branch → tympanic plexus → lesser petrosal nerve → otic ganglion → auriculotemporal nerve → parotid gland.

> *Frey's syndrome:* Its treatment includes sectioning of Jacobson's nerve. *See* Chapter 'Disorders of Salivary Glands'.

  - *Sympathetic fibers:* Caroticotympanic nerves come from the sympathetic plexus, which is present around the internal carotid artery.
- *Chorda tympani nerve:* This branch of the facial nerve enters the middle ear through posterior canaliculus. It runs on the medial surface of the tympanic membrane. It lies between the malleus and long process of incus, above the insertion of tensor tympani. It carries gustatory fibers from the anterior two-third of tongue and parasympathetic secretomotor fibers to the submaxillary and sublingual salivary glands.

Middle Ear Mucosa

Middle ear mucosa wraps ossicles, muscles, ligaments and nerves like peritoneum wraps various viscera in the abdomen. These mucosal folds divide the middle ear into various compartments. So, all the middle ear structures lie outside the mucous membrane. Mucous membrane of the nasopharynx is continuous with that of the middle ear cleft.

> - *Prussak's space:* It is bounded by pars flaccida (laterally), neck of malleus (medially), lateral process of malleus (inferiorly), and lateral malleal ligament (superiorly). Posteriorly, it opens into epitympanum.
> - *Von Troeltsch anterior pouch:* It is situated between the pars tensa and anterior malleolar fold.

Middle ear cavity is lined by ciliated columnar epithelium in its anterior and inferior part and mucosa changes to cuboidal type in the posterior part. Attic and mastoid air cells are lined by flat nonciliated epithelium. Eustachian tube is lined by ciliated pseudostratified columnar epithelium with several mucous glands in the submucosa.

MASTOID ANTRUM

This air-containing space (9 mm height, 14 mm width, and 7 mm depth) is situated in the upper part of mastoid. It has the following boundaries:

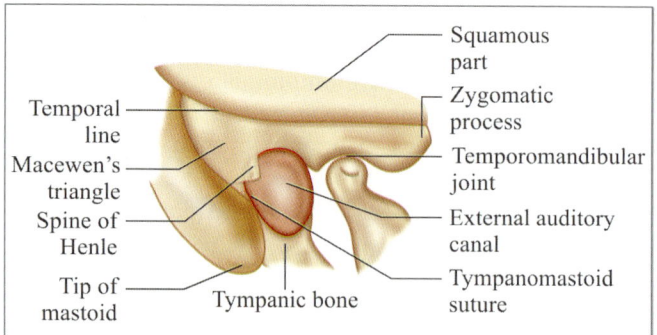

Fig. 2.17: Macewen's triangle. Surface landmark for mastoid antrum

- **Roof:** It is formed by the tegmen antri which separates mastoid antrum from the middle cranial fossa.
- **Lateral wall:** It is formed by a 1.5 cm thick plate of squamous part of temporal bone, which is marked on the lateral surface of mastoid by suprameatal (Macewen's) triangle (Fig. 2.17). It is covered by postaural skin.
  - **Boundaries of Macewen's triangle**
    - *Linea temporalis (temporal line):* A ridge of bone extending posteriorly from the zygomatic process (marking the lower margin of temporalis muscle and approximating the floor of middle cranial fossa).
    - *External auditory canal:* Posterosuperior margin of EAC.
    - *Tangent:* A tangent to the posterior margin of EAC.
- **Medial wall:** It is formed by the petrous bone and related to the following parts:
  - Posterior semicircular canal
  - Endolymphatic sac
  - Dura of posterior cranial fossa
- **Anterior:** Anteriorly, mastoid antrum communicates with the attic through the aditus ad antrum. Medial to lateral relations are as follows:
  - Facial nerve canal.
  - Aditus ad antrum and facial recess lie between tympanum and mastoid antrum (*see* 'Posterior Wall of Middle Ear' in the Section of Boundaries of Middle Ear).
  - Deep bony EAC.
- **Posterior wall:** It is formed by mastoid bone and communicates with mastoid air cells.
  - Sigmoid sinus curves downward.
- **Floor:** It is formed by mastoid bone and communicates with mastoid air cells. Other deeper relations from medial to lateral sides are.
  - Jugular bulb medial to facial canal.
  - Digastric ridge which gives origin to posterior belly of digastric muscle.
  - Origin of sternocleidomastoid muscle.

Types of Mastoid

The mastoid consists of **honeycomb** air cells, which lie underneath the bony cortex. Depending on its development, three types of mastoid are described—cellular, diploeic and acellular (Figs 2.18A, B and C).
1. **Cellular (well-pneumatized):** Mastoid cells are well developed with thin intervening septa (Fig. 2.18A).
2. **Diploeic:** Mainly there are marrow spaces with few air cells (Fig. 2.18B).
3. **Acellular (sclerotic):** There are neither cells nor marrow spaces (Fig. 2.18C).

> - **Citelli's angle (sinudural angle):** It lies between the sigmoid sinus and middle fossa dura mater.
> - **Bill's island:** This thin plate of bone left on sigmoid sinus during mastoidectomy helps in retracting the sigmoid sinus. It should not be confused with Bill's bar, which lies in the fundus of internal auditory canal.
> - **Solid angle:** This area of bony labyrinth lies between the three semicircular canals.
> - **Trautmann's triangle:** This area is bounded by the bony labyrinth anteriorly, sigmoid sinus posteriorly, and the dura or superior petrosal sinus superiorly.
> - **Donaldson's line:** This line is a surgical landmark for endolymphatic sac. It passes through horizontal bisecting the posterior semicircular canal. The endolymphatic sac that appears as thickening of the posterior cranial fossa dura is situated inferior to Donaldson's line.

Mastoid Air Cells

Mastoid antrum, which is present in all types of mastoids, is the most constant mastoid air cell. In *sclerotic mastoid*,

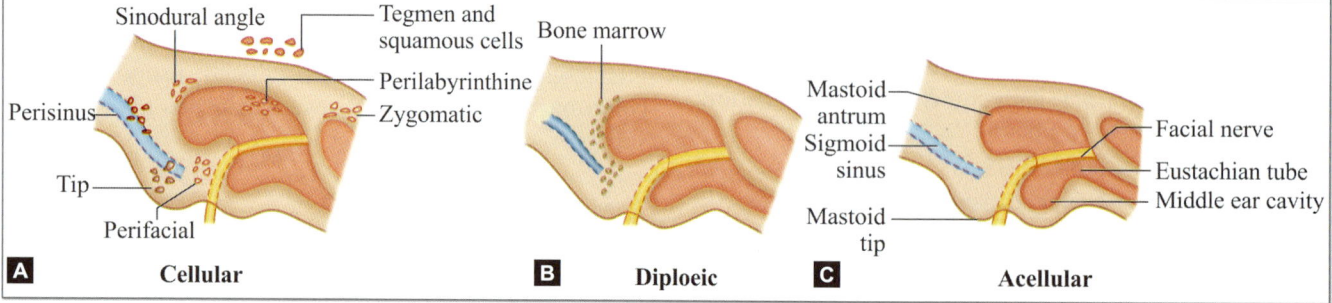

Figs 2.18A to C: Three types of mastoid. (A) Cellular; (B) Diploeic; (C) Acellular

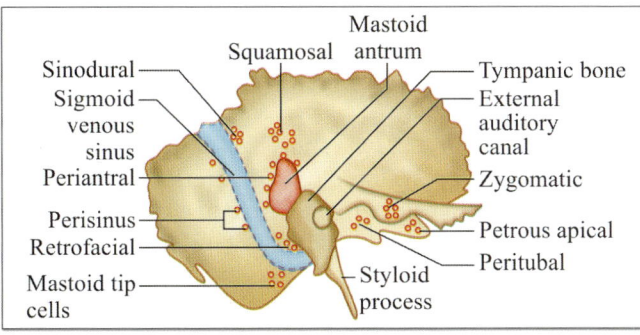

Fig. 2.19: Air cells of temporal bone

Table 2.1: Arteries supplying middle ear

• **External carotid artery**	• **Internal carotid artery**
▪ **Maxillary artery**	▪ Petrous part
▪ **Anterior tympanic artery:** Major contributor	▪ Caroticotympanic branches
▪ **Middle meningeal artery**	
– Petrosal branch	
– **Superior tympanic artery:** It traverses along the canal for tensor tympanic muscle	
– **Artery of pterygoid canal:** Branch that runs along eustachian tube	

antrum is usually small and sigmoid sinus may be anteriorly positioned. In cases of mastoiditis, abscesses may form in these air cells and result in various types of intra and extra cranial complications (*See* Chapter 'Complications of Suppurative Otitis Media').

The mastoid air cells are traditionally divided into several groups (Fig. 2.19) which include:
- ***Zygomatic cells:*** In the root of zygoma.
- ***Tegmen cells:*** In the tegmen tympani.
- ***Perisinus cells:*** Present over the sinus plate.
- ***Retrofacial cells:*** Present round the fallopian canal of facial nerve.
- ***Perilabyrinthine cells:*** They are located above, below and behind the labyrinth. The cells, which are present in the arch of superior semicircular canal, may communicate with the petrous apex.
- ***Peritubal:*** They are present around the eustachian tube. These and the hypotympanic cells communicate with the petrous apex.
- ***Tip cells:*** These large cells lie in the tip of mastoid medial and lateral to the digastric ridge.
- ***Marginal cells:*** These cells, which lie behind the sinus plate, may extend into the occipital bone
- ***Squamous cells:*** They lie in the squamous part of temporal bone.

> - ***Mastoid tip:*** It is absent at the time of birth but mastoid antrum is present. Mastoid tip does not develop till 2 years. Therefore, postaural incision for mastoid exploration in children needs modification to avoid injury to the facial nerve.
> - ***Mastoid antrum:*** In an adult, it lies 12–15 mm deep to suprameatal triangle. But at the time of birth, it lies just 2 mm deep to suprameatal triangle. The thickness of the bone increases up to puberty at the rate of 1 mm per year.

Korner's Septum

Mastoid develops from the squamous and petrous parts of temporal bone. In some cases, petrosquamous suture persists as a bony plate called **Korner's septum**, which separates superficial squamous cells from the deep petrosal cells. During the mastoid surgery, Korner's septum causes difficulty in locating the antrum and the deeper cells.

> If not recognized, Korner's septum leads to incomplete removal of disease during mastoidectomy. Mastoid antrum can be entered only after the removal of Korner's septum.

Blood Supply

Arterial Supply

The middle ear is supplied by branches of external and internal carotid arteries (Table 2.1).

Venous Drainage

Veins from the middle ear cleft drain into pterygoid venous plexus, superior petrosal sinus and sigmoid sinus.

Lymphatic Drainage

The lymphatics of middle ear drain into retropharyngeal and parotid nodes. Eustachian tube lymphatics drain into retropharyngeal group of lymph nodes (Table 2.2). Internal ear does not have any lymphatics.

Table 2.2: Lymphatic drainage of ear

Nodes	Region
Preauricular and parotid nodes	Auricle: Concha, tragus, fossa triangularis Cartilaginous EAC
Infra-auricular nodes	Auricle: Lobule and antitragus
Postauricular, deep cervical, and spinal accessory nodes	Auricle: Helix and antihelix
Retropharyngeal nodes draining into upper deep cervical nodes	Middle ear and eustachian tube

INTERNAL EAR ANATOMY

The internal ear (labyrinth), which has organs of both hearing and balance, is divided into bony and membranous labyrinth. The membranous labyrinth is filled with endolymph. Perilymph is filled in the space present between membranous and bony labyrinths.

Bony Labyrinth

Bony labyrinth (Fig. 2.20) consists of three parts: vestibule, semicircular canals, and cochlea. The lateral wall of labyrinth is medial wall of middle ear. The medial wall of labyrinth is the lateral limit of internal auditory canal (IAC) (Fig. 20.21).

Vestibule

This central chamber of the labyrinth (5 mm) has following structures:

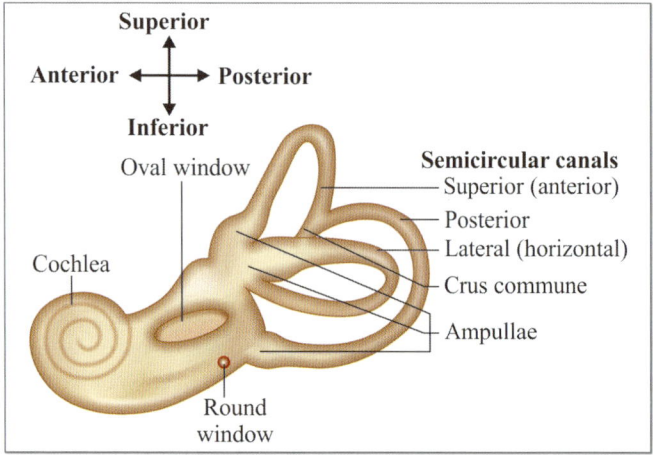

Fig. 2.20: Bony labyrinth of left side. External features seen from lateral side

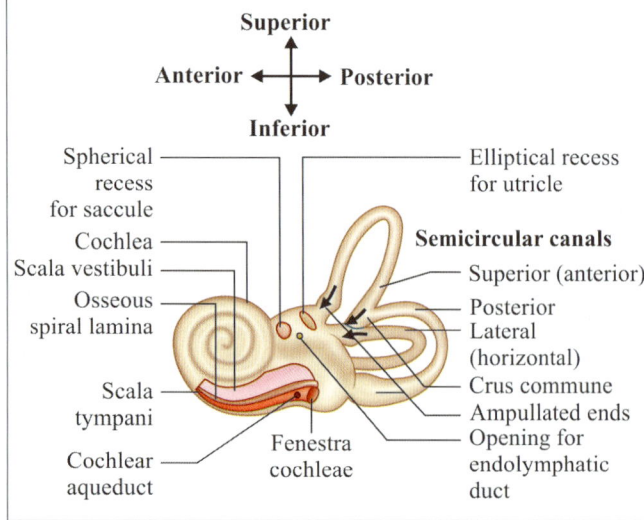

Fig. 2.21: Medial wall of left bony labyrinth seen from lateral side after the removal of its lateral wall

- *Lateral wall:* It has oval window:
  - Oval window (fenestra vestibuli): It lies in the lateral wall and closed by footplate of stapes surrounded by annular ligament.
- *Medial wall (Fig. 2.21):* It shows following structures:
  - *Spherical recess:* It is situated anteriorly and lodges the saccule. Perforations of maculae cribrosa media provides passage for fibers of inferior vestibular nerve.
  - *Elliptical recess:* It is situated posteriorly and lodges the utricle. The perforations of maculae cribrosa superior (Mike's dot) provide passage to nerve fibers that supply to utricle and ampulla of superior and lateral semicircular canals.
  - *Vestibular crest and cochlear recess:* The spherical and elliptical recesses are separated from each other by vestibular crest. Inferiorly vestibular crest splits to enclose cochlear recess for cochlear nerve fibers.
  - *Opening of aqueduct of vestibule:* It is present below the elliptical recess. Through this passes the endolymphatic duct.

Large vestibular aqueduct syndrome: An enlarged vestibular aqueduct is associated with sensorineural hearing loss, Pendred's syndrome and anatomic defects of cochlear modiolus.

- *Posterosuperior region:*
  - *Five openings of semicircular canals:* They are present in the posterosuperior part of vestibule.
- *Anterior:* Cochlea opens into the anterior region of vestibule.

Semicircular Canals (SCCs)

There are three SCCs: Lateral (horizontal), posterior, and superior (anterior). Each canal occupies two-third of a circle and has a diameter of 0.8 mm. They lie in planes at right angles to one another. Each canal has two ends, ampullated and nonampullated. All the three ampullated ends and nonampullated end of lateral semicircular canal open independently and directly into the vestibule.

1. *Superior semicircular canal:* It is 15–20 mm long and situated transverse to the axis of petrous part of temporal bone. Its anterolateral end is ampullated and opens in the superolateral part of vestibule.
2. *Lateral semicircular canal:* It is 12–15 mm long and projects as a rounded bulge into the middle ear, aditus and antrum. It makes an angle of 30° with the horizontal plane. Its anterior end is ampullated and opens into the upper part of vestibule. The posterior nonampullated end opens into the lower part of vestibule below the orifice of crus commune.

- **Posterior semicircular canal:** It is 18–22 mm long and situated parallel and close to the posterior surface of petrous part of temporal bone. Its lower end is ampullated and opens into the lower part of vestibule. Its upper limb joins the crus commune.
  - **Crus commune:** The nonampullated ends of posterior and superior canals join and form a crus commune (4 mm length), which then opens into the medial part of vestibule. So, the three semicircular canals open into the vestibule by five openings.

> **Semicircular canals:** They connect with the utricle via five openings. Semicircular canals of two sides are paired synergistically (horizontal canals of both sides: and one side posterior with opposite side superior).

Cochlea

The bony cochlea, which is a coiled tube, looks like a snail. Cochlear canal makes 2.5–2.75 turns round a central pyramid of bone called **modiolus**. The cochlear tube is 30 mm long. It is 5 mm from base to apex and 9 mm around its base.

- **Modiolus:** The base of modiolus, which is directed towards internal acoustic meatus, transmits vessels and nerves to the cochlea. The apex lies medial to tensor tympani muscle.
- **Osseous spiral lamina:** A thin plate of bone called osseous spiral lamina, winds spirally around the modiolus like the thread of a screw (Fig. 2.22). This bony lamina gives attachment to the basilar membrane and divides the bony cochlear tube into three compartments—1. scala vestibuli, 2. scala tympani and 3. scala media (membranous cochlea).
- **Rosenthal's canal:** The spiral ganglions are situated in Rosenthal's canal, which runs along the osseous spiral lamina.
- **Scala vestibuli:** This upper most channel is continuous with vestibule and closed at oval window by the stapes foot plate.
- **Scala tympani:** This lowermost channel is closed by secondary tympanic membrane of round window.

- **Promontory:** The promontory, a bony bulge in the medial wall of middle ear, represents the basal coil of cochlea.
- **Helicotrema:** This opening is situated at the apex of cochlea which provides communication between the scala vestibuli and scala tympani. They are filled with perilymph.
- **Round window (fenestra cochlea):** On the lateral wall of internal ear (medial wall of middle ear), scala vestibuli is closed by the stapes footplate, while the scala tympani is closed by secondary tympanic membrane of round window.
- **Aqueduct of cochlea:** The scala tympani is connected with the subarachnoid space through the aqueduct of cochlea. It is thought to regulate perilymph and pressure in bony labyrinth.

Membranous Labyrinth

Membranous labyrinth (Fig. 2.23) consists of cochlear duct, utricle, saccule, three semicircular ducts, and endolymphatic duct and sac.

- **Cochlear duct (membranous cochlea or scala media) (Fig. 2.23):** This blind coiled tube, which appears triangular on cross-section, is connected to the saccule through ductus reunions. It is bounded by the following three walls:
  - **Basilar membrane:** It supports the organ of Corti. Its length increases as it proceeds from the basal coil to the apical coil. So, the higher frequencies of sound are heard at the basal coil, while lower tones at the apical coil. The inner thin area is called **zona arcuata**, while outer thick area is called **zona pectinata**.
  - **Reissner's membrane:** It separates scala media from the scala vestibuli.
  - **Stria vascularis:** It contains vascular epithelium and secrets endolymph.
- **Utricle:** The utricle, which is oblong and irregular, has anteriorly upward slope at an approximate angle of 30°.

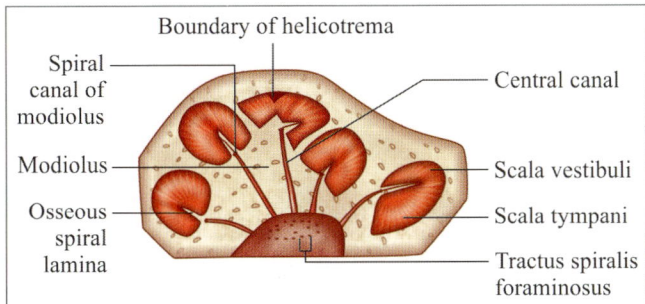

Fig. 2.22: Cross section of bony cochlea

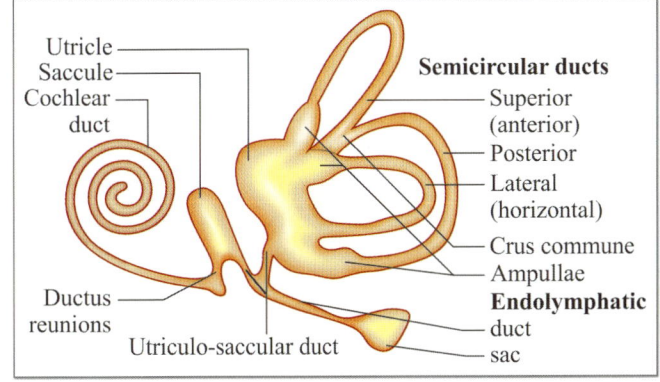

Fig. 2.23: Membranous labyrinth of left side: external features

It lies in the posterior part of bony vestibule and receives the five openings of the three semicircular ducts. The utricle (4.33 mm^2) is bigger than saccule (2.4 mm^2) and lies superior to saccule. The utricle is connected with the saccule through utriculosaccular duct. Its sensory epithelium, which is called **macula**, is concerned with linear acceleration and deceleration.

- *Saccule:* The saccule lies anterior to the utricle opposite the stapes footplate in the bony vestibule. Its sensory epithelium, macula responds to linear acceleration and deceleration. The saccule is connected to the cochlea through the thin reunion duct.

Meniere's disease: The distended saccule can be surgically decompressed by perforating the footplate because it lies against the stapes footplate.

- *Semicircular ducts:* The three semicircular ducts, which open in the utricle, correspond exactly to the three bony canals. The ampullated end contains a thickened ridge of neuroepithelium, which is called *crista ampullaris*.
- *Endolymphatic duct and sac:* The ducts from utricle and saccule unite and form utriculosaccular duct, which continues as endolymphatic duct that passes through the vestibular aqueduct. The terminal part of the endolymphatic duct is dilated and forms endolymphatic sac that is situated between the two layers of dura on the posterior surface of the petrous bone. Endolymphatic sac consists of an intraosseous and an extraosseous portion. The endolymphatic duct and sac are thought to be involved in the reabsorption and regulation of endolymph.

Endolymphatic sac: Regulate pressure of membranous labyrinth. It is decompressed and drained in the treatment of Meniere's disease.

Inner Ear Fluids

Perilymph fills the space between bony and membranous labyrinth, while endolymph fills the entire membranous labyrinth (Table 2.3).

Perilymph

It resembles extracellular fluid and is rich in sodium ions. The aqueduct of cochlea provides communication between scala tympani and subarachnoid space. Perilymph percolates through the arachnoid type connective tissue present in the aqueduct of cochlea.
- *Source:* There are two theories:
  - Filtrate of blood serum from the capillaries of spiral ligament.

Table 2.3: Differences between the composition of endolymph, perilymph and cerebrospinal fluid) (CSF)**

	Endolymph	Perilymph	CSF
Na$^+$ (mEq/L)	3	150	152
K$^+$ (mEq/L)	150	3–5	4
Cl$^-$ (mEq/L)	130	125	110–125
Protein (mg/dL)	126	200–400	20–50
Glucose (mg/dL)	10–40	85	70

**Values vary from the site of collection such as cochlea, saccule and endolymphatic sac in cases of endolymph and scala tympani and vestibuli in cases of perilymph.

- Cerebrospinal fluid (CSF) reaching labyrinth via aqueduct of cochlea.

Endolymph

It resembles intracellular fluid and is rich in potassium ions. Protein and glucose contents are lesser than perilymph.
- *Source:* They are believed to be following:
  - Stria vascularis.
  - Dark cells of utricle and ampullated ends of semicircular ducts.
- *Absorption:* There are following two opinions regarding the absorption of endolymph:
  - *Endolymphatic sac:* The **longitudinal flow theory** believes that from cochlear duct endolymph reaches saccule, utricle and endolymphatic duct and is then absorbed by endolymphatic sac.
  - *Stria vascularis:* The **radial flow theory** believes that endolymph is secreted as well as absorbed by the stria vascularis.

Organ of Corti

This sensory organ of the hearing is situated on the basilar membrane (Fig. 2.24). It is spread like a ribbon along the entire length of basilar membrane. It consists of following important components:

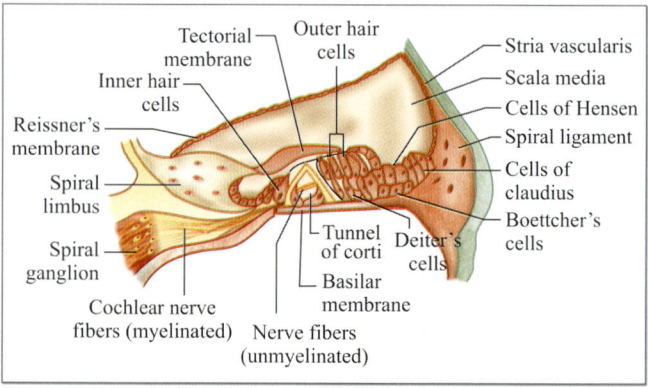

Fig. 2.24: Structure of organ of Corti

Table 2.4: Difference between inner hair cells and outer hair cells

Features	Inner hair cells	Outer hair cells
Cells numbers	3,500	12,000
Rows	One	Three or four
Shape	Flask	Cylindrical
Nerve supply	Mainly afferent fibers	Mainly efferent fibers
Development	Early	Late
Function	Transmit auditory stimuli	Modulate function of inner hair cells
Ototoxicity	More resistant	More sensitive and easily damaged
High intensity noise	More resistant	More sensitive and easily damaged
Generation of otoacoustic emissions	No	Yes

- ***Tunnel of corti:*** This tunnel, which is situated between the inner and outer rods, contains a fluid called ***cortilymph***. The functions of the rods and cortilymph are yet not clear.
- ***Hair cells:*** These important receptor cells of hearing transduce sound energy into electrical energy. There are two types of hair cells—inner hair cell and outer hair cell. At low magnification, stereocilia (evaginations of membrane on the apical surface) appear as hairs. The stereocilia have mechanically activated ion channels, which are opened by the sound stimuli.

> With the advancement of age, there is generalized reduction in the number of hair cells.

- Differences between inner and outer hair cells are given in Table 2.4.
  - ***Inner hair cells:*** Inner hair cells form a single row and are richly supplied by afferent cochlear fibers. These flask-shaped cells are very important in the transmission of auditory impulses.
  - ***Outer hair cells:*** Outer hair cells are arranged in three or four rows and mainly receive efferent innervation from the olivary complex. These cylindrical cells modulate the function of inner hair cells.
  - ***Nerve supply:*** Ninety five percent of afferent fibers of spiral ganglion of cochlear nerve supply the inner hair cells. The outer hair cells get only 5% of the cochlear nerve fibers. Efferent fibers, which are mainly for the outer hair cells, come from the superior olivary complex through the olivocochlear bundle. Hair cells are innervated by dendrites of bipolar cells of spiral ganglion. Each cochlea sends auditory information to both sides of brain
- ***Supporting cells:*** Deiter's cells are situated between the outer hair cells and provide support to outer hair cells (OHC). Cells of Hensen are situated outside the Dieter's cells.
- ***Tectorial membrane:*** The tectorial membrane, which overlies the organ of Corti, consists of gelatinous matrix and delicate fibers. The shearing force between the hair cells and tectorial membrane stimulate the hair cells.

Vestibular Receptors

Peripheral vestibular receptors are of two types—cristae and maculae.

1. ***Cristae (Fig. 2.25):*** They lie in the ampullated ends of the three semicircular ducts and respond to angular acceleration. On a crest-like mound of connective tissue lie the sensory epithelial hair cells, which are covered by cupula.
   - ***Cupula:*** The cilia of epithelial hair cells project into cupula that consists of a gelatinous mass (complex carbohydrates or glycoproteins and proteoglycans arranged in filamentous network), which extends from the surface of crista to the ceiling of the ampulla. The cupula, which is thought to be secreted by the supporting cells, forms a water tight partition. With the movements of endolymph, cupula can be displaced to any one side like a swing door. The gelatinous mass of cupula, which consists of polysaccharide, contains canals into which project the cilia of sensory hair cells.

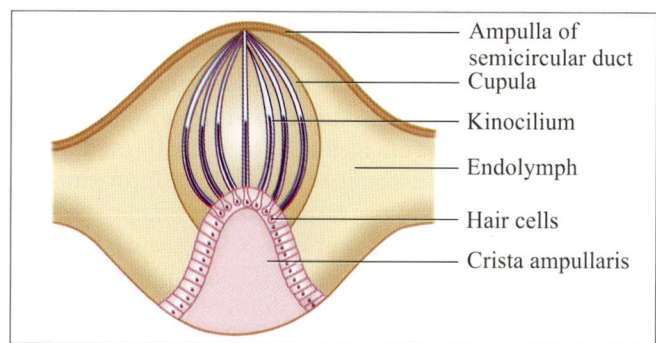

Fig. 2.25: Crista, hair cells, and cupula. Cross section of ampulla of semicircular duct

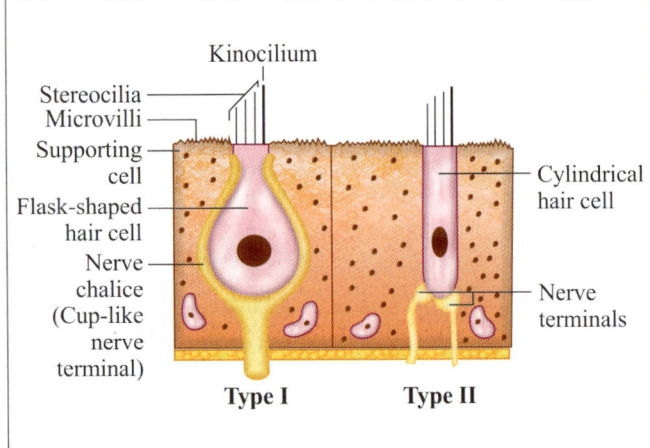

Fig. 2.26: Hair cells of vestibular organs

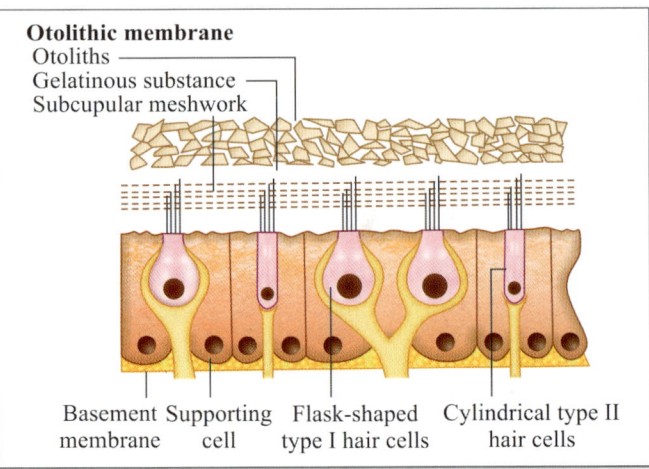

Fig. 2.27: Macula of otolith organs: utricle and saccule

The altered cupula mechanics may result in clinical manifestations of peripheral vestibular disorders such as vascular, viral or bacterial and vestibular neuronitis.

Imbalance in elderly: Similar to presbyacusis, degenerative changes occur in macular hair cells and otoconia with ageing.

- The mechanism governing caloric nystagmus under earth gravity and zero gravity in space is not clear. It seems that a direct thermal effect on the semicircular canal afferents play only a small role.
- ***Sensory epithelial hair cells (Fig. 2.26):*** The sensory hair cells are of two types: ***type 1*** and ***type 2***. From the upper surface of each cell projects a kinocilium and multiple stereocilia. The kinocilium, which is thicker than stereocilia, is located on the edge of the cell. Sensory cells are surrounded by supporting cells which have microvilli on their upper surface. Hair cells of both types may have contact with the same nerve calyce.
  - ***Type 1 cells:*** These cells are found only in birds and mammals. They are flask-shaped and correspond to the inner hair cell of organ of Corti. Each cell has a single large cup-like nerve terminal that surrounds the base.
  - ***Type 2 cells:*** They are cylindrical and have multiple nerve terminals at the base. They resemble outer hair cell of organ of Corti.
2. ***Maculae (Fig. 2.27):*** They lie in otolith organs (utricle and saccule). Macula of the utricle is situated in its floor in a horizontal plane in the dilated superior portion of the utricle. Macula of saccule is situated in its medial wall in a vertical plane. The macula utriculi (approximately 33,000 hair cells) are larger than saccular macula (approximately 18,000 hair cells). The striola, which is a narrow curved line in center, divides the macula into two areas. They appreciate position of head in response to gravity and linear acceleration. A macula consists mainly of two parts, a ***sensory neuroepithelium*** and an ***otolith membrane***.

- ***Sensory neuroepithelium:*** It is made up of type 1 and type 2 cells, which are similar to the hair cells of the crista. Type 1 cells are in higher concentration in the area of striola and change orientation (mirror-shaped) along the line of striola with opposite polarity. The kinocilia face striola in the utricular macula, whereas in saccule, they face away from the striola. The polarity and curvilinear shape of striola offer central nervous system (CNS) a wide range of neural information of angles in all the three dimensions for optimal perception and compensatory correction. During tilt, translational head movements and positioning, visual stimuli combined with receptors of neck muscles, joint, and ligaments also play an important part.
- ***Otolithic membrane:*** The otoconial membrane consists of a gelatinous mass, a subgelatinous space and the crystals of calcium carbonate called ***otoliths*** (otoconia or statoconia). The otoconia, which are multitude of small cylindrical and hexagonally shaped bodies with pointed ends, consists of an organic protein matrix together with crystallized calcium carbonate. The otoconia (3–19 µm long) lie on the top of the gelatinous mass. The cilia of hair cells project into the gelatinous layer. The linear, gravitational, and head tilt movements result into the displacement of otolithic membrane, which stimulate the hair cells lying in different planes.

Blood Supply of Labyrinth

Arterial supply: Labyrinth is supplied by internal auditory (labyrinthine) artery, which is a branch of anterior inferior cerebellar artery that arises from basilar artery. The labyrinthine artery may directly arise from the basilar artery.

Internal auditory artery divides into following two branches:
1. ***Anterior vestibular artery:*** It supplies to utricle and lateral and superior semicircular canal
2. ***Common cochlear artery:*** It further divides into two following branches:
    i. ***Main cochlear artery:*** It supplies to cochlea (80%)
    ii. ***Vestibulocochlear artery:*** It again divides into following two branches:
        a. ***Posterior vestibular artery:*** It supplies to saccule and posterior semicircular canal.
        b. ***Cochlear branch:*** It supplies to cochlea (20%).

The cochlea does not have any collateral arterial circulation.

Venous drainage: It is through internal auditory vein, vein of cochlear aqueduct, and vein of vestibular aqueduct. These veins drain into the inferior petrosal and sigmoid sinuses.

DEVELOPMENT OF EAR

The embryologic source and the time of development of external and middle ears are independent of the inner ear development. Therefore, malformed and nonfunctional inner ear can have normal external and middle ears and vice versa (Table 2.5).

Auricle

In the sixth week of embryonic life, six tubercles (Hillocks of His) appear around the first branchial cleft (Figs 2.28A and B). They progressively grow and coalesce and form the auricle. Tragus develops from the tubercle, which arise from the first branchial arch. The remaining pinna develops from the rest of the five tubercles of second arch. By the 20th week, pinna attains adult shape. Initially, pinna is located low on the side of the neck but later on, it moves to a more lateral and cranial position.

Table 2.5: Development of ear (timings shown in the week of gestation)*

Development	Beginning	Completion
Vestibule	3	20
Cochlea	3	20
Middle ear	3	30
Auricle	6	20
EAC	6	28

*Gulya AJ. Developmental anatomy of ear. Glasscock and Shambaugh. Surgery of ear. WB Saunders (1990)

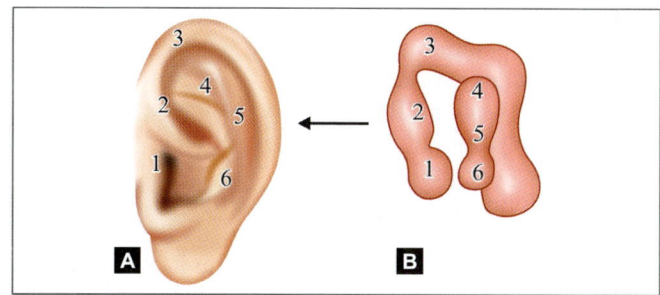

Figs 2.28A and B: Development of pinna. (A) From six hillocks of His; (B) Around the first branchial cleft (1 from first and 2–6 from second branchial arch)

Preauricular sinus or cyst: It is commonly seen between the tragus and crus of helix. It is the result of the faulty fusion between the first and the second arch tubercles.

External Auditory Canal (EAC)

EAC develops from the first branchial cleft. EAC gets fully formed by the 28th week. In the 16th embryonic week, cells proliferate from the bottom of ectodermal cleft and form a meatal plug.

Atresia of canal: The recanalization of meatal plug, which begins from the deeper part near the tympanic membrane and progresses outwards, forms the epithelial lining of the bony meatus. This is the reason why deeper meatus is sometimes developed while there is atresia of canal in the outer part.

Tympanic Membrane

It develops from all the three germinal layers.
1. ***Ectoderm:*** Outer epithelial layer
2. ***Mesoderm:*** Middle fibrous layer
3. ***Endoderm:*** Inner mucosal layer.

Middle Ear

- ***Endoderm of tubotympanic recess:*** The eustachian tube, tympanic cavity, attic, antrum and mastoid air cells are derived from the endoderm of tubotympanic recess which arises from the first and partly from the second pharyngeal pouches.
- ***First branchial arch:*** Malleus and incus develops from mesoderm of the first arch
- ***Second branchial arch:*** The stapes superstructures develop from the second arch
- ***Otic capsule:*** The stapes footplate and annular ligament are derived from the otic capsule.

Inner Ear

Development of the inner ear, which begins in third week of fetal life, is complete by the 16th week.

- **Auditory placode:** The auditory placode, which is thickened ectoderm of hind brain, gets invaginated and forms auditory vesicle (otocyst).
- **Auditory vesicle:** The auditory vesicle differentiates into endolymphatic duct and sac, utricle, semicircular ducts, saccule, and cochlea.
  - Development of pars superior (semicircular canals and utricle) takes place earlier than pars inferior (saccule and cochlea). The pars superior is phylogenetically older part of labyrinth.

> The cochlea develops by 20 weeks of gestation and the fetus can hear in the womb of the mother. The great Indian epic of Mahabharata, which was written thousands of years ago, mentions that Abhimanyu (son of great warrior Arjun) while in his mother's womb heard conversation (regarding the art of battle ground) of his mother and father.

- **Ear development:** The middle ear, malleus, incus, stapes, labyrinth, and the cochlea are fully developed by birth. Hair cells in the vestibular and cochlear end organs are derived from ectoderm. The parotid glands also develop from ectoderm.
- **Otic capsule (bony labyrinth):** It ossifies from fourteen centers. Ossification, which starts at 16th week of intrauterine life, ends by 20–21st week of gestation.

CENTRAL CONNECTIONS (NEURAL PATHWAYS)

Auditory Neural Pathways

The auditory pathway (Fig. 2.29) from peripheral to center consists of eighth CN, **c**ochlear nuclei, **o**livary

Table 2.6: Ascending auditory pathways, from below upward

Neurons order	Ascending auditory pathways
First-order neurons	Bipolar neurons of spiral ganglion in cochlear nerve
Second-order neurons	Dorsal and ventral cochlear nuclei
Third-order neurons	Superior olivary complex in pons. From here fibers travel in lateral lemniscus in pons
Fourth-order neurons	Inferior colliculus in midbrain
Fifth-order neurons	Medial geniculate body in thalamus. From here fibers go to auditory cortex in temporal lobe of the cerebrum through the auditory radiations in sublentiform part of internal capsule

complex (superior), **l**ateral lemniscus, **i**nferior colliculus, **m**edial geniculate body and **a**uditory cortex (*ECOLIMA* mnemonic) (Table 2.6).

- Axons of spiral ganglion bipolar cells form the cochlear nerve, which ends in both dorsal and ventral ipsilateral cochlear nuclei.
  - From the cochlear nuclei, some of the axons go directly to inferior colliculus (both ipsilateral and contralateral) while others go via superior olivary nucleus and lateral lemniscus (both ipsilateral and contralateral). So, the auditory fibers travel via both ipsilateral as well as contralateral routes and have multiple decussation points.

> Each side of ear is represented in both the cerebral hemispheres. The area of hearing is situated in the superior temporal gyrus (Brodmann's area 41).

CENTRAL VESTIBULAR CONNECTIONS

Vestibular Nerve

The Scarpa's ganglion, which lies in the lateral part of the internal acoustic meatus, contains bipolar cells. The peripheral processes of these bipolar cells innervate the sensory epithelium of the labyrinth. The central processes aggregate and form the vestibular nerve. A significant feature of vestibular neurons is their high frequency of resting discharge with an average of 90/sec. The majority of vestibular nerve fibers terminate in vestibular nuclei but some go directly to the cerebellum (Fig. 2.30).

> **Balance problems in elderly:** Numbers of both vestibular hair cells and nerve cells in Scarpa's ganglion are found to be reduced in the older people (18,000 in young adults, decreasing to around 12,000 at the age of 80 years).

- **Branches:** The vestibular nerve has two branches superior and inferior
  1. **Superior vestibular nerve:** It supplies the cristae of superior and lateral semicircular canal, macula of utricle, and the anterosuperior portion of the macula of the saccule.

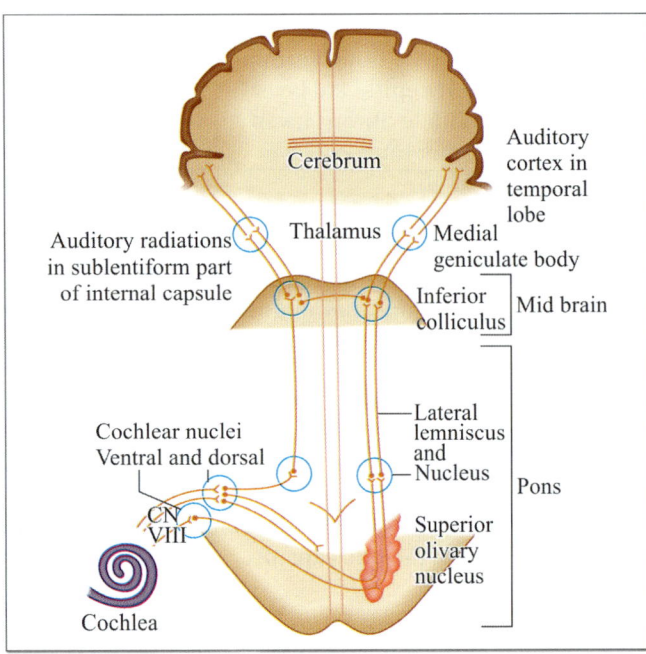

Fig. 2.29: Central auditory pathways

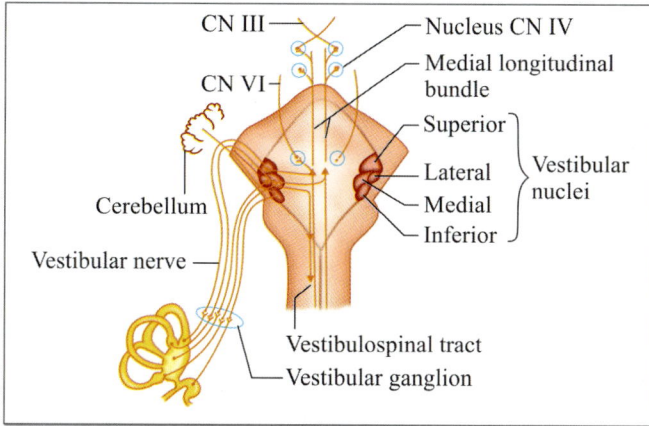

Fig. 2.30: Vestibular pathways

Table 2.7: Afferent and efferent connections of vestibular nuclei

Afferents connections	Efferents connections
Peripheral vestibular receptors (semicircular canals, utricle and saccule)	Nuclei of CN III, IV, and VI via medial longitudinal bundle
Cerebellum	Cerebellum (vestibulocerebellar fibers)
Spinal cord	Vestibulospinal tract
Vestibular nuclei of the opposite side	Vestibular nuclei of the opposite side
Reticular formation	Autonomic nervous system
	Cerebral cortex (temporal lobe) through thalamus

2. *Inferior vestibular nerve:* It innervates the crista of posterior semicircular canal and main portion of the macula of the saccule.

Vestibular Nuclei

They are four in number: 1. superior, 2. inferior (descending), 3. medial, and 4. lateral. They receive afferents not only from vestibular nerve but also from cerebellum, reticular systems, spinal cord, and contralateral vestibular nuclei (Table 2.7).

Functions of Efferents from Vestibular Nuclei

The information received from the labyrinths, eyes and proprioceptive systems is integrated in central nervous system (CNS). The efferents from vestibular nuclei perform following functions:

- *Vestibulo-ocular reflexes:* The medial longitudinal bundle is the pathway for vestibulo-ocular reflexes and explains the genesis of nystagmus. It helps in stabilizing the gaze so that image is fixed on the fovea of retina during the head movement.
- *Equilibrium:*
  - *Vestibulospinal tract:* It coordinates the movements of head, neck, and body in the maintenance of balance.
  - *Vestibulocerebellar tract:* It coordinates input information to maintain the body balance.
- *Autonomic symptoms:* Autonomic nervous system explains nausea, vomiting, palpitation, sweating and pallor seen in vestibular disorders such as Meniere's disease.
- *Motion awareness:* The temporal lobe is responsible for subjective awareness of motion.

Self-evaluation Exercises

1. Which of the following statement is not true for pinna?
   a. It has to be pulled upwards, backwards and laterally to see the tympanic membrane
   b. It attains 90–95% of adult size by 5–6 years of life
   c. Auricular cartilage gives shape to the pinna and is absent in the lobule
   d. None from the above
2. Which of the following statements are not true for external auditory canal (EAC)?
   a. Dehiscence may be seen in outer cartilaginous ear canal
   b. Foramen of Huschke is not situated in the vicinity of the "fissure of Santorini"
   c. It is 24 mm in length and shorter than Eustachian tube
   d. Outer one-third (8 mm) is bony and inner two-third (16 mm) is cartilaginous
   e. Bony EAC does not contain ceruminous glands or hair follicles
   f. The pH is acidic in normal healthy ear canals
3. Which of the following statements is not true for tympanic membrane?
   a. It develops from all the three germinal layers
   b. Red tympanic membrane may be normal in a crying child
   c. Retracted tympanic membrane shows prominent lateral process of malleus and foreshortened handle of malleus
   d. Bulging tympanic membrane loses all landmarks
   e. Supplied by branches of cervical plexus

Contd...

Contd…

4. Which of the following dimension of middle ear is not true?
   a. Vertical 15 mm
   b. Anteroposterior 25 mm
   c. Transverse 6 mm between the umbo and promontory
   d. Transverse 2 mm in epitympanum
   e. Transverse 4 mm in hypotympanum
5. _____ is a plate of bone that separates attic of middle ear from middle cranial fossa.
6. Which of the following statement is true for the development of ossicles?
   a. Malleus and incus are not derived from Meckel's cartilage of the first branchial (pharyngeal) arch
   b. Stapes superstructure and styloid process develop from Reichert's cartilage of second branchial arch
   c. Stapes footplate and annular ligament are not derived from the otic capsule
   d. None of the above
7. Which of the following statements are true for the stapes?
   a. It is smallest bone of body
   b. It weighs about 2.5 mg
   c. Stapes footplate covers oval window
   d. Area of stapes footplate is 3.2 sq mm
   e. All of the above
8. Which of the following statement is true for the stapedius muscle?
   a. It is supplied by a branch of mandibular nerve
   b. Its paralysis causes hyperacusis (phonophobia)
   c. It develops from the second branchial pouch
   d. It is larger than tensor tympani muscle
9. Which of the following boundaries are not of Prussak's space?
   a. Pars flaccida (laterally)
   b. Neck of malleus (medially)
   c. Lateral process of malleus (inferiorly)
   d. Tegmen tympani (superiorly)
   e. Posteriorly opens into epitympanum
10. Anterior pouch of _____ is situated between the pars tensa and anterior malleolar fold.
11. Which of the following statements are true for Mastoid?
    a. Mastoid tip is absent at the time of birth
    b. Mastoid antrum is absent at the time of birth
    c. Mastoid tip does not develop till 2 years
    d. Postaural incision for mastoid exploration in children is similar to adults
12. _____ triangle is a cribriform area on the lateral surface of the temporal bone that acts as surgical landmark to the mastoid antrum.
13. _____ triangle is bounded by temporal line and posterosuperior margin of bony part of external auditory meatus.
14. Which of the following statements are false for mastoid antrum?
    a. In adults it lies 12-15 mm deep to suprameatal triangle
    b. At the time of birth it lies just 2 mm deep to suprameatal triangle
    c. The thickness of the bone increases up to puberty at the rate of 1 mm per year
    d. It does not communicate with middle ear cavity
    e. Its infection cannot cause intracranial complications
15. _____ is a bony plate, which is sometimes seen during mastoid surgery and separates superficial squamous cells from the deeper petrosal air cells. Mastoid antrum lies medial to it.
16. _____ angle lies between the sigmoid sinus and middle fossa dura mater.
17. _____ is a thin plate of bone that is left on sigmoid sinus during mastoidectomy as it helps in retracting the sigmoid sinus.
18. _____ separates the facial nerve area from superior vestibular area above the crista falciformis in the fundus of internal auditory canal.
19. _____ angle is an area of bony labyrinth that lies between the three semicircular canals.
20. _____ triangle is an area that is bounded by the bony labyrinth anteriorly, sigmoid sinus posteriorly and the superior petrosal sinus superiorly.
21. _____ line is a surgical landmark that passes through horizontal semicircular canal (SCC) bisecting the posterior SCC and the endolymphatic sac is situated inferior to this line.
22. _____ is the part of membranous labyrinth that appears first during the intrauterine life.

Contd…

Contd…

23. Semicircular canals communicate with the utricle via _____ (number) openings.
24. Semicircular canals of two sides are paired synergistically (horizontal canals of both sides; and one side posterior with opposite side superior).   **T/F**
25. Which of the following statements are false for ear development?
    a. The middle ear, malleus, incus, stapes, labyrinth and the cochlea are fully developed by birth
    b. Hair cells in the vestibular and cochlear end organs are derived from ectoderm
    c. Tympanic membrane develops only from mesoderm
    d. Otic capsule ossifies from 14 centers. Ossification starts at 16th week of intrauterine life and ends by 20-21st week of gestation
26. Which of the following statements are true for cochlea?
    a. The coiled tube of this snail like structure makes 3.25 turns
    b. Cochlear tube measures 23 mm in length
    c. Modiolus, the central bony axis of cochlea measures 5 mm in length
    d. Scala tympani and vestibuli are filled with endolymph
    e. All of the above
27. Which of the following statements are true for endolymph?
    a. It is present around the membranous labyrinth
    b. It is produced by stria vascularis in scala media and dark cells of the vestibular labyrinth
    c. It is absorbed by endolymphatic sac
    d. It has more sodium than potassium
    e. All of the above
28. Which of the following statements are not true for endolymphatic sac?
    a. Endolymphatic sac appears as thickening of the cranial fossa dura during its decompression surgery for Meniere's disease
    b. It is situated posterior to the posterior semicircular canal
    c. It is situated below the Donaldson's line
    d. It is situated in the middle cranial fossa
    e. All of the above
29. _____ are key to the receptor cells of the inner ear.

Answers

1. d	2. b, d	3. e	4. b, c, d	5. Tegmen tympani
6. b	7. e	8. b	9. d	10. Von Troltsch
11. a, c	12. Macewen	13. Macewen	14. d, e	15. Korner's septum
16. Citelli's (sinudural)		17. Bill's island	18. Bill's bar	19. Solid
20. Trautmann's	21. Donaldson	22. Utricle	23. five	24. True
25. c	26. c	27. b, c	28. d	29. Stereocilia (Hairs)

Chapter 3

Physiology of Hearing and Vestibular System

> **⊙ Specific Learning Objectives**
>
> After going through the chapter, you should be able to answer the following questions:
> - Describe the impedance matching mechanism (transformer action) of middle ear that maximizes the transfer of sound stimuli to the cochlea.
> - Describe the transduction function of cochlea, tonotopic organization and "traveling wave" theory.
> - What are the functions of inner and outer cochlear hair cells?
> - Describe the electrical potentials of cochlea and cranial nerve VIII.
> - What is the neural pathway of hearing?
> - Describe the different types of vestibular receptors along with their functions.
> - Which are the afferent and efferent connections of vestibular nuclei and their importance?
> - How is the body equilibrium maintained while standing and walking?

PHYSIOLOGY OF HEARING

The pinna collects sound signal* from the environment. Sound waves pass through external auditory canal (EAC) and vibrates the tympanic membrane (Fig. 3.1). Vibrations of the tympanic membrane are transmitted to the stapes footplate through the chain of ossicles.** Vibrations of stapes footplate result in the pressure changes in the labyrinthine fluids*** that make movement of the basilar membrane and thus stimulate the hair cells of the organ of Corti. The hair cells of cochlea act as transducers and convert the mechanical energy into electrical impulses which travel along the auditory nerve.

COMPONENTS OF HEARING PHYSIOLOGY

The physiology of hearing is broadly divided into three divisions:
1. Conduction of mechanical sound energy (external and middle ear conductive apparatus).
2. Transduction of mechanical sound energy into electrical impulses (cochlear sensory system).
3. Conduction of electrical impulses to brain via cranial nerve VIII, brainstem, thalamus, and temporal lobe (neural pathways).

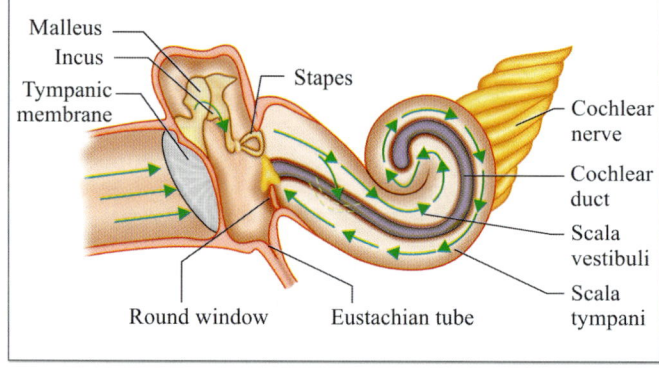

Fig. 3.1: Physiology of hearing. Arrows show sound waves

CONDUCTION OF SOUND

Pinna

Pinna serves the following functions because of its shape and location. It increases sound pressure by 6 dB (2 times).

---
* Waves of compression and rarefaction that is capable of producing sound. Speed of sound in the air at 20° C at sea level is 344 m (1120 ft).
** Sound travels faster in liquids and solids than in the air.
*** When sound energy passes from air to liquid medium, most of its energy is reflected back because of the impedance offered by the liquid.

- **Collection:** Gather sound arriving from an arc of 135°
- **Localization:** Determine the origin of sound
- **Concentration:** Horn-shaped concha acts like a megaphone and concentrates the sound at the entrance of external auditory canal (EAC).

External Auditory Canal

Along with pinna, it can increase sound pressure at the tympanic membrane by 15–22 dB at 4000 Hz.

Impedance Matching Mechanism (Transformer Action) of Middle Ear (Fig. 3.2)

When the air-conducted sound travels to the cochlear fluids, most of the sound energy is reflected away.* Middle ear compensates for this loss of sound energy.

Middle ear converts sound of greater amplitude, but lesser force, to that of lesser amplitude and greater force. This function of the middle ear is called *impedance matching mechanism* or *the transformer action*. The following are the different functions of various structures of the conducting mechanism of hearing:

- **Hydraulic action of tympanic membrane:** The area of tympanic membrane is much larger than the stapes footplate. Therefore, tympanic membrane provides large hydraulic ratio between the tympanic membrane and stapes footplate. The effective vibratory area of tympanic membrane is about two-third. The effective areal ratio between tympanic membrane and stapes footplate is about 14:1. This mechanical advantage is provided by the tympanic membrane.

- **Curved membrane effect:** Movements of tympanic membrane are more at the periphery than the center, which provide some leverage.
- **Lever action of the ossicles:** Ossicular chain conducts sound from tympanic membrane to the oval window. Lever action of the ossicles (handle of malleus is 1.3 times longer than long process of the incus) provides a mechanical advantage of 1.3.

> Wevers and laurence reports that the product of areal ratio (hydraulic action of tympanic membrane) and lever action of ossicles is 22.1 (17 × 1.3). It offers a 25 dB increase in sound energy arriving to the cochlea.

Phase Differential Between Oval and Round Window

Both oval and round windows provide free movement of cochlear fluids in scala vestibuli and scala tympani respectively. Sound waves do not reach the oval and round windows simultaneously. The preferential pathway to oval window receives sound vibrations first and round window acts as a relief window. When the oval window is receiving wave of compression, the round window is at the phase of rarefaction.

> **Otosclerosis:** If only one window is functioning, there will be no movement of cochlear fluids and the patient develops conductive hearing loss.

- **Acoustic separation of two windows:** The sound should not reach both oval and round windows simultaneously. An intact tympanic membrane with the help of intact ossicular chain provides preferential pathway to oval window. The presence of air in the middle ear delays the pathway to round window. If the sound waves strike both the windows simultaneously, they would cancel each other's effect and there will not be any movement of the perilymph. This acoustic separation of two windows is provided by the tympanic membrane and a cushion of air in the middle ear around the round window.
- **Aeration:** Patent eustachian tube provides aeration to the middle ear.

Round Window Reflex

The round window membrane moves in response to the movement of footplate of stapes. When stapes is pressed, pressure is exerted to scala vestibuli perilymph, which is transferred to scala media and then to scala tympani. The pressure is ultimately transferred to round window which bulges into the middle ear.

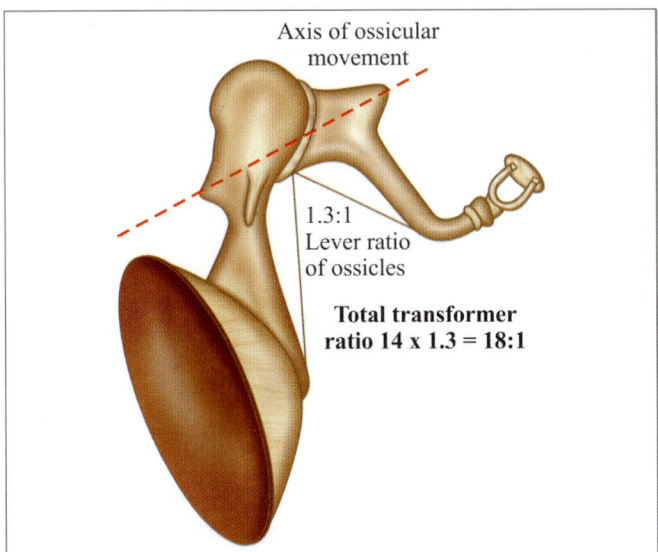

Fig. 3.2: Transformer function (ratio 18:1) of middle ear. Hydraulic effect of tympanic membrane (14:1) and lever action of ossicles (1.3:1)

---

*A person under water cannot hear any sound made in the air because 99.9% of the sound energy is reflected away from the surface of water because of the impedance offered by water.

Natural Resonance of External Ear and Middle Ear

Natural resonances* of the external and middle ear allow certain frequencies of sound to pass more easily to the inner ear. The greatest sensitivity of the sound transmission is between 500 and 3000 Hz (speech frequencies). Following are the natural resonances:
- ***External auditory canal:*** 3000–4000 Hz
- ***Tympanic membrane:*** 800–1600 Hz
- ***Ossicular chain:*** 500–2000 Hz
- ***Middle ear:*** 800 Hz

Noise-induced hearing loss: It usually occurs between 3 and 6 kHz with a peak at 4 kHz because that is the resonant frequency of EAC.

TRANSDUCTION OF MECHANICAL ENERGY TO ELECTRICAL IMPULSES

Organ of Corti

Pressure in scala media causes downward movement of basilar membrane. Along with the basilar membrane, organ of Corti moves up and down with sound stimulus. This causes a shearing action between tectorial membrane and the reticular lamina and results in bending of stereocilia.

Transduction

Transduction is the conversion of mechanical energy to electrical energy. Movements of the stapes footplate are transmitted to the cochlear fluids, which move the basilar and tectorial membranes differentially and set up shearing force that bends the stereocilia. Movement of stereocilia opens and closes ion channels and produces receptor potential in the inner hair cells. This cochlear microphonics triggers the nerve impulse by releasing neurotransmitters onto the afferent nerve fibers.

Traveling Wave Theory of von Bekesy

It hypothesizes that basilar membrane moves as traveling wave from the base of cochlea to its apex. Depending on the frequency, a particular segment of the basilar membrane achieves maximum amplitude. Each wave is weak at the onset but becomes stronger as it reaches its natural resonant frequency.

Tonotopic Gradient in Cochlea

Tonotopic map of basilar membrane determines the site of the largest peak of the wave. Higher frequencies are represented in the basal turn and the progressively lower tones towards the apex of the cochlea (Fig. 3.3). High

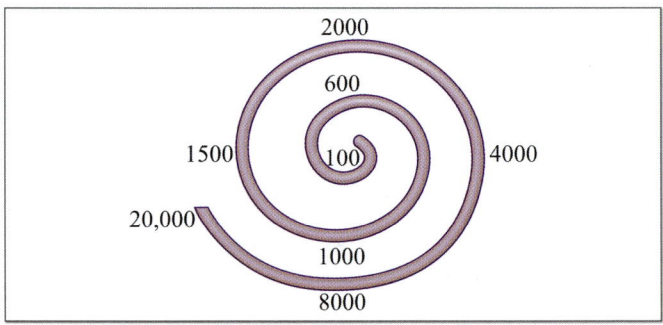

Fig. 3.3: Tonotopic gradient in cochlea. Higher frequencies are represented in the basal turn and the progressively lower tones towards the apex of the cochlea

frequency waves travel a short distance and die. Low frequency waves travel a long distance.

Functions of Hair Cells

- ***Inner hair cells:*** They are believed to be the classic auditory receptor cells, which signal the brain about the presence of specific sound.
- ***Outer hair cells:*** They have been shown to shorten and lengthen when stimulated by sound. A protein called ***prestin*** provides them ability to contract. They are thought to have the following functions:
  - ***Amplification:*** Outer hair cells amplify effect of sound stimuli of their adjacent inner hair cells.
  - ***Sharpening:*** Outer hair cells sharpen the frequency response of adjacent inner hair cells.
  - ***Inhibitory:*** Efferent stimulation of outer hair cells may be responsible for decreasing the responsiveness of cochlea.
  - ***Cochlear microphonics:*** Outer hair cells are responsible for cochlear microphonic effect of electrocochleography.
  - ***Otoacoustic emissions:*** Outer hair cells produce otoacoustic emissions that can be recorded and used to screen newborns for hearing loss. *See* Chapters 'Hearing Evaluation and Hearing Impairment in Infants and Young Children'.

Cochlear hair cells in birds regenerate after noise-induced or ototoxic loss but its significance in humans is yet to be elucidated.

Electrical Potentials

Endocochlear potential, cochlear microphonics, and summating potential are from cochlea, while the compound action potential is from the cochlear nerve fibers. Both cochlear microphonics and summating potential are receptor potentials similar to other sensory end-organs.

---
* It is the tendency of a system to oscillate with greater amplitude at some frequencies than at others.

- **Endocochlear potential:** This resting potential of +80 mV direct current is recorded from scala media. This energy source for cochlear transduction is generated from stria vascularis by Na^+/K^+ ATPase pump. Endolymph has high K^+ concentration. It acts as a battery and helps in driving the current through the hair cells when they move after exposure to any sound stimulus.
- **Cochlear microphonics:** Cochlear microphonics (CM) is an alternating current potential produced by outer hair cells. Basilar membrane moves in response to sound stimulus. Changes occur in electrical resistance at the tips of outer hair cells. Flow of K^+ through the outer hair cells produces voltage fluctuations. Cochlea has two elements—*cochlear microphonics (CM 1)*, which is oxygen-dependent and is abolished by oxygen lack or by death of the individual and *cochlear microphonics (CM 2)*, about 10 percent of the whole, which can still be elicited for several hours after total oxygen deprivation or death.

Cochlear microphonics is absent in the part of cochlea where the outer hair cells are damaged.

- **Summating potential:** It is a direct current potential, which may be either negative or positive. It is produced by hair cells. It follows the "envelop" of stimulating sound and is superimposed on cochlear nerve action potential. This is a rectified derivative of sound signal. Probably it arises from inner hair cells with a small contribution from outer hair cells.

Ménière's diseases: Summating potential of cochlea helps in the diagnosis.

- **Compound (auditory nerve) action potential:** It is the neural discharge of auditory nerve. It follows all or none phenomena so has all or none response to auditory nerve fibers. Each nerve fiber has optimum stimulus frequency for which the threshold is the lowest. Amplitude increases while latency decreases if the intensity is over 40–50 dB range. Compound potential is an example of action potential whereas both cochlear microphonics and summating potential are receptor potentials as seen in other sensory endorgans. Thus, cochlear microphonics and summating potential do not follow all or none law. The following features differentiate it from cochlear microphonics and summating potential:
  - No gradation (follows all or none law)
  - Have latency
  - Can be propogated
  - Has a post-response refractory period

AUDITORY NEURAL PATHWAYS

Details of auditory pathways have been discussed in chapter 2. Here it is worthwhile to note that the nerve impulses are transmitted by the nerve fibers to the auditory nuclei in the brainstem and from there (ipsilateral and contralateral) through the midbrain to the auditory cortex where these impulses are perceived as sound.

Medial Geniculate Body and Temporal Lobe Auditory Cortex

They are organized into isofrequency layers arranged tonotopically from low frequency to high frequency. Most cells respond to binaural stimulation. Their main function appears to be of sound localization. Neurons can either summate excitatory responses from both the ears or excitatory response from one ear and inhibitory response from the other.

PHYSIOLOGY OF VESTIBULAR SYSTEM

Vestibular system is traditionally divided into two parts—*peripheral* and *central*:
1. **Peripheral vestibular system:** It consists of semicircular ducts (dynamic labyrinth), utricle and saccule (static labyrinth), and vestibular nerve. Each vestibular receptor is precisely oriented to detect head movement in a specific direction or plane (Table 3.1). All the receptors are tonically active.
2. **Central vestibular system:** It includes vestibular nuclei and tracts that integrate vestibular impulses with other systems to maintain body balance.

SEMICIRCULAR CANALS FUNCTIONS

Semicircular canals (SCCs) respond to angular acceleration and deceleration. The three canals, which lie in three different planes, are situated at right angles to each other. Any change in position of head can be detected. The one that lies at right angle to the axis of rotation is most stimulated. For example, the horizontal canal responds maximum to rotation on the vertical axis.

Table 3.1: Vestibular receptors and direction or plane of head movement

Vestibular receptors	Direction or plane of head movement
Horizontal semicircular canal	Horizontal head turning (angular acceleration)
Superior and posterior semicircular canal	Pitching the front to back and side to side
Otolith organs (utricle and saccule)	Linear head movement (vertical and horizontal), tilting and gravity

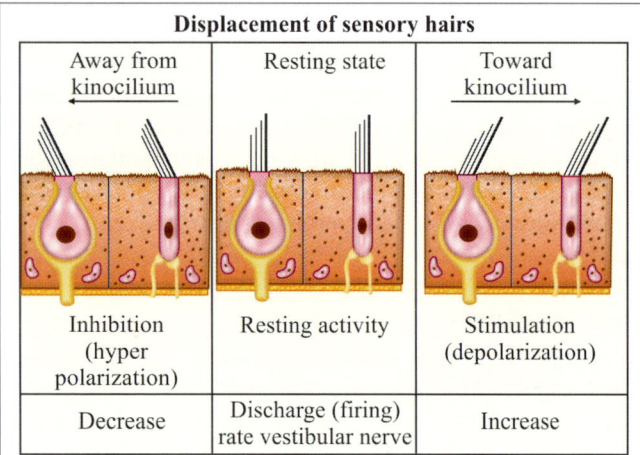

Fig. 3.4: Vestibular hair cells. Displacement of stereocilia toward kinocilium leads to depolarization (stimulation) and increases the vestibular nerve discharge rate

Nystagmus

The stimulation of semicircular canals produces nystagmus. The direction of nystagmus depends on the plane of the canal being stimulated. The nystagmus is horizontal from horizontal (lateral) canal; rotatory from the superior (anterior) canal; and vertical from the posterior canal.

- *Flow of endolymph:* The flow of endolymph displaces the cupula and stimulates the epithelial hair cells (Fig. 3.4) of crista in the ampulla of the semicircular canals. The flow of endolymph towards the ampulla or utricle is called **ampullopetal or utriculopetal**. The flow of endolymph away from ampulla or utricle is called **ampullofugal** or **utriculofugal**. The quick component of horizontal nystagmus is always opposite to the direction of flow of endolymph in the horizontal semicircular canals. In lateral semicircular canals, ampullopetal displacement of stereocilia increases (stimulatory) the firing rate, whereas ampullofugal displacement decreases (inhibitory) the firing rate. The opposite happens in posterior and superior canals.
- *Rotating chair test:* In the rotating chair test, when the patient is rotating to the right and then abruptly stopped, the endolymph continues to move to the right due to inertia. Here endolymph movement in the lateral superior semicircular canal (SCC) will be ampullopetal for the left canal and the horizontal nystagmus will be directed to the left.

Utricle and Saccule Functions

They respond to the linear acceleration and deceleration or gravitational pull during the head tilts. The sensory hair cells of the macula lie in different planes. Macula of the utricle is situated in its floor in a horizontal plane in the dilated superior portion of the utricle. Macula of saccule is situated in its medial wall in a vertical plane. During the head tilts, hair cells are stimulated by displacement of otolithic membrane. The functions of saccule and utricle are similar but the saccule is also seen to respond to sound vibrations.

- *Saccular macula* responds to the tilting of head. If the head is tilted to the left side, the left saccular macula is stimulated while the right saccular macula will remain static.
- *Utricular macula* responds to forward and backward movements of head.

Common vestibular function tests: They include head thrust test, fistula test and caloric test (*see* Chapter 'Evaluation of Vertigo').

MAINTENANCE OF BODY EQUILIBRIUM

Sensory Component

The vestibular system records changes in the head position, linear or angular acceleration and deceleration and gravitational effects. The central nervous system (CNS) receives information not only from the vestibular system but also from other sensory systems, which include visual, auditory, and somatosensory (muscles, joints, tendons, and skin) information. All this information is integrated and utilized in the regulation of equilibrium and body posture. Cerebellum, which is connected to the vestibular receptors, further helps in coordinating muscular movements, which vary in their rate, range, force, and duration.

Motor Component

The standing and walking need not only sensory integration (from vestibular, somatosensory and visual systems), but also motor commands, which are fine-tuned through the frontal cerebral lobes, cerebellum, and basal ganglia. Disorder of any of these systems can lead to dizziness.

Push and Pull System

The balance system, which includes vestibular, visual and somatosensory organs, can be compared with a two-sided push and pull system. In a neutral position, push and pull of one side is equal to that of the other side. If one side is pulling more than the other, the body balance is disturbed. During turning or tilting, a temporary change in the push and pull force of one system is taken care of by the appropriate reflexes and motor outputs to the eyes (vestibulo-ocular reflex), neck (vestibulocervical reflex) and trunk and limbs (vestibulospinal reflex), which maintains new position of head and body. If any component of push and pull system of one side is diseased, then it results in vertigo and ataxia.

Example: Turning the head to the right direction produces an increase in the resting spontaneous outflow of action potential in the nerve coming from the right horizontal semicircular canal. Simultaneously, there occurs decreased activity in the left vestibular nerve. The central nervous system (CNS) compares the input coming from each vestibule. There is no sense of movement when input is equal. The central nervous system (CNS) interprets asymmetric input not only as a head rotation but also generates compensatory eye movements and postural adjustment.

Pathophysiology of vertigo and dizziness: Imbalance due to semicircular canal-mediated vestibulo-ocular and vestibulospinal pathways results in abnormal sense of

Contd...

Contd...

rotation, while imbalance due to otolith-mediated vestibulo-ocular and vestibulospinal pathways may manifest as vertical diplopia, abnormal sense of upright, sense of tilting, and a tendency to lean or fall to the affected side.

Diseases and Evaluation of Vestibular System

For the evaluation of nystagmus, dizzy patient and diseases of vestibular system, *see* the following Chapters in this book:
- Evaluation of Vertigo
- Peripheral Vestibular Disorders
- Central Vestibular Disorders.

Self-evaluation Exercises

1. Which of the following is not a common vestibular function test?
    a. Head thrust test
    b. Fistula test
    c. Caloric test
    d. Computerized rotary chair test
2. Which of the following are not true about the physiology of hearing?
    a. Area ratio (hydraulic ratio) between tympanic membrane and stapes footplate 14:1
    b. Lever ratio is 3:1 between the handle of malleus and the long process of incus
    c. Axis of ossicular rotation passes through the anterior process of malleus and short process of incus
    d. Average loss of sound during ear transmission is 20–30 dB
    e. Cochlear microphonic occurs in the inner ear by the outer hair cells in response to sound stimulation

Answers

1. d   2. b

Pearls and Nuggets (Refresh your knowledge)

- **Abducent:** CN VI has the longest intracranial course. **Dorello's canal** transmits abducent nerve.
- **CN V₁:** The **ophthalmic division of trigeminal nerve** carries sensory fibers from cornea (sensory limb of corneal reflex), bridge of nose, forehead, and scalp (anterior to mid coronal plane). The lesion of CN V_1 will result in ipsilateral loss of corneal reflex and forehead sensations. On stimulation of opposite side of cornea with a wisp of cotton, both eyes blink.
- **Caroticotympanic artery:** It is a branch of internal carotid artery, which anastomoses with branches of external carotid system in the middle ear.
- **Dysmetria:** It is an inability to stop a movement at the proper place.
- **First pharyngeal arch:** Mandible, malleus, and incus are derived from first pharyngeal arch.
- **Glossopharyngeal nerve:** It supplies to oropharynx and stylopharyngeus muscle. It also carries preganglionic parasympathetic secretomotor axons and traverses the jugular foramen. Its tympanic branch synapses in the otic ganglion through the lesser petrosal nerve (arising from the tympanic plexus, which is formed by tympanic branch of CN IX), and provide innervation to the parotid gland.
- **Horizontal gaze:** The frontal eye field lesion would result in an inability to look towards contralateral side with both eyes. The medial longitudinal fasciculus (MLF) lesion would result in an inability to adduct the ipsilateral eye on the attempted gaze to opposite side.
- **Accessory nerve:** It innervates sternocleidomastoid and trapezius. On the lesion of CN IX, patient cannot turn head to the opposite side and has difficulty raising ipsilateral arm above the head to comb hair.
- **Ataxic gait:** The most common cause is chronic alcohol abuse, which preferentially affects Purkinje cells of anterior vermis of cerebellum that control proximal musculature.

Chapter 4

Otologic Symptoms and Examination

> ### ⊙ Specific Learning Objectives
> After going through the chapter, you should be able to answer the following questions:
> - How will you perform otoscopy and which would be the different components of your ear examination?
> - What would you look for in tympanic membrane examination and pneumatic otoscopy (siegelization)?
> - What are the differential diagnoses of a case of otalgia and what would be the components of your history taking and examination in such a case?
> - How many types of ear discharge do you know? What are their causes?
> - How will you take history and perform your examination in a case of ear polyp?
> - How would you classify and manage cases of tinnitus?

EAR SYMPTOMS

The common otologic symptoms are otorrhea, otalgia, hearing loss, vertigo and tinnitus (Table 4.1). This chapter reviews the diagnoses to be considered when evaluating these symptoms. The pain and discharge indicate inflammatory disorders while auditory disorders present with hearing loss and tinnitus. Vertigo occurs in vestibular lesions. The symptoms of hearing loss, vertigo and facial palsy are discussed in their respective chapters.

EAR EXAMINATION

Examination consists of both physical [pinna and the surrounding area, external auditory canal (EAC), tympanic membrane, middle ear, mastoid, eustachian tube, facial nerve and other cranial nerves] and functional examination (hearing and vestibular). See Table 4.2 for the general format of ear examination, which should be followed for each side of ear. The Table 4.2 also shows the findings of clinical examination as well as their causes.

The pinna needs inspection as well as palpation of its surfaces and the surrounding area including postauricular sulcus (Figs 4.1A and B). The irregularities of the mastoid are 'ironed out' in periosteal inflammation (mastoiditis).

> The external auditory canal (EAC) can be examined by pulling the pinna upward (in children, downward), backward, and laterally while the tragus is pulled forward (Fig. 4.2A). This procedure not only spreads open the meatus but also straightens it and shows tympanic membrane.

Otoscopy

For the OPD ear instruments, *see* Chapter on 'Instruments'.
- **Aural Speculum:** This is inserted into the cartilaginous portion of the EAC after retracting the pinna (Fig. 4.2B). It is used for examination and operations of the EAC, tympanic membrane and middle ear. The use of the largest ear speculum that can easily enter the canal is safe and provides a better view.
- **EAC:** Look for the abnormalities of walls of EAC and its contents, such as discharge, polyp or any other mass.

> Ear speculum should not reach into the bony part of the EAC because that is painful and patient will not allow.

Otoscope

It has its own illumination and magnification and facilitates examination of EAC and tympanic membrane (Figs 4.3A and B). It is especially useful in examining the ears and nose of infants and bedridden patients.

Table 4.1: Ear symptoms

Types	Symptoms
Common	Otorrhea, otalgia, hearing loss, vertigo, tinnitus
Other	Itching, deformities, swelling, facial palsy, injury/foreign body
Associated	Fever, headache, vomiting, convulsions

Table 4.2: Examination of ears—findings and their causes

Physical Examination

- **Pinna and surrounding area** (*see* Chapter 'Diseases of External Ear and Tympanic Membrane')
  - **Size, shape, and position:** Microtia/macrotia, cauliflower ear, bat ear
  - **Swellings:** Furuncle/hematoma/neoplasm, perichondritis, abscesses (mastoid or zygomatic abscess), lymph nodes
  - **Ulcer:** Malignancy, trauma, herpes zoster
  - **Scar:** Trauma/operation (endaural/postaural)
  - **Sinus and fistula:** Preauricular sinus, postauricular (mastoid) fistula
  - **Palpation:** Raised temperature and tenderness (perichondritis or abscess); thickness of tissues (perichondritis); fluctuation (hematoma, seroma or abscess). Painful movement of pinna (furunculosis of the external canal)
- **Examination of external auditory canal (EAC)** (*see* Chapter 'Diseases of External Ear and Tympanic Membrane')
  - **Size of meatus:** Atresia/narrow/wide
  - **Contents of lumen:** Wax, debris, discharge, polyp, and foreign body
  - **Swelling:** Furuncle, sagging of posterosuperior area (coalescent mastoiditis), granulations, exostosis, neoplasm (benign or malignant)
- **Examination of tympanic membrane (TM)** (*see* Chapter 'Diseases of External Ear and Tympanic Membrane')
  - **Color:** Red and congested (acute otitis media), bluish (secretory otitis media or hemotympanum) and a chalky plaque (tympanosclerosis)
  - **Retraction:** General retraction (tubal occlusion), attic retraction pockets or posterosuperior region/collection of epithelial flakes, deeply retracted, fixed to promontory (adhesive otitis media)
  - **Bulging:** Acute otitis media, hemotympanum or middle ear neoplasm
  - **Thickness and transparency:** Opaque/thick, translucent/semitransparent/transparent/very thin
  - **Vesicles and bullae:** Herpes zoster and myringitis bullosa; granulations (granular myringitis)
  - **Perforation (acute and chronic suppurative otitis media):** Size (small, medium, subtotal or total in pars tensa), shape (oval, round or kidney), single or multiple (tuberculosis), site: central (safe chronic suppurative otitis media) or marginal (at the periphery involving the annulus) or attic (in pars flaccida) with cholesteatoma.
  - **Mobility (siegelization):** Mobile (normal), restricted (presence of fluid), fixed (adhesions in the middle ear) or hypermobile (an atrophic segment of tympanic membrane).
- **Examination of middle ear** (through the perforation, transparent tympanic membrane, surgical exploration)
  - **Mucosa:** Normal/atrophic/hypertrophic/polypoidal/granulations/in-growth/plaques of squamous epithelium (cholesteatoma)
  - **Contents:** See for status of ossicles, growth, foreign body
  - **Normal structures:** Oval and round windows (round window reflex, perilymphatic fistula), eustachian tube opening
- **Examination of mastoid** (*see* Chapter 'Complications of Suppurative Otitis Media')
  - **Swelling:** Abscess or enlarged nodes, furuncle (obliteration of retroauricular groove), fistula (burst abscess), scar (previous operation)
  - **Palpation:** Smooth (periosteal inflammation/subperiosteal abscess)/irregular/tenderness (mastoiditis) over antrum (just above and behind the meatus), tip, and between mastoid tip and antrum.
- **Examination of eustachian tube (ET)** (*see* Chapter 'Disorders of Eustachian Tube')
  - Posterior rhinoscopy
  - Valsalva maneuver
  - Eustachian catheterization
- **Examination of facial nerve** (*see* Chapter 'Facial Nerve Disorders')
  - Lower/upper motor neuron
  - **Grade:** Complete/partial

Functional Examination

- **Auditory function** (*see* Chapter 'Hearing Evaluation')
  - Voice test
  - Tuning fork tests
    - Rinne's test
    - Weber's test
    - Schwabach's test
    - Absolute bone conduction test
  - **Audiometry:** Pure tone, speech, and impedance
- **Vestibular function** (*see* Chapter 'Evaluation of Vertigo')
  - Spontaneous nystagmus
  - Fistula test
  - Positional tests

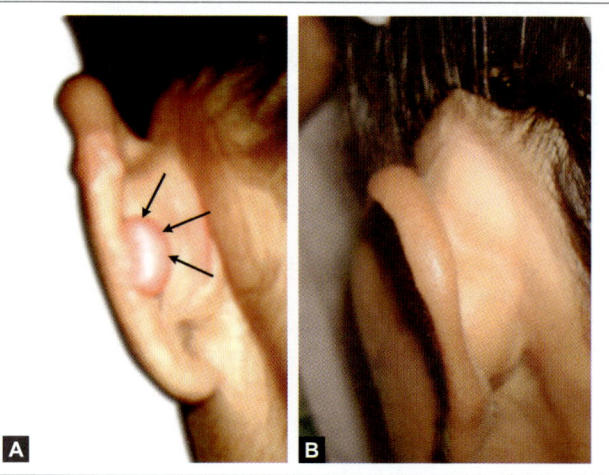

Figs 4.1A and B: (A) Keloid. Medial surface of left pinna after ear-piercing (arrows showing); (B) Cystic swelling in the upper part of retroauricular sulcus

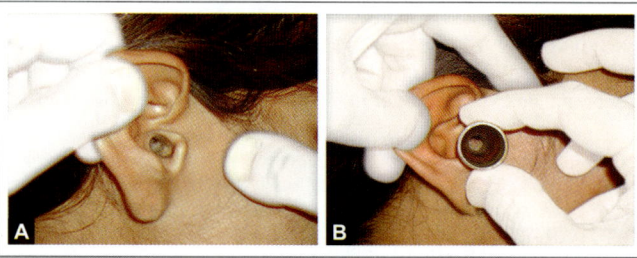

Figs 4.2A and B: (A) Pulling the pinna upward, backward and laterally and tragus forward spread and straighten external auditory canal (EAC); (B) Ear speculum insertion. With left hand, EAC is straightened and with right hand, ear speculum is inserted in the cartilaginous part of EAC

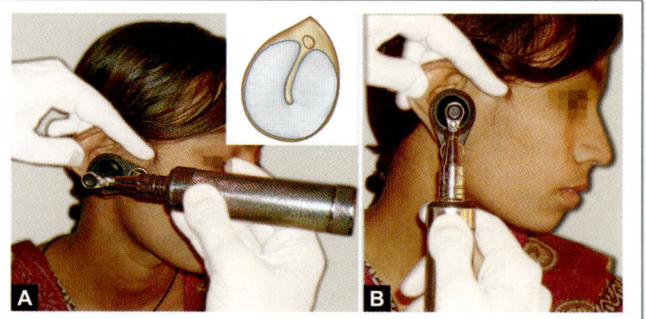

Figs 4.3A and B: Otoscopy examination. Two ways (A and B) of holding and introducing the otoscope. Note the retraction of pinna by the other hand

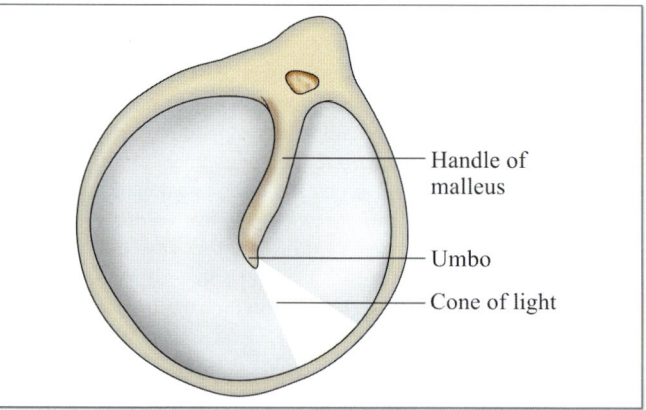

Fig. 4.4: Tympanic membrane seen on otoscopy

- *Tympanic membrane (TM):* The normal TM (Fig. 4.4) is obliquely set at the medial end of the meatus. It is semitransparent and pearly white in color. It consists of two parts—pars tensa and pars flaccida. The site and size of perforations, retraction, and granulations must be recorded. When TM is semitransparent or perforated, some structures (ossicles, windows, eustachian tube, and tumors) of the middle ear can be seen through it.

Otoscope is especially useful in examining the ears as well as the nose of infants.

Siegelization

Mobility of tympanic membrane is tested with Siegel's speculum (Chapter on 'Instruments'). The other uses of this pneumatic speculum are as follows:
- Fistula test for labyrinthine and perilymphatic fistula.
- Suction of middle ear secretions in cases of chronic suppurative otitis media (CSOM).
- Pushing of medicines through the central perforation of tympanic membrane.

Eustachian Tube (ET)

- *Inspection:* The pharyngeal opening of ET can be seen by posterior rhinoscopy mirror, nasal sinuscope, and nasopharyngoscope.
- *Patency:* See Chapter on 'Disorder of Eustachian Tube'.
    - *Valsalva maneuver:* In the presence of a hole in tympanic membrane, air can be heard escaping from the ear when patient tries to blow with mouth and nose closed.

OTALGIA (EARACHE)

Otalgia refers to pain in and around the ear. Ear pain is a very common otological complaint. For the treatment, it is essential to find its cause.

Etiology

- *Primary otalgia:* Pain in and around the ear can be caused by inflammatory, traumatic, and neoplastic conditions of the ear (primary otalgia).

- **Secondary otalgia:** The secondary otalgia is referred from the head and neck regions, which are innervated by the nerves that also supply to ear (Fig. 4.5) (Box 4.1). (*See also the Chapter 'Anatomy of Ear'*).

History and Physical Examination (Box 4.2)

History and physical examination will usually reveal the source of ear pain and indicate whether the otalgia is local or referred to in origin (Flow chart 4.1).

- **Exertional left earache:** In cases of exertional earache on left side, patient must have cardiac consultation to rule out coronary artery disease.
- **Functional:** When no cause is found, ear pain may be functional in origin. In such cases, periodic re-evaluation is important.

> If the ear pain appears to be disproportional to otological findings, especially in elderly patients, preclude the possibility of referred otalgia, especially upper aerodigestive tract malignancy.

OTORRHEA

Otorrhea*, which refers to discharge from the ear, is a very common otologic complaint.

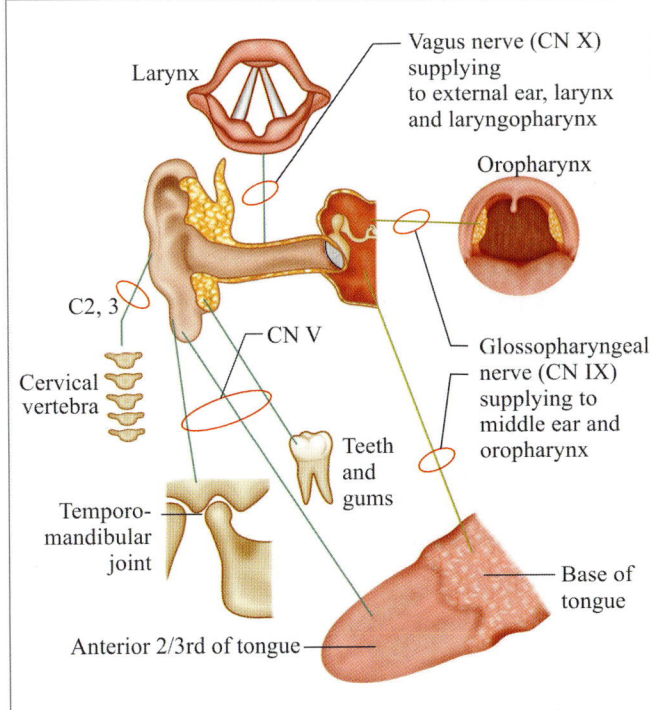

Fig. 4.5: Referred otalgia. Common causes of referred otalgia and nerve supply of ear

---
*Oto, ear + rhoia, flow

Box 4.1: Causes of otalgia

A. **Local causes (Primary otalgia)**
- **Auricle:** Skin lesion, perichondritis/chondritis, trauma
- **External auditory canal (EAC):** Furuncle*, impacted wax*, otitis externa*, trauma*, foreign bodies especially live insects*, otomycosis*, myringitis bullosa, herpes zoster oticus (Ramsay-Hunt syndrome), and malignant neoplasms.
- **Middle ear:** Acute otitis media*, Eustachian tube obstruction*, cholesteatoma*, mastoiditis*, barotrauma, and malignancy of middle ear.
- **Intracranial complications of otitis media:** Extradural abscess.

B. **Referred causes (Secondary otalgia)**
- **Area supplied by (cranial nerve) CN V (trigeminal nerve)**
  - **Dental and periodontal diseases*:** Caries tooth, apical abscess, impacted 3rd molar, malocclusion, erupting dentition in children.
  - **Oral cavity:** Infection, trauma, aphthous* or malignant ulcers of oral cavity*.
  - **Salivary glands:** Parotid and submandibular inflammatory and malignant diseases.
  - **Periauricular lymphadenopathy** from scalp or neck infections.
  - **Temporomandibular joint*:** Myofascial pain dysfunction, bruxism, osteoarthritis, recurrent dislocation, ill-fitting denture, malocclusion, Costen's syndrome.
  - **Nose and paranasal sinuses:** Trauma, infection, tumors and contact points between turbinates and septal spur.
  - **Nasopharynx:** Infection and tumors and after adenoidectomy*.
  - **Sphenopalatine (Sluder's) neuralgia.**
  - **Trigeminal neuralgia.**
  - **Headache:** Tension type, traction, and inflammatory headaches.
  - **Atypical facial pain.**
- **Area supplied by (cranial nerve) CN IX (glossopharyngeal nerve)**
  - **Oropharynx*:** Acute tonsillitis, peritonsillar abscess, post-tonsillectomy, benign and malignant ulcers of soft palate, tonsil and its pillars and base of tongue, tuberculosis.
  - **Elongated styloid process** (Eagle's syndrome).
  - **Glossopharyngeal neuralgia.**
- **Area supplied by (cranial nerve) CN X (vagus nerve)**
  - **Vallecula, larynx, laryngopharynx, esophagus:** Malignancy* or ulcerative lesions.
  - **Thyroid:** Thyroiditis.
  - **Cardiac/pulmonary:** Coronary artery disease, aneurysmal dilation of great vessels.
  - **Esophagus:** Hiatus hernia with gastroesophageal reflux.
- **Area supplied by C2 and C3 spinal nerves**
  - Cervical arthritis/disc disease
  - Cervical spondylosis*, injuries of cervical spine, caries spine.
- **Facial nerve:** Geniculate neuralgia, Bell's palsy*, and herpes zoster oticus.
- **Psychogenic**

*Common causes of otalgia

Box 4.2: Otalgia: History, physical examination and investigations

- **History**
  - **Onset and duration:** Sudden, gradual, preceding events.
  - **Quality and localization:** Vague and nonlocalizing.
  - **Associated ear symptoms:** Otorrhea, hearing loss and ear fullness, swelling, trauma, and foreign body.
  - **Whether ear pain is associated with:** Mastication, swallowing, voice change, purulent rhinorrhea or physical exertion.
  - **Past history:** Ear surgery.
- **Physical examination**
  - **Ear, nose, throat, head, and neck examination.**
  - **Dental examination.**
  - **Craniomandibular:** Palpation of temporomandibular joint (TMJ) and surrounding musculature.
  - **Cervical spines.**
  - **Neurologic examination:** Cranial nerves.
- **Investigations**
  - Flexible fiberoptic examination of nose, pharynx, and larynx (nasopharyngolaryngoscopy).
  - Esophagogram.
  - X-ray cervical spines.
  - Orthopantomogram (OPG).
  - X-rays for TMJ and styloid process

Most common causes of ear discharge: In children, they are acute suppurative otitis media (ASOM) and chronic suppurative otitis media (CSOM) while in adults, they are CSOM and otitis externa.

Otorrhea may be profuse or scanty and continuous or intermittent. Otorrhea from ASOM may be bloody, mixed with mucus, or mucopurulent and typically shortlived.

Types of Discharge and their Causes

- **Nature of discharge**
  - **Mucopurulent:** Acute suppurative otitis media (ASOM) and chronic suppurative otitis media (CSOM).
  - **Serous:** Eczematous otitis externa.
  - **Sanguinous (blood-tinged):** ASOM, granulations, trauma, tumors.
  - **Putrid (foul-smelling):** Cholesteatoma.
  - **Watery:** Watery otorrhea, which may be copious, subtle or intermittent, suggests a CSF leak.
- **Otorrhea with associated symptoms:**
  - **Pain:** Acute otitis externa.
  - **Pruritus:** Chronic otitis externa and otomycosis.
- **Recurrent otorrhea:**
  - CSOM, eczema or psoriasis of ear canal skin.

Contd...

Flow chart 4.1: Clinical diagnosis of causes of otalgia

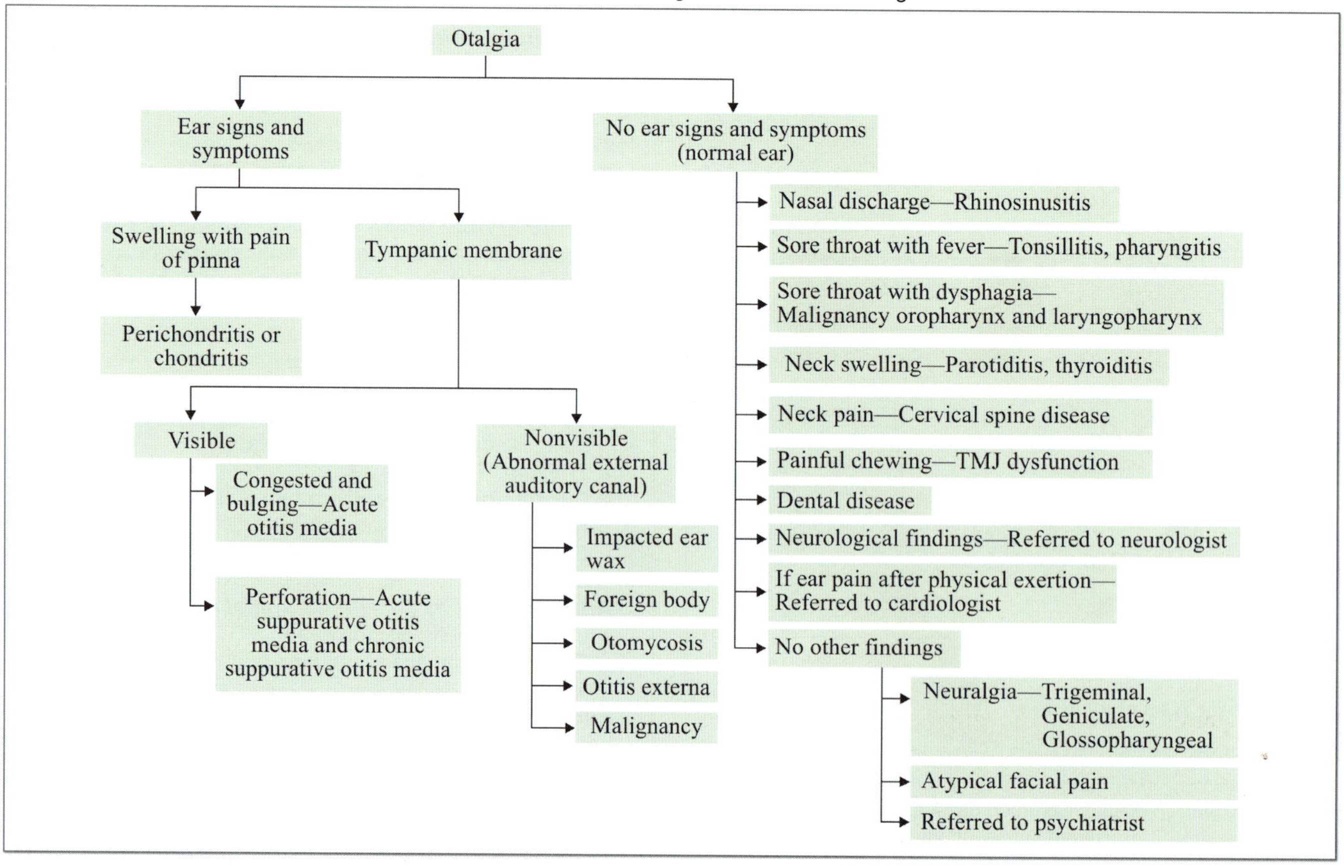

Abbreviation: TMJ—Temporomandibular joint

> **Box 4.3: Causes of polyp**
> - *External auditory canal:* Unhealed furuncle, trauma, keratosis obturans, foreign body, tumors (ceruminoma, exostosis, malignancy).
> - *Middle ear:* Chronic suppurative otitis media (CSOM) (tubotympanic and cholesteatoma), glomus tumors (tympanicum and jugulare), carcinoma.

Contd…

- **Otorrhea with specific past history:**
  - *Ear surgery:* Recurrence of middle ear disease or infection in mastoid cavity.
  - *Neurotologic surgery:* Immediate or delayed CSF otorrhea.
  - *Grommets:* Otorrhea is common after myringotomy tube insertion.

EAR POLYP

An ear polyp is a pedunculated mass, which lies in the external auditory canal (EAC). It may arise from EAC or middle ear. Granulomatous and neoplastic lesions may present as ear polyp. It is usually associated with otorrhea and hearing loss. Other associated symptoms include bleeding, pain and itching. Causes of ear polyp are shown in Box 4.3.

History and Examination

- *Associated symptoms:* Ear polyp is usually associated with otorrhea and hearing loss. Other associated symptoms include bleeding, pain and itching.
- *Consistency:* Inflammatory polyps are soft whereas tumors are firm, friable and bleed readily.
- *Probing:* It is useful in determining the site of origin of the polyp. A probe can be passed all around if it is arising from the middle ear but it cannot if polyp is arising from the external auditory canal (EAC). Glomus and malignant tumors bleed readily on probing.
- *Tuning fork tests:* They will reveal the type of hearing loss.

> *Caution:* Middle ear polyps should not be avulsed as it can damage important structures attached with them, such as ossicles and facial nerve.

TINNITUS

Tinnitus* stands for the perception of sound (ringing or noise), which has no external stimulus (Fig. 4.6). Approximately, one-third people experience tinnitus sometime in their lives. The etiology of this common ear symptom is poorly understood (Box 4.4). The severity of sound ranges from nearly undetectable to severe and debilitating. Though there is no cure for chronic tinnitus, there are various modalities of management, which significantly improve the quality of patients' life.

Auditory hallucination: It is a psychiatric disorder in which patient hears voices or other organized sounds like music or conversation.

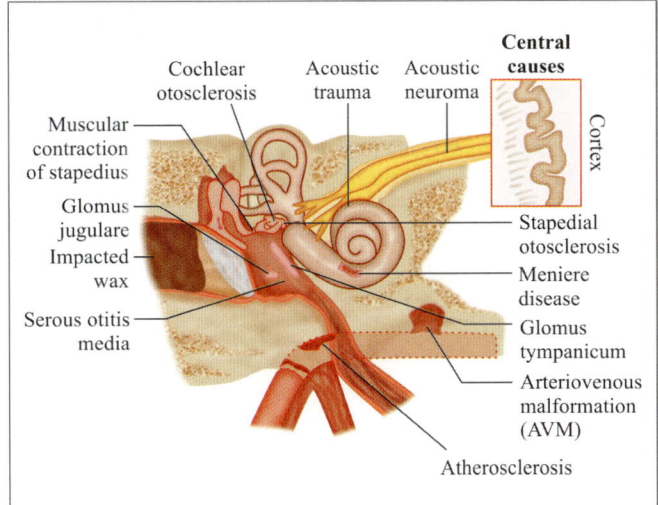

Fig. 4.6: Common causes of tinnitus

Types

Tinnitus can be categorized into different groups. *See* Box 4.4 for classification and causes:
- *Subjective and objective:* Subjective tinnitus, which is the most common, is perceived only by the patient. Objective tinnitus can be heard by the examiner also.

History and Physical Examination

Patient should describe the nature of the sound. Any change in the tinnitus that has occurred during the course of disease should be noted. Eighty-five percent of tinnitus patients have hearing loss. Most patients have normal neuro-otologic examination except for the hearing loss.
- *Otoscopy:* In cases of pulsatile tinnitus, otoscopy may reveal a middle ear mass.
- *Audiogram:* It may reveal otosclerosis, Meniere's disease, or noise-induced hearing loss.
  - *Cerebellopontine angle tumors:* The cerebellopontine angle lesions should be suspected in cases of unilateral or significant asymmetrical sensorineural hearing loss (SNHL). Ten percent of acoustic neuroma patients present with tinnitus. This rate increases to 83% with passage of time.
- *Abnormally patent Eustachian tube:* Tinnitus synchronous with respiration may occur in cases of abnormally patent Eustachian tube.

---
*Tinnitus (latin word) means 'to ring'

Box 4.4: Classification and causes of tinnitus

- **Nonpulsatile:** Subjective (most common)
  - With Hearing Loss
    - *External ear:* Wax, hair, foreign bodies, live insects
    - *Middle ear:* Otitis media, patulous eustachian tube, hemotympanum (head injury).
    - *Labyrinth:* Meniere's disease, noise exposure, ototoxic agents, presbycusis, and other causes of sensory hearing loss.
    - *CN VIII:* Acoustic neuroma and other causes of neural hearing loss.
  - Without Hearing Loss
    - Psychogenic
    - Hypotension
    - Hypoglycemia
    - Epilepsy
    - Migraine
    - Idiopathic
- **Pulsatile (noncontinuous):**
  - Vascular
    - *Arterial*
      - *Atherosclerosis:* Atherosclerotic carotid artery disease and atherosclerosis of external carotid or subclavian.
      - *Glomus tumors:* Glomus tympanicum, glomus jugulare.
      - *Vascular malformations:* Congenital arteriovenous malformations acquired arteriovenous fistulae.
      - *Arterial dissection:* Carotid, vertebral.
      - *High cardiac output:* Pregnancy, anemia, exercise, thyrotoxicosis.
      - Otosclerosis
      - Hypertension
    - *Venous*
      - Benign intracranial hypertension (BIH) syndrome (pseudotumor cerebri).
      - Venous hum
      - Jugular bulb anomalies
  - Nonvascular
    - *Myoclonus (multiple sclerosis, brainstem infarct)*
      - Palatal
      - Tensor tympani
      - Stapedius
    - *Vascular neoplasm*
      - Skull base
      - Temporal bone
    - *Temporomandibular joint disease*
  - Idiopathic

Tinnitus Management Program

In spite of treating every reasonable medical cause for tinnitus, majority of patients report little improvement. The patients, who consider their tinnitus to be a significant debilitating problem, need specialized management program.

In many cases of chronic tinnitus, there is no 'cure'. However, there is a wide array of strategies, which helps patients in getting control over their tinnitus.

- Multimodal strategies are designed as per the need of specific patient.
- Patient education, reassurance and counseling should be a part of patient's evaluation.
- Tinnitus and its coincident symptoms, such as insomnia, anxiety/stress, depression and fatigue form a vicious circle of symptoms. These coincident symptoms need effective treatment (medical and psychotherapy) because their increase would worsen the tinnitus.
- *Lifestyle changes:* Many patients observe that their tinnitus worsens when they are tired. They should get enough restful sleep.
  Though exercise may increase tinnitus problem in patients, it should be done regularly as it helps in stress reduction and in improving cardiovascular health, muscle tone, mood and sleep patterns (Box 4.5).
  - Earplugs and earmuffs protect against harmful sounds and noises, which increase not only loudness of tinnitus but also produce noise-induced hearing loss.
  - Tinnitus is less bothersome when patients are busy in their work. Retired persons should be encouraged to keep themselves busy in enjoyable and rewarding activities and volunteer work.
  - Patients are encouraged to participate in social functions and positive interactions with family members, friends and relatives.
- *Conservative management:* In conservative management, vasodilator, sedatives, vitamins, tranquilizers

Box 4.5: Factors aggravating and relieving tinnitus (lifestyle changes)

- *Factors aggravating tinnitus:*
  - Stress/fatigue
  - Excessive noise exposure
  - Upper respiratory tract infections and allergy
  - Moving jaws/clenching teeth
  - Head and neck trauma
  - Changes in altitude
  - Too much use of aspirin, alcohol, caffeine, acetaminophen, or ibuprofen
  - Changes in body position
  - Tobacco and marijuana
- *Factors relieving tinnitus:*
  - Regular exercise
  - Avoidance of noise exposure (use earplugs and earmuffs)
  - Keeping oneself busy
  - Personal relationships and socialization

and drugs like zinc therapy, carbamazepine and clonazepam have been used.

- **Acoustic therapies:** Acoustic therapies (Box 4.6) constitute a vital component of an effective tinnitus management program. This noninvasive therapy provides not only immediate relief but there also occurs tinnitus suppression or temporary disappearance of tinnitus (residual inhibition).
  - **In-the-ear devices:** For many patients, direct sounds to their ears are more effective than environmental sounds. In-the-ear devices, though comparatively expensive, are most portable, inconspicuous and efficient in obtaining relief from the tinnitus.
  - **Hearing aids:** They are beneficial for the patients who have significant hearing loss. Better hearing may relieve some patients of the frustration, isolation and depression.
  - **Combination instruments:** They are indicated in the patients who are already using the hearing aid and feel that sound generators will provide additional tinnitus relief.

> **Box 4.6: Examples of acoustic therapies**
>
> - *Pleasant environmental sounds:*
>   - Music, ocean waves, rain forest, summer night, television or relaxation CDs
>   - Tabletop sound machines
>   - Cassette tapes and CDs
>   - Tabletop water fountains
>   - Fans and air purifiers
> - *Sounds close to the ears:*
>   - Sound pillow and pillow speakers
>   - Headphones and earphones
> - *Sounds directly into the ear canal:*
>   - In-the-ear sound generators or maskers
>   - Hearing aids
>   - Combination instruments (combination of hearing aid and sound generator)

- **Surgical management:** Depending upon the causes, the surgical modalities of treatment include:
  - Endolymphatic sac decompression
  - Cryotherapy for cochlear destruction
  - Cochlear nerve section if no hearing

Self-evaluation Exercises

1. Which of the following is not the function of Siegel's pneumatic speculum?
   a. Provides magnified view of tympanic membrane
   b. Tests the mobility of the tympanic membrane
   c. Performs fistula test
   d. Introduces medicine into middle ear
   e. None from the above
2. Which of the following is not true for the nerve supply of middle ear?
   a. Lateral surface of tympanic membrane is supplied by auriculotemporal nerve (CN V_3) and auricular branch of vagus
   b. Medial surface of tympanic membrane is supplied by glossopharyngeal nerve
   c. Nerve supply of the middle ear—glossopharyngeal nerve
   d. Jacobson's nerve: This branch of vagus nerve supplies middle ear and mastoid air cells and supplies secretomotor fibers to parotid. The section of this nerve relieves gustatory sweating
3. Which of the following are common causes of referred otalgia?
   a. Peritonsillar abscess
   b. Cancer of the pyriform fossa
   c. TMJ dysfunction
   d. Ulcer tongue
   e. All of the above

True (T)/False (F)

4. Patients with Costen's syndrome usually present with referred otalgia, which may be associated with vertigo and tinnitus.
5. In cases of carcinoma base of tongue, referred ear pain is not through the glossopharyngeal nerve and otic ganglion.

Answers

1. e
2. d
3. e
4. T
5. F

Chapter 5

Hearing Evaluation

⊙ Specific Learning Objectives

After going through the chapter, you should be able to answer the following questions:
- Describe the methods and their interpretations of Rinnes, Weber, Schwabach and absolute bone conduction tuning fork hearing tests.
- What is pure tone audiometry and its uses and interpretations?
- What do you know about decibel (dB)?
- What do you know about: (1) Recruitment; (2) Tone decay; (3) Masking; (4) Pure-tone average; (5) Air-bone gap?
- What are the indications and advantages of the speech audiometry?
- What do you know about speech reception threshold test (SRT) and speech discrimination test?
- Which are the different types of tympanogram charts and their causes?
- What do you know about stapedius (acoustic) reflex and its function, neural pathways and measurement?
- What do you know about the following: (1) Electrocochleography; (2) BERA; (3) OAE; (4) Auditory steady state response

AUDIOLOGY AND ACOUSTICS

Audiology refers to the study of hearing disorders through the hearing evaluation as well as the rehabilitation of the patients with hearing impairments. *Acoustics* is the science that deals with the sounds and their perception.

Sound

Sound is a form of energy, which is produced by any vibrating object. A sound wave is produced by compression and rarefaction of molecules of the medium in which it travels such as air, liquids and solids. Velocity of sound in the air, at 20°C at sea level is 344 meters (1,120 feet) per second. Velocity of sound is faster in liquid and fastest in solid medium.

Frequency and Pitch

Frequency refers to the number of cycles per second. Its unit Hertz (Hz) is named after a German scientist Heinrich Rudolf Hertz. A sound of 500 Hz means 500 cycles per second. *Pitch* is a subjective sensation produced by frequency of sound. The higher the frequency, the greater is the pitch.

Pure Tone and Complex Sound

A single frequency sound is called *pure tone* such as 250, 500 or 1,000 Hz. In *pure tone audiometry* (PTA), thresholds of hearing in decibels for various pure tones from 250 to 8,000 Hz are measured. The sound, which has more than one frequency, is called *complex sound* such as voice and speech.

Overtones and Timbre

Overtones are frequencies which are above the fundamental frequency of the vibrating source. Overtones determine the quality or the *timbre* of sound.

Intensity and Loudness

The *intensity* is the strength of sound which determines *loudness*. The unit of intensity of sound is the decibel (dB). Loudness is a subjective sensation produced by intensity. The greater the intensity of sound more is the loudness. The intensities of different types of speech at 1 m distance are given in Table 5.1.

Table 5.1: Intensities of different types of speech

Type of speech	Intensity
Whisper	30 dB
Normal conversation	60 dB
Shouting	90 dB
Discomfort in the ear	120 dB
Pain in the ear	130 dB

Decibel

Decibel is 1/10th of a bel*. Decibel represents a logarithmic ratio between two sounds (sound being described and the reference sound). Sound can be measured in following two ways:
1. *As power (watts/cm³):* It is used in music systems and theaters.
2. *As pressure (dynes/cm³):* It is used in audiology.

The reference sound, which has a sound pressure level (SPL) of 0.0002 dynes/cm³, roughly corresponds to the threshold of normal human hearing at 1,000 Hz. Decibel notation avoids dealing with large figures of SPL.

If a sound has an SPL of 1,000 (10^3) times the reference sound, it is expressed as 20 × 3 = 60 dB. In the same way, a sound of 1,000,000 (10^6) times the reference sound SPL is expressed as 120 dB.

Several dB scales, which have a different reference scale, are used to measure sound and hearing. In audiometry, hearing is measured on a biological scale in decibels hearing level. Environmental sounds are measured on a physical scale in decibels sound pressure level. The decibel A scale (dB A) is noise level scale.

- *Audiometric zero:* According to the International Standards Organization (ISO), audiometric zero is the mean value of minimal audible intensity in a group of normally hearing healthy young adults.
- *Hearing level:* Hearing level is SPL, which is produced by an audiometer at a specific frequency. It is measured in dB with reference to audiometric zero. The 70 dB sound of audiometer is represented as 70 dB HL.
- *Sound level meter:* This instrument measures level of noise and other sounds. It has different weighting networks (A, B, C) for different sensitivities at different frequencies for describing the sound.
- *dB A scale:* Noise levels are expressed as dB A. The dB A scale is toward high frequency noises (1,000–5,000 Hz), which cause more sensorineural hearing loss (SNHL) than equivalent levels of low-frequency noise. Hearing protection for workers are required if noise exposure in the workplace is more than 90 dB A for 8 hours a day.

Sensation Level

The sensation level refers to the sound level above the threshold of hearing, which will produce a sensation. 40 dB sensation level (SL) means patient was tested at 40 dB above this threshold, which could be either zero dB (normal persons) or more in cases of hearing loss.

In cases of normal hearing it means 0 + 40 = 40 dB HL while in a case of hearing loss of say 50 dB, it would be 50 + 40 = 90 dB HL.

The discrimination scores in speech audiometry are tested at 30–40 dB sensation level (SL). Stapedial reflex is elicited at 70–100 dB SL.

Loudness Discomfort Level

This level of sound produces discomfort in the ear. It is important while prescribing a hearing aid. Normally, it is 90–150 dB SL.

Dynamic Range

Dynamic range is important while prescribing hearing aids. It refers to the difference between the most comfortable level and the loudness discomfort level. The recruitment in cochlear type of hearing loss reduces the dynamic range.

Noise

Noise is an aperiodic complex sound. Three types of noises are described—white, narrow band and speech.
1. *White noise:* It is similar to white light, which contains all the colors of the visible spectrum. White noise, contains all frequencies in the audible spectrum. This broadband noise is used for masking.
2. *Narrow band noise:* In narrow band white noise, certain frequencies above and below the given noise are filtered out. So the frequency range becomes smaller than the broadband white noise. The narrow band white noise is used for masking in PTA.
3. *Speech noise:* The speech noise has only speech range frequencies from 300 to 3,000 Hz. Other frequencies are filtered out.

> Masking of non-test ear is always done during the bone conduction tests. For air conduction tests, masking is required only when difference of hearing between two ears exceeds 40 dB.

TYPES OF HEARING LOSS

Clinically, hearing loss is traditionally divided into two types—1. conductive and 2. sensorineural. For classification of hearing loss and their causes and differences, *see* Chapter 'Conductive Hearing Loss and Otosclerosis'.

Conductive Hearing Loss (CHL)

The diseases, which interfere with the conduction of sound from the external auditory canal (EAC) to the stapediovestibular joint, result in conductive hearing loss (CHL). CHL is mostly managed successfully with medical and surgical treatment. Example includes ear wax,

---
*Alexander Graham Bell, the inventor of telephone

tympanic membrane perforation and ossicular disorders. For further details of their causes and management, *see* Chapter 'Conductive Hearing Loss and Otosclerosis'.

Sensorineural Hearing Loss (SNHL)

The diseases of the cochlea (sensory type) and CN VIII and its central connections (neural type) result in SNHL. Retrocochlear HL refers to lesions of 8th nerve and central auditory connections. For the various types of SNHL and their causes and differences, *see* Chapter 'Sensorineural Hearing Loss'. Some of the common examples include sensory (presbycusis, mumps, noise-induced) and neural (acoustic neuroma).

Mixed Hearing Loss

It has elements of both CHL and SNHL. The air-bone gap in pure tone audiometry (PTA) indicates CHL while impairment of bone conduction indicates SNHL. The most common causes of mixed hearing loss are otosclerosis and chronic suppurative otitis media (CSOM).

HEARING EVALUATION

Need of Hearing Evaluation

The hearing assessment facilitates in finding out the following features of hearing loss:
- *Type of hearing loss:* Conductive, sensorineural or mixed.
- *Severity of hearing loss:* Mild, moderate, moderately severe, severe, profound or total.
- *Site of lesion:* The diseases of external ear, tympanic membrane and middle ear result in CHL. Clinical examination and different types of audiometry are helpful in finding the site of lesion. Certain special hearing tests can differentiate between different types of SNHL such as cochlear, retrocochlear and central.
- *Cause of hearing loss:* In addition to hearing tests detailed history and laboratory investigations will indicate towards the causes of hearing loss such as congenital, traumatic, infective, neoplastic, degenerative, metabolic, ototoxic, vascular or autoimmune process.

Methods of Hearing Evaluation

- The history taking and complete ear, nose, throat, head and neck examination and general evaluation of other systems are mandatory before performing the different types hearing tests (Box 5.1).
- The most commonly employed methods of hearing evaluation are tuning fork tests (Rinne, Weber, absolute bone conduction and air conduction) and PTA. Other methods, which are routinely done in otology clinics, include speech audiometry, impedance audiometry, brainstem evoked response audiometry (BERA) and otoacoustic emission.
- Usually methods of hearing evaluation are classified into two groups subjective and objective.
  1. *Subjective methods:* These need patient's co-operation and reliability and include tuning fork test, PTA and speech audiometry.
  2. *Objective methods:* These can be done even in children and include impedance, electrocochleography, brainstem evoked response audiometry (BERA) and otoacoustic emission.
- The hearing evaluation methods employed in infants and children are discussed in Chapter 'Hearing Impairment in Infants and Young Children'.
- *Central auditory tests:* They can find the defects in the central auditory pathways and the temporal cortex. The test signals can be delivered to either one ear (monotic) or both the ears (dichotic). *Staggered spondaic words test* is widely employed.

> **Box 5.1: Different types of hearing tests**
>
> *Traditional screening tests*
> - Watch test
> - Finger friction tests
> - Voice tests (conversation and whisper)
>
> *Tuning fork tests*
> - Air conduction
> - Bone conduction
> - Rinne test
> - Weber test
> - Absolute bone conduction (ABC)
> - Schwabach's test
> - Bing test
> - Gelle's test
>
> *Audiometric tests*
> - Pure tone audiometry (PTA)
>   - Air and bone conduction thresholds
>   - Recruitment
>   - Alternate binaural loudness balance test for recruitment
>   - Short increment sensitivity index test
>   - Tone decay test
> - Speech audiometry
>   - Speech reception threshold
>   - Discrimination score
> - Impedance audiometry
>   - Tympanometry
>   - Acoustic reflex measurement
>
> *Evoked response audiometry*
> - Brainstem Evoked Response Audiometry (BERA)
> - Electrocochleography
>
> *Otoacoustic emissions*
>
> *Central auditory tests*

- **Monotic test:** Distorted speech is presented to the ear. Patients with central auditory disorders would find it difficult in understanding the message.
- **Dichotic test:** Each ear is presented with different speech messages simultaneously and patient is requested to identify them. In staggered spondaic word test, pairs of spondaic words along with digits or nonsense words are together presented to both the ears. In cases of temporal lobe lesions, contralateral ear will have difficulty in identifying these words.
- **Binaural tests:** These tests are normal in temporal lobe lesions, but pick up brainstem lesions. Binaural masking level difference test finds the disorders which are related with the integration of information from both the ears.

- *Traditional screening tests:* These tests were popular for screening before the audiometric era, but are now practically obsolete:
  - *Finger friction test* is a rough but quick method of screening. Rubbing or snapping the thumb and a finger close to the patient's ear gives rough idea of patient's hearing.
  - In *watch test*, a clicking watch is brought close to the ear and the distance when patient hears is measured.

Voice Tests

Conversation and Whisper

A normal person hears conversational voice at 12 m (40 feet) and whisper (with residual air after normal expiration) at 6 m (20 feet).

- *Method:* The test is done in quiet surroundings. The patient stands at a distance of 6 m while his test ear faces toward the examiner. Patient's eyes are closed to avoid lip-reading. The non-test ear is occluded with intermittent pressure on the tragus by an assistant. The spondee words (baseball, sunlight, daydream) or numbers with letters (AB4, X3B) are spoken by the doctor while s/he is gradually walking towards the patient. The distance at which conversational voice and the whispered voice are heard is measured.
- *Disadvantage:* Lack of standardization in intensity and pitch of voice and the level of ambient noise.
- *Interpretations:* 6 m (20 feet) distance is taken as normal for both conversation and whisper.

SUBJECTIVE HEARING EVALUATION

Tuning Forks Test (TFT)

A tuning fork consists of a base (footplate), stem and two prongs. The tuning forks of 256, 512, 1,024 and 2,048 Hz* (cycles/second) are used. The tuning fork of 512 Hz is most important. The lower frequency tuning fork produces a sense of bone vibration while higher frequencies have shorter decay time.

Methods

- *Charging:* A tuning fork may be charged with striking against the examiner's elbow, rubber heel of the shoe or special rubber pad. Tuning fork should be sounded gently. Overtones with excessive vibration lead to inaccurate results.
- *Air conduction:* For testing air conduction, a charged tuning fork is placed vertically, about 2 cm away from the EAC. The sound waves are conducted via EAC, tympanic membrane and middle ear ossicles to the inner ear. Thus, the air conduction test function of both the conducting mechanism and the cochlea.
- *Bone conduction:* For testing bone conduction, the base of charged tuning fork is placed firmly on the mastoid bone. In this way cochlea is stimulated directly by vibrations which are conducted via skull bones. Thus the bone conduction tests only the cochlear function.
- *Tests:* Normally air conduction is louder and heard twice longer than the bone conduction. The most important TFT are Rinne, Weber and absolute bone conduction (Table 5.2).

Rinne Test

- *Principle:* The Rinne test compares air conduction with bone conduction.
- *Method:* The base of a charged tuning fork is placed on the mastoid and when patient stops hearing, tuning fork is brought near the EAC. If patient still hears then air conduction is said to be more than bone conduction. Alternatively, patient is asked to compare the loudness

Table 5.2: The interpretation of tuning fork tests (TFT)

Tests	Normal	CHL	SNHL
Rinne	AC > BC (Rinne +)	BC > AC (Rinne -)	AC > BC (Rinne +)
Weber	Center (no lateralization)	Lateralized to affected ear	Lateralized to better ear
Absolute bone conduction	Normal	Normal	Reduced
Schwabach	Normal	Lengthened	Shortened
Bing	Positive	Negative	Positive
Gelle	Positive	Negative (ossicular lesions)	Positive

Abbreviations: AC—air conduction; BC—bone conduction; CHL—Conductive hearing loss; SNHL—Sensorineural hearing loss.

---

*Hertz (a German scientist) is a unit of frequency of sound. 1 Hz = 1 cycle/second

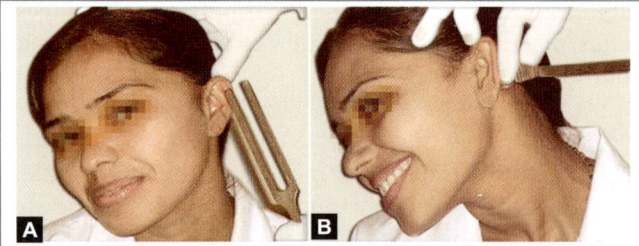

Figs 5.1A and B: Rinne Test. It compares the loudness of sound of (A) Air conduction; (B) Bone conduction

of sound of air conduction and bone conduction (Figs 5.1A and B).

Interpretations

- ***Rinne positive:*** Rinne test is said to be positive when air conduction is longer or louder than bone conduction. The positive Rinne is seen in cases of normal hearing and SNHL.
- ***Rinne negative:*** A negative Rinne (bone conduction > air conduction) is seen in cases of conductive hearing loss (CHL).
- ***Rinne equivocal:*** Here air conduction is equal to bone conduction and it indicates mild CHL.
- ***False Rinne negative:*** It is seen in profound SNHL. Here patient does not hear any sound of air conduction but responds to only bone conduction. This response to only bone conduction can be either from the opposite normal ear (through transcranial transmission) or patient considers vibration as sound. The masking of the non-test ear with Barany's noise box while testing for bone conduction usually solves the problem. Weber's test (lateralizing to opposite ear) will help in detecting the false Rinne negative.

- ***False Rinne negative:*** If Rinne is negative in one ear and Weber does not lateralize to that ear it means that test ear has severe to profound SNHL.
- A negative Rinne with 256, 512 and 1,024 Hz shows air-bone gap of approximately 15, 30 and 45 dB, respectively.

Masking

In masking, a continuous noise is presented to the better hearing ear (non-test ear) to prevent crossing over of sound from the worst ear (test ear) to the better ear. The masking of the non-test ear avoids the problem of false Rinne negative. Following types of noise may be used for masking:

- Barany's noise box generates noise and masks the better ear while testing the hearing loss.

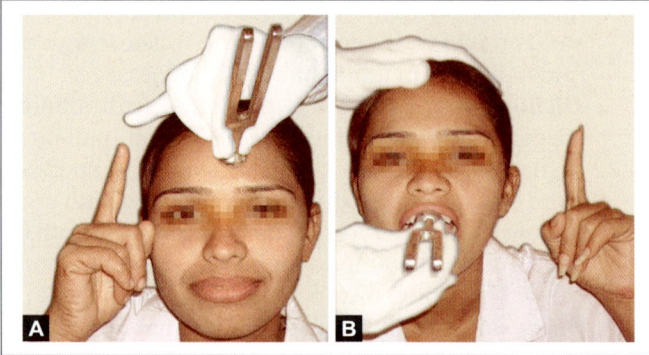

Figs 5.2A and B: Weber Test compares bone conduction of both ears simultaneously. The base of a charged tuning fork is placed in the center of the forehead (A) or upper central incisors; (B) Patient raises finger on the side of better hearing (lateralization)

- Noise with piece of paper.
- Narrow-band noise during audiometry.

Weber Test

- ***Principle:*** Bone conduction of both ears is compared simultaneously. The sound travels directly to the cochlea via bone.
- ***Method:*** The base of a charged tuning fork is placed in the center of the forehead or upper central incisors (Figs 5.2A and B). The patient is asked to tell on which side s/he hears better. The Weber test is said to be lateralized on the side on which patient hears well.

Weber test is quite sensitive as difference of only 3–5 dB hearing level can result in lateralization. Weber test readily detects the false Rinne negative.

Interpretations

- ***Normal:*** Normal person hears equally in both ears or may not hear in any ear.
- ***Conductive hearing loss (CHL):*** The test is lateralized toward the affected ear. If both the ears have CHL, Weber is lateralized to worst ear.
- ***Sensorineural hearing loss (SNHL):*** The test is lateralized towards the better ear.

- ***Tuning fork tests:*** Weber and Rinne tests are important and confirm the diagnosis of conductive hearing loss (CHL).
- ***Weber test:*** It detects a difference in hearing levels between two ears. It is more sensitive in diagnosing conductive hearing loss (CHL).

Absolute Bone Conduction Test

- *Principle:* The absolute bone conduction test compares the duration of patient's bone conduction with that of the examiner (presuming doctor's hearing to be normal).
- *Method:* EACs of the patient and examiner are occluded to prevent air-conduction of ambient noise. The charged tuning fork is put on the mastoid. When patient stops hearing, tuning fork is transferred to the examiner's mastoid.

> **Interpretations**
> - *Normal and conductive hearing loss (CHL):* Equal absolute bone conduction of both patient and doctor.
> - *Sensorineural hearing loss (SNHL):* Examiner's absolute bone conduction is longer than the patient's absolute bone conduction.

Schwabach's Test

In this TFT, bone conduction of patient is compared with that of the normal hearing examiner but EAC is not occluded. In comparison to examiner, patient's duration of hearing is reduced in SNHL and increased in CHL.

Bing Test

Bing test examines the effect of occlusion of ear canal on the bone conduction hearing. The base of a charged tuning fork is kept on the mastoid, while the examiner alternately closes and opens the EAC by pressing on the tragus.

In cases of normal hearing and SNHL, patient hears louder when EAC is occluded and softer when the EAC is open (Bing positive). In case of CHL, patient will appreciate no change in hearing (Bing negative).

Gelle's Test

Gelle's test examines the effect of increased air pressure in ear canal on the bone conduction hearing. The tuning fork is placed on the mastoid. The air pressure is increased in the EAC by Siegel's speculum, which pushes the ossicles inward and raises the middle ear pressure that results in decreased hearing (Gelle's positive) due to the immobility of basilar membrane.

There is no change in hearing (Gelle's negative) when ossicular chain is fixed (otosclerosis, tympanosclerosis) or disconnected (traumatic). Positive Gelle's test is seen in cases of normal hearing and SNHL. It is a good test when the facility of impedance audiometry is not available.

Pure Tone Audiometry

This non-invasive subjective test is a graphic recording of hearing level both quantitatively and qualitatively. An audiometer is an electronic device this generates pure tones. The intensity of these tones are either increased or decreased in 5 dB steps. The audiometer is so calibrated that the hearing of a normal person is at zero dB*level.

The air conduction thresholds are measured usually for tones of 250, 500, 1,000, 2,000, 4,000 and 8,000 Hz. (New audiometers provide further higher frequencies). The bone conduction thresholds are measured usually for 250, 500, 1,000, 2,000 and 4,000 Hz. The speech frequencies range from 500–2,000 Hz**.

- *Pure tone average:* The pure tone average is an average of the air conduction thresholds at 500, 1,000, and 2,000 Hz speech frequencies.
- *Air-bone gap:* The bone conduction thresholds are the measure of cochlear function. The difference between the thresholds of air conduction and bone conduction, called *air-bone gap*, is a feature of CHL.

Method

Audiometry is done in a soundproof room (ideal) or a quiet room (Fig. 5.3). First air conduction and then bone conduction is recorded separately for each ear. The pure tones are presented to the ears by headphone (for air conduction) and vibrator (for bone conduction). The graph on which these thresholds are charted is called an *audiogram*. For right ear red color and for left ear blue color pencils are used. For air conduction, continuous line and for bone conduction, interrupted (broken) line is used for recording (for audiograms, see Chapter 'Conductive Hearing Loss and Sensorineural Hearing Loss') (Table 5.3).

- *Masking:* Air conduction sounds "crossover" occurs when a 50 dB difference exists between air conduction thresholds of two ears. The bone conduction sounds "crossover" may occur even at 0 dB difference between

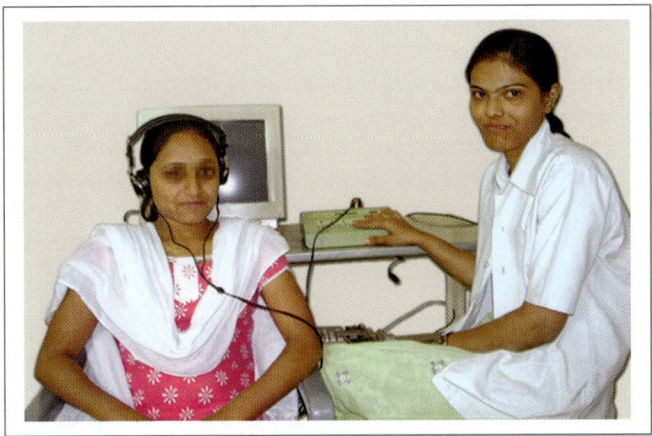

Fig. 5.3: Pure tone audiometry (PTA). See the green colored audiometer on the table

---

*The intensity of sound is measured in logarithmic units called decibel (dB), which is the smallest change in the intensity of the sound that can be appreciated by a normal human ear.
**The audible range of frequency is 20–20,000 Hz

Table 5.3: Symbols used in audiogram charting

	Right ear	Left ear
Pencil color	Red	Blue
AC without masking	O	X
AC with masking	△	□
BC without masking	<	>
BC with masking	[	]
No response	↓	↓

the thresholds of two ears. The narrow-band noise in the non-test ear (better hearing) is employed for the masking. When the difference between in air conduction of the ears is 40 dB or more, the better ear is masked. Masking avoids getting a shadow curve of the better ear. Masking of the non-test ear is necessary during the bone conduction studies.

Utility: Indications and Purposes

Measure of thresholds of AC and BC are done for following purposes and situations:

- *Degree of hearing loss:* Hearing loss may be mild, moderate, severe or profound.
- *Type of hearing loss:* Hearing loss may be conductive, sensory, neural or mixed.
- *Progress of the disease:* Hearing loss can be fluctuating, progressive and stationary.
- *Response to the treatment:* It is important to know whether the hearing loss is improving or not with the therapy.
- *Hearing aids:* The type and necessary setting of hearing aids can be determined.
- *Degree of handicap:* It is needed for compensation and certain benefits.
- *Medicolegal purposes:* It is important after accidents and fights.
- *Speech reception threshold:* It is needed for speech audiometry.
- *Etiology:* Some types of audiograms are specific for certain causes such as otosclerosis, presbycusis, noise-induced hearing loss and ototoxicity. Hearing loss can be unilateral, bilateral (symmetrical or asymmetrical), sloping, flat, with or without notches.

Interpretations

- *Normal:* Air conduction and bone conduction threshold closely follow in the range of 0–20 dB.
- *Conductive hearing loss (CHL):* Bone conduction is normal, but air conduction is reduced (especially in lower frequencies). It gives wide gap between air conduction and bone conduction called **air-bone gap**, see Chapter 'Conductive Hearing Loss and Otosclerosis'.

Contd...

Contd...

- *Sensorineural hearing loss (SNHL):* Both air conduction and bone conduction are reduced specially in higher frequencies. See Chapter 'Sensorineural Hearing Loss'.
- *Mixed hearing loss:* Both air conduction and bone conduction are reduced, but air conduction is more reduced than bone conduction which results in air-bone gap.

Severity of hearing loss:
- *Normal:* Hearing between 0 and 20 dB
- *Mild:* Hearing loss between 20 and 40 dB
- *Moderate:* Hearing loss between 40 and 60 dB
- *Severe:* Hearing loss between 60 and 80 dB
- *Profound:* Hearing loss more than 80 dB

Recruitment

- In this phenomenon of abnormal appreciation of loud sounds, a loud sound which is tolerable in normal ear may grow to abnormal levels of loudness in the recruiting ear and thus becomes intolerable. So if the patient has hearing loss, he cannot tolerate loud sounds.
- These patients are poor candidates for hearing aids.
- Recruitment is a feature of cochlear hearing loss (Meniere's disease, presbycusis). It is absent in normal, CHL (external and middle ear diseases) and nerve hearing loss (acoustic neuroma).
- The common tests for recruitment are Fowler's alternate binaural loudness balance (ABLB) test and short increment sensitivity index (SISI) test.

Fowler's Alternate Binaural Loudness Balance Test

It is done in a case of unilateral hearing loss. A tone of 1,000 Hz is played alternately to the normal and the affected ear. The intensity in the affected ear is adjusted to match the loudness in normal ear. The test begins at 20 dB above the threshold and is repeated at every 10 dB rise until the loudness is matched or the limits of audiometer reached.

Interpretations

- *Normal hearing, conductive and nerve hearing loss:* The initial difference is maintained throughout.
- *Cochlear lesions:* They show partial, complete or over-recruitment.

Short Increment Sensitivity Index Test

Due to the recruitment, patient of cochlear lesions can distinguish smaller changes in intensity of pure tone better than patients of normal hearing, conductive and nerve hearing loss.

- **Method:** A continuous tone is delivered 20 dB above the threshold and is sustained for about 2 minutes. At every 5 seconds, the tone is increased by 1dB. Twenty such blips are delivered. Patient is asked to indicate the blips heard. Short increment sensitivity index score is presented in percentage.

> **Interpretations**
> - *Score less than 20%:* Normal hearing and conductive and nerve hearing loss.
> - *Score more than 70%:* Cochlear hearing loss.

Carhart's Tone Decay Test

This simple test is a measure of nerve fatigue, which is a feature of retrocochlear hearing loss.
- *Principle:* A normal person can hear a tone continuously for 60 seconds. In nerve fatigue, patient stops hearing earlier.
- *Method:* A tone of 4,000 Hz is delivered at 5 dB above the patient's threshold for 60 seconds. When patient stops hearing, intensity is increased each time by 5 dB. The procedure is continued till patient hears the tone continuously for 60 seconds or tone's upper limit is reached.

> **Interpretations**
> A tone decay of more than 25 dB is diagnostic of a retrocochlear hearing loss.

Speech Audiometry

The patient's ability to hear and understand the speech is measured in speech audiometry. The two parameters studied are—speech reception threshold and speech discrimination score (Table 5.4).

Speech Reception Threshold (SRT)

Speech reception threshold is the minimum intensity at which 50% of spondee words are repeated correctly.
- *Spondee words:* These are two syllable words with equal stress on each syllable such as oatmeal, popcorn, shipwreck, black-night, blackboard, football, eardrum, sunset, and daydream.

Table 5.4: Relation between the speech discrimination score and ability to understand speech

Speech discrimination score	Ability to understand speech
90–100%	Normal
76–88%	Slight difficulty
60–74%	Moderate difficulty
40–58%	Poor
< 40%	Very poor

- *Method:* A set of spondee words is delivered (in the form of either recorded tapes or monitored voice) to each ear of the patient. The word lists are delivered through the headphone of an audiometer. The intensity of spondee words are changed in 5 dB steps till half of them are correctly heard.

> **Interpretations**
> The speech reception threshold is normally within the range of 10 dB of the average of pure tone threshold of 3 speech frequencies (500, 1,000 and 2,000 Hz). In cases of hearing loss, SRT is more than 10 dB better than pure tone average.

Speech Discrimination Score or Speech Recognition Score

Discrimination score is a measure of patient's ability to understand speech.
- *Phonetically balanced words:* Phonetically balanced words are single syllable words such as fish, dish, pin, sin.
- *Method:* The phonetically balanced words are delivered through the headphone to each ear at an intensity 30–40 dB above the speech reception threshold. A list of 50 phonetically balanced words is presented and the number correctly heard is multiplied by 2 (Table 5.4).
    - Speech discrimination score is the percentage of words correctly heard by the patient.

> **Interpretation**
> - *Normal hearing:* Speech discrimination score of 95–100%.
> - *Conductive hearing loss (CHL):* Speech discrimination score 90–100% but at higher intensities.
> - *Sensorineural hearing loss (SNHL):* Speech discrimination score is less. Nerve hearing loss has very poor score in comparison of cochlear hearing loss.

Modifications

There is another better method of speech audiometry, in which percentage of phonetically balanced words correctly heard by the patient at different intensity levels are charted on a graph. The following three parameters are ascertained:
1. *Optimum discrimination score:* Optimum discrimination score is the highest score irrespective of the intensity at which phonetically balanced (PB) words are delivered.
2. *Half peak level:* Half peak level represents the intensity at which 50% of the words are expected to be heard (half optimum discrimination score). This is a derived figure from the above graph.
3. *Roll over curve:* This shape of the speech audiogram is typical of retrocochlear lesion. The optimum discrimination score is maintained as a horizontal line or show a drop with increase in intensity levels.

Uses

The following are some of the uses of speech audiometry:
- *Differentiate between:*
  - Organic and functional hearing losses
  - Cochlear and retrocochlear lesions
- *Hearing aids:* The intensity level for the best discrimination score is useful for fitting and setting of hearing aids.

OBJECTIVE HEARING EVALUATION

Impedance Audiometry

It measures the impedance (resistance) which is offered by the conducting mechanism of tympanic membrane and middle ear (compliance or suppleness) to sound pressure transmission (Figs 5.4 and 5.5). This objective method of audiometry consists of tympanometry and acoustic reflex measurements.

Tympanometry

Principle

When a sound hits tympanic membrane, some of the sound energy is absorbed while the rest is reflected. A stiffer tympanic membrane reflects more of sound energy than a compliant one. The pressure in a sealed EAC is changed. The reflected sound energy is measured to find the compliance or stiffness of the tympano-ossicular system. The compliance of tympano-ossicular system against various pressure changes is charted. In this way the status of healthy or diseased middle ear is found.

Equipment

It mainly consists of a probe, which has three channels (Figs 5.4 and 5.5) with following functions. The probe snugly fits into the EAC.

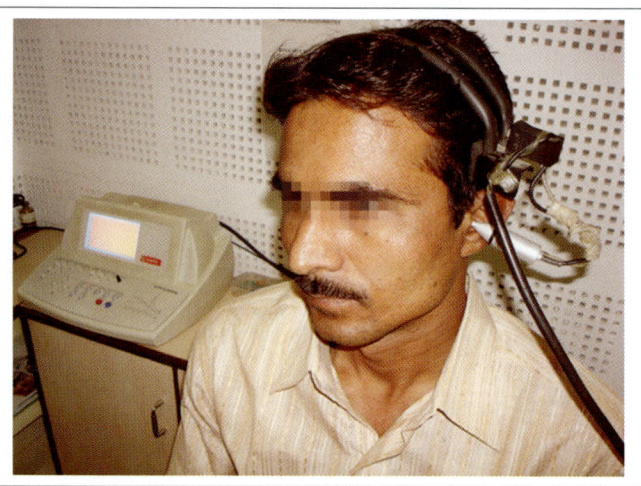

Fig. 5.5: Impedance audiometry in process. Note impedance audiometer lying on the table and the patient with ear probe with headband

- Deliver a tone of 220 Hz.
- A microphone which picks up the reflected sound.
- Bring changes in air pressure in EAC from positive to normal and then negative.

Interpretations

- Tympanometry results are represented by air pressure/compliance graphs *(tympanograms)*, that are diagnostic of certain middle ear pathologies (Table 5.5). The compliance of ear drum is maximum when air pressure on both sides is equal. The peak air pressure of tympanogram is equal to middle ear pressure.
- The middle ear pressure with normal eustachian tube function is between 0 and –150 mm H_2O.
- The middle ear pressure more negative than 150 mm H_2O suggests a poor eustachian tube function.

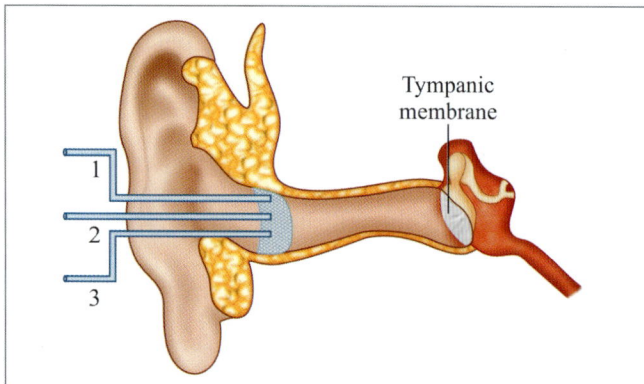

Fig. 5.4: Probe of impedance audiometer showing three channels. 1. Oscillator producing tone; 2. Air pump for increasing and decreasing of air pressure; and 3. Microphone that picks up and measures reflected sound pressure level

Table 5.5: Different types of tympanograms (Fig. 5.6)

Type	Characters of graph	Diseases of middle ear
Type A	Normal curve, compliance and pressure	Normal middle ear function
Type As	Normal curve with low compliance at or near normal ambient air pressure	Fixation of ossicles such as otosclerosis, malleus fixation
Type Ad	High compliance at or near normal ambient pressure	Ossicular discontinuity, thin and lax tympanic membrane
Type B	A flat or dome-shaped curve. No change in compliance with pressure changes	Middle ear fluid
Type C	Maximum compliance (peak) at negative pressure range < –150 mm of H_2O	Retracted tympanic membrane, negative pressure or some fluid in middle ear

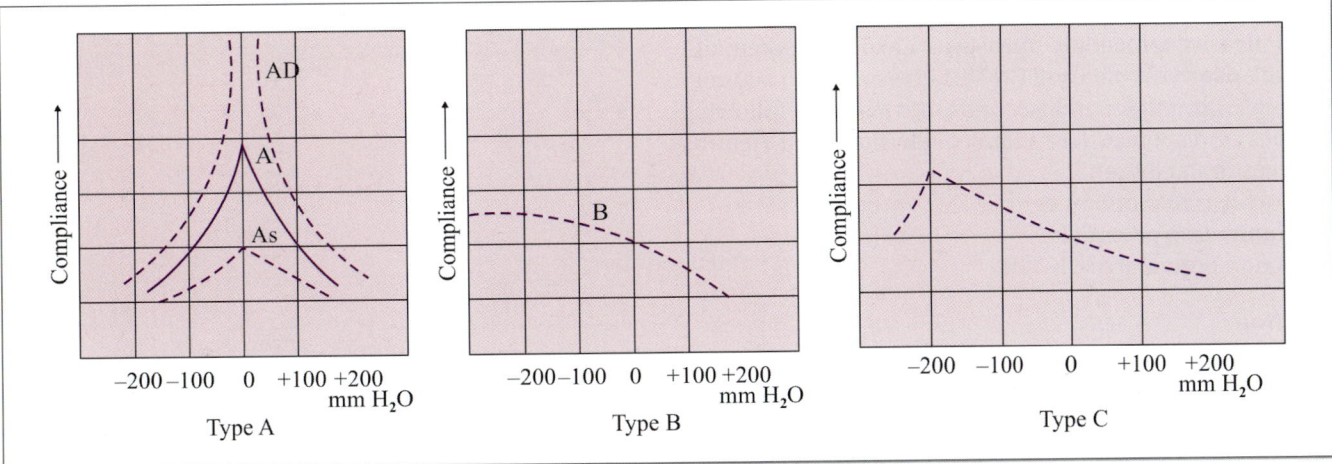

Fig. 5.6: Tympanograms (*see* Table 5.5). Type (A) A—normal; As—otosclerosis; Ad—ossicular disruption; Type (B) Flat or dome-shaped audiogram (middle ear fluid); Type (C) Maximum compliance at –200 mm of H_2O (Eustachian tube dysfunction)

- *Eustachian tube and grommet testing (inflation deflation test):* In cases of intact or perforated tympanic membrane, tympanometry can be done for testing function of eustachian tube and patency of the grommet. Grommet is placed in the tympanic membrane for the treatment of serous otitis media.

  A negative or positive pressure (–200 to +200 mm of H_2O) is created while patient is asked to swallow 5 times in 20 seconds. The ability to equilibrate the pressure suggests normal Eustachian tube function and patency of the grommet.

Acoustic Reflex

- *Principle and method:* A loud sound (70–100 dB above the threshold of hearing) causes bilateral (ipsilateral and contralateral) contraction of the stapedial muscles which are detected by tympanometry. Tone is delivered to one ear and the reflex is detected from the same and the contralateral ear.
- *Acoustic reflex neural pathways (Fig. 5.7):* Though the majority of neurons run through ipsilateral pathway, some cross the brainstem to continue to the opposite side. The pathway begins at cochlea and proceeds through CN VIII, cochlear nucleus, trapezoid body, superior olivary complex, and motor facial nucleus to the stapedial muscle. It is also called *stapedial reflex*.

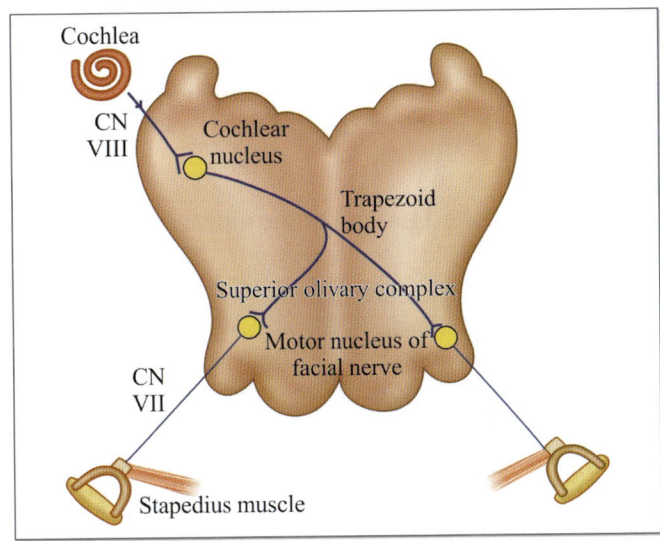

Fig. 5.7: Cut-section of the pons showing acoustic reflex pathways

Uses

The following are some of the uses of this objective method of acoustic reflex measurement:
- *Infants and young children:* Evaluation of hearing in infants and young children.
- *Malingerers* can be identified as they will show positive stapedial reflex.

Contd…

- *Differentiation between cochlear and nerve hearing losses:*
  - *Cochlear lesions:* Presence of stapedial reflex at lower intensities 40 to 60 dB (normally 70 dB) above the threshold of hearing due to *recruitment*.
  - *8th nerve lesion:* A sustained tone of 500 or 1000 Hz, 10 dB above acoustic reflex threshold, for 10 seconds, brings the reflex amplitude to 50%. This abnormal adaptation is due to stapedial reflex decay.
  - *Facial nerve palsy:* Absence of stapedial reflex in normal hearing ear indicates that the site of lesion of the facial nerve palsy is proximal to the nerve to stapedius. The appearance of reflex in cases of facial nerve palsy indicates recovery of function and a good prognosis.

Contd…

Electrocochleography

This invasive procedure measures electrical potentials, which arise in cochlea and CN VIII in response to auditory stimuli within first 5 milliseconds. It consists of following 3 types of responses (*see* Chapter 'Physiology of Hearing and Vestibular System').
- Cochlear microphonics
- Summating potentials
- Action potential of CN VIII.

Method

The recording electrode (a thin needle) is placed on the promontory through the tympanic membrane. The test can be done under local anesthesia; however, children and anxious uncooperative adults need sedation or general anesthesia, which has no effect on electrocochleography responses.

Uses

- Detection of hearing threshold in young infants and children within 5–10 dB.
- Differentiate cochlear lesions from that of CN VIII lesions.

Brainstem Evoked Response Audiometry (BERA) or Auditory Brainstem Response (ABR)

Brainstem evoked response audiometry (BERA) is a non-invasive technique that finds the integrity of central auditory pathways, which consists of CN VIII nerve, pons, midbrain, and forebrain. The electrical potentials are generated in response to several click stimuli. They are picked up from the vertex by surface electrodes. BERA measures hearing in the range of 1,000–4,000 Hz. Seven waves are generated in the first ten milliseconds (Table 5.6).

The first, third and fifth waves (among 5 waves shown in roman numbers I, II, III, IV, and V) are most stable and studied for absolute latency, inter-wave latency and the amplitude (Figs 5.8 and 5.9). The exact anatomic areas of origin of waves, though disputed, are shown in Table 5.6.

Table 5.6: Brainstem evoked response audiometry: Waves and their sites of origin

Waves	Sites of origin
Wave I	CN VIII
Wave II	Cochlear nuclei (pons)
Wave III	Superior olivary complex (pons)
Wave IV	Lateral lemniscus (pons)
Wave V	Inferior colliculus (midbrain)

Note: Current studies claim that waves I and II are from distal and proximal part of CN VIII, wave III cochlear nucleus, wave IV superior olivary complex, wave V lateral lamniscus and waves VI and VII inferior colliculus.

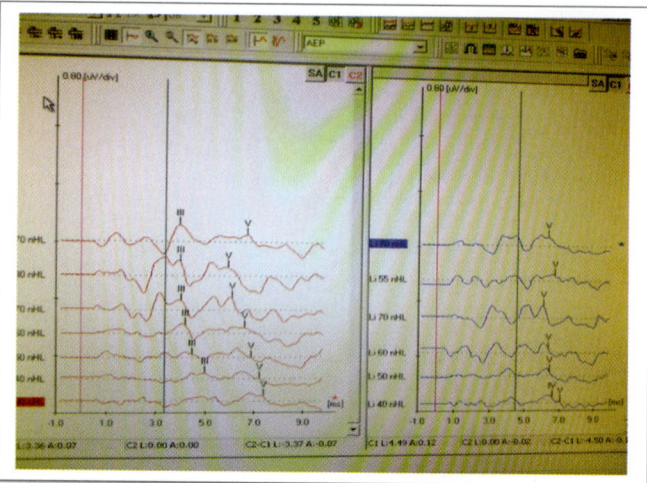

Fig. 5.8: Normal brainstem evoked response audiometry with normal latency and click stimulus from 80 to 40 dB HL
Source: Dr Amit Anand and Dr Hemant Shah, Consultant Audiologists, Anand and Ahmedabad, Gujarat (*with permission*)

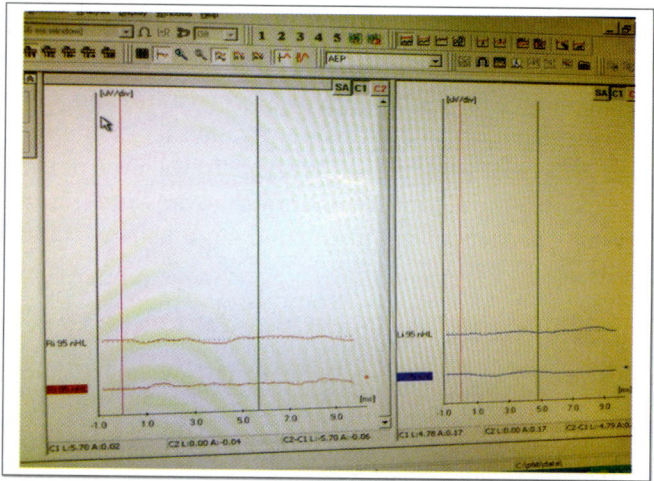

Fig. 5.9: Brainstem evoked response audiometry. Severe hearing loss. No peaks seen at 95 dBnHL
Source: Dr Amit Anand and Dr Hemant Shah, Consultant Audiologists, Anand and Ahmedabad, Gujarat (*with permission*)

Uses

- ***Threshold of hearing:*** In cases of infants and children (part of screening test), malingerer and uncooperative patients (*see* Chapter on 'Hearing Impairment in Infants and Children').
- ***Site of lesion:*** Diagnosis of lesions of nerve (acoustic neuroma) and brain-stem (multiple sclerosis and pontine tumors).
- ***Intraoperative monitoring of CN VIII:*** During the surgeries of cerebellopontine angle tumors such as acoustic neuroma.

Otoacoustic Emissions (OAE)

Otoacoustic emissions are low-intensity sounds which are produced by movement of the outer hair cells of the cochlea. They are produced spontaneously and in response to the acoustic stimuli. OAE are picked up by a miniature microphone, which is placed snugly in the EAC. Absence of OAE indicates disorders of outer hair cells.

- *Pathway:* OAE travels through basilar membrane, perilymph, oval window, ossicles, tympanic membrane, and ear canal.
- *Method:* OAE are picked up by a miniature microphone, which is placed snugly in the EAC.

Interpretations
It can diagnose damage to the outer hair cells due to acoustic trauma and ototoxic drugs. It aids in the assessment of hearing in infants. OAE are present in nerve hearing loss as the outer hair cells are normal.

- *Advantage:* This is noninvasive objective test and Sedation does not interfere with OAEs.

Types
- *Spontaneous otoacoustic emissions:* They are present in normal hearing ear or when hearing loss does not exceed 30 dB. It may be absent in about 50% of the normal persons.
- *Evoked otoacoustic emission (EOAE):* Evoked otoacoustic emission are acoustic signals generated by cochlear outer hair cells in response to auditory stimulation. EOAE measures only cochlear status and is independent of neural activity and central nervous system status. EOAE takes lesser time and uses a broader frequency range than click evoked ABR.
  - *Transient evoked otoacoustic emission (TEOAE):* It provides information over a broad frequency range (500–6000 Hz) that occurs after a brief stimulus. A series of click stimuli are presented at 80–85 dB SPL. TEOAE are observed in neonatal ears in the absence of external and middle ear disorders.
  - *Distortion evoked otoacoustic emission (DEOAE):* It provides frequency specific information and occurs in response to simultaneous presentation of two pure tones. The screening algorithms are robust in neonates and infants and use "DP grams."

Uses

- *Screening test of hearing* in neonates, uncooperative or mentally challenged patients.
- Distinguish between cochlear (acoustic trauma and ototoxic drugs) and retrocochlear hearing loss (auditory neuropathy).
- *Otoacoustic emissions (OAE)* are present in nerve hearing loss as the outer hair cells are normal.
- *Evoked otoacoustic emissions (EOAE)* takes lesser time and uses broader frequency range than click-evoked ABR.
- *Transient evoked otoacoustic emission (TEAOE)* are observed in neonatal ears in the absence of external and middle ear disorders.

Auditory Steady State Response (ASSR)

This is multiple auditory steady evoked response (MASTER) acquisition system. ASSR is an objective PTA, which assesses only air-conduction (AC). It generates multiple frequency modulated auditory stimulus and acquires electrophysiological responses to these stimuli.

Method

- The continuous sinusoid stimulus, which is amplitude or frequency modulated at relatively slow rates, is delivered to the ear via insert phones.
- The electrodes on the patient's head record the electroencephalographic activity, which is averaged by the system.
- The ASSR is converted to the frequency domain using fast Fourier transform techniques (FFT). The physiological audiogram obtained by MASTER shows air-conduction hearing threshold at each frequency.
- It needs quiet patient and better control of noise. In cases of uncooperative patients and children, it is done under sedation/general anesthesia because similar to ABR/BERA the patient's movements are not allowed.

Advantages

- *Frequency spectrum:* The frequency spectrum of the stimulus is considerably narrower than the tone burst of BERA.
- *Higher stimulation level:* Due to continuous stimulus it is possible to achieve higher stimulation level than clicks or tone bursts (transient stimulus), which are used in BERA. Therefore, it is easier to distinguish between severe and profound hearing loss. So it is possible to record ASSR in ears (especially in cochlear implant candidates) with no measurable ABR.
- *Easier analysis:* Analysis is easier than BERA and does not need much training.
- *Frequency-specific thresholds:* ASSR frequency-specific thresholds correlate with audiometric thresholds in both children and adults.

Self evaluation Exercises

1. Which is not true for the central hearing pathway?
   a. Lesions of cochlear nerve and nucleus will cause ipsilateral profound sensorineural hearing loss
   b. Central hearing pathway include superior olive, lateral lemniscus, inferior colliculus, medial geniculate body, auditory radiations, and primary auditory cortex in temporal lobe
   c. Central hearing pathway represents higher level of auditory processing
   d. Unilateral lesion of central hearing pathway would result in mild bilateral hearing loss and decreased ability to localize a source of sound
   e. None from above
2. Which of the following are not true for the Weber test?
   a. The tuning fork (usually of 512 Hz) is placed on the bridge of the nose or center of forehead
   b. Heard better (lateralization) on the side of conductive hearing loss
   c. In external ear occlusion and middle ear diseases Weber's test will be lateralized towards the normal
   d. Right side lateralization denotes right ear sensorineural hearing loss or left ear conductive hearing loss
3. Which of the following are true for the Weber test?
   a. External and middle ears are bypassed
   b. Air and bone conduction interfere with each other on the normal side and make normal ear less sensitive to bone conduction
   c. Internal ear diseases lead to decreased bone conduction
   d. All of the above
4. Which of the following are true for the Gelle's test?
   a. Gelle's test examines the effect of increased air pressure in ear canal on the bone-conduction hearing
   b. Tuning fork is placed on the frontal bone
   c. The air pressure is increased in the ear canal by Siegel's speculum
   d. In Gelle's negative there is no change in hearing. It is seen when ossicular chain is fixed (otosclerosis, tympanosclerosis) or disconnected (traumatic)
   e. Gelle's positive: Patient would appreciate change in hearing. It is seen in cases of conductive hearing loss

True (T)/False (F)

5. Quality of sound does not depend on overtones.
6. Speech frequencies include 500, 1000, and 2000 Hz.
7. Vowels are high frequency sounds while consonants are low frequency sounds.
8. dBHL is a unit for threshold of hearing in an audiogram. A sound of 20 dB is 100 fold increases in sound energy.
9. In addition to mixed hearing loss, there are two major types of hearing loss: (1) conductive and (2) sensorineural.
10. Patients with recruitment have intolerance (increased sensitivity) to loud sounds. It is seen in retrocochlear lesions such as acoustic neuroma.
11. Tone decay (auditory fatigue) is the change in auditory threshold when a continuous tone is presented.
12. Tone decay is seen in cochlear lesions such as Meniere's disease.
13. If Rinne's test is negative with a tuning fork (TF) of 512 Hz but positive for 1024 Hz, minimum predicted AB gap on audiometry would be 30 dB.
14. Tuning fork tests should confirm the results of audiometry. Never trust the audiogram alone when surgical intervention is considered. The inconsistency must be resolved with the audiologist.
15. In unilateral sensorineural hearing loss, the Rinne's test with 512 Hz tuning fork (without masking) may be false-negative but Weber's test would be lateralized towards normal ear.
16. Decreased bone conduction in an audiogram indicates involvement of middle ear.
17. Maximum conductive hearing loss is approximately 54 dB and is caused by ossicular disruption with intact tympanic membrane. Ossicular disruption with perforated tympanic membrane results in about 38 dB hearing loss.
18. Phonetically balanced (PB) words are used to measure speech reception threshold (SRT).
19. Spondee words are used to measure speech discrimination score.
20. Discrimination test measures patient's ability to understand speech.
21. Otoacoustic emissions arise from inner hair cells.
22. BERA (ABR) tracks the electrical conductivity of the hearing up to the brainstem and interpretation is not affected by the age of the child.

Answers

1. e	2. c, d	3. d	4. a, c, d	5. F	6. T
7. F	8. T	9. T	10. F	11. T	12. F
13. T	14. T	15. T	16. F	17. T	18. F
19. F	20. T	21. F	22. F		

Chapter 6

Conductive Hearing Loss and Otosclerosis

⊙ Specific Learning Objectives
After going through the chapter, you should be able to answer the following questions:
- How do you classify different types of hearing losses and what are the differences between conductive and sensorineural hearing losses?
- What are the different causes of conductive hearing losses and their line of management?
- Describe the etiopathogenesis of otosclerosis.
- How do the patients with otosclerosis present and how would you investigate and manage them?
- What are the indications, contraindications and complications of stapedectomy?

CLASSIFICATION OF HEARING LOSS (BOX 6.1)

The two broad categories of hearing loss are conductive hearing loss (CHL) and sensorineural hearing loss (SNHL). SNHL is further divided into sensory (cochlear) and neural (CN VIII and central auditory connections).

SNHL and CHL have their own characteristic features. On the basis of history, examination, tuning fork tests and audiometry, they can be easily differentiated from each other (Table 6.1).

Box 6.1: Classification of different types of hearing losses

Organic
- Conductive hearing loss (CHL)
- Sensorineural hearing loss (SNHL)
  - Peripheral
    - (Sensory) cochlear
    - (Neural) CN VIII
  - Central
    - Brainstem (medulla, pons, midbrain)
    - Thalamus
    - Temporal lobe
- Mixed hearing loss

Nonorganic
- Malingering
- Psychogenic

CONDUCTIVE HEARING LOSS

The disorders of external and middle ears up to stapediovestibular joint interfere with the conduction of sound and cause CHL (Table 6.2).

The ossicular disorders with intact tympanic membrane cause more hearing loss than ossicular diseases with tympanic membrane perforation.

Etiology

The causes may be congenital, traumatic, infectious/inflammatory, neoplasms and miscellaneous. They may lie in external ear, tympanic membrane, middle ear space, ossicles or in eustachian tube (Box 6.2).

Most common causes of CHL: They include wax, otitis media [acute suppurative otitis media (ASOM)] and chronic suppurative otitis media (CSOM), tympanosclerosis, and otosclerosis. In children, the most common cause is otitis media with effusion.

History and Physical Examination

In the evaluation of a CHL, history taking and physical examination (Flow chart 6.1) are very important.

Table 6.1: Differences between conductive hearing loss and sensorineural hearing loss

Features	Conductive hearing loss	Sensorineural hearing loss
Speech understanding	Good	Poor
Intolerance to loud sounds	Absent	Present in cochlear lesions
Speech of the patient	Low voice	Loud voice
Paracusis Willisii	Common	Absent
Common associated symptom	Otorrhea/earache	Tinnitus
Profound hearing loss	Never	Common
Rinne's test	Negative (BC > AC)	Positive (AC > BC)
Weber's test	Lateralized toward worst ear	Lateralized toward better ear
Absolute bone conduction	Normal	Reduced
PTA: Air-bone gap	Present	Absent
Recruitment	Absent	Present in cochlear lesions
Tone decay	Absent	Present in retrocochlear hearing loss
Frequencies	Usually low tones involved	Usually higher tones involved
Thresholds	Never > 60–70 dB	Can be > 60–70 dB
Speech discrimination	Not affected	Poor
Site of lesion	External and middle ear	Internal ear, CN VIII and central auditory connections

Abbreviation: PTA—pure tone audiometry

Table 6.2: Common causes of conductive hearing loss and their approximate hearing loss in dB

Causes	Approximate hearing loss
Occlusion of EAC	30–40 dB
Perforation of tympanic membrane (hearing loss depends on the size and site of perforation)	10–40 dB
Ossicular disorders without eardrum perforation (fixity and discontinuity)	54 dB
Ossicular disorders with eardrum perforation (fixation and discontinuation)	38 dB
Malleus fixation	10–25 dB
Closure of oval window	60 dB
Pure and complete conductive hearing loss	60–70 dB

Abbreviation: EAC—external auditory canal

> **Box 6.2: Causes of conductive hearing loss**
>
> - **External auditory canal:** Wax, foreign bodies, otitis externa, congenital and acquired stenosis, exostoses, osteomas, tumors, cyst.
> - **Tympanic membrane:** Perforations (traumatic, ASOM, CSOM), tympanosclerosis, retraction.
> - **Ossicles:** Fixation (otosclerosis, tympanosclerosis, congenital); discontinuity (traumatic, inflammatory, cholesteatoma).
> - **Middle ear:** Eustachian tube dysfunction, otitis media with effusion, adhesive otitis media, hemotympanum, cholesteatoma, tumors (benign and malignant).

Abbreviations: ASOM—acute suppurative otitis media; CSOM—chronic suppurative otitis media

Treatment

Most cases of CHL can be managed by medical and surgical treatment and it depends on the cause of deafness. The details of the treatment of these conditions are given in their respective chapters. Table 6.3 briefly provides different modalities of treatment and their indications. Different types of mastoid and tympanoplasty operations are described in Chapter 'Middle Ear and Mastoid Surgeries'.

OTOSCLEROSIS

Otosclerosis is a common disorder of bony labyrinth with normal tympanic membrane. It is characterized by gradually progressive CHL as a result of stapes fixation. The treatment of choice is stapedectomy.

Pertinent Anatomy

Labyrinth has three parts—membranous labyrinth, perilymphatic labyrinth, and bony labyrinth. The

Chapter 6 • Conductive Hearing Loss and Otosclerosis

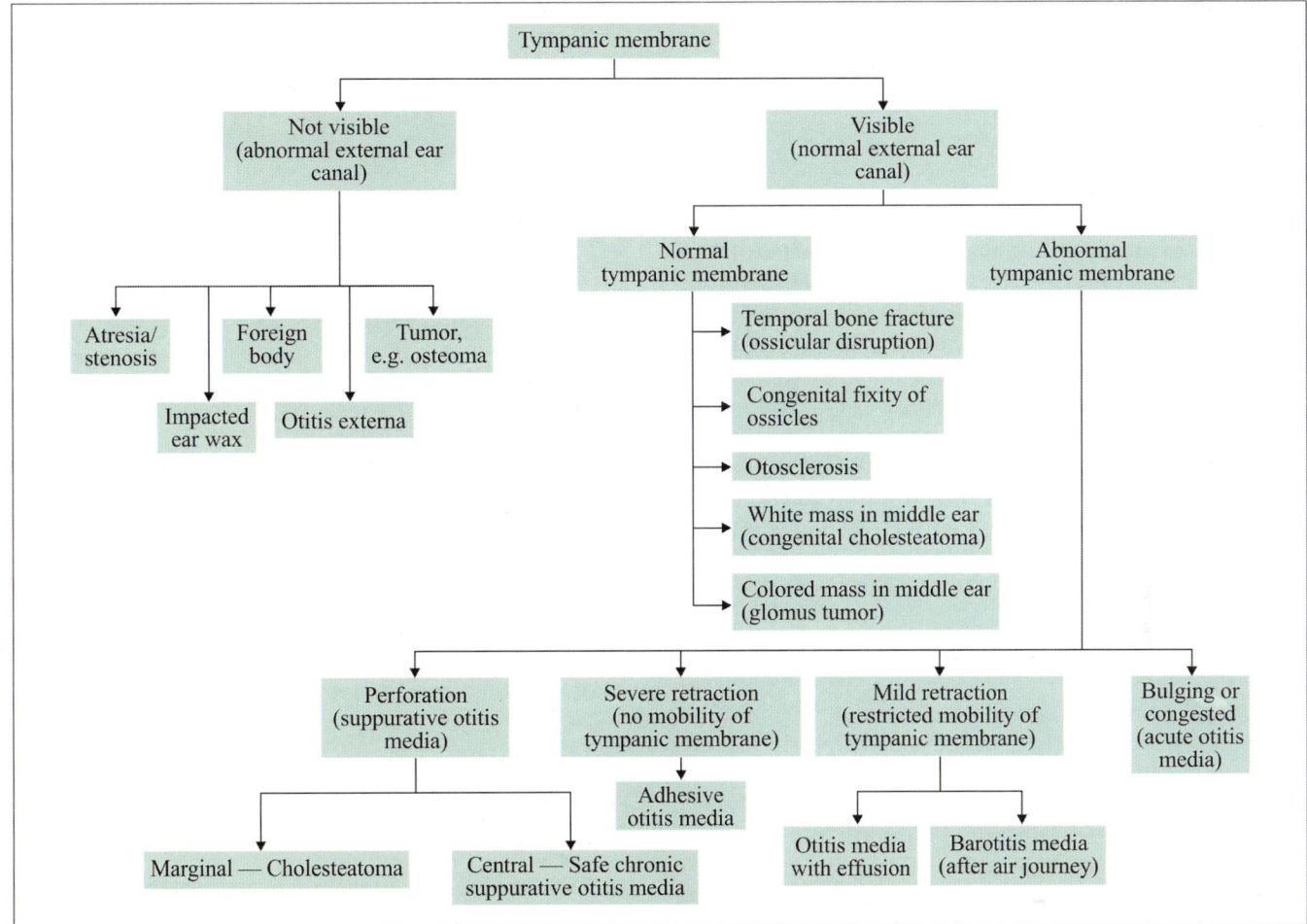

Flow chart 6.1: Clinical diagnoses of causes of conductive hearing loss

Abbreviations: OE—otitis externa; OM—otitis media; AOM—acute otitis media; CSOM—chronic suppurative otitis media

Table 6.3: Different modalities of treatment of conductive hearing loss and their indications

Different modalities	Indications
Removal of EAC occlusions	Impacted wax, foreign body, osteoma, exostosis, keratosis obturans, tumors, meatal stenosis
Myringotomy	Acute otitis media
Grommet	Otitis media with effusion
Stapedectomy	Otosclerosis (fixation of stapes footplate)
Tympanoplasty	Tympanic membrane perforations and ossicular disruptions
Hearing aids	When surgery is not possible, refused or failed

bony labyrinth has 3 layers—(1) endosteal, (2) bony (enchondral), and (3) periosteal (*see* Chapter 'Anatomy and Physiology of Ear').

1. **Membranous labyrinth (otic labyrinth or endolymphatic labyrinth):** Otic labyrinth consists of utricle, saccule, cochlear duct (scala media), semicircular ducts and endolymphatic duct and sac. It is filled with endolymph.
2. **Perilymphatic labyrinth or space (periotic labyrinth):** Periotic labyrinth surrounds the otic labyrinth and is filled with perilymph. It consists of vestibule, scala tympani, scala vestibuli and perilymphatic spaces of semicircular and endolymphatic ducts.
3. **Bony labyrinth (otic capsule):** It consists of three layers—(1) endosteal, (2) enchondral, and (3) periosteal.

Ossification of bony labyrinth: It ossifies from 14 centers. The first center appears in the cochlea at 16 weeks. The last center appears in the posterolateral part of posterior semicircular canal at 20th week.

- **Endosteal:** It is the innermost layer, that lines the internal surface of bony labyrinth.

- **Bony (enchondral) layer:** It develops from the cartilage.
- **Periosteal:** It is the outermost layer and covers the external surface of bony labyrinth (petrous part of temporal bone).

Pathogenesis

- Otosclerosis is a primary disease of the enchondral bony labyrinth. In the hard enchondral bone, some islands of cartilage remain unossified. This cartilage, due to certain nonspecific factors, is activated to form new spongy bone (*otospongiosis*).
- These irregular foci of spongy bone replace normal dense enchondral bony labyrinth. Therefore, many call this disease as *otospongiosis*. The otosclerotic focus usually involves the stapes region and results in stapes fixation and conductive deafness. The fissula ante fenestram, which lies in front of the oval window, is the site of predilection for stapedial type of otospongiosis. The otospongiosis process can involve other areas of bony labyrinth and can cause SNHL or remain asymptomatic.

Etiology

The exact cause of the disease is not yet known. The following factors have been documented in the literature:

- **Heredity:** About 50% of the cases give positive family history. Remaining cases are sporadic. An autosomal dominant inheritance with penetrance in range of 20–40 has been reported. Other studies report heterogeneity, with more than one gene defect. Some cases have been suggested to be related to COL1A1 gene, which is one of the two genes that code for type I collagen (predominant collagen of bone).
- **Osteogenesis imperfecta:** About 50% cases of type I osteogenesis imperfecta develop hearing loss, histological changes and COL1A1 gene expression that are indistinguishable from otosclerosis. Patients have history of multiple fractures.

Van der Hoeve syndrome: Patients have the triad of osteogenesis imperfecta, otosclerosis and blue sclera.

- **Viral:** Many reports suggest that otosclerosis may be related to a persistent measles virus infection of otic capsule. Perhaps it is similar to Paget's disease of bone which is related with defective paramyxovirus.

Types

- **Stapedial otosclerosis:** This most common variety causes stapes fixation and presents with conductive deafness (Figs 6.1A to E).
- **Cochlear otosclerosis:** It involves region of round window and areas in the bony labyrinth. It presents with irreversible SNHL, which is probably caused by toxic materials liberated into the inner ear fluid.

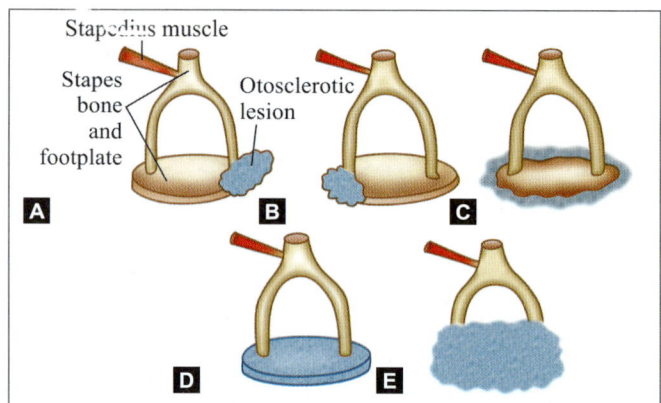

Figs 6.1A to E: Types of otosclerotic lesions causing fixation of stapes footplate. (A) *Anterior focus*, the site of predilection "fissula ante fenestram"; (B) *Posterior focus*, the lesion begins behind the oval window; (C) *Circumferential lesion* begins around the margins of footplate; (D) *Biscuit-type lesion* involves only footplate sparing the annular ligament; (E) *Obliterative lesion* completely obliterates the oval window niche

- **Histologic otosclerosis:** Histologic otosclerosis is diagnosed only on histological examination of petrous bone. Patient remains asymptomatic.

Pathology

- **Gross appearance**
  - Otosclerotic lesions appear chalky white, grayish or yellow.
  - The red color lesions indicate increased vascularity, which is the feature of active and rapidly progressive otosclerotic focus.
- **Histology:** A wave of abnormal bone remodeling occurs with resorption of enchondral bony labyrinth, which is replaced with hypercellular woven spongy bone that further remodels and results in sclerotic mosaic architecture.
  - *Immature active lesions:* Numerous narrow and vascular spaces (increased vascularity) with plenty of histiocytes, osteoblasts and osteoblast precursor cells, and mononuclear cells indicate active remodeling phase. A lot of cement substance is present, which stains blue (blue mantles) with hematoxylin-eosin stain. Acute inflammatory cells are absent.
  - *Mature lesions:* Less vascular spaces and laying off more bone and fibrillar substance than cementum. It stains red with hematoxylin-eosin stain.

Clinical Features

Otosclerosis is characterized by gradually progressive CHL with normal tympanic membrane. In most cases, the disease is bilateral.

- **Race:** White races are affected more than blacks. It is common in Indians, but rare among the Chinese and Japanese.
- **Age of onset:** Patients are usually between 20 and 30 years of age. Disease is rare before 10 years and after 40 years.
- **Sex:** In India, it occurs more in males, though the overseas studies show female preponderance.
- **Hormonal effect:** In females, deafness seems to worsen or manifest during pregnancy and menopause.
- **Trauma:** Some patients try to correlate deafness with an accident or a major operation.
- **Hearing loss:** The presenting feature is painless bilateral gradually progressive CHL.
  - **Paracusis Willisii:** In this phenomenon, the patient's hearing improves in noisy background. It happens because a normal person raises his voice in noisy surroundings and patient takes advantage of that. The speech discrimination is not affected in pure conductive hearing loss.
  - **Tuning fork tests and audiometry:** They show CHL.
- **Tinnitus:** It is usually present in cochlear otosclerosis and active lesions.
- **Vertigo:** It is an uncommon symptom. The cause of it is not well understood. Hypertension and metabolic disorders are usually present in these cases.

Stapedectomy in otosclerosis with vertigo: Some otologists consider vertigo as a contraindication to stapedectomy surgery because they feel the results are poor because of associated endolymphatic hydrops.

- **Speech:** Low, monotonous, well-modulated soft speech.
- **Otoscopy:** Tympanic membrane is normal and mobile.
  - **Schwartz sign:** It is a reddish hue seen through the tympanic membrane on the promontory. It indicates active focus, which is vascular.
- **Eustachian tube:** Its functions are normal.

Audiometry

- Pure tone audiogram shows **conductive hearing loss**, which is more on lower frequencies (Fig. 6.2).
- **Carhart's notch:** There is a dip (from 500 to 4,000 Hz) in bone conduction curve, which is maximum (15 dB) at 2,000 Hz (5 dB at 500 Hz, 10 dB at 1,000 Hz, 15 dB at 2,000 Hz and 5 dB at 4,000 Hz). The Carhart's notch disappears after successful stapedectomy surgery.
- **Air-bone gap:** The degree of footplate fixation is estimated by the size of air-bone gap. Audiometry does not predict the pattern and extent of oval window involvement. It is determined on exploratory tympanotomy during the stapedectomy surgery.
- **Mixed hearing loss:** Hearing loss with element of SNHL indicates cochlear otosclerosis.

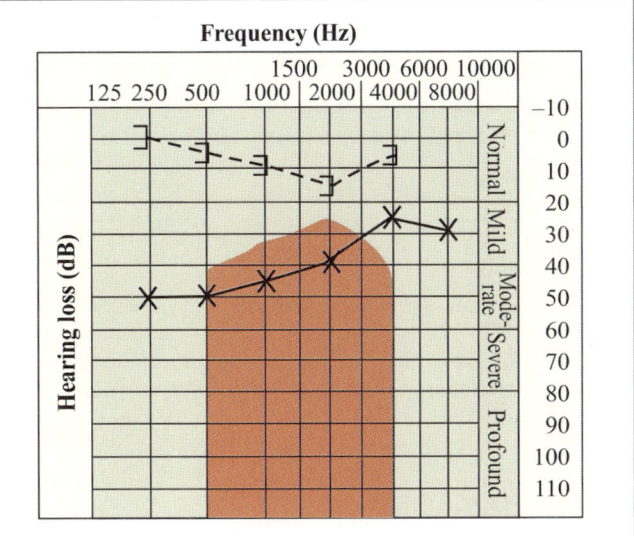

Fig. 6.2: Audiogram otosclerosis. Left ear predominantly low-frequency conductive hearing loss Carhart's notch

Differential Diagnoses

They include the following causes of CHL. They can be differentiated with the help of ear microexamination, siegalization, impedance audiometry and exploratory tympanotomy:
- Serous otitis media
- Adhesive otitis media
- Tympanosclerosis
- Attic fixation of head of malleus
- Ossicular discontinuity
- Congenital stapes fixation

Treatment

There is no curative treatment. The treatment of choice is **stapedectomy**. Other modalities of management include sodium fluoride therapy and hearing aids. Stapes mobilization and fenestration operations are performed occasionally.

- **Sodium fluoride:** Sodium fluoride hastens the maturity of active focus and arrests further SNHL.
- **Stapedectomy:** Stapedectomy operation consists of removal of the fixed stapes and insertion of prosthesis between the incus and oval window. There are various types of prostheses such as teflon piston, stainless steel piston, Tefwire or fat and stainless steel wire. Hearing improves in 90% cases.
- **Stapes mobilization:** About 1% of otosclerotic ears have fibrous fixation of stapes. Stapes mobilization provides good permanent hearing in these cases. Simple mobilization of stapes is not indicated in most of the cases as it commonly results in refixation.
- **Fenestration operation:** This operation is almost abandoned. An alternative window is created in the

lateral semicircular canal. The main disadvantage is a postoperative mastoid cavity and an inherent hearing loss of 25 dB.
- *Hearing aids:* They offer good hearing results and are indicated in patients who refuse surgery or are unfit for surgery.

Otosclerosis
Fifty per cent of patients give positive family history. Patient has CHL with normal tympanic membrane and impaired acoustic reflexes. The patients with negative Rinne (BC > AC) are candidates for stapedectomy, which provides very gratifying results.

STAPEDECTOMY

An ideal case for stapedectomy surgery is also an ideal candidate for hearing aids. So, the patient should be fully informed of the results and risks of stapedectomy.

Selection Criteria
- *Firmly fixed stapes footplate:* It is indicated by an air-bone gap of minimum 30 dB for the speech frequencies and a negative Rinne for 256 and 512 Hz magnesium tuning forks. Speech discrimination score should be minimum 60%.

The successful stapedectomy and stapes mobilization correct the CHL, remove Carhart's notch, and often lead to overclosure of air-bone gap.

Mixed profound hearing loss with sufficient speech discrimination: Stapedectomy provides better hearing with hearing aids.

Contraindications
- *The only hearing ear:* There are about 1% chances of developing dead ear.
- *Vertigo:* History of vertigo in recent months is usually associated with Meniere's disease. There is heightened risk of postoperative SNHL.
- *Young children:* Recurrent eustachian tube dysfunction commonly causes acute otitis media (AOM) in children and can displace the prosthesis. The otosclerotic focus is usually active and progresses rapidly in children and can close the oval window.
- *Certain occupations:*
  - Postoperative vertigo can interfere with the work in some professions such as athletes and high-construction workers.
  - In divers and frequent fliers, air pressure changes can damage the hearing and induce severe vertigo.
  - Industrial workers who work in noisy surroundings are more vulnerable to occupational SNHL.
- *Local diseases:* Otitis externa, tympanic membrane perforation and exostosis should be treated before the stapedectomy.
- *Pregnancy:* Stapedectomy is avoided.

Anesthesia
Surgery is preferably done under local anesthesia so that hearing can be tested on the table.

Operative Steps
- Infiltration of ear canal with lidocaine and epinephrine.
- Obtaining of the tissue graft to cover oval window—vein, temporalis fascia, perichondrium or fat.
- Endomeatal curved or triangular skin incision.
- Elevation of the posterior deep meatal skin and fibrous annulus from sulcus tympanicus.
- Removal of 2–4 mm posterosuperior bony overhang (Fig. 6.3A) of the canal rim for an adequate exposure of oval window, stapes, facial nerve canal and pyramid.
- Removal of stapes superstructure.
- Making a hole in the stapes footplate (*stapedotomy*) or remove a part of footplate (*stapedectomy*) (Fig. 6.3B).
- Tissue seal of oval window (Fig. 6.3C).
- Placement of prosthesis between the long process of incus and oval window—Shea platinum teflon cup piston, Robinson stainless steel prosthesis, Shea teflon piston, McGee piston, Fisch platinum teflon piston and house wire prosthesis.
- Repositioning the tympanomeatal flap.

Habenula perforata: The openings, through which branches of cochlear nerves enter the cochlea. If wide, they can lead to a perilymph gusher in stapes surgery. This X-linked disease can be diagnosed on CT. It is associated with congenitally enlarged internal acoustic meatus and stapes fixation.

Complications
- *Iatrogenic trauma:* Mostly trauma occurs to the following structures during the operation:
  - *Tympanic membrane:* Trauma can lead to unhealed perforation of tympanic membrane.
  - *Chorda tympani nerve:* Patient develops loss or distortion of taste sensation.
  - *Facial nerve:* Facial paresis/palsy.
  - *Incus dislocation:* Patient will have conductive hearing loss.
  - *Trauma to labyrinth:* It can lead to SNHL, dead ear, vertigo and perilymphatic fistula.

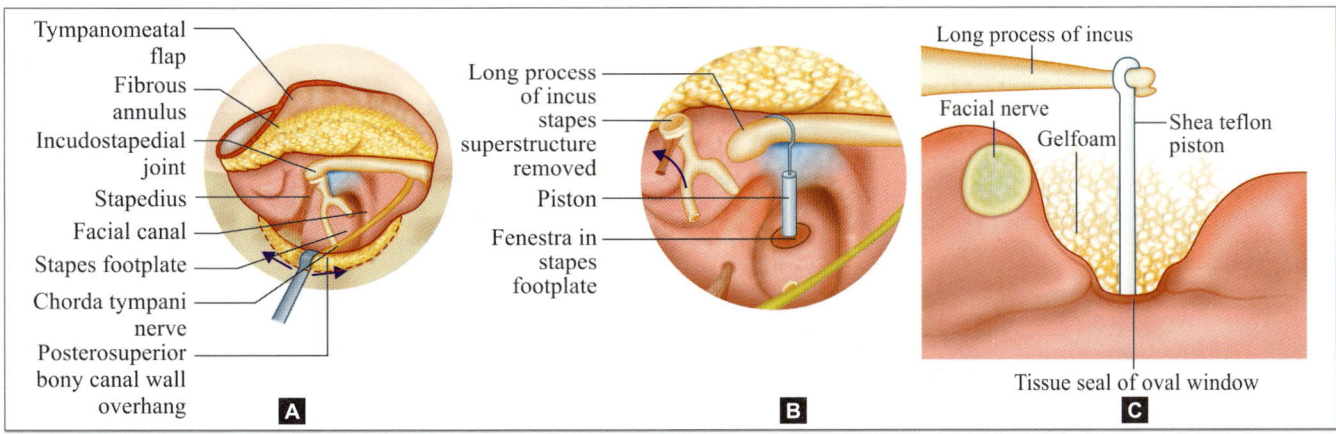

Figs 6.3A to C: Stapedectomy. (A) After elevating the tympanomeatal flap, posterosuperior bony canal wall is removed to get better view of stapes; (B) Stapedectomy piston. After creating a fenestra in the stapes footplate, piston is placed from long process of incus to the footplate fenestra. Note that the stapes superstructure is removed; (C) Shea teflon piston

- **SNHL:** 2% patients develop SNHL. Slowly progressive high-frequency loss has been seen in long-term follow-up. 0.5% patients get a "dead" ear.
- **Perilymphatic fistula:** Granuloma in oval window can occur after surgery. The symptoms of imbalance ear fullness, tinnitus and hearing loss indicate perilymph fistula (requiring tympanotomy) or endolymphatic hydrops (responding to medical treatment).
- **Conductive hearing loss:** It may occur due to short, loose and displaced piston and late erosion of long process of incus.
- **Benign paroxysmal positional vertigo.**

Self-evaluation Exercises

1. Which of the following is not the feature of Van der Hoeve syndrome?
    a. Osteogenesis imperfecta
    b. Conductive hearing loss
    c. Blue sclera
    d. None of the above
2. Patients with otosclerosis will not have:
    a. Gradually progressive bilateral conductive hearing loss
    b. Hearing loss increases during pregnancy
    c. Tympanic membrane and eustachian tube are normal
    d. Rinne's test positive
3. Which of the following statements is not related with Schwartz sign?
    a. Active otosclerosis
    b. Not seen during pregnancy and in children
    c. Pink reflex (reddish hue seen over the promontory
    d. Seen through intact tympanic membrane in the area of oval window
4. Which of the following is not true for habenula perforata?
    a. Openings through which branches of cochlear nerves enter the cochlea
    b. Even if wide, they cannot lead to a perilymph gusher in stapes surgery
    c. X-linked disease diagnosed on CT
    d. It is associated with congenitally enlarged internal acoustic meatus and stapes fixation
5. Which of the following is not the treatment of otosclerosis:
    a. Hearing aid
    b. Stapedectomy is the treatment of choice for a young stapedial otosclerosis office going patient
    c. Tympanoplasty
    d. Sodium fluoride therapy used in the treatment of cochlear otosclerosis

Mention whether the following statements are True (T)/False (F):
6. The most common causes of conductive hearing loss (CHL) are ear wax, otitis media, otomycosis and otosclerosis.
7. The prevalence of clinical otosclerosis is highest in caucasians.
8. Otosclerosis has autosomal recessive inheritance.

Contd...

Section 2 • Ear

Contd…

9. The disease process of otosclerosis starts in bone of otic capsule which develops from cartilage.
10. Fissula ante fenestram is the most common site of stapedial otosclerosis and is located at the posterior edge of oval window.
11. Carhart's notch is characteristic feature of otosclerosis and audiograms shows bone conduction (sensorineural hearing loss) dip at 4 kHz.
12. Impedance audiometry (tympanogram) of otosclerosis patients show 'A' type of curve with absent acoustic reflex.
13. Blue mantle is not associated with otospongiosis.

Answers

1. d	2. d	3. b	4. b	5. c	6. T
7. T	8. F	9. T	10. F	11. F	12. T
13. F					

Pearls and Nuggets (Refresh your knowledge)

- **Glossopharyngeal neuralgia:** The clinical features include paroxysmal attacks of pain that radiates in the area of tongue, tonsil and ear. The pain is precipitated by swallowing, talking and even laughing and responds to carbamazepine.
- **Costen's syndrome:** This disorder of temporomandibular joint, which is due to defective bite, is characterized by otalgia, feeling of blocked ear, tinnitus and sometimes vertigo. The ear pain radiates to frontal, parietal and occipital region.
- **Internuclear ophthalmoplegia:** Medial longitudinal fasciculus (MLF) lesions present with weakness of adduction during gaze and nystagmus of the abducting or normal eye. Patient can look straight ahead with both eyes. Convergence remains intact as the oculomotor nerve is normal.
- **CHARGE syndrome:** It consists of **C**oloboma, **H**eart defects, choanal **A**tresia, **R**etarded growth, **G**enital hypoplasia and **E**ar anomalies.
- **Arnold-Chiari malformation:** Cerebellar tonsils project into the vertebral canal through the foramen magnum.
- **Extraocular muscles:** The oblique muscles are tested by requesting the patient to adduct the eye first, then look up (for testing inferior oblique) or down (for testing superior oblique). The superior and inferior rectus muscles are tested by asking the patient to abduct the eye first then look up and down respectively.
- **Pneumatic otoscopy:** It is the gold standard for the diagnosis of otitis media.
- **Tinnitus:** It is a symptom and not a disease. It can be so disabling that the patient can have suicidal tendencies.

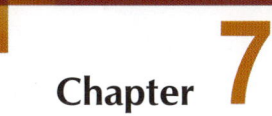

Chapter 7

Sensorineural Hearing Loss

> ### ⊙ Specific Learning Objectives
> After going through the chapter, you should be able to answer the following questions:
> - Discuss the etiology, history taking, examination, differential diagnoses and management of sensorineural hearing loss in adults.
> - What are the different internal ear manifestations of congenital and acquired syphilis and how would you manage them?
> - Mention some common ototoxic agents with their site of action and the risk factors involved.
> - What do you know about the noise trauma to ear and its prophylactic measures?
> - How will you manage cases of sudden sensorineural hearing loss and presbycusis?
> - What do you know about the following: (1) Autoimmune inner ear disease; (2) Nonorganic hearing loss; (3) Unilateral profound hearing loss?

SENSORINEURAL HEARING LOSS (SNHL)

There are characteristic features of SNHL which differentiate it from conductive hearing loss (CHL) (*see* Chapters of 'Hearing Evaluation and Conductive Hearing Loss and Otosclerosis'). The central auditory transmission has bilateral pathways from each ear. So the central defects, which cause subtle findings (such as impaired sound localization), are difficult to detect.

Etiology

The causes of sensorineural hearing loss (SNHL) lie in cochlea, CN VIII, brainstem and temporal lobe. They may be congenital, traumatic, infectious, inflammatory, iatrogenic, neoplastic, senile or miscellaneous (Box 7.1).

The congenital hearing loss is due to the anomalies of the inner ear or damage to the hearing apparatus by prenatal or perinatal factors. The causes may be divided into genetic and nongenetic. The genetic cause may have delayed onset and affect only the hearing. Other genetic causes are part of a larger syndrome affecting other systems of the body as well. *See* Chapter 'Hearing Impairment in Infants and Young Children'.

History, Examination and Investigations (Flow chart 7.1)

The essential elements of history and physical examination, which help in determining the cause and site of lesion (cochlea, nerve, central) include following:

> **Box 7.1: Common causes of sensorineural hearing loss**
> - ***Congenital:*** Genetic and nongenetic
> - ***Infections (viral, bacterial or spirochetal):*** Labyrinthitis and meningitis
> - ***Trauma*** to labyrinth and CN VIII in fractures of temporal bone and ear surgery
> - ***Ototoxic drugs:*** Streptomycin and gentamicin
> - ***Endolymphatic hydrops:*** Primary or idiopathic (Meniere's disease) and secondary
> - ***Tumors:*** CN VIII acoustic neuroma
> - ***Systemic diseases:*** Diabetes, multiple sclerosis, syphilis, hypothyroidism, kidney disease, autoimmune disorders and blood dyscrasias
> - ***Miscellaneous:*** Sudden idiopathic sensorineural hearing loss (SNHL), familial progressive SNHL, noise-induced hearing loss (NIHL) and presbycusis

- ***History:*** Congenital or acquired; unilateral or bilateral; side involved; age and mode of onset; duration and progression (stationary/progressive/fluctuating); special features (recruitment and discrimination) and severity (mild, moderate, severe, profound) of hearing loss; events preceding hearing loss, such as infection, trauma, strain, medication, surgery, noise exposure; associated ear symptoms of tinnitus, otorrhea, pain, vertigo/dizziness; family history.
- ***Physical examination:*** Complete ear (including otoscopy and tuning fork tests), nose, throat, head and

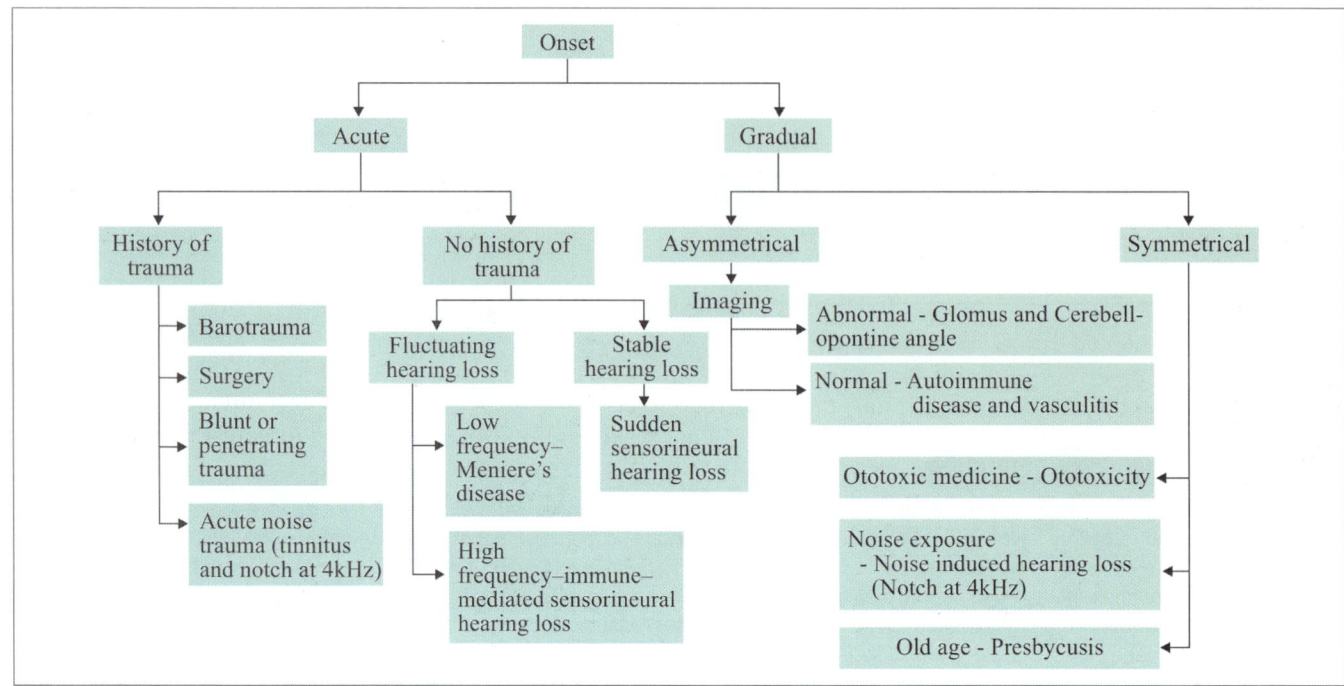

Flow chart 7.1: Differential diagnoses of sensorineural hearing loss (SNHL) in adults

neck examination including cranial nerves, neurologic and other systems to *see* any association with other syndromes.
- *Audiometry:* Pure tone audiometry (PTA) to know the severity (mild, moderate, severe, profound) and nature (high-frequency, low-frequency, or flat type); speech, impedance and evoke response audiometry and otoacoustic emission.
- *Laboratory tests:* Depending upon the suspected etiology, following investigations may be ordered: CT/MRI (congenital cholesteatoma, glomus tumor, malignancy, acoustic neuroma); CBC (leukemia); blood sugar (diabetes); serology (syphilis); T_3, T_4 thyroid-stimulating hormone (TSH) (hypothyroidism); kidney function tests.

Treatment

Hearing is an essential part of communication. Early detection of SNHL and immediate attention towards its management are of paramount importance. Measures are taken to stop and reverse the progress and for rehabilitation program. Following are some of the treatment options of different causes of SNHL:
- Syphilis is treatable with high doses of penicillin and steroids.
- Hypothyroidism needs thyroxin replacement therapy.
- Serous labyrinthitis can be reversed by active treatment of middle ear infection.
- Perilymph fistula needs surgical correction with sealing of fistula in the oval or round window with fat or other material.
- Discontinuation of ototoxic drugs.
- Rehabilitation with hearing aids and other devices. *See* Chapter 'Hearing Aids and Cochlear Implants'.

Prophylaxis

- Ototoxic drug administration should have regular monitoring. Drug should be discontinued at the right time.
- Avoidance of noisy surroundings.
- *Addiction free healthy lifestyle:* Balanced and nutritious diet and regular exercise.

LABYRINTHITIS

The infection of labyrinth may be viral or bacterial (*see* Chapter 'Peripheral Vestibular Disorders').
- *Viral labyrinthitis:* Viruses can reach the labyrinth via blood-stream and affect stria vascularis, endolymph and organ of Corti. The viruses which have been documented to cause labyrinthitis are measles, mumps and cytomegalovirus. Other viruses, which are known to cause hearing loss but lack direct proof, are rubella, herpes zoster, herpes simplex, influenza and Epstein-Barr virus.
- *Bacterial labyrinthitis:* Bacterial infections can reach inner ear through the middle ear (tympanogenic) and cerebrospinal fluid (CSF) (meningogenic). Suppurative otitis media and meningitis are common causes of labyrinthitis and SNHL.

SYPHILIS

Hearing loss (6.5% of unexplained SNHL) occurs in secondary, tertiary and congenital syphilis. Seven percent patients with Meniere's disease (see Chapter 'Vestibular Disorders') have syphilis. Saddle nose deformity, nasal septal perforation and frontal bossing are also characteristic features of syphilis.

Clinical Features

Secondary Syphilis

- *Hearing loss:* Abrupt onset, bilateral and progressive.
- *Vestibular symptoms:* They are usually uncommon. Episodes of acute vertigo are similar to Meniere's disease.
- *Hennebert's sign:* The positive fistula test in the absence of fistula may be present.
- *CNS features:* Patients may have headaches, stiff necks, cranial nerve palsies and optic neuritis.
- *Secondary syphilitic features:* Skin rashes and lymphadenopathy.
- *CSF:* Lymphocytic pleocytosis, elevated proteins and normal glucose.

Tertiary Syphilis

- *Otologic features* are similar to late congenital syphilis.
- *CSF* may have minimal pleocytosis and elevated or normal protein.
- *Electrocochleography:* Features similar to Meniere's disease.

Congenital Syphilis

- Early (birth to 3 years)
  - *Hearing loss:* Rapid bilateral profound symmetrical SNHL.
  - *Vestibular features:* They are relatively few and may vary from mild imbalance to protracted vertigo with vegetative features lasting for days.
  - *Meningo-neurolabyrinthitis:* Systemic features such as meningitis overshadow otologic symptoms.
  - *Multi-system:* Extensive damage of other organs proves fatal.
- Late (8–20 years)
  - *Hutchinson's triad:* It consists of SNHL, interstitial keratitis and notched incisors. It is an exclusive feature of congenital syphilis.
  - *Hutchinson's teeth* are peg-shaped and notched permanent upper central incisors and mulberry molars (first lower molar grinding surface has many tiny cusps).
  - *Hearing loss:* It is bilateral, asymmetric and progressive but fluctuating flat SNHL. Speech discrimination scores are disproportionately low to pure tone threshold. Recruitment is present.
  - *Tinnitus* may appear intermittently.
  - *Vestibular features:* Episodes of acute vertigo are similar to Meniere's disease.
  - *Hennebert's sign:* It is due to the softened gummatous otic capsule.
  - *Tullio's phenomenon:* Nystagmus and vertigo are often caused by loud noise.
  - *Caloric responses:* They are often decreased.
  - *Interstitial keratitis:* It occurs in 90% cases.

Diagnosis

- *Treponemal tests:* Free treponemal antigen absorption (FTA-ABS) and microhemagglutination Treponema pallidum (MHA-TP) detect organism and are more sensitive (95%).
- *Non-treponemal tests:* Screening VDRL and rapid plasma reagin (RPR) detect only 70% patients of otosyphilis.
- *Other tests:* Serum rapid plasma reagin (RPR) test and CSF-VDRL test.

Treatment

Penicillin and prednisone are the mainstay of treatment.

OTOTOXICITY

There is a long list of drugs and chemicals which are ototoxic (Box 7.2). The clinical features of ototoxicity, which may manifest during treatment or after completion of (delayed ototoxicity) the treatment, include SNHL (Fig. 7.1), tinnitus and/or dizziness/vertigo.

Pathology

Table 7.1 shows the target sites of action of common ototoxic agents.

Box 7.2: List of ototoxic agents

- *Aminoglycoside antibiotics:* Streptomycin, gentamicin, tobramycin, neomycin, kanamycin, amikacin, sisomycin
- *Analgesics:* Salicylates, indomethacin, phenylbutazone, ibuprofen
- *Antimalarials:* Quinine, chloroquin
- *Loop diuretics:* Furosemide, ethacrynic acid
- *Cytotoxic drugs:* Nitrogen mustard, cisplatin, carboplatin
- *Chemicals:* Alcohol, tobacco, marijuana, carbon monoxide poisoning
- *Topical applications:* Chlorhexidine and aminoglycoside ear drops
- *Miscellaneous:* Erythromycin, ampicillin, vancomycin, propranolol, propylthiouracil, deferoxamine

Section 2 • Ear

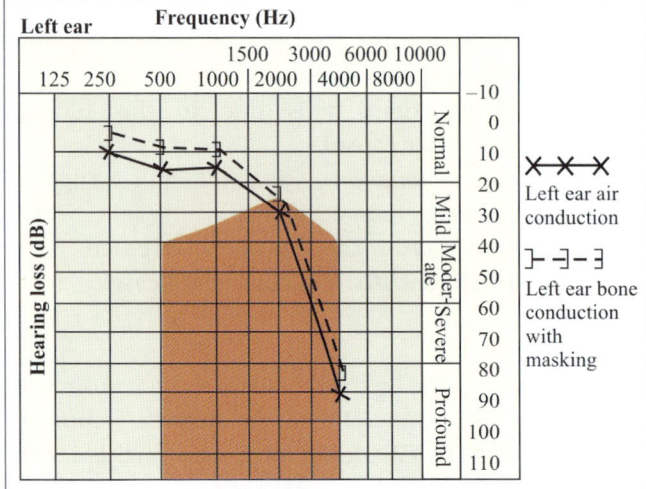

Fig. 7.1: Audiogram of a patient with ototoxicity. Bilateral symmetrical profound high-frequency SNHL

Table 7.1: The site of action of ototoxic agents

Ototoxic agent	Site of action
Aminoglycoside antibiotics	Destroy type 1 hair cells of the crista ampullaris; destruction of outer hair cells
Vancomycin	Damage to cochlear hair cells initially of basal turn (high frequency)
Loop diuretics	Edema and cystic changes in stria vascularis
Salicylates	Probably interfere at enzymatic level
Chloroquin and quinine	Vasoconstriction in the small vessels of the cochlea and stria vascularis
Cytotoxic drugs	Affect the outer hair cells

Clinical Features

- **Erythromycin:** Transient blowing tinnitus and flat type SNHL and in some cases vertigo.
  - Some patients have confusion, fear, psychiatric disturbances, visual changes, blurred speech, sensation of being drugged, or lack of control.
- **Loop diuretics:** They block transport of sodium and chloride ions in the ascending loop of Henle. Usually, the effect is reversible but permanent damage can occur.
- **Salicylates:** Patient presents with tinnitus and bilateral SNHL predominantly affecting higher frequencies. Probably, they interfere at enzymatic level. Hearing loss is reversible on cessation of the drug.
- **Chloroquin:** Ototoxic symptoms, which are reversible, include tinnitus and SNHL. The symptoms generally appear with smaller doses in the susceptible patients.
- **Quinine toxicity (cinchonism):** Deafness (reversible/permanent), vertigo, tinnitus, headache, visual loss, and nausea. If mothers receive quinine during the first trimester of pregnancy, congenital SNHL and hypoplasia of cochlea can occur.
  - **Sensorineural hearing loss:** High-frequency loss, 4 kHz notch, speech discrimination less than 30%.
- **Deferoxamine (desferioxamine):** It is an iron-chelating substance used in the treatment of thalassemic patients who receive repeated blood transfusions and, in turn, have high iron-load. The onset of SNHL may be sudden or delayed. SNHL is usually permanent. In some, SNHL is reversible on the cessation of drug.
- **Topical ear drops:** The damage to the cochlea is due to the absorption of ototoxic eardrops through oval and round windows. SNHL has been documented with the topical use of chlorhexidine and aminoglycoside antibiotics, such as neomycin, framycetin and gentamicin.
- **Cytotoxic drugs:** Nitrogen mustard, cisplatin and carboplatin can cause cochlear damage. They affect the outer hair cells of cochlea.

Caution: The patients taking ototoxic medicines must be instructed to report immediately the development of tinnitus, hearing loss, imbalance and vertigo.

AMINOGLYCOSIDE ANTIBIOTICS

- They can damage kidneys and inner ear.
- Ototoxicity usually occurs after days or weeks of these antibiotic exposures.
- Though some are more toxic to either cochlea or the vestibule, their toxicity is not selective.
  - **Vestibulotoxic:** Streptomycin, gentamicin and tobramycin are primarily vestibulotoxic. So, patient presents with dizziness/vertigo. In large doses, they can damage cochlea also.
  - **Cochleotoxic:** Neomycin, kanamycin, amikacin, sisomycin and dihydrostreptomycin are cochleotoxic.

Risk Factors

The following patients are particularly at risk:
- Bacteremia and fever.
- Hepatic and renal dysfunction.
- Elderly patients above 65 years of age.
- Combination of other ototoxic drugs—cisplatin, ethacrynic acid and furosemide, amphotericin-B and cyclosporine.
- Past history of receiving ototoxic agents.
- **Genetic susceptibility:** Mitochondrial RNA mutation may sensitize the auditory system even to single dose of drug. In genetic susceptible cases, aminoglycoside antibiotic binds to the ribosome and interferes with protein synthesis, thus causing death of the cochlear cells.

Clinical Features

- High-frequency hearing loss is detectable, which progresses to lower frequencies and speech range.
- Onset of vestibular ototoxicity is unpredictable.
    - Imbalance and ataxia worsened by motion or ambulation.
    - It may lead to oscillopsia and complete inability to walk without assistance.
- Clinical improvement is rarely complete, it may begin after 2 months.

> Incidence of ototoxicity is the highest with neomycin. Netilmycin is the weakest ototoxic.

NOISE TRAUMA

Sensorineural hearing loss caused by excessive noise is divided into two groups: (1) acoustic trauma and (2) noise-induced hearing loss (NIHL). Noise trauma (an occupational hazard) occurs in boiler makers, iron and coppersmiths and artillery men. The compensations asked for and the responsibilities thrust upon the employer and the employees are well-known.

Acoustic Trauma

A single brief exposure to a very intense sound (such as an explosion, gunfire or a powerful cracker) can result in permanent damage to hearing. Sudden loud sound has the potential to damage outer hair cells, organ of Corti, Reissner's membrane, tympanic membrane and ossicular chain. Noise level in rifle or a gun fire may reach 140–170 dB sound pressure level (SPL).

> Gunfire is a common nonoccupational cause of noise trauma. The hearing loss is in the range of 4,000 Hz.

Noise-induced Hearing Loss (NIHL)

NIHL is a major cause of preventable SNHL. SNHL may follow chronic exposure of noisy occupations, which are less intense sounds than the acoustic trauma.
- *Temporary threshold shift:* The hearing, which is impaired on the exposure to noise, recovers after an interval of time ranging from few minutes to few hours.
- *Permanent threshold shift:* The hearing loss becomes permanent and does not revert back.

Factors Affecting Noise Trauma

The SNHL caused by noise trauma depends on the following factors, which should be kept in mind for the safety of hearing:
- *Frequency:* The noise of 2,000–3,000 Hz frequencies causes more SNHL than lower and higher than these frequencies.

Table 7.2: The permissible limits of time for various intensities of noise levels

Noise level A dB	Permitted daily exposure in hours
90	8
95	4
100	2
105	1
110	½
115	¼

- *Intensity and duration:* As the intensity of noise increases, the permissible time for exposure is reduced. Table 7.2 shows the permissible limits of time for various intensities of noises. The '5 dB rule of time-intensity' maintains that any rise of 5 dB noise level will reduce the permitted noise exposure time to half.

> A noise level of 90 dB (A) SPL, 8 hours a day for 5 days per week is the highest safe limit in the factories. The exposure of more than 115 dB (A) is not permitted. The impulse noise, which is greater than 140 dB (A), is not permitted.

- *Continuous interrupted:* The continuous noise is more harmful than the interrupted one.
- *Susceptibility:* Some persons are genetically susceptible to noise trauma.
- *Pre-existing ear disease:* They can affect the impact of noise on the inner ear.

Pathology

Noise-induced hearing loss damages hair cells, which begin at the basal turn of cochlea. Outer hair cells are affected earlier than the inner hair cells.

Clinical Features

- Shouting to converse at workplace.
- Aural fullness, tinnitus, or muffled hearing after the work.

Pure Tone Audiogram (PTA)

The PTA (Fig. 7.2) shows the following characteristic findings in noise-induced hearing loss (NIHL):
- *Early stage:* A typical notch at 4 kHz is seen in both air and bone conduction. It is usually symmetrical in both the ears. Patient complains of high-pitched tinnitus and difficulty in hearing only in noisy surroundings.
- *Late stage:* The notch deepens and widens to involve lower and higher frequencies. Involvement of speech frequencies (500, 1,000 and 2,000 Hz) result in hearing difficulty even in calm surroundings also.

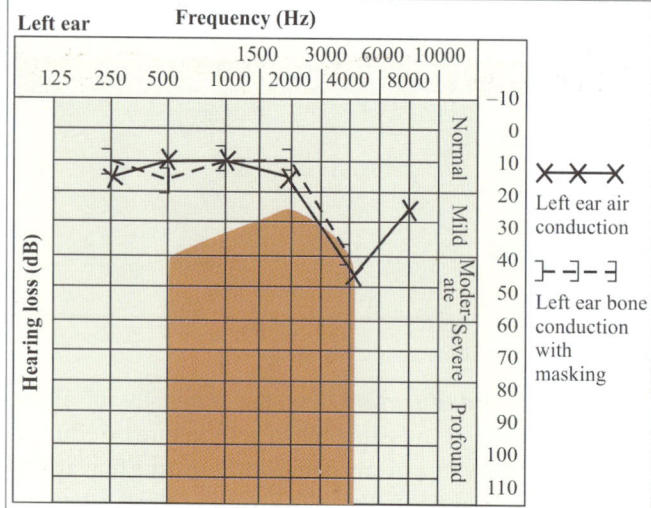

Fig. 7.2: Audiogram of a patient with NIHL. Bilateral symmetrical SNHL with notch at 4,000 Hz

Prophylaxis

Persons who work in factories where noise is above 85 dB (A) should have the following precautions:
- Pre-employment and then annual audiograms for early detection.
- Use of ear protectors (ear plugs or ear muffs) provides protection up to 35 dB.
- Rehabilitation is required in cases of NIHL.

SUDDEN SENSORINEURAL HEARING LOSS (SSNHL)

Sudden sensorineural hearing loss (SSNHL) develops over a period of hours or a few days and hearing loss may be partial or complete. Though mostly unilateral, it may affect both the ears. Patient may have associated symptoms of tinnitus and temporary spell of vertigo.

Etiology
- *Idiopathic:* Cause remains obscure in 85–90% of the cases.
- Three etiological factors speculated are viral, vascular and the rupture of cochlear membranes.
- Spontaneous formation of perilymph fistulae in the oval or round window can occur.
- The causes of sudden hearing loss, which must be ruled out in idiopathic SSNHL, are listed in Box 7.3.

The cause of sudden hearing loss should be discovered by detailed history and physical examination including audiometry (Fig 7.3).

Investigations
- *Laboratory:* The following laboratory investigations may be ordered (keeping in mind the suspected

Box 7.3: Causes of sudden sensorineural hearing loss (SSNHL)

- *Infections:* Mumps, herpes-zoster, meningitis, encephalitis, otosyphilis, Lyme disease, labyrinthitis.
- *Trauma:* Head injury, ear operations, noise trauma, barotraumas (diving and ascending) and spontaneous rupture of cochlear membranes.
- *Vascular:* Hemorrhage (leukemia), embolism, thrombosis, and spasm of labyrinthine or cochlear artery. Risk factors include diabetes, hypertension, polycythemia, macroglobulinemia and sickle-cell trait.
- *Ototoxic drugs:* See Section 'Ototoxicity'.
- *Tumors:* Acoustic neuroma, metastases in cerebellopontine angle, carcinomatous neuropathy.
- *Miscellaneous:* Meniere's disease, Cogan's syndrome, multiple sclerosis, hypothyroidism, sarcoidosis.

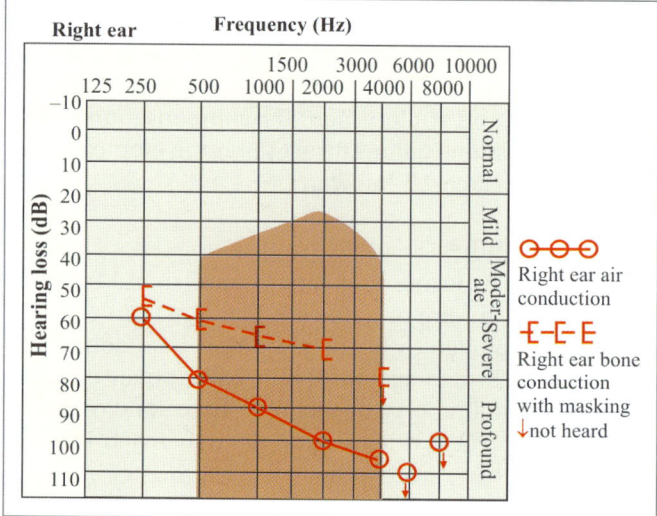

Fig. 7.3: Audiogram of a patient with SSNHL in right ear. Note high-frequency profound SNHL

cause): complete blood count (CBC), erythrocyte sedimentation rate (ESR), tests for syphilis, diabetes, hypothyroidism, blood disorders and lipid profiles, and vestibular tests.
- *Gadolinium-enhanced MRI:* It is indicated on the suspicion of acoustic neuroma.

Though only 1–3% of SSNHL is due to acoustic neuroma, about 10% of acoustic neuroma patients present with SSNHL.

- *Exploratory tympanotomy:* It may be done when perilymph fistula is suspected.

Treatment

As the cause often remains obscure, treatment also remains empirical. Though the corticosteroid therapy is the mainstay vasodilator, diuretics, anticoagulants and thrombolytic agents have also been tried.

In addition to bed rest, treatment consists of the following elements:
- **Steroid therapy:** Prednisolone 40–60 mg in a morning dose for 1 week and then tapered off in a period of 3 weeks. Steroids relieve edema as they have anti-inflammatory effect. They are of particular use in hearing loss of moderate degree.
  - *Intratympanic steroids:* They have been tried when systemic steroids failed to give satisfactory results.
- **Antivirals** such as acyclovir.
- **Inhalation of carbogen** (5% CO_2 + 95% O_2): It increases cochlear blood flow and provides better oxygenation.
- **Low molecular weight dextran:** The infusions decrease blood viscosity. It is contraindicated in cardiac failure and bleeding disorders.
- **Hyperbaric oxygen therapy:** If given in the first month of onset of hearing loss, some benefits have been seen.
- **General measures:** Low-salt diet and bed rest.
- **Other agents tried:** Vasodilator, diuretics, anticoagulants, and thrombolytic agents have also been found helpful in some studies.

Prognosis

About 50% patients recover spontaneously within 15 days. Chances of recovery are less after one month.
- **Good prognostic factors:** They include young adults, moderate and low-frequency hearing loss, lack of vertigo and early treatment.
- **Poor prognostic factors:** They include old age, profound deafness, presence of vertigo, vascular risk factors and delayed treatment.

PRESBYCUSIS

Sensorineural hearing loss, which occurs due to the aging process, is called **presbycusis**. More than one-third of elderly persons over the age of 75 have this senile hearing loss.

Predisposing Factors

Though the exact cause is not yet known, following factors have been implicated: hereditary predisposition, chronic noise exposure, vascular risk factors, ototoxicity, metabolism, arteriosclerosis and diet.

Pathology and Audiometry

The following four pathological types have been described:
1. **Sensory:** The degeneration of the organ of Corti begins at the basal coil and progresses gradually toward the apex. So, the higher frequencies are affected first. The speech discrimination remains good.
2. **Neural:** The degeneration of spiral ganglion begins at the basal coil and progresses toward the apex. Neurons of higher auditory pathways may also be affected. The PTA shows high tone loss. Speech discrimination is poor and out of proportion to the pure tone loss.
3. **Strial or metabolic:** The atrophy of stria vascularis occurs in all turns of cochlea. The physical and chemical processes of energy production are affected. This type of presbycusis pathology runs in families. Pure tone audiogram (PTA) shows flat graph. Speech discrimination remains good.
4. **Cochlear conductive:** The stiffening of the basilar membrane affects its own movements. Audiogram is sloping type.

Clinical Features

- Slowly progressive, symmetrical SNHL in people over the age of 60 years.
- **Background noise:** Great difficulty in hearing in the presence of background noise. Patients may hear well in quiet surroundings in early stage of the disease.
- **Discrimination:** Poor speech understanding. Typical complaint "I can hear but cannot understand."
- **Recruitment:** Intolerance to loud sound due to the recruitment. The patient has hearing loss but if someone speaks loudly, s/he retorts: "Why are you shouting? I am not deaf."
- **Tinnitus:** It may be bothersome and the only complaint.
- **Audiogram (Fig. 7.4):** SNHL is greatest in frequencies > 2,000 Hz with significant decrease in speech discrimination.

Treatment

Patients are advised for the following:
- Hearing aid.
- Lessons in speech reading through visual cues.

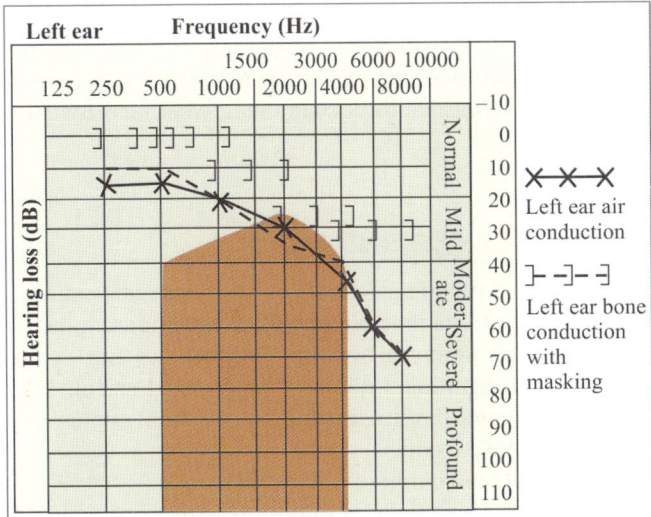

Fig. 7.4: Left ear audiogram of a patient with presbycusis. Bilateral symmetrical SNHL

- Restriction in smoking and stimulants like tea and coffee for decreasing tinnitus.
- **Cochlear implant:** It should be considered if hearing aids do not give desired benefits.

FAMILIAL PROGRESSIVE SENSORINEURAL HEARING LOSS

This genetic disorder leads to progressive degeneration of the cochlea. The disease begins in late childhood or early adult life. The SNHL (flat or basin-shaped audiogram) is bilateral with good speech discrimination.

IMMUNE-MEDIATED SENSORINEURAL HEARING LOSS

Though poorly understood and rare, the condition is treatable medically. Autoimmune disorders, which have been implicated in SNHL, include Cogan's syndrome, Wegener's granulomatosis (WG), Behçet's disease, systemic lupus erythematosus (SLE) and multiple sclerosis (MS).

Clinical Features
- Unexplained, bilateral, rapidly progressive SNHL in adults (20–50 years).
- Normal otoscopy.
- Features of coexistent autoimmune disease uncommon.
- Poor speech discrimination relative to pure tone thresholds.

Laboratory
- Serologic tests for syphilis.
- Cellular and humoral antigen-specific tests such as lymphocyte transformation testing and Western blot.

Treatment
- **Steroids:** Prednisolone 1 mg/kg/day (60 mg/day) for 4 weeks and 10-20 mg EOD maintenance dose.
- **Cytotoxic drugs:** Methotrexate 15 mg/week for 6-8 weeks.
- Injection IgG.
- Plasmapheresis.

THE ONLY HEARING EAR

Even profound unilateral loss of hearing does not produce a serious handicap. Patient may have the following complaints:
- Surprisingly many grown-up children are not aware of their congenital unilateral profound hearing loss. This accidental finding during examination comes as a shock to the parents.
- Impaired localization of the sound source.
- Difficulty in speech discrimination in noisy background.
- Difficulty in hearing when the speaker is on the side of the affected ear.

Treatment
If required, these patients can be managed with contralateral routing of signals (CROS) and bone-anchored hearing aid (BAHA) (*see* Chapter 'Hearing Aids and Cochlear Implants').

Precautions
- Patient is given instructions for the safety of the only hearing ear regarding noise trauma, ototoxic drugs, vascular risk factors and healthy food and lifestyle changes.
- Usually surgeons do not operate on the only hearing ear, until unless it has life-threatening disorder, such as cholesteatoma or acoustic neuroma.

DEGREE OF HEARING LOSS

The term *hearing loss* is preferred over the deafness. World Health Organization (WHO) recommended in 1980 that the term "deaf" should be applied when hearing impairment is so severe that patients are unable to benefit from any type of amplification. So, the cases included in the deaf category have hearing loss of more than 90 dB (profound hearing loss) in the Better ear or total loss of hearing in both the ears.

WHO Classification

The recommended WHO Classification (1980) of Degree of Hearing Loss (Table 7.3) is on the basis of average of speech frequencies (500, 1,000, 2,000 Hz) calculated from PTA with reference to ISO: R. 1970 (international calibration of audiometers). Table 7.3 also shows the disability to understand speech with different degrees of hearing loss.

Table 7.3: WHO classification of degree of hearing loss and difficulty in hearing speech

Average threshold of speech frequencies in Better ear (dB)	Degree of hearing impairment	Degree of difficulty in hearing speech
0–25	Not significant	Can hear faint speech
26–40	Mild	Difficulty with faint speech
41–55	Moderate	Difficulty with normal speech
56–70	Moderately severe	Difficulty with loud speech
71–91	Severe	Can understand only shouted or amplified speech
> 91	Profound	Cannot understand even amplified speech

WHO considers only three speech frequencies (500, 1,000 and 2,000 Hz). Currently, it is felt that frequency of 3,000 Hz is important for hearing in the presence of noise. American Academy of Ophthalmology and Otolaryngology takes into account the average of four speech frequencies 500, 1,000, 2,000 and 3,000 Hz when calculating the handicap.

Department of Personnel, Government of India

The categorization and percentage of hearing impairment recommended by Department of Personnel, Government of India is given in Table 7.4. The Indian Government has reserved certain percentage of vacancies and extended certain other benefits for groups C and D.

Degree of Hearing Handicap

The hearing impairment can affect a person's ability to hear and perform certain activities (disability) and is termed as **handicap** by the society. The degree of hearing impairment and handicap are termed in percentage for the purposes of compensation.
- Method of calculating in percentage:
  - Calculate the average of thresholds of hearing for speech frequencies of 500, 1,000 and 2,000 Hz for the ear (say = A).
  - Deduct from it 25 dB (as up to 25 dB loss is considered normal) means A-25.
  - Multiply it by 1.5, which means (A-25) × 1.5. This shows percentage of hearing impairment for the ear.
  - Percentage handicap of an individual = [(Better ear % × 5) + worse ear %]/6.
  - One example is given in Table 7.5.

NON-ORGANIC HEARING LOSS

Non-organic hearing loss (NOHL) can be either due to malingering or psychogenic.

Malingering

- The malingerer usually has motive and claim for some compensation.
- Patient has history of exposure to industrial noises, head injury or ototoxic medication.
- Patient may present with total hearing loss in both the ears, total loss in only one ear or an exaggerated loss in one or both ears.
- Patient makes exaggerated efforts to hear such as making cupped hand behind the ear.

Stenger Test

- **Principle:** When a sound of same frequency but of different intensities (one greater than the other) is presented to two ears simultaneously, only the ear which receives sound of greater intensity will hear it.

Table 7.4: Recommended categorization and percentage of hearing impairment as per the Department of Personnel, Government of India

Category	Hearing impairment	PTA speech frequencies threshold in Better ear in dB*	Speech discrimination in Better ear**	Percentage of hearing impairment
I or A	Mild	26–40	80–100%	Less than 40%
II or B	Moderate	41–55	50–80%	40–50%
III or C	Severe	56–70	40–50%	50–75%
IV or D	(a) Total	No hearing	No discrimination	100%
	(b) Near total	91 and above	No discrimination	100%
	(c) Profound	71–90	Less than 40%	75–100%

* Pure tone average of AC thresholds of three speech frequencies 500, 1,000 and 2,000 Hz in Better ear; No response to any of the three speech frequencies (500, 1,000, 2,000 Hz) is equivalent to 130 dB loss; Pure tone audiometry (PTA): calibrated at ISO R 389–1970 standards; For children, when PTA is not possible, free field testing should be employed.
** Wherever possible, the PTA results should be supplemented by the speech discrimination score.

Table 7.5: Example of calculating hearing handicap in percentage

Hearing impairment	Frequencies			
	500 Hz	1,000 Hz	2,000 Hz	Average
Right ear	50	65	80	65 dB
Left ear	20	35	50	35 dB
Right ear impairment %	(65–25) × 1.5 = 60%			
Left ear impairment %	(35–25) × 1.5 = 15%			
Total handicap (as per formula)	[(15 × 5) + 60]/6 = 22.5 = 23% (rounded off)			

- **Method:** Patient is blind-folded during the test. Take two tuning forks of same frequency. Vibrate and put them simultaneously at an equal distance (say 30 cm) from each ear. Patient will claim to hear it in the said normal ear. Now bring the tuning fork closer (say 10 cm) to the feigned ear (said deaf ear) while keeping the tuning fork on the normal side at the same distance. The patient will deny hearing in both ears though s/he must be hearing in the said normal ear. A patient with true hearing loss will continue to hear on the normal side. This can be done with a double-channel audiometer using pure tone or speech signals.

Diagnosis

In the era of objective hearing tests, it is not difficult to find a malingerer. Following findings will confirm the malingering:

- *Pure tone and speech audiometry:*
    - ***The inconsistent results of repeat pure tone audiogram (PTA) and speech audiometry:*** Readings would vary greater than 15 dB.
    - ***Absence of shadow curve*** in a patient of unilateral hearing loss is diagnostic of non-organic hearing loss (NOHL). A shadow curve is normally obtained when testing bone conduction without masking the healthy ear. The shadow curve is due to the transcranial transmission of sound to the healthy ear.
    - ***Inconsistency in PTA and speech recognition threshold indicates NOHL.*** The pure tone average of (500, 1,000 and 2,000 Hz) is normally within 10 dB of speech recognition threshold (SRT); if it is more than 10 dB, it indicates NOHL.
- *Acoustic reflex threshold:* The stapedial reflex is elicited normally at 70–100 dB SL. The presence of reflex in the feigned deaf ear will favor non-organic hearing loss (NOHL).
- *Brainstem evoked response audiometry:* Brainstem evoked response audiometry (BERA) will establish hearing acuity within 5–10 dB of actual thresholds.

Self-evaluation Exercises

1. Which of the following are not the causes of fluctuating hearing loss?
    a. Ear wax
    b. Otitis media with effusion (serous otitis media)
    c. Meniere's disease
    d. Perilymph fistula
    e. None of the above
2. The causes of sudden sensorineural hearing loss due to hemorrhage into cochlea do not include:
    a. Leukemia
    b. Sickle-cell disease
    c. Thalassemia
    d. Hypertension
3. The common ototoxic drugs are:
    a. Chloroquin
    b. Cisplatin
    c. Furosemide
    d. All of the above
4. Which of the following statements are not true for ototoxicity?
    a. The ototoxic effects of quinine, salicylates and furosemide are irreversible even if their administration is stopped.
    b. The principal site of damage in aminoglycoside ototoxicity is inner hair cells of basal turn of cochlea.
    c. Semicircular ducts and saccule are very sensitive to streptomycin sulfate therapy.
    d. Furosemide ototoxicity affects stria vascularis of scala media.
    e. None of the above

True (T)/False (F)

5. Autoimmune disorder of inner ear and syphilitic labyrinthitis are uncommon causes of fluctuating hearing loss.
6. The common vestibulotoxic drugs are streptomycin, gentamicin and minocycline.
7. Hutchinson's triad is the feature of HIV/AIDS infection.
8. Audiogram in cases of noise-induced hearing loss shows a dip at 2,000 Hz in air conduction curve.
9. In presbycusis, there occurs decreased ability to perceive high-frequency sounds in elderly people due to the loss of hair cells at the base of cochlea.

Answers

| 1. e | 2. d | 3. d | 4. a, b | 5. T | 6. T |
| 7. F | 8. F | 9. T | | | |

Chapter 8

Hearing Impairment in Infants and Young Children

⦿ Specific Learning Objectives

After going through the chapter, you should be able to answer the following questions:
- What are the prenatal, perinatal and postnatal causes of hearing loss in infants and young children?
- Describe the characteristic features of some common syndromic hearing losses in infants and young children.
- What do you know about: (1) High-risk registry and (2) Universal newborn hearing screening?
- Describe the differential diagnosis of sensorineural hearing loss in children.
- How the evaluation of universal newborn hearing screening refer infants is performed?
- What are the different methods of hearing assessment in infants and young children and how would you manage the infants and young children with hearing loss?
- Describe various rehabilitative measures of infants and young children with hearing loss.

INTRODUCTION

Bilateral severe to profound (70 dB hearing level or more) hearing loss occurs in 1 per 1,000 live births. These children fail to develop speech. Though these children have no defect in their speech producing apparatus, they become mute (dumb). Because they never hear any speech, so they are not able to develop it. The first 5 years of life are critical for the development of speech and language. Therefore, early identification and assessment of hearing loss in infants and children are vital.

Failure to manage hearing loss in infants and early childhood can affect acquisition of speech, language, cognitive and socioemotional development. Progressive, late-onset and acquired hearing loss in childhood is a diagnostic challenge. In children with less severe hearing loss, speech, though developed, may be defective. Though hearing loss happens to the child but it affects the entire family.

> ***Mild hearing loss in children:*** Address it early to prevent speech delay in children.

ETIOLOGY

Etiology of hearing loss remains obscure in about 50% children. The causes of hearing loss in children are traditionally divided into three groups—before birth (prenatal), during birth (perinatal) and after birth (postnatal).

Prenatal Causes

- ***Genetic defects:*** They may affect inner ear alone or several organs. The various genetic anomalies causing hearing loss are given in Table 8.1.

> **Types of Inner Ear Pathologies**
> - ***Michel aplasia:*** The inner ear does not develop at all.
> - ***Mondini aplasia:*** Cochlea has only 1.5 turns.
> - ***Scheibe aplasia:*** In this most common type of inner ear pathology, the membranous cochlea and saccule are abnormal, but rest of the inner ear is normal.
> - ***Alexander aplasia:*** This pathology, which affects only basal turn of cochlea, causes high-frequency sensorineural hearing loss (SNHL).

- ***Maternal infections:*** They include toxoplasmosis, rubella, cytomegalovirus and herpes simplex virus type 1 and 2 (TORCH) and syphilis.
- ***Drugs:*** They include streptomycin, gentamicin, tobramycin, amikacin, quinine and chloroquine. They cross the placental barrier and damage the cochlea. Thalidomide causes abnormalities of ears, limbs, heart, face, lip and palate.
- ***Radiation:*** Especially in first trimester.

- ***Other factors:*** They are nutritional deficiency, diabetes, toxemia and hypothyroidism.

Perinatal Causes

- ***Anoxia:*** The neonatal anoxia is caused due to placenta previa, prolonged labor, cord around the neck and prolapsed cord. It damages the cochlear nuclei and causes hemorrhage into the ear.
- ***Prematurity:*** Birth before term and birth weight less than 1,500 g are risk factors.
- ***Birth injuries:*** Forceps delivery can result in intracranial hemorrhage with extravasation of blood in the inner ear.
- ***Neonatal jaundice:*** Bilirubin levels more than 20 mg% damages the cochlear nuclei.
- ***Ototoxic drugs:*** They are used for neonatal meningitis or septicemia.
- ***Neonatal meningitis.***

Postnatal Causes

- ***Genetic:*** Though genetic, it can manifest later in childhood or adult life (Table 8.1). The child may have hearing loss alone (as in familial progressive sensorineural deafness) or with anomalies of other systems (such as Alport, Klippel-Feil and Hurler syndromes).
- ***Nongenetic:*** They are similar to adults and include the following:
  - ***Infections:*** Measles, mumps, varicella, influenza, meningitis, encephalitis and otitis media.
  - ***Ototoxic drugs:*** See Chapter 'Sensorineural Hearing Loss'.
  - ***Trauma:*** Fractures of temporal bone, middle ear surgery or perilymph leak.
  - ***Noise trauma:*** See Chapter 'Sensorineural Hearing Loss'.

CLINICAL FEATURES

The hearing loss should be suspected in the following events:
- Sudden loud sounds/noises fail to disturb the sleep and startle the child.
- Failure to develop speech in 1–2 years.
- Defective speech and poor school performance can be due to hearing loss. These children may be wrongly labeled as mentally retarded.

Syndromes with Genetic Hearing Loss (Table 8.1)

Fifty percent cases of infant hearing loss are genetic in origin. Out of them, 75–80% is autosomal recessive, 15–20% is autosomal dominant, and 1–2% is X-linked. Fewer children have mitochondrial inheritance.

Table 8.1: Syndromes with genetic hearing loss

Syndrome	System	Features
Congenital autosomal recessive		
Onchodystrophy	Nail	Dystrophy of finger and toe nails, defects of teeth, hair, sebaceous glands
Jervell and Lange-Nielson syndrome	Heart	Syncopal attacks, prolonged QT interval in electrocardiography (ECG)
Pendred's syndrome	Thyroid	Goiter, hypothyroidism
Klippel-Feil syndrome		Short neck (fusion of one or more cervical vertebrae), spina bifida, canal atresia, mixed loss
Congenital autosomal dominant		
Waardenburg's syndrome	Skin	White forelock, depigmentation of skin, heterochromia iridis, increased intercanthal distance and antimongoloid slant of eyes
Treacher-Collins (mandibulofacial dysostosis) syndrome	Craniofacial and cervical	Hypoplasia of malar bones and mandible, coloboma of lower lids, malformed external and middle ear, and conductive loss
Crouzon's syndrome		Craniofacial dysostosis (frog eyes), parrot nose, ear malformation, mixed loss
Delayed onset autosomal recessive		
Usher's	Eyes	Progressive retinitis pigmentosa
Delayed onset autosomal dominant		
Alport's syndrome	Kidney	Glomerulonephritis and corneal dystrophy
Van der Hoeve's syndrome	Skeletal	Fragile bones, blue sclera and deafness (conductive, sensorineural, or mixed)
Congenital chromosomal abnormalities		
Trisomy 21 (Down's syndrome)		Stenosis of ear canal, high incidence of serous otitis media
Trisomy 13–15		Low-set ears with malformation, cleft lip and palate, congenital heart disease
Trisomy 16–18		Cardiac abnormalities, low-set pinna, atresia of canal

Chapter 8 • Hearing Impairment in Infants and Young Children

HIGH-RISK REGISTRY

Two percent to five percent of neonates with following risk factors have moderate to profound hearing loss (Flow chart 8.1).

- Family history of hereditary childhood SNHL.
- Prenatal infections TORCH.
- Craniofacial abnormalities.
- Ototoxic drugs.
- Birth weight less than 1,500 g
- Stigmata or other findings associated with hearing loss (conductive or sensorineural) syndrome, such as deformed pinna, cleft palate and craniofacial deformities.
- Neonatal jaundice (bilirubin level more than 20 mg% requiring an exchange transfusion).
- Bacterial meningitis, especially *Haemophilus influenzae*.
- Neonatal asphyxia with seizures or coma, no spontaneous respiration in first 10 minutes; hypotonia persisting for 2 hours, mechanical ventilation lasting for 5 days or more.
- Apgar score* (0–4 at 1 minute or 0–6 at 5 minutes).

About 50% of children with moderate to profound congenital hearing loss have no risk factors. Therefore, the universal newborn hearing screening (UNHS) has evolved.

UNIVERSAL NEWBORN HEARING SCREENING (UNHS)

The UNHS is done within first 3 months of life. It detects the permanent hearing loss at an average age of 3 months. But in the absence of UNHS, average age of diagnosis was found to be 31.25 months. Reliance on physician and parent's observations were not found successful. Behavioral methods of testing do not meet the requirement of UNHS. Currently, brainstem evoked response audiometry (BERA) and evoked otoacoustic emissions (EOAE) are employed either singly or in combination.

Interpretations

The screening outcomes are either pass or refer infants:
- **Pass infants** need no further testing at this time, but progressive, late-onset and acquired hearing loss in childhood cannot be ruled out at this time.
- **Refer infants** require a diagnostic hearing evaluation. Electrocochleography measures auditory sensitivity to within 20 dB. It is an invasive procedure and avoided.

The future development of frequency-specific brainstem evoke response audiometry (BERA) and auditory steady state responses (ASSR) will probably replace current two-tiered screening protocol (EOAE and BERA).

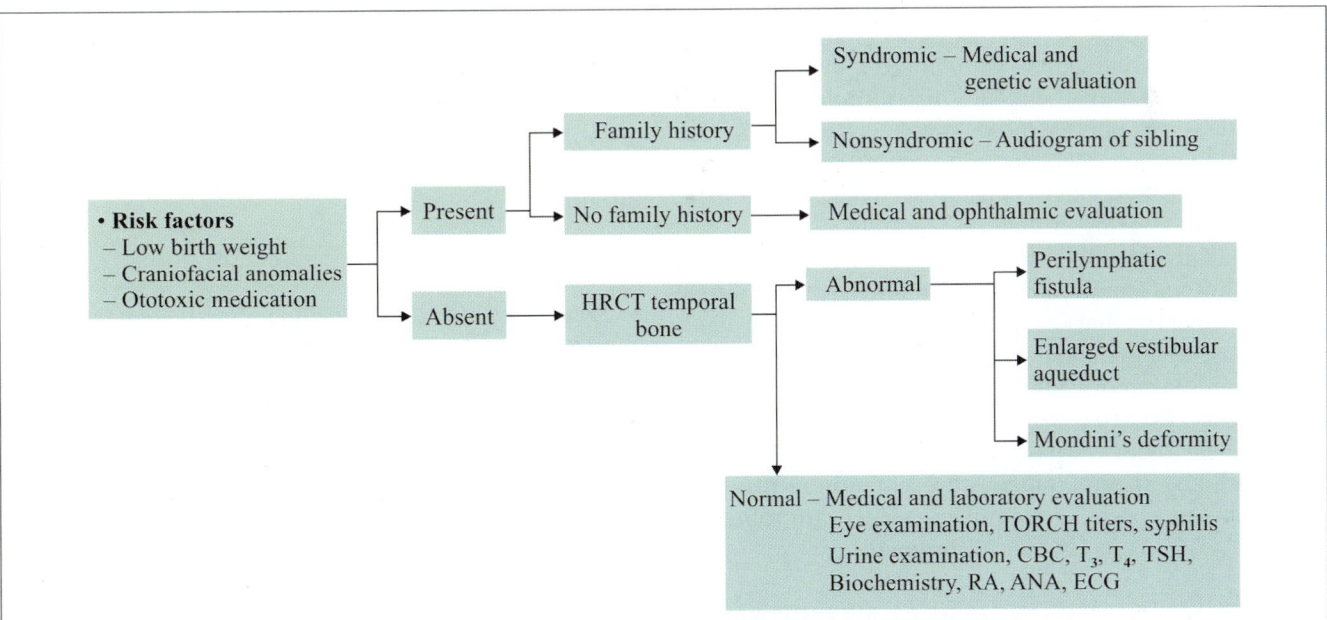

Flow chart 8.1: Differential diagnosis of sensorineural hearing loss in children

Abbreviations: HRCT, high resolution computed tomography; TORCH, toxoplasmosis, rubella, cytomegalovirus, herpes simplex; CBC, complete blood count; TSH, thyroid stimulating hormone; RA, rheumatoid arthritis; ANA, antinuclear antibody; ECG, electrocardiograph.

---

* Evaluation of a newborn's physical status by assigning numerical values (0–2) to each of five criteria: (1) heart rate, (2) respiratory effort, (3) muscle tone, (4) response stimulation, and (5) skin color; a score of 8–10 indicates best possible condition.

Limitations

No test is perfect. Regular monitoring of hearing, speech and language milestones is important even in infants who pass EOAE and BERA.
- *BERA:* Click-evoked auditory nerve and brainstem evoked potentials often miss hearing loss when hearing is normal at some frequencies.
- *Otoacoustic emissions (OAE)* screening is difficult in noisy environment, presence of vernix or debris in external auditory canal (EAC) and collapsing EAC in first 24 hours after birth. OAE may miss inner hair cell and auditory nerve hearing losses.

Brainstem Evoked Response Audiometry (BERA)

Syn: Auditory Brainstem Responses (ABR)

For hearing screening, responses are elicited by air-conducted clicks (having broadband frequency spectrum) at a level that produces response in normal hearing ears. They produce no response in ears with hearing loss of 30–35 dB HL. This evoked potential, which is present in neonates as early as 25 weeks gestational age, is unaffected by sleep, attention and sedation (*see* Chapter 'Hearing Evaluation').

BERA is affected by disorders of external, middle and internal ears and auditory nerve and brainstem. The current automated ABR detection algorithms replace the subjective impression of the examiner as to the presence or absence of ABR.

Evoked Otoacoustic Emission (EOAE)

EOAE are acoustic signals generated by cochlear outer hair cells in response to auditory stimulation. EOAE, which measures only cochlear status, is independent of neural activity and CNS status. It takes lesser time and uses broader frequency range than click-evoked ABR (*see* Chapter 'Hearing Evaluation').
- Transiently evoked otoacoustic emissions (TEOAE) provides information over a broad frequency range (500–6,000 Hz) that occurs after a brief stimulus. TEOAE are observed in neonatal ears in the absence of external and middle ear disorders.
- Delayed evoked otoacoustic emissions (DEOAE) provides frequency specific information that occurs in response to simultaneous presentation of two pure tones. The screening algorithms, which are robust in neonates and infants, use 'DP grams'.

EVALUATION OF UNIVERSAL NEWBORN HEARING SCREENING REFER INFANTS

The infants who fail UNHS should have detailed history, physical examination including ear microscopy and vestibular tests, threshold frequency-specific ABR and OAE and visual reinforcement audiometry (VRA) done.

Newborn hearing screening does not identify progressive hearing loss, which does occur in preschool children and constitute 15–20% of SNHL young children.

The ancillary testing includes laboratory and genetic testing, screening for maternally transmitted infection and temporal bone imaging.

History
- Family history for congenital hearing loss, eye and cardiac abnormalities.
- Prenatal maternal history of infection (TORCH and syphilis), diabetes, hypothyroidism, alcohol, smoking and drugs.
- Perinatal risk factors.

Physical Examination

A complete physical examination is mandatory though majority of infants do not have any positive findings. See Table 8.1 for the features of various hearing loss syndromes.

External and middle ear disorders are the most common source of failed initial hearing screening. A thorough evaluation should include following elements:
- Neurologic and developmental milestones.
- Nystagmus spontaneous and head shaking.
- *External auditory canal (EAC):* Clean it and *see* for stenosis and atresia.
- Tympanic membrane for thickness, appearance and motion and middle ear effusion.
- Pneumatic otoscopy in older children: In 0–6 months of age, both tympanometry and pneumatic otoscopy can miss middle ear effusion.

The incidence of middle ear effusion in the first year of life is quite high (61%). Tympanostomy tube insertion is done for persistent middle ear effusion. In infants with AOM, antibiotic therapy is given with close follow-up for the effusion resolution.

HEARING TESTS

- *Frequency-specific auditory brainstem response (ABR) thresholds:* Both air and bone conductions are evaluated using tone-pip ABR. Significant air-bone gap indicates external and middle ear disorders.
- *Evoked otoacoustic emission (EOAE):* See other Sections and Chapter 'Hearing Evaluation'.
- *Tympanometry using a probe-tone frequency of 1,000 Hz or more:* Provide status of middle ear. The traditional tympanometry (using 226 Hz probe tone) is invalid in 0–6 months of age.
- *Visual reinforcement audiometry (VRA):* It is a form of conditioning technique. Infants turn their heads in the direction of sound source. If this response is rewarded by activation of a lighted, animated toy, the infant usually continue to respond and an audiogram is obtained. VRA testing can be done either under earphones or sound field testing. Older infants, who

yield fewer false positive responses than 6 months infant, tend to reject earphones.
- VRA thresholds for 6 months infant are within 10 dB of adult thresholds.
- VRA detects even slight threshold elevations seen in middle ear effusion.

Other Hearing Tests

The auditory function tests in neonates, infants and young children can be classified into various groups (Table 8.2). Though currently the gold standards are auditory brainstem response (ABR) and (OAE), the following tests were done traditionally.

- *Screening procedures:* These are based on infant's behavioral response to the sound signal.
  - *Arousal test:* A high-frequency narrow band noise presented for 2 seconds to the light sleeping infant normally awakes the infant twice when three such stimuli are presented.
  - *Auditory response cradle:* The baby is placed in a cradle. The transducers monitor the infant's behavior (trunk and limb movement, head jerk and respiration) in response to auditory stimulation.
- *Behavior observation audiometry:* Auditory signal produces a change in infant's behavior, such as alerting, cessation of an activity, widening of eyes and facial grimacing.
  - *Moro's reflex:* It consists of sudden movement of limbs and extension of head in response to sound of 80–90 dB.
  - *Cochleopalpebral reflex:* A child blinks in response to a loud sound.
  - *Cessation reflex:* In response to a sound of 90 dB, an infant stops activity or starts crying.
- *Distraction techniques:* The children of 6–7 months age turn their heads to locate the source of sound.
  - *Method:* The child is seated in mother's lap. One person distracts the child's attention while the other produces a sound from behind or from one side. Note whether the child tries to locate the sound by turning head.

Table 8.2: Methods of hearing assessment in infants and young children

- Neonatal screening procedures (arousal test, auditory response cradle, electric response audiometry).
- Behavior observation audiometry (moro's reflex, cochleopalpebral reflex, cessation reflex).
- Distraction techniques.
- Conditioning techniques (visual reorientation audiometry, play audiometry).
- Objective tests (evoked response audiometry, impedance audiometry, otoacoustic emissions, heart rate audiometry).

- *Sounds:* They are high-frequency rattle (8 kHz), low-frequency hum, whispered sound as 'S, S, S', xylophone, warbled tones or narrow band noise (500–4,000 Hz).
- *Conditioning techniques (play audiometry):* The child is conditioned to perform any act on hearing a sound. The acts may be placing a marble in a box, a wooden or plastic block in the bucket, or a ring on a post. The test can be done either in the free-field or by using headphones. A frequency-specific audiogram is possible in a child of 2–4 years of age.
- *Speech audiometry:* The spondee words are presented to the child along with the pictures. The child is asked to point the appropriate picture or repeat the word. The intensity level of the spondee words is gradually lowered. The speech reception threshold is determined. To examine the expressive ability, the child is asked to name the toys and objects.

Deaf and dumb: Deaf persons are not intellectually dumb. Psychological tests usually overlook the intellectual capacity of deaf people as they consist of culturally biased material.

TREATMENT

- *Otitis media:* In infants of acute otitis media, antibiotic therapy is given with close follow-up for the effusion resolution.
  - The incidence of middle ear effusion in the first year of life is quite high (61%). Tympanostomy tube insertion is done for persistent middle ear effusion.
- *Meningitis:* Immediate broad spectrum antibiotics are given and then the regime is modified as per the report of culture and sensitivity of cerebrospinal fluid (CSF).
  - Corticosteroids administered at the earliest for 2 days reduces incidence of hearing loss, which if occurs is permanent.
- *Auditory rehabilitation:* After identifying the type and extent of hearing loss, appropriate rehabilitative measures should be initiated at the earliest. They include amplification and cochlear implantation. Hearing aids help in developing lip reading.

Hearing Aids

- Hearing aid should be fitted at the earliest. Regular follow-up appointments with audiologists is important. *See* Chapter 'Hearing Aid and Cochlear Implant'.
- *Indication:* Permanent bilateral hearing loss (conductive or sensorineural) more than 20 dB HL between 1,000 and 4,000 Hz.
- *Bone conduction hearing aids:* They are indicated in cases of atresia, stenotic ear canals and recurrent otorrhea.
- *Children less than 7 years:* They need behind-the-ear or bone conduction hearing aids.
- *Infants with 55 dB or higher hearing losses:* Personal wireless FM systems improve the speech-to-noise ratio.

Cochlear Implants

Each child should be evaluated carefully for the cochlear implant candidacy (Chapter 'Hearing Aid and Cochlear Implant').
- Younger the child better are the results of cochlear implantation. Infants younger than one year of age are also receiving cochlear implants.
- Post meningitis deafness needs early implantation to avoid later difficulties of implantation due to cochlear ossification.
- Cochlear ossification (usually post meningitis) and auditory nerve aplasia preclude this intervention.

REHABILITATIVE MEASURES

Playgroups and parent groups facilitate parents to learn how to accommodate their baby's communication needs. Services of expert professionals who deal with childhood hearing loss and early childhood education are important. It is essential to know not only the degree and type of hearing loss, but also other associated handicaps, such as blindness or mental retardation. The prelingual and postlingual hearing loss bears prognostic importance.

The broad groups of communication methodologies include American sign language (ASL), spoken and signed language and auditory oral methods. Aims of rehabilitation include development of speech and language, adjustment in society and useful vocational employment.

Parental Guidance

Hearing loss happens not just to a child, but to the whole family. The parents should be sympathetically told of child's disability and how to care for it. Parents should know regarding the following requirements:
- Care and periodic replacement of hearing aid
- Change of ear moulds as the child grows
- Follow-up visits for re-evaluation
- Education at home
- Selection of vocation

Development of Speech and Language

Reception of information occurs through visual, auditory or tactile faculties while expression is through the oral/written speech or manual sign language. The proper communication needs either the improvement in hearing through amplification or the development of visual or tactile means of communication.

- ***Auditory oral communication:*** This method of normal people communication can be used for the children of postlingual deafness. Hearing aids augment auditory reception. Training is imparted in speech reading, which encourages attention towards the movements of lips, face and natural gestures of hand and body. Expressive skill should be encouraged through verbal speech.
- ***Manual communication:*** It uses the sign language and fingerspelling method. The abstract ideas are difficult to express because general public does not understand it.

Total Communication

This form of communication, which is good for children with prelingual severe to profound deafness, employs all the sensory inputs such as auditory, visual, tactile and kinesthetic. These children are taught to develop oral speech, lip-reading and sign language.

Vibrotactile Aids

These are useful in children who are both deaf, as well as blind. The aids are fitted to the child's hand or sternum. The vibrations of speech are perceived by the child through tactile sensation (Have you seen film 'Black' of Amitabh and Rani Mukherji?).

Education and Vocation of Deaf

- The residential and day schools for the deaf children are available.
- The children with moderate hearing loss can be integrated into normal schools with preferential seating arrangement in the class.
- In radio hearing aids, the microphone and transmitter are with the teacher and the receiver and amplifier are worn by the child. The child can hear the teacher's voice in a better way, avoiding the environmental noises.
- Given the opportunity, commensurate with their ability, the deaf people, who are sincere and good workers, can be successfully employed in several vocations.

Chapter 8 • Hearing Impairment in Infants and Young Children

Self-evaluation Exercises

1. Inner ear malformation in fetus can occur when pregnant mother is exposed to:
   a. Radiation
   b. German measles
   c. Cytomegalovirus
   d. Thalidomide
   e. All of the above

Match the following

2. Michel aplasia
3. Mondini's malformation
4. Scheibe aplasia
5. Alexander aplasia

   a. Cochlea lacks bony partitions between the coils
   b. Total lack of inner ear development
   c. Only basal turn of cochlea abnormal
   d. Membranous cochlea and saccule are abnormal

True (T)/False (F)

6. Brainstem evoked response audiometry is indicated in assessing hearing loss in neonates.

Match the following

7. Waardenburg's syndrome
8. Pendred's syndrome
9. Alport's syndrome
10. Klippel-Feil syndrome
11. Usher's syndrome

   a. Abnormality of thyroxine synthesis and goiter
   b. Glomerulonephritis
   c. Retinitis pigmentosa
   d. White forelock, depigmentation of skin
   e. Congenital spinal deformities

Answers

1. e   2. a   3. b   4. c   5. d   6. T
7. d   8. a   9. b   10. e   11. c

Pearls and Nuggets (Refresh your knowledge)

- **Reversible causes of sensorineural hearing loss:** They must be ruled out even in patients with presbycusis and noise induced hearing losses, which constitute the most common causes of hearing loss.
- **Hypothyroidism:** The ENT symptoms include hoarseness of voice, nasal stuffiness, vertigo, and hearing loss.
- **"Locked in" syndrome:** It occurs in elderly people due to the occlusion of basilar artery in the caudal pons. It has following lesions and features:
  - **Bilateral abducens and horizontal gaze centers:** Patient can only move eyes vertically and is able to blink bilaterally. Patient can read and understand speech and remains aware of surroundings. Patient responds by blinking as s/he has quadriplegia.
  - **Bilateral corticobulbar fibers to nucleus ambiguus and hypoglossal nuclei:** Patient becomes unable to speak and swallow.
  - **Bilateral corticospinal tracts:** Patient becomes tetraplegic (quadriplegia).
- **Marcus-Gunn pupil:** When light is put on the blind eye, the pupils of both eyes remain dilated. But when the light is put on the normal eye, pupils of both eyes constrict. It happens due to the consensual pupillary light reflex because the efferent pathway on diseased side is normal. This interruption of afferent papillary pathway occurs in retrobulbar neuritis or optic nerve lesions (such as injury to the optic nerve during endoscopic sinus surgery).
- **Trigeminal nerve:** CN V is the largest cranial nerve. Muscles supplied by trigeminal nerve include muscles of mastication (masseter, temporalis, and medial and lateral pterygoids), mylohyoid, anterior belly of digastric, tensor tympani, tensor veli palatini.
- **Trigeminal neuralgia:** Carbamazepine is the drug of choice.

Chapter 9

Hearing Aids and Cochlear Implants

⊙ Specific Learning Objectives

After going through the chapter, you should be able to answer the following questions:
- What are the different types of hearing aids and their advantages and disadvantages? Mention major components and their functions.
- What do you know about the assistive listening devices and CROS type and implantable hearing aids and their indications?
- What are the different components of cochlear implant (CI) and their function? Mention the indications and postoperative complications.
- What are the differences between hearing aids and cochlear implants? What is auditory brain stem implant?

INTRODUCTION

Patients with impaired hearing need auditory rehabilitation for better communication. The auditory rehabilitation includes not only instrumental devices but also training.

The various types of instruments are—hearing aids, assistive devices and cochlear implants (Table 9.1). The heightened volume increases audibility and reduces the strain of understanding sound in daily listening situations.

TRAINING

- **Speech reading (lip reading):** This integrated process for understanding the speech studies the movements of lips, facial expression, gestures and the probable context of conversation. This skill is useful for individuals with impaired hearing who have high frequency loss and difficulty in hearing in noisy surroundings.
- **Auditory training:** Auditory training is useful for those using hearing aids and cochlear implants. It is used along with the skill of speech reading. The patient is exposed to various listening situations with different degrees of difficulty. They are taught selectively to concentrate on speech sounds.
- **Speech conservation:** Patients with profound hearing loss, lose the ability to monitor their own speech production. The defects appear in articulation, response, pitch and the volume of voice. Speech conservation educates such persons to use their tactile and proprioceptive feedback systems so that they can monitor their speech production.

Table 9.1: Instrumental devices for impaired hearing

Hearing aids
• Body-worn
• Behind-the-ear (BTE)
• Spectacle
• In-the-ear (ITE)
• Canal types
▪ In the canal (ITC)
▪ Completely in canal (CIC)
Assistive devices
• Assistive listening devices and systems
• Alerting devices
• Telecommunication devices
Implantable hearing aids
• Bone-anchored hearing aid (BAHA): Entific BAHA, RetroX
• Implantable middle ear hearing aids
▪ Piezoelectric actuator: Rion-E, Otologics MET, Implex TICA
▪ Piezoelecric sensor and actuator: St. Croix Envoy
▪ Magnetic actuator: Vibrant MED-EL Soundbridge, Soundtec DDHS
Cochlear implants
• Advanced bionics corporation: HiRes 90K
• Cochlear corporation: Nucleus 5 System
• MED-EL corporation: C40 + device

Abbreviations: TICA, totally implantable communication assistant; DDHS, direct drive hearing system; MET, middle ear transducer.

HEARING AIDS

Any patient of hearing loss, conductive or sensorineural who cannot be helped by medical and surgical means, is a candidate for hearing aids (Figs 9.1 and 9.2A to E).

Chapter 9 • Hearing Aids and Cochlear Implants

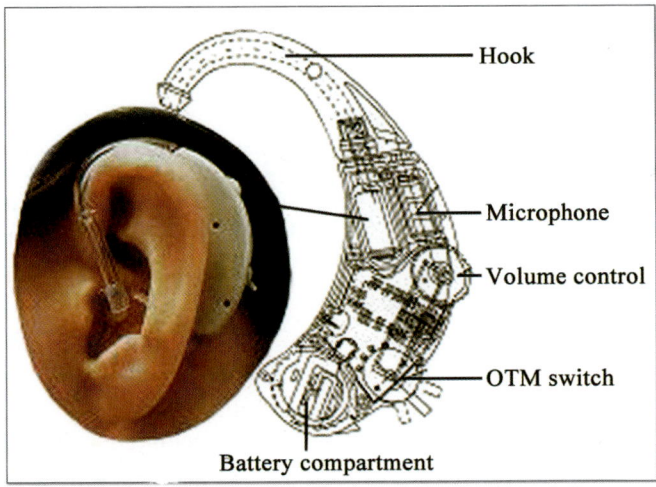

Fig. 9.1: Parts of behind-the-ear hearing aid
Source: Siemens

Parts

A hearing aid machine presents amplified sound to the ear. It has the following parts (Fig. 9.1):
- *Microphone:* It picks up sound and converts them into electrical impulses.
- *Amplifier:* It amplifies electrical impulses.
- *Receiver:* It converts electrical impulses back to sound.
- *Volume control*
- *Battery power source*
- *Earmold:* The amplified sound is carried to the ear through the earmold. Poor earmold fitting results in annoying acoustic feedback, amplification of background noise and distortion of sound.

Types

There are mainly two types of hearing aids—air conduction and bone conduction. Most of the hearing aids are air conduction type:
1. *Air conduction hearing aid:* The amplified sound is transmitted to the external auditory canal (EAC) in which the receiver is situated.
2. *Bone conduction hearing aid:* The amplified sound is transmitted to the mastoid bone through a bone vibrator which snugly fits on the mastoid. So the vibrator acts as a receiver and directly stimulates the cochlea. This type of aid is indicated in patients who suffer from active ear discharge, otitis externa (OE) and atresia of the ear canal.

Shapes and Sizes

On the basis of shapes and sizes (Fig. 9.2), hearing aids can be classified into following groups:
- *Body-worn:* Microphone, amplifier and the battery are in one small box, which is worn at the chest level. The receiver is situated in the EAC. It allows a high degree of amplification and minimal feedback. These aids are rarely used now because of their size. Clothes rub against the microphone cause excessive and unusual sounds (Fig. 9.2A).
- *Behind-the-ear:* Microphone, amplifier, receiver and battery lie in one small unit which is worn behind the ear by a hook-shaped rigid tube that fits over the auricle. Through a soft polyethylene tube and an earmold, it is coupled to the ear canal (Fig. 9.2B).
- *Eye-glass-aid or spectacle types:* In this modification of behind-the-ear, the unit is housed in the auricular part of the spectacle frame. Though not very popular now, it can be used by patients who wear eye glasses.
- *In-the-ear:* All the parts of hearing aid are housed in a small box, which resembles earmold in size and shape and is worn in the ear (Fig. 9.2C).
- *Canal aids:* This type of hearing aid is small and worn in the ear canal. They are preferred because of their small size. The ear canal should be large and wide. The patient should have the dexterity to manipulate the minute controls in the aid. Small size limits number of controls for adjustment. Two types of hearing aids are available in this category (Figs 9.2D and E):
1. *In-the-canal:* They have limited venting options.
2. *Completely-in-canal:* It is the smallest and invisible type. Only a clear filament protrudes from the ear canal that helps in removing the hearing aid. They provide full or partial resolution of the occlusion effect. Telephones can be used as they do not need

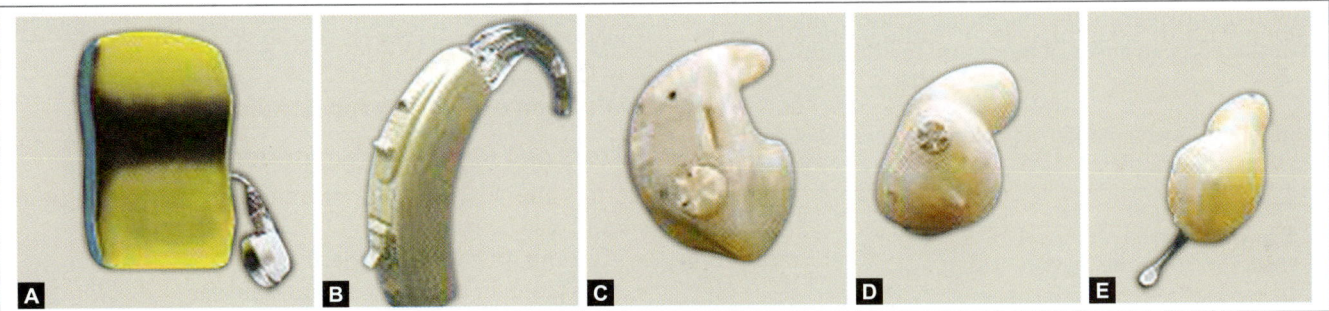

Figs 9.2A to E: Hearing aids. (A) Body-worn; (B) Behind-the-ear; (C) In-the-ear; (D) In-the-canal; (E) Completely in canal
Source: Siemens

a vent. They resolve wind-noise problem. They can develop feedback with jaw movement (Fig. 9.2E).

Features of Behind-the-ear and Canal Aids

They are the most commonly used hearing aids:
- Canal aids are one shell hearing aids and improve localization of sounds.
- Smaller the size higher is the cost and cosmetic appearance.
- Increased amplification provided by the pinna boosts gain in higher frequencies.
- Amount of gain is limited due to problems with acoustic feedback.
- Patients need to have good vision and manual dexterity to manipulate smaller size hearing aid. This is a problem for older patients. Now remote controls are available.
- The canal length and bore size and vent size of behind-the-ear earmold or in-the-ear shell may be used to alter the acoustic output.
- A relatively large vent is required if less output at low frequency is desirable as in cases of high frequency hearing loss.

The disadvantages of using behind-the-ear and canal aids are given in Table 9.2.

Contralateral Routing of Signals

In this special hearing aid, microphone fits in the profoundly deaf ear and the receiver is placed in the better ear. The microphone in the deaf ear picks up sounds, which are passed to the receiver placed in the better ear. This type of arrangement, which is useful in patients with unilateral profound hearing loss, helps in localizing the sound coming from the side of the deaf ear.

The contralateral routing of signals can be accomplished through wiring or through radio frequency transmission. A nonoccluding or open earmold is used in better ear to allow detection of sounds without amplification. If the better ear also has hearing loss, a microphone can be made available on that side.

Monaural/Binaural Amplification

In cases of bilateral hearing loss, binaural hearing aid amplification eliminates the head shadow effect and is advantageous. In cases of monaural hearing aid, the other ear suffers a reduction in word recognition score. The other benefits of binaural amplification include better speech discrimination and localization. The improved ease of listening avoids sensory deprivation.

> **Head shadow effect**: When sound has to cross the head to reach other side of the ear, 6 dB loss in sound intensity occurs.

Hearing Aids in Children

An infant should be fitted with a hearing aid based on available audiometric information. More reliable hearing tests can be done later on. The amplification is adjusted as the child grows. Overamplification is avoided as it can damage the inner ear. In infants with congenital atresia or microtia, hearing aid can be fitted at the age of 2 months.

> - *Prelingual deafness* is the hearing loss that occurs prior to the development of basic spoken language skills, which usually occurs at 2–3 years of age.
> - *Postlingual deafness* is the hearing loss that occurs after the development of basic spoken language skills. It has prognostic importance in candidates of cochlear implants.

Analog, Hybrid and Digital Hearing Aids

- *Analog hearing aids:* Traditional hearing aids are analog machines. They convert the acoustic energy to electric signals (similar in shape or analogous to actual sound waves), which are amplified and delivered to transducer that converts electrical signal back to acoustic energy.
- *Hybrid hearing aids:* They use digital components that control and modify the operation of the analog components in the signal-processing stage.
- *Digital hearing aids:* In these types of hearing aid, an electric signal is modified to a digital signal, which is composed of discrete signals coded by binary numbers. These have not only the higher fidelity signal but can also modify the output in many ways. They can be thus programed for an individual's specific needs. Though they are expensive, they can contain several frequency responses, which can be selected by the patients depending on their auditory needs.

Evaluation of Hearing Aid Candidates

History and Physical Examination

During the history and examination following points should also be included:
- Age and dexterity of patient
- Condition of the outer and middle ear
- Cosmetic concerns of the patient
- Type of earmold

Table 9.2: Disadvantages of behind-the-ear and canal hearing aids

- Acoustic feedback
- Spectral distortion
- Occlusion of external auditory canal (EAC)
- Blockage of EAC and insert by ear wax
- Earmold skin reaction
- Not suitable in discharging ears

Audiogram

The audiograms determines following parameters and helps in selecting the type of hearing aids:
- Degree of hearing loss
- Frequencies affected
- Type of hearing loss (conductive or sensorineural)
- Presence of recruitment
- Uncomfortable loudness level
- Type of fitting, monaural, binaural (separate aid for each ear), binaural Y-connection (one aid with two receivers) or CROS type.

ASSISTIVE DEVICES

Assistive devices help the patients with impaired hearing in special difficult situations, warn them of danger signals and help in telecommunication. These devices are divided into three groups:

1. *Assistive listening devices and systems:* These devices help the patients to listen efficiently in the presence of background noise, over the telephone, in auditoriums or theaters. They can be used by either individual person or by a group. The technology employed includes hard-wired system, induction loops, amplitude modulation, frequency modulation or infrared signals.
2. *Alerting devices:* They produce an extra loud sound signal so that patients can hear a telephone or a doorbell, a baby crying in another room, an alarm clock or the noise of a smoke detector.
   - *Hearing dog:* It is trained to bark loudly at the sound of a doorbell and cry of a baby.
   - *Light signal or vibrations:* Patients with profound or total hearing loss need devices where the sound is changed into a light signal or vibrations. Alarm clock with flashing lights and devices producing strong vibrations can awaken the individual and even shake the bed.
3. *Telecommunication devices:* An amplifier added to the hand set of a telephone can amplify the sound. A telephone coupler can be connected to the telephone and the signal produced is picked up by the hearing aid.
   - *Telecommunication devices for the deaf (TDD)* are meant for the profoundly or totally deaf patients. They convert typed message into sounds which is transmitted over the standard telephone lines. The other end TDD converts these sound signals back into the written messages.
   - Closed caption television decoder provides cues to the hearing impaired patients so that they can enjoy news, movies and other TV programs.

IMPLANTABLE HEARING AIDS

Implantable hearing aids can be totally or partially concealed. The transducer of the aid is coupled directly to the bone or ossicular chain (malleus or stapes).
- *Advantages:* These devices offer:
  - Better acoustic gain
  - No feedback
  - Low battery consumption
- *Indications:* In addition to sensorineural hearing loss (SNHL), they are indicated in conductive hearing loss (CHL) (congenital or acquired) which are not amenable to surgical treatment.

Classification

Implantable hearing aids can be classified into following categories:
- *Bone-anchored hearing Aid (BAHA):* Entific BAHA and RetroX.
- *Implantable middle ear hearing aids:*
  - *Piezoelectric:* An electric current is passed into a piezoceramic crystal which changes its volume and produces vibratory signals. The piezoelectric transducer is coupled to ossicles and drives the ossicular chain by vibration. There are two types of piezoelectric devices:
    1. *Piezoelectric actuator:* Rion-E, Otologics middle ear transducer (MET), Implex totally integrated cochlear amplifier (TICA).
    2. *Piezoelectric sensor and actuator:* St. Croix Envoy.
  - *Magnetic actuator:* An electric current is passed into a coil, which creates a magnetic flux and drives an adjacent magnet. The magnet is attached to the ossicle, which conveys vibrations to the cochlea. The examples of this aid include vibrant MED-EL Soundbridge and Soundtec direct drive hearing system (DDHS).

Bone-Anchored Hearing Aid (BAHA)

Bone-anchored hearing aid is based on the principle of bone conduction. It uses surgically implanted abutment to transmit sound by bone conduction directly to cochlea. Thus, BAHA bypasses EAC and middle ear.
- *Components:* Bone-anchored hearing aid has following three components (Figs 9.3A to C):
  1. *Titanium fixture:* It is surgically embedded in the skull bone. The process of osseointegration, whose completion usually takes 2–6 months, binds the titanium fixture with the surrounding tissue.
  2. *Titanium abutment:* The abutment is attached to the titanium fixture. It remains exposed outside the skin.
  3. *Sound processor:* After the completion of osseointegration, it is attached to the abutment.

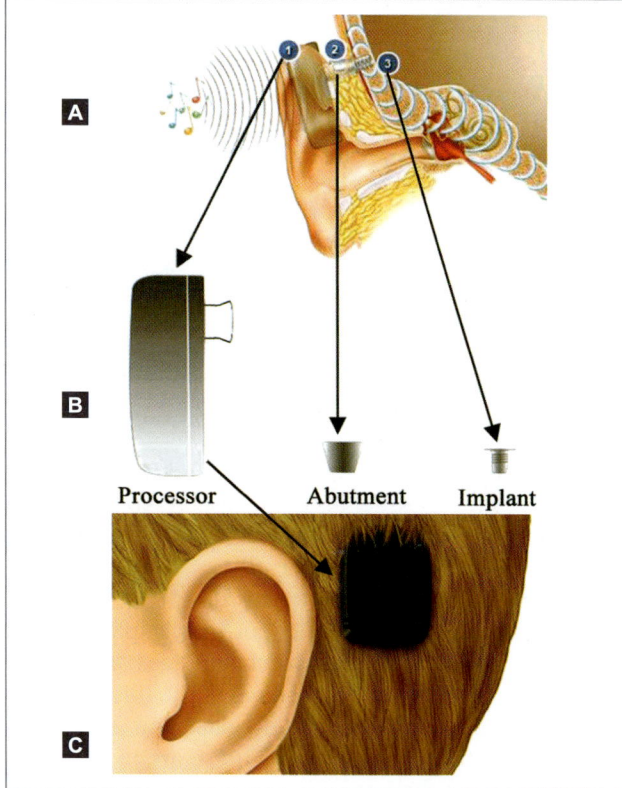

Figs 9.3A to C: BAHA. (A) BAHA system; (B) BAHA parts; (C) BAHA processor in position
Source: Cochlear Limited

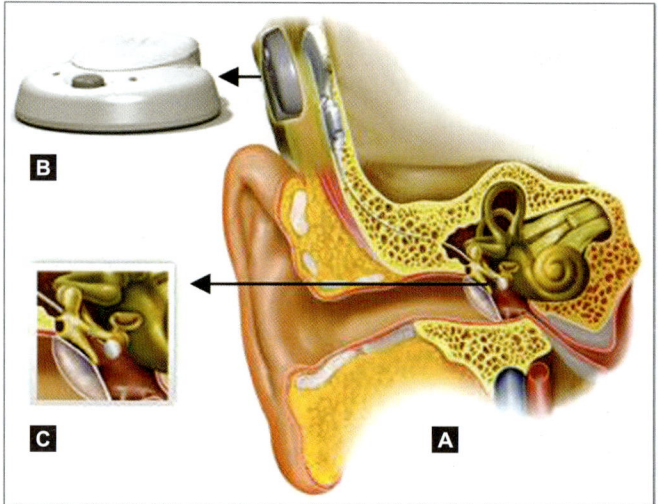

Figs 9.4A to C: Vibrant MED-EL soundbridge. (A) Implant in position; (B) External audio processor worn on head; (C) Internal implantable part FMT
Source: MED-EL Corporation

- **Indications:** Bone-anchored hearing aid is suited to following category of patients who cannot use or be benefited by behind-the-ear and canal hearing aids:
  - Chronic otitis media and externa (chronic otorrhea not amenable to treatment).
  - Congenital anomalies of ear such as microtia.
  - Canal atresia (congenital and acquired) not amenable to treatment.
  - Otosclerosis and tympanosclerosis, when surgery is contraindicated or patient is not willing for surgery.
  - **Unilateral profound hearing loss:** BAHA offers better result than CROS and substantially improves speech recognition even in a noisy background. BAHA is implanted on the side of hearing loss. It transmits the sound to normal side cochlea through the bone conduction. This process eliminates the head shadow effect.
- **Surgical technique:** Surgery is performed in a single stage in adults but children need two stages. On first stage, the titanium fixture is placed into the skull bone. In second stage, which is performed after the 6 months (period of osseointegration), titanium abutment is connected through the skin to the fixture.
- **Complications:** They are very few and includes.
  - Failure of osseointegration
  - Local infection and inflammation.

Vibrant MED-EL Soundbridge

- **Components (Fig. 9.4):** This semi-implantable hearing aid has two components—external and internal.
  1. **External component:** Audio processor is worn behind the ear. It contains a microphone and transmits sound across the skin by radiofrequency to the internal receiver VORP.
  2. **Internal component:** Vibrating ossicular prosthesis (VORP) is made up of three parts (1) receiver, (2) floating mass transducer (FMT) and (3) conductor link between receiver and FMT (connected to incus).
- **Indications:** Adult and elderly patients with moderate-to-severe hearing loss who are not satisfied with behind-the-ear and canal hearing aids (Table 9.2).
- **Surgical procedure:** The receiver of the internal device is positioned under the skin over the mastoid bone. After performing mastoidectomy, the ossicular chain is visualized through a posterior tympanotomy approach. Floating mass transducer (FMT) is attached to the long process of incus. The residual hearing is not affected as the middle ear ossicular chain is not disturbed. The external audio processor is fitted and programed 6–8 weeks after the surgery. It attaches magnetically behind the ear.
- **Advantages:** The mechanical energy is directly passed to ossicles. Bypassing of EAC and tympanic membrane eliminates problems of occlusion, feedback, discomfort and wax which are faced in external hearing aids. It provides improved sound quality even in noisy surroundings.

COCHLEAR IMPLANTS

Cochlear implants, which are becoming popular these days, are relatively recent development. These electronic devices convert sound signals into electrical impulses which directly stimulate the cochlear nerve.

They are indicated for patients of profound binaural SNHL (with nonfunctional cochlear hair cells) who have intact auditory nerve functions and show little or no benefit from hearing aids. Other prognostic findings include general health, level of motivation, expectations and patient's support group.

Depending on whether the child was deafened before or after the acquisition of speech and language, hearing loss could be *prelingual* or *postlingual*. Children with congenital and early childhood hearing loss need early intervention with hearing aids or cochlear implants. Auditory deprivation during the early developmental period results in degeneration in central auditory pathways which limits the speech and language acquisition following cochlear implantation.

Available Devices

The three devices, which are approved by the US Food and Drug Administration (FDA), are manufactured by following companies:
1. **Advanced Bionics Corporation:** Clarion C-II/HiRes 90K (Fig. 9.5A to D)
2. **Cochlear Corporation:** Nucleus 5 System (Figs 9.6A to D)
3. **MED-EL Corporation:** Pulsar and Sonata (Figs 9.7A and B)

Components and their Functioning

Cochlear implant consists of following internal and external components:
- **External components:** Microphone, speech processor and transmitter are connected by wires. Current models have one integrated piece.
  - *Microphone* placed behind the ear picks up the acoustic signals and converts it into electrical signals which are delivered to the speech processor.
  - *Speech processor* can be body-worn or behind-the-ear. It modifies the signal and delivers it to the transmitter. It uses specific speech coding strategy to translate acoustic information into electric stimulation.
  - *Transmitter* is secured over the mastoid to the magnet in the implanted portion of machine. It delivers the signal to the implanted receiver/stimulator via FM radio frequency or magnetic coil.
- **Internal components:** It is surgically implanted and comprises following:
  - *Receiver/stimulator, magnet and antenna:* It is placed under the skin. It decodes and further modifies the signal and delivers to an electrode.
  - *Electrode* is placed into the scala tympani through round window cochleostomy. The electrode has multiple channels. The electrodes stimulate the remaining cochlear nerve tissue, usually spiral ganglion cells in cochlea.

Outcomes

The sound produced by cochlear implants is perceived as auditory sensation (not like normal hearing) which vary in pitch and loudness. The speech processor selects specific characteristics of sound which are important for understanding the speech. Some patients become enabled to understand speech without visual cue. Some patients even enjoy music and can talk on the phone. Children can attend normal schools.

Children and adults with postlingual short duration deafness achieve very good results. If implanted early (12 months of age) even prelingual deafened children develop better understanding of speech and acquisition of language over a couple of years. They need constant auditory-verbal training. Prelingually deafened adults obtain very limited benefit from cochlear implants. They just develop sound awareness.

Factors Improving Outcomes of Cochlear Implants in Children

They include:
- Postlingual hearing loss in children.
- Early implantation (1 year of age) in prelingual children.
- Shorter duration of postlingual hearing loss.
- Neural plasticity within central auditory pathway and area.

Indications for Cochlear Implant Evaluation

The following referral criteria are for evaluating the patient to know whether h/she will be benefited by the cochlear implant or not:

Adults

- Thresholds of 70 dB or more at 1,000 Hz and above in the better ear.
- Word discrimination less than 70%.
- Communication difficulties even with appropriate hearing aid use.

Children

There is no lower age limit for evaluation.
- Thresholds of 90 dB hearing loss or more at 2,000 Hz and above in better ear.

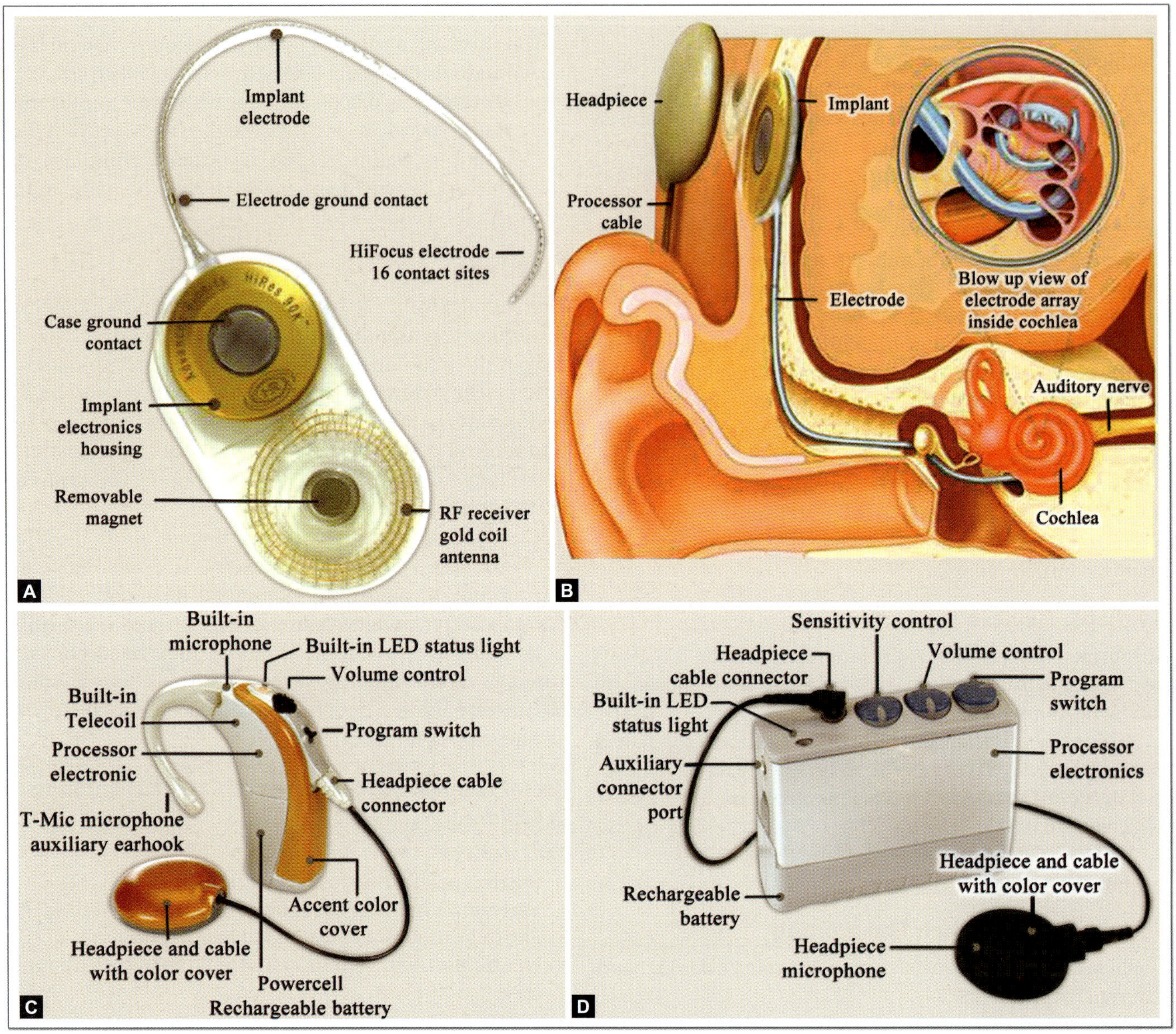

Figs 9.5A to D: HiRes 90K cochlear implant. (A) Internal parts; and (B) Implant in position; (C) External Parts (harmony behind-the-ear); (D) External parts (platinum body-worn)
Source: Advanced Bionics Corporation

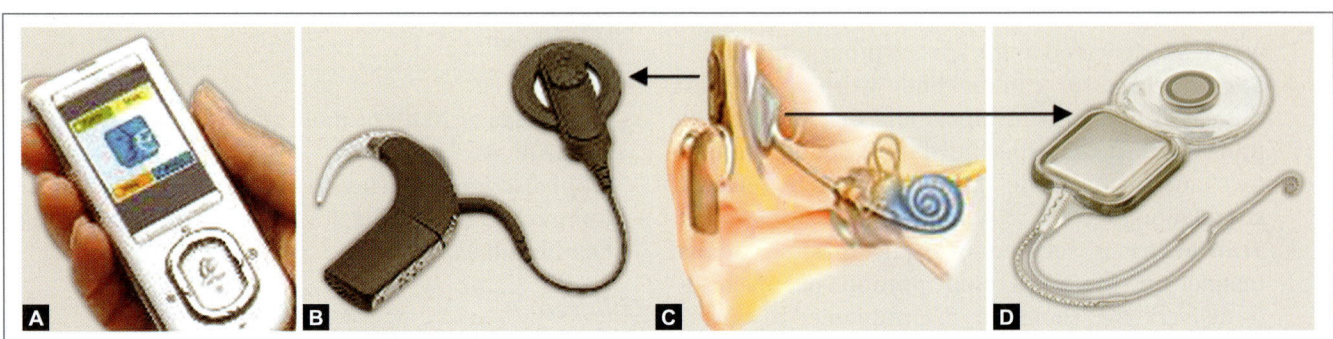

Figs 9.6A to D: Nucleus 5 cochlear implant. (A) Bidirectional remote assistant, which monitors, controls and manages the functions of implant; (B) External parts (behind-the-ear); (C) Implant in position; (D) Internal parts
Source: Cochlear Corporation

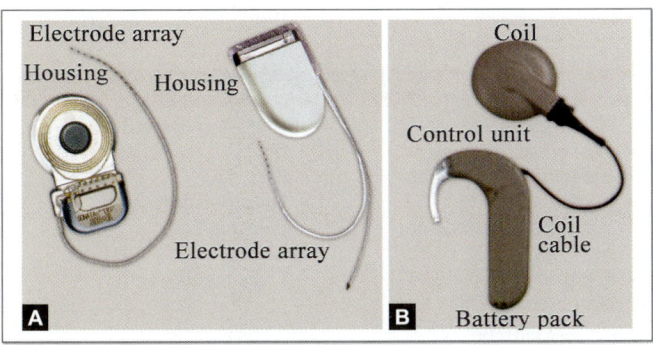

Figs 9.7A and B: MED-EL Cochlear Implant. (A) Internal part (Sonata and Pulsar); (B) External parts (Opus 2)
Source: MED-EL Corporation

- Aided levels poorer than 35 dB hearing loss (especially at 4,000 Hz) in better ear.
- Brainstem evoked response audiometry (BERA):
  - No response in both ears.
  - No response in one ear and elevated responses in other ear.
- Poor development of auditory or communication skills.
- Severely impairing auditory neuropathy/dyssynchrony.

Evaluation of Cochlear Implant Candidates

The cochlear implant candidates are assessed carefully for the following elements:

- ***History and examination*** in detail to determine the medical fitness and predict expected outcomes.
- ***Audiologic evaluation*** to determine suitability for the implant (depending on the age) include:
  - Pure tone audiogram (PTA)
  - Speech discrimination tests
  - Tympanometry
  - Otoacoustic emissions (OAE)
  - Auditory brainstem responses (ABR)
  - Auditory steady state responses (ASSR)
- ***Imaging*** of temporal bone and brain especially for cochlea and auditory nerve by CT and MRI.
- ***Hearing aid fitting and performance:*** A hearing aid trial and evaluation is mandatory. To determine the performance, it needs:
  - Aided free-field sound detection thresholds
  - Aided speech perception and discrimination scores
- ***Communicative status*** or speech and language evaluation to determine any developmental language or articulation disorders. During the postoperative mapping of the device, it helps in identifying areas of deficit in speech perception and necessary programming of the implant.
- ***Psychological evaluation*** to determine the cognitive status or mental disabilities other than hearing loss.
- ***Comparison*** between the performance of the patient and implant recipients.

- ***Decision*** for or against the implant.
- ***Selection*** of the ear.
- ***Expectations*** of prospective patients/parents.
- ***Vaccination*** against meningitis especially *Haemophilus influenzae* type B, *Pneumococcus* and in some areas *Meningococcus*.

Selection Criteria

The guidelines vary and change overtime. The generally accepted selection criteria include:

General

- No evidence of central auditory lesions and absence of auditory nerve.
- No contraindications for surgery.
- Realistic expectations by the patient and family members.
- Willingness to comply with follow-up procedures.

Adults

- Hearing loss with pure tone average of 70 dB HL.
- Hearing aid fitting and performance (1–3 months of hearing aid use).
- Aided scores on open-set sentence tests less than 50%.

Children

- Age: 1–17 years
- Pure tone average thresholds of 90 dB HL or more.
- Minimal benefit from hearing aids: 3–6 months of hearing aid use.

Surgical Procedure

The surgery is done under general anesthesia. The position of the device is marked and the incision is planned. With the postaural/endaural approach, the site is prepared for the location of receiver/stimulator. Flaps are elevated using a two-layered approach. First layer flap is of skin and subcutaneous tissue and second layer is of musculoperiosteal flap. After creating a pocket under the second flap, a "well" is drilled in the skull bone that would house the receiver/stimulator.

Depending upon the type of electrode, 1.0–1.6 mm cochleostomy opening is made anteroinferior to the round window in the basal turn of cochlea. The electrode array is gently and gradually entered into the scala tympani through the cochleostomy till its complete insertion. The receiver/stimulator is fixed in the created "well" with ties.

Electrophysiological tests are performed to determine the electrode impedance and telemetry responses.

Introduction of Electrode

The two popular methods of introducing the electrode array are posterior tympanotomy facial recess approach and Varia technique.

- ***Posterior tympanotomy facial recess approach:*** A simple mastoidectomy is performed. Round window is approached by opening the facial recess, through which the electrode array is passed to cochleostomy.
- ***Varia technique:*** The posterior tympanomeatal flap is elevated to expose the round window. A tunnel is drilled in the posterior bony meatal wall directed from 11 o'clock position for right ear and 1 o'clock position for left ear. The electrode array is passed to the cochleostomy through the tunnel created in posterior meatal wall.
  - ***Advantages:*** The advantages of this technique include:
    - No need of mastoidectomy
    - Takes less time
    - Minimal chances of injury to facial nerve

Postoperative Complications

Though occuring in less than 1–2% of cases, facial nerve injury during the surgery is feared most. The alteration of taste due to the irritation or injury to chorda tympani is quite common after surgery. Postoperative bleeding or hematoma formation occurs occasionally. The extrusion or exposure of the device, though uncommon is one of the most feared late complications. Other early and late complications are listed in Table 9.3.

Postoperative Mapping

Activation of the device is done 3–4 weeks after the surgery and the implant is programmed or mapped. Mapping continues during the period of rehabilitation and finely tunes the processor to get better hearing with the implant. All patients need auditory-verbal therapy, in which emphasis is laid on making the patient listen and speak without using lip reading and visual cues. The rehabilitation period is a task that needs concerted efforts of patient, family and the professionals concerned.

Table 9.3: Early and late complications of cochlear implant surgery

Early complications	Late complications
• Facial palsy • Taste disturbances • Bleeding or hematoma • Infection • Wound dehiscence/flap necrosis • Early device failure • Cerebrospinal fluid leak • Vertigo and dizziness • Meningitis	• Extrusion or exposure of device • Pain • Device migration or displacement • Late device failure • Otitis media

AUDITORY BRAINSTEM IMPLANT

Auditory brainstem implant directly stimulates the cochlear nuclei in the brainstem and bypasses the auditory nerve.

- ***Indications:*** It is indicated in cases of bilateral auditory nerve lesions. This implant is ideal in the cases of bilateral acoustic neuroma (neurofibromatosis type 2) when auditory nerve is severed during the surgery.
- ***Device:*** It is placed in the lateral recess of the fourth ventricle. The multielectrode array of "nucleus" auditory brainstem implant, which is similar to cochlear implant, is attached to a decron mesh that is placed on the brainstem. The facility of removable magnet of receiver/stimulator makes the device MRI compatible.
- ***Outcomes:*** Auditory brainstem implant helps in communication, awareness and recognition of environmental sounds. Its efficiency is not similar to cochlear implant.

Self-evaluation Exercises

1. Which of the following parts are not of hearing aids?
   a. Microphone
   b. Amplifier
   c. Receiver
   d. Speech processor
   e. Electrode array
2. Cochlear implant consists of:
   a. Microphone
   b. Speech processor
   c. Electrode array
   d. Receiver
   e. All of the above
3. Cochlear implant can be used in cases of bilateral severe to profound hearing loss caused by:
   A. Meningitis
   b. Otosclerosis
   c. Ototoxic drugs
   d. Mumps
   e. All of the above

True (T)/False (F)

4. Cochlear implant will not be of any use in children with bilateral severe sensory hearing loss who are not benefited by hearing aids.
5. Cochlear implant is contraindicated in cases of retrocochlear hearing loss.
6. Auditory brainstem implant is not indicated in cases of bilateral profound neural hearing loss following surgery for bilateral acoustic schwannoma.

Answers

| 1. d, e | 2. e | 3. e | 4. F | 5. T | 6. F |

Chapter 10

Diseases of External Ear and Tympanic Membrane

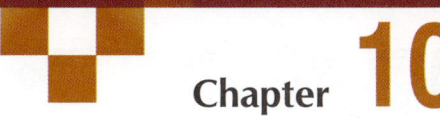

Specific Learning Objectives

After going through the chapter, you should be able to answer the following questions:
- Describe various types of otitis externa including their management.
- What do you know about the following: (1) Preauricular sinus; (2) Perichondritis; (3) Otomycosis; (4) Keratosis obturans; (5) Ear syringing; (6) Malignant otitis externa; (7) Retracted tympanic membrane and retraction pocket; (8) Tympanosclerosis; (9) Granular myringitis; (10) Myringitis bullosa (otitis externa bullosa); (11) Causes of traumatic tympanic membrane perforations; (12) Microtia and aural atresia?
- How will you manage the following: (1) Auricular hematoma; (2) Frostbite to external ear?

INTRODUCTION

The diseases of external ear may be categorized into congenital, traumatic, inflammatory, neoplastic and miscellaneous groups (Table 10.1).

DISORDERS OF AURICLE

CONGENITAL DISORDERS

The developmental abnormalities of the external ear may be minor or major.
- **Bat ear (lop ear)** is an abnormally protruding ear, which has large concha and poorly developed antihelix and scapha. If the child or parents are concerned, the deformity can be corrected surgically after the age of 6 years.
- **Preauricular appendages** are skin-covered tags that appear between the tragus and the angle of mouth (Fig. 10.1A). They usually contain small piece of cartilage.
- **Macrotia** is an abnormally large pinna.
- **Anotia** refers to complete absence of auricle. The anomaly is usually a part of the first arch syndrome.
- **Microtia** is a major developmental anomaly which varies in severity (Fig. 10.1B). It may be unilateral or bilateral. It is frequently associated with deafness and anomalies of external, middle and internal ears.
- **Other abnormalities:** Cryptotia (pocket ear—upper third of pinna embedded in scalp); coloboma (middle transverse cleft in auricle); absence of tragus and Darwin's tubercle; Stahl's ear (flat helix with duplication of upper part of antihelix) and abnormalities of lobule (absence, large, bifid and pixed attached).

Table 10.1: Diseases of external ear and tympanic membrane

Causes	Diseases
Congenital	Bat or lop ear*, preauricular appendages, preauricular pit or sinus*, anotia, microtia, macrotia, atresia of EAC, collaural fistula, Treacher-Collins syndrome
Trauma	Hematoma*, lacerations*, avulsion of pinna, frostbite*, foreign bodies*, perforation of tympanic membrane*
Inflammatory	Perichondritis*, chondritis, chondrodermatitis nodularis chronica helicis, acute OE*, furuncle*, cellulitis, erysipelas, chronic OE* (allergic, contact dermatitis, seborrheic or psoriasis, neurodermatitis, granulations), otomycosis*, OE hemorrhagica or bullous myringitis, herpes zoster oticus (Ramsay-Hunt syndrome), malignant OE, necrotizing OE, perforation of tympanic membrane*
Tumors	• **Benign:** Preauricular cyst, sebaceous cyst, dermoid cyst, keloid, hemangiomas, papilloma, cutaneous horn, keratoacanthoma, neurofibroma, osteoma, exostoses, ceruminoma, sebaceous adenoma • **Malignant:** Squamous cell carcinoma, basal cell carcinoma, melanoma, adenocarcinoma, malignant ceruminoma, malignant melanoma (see Chapter 'Tumors of Ear and Cerebellopontine Angle')
Miscellaneous	Ear wax*, keratosis obturans, stenosis of EAC, retracted tympanic membrane* (general, retraction pockets, atelectasis), tympanosclerosis*, atrophic tympanic membrane, healed otitis media*, cholesteatoma

Common disorders

Abbreviations: EAC—external auditory canal; OE—otitis externa

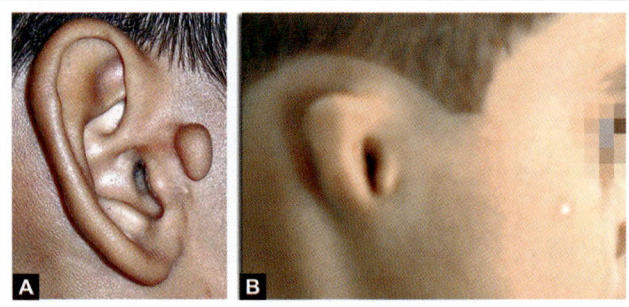

Figs 10.1A and B: (A) Preauricular appendages; (B) Microtia

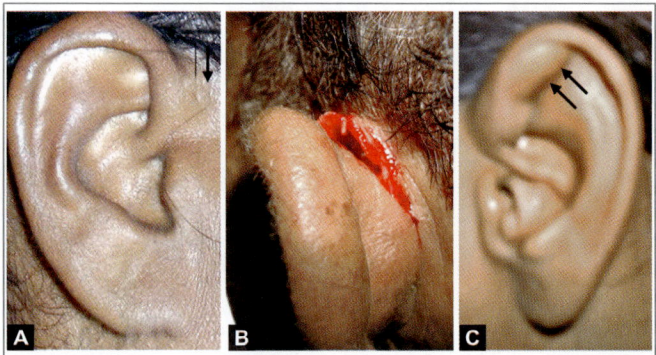

Figs 10.2A and B: (A) Preauricular sinus/pit (arrow showing); (B) Avulsion of upper part of pinna; (C) Auricular hematoma (arrows showing)

Preauricular Sinus and Cyst

Preauricular sinus is a commonly seen congenital anomaly (Fig. 10.2A). The faulty union of hillocks of the first and second branchial arches during the development of pinna results in a sinus at the root of helix. The sinus has a branching tract which is lined by squamous epithelium. When sinus gets blocked, it results in a retention preauricular cyst.

- *Clinical feature:* Preauricular cyst usually is infected and presents as a painful swelling.
  - The sinus presents as a small opening in front of the crus of helix.
  - The sinus may get repeatedly infected (abscess formation) and present with painful swelling and purulent discharge.
- *Treatment:* Surgery is indicated if there is unsightly swelling or infection.
  - The cyst or sinus track needs complete surgical excision to avoid recurrence.
  - If abscess does not respond to antibiotics, incision and drainage is required.

TRAUMATIC DISORDERS

- *Lacerations:* They are repaired at the earliest and the perichondrium is stitched with absorbable sutures under the cover of broad-spectrum antibiotics.
  The stripping of perichondrium from cartilage must be avoided as it results in avascular necrosis. The fine nonabsorbable sutures are employed for the skin closure.
- *Avulsion of pinna (Fig. 10.2B):* When the pinna remains attached to the head by a small skin pedicle, primary reattachment is usually successful. Completely avulsed pinna may be either reimplanted by the microvascular surgery or the skin of the avulsed segment of pinna is removed and the cartilage implanted under the postauricular skin for later reconstruction.
- *Hematoma of auricle (Fig. 10.2C):* It refers to collection of blood between the auricular cartilage and perichondrium due to blunt trauma.
  - *Occupations:* Common in boxers, wrestlers and rugby players.
  - *Cauliflower ear:* This auricular deformity occurs when extravasated blood clots get organized.
  - *Complications:* Infection of hematoma leads to severe perichondritis. Prophylactic antibiotic course is given.
  - *Treatments:* Aspiration of hematoma under strict aseptic conditions followed by a pressure dressing, packing all concavities of the auricle to prevent reaccumulation of blood. Aspiration may need to be repeated.
    - Incision and drainage is done when aspiration fails. Pressure is applied by dental rolls which are tied with through-and-through sutures.

Frostbite

Depending upon the severity, patients may present with erythema, edema, bullae, necrosis of skin and subcutaneous tissue or complete loss of the affected part.

Treatment

It consists of the following:
- *Rewarming of pinna* at a temperature of 38–42°C with moist cotton pledgets.
- *Application of 0.5% silver nitrate soaks:* Superficial infection is controlled.
- *Analgesics:* Considerable pain occurs during the rapid rewarming of the ear.
- *Bullae:* They are protected from rupturing.
- *Systemic antibiotics* take care of deep infection.
- *Surgical debridement:* It is considered after several months when true demarcation between the dead and living tissues appears.

PERICHONDRITIS AND CHONDRITIS

The condition is the result of secondary infection. The formation of abscess between the perichondrium and cartilage cuts off the blood supply of the cartilage and result in its necrosis.

Etiology

- ***Infected hematoma:*** Blunt trauma in boxers, wrestlers, and fist-fighting.
- ***Penetrating trauma:*** Ear piercing, assaults, bites and after ear surgery.
- ***Otitis externa (OE):*** Direct extension from an OE.
- ***Causative organism:*** Pseudomonas.

Clinical Features

- Tender, erythematous, indurated pinna (Figs 10.3A and B).
- Fluctuance occurs in presence of abscess and chondritis.

Treatment

- ***Antibiotics:*** Oral quinolone antibiotic (such as ciprofloxacin) and local application of 4% aluminium acetate compresses.
- ***Surgical:*** Elimination of any piercing foreign body.
  - Prompt incision and drainage of abscess is recommended. Pus is submitted for culture and sensitivity. Wound is packed with antibiotic-impregnated ribbon gauze.
  - Resection of necrotic cartilage and placement of through-and-through Penrose or catheter drain.
  - Postoperative course of antibiotic for 7–10 days.

Complications

Cauliflower ear deformity.

CHONDRODERMATITIS NODULARIS CHRONICA HELICIS

Middle aged men of 50 years are the common victims of this auricular disease.

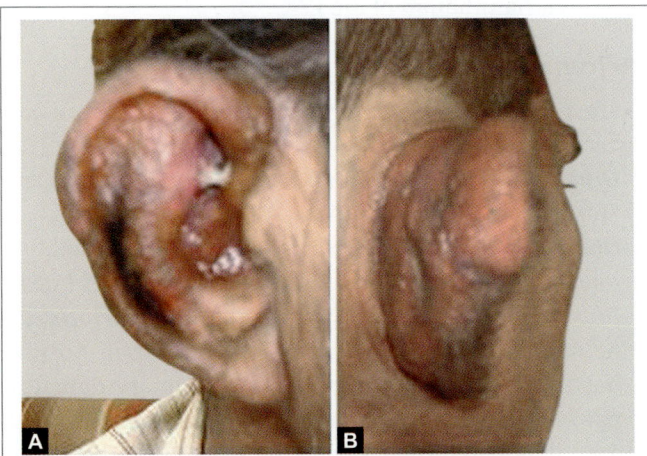

Figs 10.3A and B: Perichondritis. (A) Lateral surface showing pus coming out; (B) Medial surface showing healed suture site of injury

- ***Clinical features:*** The condition presents with small painful nodules which appear near the free border of helix. Nodules are so tender that the patient is not able to sleep on the affected side.
- ***Treatment:*** Excision of the nodule with its skin and cartilage.

RELAPSING POLYCHONDRITIS

It is a rare autoimmune disease, which involves cartilages of ear, nose, larynx, trachea and chest. In cases of recurrent bilateral auricular swelling, rheumatologic workup for relapsing polychondritis must be done at the earliest.

- ***Clinical features:*** The auricle becomes inflamed and tender. EAC becomes stenotic. Lobule of the ear is spared as it does not have any cartilage.
- ***Treatment:*** High doses of systemic steroids.

DISORDERS OF EXTERNAL AUDITORY CANAL (EAC)

CONGENITAL DISORDERS OF EAC

- ***Atresia of EAC:*** It may occur alone or in association with microtia.
  - ***Atresia with microtia:*** It is more common and may be associated with anomalies of the middle and internal ears and other structures.
  - ***Isolated atresia:*** It is due to failure of canalization of the first branchial cleft. The outer meatus is obliterated with fibrous tissue or bone. The deep meatus and the tympanic membrane are normal in these isolated cases of atresia.
- ***Collaural fistula:*** It is an abnormality of the first branchial cleft. The one opening of fistula is situated in the neck just below and behind the angle of mandible while second opening is in the external canal or the middle ear. The track of the fistula passes through the parotid gland in close relation to the facial nerve.

TRAUMA OF EAC

- Minor lacerations of EAC occur while (Q-tip injury) scratching the ear with hair pins, needles or matchstick or unskilled instrumentation. They generally heal without any complications.
- Major lacerations of EAC usually result from gunshot wounds, automobile accidents or fights. In some cases, the condyle of mandible injures the anterior wall of EAC.

Table 10.2: Types of ear foreign bodies

Non-living	Living
• **Hygroscopic:** Grain seeds such as rice, peas, wheat, maize • **Non-hygroscopic:** Slate pencil, chalk, metallic ball bearings, matchstick, cotton swab, paper, sponge, plastic	**Living:** Flying or crawling insects, such as mosquitoes, beetles, cockroaches and ants

Treatment: These cases of major lacerations are managed surgically to have skin-lined EAC of adequate diameter as the stenosis of the canal is a common complication.

FOREIGN BODIES OF EAR

Children may insert a variety of non-living items in their ears (Table 10.2).

Types and Features of Foreign Bodies

- Adults, who are fond of scratching their ears, can have a broken end of matchstick or an overlooked cotton swab.
- Vegetable foreign bodies swell up with time and get impacted in the ear canal. They may even result in suppuration.
- Living foreign bodies cause intense irritation and pain. No attempt should be made to catch them alive.
- Injury to tympanic membrane middle ear structures, inner ear (subluxation of stapes into vestibule) can occur due to the introduction of hairpin or a bullet.

Treatment

- *Antibiotics:* Antibiotics facilitate in controlling infection and edema.
- *Ear drops:* Hygroscopic foreign body can be shrunk with glycerin and absolute alcohol drops.
- *Removal of foreign body:* The best way is to remove them under operative microscope. Unskilled attempts may lacerate not only the meatal lining, but can also damage the tympanic membrane and the ear ossicles. Methods of removing a foreign body include:
    - *Forceps removal:* Soft and irregular foreign bodies, such as a piece of paper, swab or a piece of sponge can be removed with forceps. Smooth and hard objects, such as steel ball bearing tend to slip from the forceps and move inwards and may injure the tympanic membrane while grasping with forceps.
    - *Syringing:* Seed grains and smooth objects can be removed with syringing.
    - *Hooking out:* Wax hook or vectis is passed beyond the foreign body and pressed against either floor or posterior wall and foreign body is hooked out.
- *Insects:* First, they are killed by instilling oil, spirit, chloroform or water and then removed.
- *Postaural approach:* Foreign bodies impacted in deep meatus, medial to the isthmus and pushed into the middle ear may need postaural incision for their removal.
- *Removal under general anesthesia:* In cases of impacted foreign body, uncooperative children, and foreign body that failed to come out with earlier attempts are removed under general anesthesia.

Complications

They include the following:
- Injury to tympanic membrane and middle ear structures.
- Secondary infection: Otitis externa and otitis media.

Live insect in external ear: Never remove live insect from external ear. First either drown or anesthetize the insect. Live angry insect can further damage the canal.

EAR MAGGOTS

Ear maggots are mostly seen in the months of August, September and October. Flies are attracted to the foul-smelling ear discharge and lay their eggs which hatch out into larvae (maggots).

- *Clinical features:* Severe pain with swelling round the ear and blood-stained discharge.
    - Maggots in the EAC.
    - Perforation of the tympanic membrane.
- *Treatment:* Chloroform water ear drops kill the maggots which are then removed by forceps.

OTITIS EXTERNA (OE)

OE is an inflammation of the EAC.

Microorganisms

- *Most common microorganism:* Pseudomonas aeruginosa.
- *Other common organisms:* Staphylococcus aureus and Staphylococcus epidermidis.
- *Uncommon microorganisms:* Coryneform (diphtheroids), Gram-negative rods (Enterobacter, Klebsiella, Proteus, Escherichia coli), Streptococcus and Enterococcus.
- *Actinomyces israelii* is an anaerobic Gram-positive bacterium that can cause OE from primary dental or parotid infection. This refractory OE presents with granulation tissue in EAC and thick yellow ear discharge. It needs surgical debridement and prolonged antibiotic therapy.

- Cultures for bacteria and fungus are indicated in persistent or refractory infection.

Treatment
- Debridement of EAC clears the infected material and allows topical antibiotics to reach the infected site.
- Acidification of EAC (acetic acid solution and antibiotics in acidic suspensions and solutions) kills many bacteria and fungus.
- Topical antibiotics provide a concentration of many times greater than systemic antibiotics. Thus, usually it is not necessary to start systemic antibiotics even in resistant infection.
  - Antibiotic impregnated ear wicks (cotton, merocel, ribbon gauze) offers better absorption through an edematous canal skin.
  - Quinolone antibiotic drops (ofloxacin, ciprofloxacin) with dexamethasone (hydrocortisone avoided as it leaves a precipitate) in an acidic vehicle are the best as they have no ototoxicity and no potential for allergic reactions.
- Oral antibiotics are reserved for complications of OE, such as cellulitis, perichondritis, chondritis and malignant OE.

ACUTE OTITIS EXTERNA

An abrogation of hydrophobic ceruminous coating of EAC exposes the underlying epithelium to water, infection and other contaminants and leads to progressive erythema and edema.

Predisposing Factors
- **Warm humid environment:** Excessive sweating changes the canal pH to alkaline, which favors bacterial growth.
- **Obstruction of EAC:** Stenosis, exostoses, impacted wax.
- **Ear trauma:** Use of cotton-tip swabs, irrigators for wax removal, in-the-canal hearing aids, digital ear thermometers, unskilled instrumentation.
- **Water contamination of EAC:** Usually swimming related.

Clinical Features
- **Presenting complaints:** Otalgia and otorrhea.
  - Ear pain may be aggravated with jaw movements.
  - Itching is present in some cases.
- **Early stage:** An erythematous canal with scanty discharge.
- **Later stage:** Edematous and exquisitely tender canal occluded with purulent squamous debris.
- **In severe cases:** Enlarged and tender regional lymph nodes and periauricular cellulitis.
- No additional systemic signs and symptoms.

CHRONIC OTITIS EXTERNA
- No prior history of trauma or water contamination.
- Usually not painful.
- Examination may reveal fungal hyphae in the canal or keratin debris from chronic dermatitis.
- Acute exacerbation is usually preceded by itching.

Types
The four different disease states with distinct etiologies are allergic, contact dermatitis, seborrhea and granular OE.

1. **Allergic otitis externa**
   - *Clinical features:* Edema and purulent discharge secondary to topical antibiotic (most commonly neomycin) ointment or drops.
     - Maculopapular eruption in concha and EAC.
     - A thickened and erythematous canal.
   - *Treatment:* Elimination of offending agent, debridement and topical steroid drops.
2. **Contact dermatitis**
   - *Clinical features:* It can result from a variety of agents, such as hairsprays, shampoos and hearing aid molds. It is characterised by a thickened and erythematous canal.
   - *Treatment:* Elimination of offending agent by debridement and topical steroid drops.
3. **Psoriasis or seborrhea**
   - *Clinical features:* Hyperkeratosis and lichenification of EAC skin.
     - Seborrheic OE is associated with seborrheic dermatitis of the scalp. Itching is the presenting complaint. Greasy yellow scales may be seen in the canal, over the lobule and in postauricular sulcus.
     - Secondary bacterial or fungal infections may occur.
   - *Treatment:* Treatment of scalp seborrhea and ear toilet, salicylic acid and sulphur cream.
4. **Granular otitis externa**
   - *Clinical features:* It results from chronic bacterial or fungal infection of EAC. Granulation and excoriation are seen on tympanic membrane and EAC skin.
   - Culture for bacteria and fungus may show causative organisms.
   - *Treatment*
     - Repeated debridement.
     - Cauterization of granulations.
     - Topical antibiotic or antifungal creams.
     - Topical gentian violet facilitates at drying the EAC.
     - Topical steroid or 5-fluorouracil.
     - De-epithelialization of tympanic membrane: If it does not respond to drying agent (Burow's solution), it may need spilt-thickness skin graft.

Complications

- **Cellulitis:** It presents as an erythematous ear. There is no induration like perichondritis. Treatment is usually with systemic antistaphylococcal agent.
- **Perichondritis or chondritis**
- **Medial EAC fibrosis:** In chronic OE, thick fibrous scar may obstruct deep aspect of EAC. Tympanic membrane appears lateralized with absence of typical landmarks. Surgical treatment consists of excision of the fibrous scar followed by canaloplasty with split thickness skin graft and if needed tympanoplasty.
- **Malignant OE:** See next section.

> *Otitis externa treatment:* First line treatment for OE is topical antibiotics. Systemic antibiotics are given only for severe infections.

OTOMYCOSIS

Fungal infection of ear is frequently seen in hot and humid climate of tropical and subtropical countries.

- Superficial fungal infection is the most common and limited to EAC. Invasive type is rare and involves temporal bone.
- In cases of associated bacterial infection, the fungal infection may not be immediately evident.
- Common fungal species are *Aspergillus niger* and *Candida albicans*.

Clinical Features

- Intense itching, discomfort, or ear pain.
- Discharge with musty odor and ear blockage.
- Sodden, red and edematous meatal skin.

Treatment

- **Antifungal agents:** Antifungal treatment (Povidine iodine, 2% salicylic acid in alcohol) should be continued for a week after the apparent cure.
- **Dry ear:** Ear should be kept dry.
- **Antibiotic/steroid ear drops** in cases of associated bacterial infection help in reducing edema and inflammation and better penetration of antifungal agents.

Aspergillus Niger

- **Clinical features:** Pigmented fungal tufts atop a tangle of hyphal threads resembling moist white plug dotted with black debris (wet newspaper). Aggressive infection involves epithelial and subcutaneous tissues and may result in tympanic membrane perforation, which heals spontaneously following medical treatment.
- **Treatment:** Frequent debridement and acidic drops (acetic acid) and gentian violet painting of EAC are effective. Persistent infection needs oral itraconazole.

Candida Albicans

- **Clinical features:** This opportunistic fungal infection is common in patients getting prolonged course of antibiotic ear drops.
  - The EAC appears wet and macerated and is filled with soft, curd-like debris sprouting hyphae.
- **Treatment:** Antifungal solutions or creams, such as clotrimazole, nystatin (100,000 units/mL of propylene glycol) are effective.

FURUNCULOSIS

- This localized form of acute OE is a staphylococcal infection of the hair follicles, which are present only in the outer cartilaginous part of EAC.
- Nasal vestibule may harbor staphylococci and fingering in the nose transfers the infection to other sites of the body.

Clinical Features

- Though usually single, the furuncles may be multiple.
- Severe pain and tenderness are out of proportion to the size of the furuncle.
- A small nodular swelling proceeds to fluctuance.
- Movements of the pinna and lower jaw (chewing) become painful.
- Posterior meatal wall furuncle causes edema over the postauricular region with obliteration of the retroauricular groove. For DD with mastoiditis *see* Chapter 'Complications of Suppurative Otitis Media'.
- Periauricular lymph nodes (anterior, posterior, and inferior) may get enlarged and tender.
- In cases of recurrent infection, blood should be tested for diabetes.

Treatment

- Oral antistaphylococcal antibiotics, analgesics, local heat and antibiotic ointment can be administered.
- Ten percent ichthammol glycerin ear wick provides splintage and reduces pain. Hygroscopic action of glycerin reduces edema, while ichthammol is mildly antiseptic.
- Incision and drainage is done if the abscess has formed.

KERATOSIS OBTURANS

In this EAC disorder, a dense plug of keratin, which gets accumulated in the deep bony ear canal, completely occludes the EAC. A faulty epithelial migration pattern of EAC has been documented.

Clinical Features
- Both ears are frequently involved.
- Adults between 30 years and 60 years are affected.
- Severe otalgia from an aggressive secondary OE.
- Deafness, tinnitus and in some cases, ear discharge.
- Pearly white mass of keratin material filling the ear canal.
- Thickening and mucosalization of tympanic membrane.
- Blunting of periannular canal skin from scarring.
- The pressure absorption of canal bone results in widening of the canal. It can cause facial nerve palsy.

Treatment
- Treatment of secondary OE.
- Removal of the epithelial debris under ear microscopy.
- Use of keratolytic agent, such as 2% salicylic acid in alcohol.
- *Prophylaxis:* Cleaning of the canal before the occurrence of inflammation and infection.

PRIMARY CHOLESTEATOMA OF EAC

Squamous epithelium of EAC starts getting collected with its keratin in EAC and invades its own bone.
- *Predisposing factors:* Trauma and surgery of EAC.
- *Clinical features:* Ear pain and purulent discharge.
- *Differential diagnoses:* Carcinoma, sequestrum and necrotizing otitis externa.
- *Diagnosis:* Histopathology of the removed specimen.
- *Treatment:* Removal of the cholesteatoma and necrotic mass.

EAR WAX

Anatomy and Physiology
Sebaceous and ceruminous (modified sweat glands) glands open into the space of the hair follicle. Secretion of both these glands mixes with the desquamated epithelial cells and keratin and form wax. This lubricates the ear canal and entraps the foreign material that enters into the canal.

Usually a small amount of wax is formed which dries up and is expelled from the meatus by movements of the jaw. Excessive wax secreted by the glands is deposited as a plug in the outer EAC.

Components of Ear Wax
The ear wax is made up of the following components:
- Sebaceous gland's secretion rich in fatty acids.
- Ceruminous gland's secretion rich in lipids and pigment granules.
- Hairs.
- Desquamated epithelial debris and keratin shed from the tympanic membrane and bony EAC.
- Dirt.

Factors Facilitating Ear Wax Problem
Following are the factors, which facilitate wax problems:
- Narrow and tortuous ear canal, stiff hair and exostosis facilitate retention of wax, which may dry up and form a hard impacted mass.
- Excessive secretion of wax and dusty occupations result in increased amounts of wax.
- Self-cleaning of ear wax may push wax into the deeper bony EAC.

Clinical Features
- *Hearing loss or sense of blocked ear:* Sudden hearing loss may occur when water enters into the EAC (wax swells up) while bathing or swimming.
- *Tinnitus and giddiness* due to impaction of wax against the tympanic membrane.
- *Reflex cough* can result from the stimulation of auricular branch of vagus nerve.
- *Wax granuloma:* The impacted wax ulcerates the meatal skin and results in granuloma formation.

Treatment
It consists of removal of wax by either syringing or other ear instruments.
- *Wax softening agents:* Hard impacted mass usually needs prior softening with any of the following wax softening agents:
  - 5% sodabicarb in equal parts of glycerin and water
  - Hydrogen peroxide
  - Liquid paraffin
  - Olive oil
  - Paradichlorobenzene 2%
- *Removal:* Instrumental manipulation should always be done by skilled hands preferably under ear microscopy. Cerumen hook, scoop and Jobson-Horne probe are usually employed. Wax hook and vectis are used for removing wax, foreign bodies and debris from the external ear canal. They may be used for removing foreign body nose. In cases of impacted wax, a space is created between the wax and canal wall. The instrument is then passed beyond the wax and the lump of wax is then dragged out. If the lump breaks, syringing or suctioning may be used to remove the fragment.

EAR SYRINGING

Aural Syringe: This metal syringe consists of a cylinder with a well fitting piston and a nozzle (Fig. 10.4A).

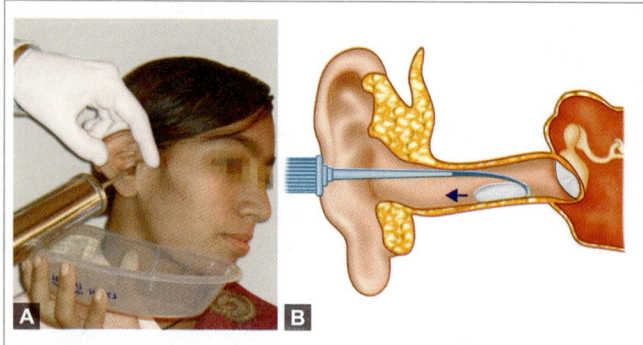

Figs 10.4A and B: Ear syringing. (A) The auricle is pulled upwards and backwards and the direction of the ear syringe is posterosuperior; (B) Water jet of ear syringe taking out lump of wax

Method

Patient is seated comfortably and the diseased ear faces towards the doctor. A towel is placed on the shoulder. Patient's head is slightly tilted toward the shoulder. A kidney tray is held snugly well below the ear to collect the return fluid. Boiled tap water cooled to body temperature (or normal saline) is used.

The auricle is pulled upwards and backwards while the direction of the stream of ear syringe is towards the posterosuperior wall of the meatus. Pressure of water that builds up deeper to the wax expels the wax out (Fig. 10.4B). In cases of impacted wax, some space is created between the wax and the meatal wall so that stream of water passes through that. Otherwise wax would be pushed deeper. After the procedure, ear canal and tympanic membrane are dried up with cotton.

Cautions

- Too much force of the syringing can rupture the tympanic membrane and leads to intense pain and dizziness and fainting.
- Past history of ear discharge or an existing perforation must be asked before venturing for the syringing. A quiescent otitis media can get reactivated after syringing.
- Too cold or too hot water would stimulate the labyrinth and result in vertigo.
- Ulceration in meatal wall needs application of broad-spectrum antibiotic ointment.

HERPES ZOSTER OTICUS-RAMSAY HUNT SYNDROME (VARICELLA-ZOSTER VIRUS)

See Chapter 'Facial Nerve Disorder'.

BULLOUS (HEMORRHAGIC) OTITIS EXTERNA AND MYRINGITIS BULLOSA

This inflammatory/infectious disease is believed to be primarily viral.
- *Cause:* Viral infection, *Mycoplasma pneumoniae* and *Haemophilus influenzae.*
- *Predisposing Factors:* Upper respiratory tract infection and winter season.

Clinical Features

- Exquisite (severe) ear pain with bloody or serous ear discharge.
- Hemorrhagic vesicle(s) or bulla(e) on the deep bony ear canal and tympanic membrane rupture spontaneously and result in serosanguineous discharge.
- Associated middle ear effusion is common.
- Conductive or mixed hearing loss with significant sensorineural element.

Treatment

- Analgesics
- Topical antibiotic/steroid ear drops to prevent bacterial superinfection.
- Macrolide or quinolone antibiotics for associated mycoplasma.
- Rupturing of the bullae may relieve pain.

MALIGNANT OTITIS EXTERNA

This rare OE of immunocompromised patients is an aggressive and potentially fatal infection, which progressively spreads to skull base and intracranial structures.
- *Causative microorganisms: Pseudomonas aeruginosa* is most common. *Staphylococcus aureus* and *Staphylococcus epidermidis* are uncommon.
- *Immunocompromised patients:* Elderly diabetics, HIV/AIDS, myeloid malignancies, anticancerous drugs and organ transplant recipients are at more risk.

Clinical Features

- *Severe otalgia and otorrhea.*
- *Granulations* in the floor of EAC at the bony-cartilaginous junction is the *hallmark* finding.
- *Facial nerve* is the most commonly involved cranial nerve.
- *Advanced stage:* CN IX, X and XI palsies can occur.
- *Intracranial spread:* Headache, fever, neck stiffness and altered levels of consciousness can occur.
- *Spread of infection to neighboring structures:* Temporomandibular joint, mastoid, middle ear and petrous bone can be involved.

Chapter 10 • Diseases of External Ear and Tympanic Membrane

- **Children:** Acute onset of painful otorrhea in children with immunosuppression, diabetes or Stevens-Johnsons syndrome and poor general health has been reported. Prognosis is better than adult form of disease.

Investigations
- Bacterial and fungal culture
- High-resolution computed tomography (HRCT) scan
- Single-photon emission tomography (SPECT) with radionuclide tracers.

Treatment
The success of aggressive medical treatment will predict the prognosis.
- **Antipseudomonal antibiotics:** Oral or parenteral (depending upon the severity) ciprofloxacin for 6–8 weeks or longer. In ciprofloxacin resistance cases other antibiotics such as tobramycin, ticarcillin and third generation cephalosporins may be used.
- Hyperbaric oxygen therapy.
- The treatment of the cause of immunosuppression, such as diabetes and HIV/AIDS.
- Surgical debridement of nonviable sequestra of bone is required when bone involvement is resistant to antibiotic therapy.

DISORDERS OF TYMPANIC MEMBRANE (TM)

GRANULAR MYRINGITIS
- It is an idiopathic inflammatory process of tympanic membrane.
- Patches of granulation tissue and mucosalized epithelium on the tympanic membrane are seen.
- In advanced cases, complete tympanic membrane gets thickened. Granulation tissue exudes thin transudate and may become secondarily infected.
- Secondary granulations may be associated with impacted wax, long-standing foreign body (such as myringotomy tube) or external ear infection.

RETRACTED TYMPANIC MEMBRANE
The retraction of TM is the result of negative middle ear pressure, which occurs due to the blockage of Eustachian tube (*see* Chapters 'Disorders of Eustachian Tube' and 'Chronic Suppurative Otitis Media and Cholesteatoma').

Otoscopy
Following otoscopic findings indicate that tympanic membrane is retracted towards the middle ear:
- Dull and lusterless tympanic membrane
- Absent or interrupted cone of light
- Apparent foreshortening of the malleus handle
- Extra prominent lateral process of malleus
- Sickle-shaped prominent anterior and posterior malleal folds.

ATROPHIC TYMPANIC MEMBRANE
This thin tympanic membrane easily gets collapsed with Eustachian tube insufficiency (*see* Chapter 'Disorders of Eustachian Tube'). It can be present in following conditions:
- In cases of otitis media with effusion, the middle fibrous layer of tympanic membrane gets absorbed.
- When a central perforation of tympanic membrane heals, only epithelial and mucosal layers grow and the intervening fibrous layer remains absent in healed drum.

RETRACTION POCKETS AND ATELECTASIS OF TM
- A segment of thin and atrophic tympanic membrane or the entire membrane may collapse inwards due to Eustachian tube insufficiency (*see* Chapter 'Disorders of Eustachian Tube').
- The membrane may get plastered onto promontory and also wraps round the ossicles.
- A deep retraction pocket (usually in posterosuperior and attic region) may accumulate keratin debris and form a cholesteatoma.
- **Sade classification:** *See* Chapter 'Chronic Suppurative Otitis Media and Cholesteatoma'.

TYMPANOSCLEROSIS
This hyalinization (and later calcification) in the fibrous layer of tympanic membrane appears as chalky white plaque.
- **Causes:** Generally, it is the result of safe chronic suppurative otitis media (CSOM), serous otitis media and ventilation tube.
- **Clinical features:** If the ossicles and middle ear are not involved, the condition may remain asymptomatic.
  - It generally affects tympanic membrane. It can involve ligaments, joints of ossicles, muscle tendons and submucosal layer of middle ear cleft and results in conductive hearing loss (CHL).

PERFORATION OF TYMPANIC MEMBRANE
They may be central, attic or marginal and are usually seen in cases of CSOM (*see* Chapter 'Chronic Suppurative Otitis Media and Cholesteatoma').

Traumatic Rupture of Tympanic Membrane
- **Etiology:** The modalities of injuries are following:
  - **Q-tip injury:** Scratching the ear with hair pins, needles or matchstick or unskilled instrumentation.

- **Air pressure:** An open handed slap, a kiss on the ear, blast and forceful valsalva. Explosive blasts can produce more than 200 dB sound pressure level.
- **Fluid pressure:** Diving, water sports and forceful syringing.
- **Fracture of temporal bone.**
- **Clinical features:** Sudden deafness, tinnitus or dizziness after the injury.
  - **Ear microscopic examination:** Perforation with the edges turned either outward or inward.
- **Treatment:** The edges of perforation are repositioned and splinted under ear microscopic examination.
- **Complications:** Rupture of the tympanic membrane may be associated with following complications:
  - Facial paralysis
  - Subluxation of stapes
  - Vertigo and nystagmus
  - Sensorineural hearing loss (SNHL)

Self-evaluation Exercises

1. The treatment of otomycosis includes:
   a. 2% salicylic acid
   b. 1% gentian violet
   c. Clotrimazole
   d. All of the above
2. Which of the following are not true for ear wax?
   a. Secretions of sebaceous and apocrine glands
   b. Bactericidal enzyme
   c. Desquamated skin with keratin
   d. Needs removal in all patients
3. Which of the following are not true for malignant otitis externa?
   a. *Pseudomonas aeruginosa* infection
   b. Elderly patients
   c. Diabetic or immunocompromised
   c. Spread to skull base
   d. Involves facial nerve at stylomastoid foramen
   e. None from above
4. Tympanic membrane appears blue (blue drum) in cases of:
   a. Hemotympanum (temporal bone fracture)
   b. Glue ear
   c. Glomus tumor
   d. Hemangioma of middle ear
   e. All of the above

Filling the blanks

5. _____ is the most common congenital deformity of the ear.
6. _____ is the rarest congenital anomaly of the ear.

True (T)/False (F)

7. Asymptomatic patients with preauricular sinus (no discharge or inflammation) need surgical excision of the complete tract to prevent future developments and complications.
8. The treatment of recurrent swimmer's otitis externa includes 2% acetic acid ear drops after swimming.
9. Most common causative fungus in otomycosis is *Candida*.
10. Reflex cough response while cleaning the ear canal is mediated by stimulation of the tympanic branch (Jacobson nerve) of CN IX.
11. The treatment of dry traumatic rupture of tympanic membrane includes protection of ear against water and ear drops.

Answers

1. d   2. d   3. e   4. e   5. Bat ear   6. Polyotia
7. F   8. T   9. F   10. F   11. T

Chapter 11

Disorders of Eustachian Tube

⊙ Specific Learning Objectives
After going through the chapter, you should be able to answer the following questions:
- Describe the anatomy and physiology of Eustachian tube.
- What are the differences between the Eustachian tube of adults and infants?
- How will you examine and test functions of Eustachian tube?
- What are the different causes of Eustachian tube malfunctioning and its consequences?
- What do you know about: (1) Atelectasis and retraction pocket; (2) Patulous Eustachian tube?

ANATOMY OF EUSTACHIAN TUBE (ET)

Eustachian* tube (auditory or pharyngotympanic tube) connects nasopharynx with the tympanic cavity. It is about 36 mm long and runs downwards, forwards and medially from its tympanic end, forming an angle of 45° with the horizontal.

Parts

Eustachian tube consists of two parts—bony and fibrocartilaginous (Fig. 11.1). The area where two parts meet is the narrowest part of the tube and called *isthmus*.
1. **Posterolateral bony part:** It forms one-third of the (12 mm) of the total length.
2. **Anteromedial fibrocartilaginous part:** It forms two-third of the (24 mm) of the tube. This is made of a single piece of cartilage, which is folded upon itself and forms the medial lamina, roof and a part of the lateral lamina. The rest of the lateral lamina is made of fibrous membrane.
    - *Elastin hinge:* It is rich in elastin fibers and is situated in the roof at the junction of medial and lateral lamina. By its recoil it keeps the tube closed when dilator of ET (tensor veli palatini) is not in action.
    - *Ostmann's pad of fat:* It keeps the tube closed and is related laterally to the membranous part of the cartilaginous tube. The closed tube protects itself and middle ear from the reflux of nasopharyngeal secretions.

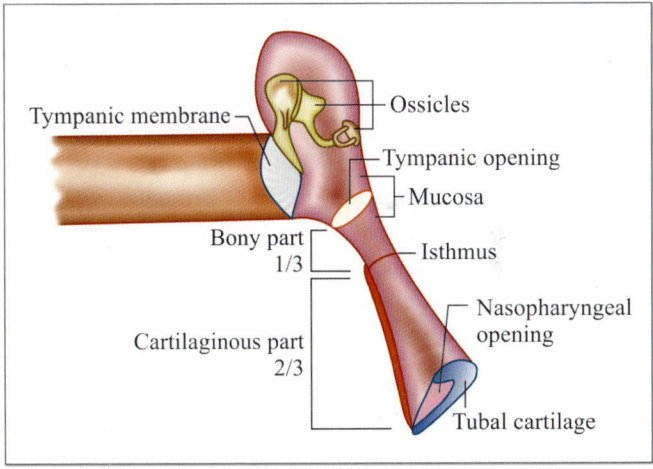

Fig. 11.1: Eustachian tube anatomy (horizontal section)

Openings

Eustachian tube has two openings—tympanic and pharyngeal.
1. **Tympanic opening:** This bony part measures 5 mm × 2 mm. It is situated in the anterior wall of middle ear, a little above the middle ear floor.
2. **Pharyngeal end:** This is slit-like and situated in the lateral wall of nasopharynx. It is about 1.25 cm behind the posterior end of inferior turbinate.
    - *Torus tubarius:* Posteriorly, the cartilage produces an elevation, which is called *torus tubarius.*

---
* Bartolomeo Eustachio (1524-1574)

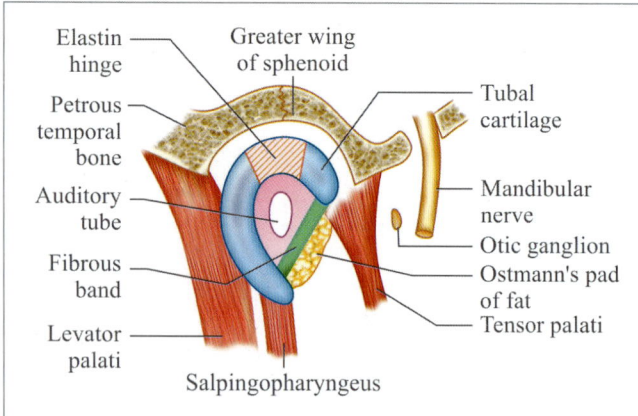

Fig. 11.2: Relations and structure of the cartilaginous part of Eustachian tube

- *Fossa of Rosenmuller:* Posterior to torus tubarius is situated the *fossa of Rosenmuller*, which is a common site for malignancy of nasopharynx.

Muscles in Relation to Eustachian Tube

The three muscles, which are related to the Eustachian tube, are—***tensor veli palatini*** (tensor palati), ***levator veli palatini*** (levator palati) and ***salpingopharyngeus*** (Fig. 11.2).

1. ***Tensor veli palatini muscle:*** The medial fibers of the tensor veli palatini muscle, which are attached to the lateral lamina of the tube, when contract open the tube.
2. ***Levator veli palatini muscle:*** It runs inferior and parallel to the cartilaginous part of the tube and forms a bulk under the medial lamina. This muscle during contraction pushes the tube upward and medially, thus assisting in opening the tube.

Mucosa of Eustachian Tube

- The pseudostratified ciliated columnar epithelium is interspersed with mucous secreting goblet cells.
- The submucosa, especially in the cartilaginous part, is rich in seromucinous glands.
- The cilia beat in the direction of nasopharynx.
- The ciliary movements drain middle ear secretions and fluid into the nasopharynx.

- The lymphoid tissue of Eustachian tube is called Gerlach tonsil.
- Mucosa of auditory tube and middle ear is derived from an outgrowth of the endoderm of the first pharyngeal pouch.

Nerve Supply

- Tympanic branch of cranial nerve IX carries sensory and parasympathetic secretomotor fibers to the tubal mucosa.
- Mandibular branch of trigeminal (cranial nerve V_3) supplies tensor veli palatini and tensor tympani.
- Cranial part of cranial nerve XI through vagus supplies the levator veli palatini and salpingopharyngeus.

Differences between Infant and Adult Eustachian Tube

In infants, infections from the nasopharynx can easily reach the middle ear because the Eustachian tube is wider, shorter and more horizontal in children (Table 11.1). The milk can also regurgitate into the middle ear, when infants are not fed in head-up position. The tube attains adult morphology and functions by the age of 7–10 years.

Retrograde reflux of nasopharyngeal secretion occurs in infants because tubal cartilage is flaccid, whereas it is comparatively rigid in adults and remains closed and protects the middle ear from the reflux.

PHYSIOLOGY OF EUSTACHIAN TUBE

- Eustachian tube usually remains closed. It opens during swallowing, yawning and sneezing.
- The poor tubal functions are responsible for middle ear infections. They are more common in infants and young children.
- Posture can affect the tubal function. The tubal mucosa gets congested in recumbent position and during sleep due to venous engorgement.

Table 11.1: Differences between infant and adult Eustachian tube (ET)

Characteristics	Infant	Adult
Length	13–18 mm at birth	31–38 mm
Direction	More horizontal. Forms an angle of 10°	Forms an angle of 45° with the horizontal
Angulation at isthmus	Absent	Present
Bony part	Relatively longer and wider	Relatively short and narrow
Tubal cartilage	Flaccid	Comparatively rigid and keeps ET closed
Density of elastin at the hinge	Less dense	More dense and keeps ET closed
Ostmann's pad of fat	Less in volume	Large in volume and keeps ET closed

Chapter 11 • Disorders of Eustachian Tube

- The three main functions of the ET are as follows:
  1. Ventilation and regulation of middle ear pressure.
  2. Protection of middle ear against nasopharyngeal sound pressure and reflux of nasopharyngeal secretions.
  3. Middle ear clearance of secretions.
- High pressures in the nasopharynx during forceful nose blowing and closed-nose swallowing (due to big adenoids and bilateral nasal obstruction) force nasopharyngeal secretions into the middle ear.

Ventilation and Regulation of Middle Ear Pressure

During normal hearing, the pressure on two sides of the tympanic membrane remains equal. The increase and decrease in middle ear pressure affects hearing. Eustachian tube opens periodically and maintains the equilibrium of the air pressure in the middle ear with that of ambient pressure.

Ventilation Pathway of Middle Ear Cleft

Ventilation of middle ear cleft occurs through ET.
- From the mesotympanum, air passes to attic, aditus, antrum and mastoid air cells.
- Mesotympanum communicates with the attic through the anterior and posterior isthmi, which are situated in membranous diaphragm that lies between the mesotympanum and the attic.
  - Anterior isthmus lies between the tendon of tensor tympani and the stapes.
  - Posterior isthmus lies between the tendon of stapedius, pyramid and the short process of incus.
  - The middle ear can communicate directly with the mastoid air cells through the retrofacial air cells.

Protective Functions

- The Eustachian tube remains closed and protects the middle ear against abnormally high sound pressures of the nasopharynx, which if transmitted to the middle ear can interfere with normal hearing.
- A functioning Eustachian tube protects middle ear from reflux of nasopharyngeal secretions. The reflux occurs if the tube is wide (patulous tube), short (as in infants), or the tympanic membrane is perforated.

Clearance of Middle Ear Secretions

- Mucosa of the Eustachian tube and anterior part of the middle ear is ciliated columnar.
- The cilia beat towards the nasopharynx and thus clear the middle ear secretions and debris into the nasopharynx.
- The clearance function is further enhanced by active opening and closing of the tube.

EXAMINATION OF EUSTACHIAN TUBE

ET can be examined with the following means:
- *Posterior rhinoscopy* (see Chapter 'Nasal Symptoms and Examination').
- *Rigid nasal endoscope (sinuscope)* (see Chapter 'Operations of Nose and Paranasal Sinuses').
- *Flexible nasopharyngolaryngoscope* (see Chapter 'Laryngeal Symptoms and Examination').
- *Eustachian tube endoscopy* or middle ear endoscopy is performed with a very fine flexible endoscope that is passed into Eustachian tube.
- *Microscope/endoscope* retraction pockets, fluid in the middle ear, movements of tympanic membrane with respiration may be seen.

In cases of preexisting perforation of tympanic membrane, the tympanic end of Eustachian tube can be examined by a microscope, as well as an endoscope.

- *Allergy testing* may reveal the allergic cause.
- *CT scans* of temporal bones and of paranasal sinuses may reveal the cause of Eustachian tube obstruction. MRI excludes the multiple sclerosis in cases of patulous ET.

TESTS FOR EUSTACHIAN TUBE FUNCTION

Tests for the function of ET are listed in Table 11.2.

Maneuver Building Positive Pressure in Nasopharynx

- *Principle:* To build positive pressure in the nasopharynx so that air enters into the ET. These methods can be employed therapeutically to ventilate the middle ear.
- *Method:* Air is pushed into the middle ear and tympanic membrane (TM) moves outwards which can be seen by an otoscope/microscope.
  - In cases of tympanic membrane perforation, a hissing sound and in cases of middle ear discharge, a cracking sound can be heard with the help of

Table 11.2: Tests for Eustachian tube function

Characteristics
• Maneuver building positive pressure in nasopharynx
▪ Valsalva test
▪ Politzer test
▪ ET catheterization
• Maneuver building negative pressure in nasopharynx
▪ Toynbee's test
• Tympanometry (see Chapter 'Hearing Evaluation')
• Mucociliary drainage/clearance
▪ Saccharine
▪ Methylene blue
▪ Antibiotic/steroid ear drops
• Sonotubometry

stethoscope. An auscultation tube can connect the patient's ear under test to that of the examiner.
- **Complications/contraindications:** The following are the relative contraindications:
  - *Atrophic scar:* Healed or thin TM can rupture.
  - *Infection of nose and nasopharynx:* Infected secretions are pushed into the middle ear and can cause otitis media.

Valsalva Test

About 65% of the patients can successfully perform this test. Patient pinches his nose and takes a deep breath through mouth and then closes his mouth. He tries to blow his cheeks and pushes air into the ears.

Politzer Test

This test is good for children who cannot perform Valsalva test (Fig. 11.3A).
Method: An olive-shaped tip of the Politzer's bag is introduced into the child's ipsilateral nose (side of ET to be tested). Other nose is also closed/pinched. Politzer bag is compressed while the child swallows sips of water or says "ik, ik".

> **Frenzel maneuver:** It opens the ET and ventilates the middle ear. Muscles of the floor of mouth and pharynx are contracted while nose, mouth and glottis are closed. In comparison to Valsalva maneuver, it is difficult to learn.

Eustachian Tube Catheterization

- **Method:** Nose is anesthetized by topical spray of lignocaine. Eustachian catheter (*see* Chapter 'Instruments') is passed along the floor of nose till it reaches the nasopharynx. The catheter is then rotated 90° medially and then gradually pulled outward so that it touches the posterior border of nasal septum. The catheter is then again rotated 180° laterally so that tip lies in the pharyngeal opening of ET (Fig. 11.3B). A Politzer bag is connected to the catheter and air is insufflated. The procedure should be done gently.

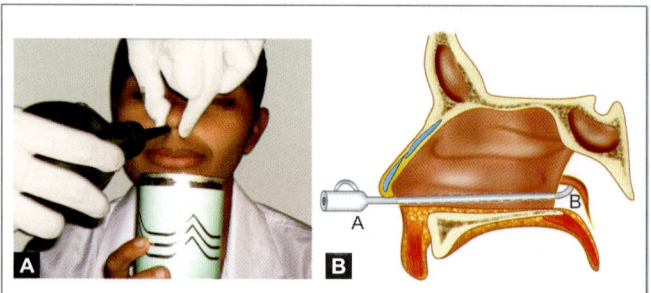

Figs 11.3A and B: (A) Politzer test; (B) Eustachian catheter
Key: A—Eustachian catheter; B—ET opening

- **Complications:** Complications include:
  - Injury to ET opening can result in scarring.
  - Bleeding from the nose.
  - Perforation of the ear drum is possible if air is squeezed with a great force.
  - Vasovagal syncope may occur.
- **Difficulties:** Adenoids and nasal obstructions (deviated septum and nasal mass) prevent the tip of the catheter from reaching the Eustachian tube.
- **Therapeutic indications of Eustachian catheter:**
  - Relieving the blockage of the Eustachian tube.
  - Insufflations of medicine into the middle ear.
  - Removal of nasal foreign bodies.

Maneuver Building Negative Pressure in Nasopharynx

Toynbee's Test

It is a physiological test. The patient is asked to swallow while he/she keeps the nose pinched. The maneuver draws air from the middle ear into the nasopharynx and causes inward movement of tympanic membrane, which can be seen through an otoscope/microscope.

Tests for Mucociliary Drainage/Clearance

These tests are conducted in cases of TM perforation. The time taken by materials to reach the pharynx and impart its taste provides an idea about the functioning of the ET and a measure of clearance function.

- **Saccharine solution** drops are instilled in the ear. The time taken by saccharine to reach the pharynx and impart a sweet taste is noted.
- **Methylene blue dye** is instilled into the ear. The time taken by the dye to stain the pharyngeal secretions is noted.
- **Antibiotic/steroid ear drops** are instilled into the ear. The time taken by drops to impart its bad taste is noted.

Sonotubometry

This noninvasive technique provides the information on active tubal opening. A tone, which is delivered to the nose, is recorded from the external auditory canal (EAC). The tone is heard louder if the Eustachian tube is patent. The duration for which the tube remains open can also be noted. The accessory sounds produced during swallowing interfere with the test results.

OBSTRUCTION OF EUSTACHIAN TUBE

The hallmark of ET obstruction is middle ear effusion. Though the child may remain asymptomatic.

Etiology

The common causes of tubal obstruction can be divided into two groups—mechanical and functional.
1. *Mechanical obstruction:*
   - *Intrinsic causes:* Upper respiratory infection (viral or bacterial), allergy, sinusitis and barotrauma.
   - *Extrinsic causes:* Hypertrophic adenoids, nasopharyngeal tumors/mass, deviated nasal septum, nasal polyp.
2. *Functional obstruction:* The common causes in this category include cleft palate, submucous cleft palate and Down's syndrome.
   - Increased cartilage compliance resists opening of the tube.
   - Poor function of tensor veli palatini results in the failure of active tubal opening.

Adenoids

- Big adenoids can result in otitis media with effusion or recurrent acute otitis media because of the following elements:
  - Mechanical obstruction of Eustachian tube.
  - Reservoir for pathogenic organism.
  - Mast cells of the adenoid tissue release inflammatory mediators that lead to tubal obstruction.
- Treatment consists of adenoidectomy.

Cleft Palate

- Otitis media with effusion is common in cases of cleft palate. The reasons are following:
  - High elastin density in the abnormalities of torus tubarius makes the tube opening difficult.
  - In 40% cases of cleft palate, tensor veli palatini muscle has poor function and does not insert into the torus tubarius.
- Even after the repair of cleft palate, many children need grommets to ventilate their middle ear.

Down's Syndrome

The poor tone of tensor veli palatini muscle and abnormal shape of nasopharynx result in defective function of ET in children suffering from Down's syndrome.

After-effects of Eustachian Tube Obstruction

The ET opens intermittently during swallowing, yawning and sneezing through the active contraction of tensor veli palatini muscle. Air (mixture of oxygen, carbon dioxide, nitrogen and water vapor) fills the spaces in middle ear and mastoid. If the ET remains blocked for long time, first oxygen and later other gases diffuse out into the blood and create negative middle ear pressure, which results in retraction of TM. It leads to "locking" of the ET. The ET can be blocked suddenly and may remain blocked for a long time.

- *Acute tubal blockage* can result into collection of transudate and later exudate (acute otitis media) and even hemorrhage (barotitis media) in the middle ear.
- *Prolonged tubal blockage/dysfunction* can lead to a chain of events beginning from otitis media with effusion, atelectatic ear and retraction pocket, which may lead to erosion of incudostapedial joint and cholesteatoma formation.

Clinical Features

Symptoms and signs of tubal occlusion vary depending upon the acuteness of the condition and severity.
- Otalgia varying from mild to severe.
- Hearing loss.
- Popping sensation or tinnitus.
- Disturbances of equilibrium or vertigo.
- Retracted tympanic membrane.
- Congestion along the handle of malleus and pars tensa.
- Transudate behind the tympanic membrane imparts an amber color and may show fluid level.
- Conductive hearing loss (CHL).
- In severe barotraumas, markedly retracted tympanic membrane with hemorrhages in subepithelial layer (hemotympanum). Perforation is uncommon.

Retraction Pockets and Atelectasis

The obstruction in different pathways of middle ear cleft ventilation can result in retraction pockets or atelectasis of the TM (*see* Chapter 'Diseases of External Ear and Tympanic Membrane'). A retraction pocket is an invagination of the TM. The negative middle ear pressure can cause retraction pocket and otitis media.
- *Sites:* The common sites are pars flaccida and posterosuperior quadrant of pars tensa. Retraction pockets or atelectasis of the following parts of tympanic membrane can occur:
  - Total atelectasis of tympanic membrane occurs due to the obstruction of Eustachian tube.
  - Retraction pocket in posterior part of middle ear occurs due to obstruction in middle ear while the anterior part is ventilated.
  - Attic retraction pocket occurs due to the obstruction of isthmi.
- *Sequelae:* As a retraction pocket deepens, desquamated keratin cannot be cleared and a **cholesteatoma** is formed. Other changes, which depend on the location of pathology, include **thin atrophic TM** (due to the absorption of middle fibrous layer), **ossicular necrosis** and **tympanosclerosis**. **Cholesterol granuloma** and collection of mucoid discharge in mastoid air cells occur due to the obstruction at aditus. Middle ear and attic appear normal.
- *Treatment:* It consists of correction/repair of the cause and establishment of ventilation.

PATULOUS EUSTACHIAN TUBE

Eustachian tube becomes undue patent.

Etiology

Mostly it is idiopathic, but following predisposing factors may be present:
- Rapid weight loss
- Pregnancy especially third trimester
- Multiple sclerosis.

Clinical Features

- *Presenting complaints:* Hearing of own voice (autophony) and breath sounds.
- *Otoscopy/microscopy:* The movements of TM can be seen with inspiration and expiration especially when patient breathes after closing the opposite nostril. Due to undue patency of ET, pressure changes in the nasopharynx are easily transmitted to the middle ear.

Treatment

Acute condition is generally self-limiting. In chronic cases treatment consists of the following:
- Weight gain
- Oral administration of potassium iodide
- Cauterization of the tubes
- Insertion of a grommet.

Self-evaluation Exercises

1. Which of the following is not true for Eustachian tube?
    a. Provides communication between middle ear and nasopharynx
    b. 36 mm in length
    c. Lateral one-third bony and medial two-third cartilaginous
    d. Remains open at rest
2. Frenzel maneuver:
    a. Opens the Eustachian tube and ventilates the middle ear
    b. Muscles of the floor of mouth and pharynx are contracted while nose, mouth and glottis are closed
    c. In comparison to Valsalva maneuver, it is difficult to learn
    d. All of the above
3. Which of the following is not true for Patulous Eustachian tube?
    a. Common in third trimester of pregnancy
    b. Patient becomes aware about their own breathing sounds
    c. Movements of tympanic membrane are synchronous with breathing and are decreased when patient breaths only through the affected side of nose
    d. None from above

True (T)/False (F)

4. Opening of the Eustachian tube is an active process and occurs due to relaxation of tensor veli palatini muscle while closure occurs due to recoiling of the cartilaginous part.
5. Mucosa of auditory tube and middle ear is derived from an outgrowth of the endoderm of the second pharyngeal pouch.
6. The lymphoid tissue of Eustachian tube is called Gerlach tonsil.

Answers

1. d   2. d   3. c   4. F   5. F   6. T

Chapter 12

Acute Otitis Media and Otitis Media with Effusion

> **Specific Learning Objectives**
>
> After going through the chapter, you should be able to answer the following questions:
> - Describe etiopathology, clinical features and management of acute otitis media.
> - Describe etiopathology, clinical features and management of otitis media with effusion.
> - What do you know about: (1) Recurrent acute otitis media; (2) Acute necrotizing otitis media; (3) Aerotitis (Barotitis) media?

INTRODUCTION

Otitis media (OM) refers to inflammation of middle ear cleft. OM is not only the most common bacterial infection in children, but also a leading cause of hearing loss in children. OM is the most common disease of childhood, with the exception of viral upper respiratory infection. Most of the children have at least one incidence of middle ear infection. Fifty percent of the children get three or more episodes of OM and twenty five percent have six or more episodes. The highest prevalence occurs in the first 2 years and decreases thereafter. Otitis media is more frequent in winter months.

The two major classes of otitis media are—acute otitis media (AOM) and chronic otitis media with effusion. AOM consists of middle ear effusion and features of acute infection (fever, ear pain and red bulging eardrum). Otitis media with effusion (OME) is middle ear effusion without features of inflammation. AOM and OME represent the two stages of the same disorder.

Risk Factors

Most of the causes of OM are related to Eustachian tube (ET), which are described in detail in Chapter 'Disorders of Eustachian Tube'. The risk factors, which are same for AOM and otitis media with effusion, include following:
- Male children
- Bottle feeding (breastfeeding is protective)
- Allergy
- Crowded living conditions and poor socioeconomic status
- Smoking by family members in the home
- Siblings having otitis media (OM)
- Viral infections in the home and daycare centers
- Heredity and genetic factors
- Associated conditions:
  - Cleft palate
  - Immunodeficiency
  - Ciliary dyskinesia
  - Cystic fibrosis
  - Down's syndrome.

Prophylactic Measures

Factors which can reduce the morbidity of otitis media, include:
- Proper vaccination
- Breastfeeding
- Better general health and nutrition
- Public awareness.

> Eustachian tube dysfunction is the key to the pathogenesis of otitis media.

ACUTE OTITIS MEDIA (AOM)

AOM implies an acute pyogenic inflammation of the middle ear cleft, which includes Eustachian tube, middle ear, attic, aditus, antrum and mastoid air cells.

Though AOM can occur in all ages, it is mainly the disease of children as the Eustachian tube (ET) is shorter, wider and more horizontal and opens at the lower level in children. Both ears may be involved.

ETIOPATHOLOGY

Routes of Infection
- *Eustachian tube (ET):* The infection in the middle ear usually reaches through the ET. Reflux from the nasopharynx into the middle ear occurs during the swallowing; nose blowing and closed-nose swallowing (Toynbee's maneuver). It is the result of negative middle ear pressure (sniffing). Following conditions can cause AOM:
  - *Anatomical obstruction:* Big adenoids and nasopharyngeal tumors. Currently, it is believed that it is not the obstruction but the bacterial entry into the middle ear due to the failure of protection (abnormally patent tube), which is more important. Big adenoids, which are elevated during swallowing, may obstruct the posterior choanae and increase nasopharyngeal pressure that results into reflux.
  - *Infections:* Adenoiditis, tonsillitis, rhinitis, sinusitis, pharyngitis. Adenoids serve as a bacterial reservoir in nasopharynx in children with AOM.
  - *Forceful blowing of nose:* The forcible blowing of the nose can push the infection into middle ear through the ET.
  - *Swimming:* Especially during diving, water enters in the nose under pressure. If water is infected it can spread infection to nose, sinuses and the middle ear.
  - *Iatrogenic:* Postnasal packing and after adenoidectomy.
  - *Feeding bottle:* In the supine position, bottle feeding may lead milk to enter middle ear via ET.
- *Pre-existing tympanic membrane (TM) perforation:* The causes include trauma while cleaning the external auditory canal (EAC), an open hand slap on the ear and past chronic suppurative otitis media (CSOM).
- *Fracture of temporal bone:* In cases of head injury, middle ear may be involved with the fracture of the temporal bone.
- *Blood borne infection:* Rare.

Predisposing Factors
- *Reduced immunity:* Malnourishment, poor dietary habits, too much physical and mental exertion, exposure to extremes of climate and temperatures, can affect the overall resistance of the persons and infections can occur easily.
- *Barotrauma:* Atmospheric pressure changes especially during flying and deep water diving can affect ET.
- *Exanthematous fevers:* Measles, diphtheria and whooping cough.
- *Palatal disorders:* Cleft palate and palatal palsy.
- *Nasal allergy:* Common allergens inhalants and foods.

Causative Microorganisms
Generally, viral nasal infection precedes the ear bacterial infection. The adenoids of children with recurrent AOM contain pathogenic bacteria in clinically significant amounts.
- *Most common: Streptococcus pneumoniae, Haemophilus influenzae, Branhamella catarrhalis (Morexella catarrhalis).*
- *Other common: Pyogenes, Staphylococcus aureus.*
- *Uncommon:* Gram-negative bacilli from skin (after trauma) such as *Bacillus proteus, pyocyaneus* and *E. coli.*
- In some cases no organisms are found.

CLINICAL FEATURES

Pathology and Clinical Features
The course of disease is usually divided into the 5 stages, which begin from tubal occlusion, pre-suppuration and suppuration and ends with either resolution or complications. If the proper antibiotic therapy is started early during the course of AOM, the the disease process may revert back from any stage. The resolution may start even without the rupture of TM.

Most of the children will have a preceding history (cold and cough) of upper respiratory tract infection. Infants become fussy, sleep poorly and often pull or tug at the affected ear and fever heralds the onset of AOM.

1. **Stage of tubal occlusion:** The edema and hyperemia of nasopharynx and ET occludes the ET. It leads to absorption of air and creation of negative middle ear pressure. Some middle ear effusion may occur, but is not clinically appreciable.
   - *Symptoms:*
     - Mild deafness
     - Ear fullness and ear pain
     - No fever
   - *Signs:*
     - Retracted tympanic membrane—findings include relative shortening and more horizontal position of malleus handle, prominent lateral process of malleus and loss of light reflex.
     - Conductive hearing loss (CHL).
2. **Stage of pre-suppuration:** Prolonged tubal occlusion facilitates invasion of pyogenic organism into middle ear and results in mucosal hyperemia. Inflammatory exudates appear in the middle ear.
   - *Symptoms:*
     - Marked throbbing ear pain, which can awake the child from sleep in night.
     - High degree of fever and restlessness.
     - Bubbling sound in the ear.
     - Deafness though present does not get child's attention due to the severe ear pain.

- **Signs:**
  - Pars tensa congested and bulging out with cart-wheel appearance (leash of blood vessels along the handle of malleus and at the periphery of tympanic membrane) and loss of light reflex.
  - Later on complete tympanic membrane including pars flaccida get uniformly congested and red.
  - Tuning fork tests show CHL.
3. **Stage of suppuration:** There occurs formation of pus in the middle ear and somewhat in mastoid air cells. Tympanic membrane starts bulging.
   - **Symptoms:**
     - Excruciating ear pain
     - Increasing deafness
     - Constitutional symptoms due to absorption of toxins include rising fever, which may be accompanied with vomiting, diarrhea and even convulsions.
   - **Signs:**
     - Tympanic membrane appears red and bulging to the point of rupture with loss of landmarks.
     - Handle of malleus engulfed by the swollen and protruding tympanic membrane.
     - A yellow spot on the tympanic membrane where rupture is imminent (a nipple like protrusion of tympanic membrane with a yellow spot on its summit).
     - Tenderness over the mastoid antrum in the region of suprameatal triangle due to mastoidism.
     - Clouding of air cells in X-ray of mastoid because of exudates.
4. **Stage of resolution:** The tympanic membrane ruptures (due to pressure necrosis) and results in otorrhea and subsidence of other symptoms. Inflammatory process begins resolving.
   - **Symptoms:**
     - Otorrhea: Blood tinged ear discharge (serosanguinous) later becomes mucopurulent.
     - Ear pain and fever subside.
   - **Signs:**
     - External auditory canal (EAC) filled with blood tinged or mucopurulent discharge, which may be pulsatile (**Lighthouse sign**; pus coming out under pressure and synchronizing with each arterial dilatation of heartbeat).
     - Perforation of pars tensa usually in anteroinferior quadrant.
- **Stage of complication:** In majority of the children, AOM is self limiting and responds well to medical treatment. If the virulence of organism is high and resistance of the child is poor, infection may spread beyond the middle ear space. Complications occur in the second week and constitutional and infectious sign and symptoms reappear.

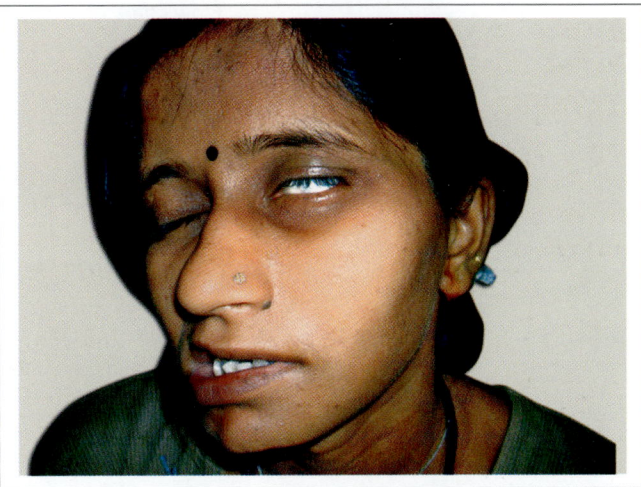

Fig. 12.1: Left side facial palsy in a case of acute suppurative otitis media. Note the blood tinged discharge from left ear. Otoscopy showed subtotal central perforation

The complications (see Chapter 'Complications of Suppurative Otitis Media') include acute mastoiditis, subperiosteal abscess, facial paralysis (Fig. 12.1), labyrinthitis, meningitis, extradural abscess, brain abscess and lateral sinus thrombophlebitis. Infants are at greater risk because AOM and meningitis usually coexist.

DIAGNOSIS

The AOM is a clinical diagnosis.
- **Tests for hearing:** They show CHL.
- **CT temporal bone:** It is indicated only in cases of refractory mastoiditis. The clouding of air cells (because of exudates) and their pressure necrosis (coalescent mastoiditis) may be seen. Demineralization of the air cell septa is the key radiographic sign of mastoid osteitis.
- **Bacteriological examination:** The ear discharge is submitted for the culture and sensitivity to know the type of causative microorganism and the antibiotic to which they are sensitive.

Differential Diagnoses

- **Causes of otalgia:** See Chapter 'Otologic Symptoms and Examination'.
- **Causes of otorrhea:** See Chapter 'Otologic Symptoms and Examination'.
- **Otitis externa, myringitis and bullous myringitis:** See Chapter 'Diseases of External Ear and Tympanic Membrane'.
- **Crying child:** The tympanic membrane may look red and congested, but is never edematous. The light reflex is always present.

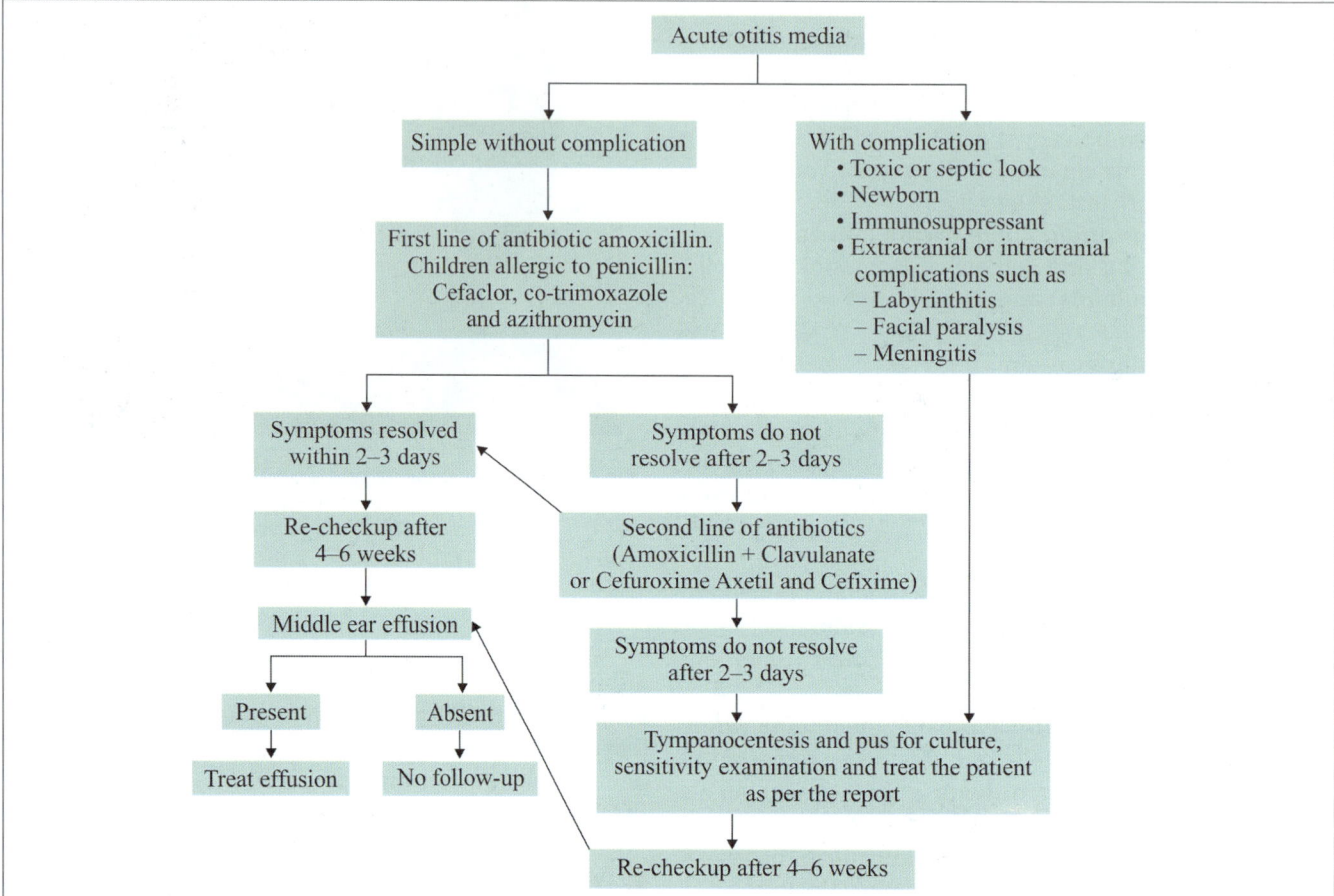

Flow chart 12.1: Management of acute otitis media

TREATMENT (FLOW CHART 12.1)

Medical Treatment

There has been considerable debate on the usefulness of antibiotics for the treatment of AOM. There are no evidences which show that antihistamine, decongestants, or any other form of adjunct medical therapy result in shortening the course of AOM.

- **Antibiotics:** Traditionally antibiotic therapy is continued till tympanic membrane and hearing become normal. Different antibiotic regimes have been suggested such as:
  - A single intramuscular dose of ceftriaxone.
  - A 5-day course or 10–14 days course of oral antibiotics.
  - The first line of antibiotic is amoxicillin (40 mg/kg/day in 3 divided doses).
  - The children who are allergic to penicillin can be given cefaclor, cotrimoxazole and erythromycin.
  - Beta-lactamase-producing *H. influenzae* or *catarrhalis* need amoxicillin-clavulanate, cefuroxime axetil or cefixime.

- **Decongestants:** Topical ephedrine (1% in adults and 0.5% in children), oxymetazoline (nasivion) and xylometazoline (otrivin) nasal drops and oral pseudoephedrine 30 mg BID and phenylephrine hydrochloride with or without antihistaminic are said to relieve ET edema and promote ventilation of middle ear.
- **Analgesics and antipyretics:** Paracetamol takes care of pain and fever.
- **Ear drops and aural toilet:** Ear discharge must be cleaned. Water is prevented from entering the ear. Quinolone/steroids ear wick/drops take care of local infection and inflammation.
- **Dry local heat:** It relieves pain.

Surgical Treatment

- **Tympanocentesis:** It is needle aspiration of fluid from middle ear. The culture and sensitivity of ear fluid for knowing the organism and selecting the antibiotics is indicated in following conditions:
  - Premature newborns
  - Immunocompromised patients

- Failure of previous antibiotic therapy
- Intracranial complications.
- *Myringotomy:* An incision is put in the tympanic membrane to evacuate middle ear fluid. It is usually preceded by tympanocentesis. The indications are followed:
  - Bulging eardrum
  - Acute excruciating pain
  - Unresponsiveness to antibiotics
  - Facial palsy
  - Intracranial complications
- *Mastoidectomy:* Diagnosis of osteitis on computed tomography (CT) warrants mastoidectomy to remove the necrotic and infected bone.
- *Incision and drainage* of subperiosteal postauricular abscess.
- *Tympanoplasty:* In cases of permanent tympanic perforation and ossicular necrosis.

RECURRENT ACUTE OTITIS MEDIA

Infant and children may get recurrent episodes of acute otitis media (AOM), which may be 4–5 or more in a year.
- Usually, episodes of AOM follow acute upper respiratory tract infections.
- The recurrent AOM may be superimposed upon pre-existing maximal expiratory flow.
- Feeding the babies in supine position without propping up the head can cause the milk to enter into the middle ear.

Treatment

Try to find the predisposing factor and the cause of the recurrent infection and treat them. Generally, treatment includes the following:
- *Antimicrobial prophylaxis:* Many use single daily doses of amoxicillin (20 mg/kg) for 3–6 months to prevent recurrent attacks of AOM. Prophylaxis with long-term use of an antibiotic is currently discouraged. Surgical therapy reduces the number of new episodes of AOM and removes persistent effusion in a better way.
- *Surgical prophylaxis with tympanostomy tubes (grommet):* In recurrent and chronic cases, ventilation of middle ear is provided by inserting a ventilatory tube (grommet) through the eardrum.
  - *Indication:* Four bouts of AOM in 6 months or 6 bouts in an year.
- *Adenoidectomy:* With or without tonsillectomy in cases of adenoid hypertrophy and infection.
- *Management of allergy:* In cases of inhalant or food allergy.

ACUTE NECROTISING OTITIS MEDIA

This type of AOM is seen in children, who are suffering from measles, scarlet fever and influenza.
- Causative organism is β-*Haemolyticus streptococcus*.
- Rapid destruction of complete tympanic membrane along with its annulus, mucosa of promontory, ossicular chain and mastoid air cells occurs.
- Profuse otorrhea is there.
- *Sequel:* Secondary acquired cholesteatoma. Ingrowth of squamous epithelium from the external auditory canal (EAC).
- *Treatment:*
  - Antibacterial therapy is started at the earliest and continued for minimum 7–10 days.
  - Cortical mastoidectomy is needed in refractory cases and acute mastoiditis.

OTITIS MEDIA WITH EFFUSION (OME)

Syn: Chronic secretory otitis media; chronic serous otitis media; mucoid otitis media; glue ear

In OME, there occurs collection of non-purulent nearly sterile effusion in the middle ear cleft. The effusion is usually thick and viscid but may be thin and serous.

In younger children, OME is most often the unresolved stage of AOM. In older children, OME has a silent onset without a clinically evident antecedent AOM.

ETIOLOGY

The ET dysfunction is nearly always present in children with otitis media with effusion. The obstruction, which is usually functional and due to edema and viscous secretions, is believed to be secondary to disease process rather than that of the cause.

Current evidence suggests that effusion is not sterile. Polymerase chain reaction (PCR) studies have found metabolically active bacteria in culture-negative middle ear effusions.
- *Malfunctioning of ET:* It fails to ventilate and drain the middle ear. Factors affecting the middle ear clearance mechanism include following:
  - Ciliary dysfunction
  - Mucosal edema and hyperplasia
  - Viscous secretions
  - Middle ear/nasopharyngeal pressure gradient
  - Adenoid hyperplasia and infection.
  - Chronic rhinitis, sinusitis and tonsillitis
  - Benign and malignant tumors of nose, paranasal sinuses and nasopharynx
  - Cleft palate and palatal paralysis.

Currently it is felt that tubal obstruction along with failure of clearance, which are common findings in children with otitis media with effusion, maybe secondary rather than the primary process.
- **Allergy** to inhalants and foodstuffs is present.
- **Unresolved acute otitis media (AOM):** Inadequate antibiotic course, just inactivates infection but does not resolve it completely. Low grade infection acts as a stimulus for mucosa to secrete more fluid.
- **Viral infections:** Adenoviruses and rhinoviruses for upper respiratory tract are responsible.
- **Increased secretory activity of middle ear mucosa:** Increased number of mucous and serous secreting cells results in more secretions.

CLINICAL FEATURES

- Maybe completely asymptomatic.
- The child turns up the volume of television and is not attentive during normal conversation.
- Insidious conductive hearing loss (CHL) (rarely exceeds 40 dB), which may be unnoticed by the parents and is accidentally discovered during audiometry.
- Delayed and defective speech in children due to the hearing loss.
- Mild earache accompanies the other symptoms.

Otoscopy/Microscopy (Fig. 12.2A)

- Retracted, less mobile or immobile tympanic membrane; outward brisk movement of tympanic membrane on reducing pressure in external auditory canal (EAC) with pneumatic otoscope.
- Dark, fluid-filled middle ear obscures the vision of long process of incus.

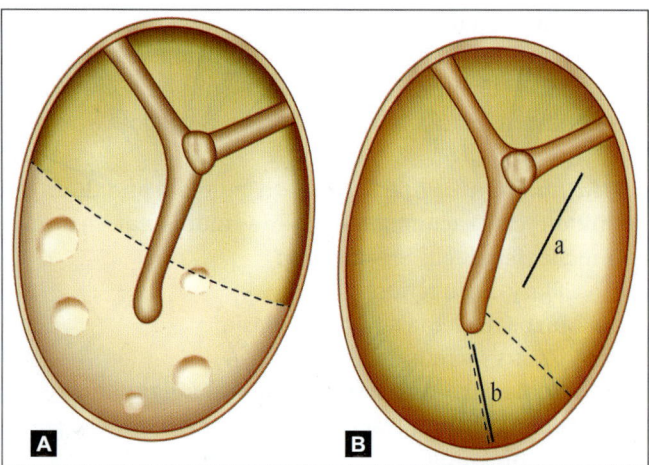

Figs 12.2A and B: (A) Otitis media with effusion. Otoscopy shows fluid level and air bubbles; (B) Incisions for middle ear effusion. **Key:** Two incisions: a, anterosuperior quadrant and b, anteroinferior quadrant

Pneumatic otoscopy is the gold standard for the diagnosis of otitis media with effusion.

DIAGNOSIS

In infants and young children otoscopy and tympanometry findings are sufficient for the diagnosis.
- **Tympanometry:** When the middle ear is filled with effusion, compliance is low and the tympanogram is flat because reflected energy does not vary with the pressure change.

Caution: The ear canals of infants younger than 7 months are hypercompliant and normal tympanograms are possible in cases of otitis media with effusion.

- **Audiometry:** Mild to moderate conductive hearing loss (CHL) is the most common finding. Because of excellent cochlear sensitivity in children, bone conduction thresholds are usually less than audiometric zero.

TREATMENT

If the predisposing and causative factors are known they should be addressed. Considering the long-term impact, surgical therapy is more cost effective than the medical for the severe cases.

Medical

- **Antibiotic therapy:** The efficacy of antibiotic therapy has been shown by many reports. Like AOM, otitis media with effusion is a bacterial disease. Following antibiotics have been suggested:
  - Combination of erythromycin ethylsuccinate and sulfisoxazole
  - Trimethoprim-sulfisoxazole
  - Amoxicillin
  - Amoxicillin-clavulanate
- **Antihistamines and decongestants:** Currently, routine use of decongestants in children with otitis media with effusion has been abandoned.
- **Inflation of middle ear (valsalva's maneuver, politzerization or Eustachian catheterization):** Though popular these maneuvers are not generally used in USA.
- **Corticosteroids:** The effects of steroids are equivocal and not clear.

Surgical

Surgical treatment is considered when effusion persists and is associated with hearing loss. The insertion

of tympanostomy tube (grommet) with or without adenoidectomy is preferred over myringotomy alone.
- *Myringotomy (Fig. 12.2B):* Aspiration of "glue" or middle ear effusion.
- *Tympanostomy tube (grommet):* Most widely used treatment option for otitis media with effusion when present for more than 3 months with associated hearing loss of more than 30 dB in better ear.
- *Adenoidectomy:* This surgery is being increasingly used for the management of otitis media with effusion in children of 4 years of age or older.

SEQUELAE AND COMPLICATIONS

A chronically and frequently ill, irritable, and inattentive child affects entire family. The sequelae of OME are following:
- Atrophic tympanic membrane
- Atelectasis of the middle ear
- Tympanic membrane perforation
- Ossicular necrosis
- Tympanosclerosis
- Adhesive otitis media
- Retraction pockets
- Chronic suppurative otitis media and cholesteatoma
- Cholesterol granuloma
- Sensorineural hearing loss (SNHL).

> **Unilateral Otitis Media with Effusion in Adults**
> In cases of unilateral otitis media with effusion in adults and elderly patients, nasopharynx must be examined with the help of endoscope for the presence of nasopharyngeal mass, which may be obstructing the ET.

AERO OTITIS MEDIA (OTITIC BAROTRAUMA)

In this type of otitis media with effusion, ET fails to maintain middle ear pressure at ambient atmospheric level.

Etiopathology

- *Pressure changes:* When the pressure is relatively high in the middle ear (during ascent), air escapes via the ET passively. But when the pressure is low (during descent), the equalization of pressure may not occur due to the locking of the tube. ET is actively opened by swallowing and yawing. A descent (during a flight and deep water diving) produces a relative negative middle ear pressure.
- *ET dysfunction:* Edema or obstruction of the ET due to adenoids, rhinitis or deviated nasal septum aggravates the problem of locking of the tube.

Clinical Features

- Hearing loss may get relieved by swallowing and yawning.
- Earache may be severe.
- Tinnitus may be present.
- Vertigo is not common.
- Middle ear may have air bubbles or effusion.

Treatment

- Repeated swallowing, yawning and Valsalva maneuver.
- Antibiotics, analgesics, decongestants (topical nasal drops and oral tablets).
- Myringo puncture with injection of air into the middle ear.
- Myringotomy with grommet insertion in refractory cases.

Prophylaxis

- Avoid flying and diving during rhinitis.
- Decongestion of the nose before the flight, especially before the descent. Take decongestant nasal drops/spray and tablets.
- Repeated swallowing during descent, e.g. sipping of water/drinks; sucking of sweets/chocolates/chewing gum.
- Never sleep during the descent.
- Perform intermittently Valsalva maneuvers.
- Treatment of the cause of ET dysfunction such as nasal polyps, septal deviation, adenoids, allergy, and chronic rhinosinusitis.

Self-evaluation Exercises

1. Which of the following is not true about acute otitis media?
    a. Preceding history of cough and cold
    b. Antibiotics for 10 days control pain and fever
    c. Conductive hearing loss may persist for long time and needs observation for 3 months for the fluid to drain spontaneously
    d. Adults are affected more than the children
2. Which of the following is not the common causative organisms of acute otitis media?
    a. *Streptococcus pneumonia*
    b. *Haemophilus influenza*
    c. *Staphylococcus aureus*
    d. *Moraxella catarrhalis*

Contd...

Section 2 • Ear

Contd…

3. Which of the following is not the predisposing condition for otitis media with effusion?
   a. Cleft palate
   b. Down's syndrome
   c. Carcinoma nasopharynx
   d. Adenoidal hypertrophy
   e. None of the above
4. Which of the following is not true for otitis media with effusion?
   a. Conductive hearing loss is the presenting clinical feature
   b. Tympanometry shows evidence of positive pressure and fluid in the middle ear
   c. Treatment of choice is myringotomy with grommet insertion
   d. Rule out nasopharyngeal pathology in elderly patients
   e. None of the above
5. Which of the following are sequel of otitis media with effusion?
   a. Retraction pockets
   b. Middle ear atelectasis
   c. Cholesterol granuloma
   d. Cholesteatoma
   e. All of the above

True (T)/False (F)

6. Otitis media with effusion is not the most common cause for bilateral conductive hearing loss in children.
7. The persistent negative pressure can lead to deposition of cholesterol crystals and granuloma formation in the middle ear and mastoid.
8. In cases of unilateral otitis media with effusion in adults, rule out nasopharyngeal pathology especially the carcinoma in elderly patients.

Answers

| 1. d | 2. c | 3. e | 4. b | 5. e | 6. F |
| 7. T | 8. T | | | | |

Chapter 13

Chronic Suppurative Otitis Media and Cholesteatoma

> **Specific Learning Objectives**
>
> After going through the chapter, you should be able to answer the following questions:
> - What are the differences between atticoantral and tubotympanic types of CSOM?
> - Describe the microbiology and different types and stages of CSOM.
> - Describe the clinical features and management of safe CSOM.
> - How do the different types of cholesteatoma arise and spread?
> - Describe the clinical features and management of unsafe CSOM.

INTRODUCTION

Chronic suppurative otitis media (CSOM) is the most common cause of otorrhea. In most children, acute otitis media (AOM) and otitis media with effusion subside either spontaneously or after treatment. CSOM could be one of the sequelae of AOM and otitis media with effusion.

CHRONIC SUPPURATIVE OTITIS MEDIA

Chronic suppurative otitis media (CSOM) is a long-standing infection of the middle ear cleft. It is characterized by ear discharge and a permanent perforation of tympanic membrane. The perforation's edges are covered by squamous epithelium. It does not heal spontaneously and become, a sort of an epithelium-lined fistulous track.

Epidemiology
- Incidence is higher in poor socioeconomic standards, poor nutrition and lack of health education.
- It affects both sexes and all age groups.
- In India, prevalence rate is higher in rural area (46/1,000 persons) and lesser in urban area (16/1,000 persons).
- CSOM is the leading cause of hearing impairment in rural population.

Types
Traditionally, CSOM is divided into two types—*tubotympanic* and *atticoantral*. Table 13.1 shows the differences between atticoantral and tubotympanic types of CSOM.

Table 13.1: Differences between atticoantral and tubotympanic types of CSOM

Characteristics	Tubotympanic CSOM	Atticoantral CSOM
Nature	Safe and benign	Unsafe and dangerous
Otorrhea (ear discharge)		
• Odor	Odorless	Malodorous (putrid)
• Amount	Usually profuse	Usually scanty
• Type	Usually mucoid	Usually purulent
• Periodicity	Usually intermittent	Usually continuous
Perforation (Fig. 13.1)	Central	Attic or marginal
Granulations	Uncommon	Common
Polyp (Fig. 13.2A)	Pale	Red and fleshy
Cholesteatoma	Absent	Present
Intracranial complications	Never	Not uncommon

1. ***Tubotympanic type (safe or benign):*** This type of CSOM involves anteroinferior part of middle ear cleft and is associated with a permanent central perforation (Figs 13.1A to C). As there is no risk of serious complications, it is also called ***safe*** or ***benign CSOM***.
   - ***Active (wet perforation):*** In the presence of inflammation of mucosa and mucopurulent discharge, the disease is called ***active***.
   - ***Inactive (dry perforation):*** In the absence of inflammation of mucosa and mucopurulent discharge, the disease is called ***inactive***.

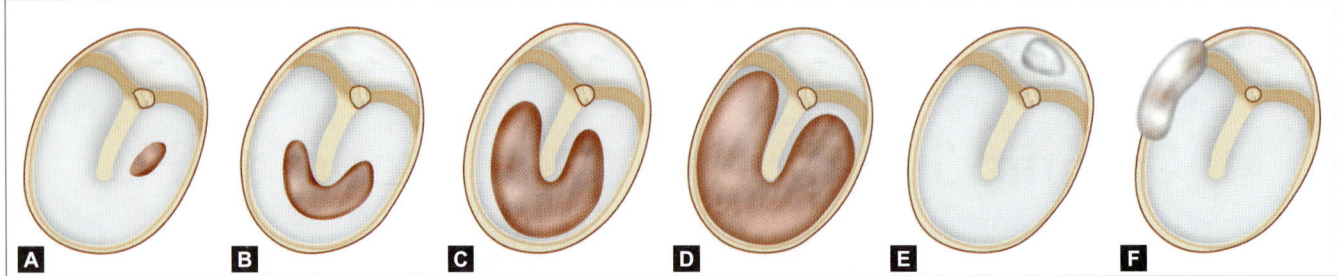

Figs 13.1A to F: Types of perforations of tympanic membrane in cases of CSOM. (A) Small central perforation in anterosuperior quadrant; (B) Medium-size kidney-shaped central perforation; (C) Subtotal central perforation; (D) Total perforation with destruction of fibrous annulus; (E) Attic perforation of pars flaccida; (F) Posterosuperior marginal perforation. **Note:** A, B and C occur in tubotympanic CSOM. D, E and F are seen in CSOM with cholesteatoma

- *Permanent perforation:* Long duration nonhealing dry central perforation indicates that external squamous epithelium is fused with the internal mucosa at the margins of the perforation.
- *Healed chronic otitis media:* Healing of perforation leads to its closure with thin membrane (fibrous layer absent). It may be associated with tympanosclerosis or some conductive hearing loss.

2. *Atticoantral type (unsafe, dangerous, posterosuperior lesion or cholesteatoma):* This type of CSOM involves attic and posterosuperior regions of the middle ear cleft. It is associated with an attic or marginal perforation in posterosuperior quadrant of the pars tensa (Figs 13.1D to F). As it is often associated with risk of serious complications due to the bone erosion nature of cholesteatoma, it is called *unsafe or dangerous CSOM*. Granulations and osteitis are present in many cases.
   - *Inactive:* Self-cleaning retraction pocket in posterosuperior pars tensa or an attic region with potential chances of cholesteatoma is called *inactive disease*.
   - *Active:* Active cholesteatoma erodes bone, forms granulations and presents with putrid continuous ear discharge.

> *Examination:* Suction clearance and examination under operating microscope forms an important part of the clinical examination and assessment of any type of CSOM.

Microbiology

The incriminating microorganisms are identical in both the types of CSOM. The culture (aerobic and anaerobic) may show multiple organisms.
- *Aerobic organisms:* Pseudomonas aeruginosa (most common), Proteus, Escherichia coli and Staphylococcus aureus.
- *Anaerobes:* Bacteroides fragilis (most common) and anaerobic streptococci.

ATTICOANTRAL CHRONIC SUPPURATIVE OTITIS MEDIA OR CHRONIC OTITIS MEDIA WITH CHOLESTEATOMA

The term **cholesteatoma** is a misnomer as it is neither a tumor nor contains cholesterol. It has destructive nature and erodes bone. Infected cholesteatoma causes rapid bone destruction.

The ciliated columnar epithelium in the anterior and inferior part, cuboidal epithelium in the middle part and pavement-like epithelium in the attic region line the middle ear cleft. In normal persons, there is no keratinizing squamous epithelium in the middle ear cleft and its presence (skin in the wrong place) is called **cholesteatoma** (epidermosis or keratoma).

The cholesteatoma is seen in sclerotic mastoid but whether the latter is the cause or the effect of the former is not yet clear.

Structure of Cholesteatoma

Cholesteatoma is an epidermal inclusion cyst, which opens into the external auditory canal (EAC). It contains desquamated debris (mainly white-yellow keratin flakes

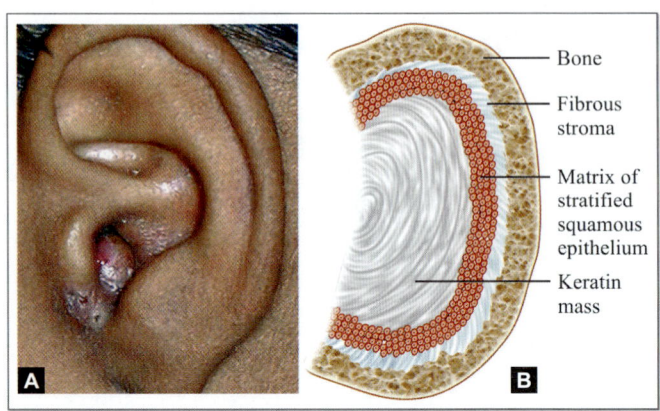

Figs 13.2A and B: (A) A ear polyp; (B) Cholesteatoma structure: stroma, matrix and keratin mass

resembling cholesterol crystals) from its keratinizing squamous epithelial lining.

Cholesteatoma has two parts—matrix and central white mass.
1. *Matrix:* It is made up of keratinizing squamous epithelium, which rests on a thin stroma of fibrous tissues (Fig. 13.2B).
2. *Central white mass:* It consists of keratin debris, which is produced by the matrix (Fig. 13.2B).

Types of Cholesteatoma

Cholesteatoma of temporal bone is classified into two categories—congenital and acquired (Table 13.2).
1. *Congenital cholesteatoma:* It arises from the embryonic epidermal cell rests (keratinizing epithelium) entrapped in the middle ear cleft or temporal bone. The three important sites are—middle ear, petrous apex and the cerebellopontine angle.
    - *Clinical features:* A middle ear congenital cholesteatoma presents with conductive hearing loss (CHL) and a white mass that can be seen behind an intact tympanic membrane. It may rupture through the tympanic membrane and present with a discharging ear. Then it becomes indistinguishable from CSOM.
2. *Acquired cholesteatoma:* They are the most common varieties of cholesteatomas and result from AOM and otitis media with effusion (Flow chart 13.1). Acquired cholesteatoma is also called **unsafe CSOM**. Acquired cholesteatomas are further divided into two types, primary and secondary acquired cholesteatoma (Table 13.2).
    i. *Primary acquired cholesteatoma:* In primary acquired cholesteatoma, there is neither a history of a pre-existing tympanic membrane perforation nor otorrhea.
    ii. *Secondary acquired cholesteatoma:* This cholesteatoma occurs in pre-existing perforation of pars tensa, which is usually posterosuperior marginal perforation or sometimes large central perforation.

Pathogenesis of Acquired Cholesteatoma

The pathogenesis of acquired cholesteatoma is yet a matter of debate. The four basic theories are invagination, hyperplasia, migration and metaplasia. Attempts have been made to explain the pathogenesis on the basis of combination of these theories.

Table 13.2: Types of cholesteatoma

Congenital	Acquired

• Middle ear
• Petrous apex
• Cerebellopontine angle
	• Primary
	  ▪ Attic region
	  ▪ Posterosuperior region
	• Secondary

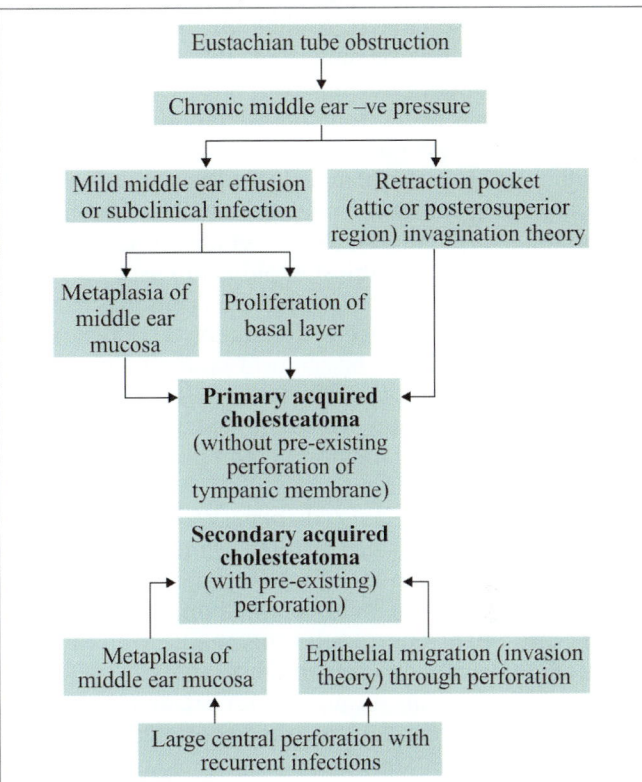

Flow chart 13.1: Etiopathogenesis of primary and secondary acquired cholesteatoma

1. *Invagination theory (Wittmaack):* This theory explains primary acquired cholesteatoma. Invagination of tympanic membrane from the attic or posterosuperior part of pars tensa occurs in the form of retraction pockets. The outer surface of tympanic membrane is lined with stratified squamous epithelium, which after invagination forms the matrix of cholesteatoma and lays down keratin in the pocket.

    As the retraction pocket deepens because of negative middle ear pressure and repeated inflammation, desquamated keratin cannot be cleared from the recess and results in cholesteatoma. Bacteria can infect the keratin matrix, forming biofilms resulting in chronic infection and epithelial proliferation.

    The most common sites for this primary acquired cholesteatoma are pars flaccida or attic (being less fibrous and less resistant to displacement) and posterosuperior quadrant of pars tensa. The attic perforation is simply the proximal end of an expanding invaginated sac.

2. *Epithelial invasion or migration theory (Habermann):* This theory explains secondary acquired cholesteatoma. The keratinizing squamous epithelium of tympanic membrane or deep canal wall migrates into the middle ear through a tympanic membrane perforation. The pre-existing perforation is especially of the marginal type where part of annulus tympanicus has been destroyed.

The damaged (due to inflammation) inner mucosal lining of tympanic membrane, allows the outer keratinizing squamous epithelium to migrate inward and produce this secondary acquired cholesteatoma. Cholesteatomas, which arise after temporal bone fractures, may result from this migration.

3. **Basal cell hyperpalsia theory (Lange and Ruedi):** Under the influence of infection, basal cells of germinal layer of skin can proliferate and lay down keratinizing squamous epithelium. Prickle epithelial cells of pars flaccida can invade the subepithelial tissue by means of proliferating columns of epithelial cells. Basal lamina disruptions have been documented. These basal lamina breaks allow invasion of epithelial cones into the subepithelial connective tissue and the formation of microcholesteatomas, which may enlarge and perforate an intact tympanic membrane and present as primary acquired cholesteatoma.

4. **Squamous metaplasia theory (Wendt and Sade):** Middle ear mucosa, like respiratory mucosa elsewhere, can undergo metaplasia due to repeated infections and transform into squamous epithelium. Such a change has also been reported in otitis media with effusion. Middle ear mucosa can undergo metaplasia due to repeated infection through a pre-existing perforation and result in secondary acquired cholesteatoma.

The simple squamous or cuboidal epithelium of middle ear cleft can undergo a metaplastic transformation into keratinizing epithelium. The pluripotent epithelial cells, stimulated by inflammation can become keratinizing. The mass gradually enlarges because of accumulated debris and come in contact with tympanic membrane. With infection and inflammation, cholesteatoma results in perforation of the tympanic membrane and present as primary acquired cholesteatoma.

Spread of Cholesteatoma

In the middle ear cleft, cholesteatoma follows the path of least resistance and causes enzymatic bone destruction. The growth of attic cholesteatoma is limited by the mucosal folds and suspensory ligaments of the ossicles.

Attic cholesteatoma first invades Prussak's space (lateral most portion of epitympanum) and then into the recesses of epitympanum posteriorly, lateral to the body of incus. Inferiorly, it goes into the middle ear via pouch of Von Troeltsch. Anteriorly, cholesteatoma enters into the protympanum. An attic cholesteatoma thus extends posteriorly into the aditus, antrum and mastoid, inferiorly into the mesotympanum and medially surrounds the incus and head of the malleus.

Destruction of Bone

Cholesteatoma destroys the bones, which come in its way such as ear ossicles, bony labyrinth, canal of facial nerve, sinus plate and tegmen tympani. This bone destruction results in several complications.

Formerly bone destruction was believed to be due to pressure necrosis. Currently, bone destruction has been attributed to enzymes. They are liberated by osteoclasts and mononuclear inflammatory cells (associated with cholesteatoma) and include collagenase, acid phosphatase and proteolytic enzymes.

Clinical Features

- **Symptoms**
  - **No symptoms:** Patient with primary acquired cholesteatoma may remain asymptomatic in initial stages.
  - **Ear discharge:** The persistent malodorous (putrid due to anaerobic bacteria) ear discharge is usually purulent and scanty in amount. It can be so scanty that the patient may not be aware of it.

> The cessation of discharge in a continuously discharging ear is an ominous sign. The perforation might be sealed by crusted discharge, mucosa or polyp. The obstruction of the free flow of purulent discharge has the potential to result in complications.

  - **Slowly progressive hearing loss:** The severity of hearing loss, which is conductive, varies. Hearing is normal when ossicular chain is intact. The cholesteatoma, destroys the ossicles. It may bridge the gap caused by destroyed ossicles. The sensorineural element may be added to hearing loss.
  - **Bleeding:** It can occur from granulations and red fleshy polyp, especially while cleaning the ear by patient or doctor.
  - **Symptoms of sequelae:** Pain, vertigo, facial palsy, headache, vomiting, ataxia and fever.
- **Otoscopy/microscopy/endoscopy**
  - **Perforation:** The most common sites of the perforation, which is marginal, are attic and posterosuperior region (Fig. 13.1). An attic perforation may be hidden behind a small amount of crusted discharge.
  - **Retraction pocket:** The degree of an invagination and retraction in the attic and posterosuperior pars tensa varies from shallow and self-cleansing pocket to deep pocket with accumulation of keratin and infected debris.
  - **Cholesteatoma:** Pearly-white flakes of cholesteatoma can be seen in the retraction pockets. The most common sites are attic and posterosuperior region, but cholesteatoma may extend and present in other parts of middle ear cleft.

- *Primary acquired cholesteatoma:* Defect of variable sizes in attic or posterosuperior region containing keratin debris.
- *Secondary acquired cholesteatoma:* Keratinizing epithelium migrating through a pre-existing perforation into middle ear.
- *Congenital cholesteatoma:* Pearl-like mass appears behind an intact tympanic membrane.
■ *Granulation tissue:* It surrounds the area of osteitis, especially attic and posterosuperior region and may be present in the attic, antrum, posterior tympanum and mastoid.
■ *Polyp:* A fleshy red polyp may be seen filling the meatus.

Ear polyp: In a chronic case of otorrhea it should be considered due to cholesteatoma until proven otherwise.

■ *Ossicular necrosis:* Bony destruction may involve the long process of incus, stapes and handle of malleus or the entire ossicular chain.
■ *Cholesterol granuloma:* This mass of granulation tissue appears blue in color. It may be present in association with cholesteatoma or in the mesotympanum behind an intact drum. Cholesterol granuloma is a mass of granulation tissue with foreign body giant cells surrounding the cholesterol crystals. It is a reaction to the retained secretions and hemorrhage.
● *Fistula test:* The positive fistula test indicates an erosion of lateral semicircular canal.

Congenital cholesteatoma: A whitish mass behind a child's intact tympanic membrane with hearing loss indicates congenital cholesteatoma.

Complications

The sign and symptoms of complications (Table 13.3) which need immediate referral to specialist for urgent management, include, pain, vertigo, headache, facial palsy, listless, drowsiness, loss of appetite, fever, nausea and vomiting, irritability, neck rigidity, diplopia, ataxia and painful swelling around the ear.

Pain in cases of CSOM is an ominous sign and needs special attention to rule out intracranial complications.

Investigations

- *Tuning fork tests and audiogram:* They are essential for pre-operative assessment and to confirm the degree and type of hearing loss.
- *Imaging:* The extent of bone destruction, degree of mastoid pneumatization or sclerosis, a low lying

Table 13.3: Sign and symptoms of complications of CSOM and their causes

Signs	Symptoms
Pain	Otitis externa, extradural abscess, perisinus abscess
Vertigo	Labyrinthitis, cerebellar abscess
Facial weakness	Facial palsy due to erosion of facial canal
A listless child with insomnia and anorexia	Extradural abscess
Headache, nausea and vomiting	Raised intracranial pressure
Fever, irritability and neck rigidity	Meningitis
Diplopia	Gradenigo's syndrome
Drowsiness and bradycardia	Brain abscess
Ataxia	Cerebellar abscess
Nominal aphasia	Temporal lobe abscess
Painful swelling around the ear	Mastoid abscess

dura and an anteriorly placed sigmoid sinus can be seen. These findings help in the planning of surgery. High-resolution computed tomography (HRCT) and magnetic resonance imaging (MRI) are recommended for revision mastoid operations. They help in:
■ Establishing the presence of cholesteatoma.
■ Operative planning.
● *Culture and sensitivity:* It is done to identify the causative microorganisms and antibiotic sensitivity.

Surgical Treatment

The mainstay of treatment is surgical removal of cholesteatoma and rendering the ear safe. The secondary part of the surgery includes preservation and reconstruction of hearing system. In presence of complications, surgery should be performed at the earliest possible.
● *Types of surgery:* The two types of surgical procedures are done to remove the cholesteatoma. They are canal wall-down and canal wall-up procedures (Table 13.4). See Chapter 'Middle Ear and Mastoid Surgeries'.
■ *Atticotomy:* Transcanal.
■ *Canal wall-up procedure (intact posterior meatal wall or closed procedure):* This procedure employs combined approach. Cholesteatoma is approached through the EAC and mastoid cavity. The posterior canal wall remains intact and keeps the EAC and mastoid cavity separate (closed). Though it gives dry ear, better hearing and less postoperative care, patients need long postoperative follow-up. The chances of residual and recurrent cholesteatoma are high. The approaches for this procedure include:
- With facial recess approach
- Without facial recess approach

Table 13.4: Differences between canal wall-up and canal wall-down procedures

	Canal wall-up	Canal wall-down
Examples	• Combined approach tympanoplasty • Posterior tympanotomy	• Radical mastoidectomy • Modified radical mastoidectomy • Bondy operation
Posterior canal wall	Not removed	Removed
Mastoid and ear canal	Remains separate	Merge with each other
Meatoplasty	Not required	Required
Postoperative regular cleaning under microscope	Usually not needed	Usually required
Rate of recurrence/residual cholesteatoma	High	Low
Second look surgery	Required after 6 months	Not required
Swimming	Allowed	Usually discouraged
Hearing aid fitting	Easy	Problematic

- **Canal wall-down procedure (open procedure):** The cholesteatoma is fully exteriorized and mastoid cavity and EAC become one big cavity. The commonly performed procedures include:
    - Radical mastoidectomy
    - Modified radical mastoidectomy
    - Bondy procedure
- **Tympanoplasty:** Reconstructive surgery
    - During the primary surgery
    - Second stage
- Factors determining extent and type of surgery: These are:
    - Hearing status of both the ears
    - Extent of cholesteatoma
    - Mastoid pneumatization
    - Function of eustachian tube
    - Presence of complications
    - Patient factors like age, occupation and general medical status.

Conservative Treatment

- Though it has a limited role, it should be considered in the critically ill patient and only-hearing ear, where risk of surgery may not outweigh benefits.
- In small and limited cholesteatoma or having fairly large opening in the EAC, entrapped keratin may be removed directly or by irrigation with saline or 1:1 distilled white vinegar and 70% isopropyl alcohol for stabilization.

TUBOTYMPANIC (SAFE) CHRONIC SUPPURATIVE OTITIS MEDIA

The tubotympanic disease remains localized to the mucosa of anteroinferior part of the middle ear cleft. The processes of healing and destruction go together and depend upon the virulence of organism and resistance of the patient.

Acute exacerbations occur frequently. The cochlea may be damaged due to absorption of toxins from the oval and round windows and hearing loss becomes a mixed type.

Etiology/Predisposing Factors

- **Permanent perforation:** This benign type of CSOM is mostly the sequela of a large central perforation of childhood acute otitis media (AOM), which usually follows after exanthematous fever. The permanent perforation allows repeated infection through the external ear canal causing otorrhea. The middle ear mucosa, which is exposed to the environment, gets sensitized to dust, pollen and other aeroallergens from the environment.
- **Eustachian tube:** Ascending infection of the tonsils, adenoids and sinuses may result in persistent or recurring otorrhea.
- **Allergy:** This may be from foods (such as milk, eggs, fish) and inhalants (pollen, fungi, dust).

Clinical Features

- **Symptoms**
    - **Ear discharge:** The odorless ear discharge may be mucoid or mucopurulent, profuse or scanty and intermittent. The ear discharge is common at the time of upper respiratory tract infection and when water enters into the ear.
    - **Hearing loss:** The severity of conductive hearing loss varies, but is rarely profound. The hearing may improve in the presence of discharge due to **round window shielding effect,** because the discharge helps to maintain the phase differential. In the dry ear, sound waves reach both the oval and round windows simultaneously and cancel each other's effect.
- **Otoscopy/microscopy/endoscopy**
    - **Central perforation of pars tensa (Fig. 13.1):** Note the following points:
        - **Size:** Small, medium, large, or subtotal (extending up to annulus).
        - **Shape:** Round, oval or kidney-shaped.
        - **Position:** Anterior, posterior, or inferior to the handle of malleus.
- **Middle ear mucosa:** It is normal (pale pink and little moist) when the disease is inactive, but looks inflamed red edematous and velvety when disease is active.

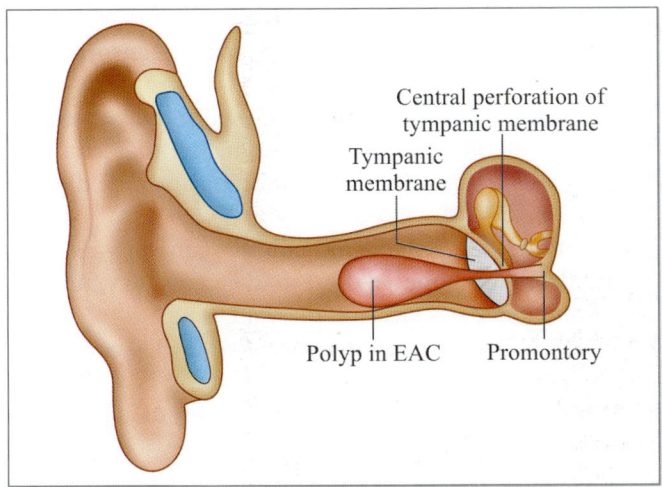

Fig. 13.3: Ear polyp in tubotympanic CSOM, arising from the promontory and coming to EAC through the central perforation of tympanic membrane

- ***Polyp (Fig. 13.3):*** An edematous and inflamed mucosa protrudes through the perforation and presents in the external canal as polyp. It is usually pale (pink and fleshy polyp in cases of atticoantral cholesteatoma).
- ***Tympanosclerosis:*** The hyalinization and subsequent calcification occurs in the subepithelial connective tissue of tympanic membrane and middle ear mucosa. It appears as white chalky deposits on the promontory, ossicles, joints, tendons and oval and round windows and may interfere with the mobility of these structures.
- ***Ossicular chain:*** Ossicular chain usually remains intact and mobile but may show some degree of necrosis, particularly on the long process of incus.
- ***Fibrosis and adhesions:*** They result from the healing process and may impair mobility of ossicular chain or block the Eustachian tube.
- ***Granulations:*** They may be seen over the remnant of tympanic membrane.
- ***Rule out in-growth of squamous epithelium:*** In growth of squamous epithelium should be ruled out from the edges of perforation. Though rare, cholesteatoma can coexist with a central perforation.

Investigations

- ***Hearing tests (tuning fork and audiogram):*** They give an idea regarding the degree and type of hearing loss. The severity of hearing loss, which is usually conductive, varies, but rarely exceeds 50 dB. The cochlea may get damaged due to absorption of toxins from the oval and round windows and results in sensorineural element in CHL (mixed type).
- ***Culture and sensitivity:*** Culture and sensitivity of ear discharge helps in identifying the microorganisms and selecting the proper antibiotics.
- ***Imaging:*** Mastoid is usually found sclerotic. The pneumatized mastoid may show clouding of air cells. There is no evidence of bone destruction, which is a feature of atticoantral cholesteatoma.

Treatment

In the presence of otorrhea, the aim is to clean the ear discharge and control infection. In cases of dry ear, perforation may be repaired by tympanoplasty, which not only improves hearing, but also prevents recurrent infection and acute exacerbations.

- ***Medical therapy***
  - ***Aural toilet:*** Removal of discharge and debris from the external auditory canal (EAC) can be done by dry mopping with absorbent cotton buds and suction clearance under microscope.
  - ***Antibiotic/steroid ear drops:*** Antibiotic/steroid ear drops 3–4 times a day in wet and running ears have local antimicrobial and anti-inflammatory effects.
    * An acid pH of ear drops helps in eliminating pseudomonas infection.
    * Ear drops of 1.5% acetic acid are useful for acidifying ear canal.
    * Ototoxic antibiotic ear drops are not used.
    * The most preferred antibiotics and steroids are quinolone group (ciprofloxacin and ofloxacin) and dexamethasone.
    * After instilling drops, the ear is kept upward when the patient is in supine position. Intermittent pressure on the tragus facilitates the drops to reach in the middle ear.
    * The ear drops are stopped once the ear becomes dry. They should never be used in dry ears as it can make the ear wet and discharging.
    * The ear should be examined regularly as ear drops can cause maceration of canal skin, local allergy, growth of fungus and resistance of organisms.
  - ***Systemic antibiotics:*** They are prescribed only in cases of acute exacerbation. There is no role of systemic antibiotics in the treatment of uncomplicated safe CSOM.
  - ***Patient's instructions:***
    * Water should not enter into the ear while bathing, swimming and hair-wash. The ear plugs and rubber inserts may be employed.
    * Avoid hard nose-blowing as it can push the infection from nasopharynx to middle ear.
    * Avoid self-cleaning of the ear.
    * Stop the ear drops once the ear becomes dry.
    * Take treatment of upper respiratory infections at the earliest.
  - ***Treatment of source of infection:*** Treatment of contributory diseases (infections of tonsils,

adenoids, nose and paranasal sinuses and allergy) is important.
- **Surgical treatment**
  - *Removal of ear polyp or granulations:* They facilitate ear toilet and treatment with local antibiotics.

> *Ear polyp:* It is never avulsed because it may be attached to the stapes, facial nerve and horizontal semicircular canal and can injure these important structures and lead to complications such as facial paralysis and labyrinthitis.

  - *Tympanoplasty:* In a dry ear, myringoplasty/tympanoplasty restore hearing and check repeated infection from the external ear canal (*see* Chapter 'Middle Ear and Mastoid Surgeries').

TUBERCULAR OTITIS MEDIA

It is not common now, but must be kept in mind when CSOM cases do not respond with necessary medical and surgical treatment and complications like facial palsy appears.

Etiopathology

- *Primary:* Very rare.
- *Secondary:* From pulmonary tuberculosis, infection enters via Eustachian tube. Blood-borne spread can occur from tubercular lesions of lungs, tonsils and cervical and mesenteric nodes.
- *Age:* Most of the patients are children and young adults.
- *Tubercles:* They occur in submucosa and lead to painless necrosis.

Clinical Features

- *Foul smelling ear discharge:* Due to underlying bone destruction.
- *Hearing loss:* It is severe and conductive to start with but once labyrinth involvement occurs sensorineural component appears.
- *Tympanic membrane perforations:* Initially there are multiple perforations (2-3) but later on they coalesce and give rise to single large perforation and then disease looks like CSOM.
- *Granulations:* Pale granulations can be seen in middle ear and operated mastoid cavity. They indicate destruction of ossicles and mastoid bone.
- *Mastoiditis and postauricular fistula:* Osteomyelitis and bony sequestrum occur.
- *Facial nerve palsy:* Patient may present with facial palsy.

Diagnosis

- *X-ray Chest:* Shows pulmonary tuberculosis.
- *Ear discharge:* Culture for *Mycobactrium tuberculosis* take longer time but DNA probe and polymerase chain reaction (PCR) provide early results.
- *Histopathology of granulations:* Confirm the diagnosis.

Treatment

- Multi-drugs antitubercular therapy (AKT).
- Local aural toilet and control of secondary infections.
- Mastoidectomy and tympanoplasty are done under the cover of AKT to avoid delayed healing, wound breakdown and fistula formation.

SYPHILITIC OTITIS MEDIA

It is very rare and infection enters middle ear through either blood-borne or Eustachian tube from the syphilitic lesions of nose and nasopharynx. Bone necrosis and sequestrum formation lead to foul smelling ear discharge and mimic CSOM. The topic is covered in detail in Chapter 'Sensorineural Hearing Loss'.

Self-evaluation Exercises

1. Which of the following is not true for cholesteatoma?
   a. Erodes bone
   b. Attic perforation
   c. Primary treatment of cholesteatoma is canal wall-down mastoidectomy, which may be combined with tympanoplasty
   d. None of the above

True (T)/False (F)

2. The posterosuperior retraction pocket can progress and lead to primary cholesteatoma.

Answers
1. d   2. T

Chapter 14

Complications of Suppurative Otitis Media

> **Specific Learning Objectives**
>
> After going through the chapter, you should be able to answer the following questions:
> - Describe the factors affecting and routes of spread in the development of complications of suppurative otitis media.
> - Classify the complications of suppurative otitis media.
> - Describe the clinical features and management of acute mastoiditis and its differences from masked (latent) mastoiditis.
> - What do you know about petrositis and its management?
> - Describe the various abscesses in relation to mastoid infections.
> - Describe the differential diagnoses of intracranial complications of suppurative otitis media? What are their early warning and characteristic features?

INTRODUCTION

The otitis media (OM) is one of the most commonly treated infections. In acute otitis media (AOM) and cholesteatoma, disease process is usually limited only to the mucoperiosteal lining of the middle ear cleft. When it breaks into the bony walls of the cleft, various complications can arise (Fig. 14.1). Complications can occur as the result of bony destruction from either hyperemic decalcification in AOM or chronic bioenzymatic activity in cholesteatoma.

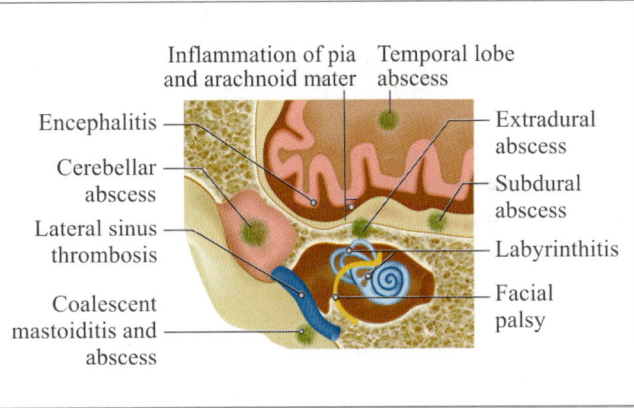

Fig. 14.1: Complications of suppurative otitis media (SOM) and their sites

- **Most common complications of suppurative otitis media (SOM):** Purulent meningitis and brain abscesses (temporal lobe more common than cerebellar) are the most frequent intracranial complications these days. The sinus thrombosis, which was common before this antibiotic era, has nearly disappeared as a cause of death. In majority of the patients, the cause is cholesteatoma.
- **Early symptoms of intracranial complications of suppurative otitis media (SOM):** Appearance of ear pain in cases of chronic otorrhea indicates impending intracranial complications until unless proved otherwise. Foul-smelling, creamy ear discharge indicates a fulminant, destructive process. Headache and drowsiness are danger signs. One of the earliest signs of brain abscess is a visual field defect. Fever is mostly due to either meningitis or sinus thrombosis.

In the current era of new range of antibiotics although the incidence of complications has significantly declined, they do occur and must be kept in mind as the early diagnosis and prompt treatment reduces mortality. Complications of SOM can be categorized into three groups—intratemporal, extratemporal and intracranial (Table 14.1).

FACTORS INFLUENCING DEVELOPMENT OF COMPLICATIONS

Complications usually occur when ear infections are either uncontrolled or inadequately controlled. The factors which influence complications of SOM, include:

Table 14.1: Three groups of complications of suppurative otitis media (SOM)

Intratemporal	Extratemporal	Intracranial

• Persistent tympanic membrane perforation
• Mastoiditis
  ▪ Acute coalescent mastoiditis
  ▪ Masked (latent) mastoiditis
• Acute petrositis
• Facial paralysis
• Labyrinthitis
  ▪ Labyrinthine fistula
  ▪ Serous labyrinthitis
  ▪ Suppurative labyrinthitis
	• Postauricular abscess
	• Zygomatic abscess
	• Bezold's abscess
	• Meatal abscess (Luc's abscess)
	• Behind the mastoid abscess (Citelli's abscess)
	• Parapharyngeal and retropharyngeal abscesses
		• Extradural (epidural) abscess
		  ▪ Middle cranial fossa
		  ▪ Posterior cranial fossa
		• Subdural empyema
		• Meningitis
		• Brain abscess
		  ▪ Temporal lobe of cerebrum
		  ▪ Cerebellum
		• Lateral sinus thrombophlebitis
		• Cerebrospinal fluid (CSF) otorrhea
		• Otitic hydrocephalus

- ***Microorganisms:*** High virulence of organisms.
- ***Host:*** Poor nutrition and resistance and immunosuppression.
- ***Antibiotics:*** Inadequate course and dose of antibiotic in treating acute middle ear and mastoid infections and resistance of organisms to antibiotics.
- ***Chronic systemic diseases:*** Diabetes mellitus, tuberculosis, nephritis and leukemia, etc.
- ***Pneumatization of temporal bone:*** Intracranial complications of AOM are common in poorly pneumatized temporal bone.

PATHWAYS OF SPREAD

The uncontrolled or poorly controlled middle ear cleft infections can cause complications through any of the following three routes.

1. ***Bone erosion:*** This is the most common route of spread. The process of hyperemic decalcification occurs in acute infections. Chronic infection results in osteitis and granulation tissue and in some cases, osteomyelitis. Bony erosion is caused by chronic bioenzymatic activity in cases of cholesteatoma.
2. ***Progressive retrograde thrombophlebitis of small venules:*** The rich network of veins within the temporal bone is in direct communication with extracranial, intracranial and cranial diploeic veins. Haversian canal veins communicate with intracranial dural venous sinuses and superficial veins of brain. The mastoid bone infection can result in thrombophlebitis of venous sinuses (usually sigmoid sinus) and even cortical vein thrombosis. The bony walls of middle ear and mastoid air cells are found intact in this type of spread. It is common in acute infections.
3. ***Preformed pathways:***
   - ***Congenital dehiscence:*** Dehiscence in facial canal (facial palsy) and floor of hypotympanum over the jugular bulb (thrombophlebitis).
   - ***Patent sutures:*** Such as petrosquamous suture.
   - ***Temporal bone fractures:*** The fibrous scar permits infection.
   - ***Surgical defects:*** Stapedectomy, fenestration and exposure of dura.
   - ***Perilymphatic fistula:*** Congenital or acquired.
   - ***Normal anatomy openings:*** Infection of labyrinth and from labyrinth to the meninges:
     - Oval and round windows
     - Internal acoustic meatus
     - Cochlear aqueduct
     - Endolymphatic duct and sac.

Hyrtl's fissure (tympanomeningeal hiatus): This is an embryonic remnant that runs parallel to cochlear aqueduct and connects subarachnoid space to middle ear just anterior and inferior to the round window. It can be a source of congenital CSF otorrhea or meningitis in cases of middle ear infections. Normally it is obliterated.

ACUTE MASTOIDITIS

The inflammation of mucosal lining of mastoid antrum air cells invariably occurs in AOM. However, in "mastoiditis," which is now relatively rare, infection involves bony walls of the mastoid air cells.

Characteristic features of acute mastoiditis: Ear pain and tenderness extending into the postauricular region and fever are hallmark symptoms. Protrusion of pinna and postauricular erythema and swelling are classic findings.

Etiology and Predisposing Factors

- AOM especially in cases of measles, exanthematous fevers, poor nutrition and diabetes.
- β-hemolytic streptococci (most common) and other organisms causing AOM. Anaerobic organisms are also common.

- Mastoids with well-developed mastoid air cells.
- Children are affected more.

Pathology

Acute mastoiditis can manifest in two ways:

1. *Acute periostitis (inflammation of periosteum):* Spread of infection occurs via venous channels.
2. *Acute osteitis (coalescent mastoiditis):* Destruction of mastoid air cells trabeculae.

The pathological processes include production of pus, hyperemic decalcification and osteoclastic resorption of bony walls.

- *Pus under tension:* The inflammatory process to mucoperiosteal lining increases the amount of pus. The drainage of pus through a small perforation of tympanic membrane and eustachian tube cannot keep pace with the amount of pus production. Swollen mucosa of the antrum and attic impede the drainage and result in further accumulation of pus.
- *Hyperemic decalcification and osteoclastic resorption:* Hyperemia causes dissolution of calcium from the mastoid air cells (hyperemic decalcification).

The destruction and coalescence of mastoid air cells convert mastoid into a single large cavity, which is filled with pus and also called *empyema mastoid*. The mastoid cortex may be broken leading to subperiosteal abscess which can burst the overlying skin and result in discharging fistula.

Clinical Features

The change in the character and reappearance of clinical features during the resolving AOM points to the development of acute mastoiditis.

- *Pain:* Behind the ear in mastoid region.
- *Fever:* Usually low grade. In children, fever is high with a rise in pulse rate.
- *Ear discharge:* Profuse and increases in purulence.

The persistence of otorrhea beyond 3 weeks in a case of AOM indicates mastoiditis.

The discharge may cease (due to obstruction in its drainage) with progressive worsening of clinical features. Mucopurulent or purulent discharge is often pulsatile *(light-house effect)*. It comes through the perforation of pars tensa.

- *Mastoid tenderness:* Tenderness may be present over the middle of mastoid process, mastoid tip, posterior border or the root of zygoma. Tenderness over the suprameatal triangle may be seen in AOM due to inflammation of mastoid antrum. Tenderness may be compared with that of the healthy side.
- *Sagging of posterosuperior meatal wall:* It indicates periostitis of bony wall that lies between the antrum and deep bony canal.
- *Perforation of tympanic membrane (TM):* A small central perforation or nipple-like protrusion can be seen in pars tensa with congestion of remaining TM. The TM may remain intact (inadequate antibiotics treatment) but looks dull and opaque.
- *Swelling over the mastoid region:* Edema of periosteum imparts a smooth "ironed out" feeling over the mastoid. If pus bursts bony cortex, a subperiosteal fluctuant abscess is seen. The pinna is pushed forward and downwards.
- *Conductive hearing loss (CHL)*
- *General appearance:* Ill and toxic look.

Investigations

- *Complete blood count (CBC):* Polymorphonuclear leukocytosis and raised ESR.
- *HRCT temporal bone:* Loss of bony trabeculae indicates coalescent mastoiditis. CT can also identify other intracranial or neck abscesses.
- *Culture and sensitivity of ear discharge:* To know the organism and the antibiotics to which they are sensitive.

Differential Diagnoses

- *Suppuration of mastoid lymph nodes:* Scalp infection can lead to postauricular lymphadenopathy, which though suppurates rarely and leads to abscess formation. There is no history of preceding OM and TM is normal. The abscess is quite superficial.
- *Furunculosis of EAC:* It should be differentiated from acute mastoiditis (Table 14.2).

Treatment

Majority of the cases of acute mastoiditis usually respond to culture-directed intravenous antibiotics and myringotomy with or without tympanostomy tube.

- *Hospitalization and antibiotics:* These patients need intravenous antibiotics in high doses. Till the report of culture and sensitivity, amoxicillin or ampicillin is given. As the anaerobic organisms are often present, metronidazole is added.
- *Myringotomy:* Small TM perforation is insufficient and wide myringotomy facilitates pus drainage.
- *Cortical mastoidectomy:* The cortical mastoidectomy exenterates all mastoid air cells along with the removal of pockets of pus. Adequate antibiotic treatment is continued for 5–10 days postoperatively. The *indications* include the following:

Table 14.2: Differentiating features between acute mastoiditis and furuncle of external audiotory canal (EAC)

	Acute mastoiditis	Furuncle of external auditory canal
Preceding history	Ear discharge and acute otitis media	Self cleaning of ear
Ear discharge	Mucoid or mucopurulent	Pain and swelling subside after purulent (mixed with blood) discharge
Conductive hearing loss (CHL)	Always present	Only on canal occlusion
Tenderness	On mastoid region	Tragal or inferior to pinna movement
Auricle movement	Usually painless	Always painful
Displacement of auricle	Inferior, anterior and lateral	Only anterior and lateral
Retroauricular sulcus	Not obliterated	May be obliterated
Tympanic membrane	Perforation	Normal
EAC swelling	Sagging of posterosuperior deep canal wall	In outer cartilaginous part
Pre-or postauricular lymph nodes	Absent	May be present and tender
Imaging temporal bone	Destruction of mastoid air cells	Normal

- Subperiosteal abscess
- Sagging of posterosuperior meatal wall.
- Positive reservoir sign: EAC fills with pus immediately after it has been cleaned.
- No improvement or worsening of condition in spite of adequate medical treatment for 48 hours.
- Complications: Facial paralysis, labyrinthitis and intracranial complications.

Complications

They include subperiosteal abscess, labyrinthitis, facial paralysis, petrositis, extradural abscess, subdural abscess, meningitis, brain abscess, lateral sinus thrombophlebitis, and otitic hydrocephalus.

MASKED (LATENT) MASTOIDITIS

It refers to slow destruction of mastoid air cells without the acute sign and symptoms of acute mastoiditis, such as pain, ear discharge, fever and mastoid swelling.
- *Etiology:* Inadequate dose, frequency and duration of antibiotic therapy are the most incriminating factors. Oral penicillin in AOM controls acute symptoms but smoldering infection continues in the mastoid.
- *Pathology:* Mastoidectomy in latent mastoiditis shows extensive destruction of the air cells with granulation tissue and dark gelatinous material filling the mastoid. Erosion of the tegmen tympani and sinus plate can result in extradural and perisinus abscess, respectively.
- *Clinical features*
  - Mild mastoid pain and tenderness.
  - Persistent CHL.
  - TM looks thick and loses its translucency.
- *Imaging:* Mastoid will reveal clouding of air cells with loss of cell outline.
- *Treatment:* Treatment consists of cortical mastoidectomy with full doses of antibiotics.

EXTRATEMPORAL COMPLICATIONS (ABSCESSES)

About 50% patients of mastoiditis develop subperiosteal abscess (Fig. 14.2).
- *Postauricular abscess:* This common abscess forms over the Macewen's triangle of the mastoid. The pus travels along the vascular channels of lamina cribrosa. Auricle is displaced forward, outward and downward. It is common in children.
- *Zygomatic abscess (Fig. 14.3):* Infection of zygomatic air cells, which are situated at the posterior root of zygomatic arch, results in zygomatic abscess. The pus can present either superficial or deep to the temporalis muscle. Swelling occurs in front of and above the auricle. Associated edema of the upper eyelid is common.

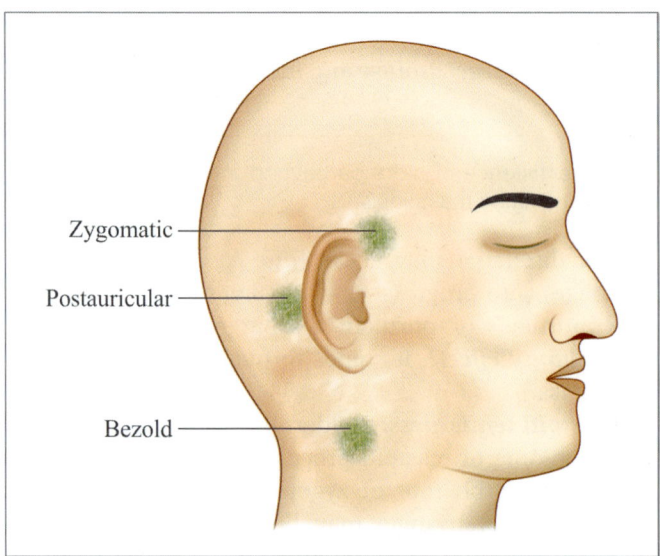

Fig. 14.2: Types of mastoid abscesses

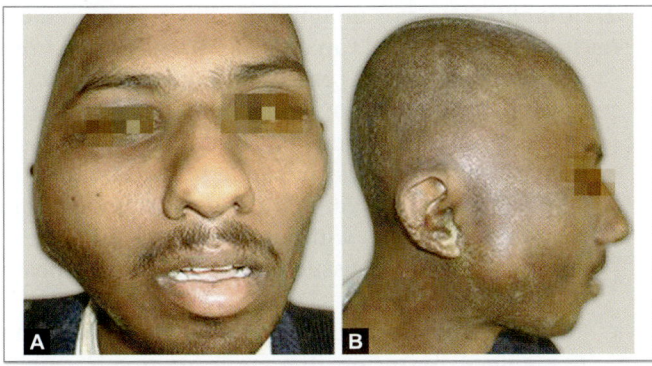

Figs 14.3A and B: Zygomatic abscess. (A) Front view; (B) Lateral view

- *Meatal abscess (Luc's abscess):* Mastoid abscess breaks the bony wall that lies between the antrum and external bony canal and may burst into the meatus. Swelling becomes visible in the deep part of bony meatus.
- *Behind the mastoid (Citelli's abscess):* Pus can travel either along the mastoid emissary vein or occipitotemporal (also called occipitomastoid) suture. Citelli's abscess is situated posterior to the mastoid. The postauricular mastoid abscess forms over the mastoid.
- *Parapharyngeal and retropharyngeal abscesses:* Infection of the peritubal cells in cases of acute coalescent mastoiditis can result into these abscesses (*see* Chapter 'Deep Neck Abscesses').

Bezold's Abscess (Fig. 14.4)

- In acute coalescent mastoiditis, pus can break the thin medial side of the tip of the mastoid and present as upper neck swelling. The abscess may follow any of the following course:
  - Lie deep to sternocleidomastoid muscle and pushing it laterally.

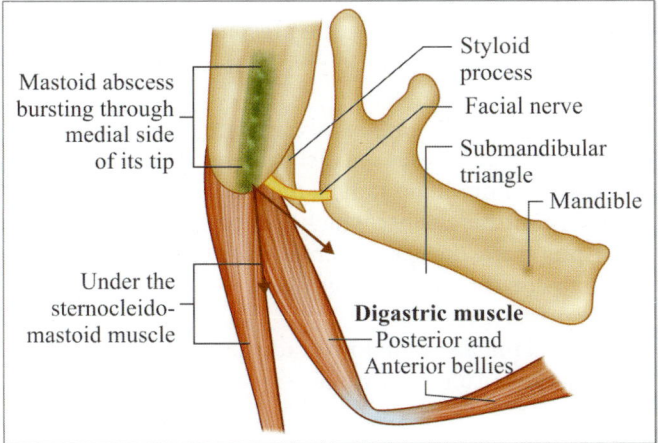

Fig. 14.4: Bezold's abscess. Through the mastoid tip abscess extends either deeper to sternocleidomastoid muscle or into the submandibular triangle

  - Lie in the digastric triangle (follow the posterior belly of digastric and present between the tip of mastoid and angle of jaw).
  - Lie in the upper part of posterior triangle.
  - Lie in the parapharyngeal space.
  - Lie along the carotid vessels.
- *Clinical features:* Sudden onset of pain, fever, a tender swelling in the neck and torticollis in cases of purulent otorrhea.
- *Differential diagnoses:*
  - Acute upper deep cervical lymphadenitis
  - Abscess of the lower part of the parotid gland
  - Infected branchial cyst
  - Parapharyngeal abscess
  - Jugular vein thrombosis
- *CT scan:* It will establish the diagnosis.
- *Treatment:* It is surgical. Intravenous antibiotics are given as per the report of culture and sensitivity of the pus taken at the time of surgery.
  - Cortical mastoidectomy with exploration of mastoid tip for a fistulous opening into the soft tissues of the neck.
  - Incision and drainage of the neck abscess is done through a separate incision and putting a drain.

PETROSITIS OR PETROUS APICITIS

Infection of the petrous part of temporal bone is called **petrositis**. It is usually associated with acute coalescent mastoiditis, latent mastoiditis and cholesteatoma.

Pertinent Anatomy

The petrous bone is pneumatized in about 30% individuals. The CN VI (abducens) and CN V (trigeminal) ganglion are closely related to petrous apex. There are two groups of air cells' tracts that communicate mastoid and middle ear to the petrous apex. Infection may pass through these cell tracts and reach petrous apex.

- *Posterosuperior tract:* From the attic and antrum the tract passes around semicircular canals to petrous apex. This tract begins in the Trautmann's triangle or the attic.
- *Anteroinferior tract:* From the hypotympanum, the tract passes around the Eustachian tube and cochlea to the petrous apex. Tract is situated near the tympanic opening of Eustachian tube anterior to the cochlea and passes above the carotid artery.

Clinical Features

- Gradenigo's syndrome or triad:
  - CN VI (abducens) palsy (palsy of lateral rectus causing squint).

- Deep seated ear or retro-orbital pain (due to the involvement of CN V ganglion).
- Persistent ear discharge.
- Fever, headache, vomiting and neck rigidity may be present.

> **Petrositis:** Persistent ear discharge in cases of cortical or modified radical mastoidectomy may be due to petrositis.

- CT scan of temporal bone confirms the diagnosis.

Treatment

- *Antibiotic therapy:* It should precede and follow the surgery. Most patients respond well to antibacterial therapy alone, which is given in high doses and continued for 4–5 days after the disappearance of symptoms.
- *Radical or modified radical mastoidectomy:* The fistulous tract is curetted and enlarged to provide free drainage. The anteroinferior tract cells need radical mastoidectomy.

FACIAL NERVE PARALYSIS

It can occur in cases of both AOM as well as cholesteatoma (*see* Chapter 'Facial Nerve Disorders').

Acute Otitis Media (AOM)

- *Clinical features:* In cases of dehiscent fallopian bony canal, facial nerve lies just under the middle ear mucosa. Inflammation of middle ear easily spreads to epineurium and perineurium and results in facial paralysis, which usually manifests within 10 days. Facial palsy after 2 weeks of AOM indicates erosion of bony facial canal.
- *Treatment:* Facial nerve function usually recovers with systemic antibiotics and wide myringotomy or tympanostomy tube. Some prefer concomitant corticosteroids. Cortical mastoidectomy is required occasionally.

Cholesteatoma

Facial paralysis can result from either cholesteatoma or penetrating granulation tissue. Cholesteatoma destroys bony facial canal and involves facial nerve.

- *Clinical features:* Facial nerve paralysis is insidious and progressive.
- *HRCT temporal bone:* It is essential in the evaluation of facial nerve palsy. It delineates extent of disease and identifies cholesteatoma and neoplasms.
- *Treatment:* It is urgent modified or radical mastoidectomy. Facial canal should be examined from the geniculate ganglion (processus cochleariformis) to the stylomastoid foramen.
  - In cases of granulation tissue and cholesteatoma, bony facial canal is uncapped in the area of involvement. Granulation tissue surrounding the nerve is removed without damaging the nerve sheath. Granulation tissue invading the nerve sheath is left in place.
  - The nerve segment destroyed by the granulation tissue needs resection. The nerve grafting is usually preferred in the second stage when infection is controlled.

LABYRINTHITIS

It is described in detail in the Chapter 'Peripheral Vestibular Disorders'.

EXTRADURAL (EPIDURAL) ABSCESS

This collection of pus between the bone and dura can occur in both AOM as well as cholesteatoma. An extradural abscess frequently coexists with sinus thrombophlebitis and precedes brain abscess.

Pathology

- The overlying dural bone can be destroyed by hyperemic decalcification (in AOM) and bioenzymatic activity (in cholesteatoma). Pus collects in epidural space.
- In venous thrombophlebitis mode of spread, overlying dural bone remains intact.
- The affected dura gets covered with granulations and appears unhealthy and discolored.
- An extradural abscess may lie in
  - Middle cranial fossa
  - Posterior cranial fossa
  - Perisinus abscess may be present outside the dura of lateral venous sinus in posterior cranial fossa.

Clinical Features

- Asymptomatic cases are discovered incidentally during cortical or modified radical mastoidectomy.
- Persistent headache, which disappears with free flow of pus from the ear (spontaneous abscess drainage), occurs on the side of otitis media.
- Severe earache.
- General malaise with low-grade fever.
- Pulsatile purulent otorrhea.

Diagnosis

Contrast enhanced CT (CECT) or MRI show dural elevation which is indicative of extradural abscess.

Treatment

- *Antibiotic therapy:* An antibiotic cover before and after the surgery is mandatory.
- *Mastoidectomy (cortical, radical or modified radical):* The overlying bone is removed until the healthy dura appears. In cases of strong suspicion, overlying intact tegmen tympani or sinus plate is deliberately removed to evacuate any collection of pus.

Follow-up

Patient should be closely observed for further intracranial complications, such as sinus thrombosis, meningitis or brain abscess.

SUBDURAL ABSCESS OR EMPYEMA

It refers to collection of pus in subdural space that lies between dura and arachnoid mater. The subdural space is divided into several large compartments, which are anatomically confined by foramen magnum, tentorium cerebelli, base of the brain and falx cerebri.

The subdural empyema is the rarest complication now and used to be fatal in preantibiotic era.

Pathology

Infection can spread either by erosion of bone and dura or by thrombophlebitic process (intervening bone remains intact). Pus in the subdural space lies against the convex surface of cerebral hemisphere and results in pressure symptoms. Later on the pus gets loculated at various places in subdural space. The developing subdural empyema quickly evolves into a fatal mass.

Clinical Features

Sudden unusually severe headache, which is usually associated with fever and vomiting and rapid deterioration of patient, points towards subdural abscess.

The clinical features are due to meningeal irritation, thrombophlebitis of cortical veins of cerebrum and raised cerebrospinal fluid (CSF) pressure.

- *Meningeal irritation:* Headache, fever (102° F or higher), malaise, progressive drowsiness, neck rigidity and Kernig's sign.
- *Thrombophlebitis of cortical veins of cerebrum:* Aphasia, contralateral hemiplegia and hemianopia. The Jacksonian type of epileptic fits may progress to status epilepticus.
- *Raised CSF pressure:* Papilledema, ptosis and dilated pupil due to CN III involvement. Other CNs may also be involved.

Diagnosis

- *MRI:* It is superior to CT. It can distinguish between epidural and subdural abscesses. Multiple, discrete, lobulated subdural collections may be seen. MRI allows differentiation of sterile, bloody and infected collections. The advantages of MRI include absence of bone artifact, increased contrast between bone, CSF and brain parenchyma and multiplanar imaging capabilities.
- *CT:* Loculated subdural abscess can be seen.

Lumbar puncture is contraindicated as it can result in herniation of cerebellar tonsil.

Treatment

It is a neurosurgical emergency.

- Series of burr holes are made to drain subdural space abscess.
- High dose intravenous antibiotics are administered.
- Radical mastoidectomy is done once the subdural abscess is treated.

MENINGITIS

It refers to the inflammation of leptomeninges (pia-arachnoid) and CSF of subarachnoid space, which surrounds brain, spinal cord and optic nerves. Mortality rate is very high.

Meningitis: It is the most common intracranial complication of suppurative otitis media. In infants and children, meningitis is often the complication of AOM, while in adults it occurs due to cholesteatoma. The one-third cases of meningitis are otogenic in origin.

Causes

- Suppurative otitis media (AOM and cholesteatoma)
- Temporal bone fracture
- CSF leak
- Middle ear and mastoid surgery.

Pathways of Infection

The middle ear and mastoid infection can reach meninges via following pathways:

- Preformed pathways like patent petrosquamosal suture and perineural spaces to the internal auditory canal (uncommon via endolymphatic ducts) via labyrinth (through round and oval windows).
- Retrograde venous thrombophlebitis.
- Direct erosion of bone (mastoiditis and petrositis) and dura.

Microbiology

- Major pathogens are *Hemophilus influenzae* and *Streptococcus pneumoniae*.
- Anaerobic organisms indicate interventricular rupture of brain abscess.
- Polymicrobial infection of CSF occurs in less than 1% of cases.

Clinical Features

The severity of symptoms and signs depends on severity of infection. The raised intracranial tension and meningeal and cerebral irritations vary with the extent of disease.

- Earliest symptoms include:
  - Fever (102–104° F) often with chills and rigors
  - Headache
  - Vomiting (sometimes projectile)
  - Photophobia
  - Irritability and restlessness
- Seizures (may be present in infants).
- Neck rigidity.
- Kernig's sign (extension of leg with thigh flexion on abdomen is painful).
- Brudzinski's sign (flexion of neck results in flexion of hip and knee).
- Motor deficit (cranial nerve palsies and hemiplegia).
- Deep tendon reflexes are exaggerated initially but later become sluggish or absent.
- Papilledema is a late feature.
- Drowsiness that may progress to delirium or coma.

Diagnosis

- **HRCT temporal bone:** It is the imaging modality of choice. It provides not only the bony details but also rules out congenital ear malformations, which permit CSF leak through an inner ear fistula.
- **MRI:** It shows middle ear fluid and inflammatory changes in brain and meninges.
- **Fundoscopy:** Indistinct disk margin and choking of vessels.
- **Lumbar puncture:** *Imaging usually precedes lumbar puncture to identify mass effect that can lead to herniation on LP.* CSF shows following features:
  - Cloudy (turbid) or yellow (xanthochromic).
  - Raised cell count with predominance of polymorphs.
  - Raised protein level.
  - Low level of sugar and chlorides.
  - Gram-staining to identify organisms.
  - Culture and sensitivity to find the causative organisms and their antibiotic sensitivity.
- **Ear pus for culture and sensitivity:** To find the causative organisms and their antibiotic sensitivity.

Treatment

Medical treatment always takes precedence over surgery. Surgery is done when general condition of patient permits. If there is no satisfactory response to medical treatment, early surgery is required.

- **Antibiotics:** Crystalline penicillin, ampicillin, chloromycetin or third generation cephalosporin (drugs of choice) should be given intravenously for 7–10 days. Antibiotics are changed according to the culture and sensitivity report.
- **Surgical:**
  - **Acute otitis media:** Myringotomy and/or cortical mastoidectomy.
  - **Cholesteatoma:** Radical or modified radical mastoidectomy.

OTOGENIC BRAIN ABSCESS

Brain abscess is a focal suppurative process of brain parenchyma. It is surrounded by an area of inflammation (encephalitis).

> **Brain Abscess**
> - Fifty percent cases of brain abscesses in adults and twenty five percent in children are otogenic. In adults, cholesteatoma and in children AOM are the most common causes.
> - Cerebral abscess occurs more frequently than cerebellar abscess. Most cerebellar abscesses are due to suppurative otitis media.

- **Bimodal age distribution:** Peak incidences are in early childhood and 4th decade of life.
- **Sex:** Male-to-female ratio is 3:1.
- Mortality is greater in cerebellar abscesses (about 25%).

Route of Infection

Otogenic brain abscesses are usually the result of venous thrombophlebitis rather than direct dural extension. Retrograde thrombophlebitis of dural vessels, which terminate in white matter (Fig. 14.5), is usually caused by the osteitis and granulation tissue.

- **Cerebral abscess:** It is often associated with extradural abscess that occurs due to erosion of the tegmen. In cases of retrograde thrombophlebitis the tegmen remains intact.
- **Cerebellar abscess:** It usually develops through the Trautmann's triangle. It is often associated with extradural abscess, perisinus abscess, sigmoid sinus thrombophlebitis and labyrinthitis. The retrograde thrombophlebitis is uncommon.

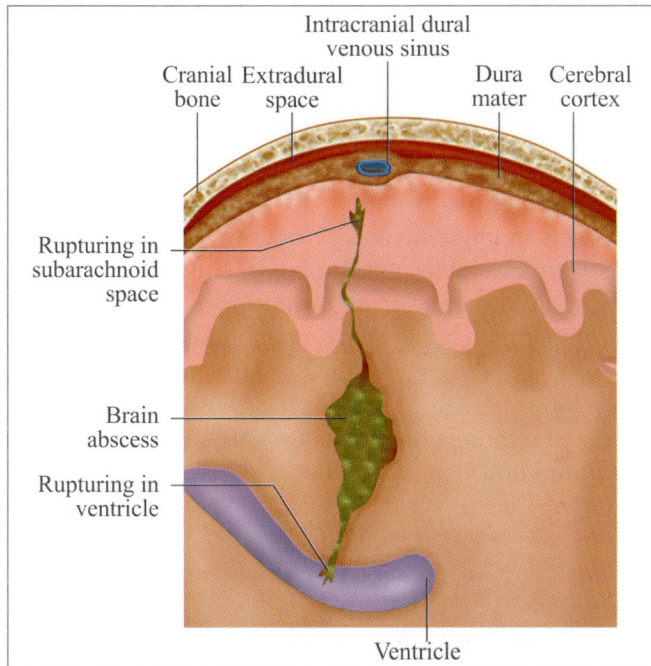

Fig. 14.5: Brain abscess rupture in ventricle and subarachnoid space. Rupture usually occurs in the ventricle because encapsulation of abscess is more on outer side

Bacteriology

Multiple organisms with high incidence of anaerobes are usually seen. Polymicrobial cultures are influenced by host immune status. *H. influenzae* is very rare.
- **Aerobic:**
  - *Gram-positive:* Pyogenic staphylococci, *Streptococcus pneumoniae* and *Streptococcus haemolyticus*.
  - *Gram-negative:* *Proteus mirabilis*, *Escherichia coli*, *Klebsiella* and *Pseudomonas aeruginosa*.
- **Anaerobic:** *Peptostreptococcus* and *Bacteroides fragilis*.

Pathogenesis and Pathology

There are four stages of brain abscess development:
1. *Stage of invasion (initial encephalitis) of 1–3 days:* The mild symptoms include headache, low-grade fever, malaise and drowsiness. They often pass unnoticed.
2. *Stage of localization (latent abscess) of 4–10 days:* In this asymptomatic stage, which may last for several weeks, pus is getting localized by the formation of a capsule.
3. *Stage of enlargement or early capsule formation (manifest abscess) of 10–13 days:* The enlarging abscess surrounded by a zone of edema aggravates the severity of clinical manifestations, which are due to raised intracranial tension and the focal involvement of brain.
   - Raised CSF pressure
   - Cerebrum and cerebellum show focal symptoms and signs.
4. *Stage of termination or late capsule formation (rupture of abscess) of 14 days:* The enlarging abscess ruptures into either the ventricle or subarachnoid space (Fig. 14.5) and results in fatal meningitis.

Clinical Features

The patient often appears toxic and drowsy and complains of deep cranium pain. Dizziness, ataxia, vomiting and nystagmus indicate cerebellar abscess. Temporal lobe abscess results in seizures.

As the brain abscess is often associated with extradural abscess, perisinus abscess, meningitis, sinus thrombosis and labyrinthitis, the clinical picture may be overlapping.

Clinical features are mainly due to raised intracranial tension and the area of brain affected.
- *Raised intracranial tension*
  - Headache is severe and generalized, worse in the morning.
  - Nausea and vomiting (usually projectile) is more common in cerebellar abscess.
  - Lethargy progresses to drowsiness, confusion, stupor and finally coma.
  - Papilledema usually appears after 2–3 weeks; however, it appears early in cerebellar abscess.
  - Slow pulse.
  - Subnormal temperature.
- *Localizing features of temporal lobe abscess*
  - *Nominal aphasia:* It occurs if the lesion is of dominant cerebral hemisphere. It is left side in right handed persons. Patient cannot name the common objects, such as key, pen and phone. However patient explains the utility of that object.
  - *Contralateral homonymous hemianopia:* It indicates pressure on the optic radiations. The visual field defect is usually in the upper quadrants. It can be recorded by perimetry.

> *Confrontation test:* The examiner stands in front of the patient and compares his visual field with that of the patient.

  - *Contralateral motor paralysis:* They are:
    - *Upward spread:* Facial palsy is followed by palsy of arm and leg.
    - *Inward spread towards internal capsule:* Paralysis of leg is followed by the paralysis of arm and face.
  - *Epileptic fits:* Small and involuntary smacking movements of lips and tongue. Generalized fits can also occur.
  - *Pupillary changes and oculomotor palsy:* It suggests transtentorial herniation.
- *Localizing features of cerebellar abscess*
  - Suboccipital headache associated with neck rigidity.
  - Spontaneous nystagmus.
  - Ipsilateral ataxia (patient staggers to the side of lesion).

- Finger nose test (past pointing and intention tremor).
- Dysdiadokokinesia (rapid pronation and supination movements become slow and irregular on the affected side).

Investigations

- **CT scan:** It reveals not only the site and size of an abscess but also shows other associated complications (extradural abscess, sigmoid sinus thrombosis). Temporal bone is better evaluated by CT than MRI.

> **"Ring" sign:** Brain abscess appears hypodense area surrounded by an area of edema.

- **MRI:** MRI is superior to CT. It detects not only the subtle changes in brain parenchyma but also spread of abscess into the subarachnoid space or into the ventricle.
- **Lumbar puncture:** *There is risk of coning and LP is usually not done.* CSF shows following features:
  - Rise in pressure.
  - Increase in protein with normal glucose.
  - White cell count is raised (polymorphs or lymphocytes depending on the acuteness of infection) but is much less than meningitis.

Treatment

It is controversial.
- **Medical:** The different medical treatments are:
  - Parenteral broad spectrum antibiotics, penicillin or its derivatives can be given. Anaerobes respond to metronidazole. Aminoglycoside such as gentamicin covers *Pseudomonas* and *Proteus*. As per the report of culture and sensitivity, antibiotics are changed. Newer and more effective antibiotics can obviate the neurosurgical intervention.
  - For raised intracranial tension, dexamethasone 4 mg intravenous 6 hourly or mannitol 20% in doses of 0.5 g/kg body weight can be administered.
  - Suction clearance of ear and use of topical ear drops.
- **Neurosurgical:** Life saving neurosurgical intervention takes precedence over the otologic management. Aspiration (pus sent for culture and sensitivity) is followed by repeat CT or MRI scans to *see* whether it is diminishing in size. Excision is required if abscess is expanding or not decreasing in size. Penicillin is instilled into the abscess after its aspiration. Neurosurgeon may consider any of the following procedures:
  - Burr hole (repeated aspiration of pus).
  - Excision of abscess.
  - Open incision of the abscess and evacuation of pus.
- **Otologic:** Only neurologically stabilized patients are taken for tympanomastoid surgery. Ear surgery is planned only after the abscess has been managed by antibiotics and neurosurgery. Cholesteatoma needs radical mastoidectomy, which removes the irreversible disease and exteriorizes the infected area.

LATERAL SINUS THROMBOPHLEBITIS

Syn: Sigmoid sinus thrombosis or otogenic suppurative thrombophlebitis

It refers to inflammation of inner wall of lateral venous sinus with formation of a thrombus, which gets infected. With the advent of new range of antibiotics, the incidence of this complication has declined yet mortality remains high.

Etiology

It is a complication of acute coalescent mastoiditis, masked mastoiditis and cholesteatoma.

Pathology

The pathological process is divided into the following four stages:
1. **Perisinus abscess:** Extradural abscess is formed outer to the dural wall of the sinus.
2. **Endophlebitis and mural thrombus:** Inflammation of the inner wall of the venous sinus results in thrombus formation (deposition of fibrin, platelets and blood cells) within the lumen of sinus.
3. **Obliteration of sinus and intrasinus abscess:** Expanding mural thrombus occludes the sinus lumen. Organisms invade the thrombus and form intrasinus abscess that releases infected emboli into the blood stream (septicemia).
4. **Extension of thrombus:** Thrombotic process continues both proximally and distally. It may spread to confluence of sinuses, superior sagittal sinus, cavernous sinus, mastoid emissary vein, jugular bulb or internal jugular vein.

Bacteriology

- **Acute otitis media:** β-hemolytic streptococci, Pneumococci.
- **Cholesteatoma:** *Bacillus proteus, Pseudomonas pyocynea, Escherichia coli* and *Staphylococci*.

Clinical Features

High-grade fever, toxic look, deep ear pain, restlessness, neck stiffness and papilledema are typical features of suppurative thrombophlebitis.
- **Fever:** Hectic type of fever with chills and rigors coincides with the release of septic emboli into blood stream. Fever has one or more peaks a day. Profuse sweating follows during the fall of temperature and patient becomes alert with a sense of well-being. This fever pattern resembles malaria but lacks regularity. Antibiotics may mask this classic pattern.

- **Headache:** During perisinus abscess, it is mild. Headache becomes severe when venous obstruction increases the intracranial pressure.

> **Griesinger's sign:** Tenderness and edema over the posterior part of mastoid, which is due to thrombosis of mastoid emissary vein, are pathognomonic for thrombophlebitis of sigmoid sinus.

- **Tenderness along jugular vein:** It indicates thrombophlebitis along the jugular vein.
- **Enlarged and tender jugular lymph nodes:** It may lead to torticollis.
- **Anemia and pallor:** They occur due to β-*hemolytic streptococci*. They are progressive.
- **Papilledema:** It is seen when clot extends to superior sagittal sinus, which is the continuation of right sigmoid and transverse sinus. Fundus shows blurring of disk margins, retinal hemorrhages or dilated veins.

> **Crowe-Beck test:** Pressure on opposite side internal jugular vein produces engorgement of retinal veins and supraorbital veins and subside on release of pressure.

- **Cavernous sinus thrombosis:** Proptosis, ptosis, chemosis and ophthalmoplegia.

Investigations

- **Blood culture** helps in finding the causative organisms.
  - Blood sample is taken when patients have chills and rigor because at that time organisms enter the blood stream.
  - Repeated cultures are required to identify the organisms.
- **Peripheral blood smear:** Absence of malarial parasites rules out malaria.
- **Culture and sensitivity** of ear discharge.
- **Lumbar puncture:** CSF examination is normal except for rise in pressure. It helps to exclude meningitis.

> **Queckenstedt's test or Tobey-Ayer test:** In this test CSF pressure is recorded by manometer when one or both jugular veins are compressed manually. Compression of affected (thrombosis) side of vein produces no effect. Compression of opposite side internal jugular vein produces rapid rise in CSF pressure.

- **Contrast enhanced CT scan (CECT):** Though not seen always, "delta sign" in axial cuts is typical of sinus thrombosis on CECT scan. It is an empty triangular area having rim enhancement and central low density area that is seen at the level of sigmoid sinus.
- **MRI** is more sensitive than CT. MRI shows blood flow, sinus obstruction, subsequent reversal of flow and higher resolution in detailing nerve tissue. On gadolinium-enhanced MRI, thrombus appears as a soft tissue signal associated with a vascular and bright appearance of dural walls (delta sign).

Complications

- Septicemia.
- Pyemic abscesses in lung, bone, joints or subcutaneous tissue.
- Meningitis and subdural abscess.
- Cerebellar abscess.
- Thrombosis of jugular bulb and jugular vein with involvement of CN IX, X and XI.
- Cavernous sinus thrombosis (chemosis, proptosis, fixation of eyeball and papilledema).
- Otitic hydrocephalus (thrombus extends to superior sagittal sinus through the transverse and confluence of sinuses).

Treatment

- **Antibiotic therapy:** Injection crystalline penicillin 1 million units intramuscularly 6 hourly cover pyogenic cocci. Antibiotic is changed as per the report of culture and sensitivity. Antibiotics are continued postoperatively for a week.
- **Mastoidectomy:** A complete cortical mastoidectomy in cases of AOM and modified radical mastoidectomy in cases of cholesteatoma is performed. Sinus bony plate must be removed to expose the dura and drain the perisinus abscess.

  Destruction of sinus dura, unhealthy and discolored dura with granulations on its surface indicate infected clot or intrasinus abscess, which must be drained. After packing the sinus above and below with a pack that lies between the bone and dura of sinus to control bleeding, dura of the sinus is incised and the infected clot and abscess is drained.

  Healthy red clot beyond the abscess at either end of sinus is not disturbed. Pack is removed after 5–6 days. The wound is closed secondarily.
- **Ligation of internal jugular vein:** Though rarely required, it is needed when antibiotic and surgical treatment fails to control embolic phenomenon and rigors and tenderness and swelling of internal jugular vein is spreading into the heart.
- **Supportive treatment:** Repeated blood transfusions combat anemia and improve patient's general condition.

OTITIC HYDROCEPHALUS

Otitic hydrocephalus consists of raised intracranial pressure and normal CSF. It is seen in both children as well as adolescents. Some prefer the term "benign raised intracranial tension" because there is no associated ventricular dilation.

In this rare complication spontaneous recovery occurs in some cases.

Mechanism

The following two factors result in raised intracranial tension.
1. The thrombosis of the sigmoid sinus, which continues as internal jugular vein, causes obstruction to venous return.
2. When thrombosis extends to superior sagittal sinus, which generally continues as right sigmoid sinus, it will impede the functioning (absorption of CSF) of arachnoid villi.

Clinical Features

The following clinical sign and symptoms are due to raised intracranial tension.
- ***Severe headache:*** It is the presenting complaint and may be associated with nausea and vomiting.
- ***Diplopia:*** It is due to paralysis of lateral rectus, which is supplied by CN VI.
- ***Blurring of vision:*** It is because of papilledema and optic atrophy.
    - ***Papilledema:*** The 5-6 diopters papilledema may be accompanied with patches of exudates and hemorrhages.
- ***Nystagmus***.

Diagnosis

- ***MRI:*** MRI allows better evaluation of venous sinuses.
- ***Lumbar puncture:*** *It should be done with caution lest herniation of cerebellar tonsil occur.* The pressure of CSF, which is sterile and normal in cell, protein and sugar content, exceeds 300 mm of water (normal 70–120 mm H_2O).

Treatment

- ***Medical***
    - Medical treatment includes corticosteroids, mannitol, diuretics and acetazolamide.
    - Middle ear infection requires antibiotic therapy.
- ***Surgical***
    - The raised CSF pressure must be reduced to prevent optic atrophy and blindness. This can be done with the following procedures:
        - Repeated lumbar puncture or placement of a lumbar drain.
        - Lumboperitoneal shunt drains CSF into the peritoneal cavity.
    - Mastoidectomy is done for managing the sinus thrombosis. Decompression of sigmoid sinus is recommended.
    - Optic sheath decompression prevents optic atrophy.

Self-evaluation Exercises

1. Which of the following statements are not true for Hyrtl's fissure (tympanomeningeal hiatus)?
    a. This embryonic remnant runs parallel to cochlear aqueduct
    b. It connects subarachnoid space to middle ear just anterior and inferior to the oval window
    c. It can be a source of congenital CSF otorrhea or meningitis in cases of middle ear infections
    d. Normally it is obliterated
    e. None from the above
2. Two weeks later the child of an acute otitis media develops a swelling over the mastoid, pain in the ear, fever and pulsatile ear discharge. What is your provisional diagnosis?
3. Which of the following are not the extracranial complications of suppurative otits media?
    a. Facial nerve palsy
    b. Hearing loss
    c. Labyrinthitis
    d. Extradural abscess
    e. None of the above
4. Which of the following are not the features of Gradenigo's syndrome?
    a. Mastoid air cells responsible for Gradenigo's syndrome are zygomatic cells
    b. Patient presents with the triad of ear discharge, CN VII paralysis and retro-orbital pain (involvement of trigeminal ganglion)
    c. It is seen in cases of petrositis (an abscess in the petrous apex), which is a complication of CSOM (coalescent mastoiditis and cholesteatoma)
    d. Egleton, Almoor, Ramadier and Frenker operations are done for drainage of petrositis abscess
    e. None of the above
5. Which of the following are the features of Bezold's abscess?
    a. Torticollis
    b. Tender swelling behind the angle of mandible
    c. Fever
    d. Chronic ear discharge with granulations in the ear canal
    e. All of the above

Contd...

Contd…

True (T)/False (F)

6. The treatment of coalescent mastoiditis includes intravenous antibiotics and radical mastoidectomy.
7. MRI is the investigation of choice in extradural, Bezold's and cerebral abscesses.
8. CT is the investigation of choice in cases of coalescent mastoiditis.
9. The treatment of postauricular mastoid abscess includes incision and drainage, antibiotics and mastoidectomy.
10. Sigmoid sinus thrombosis cannot be seen during mastoid exploration.
11. Griesinger's sign is the edema over the tragus seen in patients of lateral sinus thrombosis. The thrombosis of pterygoid emissary vein impedes venous drainage and causes edema over the tragus.
12. Picket-fence graph of temperature is the diurnal spikes of fever of 104° or 105° F and is the feature of sigmoid sinus thrombosis. The antibiotics use will not alter the pattern.

Answers

1. b
2. Coalescent mastoiditis
3. d
4. a, b
5. e
6. F
7. T
8. T
9. T
10. F
11. F
12. F

Pearls and Nuggets (Refresh your knowledge)

- **Congenital cholesteatoma:** A whitish mass behind a child's intact tympanic membrane with hearing loss indicates congenital cholesteatoma.
- **Facial nerve:** The regeneration and degree of return to normal is dependent on the degree of initial injury (neuropraxia vs. neurotmesis). The most important factor in history is whether the palsy develops slowly over days or immediately at the time of the injury.
- **Clinical features of temporal bone fracture:** Clinical features include hearing loss, dizziness, facial weakness, ear bleeding, hemotympanum, raccoon eyes, and/or bruising over the mastoid cortex (Battle's sign).
- **Radiological investigation for temporal bone fracture:** The best radiologic examination is a fine cut, axial and coronal, temporal bone high resolution CT scan.
- **Indications for surgical exploration of the facial nerve in temporal bone fracture:** They include:
  - Immediate onset of complete facial paralysis.
  - Delayed onset of complete facial paralysis associated with
    - Radiologic evidence of a fracture through the fallopian canal of facial nerve.
    - Poor prognostic testing with electroneuronography (EnoG) or electromyography (EMG).
- **CT and MRI temporal bone:** Thin sectioned high resolution CT is ideal for looking temporal bone abnormalities or fractures, but MRI is gold standard for acoustic neuroma.

Chapter 15

Evaluation of Vertigo

> ### ⊙ Specific Learning Objectives
> After going through the chapter, you should be able to answer the following questions:
> - How will you take the history of a dizzy patient?
> - Describe the commonly performed vestibular function tests.
> - What are the different types of spontaneous nystagmus and their clinical importance?
> - Which are the distinguishing characteristics of peripheral and central vertigo?
> - What do you know about: (1) Fistula test; (2) Dix-Hallpike test?

EVALUATION–GENERAL OUTLINE

The history (Box 15.1) and examination provide important clues to the diagnosis. A patient's history, which is of paramount importance in cases of balance disorders, often provides enough information to diagnose causes for various types of dizziness.

Audiogram

Audiometry is usually performed in all the cases of vertigo. It helps in establishing the diagnoses of peripheral vestibular disorders, which are accompanied with hearing loss, such as Ménière's disease.

SPONTANEOUS NYSTAGMUS

Nystagmus consists of involuntary, rhythmical and oscillatory movement of eyes. It may be horizontal, vertical or rotatory. Vestibular jerky nystagmus has a slow and a fast component. The direction of nystagmus is indicated by the direction of the fast component.

Method of Eliciting Nystagmus

The patient is either seated or lies supine on the bed. The examiner's finger is about 30 cm from the patient's eyes in the central position. The finger is moved to the right or left, up or down 30° from the central position, while the patient's eyes follow the finger. If the eye is moved more than 30° from central position it results in gaze nystagmus.

> **Box 15.1: Elements in the history of dizzy patients**
> - Description of the dizziness:
>   - Vertigo and oscillopsia
>   - Disequilibrium and unsteadiness
>   - Lightheadedness
>   - Presyncope
> - Episodic or continuous.
> - Duration of the individual attacks (seconds, minutes, hours, days or months).
> - Associated/concomitant symptoms:
>   - Ear: Discharge, pain, hearing loss, tinnitus, ear fullness
>   - Eye: Diplopia, vision loss
>   - Headache
>   - CNS: Paralysis and paresthesias, dysarthria, dysphagia
>   - Sweating, dyspnea and palpitation.
> - Effect of head movements (worse, better or no effect).
> - Specific positions that induce vertigo.
> - Preceding history of:
>   - Trauma (physical, barotraumas, surgical)
>   - Medicines for infections, hypertension, hyperglycemia and cardiac arrhythmias and CNS disorders.
> - Triggering events like stimuli (sound, pressure, or movements), rolling onto the side in bed.
> - Medical conditions: hypothyroidism, diabetes mellitus, anemia, autoimmune diseases and hypoperfusion of brain from postural hypotension or cardiac arrhythmia.
> - Psychogenic disorders: anxiety panic disorders and agoraphobia.

Interpretations
- Presence of spontaneous nystagmus usually indicates an organic lesion.

- Peripheral vestibular nystagmus is due to lesions of labyrinth and CN VIII while central vestibular nystagmus is due to lesions in the central neural pathways (vestibular nuclei, brainstem, and cerebellum).
- In irritative lesions or stimulation of the labyrinth (serous labyrinthitis and paroxysmal benign positional vertigo) the direction of the nystagmus is towards the side of lesion.
- In paretic lesions (purulent labyrinthitis, trauma to labyrinth, and damage of CN VIII) nystagmus is in the opposite direction.
- Nystagmus of peripheral origin is suppressed by optic fixation (by looking at a fixed point) and enhanced in darkness and on closing the eyes. The use of Frenzel glasses (20 diopter glasses) abolishes optic fixation. Central nystagmus is not suppressed by optic fixation.
- Purely down beating vertical (Arnold Chiari malformation or degenerative lesion of cerebellum), up-beating vertical (lesions of pontomedullary junction, pons and mibrain) rotatory (syringomyelia), pendular (multiple sclerosis), dysconjugate and monocular nystagmus indicates central vestibular lesions.

Degree of Nystagmus (Alexander Law for Peripheral Vestibular Nystagmus)

The intensity of nystagmus is indicated by its degree.
- *First degree:* This weak nystagmus is present only when patient looks in the direction of fast component.
- *Second degree:* This moderate nystagmus is present when patient looks straight ahead.
- *Third degree:* This strong nystagmus is present even when patient looks in the direction of slow component.

Ewald's Law

It has following three major components:
1. Head and eye movements in the plane of canal being stimulated decide direction of endolymph flow.
2. Ampullopetal flow of endolymph is excitatory in horizontal (lateral) semicircular canal.
3. Ampullofugal flow of endolymph is excitatory in vertical (anterior and posterior) semicircular canals.

PAST-POINTING AND FALLING

The past-pointing and falling occur toward the slow component of nystagmus, which indicates the side of vestibular weakness. In case of left side acute vestibular failure, fast component of the nystagmus will be towards right side whereas the past-pointing and falling will be towards the left (side of the slow component).

FISTULA TEST

Principle

The pressure changes in the external canal are transmitted to the labyrinth. In cases of labyrinthine and perilymphatic fistula, it stimulates labyrinth and results in nystagmus and vertigo. When pressure is increased in external canal, ampullopetal flow of endolymph or displacement of cupula results in nystagmus of the same side.

If pressure is decreased in external ear canal, ampullofugal displacement of cupula or endolymph occurs. The quick component of induced nystagmus would be directed to the opposite side.

Method

It can be performed in two ways:
1. *Pressure on tragus:* Sudden inwards pressure on the tragus increases air pressure in the ear canal and stimulates the labyrinth.
2. *Siegel's speculum:* The increased pressure in the ear canal produces vertigo and nystagmus.

Interpretation

- *Negative fistula test:* Normally, the pressure changes in the external auditory canal (EAC) do not stimulate the labyrinth. It is absent in following conditions:
  - Normal persons
  - Dead labyrinth
- *Positive fistula test:* A positive fistula test also implies that the labyrinth is still functioning. It produces vertigo and nystagmus and is present in the following conditions:
  - *Labyrinthine fistula*: Erosion of horizontal semicircular canal as in cholesteatoma.
  - *Perilymphatic fistula:* Abnormal opening in the oval window (post-stapedectomy fistula) or the round window (rupture of round window membrane).
  - *Fenestration operation:* Surgically created window in the horizontal canal.
- *False negative fistula test:* It occurs when cholesteatoma covers the site of fistula and does not allow pressure changes to be transmitted to the labyrinth.
- *A false positive fistula test (Hennebert's sign):* It is the positive fistula test in the absence of a fistula. It is seen in following conditions:
  - *Congenital syphilis:* Stapes footplate becomes hypermobile.
  - *Meniere's disease:* It occurs in about 25% cases due to fibrous bands connecting utricular macula to the stapes footplate. Movements of stapes result in stimulation of the utricular macula.

VALSALVA MANEUVER

- *Forced exhalation with closed nose and mouth* increases pressure in the middle ear through Eustachian tube. It causes vertigo in some cases of perilymphatic fistulae.
- *Forced exhalation with closed glottis* raises intracranial pressure, which can cause dizziness in cases of anterior semicircular canal dehiscence and Arnold Chiari malformations.

> **Tullio's phenomenon:** In this vertigo is induced by loud sounds. The causes include perilymphatic and labyrinthine fistulae and congenital syphilis. Additional third labyrinthine window occurs in cases of fistula of semicircular canal and fenestration operation in the presence of mobile footplate of stapes.

DIX-HALLPIKE MANEUVER

Dix-Hallpike maneuver has a positive predictive value for the diagnosis of benign paroxysmal positional vertigo and differentiate it from central causes of vertigo.

Method

From the sitting position with head turned 45° to one side, patient is rapidly lowered and placed in supine position and head extends over the edge of the examination couch (Figs 15.1A and B). Eye movements are observed for 45 seconds and patient is brought back to upright position. The process is repeated with the head turned opposite side and then with the head extended supine. The classic eye movements are enhanced by the use of Frenzel lenses.

> **Frenzel glass:** Nystagmus is best observed in the darkened room by illuminated Frenzel glass, which is nothing but a 20 diopter lens.

Interpretations

The intensity of induced vertigo and nystagmus wanes with repeated maneuvers in peripheral vertigo, but is not affected in central vertigo. Purely vertical (usually downbeat) or torsional nystagmus without a latent period and unfatigable (does not wane with repeated maneuvers) suggests central causes for vertigo, such as a posterior fossa tumor or hemorrhage.

- **Features of peripheral vestibular lesions:** Presence of latency of onset of nystagmus, duration less than 1 minute, induced vertigo and nystagmus disappears with repeated testing (fatigable), and vertigo may recur with nystagmus in the opposite direction on return of head to upright position.
  - Combined vertical upbeating and rotary (torsional) component beating toward downward eye (superior poles of eyes beat toward the downward ear): This most common finding indicates:
    - Benign paroxysmal positional vertigo (BPPV) of posterior semicircular canal (canalithiasis).
  - Combined vertical downbeating and rotary (torsional) component beating toward upward eye (superior poles of eyes beat toward the upward ear):
    - Benign paroxysmal positional vertigo (BPPV) of superior semicircular canal (Canalithiasis). It is very rare.
  - Nystagmus present with patients head turned to both right and left sides:
    - Bilateral benign paroxysmal positional vertigo.
    - Head injury or brainstem ischemia.
- **Features of central vestibular lesions:** In head hanging position nystagmus begins without a latent period and persists with a constant slow-phase velocity for as long as the head position is maintained. Subjective vertigo is much less than expected from the intensity of nystagmus.

Pure vertical nystagmus is usually downbeating with respect to the head. It is the most common type in central vestibular lesions (Table 15.1).

HEAD THRUST TEST (VESTIBULO-OCULAR REFLEX) OR DOLL'S-EYE TEST

From the primary neutral position, brief, high-acceleration horizontal head thrusts are applied while patient is instructed to look at the examiner's nose. In normal persons, compensatory eye movements keep the patient's eyes remain stable on the examiner's nose. When the head is rotated on the side of hypoactive labyrinth it results in a delayed catch-up saccade to maintain gaze.

OPTOKINETIC TEST

- **Method:** Patient's eyes follow a series of vertical stripes on drum, which moves first from right to left and then left to right.
- **Interpretations:**
  - **Normal:** Nystagmus with slow phase in the direction of moving stripes.
  - **Abnormalities:** Brainstem and cerebral hemisphere lesions.

ROTATION TESTS

- **Method:** Patient sits with head flexed 30° in Barany's revolving chair, which is rotated 10 times in 20 seconds first in clockwise direction and then in anticlockwise

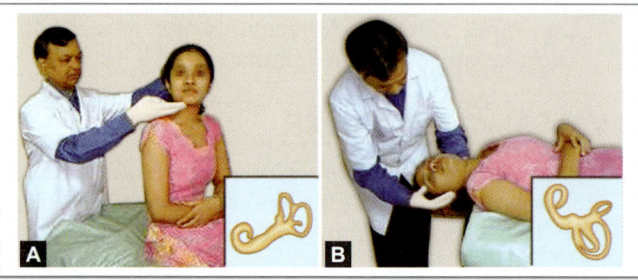

Figs 15.1A and B: Dix-Hallpike test for right side posterior canal BPPV. (A) First sitting position (inset shows debris near ampulla of posterior canal); (B) Second supine head hanging position (Inset shows debris moving away from the ampulla in the posterior canal)

Table 15.1: Distinguishing characteristics of peripheral and central vertigo

Features	Peripheral vertigo	Central vertigo
Nystagmus		
Type	Combined horizontal and torsional	Purely vertical (most common), horizontal, or torsional
Direction	One direction	May change direction
Visual fixation	Inhibits	No change
Fatigable	Yes	No
Latency	Present	Absent
Imbalance	Mild to moderate but able to walk	Severe and unable to stand or walk
Nausea and vomiting	Usually present and severe	Varies
Hearing loss, tinnitus	Common	Rare
Neurologic symptoms (motor and sensory deficiencies, ataxia, Horner's syndrome)	Absent	Common
Recovery	Begins within days	Slow
Head thrust sign	Present	Absent
Common causes	Benign paroxysmal positional vertigo, vestibular neuritis, Meniere's disease, trauma to labyrinth, infection and drugs	Vertebrobasilar insufficiency, cerebrovascular accidents, multiple sclerosis, brain tumors and cerebellar disorders

direction. The rotating Barany's chair is stopped suddenly and nystagmus is observed.
- *Advantage:* It can be done in cases of atresia of external auditory canal.
- *Disadvantge:* Both the labyrinths are stimulated simultaneously.
- *Interpretations:* Twenty-five to forty seconds nystagmus is normal.

CALORIC TEST

It compares the labyrinthine (lateral semicircular canal) functioning of both the ears, however there are no absolute figures for normality.

Fitzgerald-Hallpike Bithermal Caloric Test

The patient lies in supine position with head flexed 30° (to bring horizontal semicircular canal in vertical position) (Fig. 15.2). Ears are alternately irrigated for 40 seconds with water that is 7°C above and below the normal body temperature, i.e. 30° C and 44° C. The eyes are observed for nystagmus. A gap of 5–10 minutes is kept between each ear test. The time is recorded from the start of irrigation to the end of nystagmus on a calorigram. It is easy to remember the mnemonic COWS, which says that *"cold water will produce nystagmus on the opposite side while warm water on the same side."*

Interpretations

- *Canal paresis:* Lesser response than normal indicates depressed function of labyrinth as occurs in Meniere's disease.
- *Dead labyrinth:* No response indicates absence of labyrinthine functions as occurs in purulent labyrinthitis, ototoxicity and acoustic neuroma.
- *Directional preponderance:* The total duration of right side of nystagmus (not the side of ear), which is produced by cold water in left ear and warm water in right ear, is compared with the left side nystagmus that is generated by cold water in right ear and warm water in left ear. Twenty five to thirty percent more nystagmus on any one side is called *directional preponderance* to that particular side. It indicates side of the central lesion that is away from the side in a peripheral lesion. It does not localize the site of lesion in central vestibular pathways.
  - Ipsilateral canal paresis and contralateral directional preponderance (Meniere's disease).
  - Ipsilateral canal paresis and directional preponderance (acoustic neuroma).

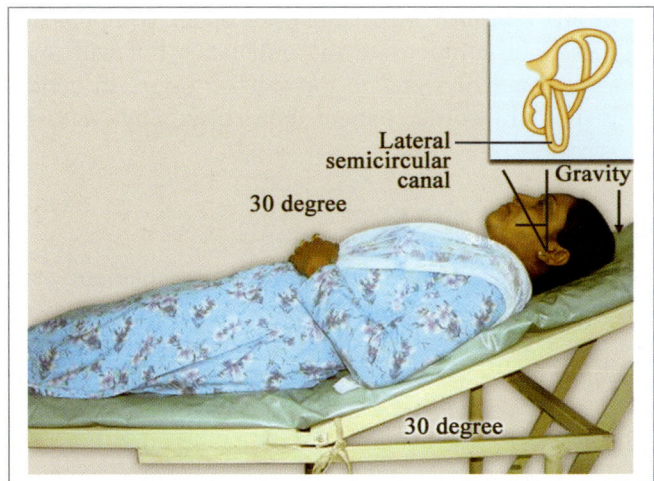

Fig. 15.2: Caloric testing. In reclined position, 30° elevation of head end of table brings the lateral semicircular canal in vertical plane (inset)

Modifications
- *Screening test:* In certain cases only when genuinely needed, a strong stimulus (2 mL ice water) is used to know the presence or absence of vestibular function.
- *Modified Kobrak test:* Ear is irrigated with ice cold water (5, 10, 20 and 40 mL) for 1 minute. Patient sits in a chair with extended head at 60° and this brings lateral canal in vertical position. Normally opposite side nystagmus appears with 5 mL ice water. No nystagmus with 40 mL ice water indicates dead labyrinth.
- *Cold air caloric test:* It is indicated when patient has chronic suppurative otitis media (CSOM). Through Dundas-Grant tube (coiled copper tube wrapped with cloth) air is blown into the ear. The tube is cooled by moistening the cloth with ethyl chloride.

TANDEM WALKING

The patient walks (first with eyes open and then closed) along a straight line. In uncompensated peripheral vestibular lesions, with eyes closed, the patient deviates to the diseased side. Patients with peripheral vertigo may have some impaired balance, but are still able to walk. But patients with central vertigo often cannot walk or even stand without falling.

ROMBERG'S TEST

Although Romberg's sign is usually done in cases of vestibular and proprioceptive disorders, it was found only 19% sensitive for peripheral vestibular disorders.
- *Method:* The patient stands with feet together and arms by the side. First the eyes are open and then close. In sharpened Romberg test, the patient stands with one heel in front of toes and arms folded across the chest.
- *Interpretations:* With the eyes open, compensated cases can compensate the imbalance but with eyes closed patient sways to the side of lesion. In central vestibular disorder, patient shows instability even with eyes open.

CEREBELLAR TESTS

Gaze evoked, rebound and abnormal optokinetic type nystagmus are present in cerebellar lesions. Depending on the site of lesion, cerebellar disorders can have following features:
- *Cerebellar hemisphere*
  - *Asynergia:* Finger nose test becomes abnormal.
  - *Dysmetria:* Patient is not able to control range of motion.
  - *Adiadochokinesia:* Patient is unable to perform rapid pronation and supination.
  - *Rebound phenomenon:* Patient is not able to control movement when opposing force is suddenly withdrawn.
- *Vermis*
  - Wide base gait and inability to make sudden turns on walking
  - Falls
  - Truncal ataxia

HYPERVENTILATION

Hyperventilation for 30 seconds helps in ruling out hyperventilation syndrome in psychogenic causes of vertigo. One should be aware that rarely it can cause true vertigo in patients with perilymphatic fistula and acoustic neuroma.

ORTHOSTATIC HYPOTENSION

Orthostatic hypotension upon standing (systolic blood pressure drops 20 mm Hg or more and pulse increase 10 beats per minute) is seen in cases of dehydration or autonomic dysfunction.

SPECIAL VESTIBULAR INVESTIGATIONS

A wide range of vestibular investigations (such as electronystagmography, caloric and rotating chair tests) is available but they have few clinical uses. The following tests are rarely of clinical value and are usually not done.
- *Rotating chair test:* The rotating chair stimulates both sides of labyrinth concurrently and can test each pair of semicircular canals separately in each of the 3 different planes.
- *Electronystagmography (ENG):* It records eye movements and detects nystagmus. The torsional component of nystagmus cannot be recorded with electronystagmography. Currently videonystagmography (VNG) has become more popular.
- *Computerized tests (such as posturography):* The computerized system such as force plate, records all changes in the position of the center of gravity of the patient, who stands on a small platform. The amount of sway in various situations such as with eyes closed and standing on one leg is recorded. It is difficult to justify the use of these tests for routine clinical work.
- *Galvanic test:* It distinguishes labyrinth lesions from the vestibular nerve. A current of 1 mA is passed to ear. A normal person would sway towards the side of test ear. Patient is blind folded and standing with out-stretched arms. Body sway is analyzed by a special platform.

Self-evaluation Exercises

1. Which of the following are not true for Tullio's phenomenon?
   a. Vertigo is induced by pressure changes
   b. The causes include perilymphatic and labyrinthine fistulae and congenital syphilis
   c. Additional third labyrinthine window in cases of fistula of semicircular canal and fenestration operation in the presence of mobile footplate of stapes
   d. None of the above
2. Which of the following are true for fistula test?
   a. Performed by applying intermittent pressure on the tragus or by using Siegle's speculum
   b. Positive in cases of labyrinthine fistula, hypermobile stapes footplate, following fenestration surgery and erosion of the horizontal semicircular canal in cholesteatoma
   c. Positive fistula indicates that labyrinth is still active and alive
   d. The test is negative when labyrinth is dead
   e. All of the above
3. What are the causes of ipsilateral (same direction) nystagmus?
   a. Irrigation of ear with warm water
   b. Serous labyrinthitis
   c. Irrigation of ear with cold water
   d. Purulent labyrinthitis
4. What are the causes of contralateral (opposite direction) nystagmus?
   a. Purulent labyrinthitis
   b. Labyrinthectomy
   c. Irrigation of ear with warm water
   d. Serous labyrinthitis
5. Which of the following are not true for Fitzgerald-Hallpike bithermal caloric test?
   a. The posterior semicircular canal is stimulated by irrigating cold (30°C) and warm (44°C) water in the EAC
   b. Cold water induces opposite side nystagmus while warm water results into the same side nystagmus
   c. To bring the lateral semicircular canal in vertical position, patient's head is raised 30° forward if s/he is in supine position but in a sitting position the head is tilted 60° backward
   d. None of the above

True (T)/False (F)

6. Utricle is the first part of membranous labyrinth to appear during the intrauterine life.
7. Semicircular canals connect with the utricle via 6 openings.
8. Semicircular canals of two sides are paired synergistically (horizontal canals of both sides and one side posterior with opposite side superior).
9. Hennebert's sign is positive fistula test in the absence of fistula. The causes include congenital syphilis (utricular adhesions to stapes) and some cases of Meniere's disease.
10. Romberg's sign is indicative of the dorsal column (somatosensory) lesions and not the cerebellar lesions.
11. Nystagmus is best observed in the darkened room by illuminated Frenzel glass, which is nothing but a 40 diopter lens.
12. Dix-Hallpike test is used in patients with episodic positional vertigo.
13. On Dix-Hallpike testing, peripheral nystagmus appears immediately without a latent period as soon as head is in critical position.

Answers

1. a
2. e
3. a, b
4. a, b
5. a
6. T
7. F
8. T
9. T
10. T
11. F
12. T
13. F

Chapter 16

Peripheral Vestibular Disorders

Specific Learning Objectives

After going through the chapter, you should be able to answer the following questions:
- Describe the etiopathogenesis, clinical features and management of benign paroxysmal positional vertigo.
- What do you know about the acute vestibular neuritis?
- Describe the etiopathogenesis, clinical features and management of Meniere's disease.
- What are the differences between perilymphatic and labyrinthine fistula?
- What are the differences between serous and purulent labyrinthitis?

INTRODUCTION

Benign paroxysmal positional vertigo (BPPV), acute vestibular neuritis and Ménière's disease are the most common causes of vertigo. Otitis media is the most common cause of vertigo in children. Some of the other common causes of peripheral vertigo include:
- Delayed endolymphatic hydrops
- Recurrent vestibulopathy
- *Fistulas:* Labyrinthine and perilymphatic
- *Labyrinthitis:* Serous and suppurative
- Syphilis

BENIGN PAROXYSMAL POSITIONAL VERTIGO (BPPV)

BPPV is the most common cause of vertigo. The mean age of onset is fourth to fifth decades. Incidence increases with age.

Etiological Factors
- Most common are closed head injury and vestibular neuronitis (vertigo lasting days).
- Infections
- Old age
- Surgery (stapedectomy or nonotologic)
- Prolonged bed rest and inactivity

Pathogenesis

Otoconia gets displaced from utricle to posterior semicircular canal.

- *Cupulolithiasis:* Deposition of otoconia on the cupula of posterior semicircular canal.
- *Canalithiasis:* Free floating otoconia within the lumen of posterior semicircular canal.

Clinical Features

- Sudden brief (lasting for seconds) spells of severe whirling/spinning vertigo associated with change in head position, so the triggers are:
  - Rolling over in the bed
  - Getting into bed and assuming a supine position
  - Arising from a bending position
  - Extending the neck
  - Turning rapidly
- Vertigo spell lasts for seconds and never more than a minute. However, patients usually complain of longer subjective feeling of dizziness.
- Bouts of vertigo are clustered in time. Remissions may last for months or more.
- The active spells may be associated with the feeling of light headedness or mild imbalance, which is worsened by head movement.
- Some patients have chronic balance problem, which may be worse at the time of awakening from the sleep.

Diagnosis

Dix-Hallpike test: Nystagmus and/or vertigo is elicited by Dix-Hallpike test. For details of the test method and interpretations, *see* Chapter 'Evaluation of Vertigo'.

Chapter 16 • Peripheral Vestibular Disorders

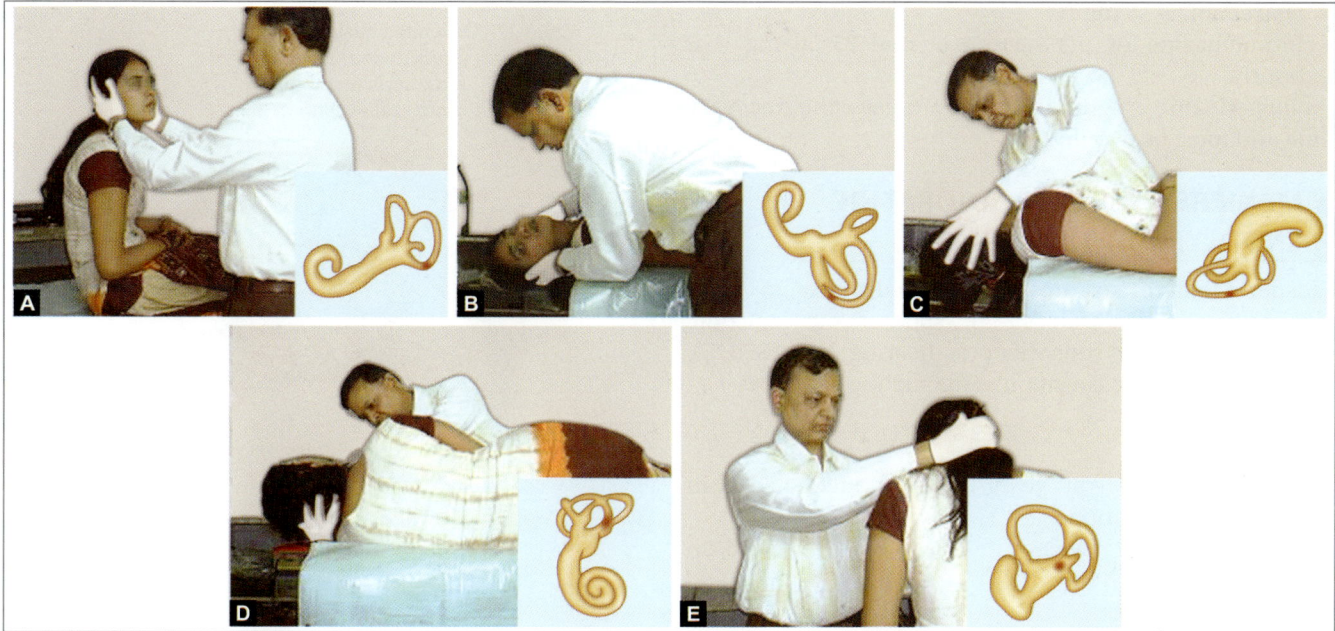

Figs 16.1A to E: Canalith repositioning for right posterior canal benign paroxysmal positional vertigo. (A) Patient sitting with head turned right and debris near ampulla (inset); (B) Patient in supine position with extended neck and debris move away from the ampulla in the posterior canal (inset); (C) Head moved 90° to left and debris comes near the common crus (inset); (D) Patient rolled onto left and head faces down and debris starts entering into the utricle from the common crus (inset); (E) Patient in upright position and debris collects in utricle (inset)

Differential Diagnoses

- Vascular compression of cranial nerve VIII complex.
- Multiple sclerosis.
- Acoustic neuroma.

Treatment

Treatment consists of repositioning maneuvers. There is no role of any medicine. The following maneuvers are effective in majority of the BPPV patients.

Repositioning Maneuvers (Figs 16.1A to E)

After the maneuver, patients are told to sleep with 45° elevated head and avoid bending. En bloc movement of the head and body is preferred during these maneuvers. Mastoid vibrator gives slightly better results.

Epley maneuver (Fig. 16.1): It is effective in 90% cases of posterior canal BPPV. Meclizine or benzodiazepine 1 hour before may be given in anxious patients. First 2 positions (upright and supine position with extended neck turned 45°) are similar to Dix-Hallpike maneuver (*see* Chapter 'Evaluation of Vertigo'). Then head is rolled 180° in two 90° increments so that the offending ear is up. From this position, patient is brought to the sitting position. The repositioning maneuver is repeated again and again until no nystagmus is produced. Head remains in that particular position until any nystagmus resolves.

ACUTE VESTIBULAR NEURITIS

Syn: Vestibular neuronitis, acute viral labyrinthitis

This is the second most common cause of peripheral vestibular vertigo after the BPPV.

Etiology

The exact cause of the disease is yet not known. Fifty percent patients have preceding history of upper respiratory viral infections and sinusitis.

Clinical Features

- Often patients have dramatic sudden onset of vertigo and attendant vegetative symptoms (such as nausea, vomiting and sweating) with gradual but definite improvement throughout the course.
- Occasionally, patients have bouts of attacks over several weeks. Few patients complain of stuffiness in their ear.
- The direction of horizontal or horizontal-rotary nystagmus is towards the healthy ear.

Prognosis

Vertigo usually lasts many hours to 1–2 weeks and then spontaneously disappears over weeks to months.

Treatment

The treatment is nonspecific and includes:
- Hospitalization and intravenous (IV) fluids.

- Diazepam, 5–10 mg IV
- Promethazine IV, per rectum or oral 25–50 mg, 4–6 hourly.

Prolonged antivertiginous therapy delays the recovery time and must be avoided.

MÉNIÈRE'S DISEASE (IDIOPATHIC ENDOLYMPHATIC HYDROPS)

Prosper Ménière first described this disorder in 1861. Symptom complex consists of spontaneous episodic vertigo, fluctuating sensorineural hearing loss (SNHL), tinnitus and often a sensation of fluctuating ear fullness.

Incidence
- Age of onset is 4–90 years but peak incidence is in 40–60 year age group.
- Bilateral disease develops in 47% of cases followed up for 20 years.

Etiology
Exact cause of the disease is not yet known.
- ***Viral:*** The causative roles of viruses (herpes simplex virus, cytomegalovirus or varicella-zoster virus) remain uncertain.
- ***Hereditary:*** Familial occurrence in 10–20% cases. There is an autosomal dominant mode of inheritance.
- ***Autoimmune:*** Certain genetically acquired major histocompatibility complexes specifically human leukocyte antigens B8/DR3 and Cw7 have been associated with Meniere's disease.

Pathogenesis
- ***Inadequate absorption of endolymph by the endolymphatic sac*** due to perisaccular ischemia and fibrosis.
- ***Overaccumulation of endolymph*** at the expense of perilymphatic space results in the distortion of membranous labyrinth (Fig. 16.2). Alterations in the size of endolymphatic duct and sac along with reductions in tubular specializations of the lining of these structures have been observed.
- ***Endolymphatic hydrops*** mainly occurs in pars inferior (cochlea and saccule) and changes in pars superior (utricle and semicircular canal) are usually less obvious.
- ***Basilar membrane*** gets distended into scala tympani.
- ***Hennebert's sign:*** Saccular distension can distort not only utricle and semicircular canals but can also come in contact with stapes footplate. That can cause Hennebert's sign.
- ***Hair cells and their neurons*** are usually spared.
- ***Acute attack:*** Rupture of membranous labyrinth allows leakage of potassium-rich endolymph into perilymph.

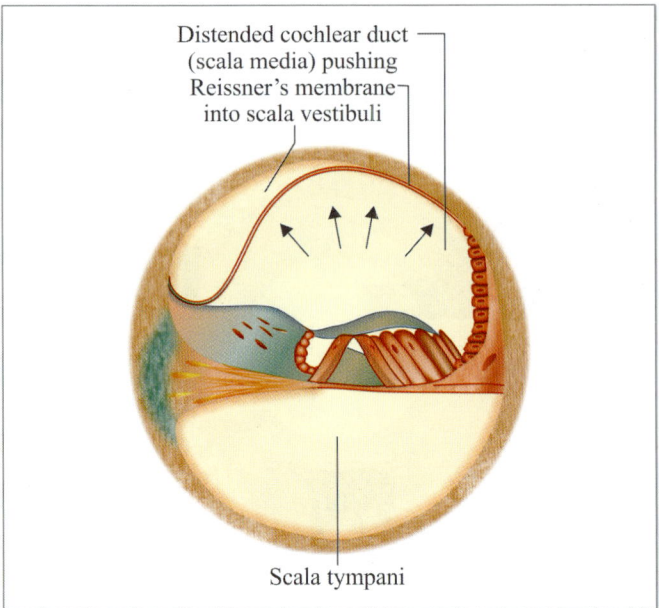

Fig. 16.2: Ménière's disease

The high concentration of K^+ depolarizes the neurons and inactivates both vestibular and auditory neurons that result in vertigo (paralytic nystagmus) and deafness.
- ***Remission:*** Healing of membranes allows restitution of normal chemical and clinical status.
- ***Progressive hearing loss:*** Repeated membranous rupture and potassium exposure leads to chronic deterioration in the functions of inner ear.

Clinical Features
- The typical presentation consists of recurring attacks (3–11 per year) of spinning vertigo in horizontal axis (usually for minutes to 2–3 hours) with tinnitus and hearing loss. Attack lasting more than a day is inconsistent with the diagnosis.
- ***Vertigo attacks*** are usually preceded by an aura consisting of fullness in the ear, increasing tinnitus and decrease in hearing. Attacks may be sudden without any warning or may awaken patient from sleep.
  - Attacks may cease spontaneously after 2 years or may occur for 20–40 years.
  - ***Vestibular and cochlear Ménière or hydrops:*** In the early phases of disease, patient may have either vestibular (recurrent vestibulopathy) or auditory symptoms. The terms vestibular Ménière or cochlear Ménière are considered inappropriate by American Academy of Otolaryngology-Head and Neck Surgery Committee on Hearing and Equilibrium (Box 16.1).
  - Attacks are often accompanied by nausea, vomiting, diarrhea or sweating. Vertigo is exacerbated with any head movement.

> **Box 16.1: Classification and diagnosis of Ménière's disease. Committee of hearing and equilibrium. American Academy of Otolaryngology-Head and Neck Surgery**
>
> - **Certain:** Confirmed by histopathology.
> - **Definite:** Two or more episodes of spontaneous whirling vertigo lasting for 20 minutes or more.
>   - Documented sensory hearing loss (HL) on audiometry on at least one occasion.
>   - Tinnitus or aural fullness.
>   - Other causes excluded.
> - **Probable:**
>   - One episode of spontaneous whirling vertigo.
>   - Documented sensory HL.
>   - Tinnitus or aural fullness.
>   - Other causes excluded.
> - **Possible:**
>   - **Vestibular variant:** Episodes of spontaneous whirling vertigo without documented HL.
>   - **Cochlear variant:** Fluctuating or fixed sensory HL with disequilibrium but without episodes of spontaneous whirling vertigo.
>   - Other causes excluded.

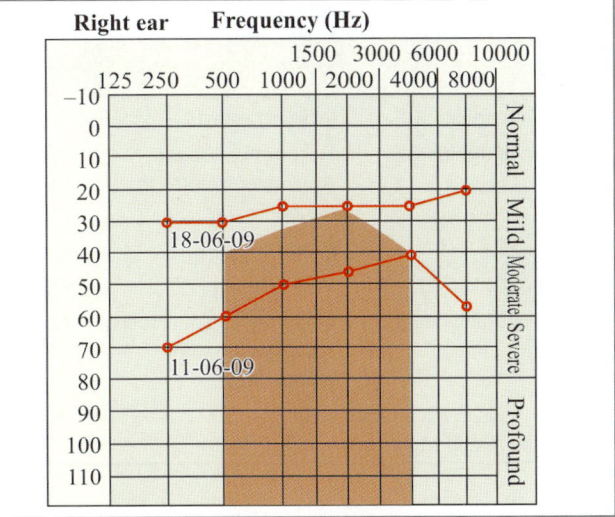

Fig. 16.3: Audiogram Ménière's disease right ear. Low-frequency fluctuating (improvement after 1 week) sensorineural hearing loss in right ear

- Between the attacks patient may be totally symptom-free or feel disequilibrium, light headedness or tilt.
- *Hearing loss* is fluctuating and progressive. Diplacusis (a difference in the perception of pitch between the ears) and recruitment (intolerance to loud sounds) may be present.
- *Tinnitus* is nonpulsatile and may be whistling or roaring, continuous or intermittent. It becomes louder or changes pitch as an attack approaches and improves after the attack.
- *Lermoyez attack:* In this, increased tinnitus and hearing loss precedes the vertiginous episode and dramatically resolves with onset of vertigo.
- *Drop attacks (otolithic crises of Tumarkin)*
  - Occasionally sudden unexplained falls without loss of consciousness or associated vertigo occur. Patient feels pushing or moving during this short-lived spells.
  - Acute utriculosaccular dysfunction leads to inappropriate postural adjustment via vestibulospinal pathway.
  - Other causes of drop spells which must be kept in mind, include cardiogenic, vertebral basilar insufficiency and migraine.

Nystagmus

The diseased ear cannot be determined just on the basis of direction of nystagmus. The direction of horizontal nystagmus, which is the cardinal finding, varies over the course of the attack.
- Early irritative nystagmus (ipsilateral)
- Later paralytic nystagmus (contralateral)
- Late recovery nystagmus (ipsilateral)

Audiogram (Fig. 16.3)

- Low frequency fluctuating and progressive SNHL and a coincident nonchanging high frequency loss occurs. Average pure tone loss is of 50 dB. Profound hearing loss is rare.
- It is peaked at 2 kHz (tent-like audiogram).
- In early disease, it shows a rising curve (lower frequencies are affected more). Overtime hearing loss flattens.
- *Recruitment* is present in 56% cases.
- *Staging* is done on the basis of pure tone average (500, 1,000, 2,000 and 3,000 Hz) in dB of the worst hearing loss (audiogram) in the interval of 6 months before treatment. Ménière's disease has been graded into following 4 stages:
  - *Stage I:* Less than 25 dB
  - *Stage II:* 26–40 dB
  - *Stage III:* 41–70 dB
  - *Stage IV:* More than 70 dB
- *Speech audiometry:* A mean speech discrimination score of 53%.

Differential Diagnoses

Ménière's disease, which is an idiopathic lesion, is a clinical diagnosis. The differences between various causes of dizziness are given in Table 16.1.

Investigations

Findings observed in different investigations include:
- *Glycerol test:* Ingestion of glycerin 1.5 g/kg mixed with equal volume of juice is followed by serial audiograms over 3 hours.
  - *Positive test:* 25 dB shift at 3 consecutive frequencies, or 16% improvement in speech discrimination.
- *Dehydrating agents:* Urea, glycerol and furosemide produce measurable improvement in audiometric

Table 16.1: Differential diagnoses of common causes of dizziness

Clinical features	Meniere's disease	Vestibular neuritis	Benign paroxysmal positional vertigo	Acoustic neuroma
Type of dizziness	Whirling vertigo	Whirling vertigo	Whirling vertigo	Unsteadiness
Duration of dizziness	Recurrent episodes (lasting for minutes to hours)	Acute prolonged attack (lasting for days)	Short spells (lasting for seconds) in certain positions	Recurrent momentary or chronic
Tinnitus	Present	Absent	Absent	Present
Vomiting	Very common	Always	Uncommon	Rare
Sensorineural hearing loss	Moderate and fluctuating sensory type with recruitment	Absent	Absent	Progressive neural type with tone decay
Cranial nerve involvement (V, VII, IX, X and XI)	Absent	Absent	Absent	Present in late stages

score, reduction in summating potential negativity (electrocochleography) and change in gain of vestibulo-ocular response to rotational stimulation. Sensitivity and specificity vary widely.

- **Electronystagmography:** Caloric response is significantly reduced in 48–73.5% cases. Complete loss occurs in 6–11%.
- **Electrocochleography:** It is infrequently used. Ratio of summating potential and action potential increases.
    - **Summating potential:** It is larger and more negative due to the distension of basilar membrane into scala tympani.
    - **Action potential (AP) of CN VIII:** Reduction in amplitude.

Medical Treatment

There is no curative therapy for Ménière's disease. Following conservative measures are usually taken:

- **General measures**
    - **Reassurance:** Explaining the benign nature of disease relieves the patient's anxiety.
    - **Lifestyle changes**
        - Cessation of smoking should be recommended.
        - Avoid excessive intake of water and salt.
        - Avoid too much tea, coffee and alcohol.
        - Avoid stress, practice mental relaxation exercises, meditation and yoga.
        - Avoid flying, diving and working at great heights to prevent accident in cases of sudden episode.
- **Acute attack**
    - **Reassurance and bed rest**
    - **Vestibular sedatives** are given parenterally if vomiting precludes oral use. They take care of vertigo and anxiety and include prochlorperazine (stemetil), promethazine theoclate (avomine), dimenhydrinate (dramamine), and diazepam. Atropine can also be very effective.
    - **Vasodilators:**
        - Inhalation of carbogen (5% CO_2 with 95% O_2) causes cerebral vasodilatation and improves labyrinthine circulation.
        - Histamine diphosphate 2.75 mg in 500 mL glucose, slow IV drip helps in managing acute episodes but is contraindicated in asthmatics and should not be given empty stomach. The adverse side effects include tachycardia, disturbed cardiac rhythm, hypotension, hyperthermia and bronchospasm.
- **Chronic phase**
    - **Dietary modifications**
        - Salt restriction
        - Intermittent dehydration
        - Hyperosmolar dehydration
    - **Diuretics**
        - Hyperosmotic diuretic isosorbide.
        - Acetazolamide (carbonic anhydrase inhibitor).
        - Furosemide 40 mg on alternate day with potassium supplement.
    - **Vasodilators:** Quantitative improvement was not seen consistently with these medications.
        - Histamine, betahistine, papaverine analog, eupavarine, nicotinic acid, adenosine triphosphate and dipyridamole.
    - **Symptomatic medications:** They are beneficial in reducing the symptoms and in improving tolerance.
        - Antivertiginous, antiemetics, sedatives, antidepressants and psychiatric treatment.
    - **Propantheline bromide:** Pro-Banthine 15 mg, 3 times a day is found effective in some cases.
    - **Elimination of allergen:** In cases of allergy, the causative allergen should be eliminated or desensitized.
    - **Hormones:** Endocrinal hypofunctioning, such as hypothyroidism, need appropriate replacement therapy.

- *Other therapies*
  - Acupuncture
  - Herbal remedies
- *Pulsed positive pressure in external auditory canal (EAC) and pressure equalization tube (Meniett device therapy):* This has been approved by FDA. Through the ventilation tube (grommet) pressure waves are delivered to round window. As the device is coupled to EAC it can be used by patient at home.
- *Bilateral Ménière's disease.*
  - *Parenteral streptomycin:* Streptomycin is primarily vestibulotoxic and usually leaves hearing unchanged. It is indicated only for incapacitating bilateral Ménière's disease.
- *Immunosuppressant therapy*
  - Chronic steroids
  - Nonsteroidal immunosuppressant (methotrexate)

Surgical Treatment

The patients who do not respond to medical treatment, following surgical procedures should be considered.
- *Hearing-conservative nonvestibular ablative surgery*
  - *Endolymphatic sac decompression:* The drainage pathway is routed to the epidural space by incision of the back wall of the sac. Fifty to seventy-five percent of patients have complete resolution of the vertigo.
  - *Cochleosacculotomy:* Perforation of the saccule is done behind the oval window with a pick through the round window. Seventy percent of patients have complete control of vertigo. Major drawbacks include recurrence and high incidence of hearing loss.
  - *Fick and Cody tack procedures:* Fick operation creates fistulas in the saccule via the oval window. Cody's tack procedure places a stainless steel tack through the stapes footplate. These techniques are rarely practiced today.
  - *Transtympanic corticosteroid infusion of middle ear.*
- *Hearing-conservative vestibular ablative surgery*
- *Vestibular neurectomy:* About 95% patients have complete resolution of vertigo.
- *Intratympanic injections of gentamicin:* Seventy to ninety percent patients have complete control of vertigo. Profound HL occurs in 0–4%. It is considered first line of treatment among the invasive vestibular procedures when medical measures fail.
  - *Microwick:* A microwick of polyvinyl acetate is passed through the grommet. When gentamycin or steroid drops are instilled in the ear microwick soaks it and delivers the same to the round window.
  - Cryosurgery
  - Ultrasound
  - Cochlear dialysis
  - Cochlear implantation for bilateral severe-to-profound hearing loss.
- *Non-hearing conservative vestibular ablative surgery*
  - *Labyrinthectomy:* It is indicated when serviceable hearing is absent, pure tone average more than 60 dB, speech discrimination less than 50%.
    - Ablation with hypertonic saline
    - Transcanal
    - Transmastoid
  - Translabyrinthine cochleovestibular neurectomy
  - Destruction of Scarpa's ganglion.

- *Cogan's syndrome:* The features include episodic vertigo, interstitial keratitis, SNHL and negative serology for syphilis.
- *Leukemia:* Hemorrhage into the inner ear can occur in cases of leukemia.

LABYRINTHINE FISTULA

Syn: Circumscribed labyrinthitis, paralabyrinthitis and perilabyrinthitis

There occurs loss of endochondral bone without loss of perilymph usually due to cholesteatoma (mainly horizontal semicircular canal). Inflammation of a discrete portion of bony labyrinth and endosteum occurs without the involvement of membranous labyrinth.

Causes
- Chronic suppurative otitis media (CSOM) with cholesteatoma is most common cause
- Congenital syphilis
- Carcinoma
- Glomus jugulare tumors
- Fenestration operation for otosclerosis—no inflammation.

Clinical Features
- Patient may remain asymptomatic.
- Brief periods of imbalance, disequilibrium, or vertigo. Patient has normal equilibrium most of the time.
- *Fistula sign:* Momentary imbalance on pushing external ear canal with tragus. Transient vertigo induced by washing the ear.
- *Tullio's phenomenon:* Loud sounds provoke brief imbalance.

Investigations
- *Fistula test positive:* See Chapter 'Evaluation of Vertigo'.
- *HRCT temporal bone:* Bone erosion of lateral semicircular canal.

Treatment

Surgery
Complete removal of cholesteatoma matrix is done from the fistula site. Labyrinthine fistula is usually accompanied by erosion of bony fallopian canal and tegmen. So surgeon

should be careful. The blue line of actual fistula is identified along with the adjacent thinnest layer of bone. A small piece of tissue is placed over the site. Large fistula may be left covered by cholesteatoma matrix, which would form the lining of mastoid cavity. Fistula sign persists until the regrowth of bone.

SEROUS LABYRINTHITIS

This refers to a transient nonpurulent inflammation or chemical irritation of the inner ear, which usually does not result in any permanent damage.
- If diagnosed and treated successfully before the development of suppurative labyrinthitis, the prognosis is excellent.
- Hearing and vestibular dysfunction are entirely reversible.
- The perilymph is involved but not the endolymph.

Causes
- All the causes of *labyrinthine fistula.*
- *Bacterial or viral toxin invasion through round or oval window:* All types of otitis media and mastoiditis.
- *Blood-borne infection*
- *Meningeal inflammation*
- *Ear surgery:* Fenestration and stapedectomy.

Clinical Features
- *Spontaneous vertigo* in cases of middle ear infection usually indicates serous labyrinthitis. Vertigo is more severe than labyrinthine fistula, but less severe than suppurative labyrinthitis.
- *Irritative type of nystagmus (hyperactive labyrinthitis):* Quick component is directed toward the affected ear.
- *Worsening of labyrinthine fistula symptoms:* If the condition is secondary to labyrinthine fistula, fistula sign will be positive. Vertigo is less severe because some compensation develops during the inflammation of labyrinthine fistula.
- *Hearing* may be impaired but not markedly. If useful hearing is present, then suppurative labyrinthitis has not developed. Insidious high-tone sensorineural hearing loss (SNHL) is a frequent accompaniment of chronic suppurative otitis media (CSOM) even without vertigo.
- *Caloric tests* usually reveal diminished vestibular response.

Treatment
- *Active and prompt treatment* prevents development of suppurative labyrinthitis (permanent and complete damage of the labyrinth) and spread to meninges.
- *Acute otitis media (AOM):* Parenteral broad-spectrum antibiotics and wide myringotomy. Culture and sensitivity should be done quickly.
- *CSOM:* Modified radical mastoidectomy (without entering into the labyrinth) under the full cover of antibiotics should be done at the earliest.

SUPPURATIVE (PURULENT) LABYRINTHITIS

It is characterized by complete hearing loss (permanent) and acute vertigo. Vertigo slowly resolves over weeks to months. Patients usually give history of ear discharge, ear pain, preceding cold and cough or meningitis.

Routes of Infection
- *Tympanogenic:* Suppurative otitis media, mastoiditis, petrositis, temporal bone fracture, penetrating injury, middle ear surgery and tumors.
- *Meningogenic:* Meningitis.
- *Hematogenic:* From distant or systemic infection or from adjacent areas, such as meningitis, encephalitis or brain abscess.

Etiology

All the causes of serous labyrinthitis can result in suppurative labyrinthitis. The most common causes are AOM, CSOM with cholesteatoma and meningitis.

Clinical Features

Rapid onset (0.5-1 hour) of tinnitus, whirling vertigo, pallor, diaphoresis (sweating), nausea and vomiting occur. Symptoms remain unrelenting and may not respond to any treatment for 8-12 hours. Dizziness improves during next few days but head motion evokes severe vertigo and nausea. Central nervous system (CNS) compensation occurs over next 2-3 weeks.
- *Brisk jerky nystagmus:* Horizontal rotary nystagmus has the quick component on affected side for the first day (irritative) but than toward the opposite side (paralytic).
- Patient lies quietly on the affected ear and cannot stand or sit.
- Even slight head movements produce vomiting.
- Complete hearing loss, past pointing and fall occur toward the diseased side.
- Unilateral labyrinthitis produces more severe vestibular upset than bilateral meningogenic labyrinthitis.

Treatment

It is similar to serous labyrinthitis.

PERILYMPHATIC FISTULA

Syn: Inner ear fistula, round or oval window fistula

These inner ear fistulae provide communication between the perilymphatic space and the middle ear or intramembranous communication between endolymphatic and perilymphatic spaces. The common sites are oval and round windows.

Etiology

- Barotrauma
- Penetrating trauma
- Surgery (stapedectomy)
- Head trauma
- Explosive blast
- Physical exertion (heavy weight lifting or straining)
- Spontaneous in cases of congenital hearing loss (such as Mondini's deformity).

Perilymphatic fistula should be ruled out in cases of vertigo congenital SNHL.

Clinical Features

Auditory and vestibular symptoms are variable.
- *Dizziness:* Variable and include episodic incapacitating vertigo like Ménière's, positional vertigo, motion intolerance, to occasional disequilibrium. Spontaneous inner ear fistula in cases of congenital hearing loss.
- *Tullio's phenomenon:* Vertigo occurs after exposure to loud noises.
- *Hearing loss (fluctuating/progressive):* Usually present but not must.

Self-evaluation Exercises

1. Which of the following are not the features of benign paroxysmal positional vertigo?
    a. Most common cause of peripheral vertigo
    b. Predisposing factors include age > 40 years, vestibular neuronitis, head trauma and ear surgery
    c. Lateral semicircular most commonly affected
    d. Whirly vertigo spell last for couple of minutes
    e. None of the above
2. Which of the following are the features of Ménière's disease?
    a. Raised endolymphatic pressure
    b. Fluctuating SNHL, episodic vertigo, roaring tinnitus and ear fullness
    c. Idiopathic
    d. Recruitment causes intolerance to loud sounds
    e. All of the above
3. Which of the following are not the features of Cogan's syndrome?
    a. Episodic vertigo
    b. Interstitial keratitis
    c. SNHL
    d. Syphilis
4. The treatment of the Meniere's disease patients, who have failed medical treatment but retain a serviceable hearing, includes:
    a. Endolymphatic sac decompression
    b. Intratympanic gentamicin
    c. Vestibular nerve section
    d. All of the above

True (T)/False (F)

5. Pulsatile tinnitus and unconsciousness can occur in Ménière's disease.
6. In early Ménière's disease, audiogram shows a declining curve.
7. Cody tack operation is one of the surgical options in the treatment of Ménière disease.
8. In Lermoyez syndrome (variant of Ménière's disease), patient first gets hearing loss and tinnitus, which are relieved following the episode of vertigo.
9. In cases of perilymphatic fistula, patient develops disequilibrium after nose blowing or heavy weight lifting.
10. Hemorrhage into the inner ear cannot occur in cases of leukemia.

Answers

1. c, d 2. e 3. d 4. d 5. F 6. F
7. T 8. T 9. T 10. F

Chapter 17

Central Vestibular Disorders

> ### ⊙ Specific Learning Objectives
> After going through the chapter, you should be able to answer the following questions:
> - Describe the differential diagnoses of central vestibular vertigo.
> - What do you know about the following?
>   - Wallenberg's syndrome
>   - Motion sickness
>   - Hyperventilation
>   - Cervical vertigo

MIGRAINE

Migraine is the most common cause of central vestibular disorders. Some of the other common causes of central vertigo are enumerated in Box 17.1.

> **Most common cause of central vertigo:** Migraine has been reported the most common cause of dizziness in many neuro-otologic clinics.

- It usually begins in first three decades of life and prevalence peaks in the fifth decade.

Box 17.1: Common causes of central and peripheral vertigo

Central vestibular disorders
- Migraine
- Basilar migraine
- Vertebrobasilar insufficiency
- Subclavian steal syndrome
- Wallenberg's syndrome
- Cerebellar infarction
- Cerebellar hemorrhage
- Multiple sclerosis (MS)
- Motion sickness
- Phobic postural vertigo
- Hyperventilation
- Agoraphobia
- Cervical vertigo

- Family history is often present.
- Migraine without aura is the most common variety.
- The usual migraine headache is unilateral, throbbing, moderate to markedly severe and aggravated by physical activity. Sensitivity to light and noise are common.
- Migraine headache may be associated with episodic vertigo, motion sensitivity and nonspecific dizziness, such as swimming or rocking sensation inside the head.
- Episodic vertigo (rotational or to-and-fro) usually lasts for few minutes to several hours.
- Vertigo is associated with postural imbalance and unsteadiness with motion sensitivity or visual hallucinations.
- Vertigo can also occur after taking certain food.
- Multiple attacks may occur.
- Vertigo usually occurs during the headache but may also occur during the headache free interval or preceding the headache.

Basilar Migraine

It is a subtype of migraine with aura.
- It is characterized by recurrent headache that is usually occipital.
- This is associated with minimum two of the multiple neurologic symptoms of brainstem, cerebellum and occipital lobe (supplied by basilar artery).
- Consciousness is impaired quite often.
- Symptoms of vertigo, fluctuating hearing loss and tinnitus may make basilar migraine difficult to

distinguish from Ménière's disease and vertebrobasilar transient ischemic attacks.
- Tinnitus is common.
- Low frequency fluctuating hearing loss is common. Sudden profound unilateral sensorineural hearing loss (SNHL) occurs occasionally. Migraine related vasospasm can cause cochlear infarction.

Vertigo spells in children: Migraine is not uncommon in children. It must be considered when vertigo spells are not associated with ear malformations or middle ear infections.

VERTEBROBASILAR INSUFFICIENCY

This is a common cause of central vertigo. Transient ischemic attacks are common in elderly and usually last for minutes and completely resolve within 24 hours. Presentation can mimic acute peripheral vestibular disorder.

Etiology

- *Common:* Atherosclerosis, embolism and dissection of the vertebral artery (in young persons).
- *Uncommon:* Arteritis and other inflammatory conditions, hypercoagulation disorders and hyperviscosity syndromes.

Clinical Features

Vertigo lasts more than a minute to couple of hours. Vascular risk factors such as smoking, hypertension, diabetes and high cholesterol are usually present in these patients.
- Abrupt isolated vertigo is a common presentation of transient ischemic attacks of labyrinth and/or brain.

Transient ischemic attack (TIA): Isolated spells of vertigo continuing for more than 3 months usually rule out TIA.

- *Other features:*
  - Visual symptoms (diplopia, visual field defects, blindness and visual illusions and hallucinations) may be followed by drop-attacks, unsteadiness-incoordination and weakness in limbs.
  - Confusion, headache, hearing loss, loss of consciousness, numbness in limbs, dysarthria, tinnitus and perioral numbness are rarely accompanied with episodes of vertigo.

WALLENBERG'S SYNDROME

(Lateral medullary infarction)

Occlusion of vertebral artery is more frequently seen than the posteroinferior cerebellar artery in this syndrome.

Clinical Features

- *Partial syndrome:* It presents with only disequilibrium and a tendency to fall to one side.
- *Complete syndrome:* It presents with
  - Vertigo, nausea, vomiting, diplopia, severe gait and ipsilateral limb ataxia.
  - Ipsilateral Horner's syndrome and facial anesthesia and contralateral hemianesthesia.
  - Bizarre sensations of body and environment.
  - *Localizing features:* Dysphagia, hoarseness and dysphonia; decreased gag and ipsilateral vocal cord weakness.

CEREBELLAR INFARCTION

Twenty-five percent elderly patients suffering from acute isolated vertigo have a cerebellar infarction.

Clinical Features

- Vertigo and vomiting, ipsilateral limb ataxia, Horner's syndrome and facial hemianesthesia and contralateral body anesthesia.
- Brainstem features help in localizing feeding vessels:
  - *Superior cerebellar artery:* Impaired vibration and position sense of contralateral side.
  - *Anteroinferior cerebellar artery:* Unilateral paresis of muscles of mastication.
  - *Posteroinferior cerebellar artery:* Dysphagia, dysphonia.

CEREBELLAR HEMORRHAGE

Headache or stiffness of the neck in cases of brain stroke suggest hemorrhage. Sudden vertigo with multiple neurological findings (localizing signs and symptoms) often rapidly progresses to coma and death.
- The condition often begins with vertigo, headache, vomiting and an inability to stand and walk. Severe ataxia, dysmetria, gaze-evoked nystagmus, stiff neck also accompany the above symptoms.

Absence of head thrust sign will differentiate cerebellar hemorrhage from acute peripheral vestibular disease.

- Abducens and facial palsies can occur from hematoma compression.

MULTIPLE SCLEROSIS

Multiple sclerosis is a demyelinating disorder of central nervous system (CNS), where myelin is formed from oligodendroglia. Demyelinating plaque affects vestibular nuclei, cerebellum and its peduncles and cranial nerves.

Etiology

- **Cause:** It is not yet known but autoimmunity, infection and heredity may play a role.
- **Age:** 15–50 years. Peak incidence is at the age of 24 years.
- **Sex:** Females are more affected than males (2:1).

Clinical Features

- It usually manifests as relapsing and remitting or progressive disease. CNS dysfunctions are disseminated in time and space.
- The most common symptoms are vision loss (optic neuritis) and diplopia (bilateral internuclear ophthalmoplegia). Other common findings include weakness, ataxia or sudden hearing loss.
- Vertigo occurs in 50% cases, but is initial symptom in only 5% cases.
  - Sustained over days to weeks.
  - Positional nystagmus with vertigo may be the first manifestation of multiple sclerosis. Confirmation with Dix-Hallpike maneuver can be done (*see* Chapter 'Vertigo Evaluation').
  - ***Involvement of an intrapontine portion of vestibular nerve or nucleus:*** It presents with vertigo (hours to days), vomiting, imbalance, direction-fixed (toward normal side) horizontal-torsional nystagmus and canal paresis (caloric test). Though it mimics peripheral lesion, this central nystagmus is not suppressed by visual fixation.
- Sudden hearing loss may accompany vertigo.
- Demyelinating plaque involving vestibular nuclei, cerebellum and its peduncles presents as severe ataxia, direction-changing nystagmus, intention tremor or pyramidal signs.
- **Eyes:** Pendular nystagmus often causes oscillopsia and poor vision. It is a common feature.

MOTION SICKNESS

This common form of physiological dizziness occurs in susceptible individuals, usually with prolonged vestibular stimulation. It may also be caused by visual stimulation. This may be induced by real or apparent motion. The condition is the result of the mismatch of information that is reaching the vestibular nuclei and cerebellum from the visual, labyrinthine and somatosensory systems. It is usually managed effectively by labyrinthine sedatives.

> Complete bilateral vestibular loss makes the patient resistant to motion sickness.

> **Migraine and Motion Sickness**
> - Migraine patients are more prone to motion sickness.
> - Motion sickness in children may be the starting feature of migraine.

Dizziness, fatigue, pallor, cold sweats, salivation, nausea and vomiting develop when the person is aboard a ship, in a car, on an airplane, or in space.

PHOBIC POSTURAL VERTIGO

Phobic postural vertigo patients are obsessively preoccupied with their psychophysiologic dizziness, which is predominantly subjective postural imbalance without falls.

HYPERVENTILATION

Though hyperventilation usually induces dizziness in anxious or phobic individuals, it can also cause dizziness in peripheral or central vestibular disorders.

Rapid drop in partial pressure of CO_2 (pCO_2) is presumed to result in cerebral vasoconstriction.

- Symptoms include giddiness, lightheadedness, feelings of suffocation, perioral and acral (extremities such as limbs, fingers, or ears) paresthesias (sensation of burning, pricking, tickling, numbness or tingling).
- Voluntary hyperventilation can reproduce symptoms but may also provoke symptoms from peripheral or central vestibular disorders.

AGORAPHOBIA

(Agora-market place; phobo-fear)

- Irrational fear of leaving the familiar setting of home and venturing into the open are often associated with panic attacks.
- Patients of this type of panic disorder avoid or endure with great distress the feared situation.

CERVICAL VERTIGO OR WHIPLASH VERTIGO

(Musculoskeletal vertigo)

Vertigo provoked by changes in neck position in patients with neck pain or occipital headache without any otological or neurological disease is diagnosed musculoskeletal vertigo.

Vertigo is usually provoked by movements of neck to the side of injury. It may develop 7–10 days after the accident. Examination reveals tenderness of neck, spasms of cervical muscles and limitation of neck movements.

The exact mechanism of cervical vertigo is not known. It is said to be due to disturbed vertebrobasilar circulation, involvement of sympathetic vertebral plexus and alteration of tonic neck reflexes. Currently, it is believed that the vertigo in these patients is due to following conditions:

- Post-traumatic benign paroxysmal positional vertigo
- Concussion

- Deceleration injury
- Direct trauma to labyrinth.

Cervical spondylosis is common in older people and too often blamed for symptoms. It should be considered only when vertigo is clearly associated with movements of the neck (not the head) and appreciable radiological changes.

After ruling out the cervical fracture, Dix-Hallpike examination and audiogram usually clinch the diagnosis. Some patients may need electroneurograph (ENG) and MRI studies.

Self-evaluation Exercises

1. Which of the following are not the features of lateral medullary syndrome?
   a. Thrombosis of posterior inferior cerebellar artery
   b. Vertigo, dysphagia, dysphonia, ataxia and tendency to fall on same side
   c. Ipsilateral Horner's syndrome
   d. Loss of pain and temperature sensation on ipsilateral face and contralateral limbs
   e. None of the above
2. Which of the following are the features of Wallenberg syndrome?
   a. Ipsilateral sensorineural hearing loss, vertigo and horizontal nystagmus with fast component on opposite side (vestibular and cochlear nuclei lesions)
   b. Analgesia and thermal anesthesia of opposite side of body (spinothalamic tract lesion) and ipsilateral side of face (spinal nucleus of trigeminal nerve)
   c. Dysphagia and drooping of palate (nucleus ambiguus lesion)
   d. Ipsilateral Horner's syndrome (lesion of descending hypothalamic tract) dryness of face and constriction of pupil
   e. All of the above

True (T)/False (F)

3. Migraine headache may last for hours and can cause neuralgic symptoms. Females are affected more than males.
4. Patients with multiple sclerosis (MS) may present with symptoms such as vertigo, sudden hearing loss or facial palsy. Optic nerves are most commonly affected because they are direct outgrowths of the CNS and their axons have myelin sheaths formed by oligodendrocytes.

Answers

1. e   2. e   3. T   4. T

Pearls and Nuggets (Refresh your knowledge)

- **Dix-Hallpike examination:** It is the most important clinical test for dizzy patients because 25% of all dizzy patients have benign paroxysmal positioning vertigo.
- **Downbeating nystagmus:** A pure downbeating nystagmus during Dix-Hallpike testing suggests Chiari malformation or other posterior fossa lesions. MRI must be done.
- **Peripheral and central vertigo:** Patient with central dizziness complaints few symptoms but have many findings (sensory/motor deficits). Patients with peripheral vertigo have many symptoms (severe whirling vertigo with or without otological symptoms) but few findings.
- **Multisensory imbalance:** It is suggested when dizziness appears on walking but is relieved by pushing a grocery store cart.
- **Vertigo spells in children:** Migraine is not uncommon in children. It must be considered when vertigo spells are not associated with ear malformations or middle ear infections.
- **Horner's syndrome:** It consists of partial ptosis, miosis (constriction of pupil), anhidrosis and apparent enophthalmos. It occurs due to an ipsilateral lesion of cervical sympathetic chain or its central pathways.
- **Mesencephalic nucleus of CN V:** Lesion results in a loss of touch sensations in the face. Facial sensations of pain and temperature remain intact and there is no jaw weakness.
- **Schaumann's bodies:** These are seen in sarcoid granuloma.
- **Schwann cells:** They are derived from neural crest.

Chapter 18

Facial Nerve Disorders

> **Specific Learning Objectives**
>
> After going through the chapter, you should be able to answer the following questions:
> - Name the various functional components and branches of facial nerve and the structures supplied by them.
> - Describe the course of different segments of facial nerve and their important relations and applied anatomy.
> - Which are the different surgical landmarks that surgeon should be aware of to avoid injury to the facial nerve while performing surgery of middle ear, mastoid and parotid gland?
> - Describe the pathophysiology of nerve injury and Sunderland classification.
> - How will you differentiate between upper and lower motor neuron facial palsy and its anatomical explanation?
> - What are different electrical tests performed in patients with facial palsy and their importance?
> - Which are various topodiagnostic tests of facial nerve and how they help in localizing the site of lesion?
> - What are the various causes and sequelae/complications of facial nerve palsy?
> - Describe the etiopathology and clinical features and management of Bell's palsy.
> - What do you know about the following conditions: (1) Recurrent facial palsy; (2) Melkersson's syndrome; (3) Ramsay Hunt syndrome or Herpes-zoster oticus (Varicella-zoster virus)?
> - What are the differences between longitudinal and transverse temporal bone fractures?
> - Describe hyperkinetic disorders of facial nerve.

PERTINENT ANATOMY

The facial nerve (CN VII) is the nerve of second branchial arch. Its sensory root is also called **nerve of Wrisberg** and carries both secretomotor as well as gustatory fibers.

Functional Divisions

It is a mixed nerve and consists of following types of fibers:
- **Branchial motor fibers:** They supply muscles of facial expression (develop from the second branchial arch) and arise from the motor facial nucleus that is situated on the medial side of floor of the IV ventricle in the pons.
- **Parasympathetic preganglionic secretomotor fibers:** They supply to the lacrimal gland, submandibular and sublingual salivary glands and the glands in the nose and palate. They arise from the superior salivary and lacrimatory nuclei that are situated near the motor facial nucleus in pons.
- **Gustatory fibers:** They carry taste sensation from the anterior two-third of tongue and hard palate and go to the nucleus of solitary tract.
- **General sensations:** They are carried from the posterior part of external ear and retroauricular skin.

Motor Nucleus of Facial Nerve (Fig. 18.1)

Motor nucleus of facial nerve is situated in the pons near the nucleus of abducens. **Upper part of the nucleus**, which innervates forehead muscles, receives corticonuclear fibers from both the cerebral hemisphere, while the **lower part of nucleus** that supplies lower face gets only crossed fibers from opposite side of cerebral hemisphere. Facial motor nucleus also receives fibers from the thalamus by alternate routes and provides involuntary emotional expressions such as happy, sad, depressed and angry faces. This explains why frontalis muscle and emotional facial expressions remain intact in supranuclear lesions.

Course of Facial Nerve

The course of facial nerve is divided into three parts—intracranial, intratemporal and extracranial.
1. **Intracranial course (15-17 mm):** Motor fibers first hook round the nucleus of CN VI and then are joined by

Chapter 18 • Facial Nerve Disorders

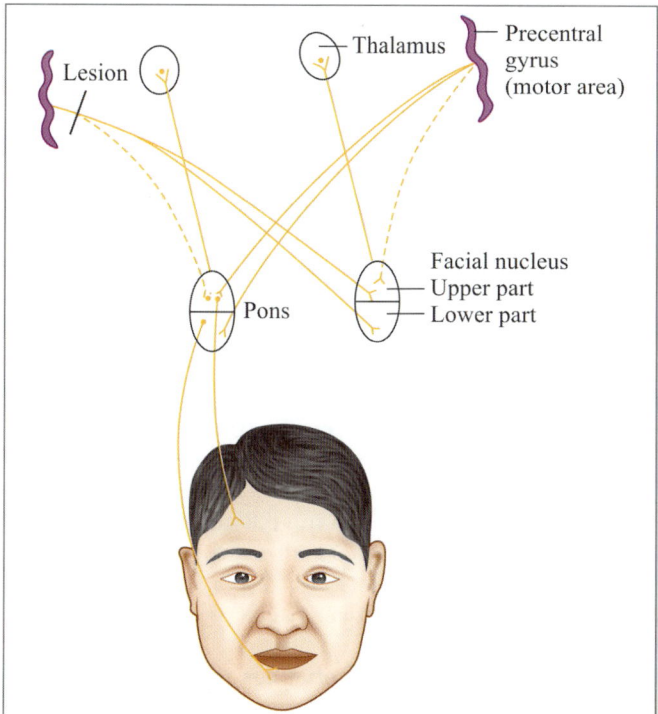

Fig. 18.1: Facial nerve nucleus. Upper part of nucleus, which supplies frontalis muscle of forehead, receives corticonuclear fibers from both the sides. Therefore, in unilateral supranuclear facial palsy frontalis muscle is spared

the sensory root (nerve of Wrisberg). Facial nerve along with the vestibulocochlear and abducens nerves leaves the brainstem at pontomedullary junction. It travels through the cerebellopontine angle and along with vestibulocochlear nerve enters the internal auditory canal. At the fundus of internal auditory canal, facial nerve enters into the bony fallopian canal.

2. *Intratemporal course (Fig. 18.2):* The part of the facial nerve, from internal acoustic meatus to stylomastoid foramen, is further divided into four segments—meatal, labyrinthine, tympanic and mastoid.
   i. *Meatal segment (8–10 mm):* It lies within internal auditory canal. The meatal foramen is the narrowest aperture of facial canal. The length of facial nerve from brainstem to meatal foramen is 23–24 mm.
   ii. *Labyrinthine segment (3–5 mm):* It extends from internal auditory canal fundus (meatal foramen) to the geniculate ganglion (may be dehiscent) where facial nerve takes a posterior turn forming the first 'genu'.

The bony Fallopian canal in the labyrinthine segment is narrowest and more prone to compression in Bell's palsy.

   iii. *Tympanic or horizontal segment (8–11 mm):* It extends from geniculate ganglion, to just above the pyramidal eminence, where it turns inferiorly and makes the second genu. The tympanic segment lies above the oval window (dehiscence in 15–30%) and below the lateral semicircular canal.
   iv. *Mastoid or vertical segment (10–14 mm):* It extends from the pyramid to the stylomastoid foramen.
3. *Extracranial course:* The facial nerve comes out of the temporal bone through the stylomastoid foramen. Here, it crosses the styloid process and enters into the parotid gland. This extracranial part from stylomastoid foramen to the termination of its peripheral branches (Fig. 18.3) is situated in the substance of parotid gland.

Branches of Facial Nerve

- *Greater superficial petrosal nerve:* This first branch of the facial nerve arises from geniculate ganglion and carries preganglionic secretomotor fibers to lacrimal gland and the glands of nasal mucosa.
- *Nerve to stapedius:* This branch arises at the level of second genu and carries motor fibers to the stapedius muscle.

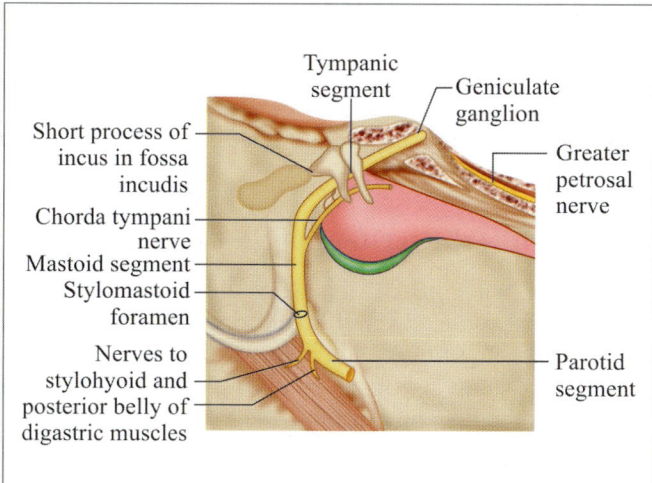

Fig. 18.2: Intratemporal course of facial nerve

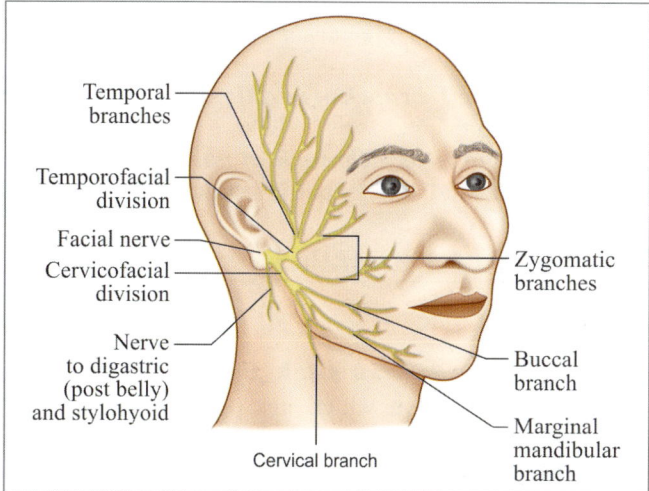

Fig. 18.3: Branches of facial nerve after emerging from stylomastoid foramen

- **Chorda tympani:** It arises from the middle of mastoid vertical segment and passes between the incus and neck of malleus. It leaves the middle ear cavity through petrotympanic fissure. It carries preganglionic parasympathetic secretomotor fibers to submandibular and sublingual salivary glands and gustatory fibers (taste sensation from anterior two-third of tongue).
- **Communicating branch:** It joins auricular branch (Arnold's nerve) of vagus and supplies the concha, retroauricular groove, posterior of meatus and tympanic membrane.
- **Posterior auricular nerve:** It supplies muscles of pinna and occipital belly of occipitofrontalis muscle.
- **Muscular branches:** They supply to stylohyoid and posterior belly of digastric, which are developed from the second branchial arch.
- **Terminal branches:** The facial nerve, after crossing the styloid process, is divided into two terminal divisions **upper temporofacial** and a **lower cervicofacial**. The smaller terminal branches from these two divisions are temporal, zygomatic, buccal, mandibular and cervical. This network of terminal divisions and branches of facial nerve supply all the muscles of facial expression (except levator palpabri superioris) and form pes anserinus (goose-foot).

> **Congenital anomalies:** Facial canal may be dehiscent over oval window (common) and geniculate ganglion and retrofacial mastoid air cells regions and the facial nerve is at greater risk of injury during the middle ear and mastoid surgery. The nerve may prolapse from these dehiscent areas.

Blood Supply

Following are the arteries and areas of facial nerve supplied by them:
- **Labyrinthine artery (branch of anterior inferior cerebellar artery):** Meatal segment within the internal auditory canal.
- **Petrosal artery (branch of middle meningeal artery):** Perigeniculate area.
- **Stylomastoid artery (branch of posterior auricular artery):** Mastoid and tympanic segments.

SURGICAL LANDMARKS

Middle Ear Cleft

- **Processus cochleariformis:** It presents the site of the geniculate ganglion which lies just anterior to it. It shows the beginning of horizontal tympanic segment.
- **Oval window and horizontal semicircular canal:** The tympanic segment is situated above the oval window and below the horizontal semicircular canal.
- **Short process of incus:** Facial nerve lies medial and inferior to the short process of incus at the level of aditus ad antrum.
- **Pyramid:** Facial nerve is situated posterior to the pyramid and the tympanic sulcus.
- **Tympanomastoid suture:** The vertical mastoid segment of facial nerve lies about 6–8 mm deep to this suture and always runs behind the level of this suture.
- **Digastric ridge:** Facial nerve leaves the mastoid through the stylomastoid foramen, which is situated at the anterior end of digastric ridge.

Parotid Gland

- **Tragal cartilage pointer:** The tragal cartilage ends in a point. It is a sharp triangular extension of tragal cartilage, which seems to point towards facial nerve. Facial nerve lies 1–1.5 cm medial and inferior to tragal point surrounded by a small aggregation of fat and overlain by a small vessel.
- **Tympanomastoid suture:** Facial nerve lies 6–8 mm deep to the suture.
- **Styloid process:** Facial nerve lies in the posterolateral aspect of the styloid process near its base.
- **Posterior belly of digastric:** Follow the posterior belly of digastric up to 5 mm below the bony meatal edge. The facial nerve lies between the mastoid and the posterosuperior part of the posterior belly of digastric muscle. The facial nerve passes downwards, forwards and laterally immediately above the upper border of digastric posterior belly.
- **Mastoid process:** Follow the anterior border of mastoid process up to the vaginal process of tympani bone. Facial nerve bisects the tympanomastoid angle at the tympanomastoid suture.

HOUSE-BRACKMANN SYSTEM OF GRADING FACIAL NERVE PALSY

Facial weakness can be subtle, moderate, near total or total. House-Brackmann system of grading facial nerve palsy (Table 18.1) has been widely used (endorsed by the American Academy of Otolaryngology-Head and Neck Surgery).

PATHOPHYSIOLOGY OF NERVE INJURY

A nerve fiber consists of axon, myelin sheath and neurilemma and is covered by endoneurium (Figs 18.4A to C). A bundle of nerve fibers forms a fascicle, which is enclosed in a sheath called **perineurium**. The fascicles are bound together by epineurium.

The degree of nerve injury determines the degeneration and regeneration of nerve and its function. Traditionally, nerve injuries are divided into three types—neuropraxia, axonotmesis and neurotmesis.

Chapter 18 • Facial Nerve Disorders

Table 18.1: House-Brackmann system of grading facial nerve palsy

Grade	Dysfunction	Symmetry at rest	Frontalis motion	Effort in eye closure	Motion of mouth angle
I	Absent	Normal facial functions in all areas	—	—	—
II	Mild	Normal	Moderate to good	Minimum	Slight asymmetry
III	Moderate	Normal	Slight to moderate	Moderate	Moderate asymmetry
IV	Moderately severe	Normal	None	Incomplete closure	Moderate with great effort
V	Severe	Absent	None	Incomplete closure	Slight
VI	Total	Absent	No movement in any area		

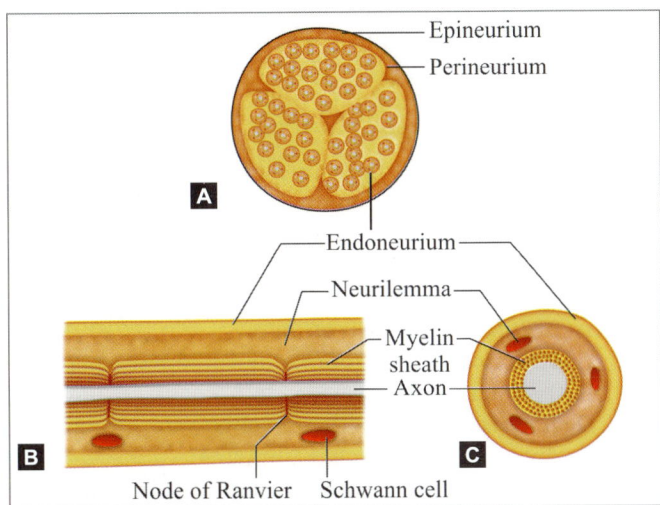

Figs 18.4A to C: Nerve structure. (A) Cross-section of nerve; (B) Longitudinal section of nerve fiber; (C) Cross-section of nerve fiber

SUNDERLAND CLASSIFICATION

Based on anatomical structure of the nerve, Sunderland classified the severity of nerve injuries into 5 degrees (Fig. 18.5). This classification is now widely accepted. The third, fourth and fifth degrees are types of neurotmesis.

1. ***First degree (obstruction to axoplasm, neuropraxia):*** In this conduction block, flow of axoplasm through the axons is obstructed. No morphological changes are seen. In this type of injury, recovery of function is complete. Nerve excitability test and maximum stimulation test are normal. Electromyography fails to show voluntary motor action potential as they are not conducted across the blockade (Fig. 18.5A).
2. ***Second degree (injury to axon, axonotmesis):*** There is loss of axons, but endoneurial tubes remain intact. Wallerian degeneration occurs distal to the lesion. Electrical tests show rapid and complete degeneration, with loss of voluntary motor units. During regeneration, axons will grow into their respective tubes. Recovery is good (Fig. 18.5B).
3. ***Third degree (injury to endoneurium, neurotmesis):*** It is an injury to nerve fiber along with both Wallerian degeneration and loss of endoneurium. Electrical tests show complete nerve degeneration. During regeneration, axon of one tube can grow into another. There are chances of synkinesis (Fig. 18.5C).
4. ***Fourth degree (injury to perineurium):*** Partial transection of nerve occurs. Scarring occurs and impairs regeneration of axons (Fig. 18.5D).
5. ***Fifth degree (injury to epineurium):*** There occurs complete nerve transaction (Fig. 18.5E).

The first three degrees are seen in viral and inflammatory lesions of the nerves. The fourth and fifth degrees happen in surgical and accidental traumas and in neoplasms.

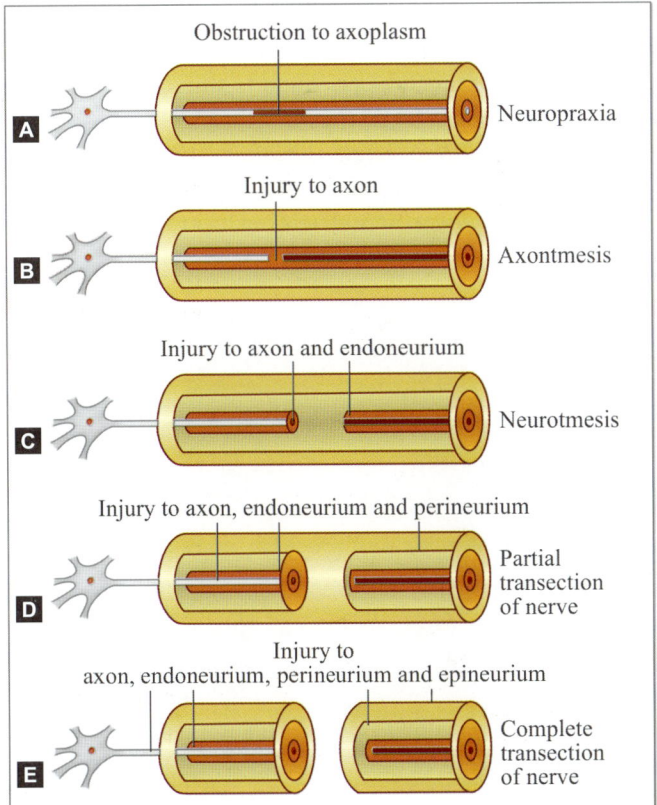

Figs 18.5A to E: Sunderland histologic classification of peripheral nerve injury is helpful in understanding the results of electrical tests

Facial nerve regeneration: The regeneration and degree of return to normal is dependent on the degree of initial injury (neuropraxia vs. neurotmesis). The most important factor in history is whether the palsy developed slowly over days or immediately at the time of the injury.

DIFFERENCES BETWEEN UPPER AND LOWER MOTOR NEURON PALSY

Upper Motor Neuron Facial Paralysis

The paralysis occurs only in the lower half of face (Fig. 18.6) on the contralateral side. Frontalis muscle movements are retained due to bilateral innervation of upper part of motor facial nucleus.
- Involuntary emotional expressions and the tone of facial muscles remain intact.
- Central facial paralysis is caused by cerebrovascular accidents (hemorrhage, thrombosis or embolism), tumor or an abscess.

Lower Motor Neuron Facial Paralysis

In the peripheral facial paralysis, all the ipsilateral muscles of the face become paralyzed. Patient is unable to frown, close the eye, purse the lips and whistle.
- *Nuclear palsy:* It is identified by associated paralysis of CN VI, the nucleus of which is situated near to the motor nucleus of facial nerve.
- *Cerebellopontine angle lesions:* They are usually associated with vestibular and auditory defects such as vertigo and sensorineural hearing loss (SNHL).

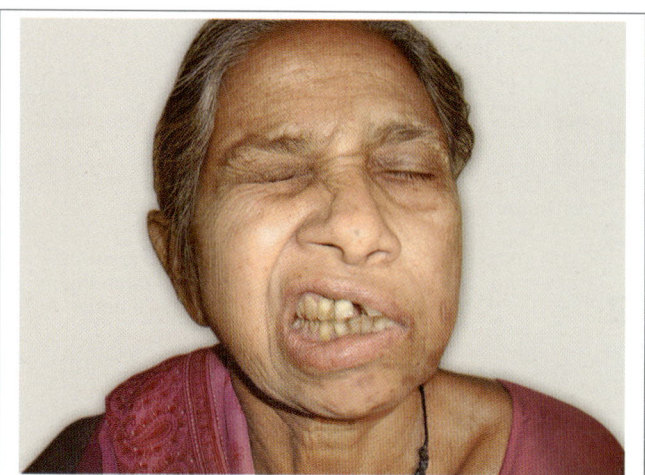

Fig. 18.6: Left facial palsy of lower half of the face. Note patient can close her both eyes. This patient also had associated left side abducent nerve lateral rectus palsy

- *Lesion in the bony Fallopian canal:* From internal acoustic meatus to stylomastoid foramen the lesions can be localized with the help of topodiagnostic tests.
- *Lesion in the parotid area:* It affects only the terminal branches of the nerve, which may be involved by the tumor or injury.

INVESTIGATIONS

Electrical Tests

These tests are useful not only in differentiating between the neuropraxia and degeneration of the nerve, but also help in predicting prognosis and indicating the time for surgical decompression.

Nerve Excitability Test

This test measures the threshold of stimulation of both sides of facial nerve and compares them. A $1/sec^2$ wave pulse, which is 1 msec in duration, is applied. The steadily increasing intensity till facial twitch appears tells the threshold.
- *Interpretations:* They are as follows:
  - *Conduction block:* There is no difference between the normal and paralyzed side.
  - *Degeneration:* The difference between normal and paralyzed sides exceeds 3.5 mA.
- *Limitations:* Degeneration of nerve fibers cannot be detected earlier than 3 days. When degeneration sets in, nerve excitability is gradually lost. So, the patient should come after 3 days and before 3 months.

Maximal Stimulation Test (MST)

Instead of measuring the threshold of stimulation, MST measures the current that gives maximum facial movement. The levels are compared the normal side. Maximal stimulation indicates degeneration and incomplete recovery.
- *Advantage:* MST becomes abnormal earlier than nerve excitability test. So it is a better prognostic indicator.
- *Disadvantage:* Response is subjectively graded as equal, decreased or absent.

Electroneurography (ENoG)

In this evoked electroneurography, the facial nerve is stimulated and the compound action potentials (amplitudes of the summation potentials) from the facial muscles are recorded and measured objectively. Supramaximal level of current is applied over the main trunk of facial nerve. The readings are compared with the normal side.

The peak-to-peak amplitude is directly proportional to the number of intact motor axons. So the test assesses extent of neuronal degeneration. The response of paralyzed side is reported as a percentage of response on

normal side, thus telling the proportion of fibers that have degenerated.
- *Interpretation:* Fall of summating potential to 10% of the normal value is an indication (90% degeneration) for the surgical decompression.
- *Limitation:* It must be done within 2 weeks of the onset of palsy.

Electromyography (EMG)

It records spontaneous activity of facial muscles at rest and on voluntary contraction. Electrode is directly inserted into the muscle. The test provides information regarding intact motor units in acute phase and detects reinnervation potentials.

Interpretations

- *Normal:* At rest, normal muscle does not show any electrical activity. On voluntary contraction, normal volitional motor unit potentials are observed.
- *Denervated muscle:* Fibrillation potentials appear within 14–21 days after denervation.
- *Earliest signs of recovery:* Reinnervation potentials can be seen much before (up to 12 weeks) any visible facial movement.
- *Limitation:* It cannot assess the degree of degeneration or prognosis for recovery.

Nerve Conduction Velocity

Nerve conduction can be measured between the stylomastoid foramen and the ramus mandibularis. A strong correlation exists between decrease in nerve conduction and decrease in compound nerve action potential eletroneurography during the first two weeks of facial palsy.

Interpretations

They are as follows:
- *Normal:* 37–58 m/sec
- *Fifty percent chance of residual paresis:* 20–30 m/sec
- *Poor prognosis:* < 10 m/sec

TOPODIAGNOSTIC TESTS

These tests are done to find the site of lesion in the intratemporal segment of facial nerve (Figs 18.7A to D).
- *Schirmer's test (Fig. 18.8):* A strip of filter paper (5 mm x 35 mm) is hooked in the lower fornix of each eye and kept for 5 minutes. The length of wetting of strip is measured. The lacrimation of the two sides is compared.
  - *Interpretations:* 25–30% decrease in lacrimation indicates that lesion is proximal to the geniculate ganglion. The greater superficial petrosal nerve carrying secretomotor fibers to lacrimal gland arises from the geniculate ganglion.

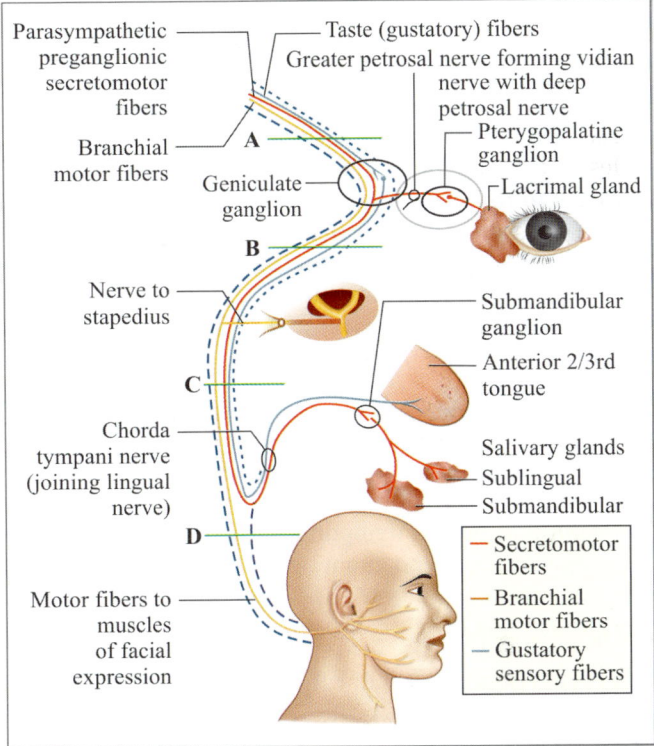

Figs 18.7A to D: Topographical lesions of facial nerve. (A) Lesion above the geniculate ganglion damages the motor fibers to facial muscles and stapedius, secretomotor fibers to lacrimal and submandibular salivary glands, and taste fibers; (B) Lesion between the geniculate ganglion and nerve to stapedius spare secretomotor fibers to lacrimal gland; (C) Lesion between the nerve to stapedius and chorda tympani nerve spares stapedial reflex and lacrimation; (D) Lesion below chorda tympani nerve affects only muscles of facial expression

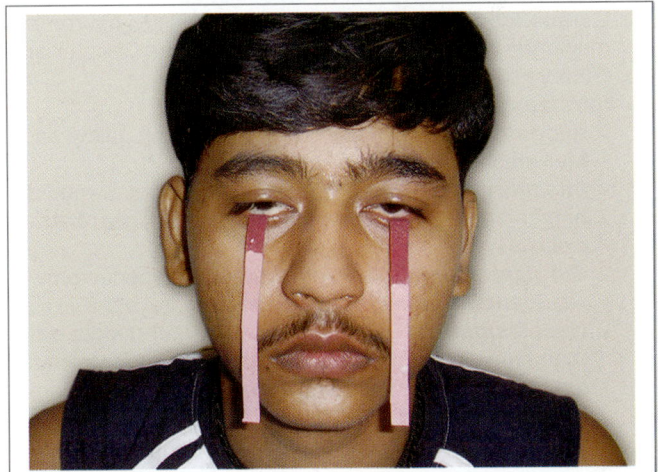

Fig. 18.8: Schirmer's Test. A strip of filter paper hooked in the lower fornix of each eye. The length of wetting of strip measures lacrimation of the two sides

- *Stapedial reflex:* It is lost in the lesions that lie above the nerve to stapedius. It is tested by tympanometry (*see* Chapter on 'Hearing Evaluation').

- **Taste test or electrogustometry:** It measures function of chorda tympani. A drop of salt or sugar solution is placed on one side of the protruded tongue. The electrogustometry is another method of testing taste sensations. Impairment of taste sensation indicates that lesion is above the origin of chorda tympani.
- **Submandibular salivary flow:** Polythene tubes are passed into both sides of Wharton's ducts. The drops of saliva are counted during 1 minute period. It also measures function of chorda tympani. Decreased salivation indicates that lesion is above the origin of chorda tympani.

CAUSES OF FACIAL NERVE PARALYSIS

The cause may be central or peripheral. The peripheral lesion may involve the nerve in its intracranial, intratemporal or extratemporal parts. Peripheral lesions are more common and about two-third of them are of the idiopathic variety. The various causes of facial nerve palsy are listed in Box 18.1.

Bilateral Facial Nerve Paralysis

The causes of bilateral facial nerve paralysis include:
- Guillain-Barre syndrome
- Lyme disease
- Mobius syndrome
- Sarcoidosis
- Bilateral temporal bone fractures in head injuries.

Box 18.1: Causes of facial nerve palsy

- **Central:** Brain abscess, pontine gliomas, poliomyelitis, multiple sclerosis and cerebrovascular strokes.
- **Cerebellopontine angle tumors:** (Acoustic neuroma, meningioma, congenital cholesteatoma) see Chapter on 'Tumors of Ear and Cerebellopontine Angle'.
- **Intratemporal part**
  - *Idiopathic:* Bell's palsy, recurrent facial palsy and Melkersson's syndrome.
  - *Infection:* Acute and chronic suppurative otitis media, herpes zoster oticus, tuberculosis and malignant otitis externa.
  - *Surgical trauma:* Mastoidectomy and stapedectomy.
  - *Accidental trauma:* Fractures of temporal bone.
  - *Neoplasms:* Malignancy of external and middle ear, rhabdomyosarcoma, histiocytosis, leukemia, glomus tumors, facial nerve neuroma, metastasis to temporal bone (from cancer of breast, bronchus, prostate).
- **Parotid:** Malignancy, surgery, accidental injury and birth trauma.
- **Congenital:** Compression injury, Mobius syndrome, lower lip paralysis.
- **Systemic diseases:** Diabetes mellitus, hypothyroidism, uremia, polyarteritis nodosa, Wegener's granulomatosis, sarcoidosis (Heerfordt's syndrome), leprosy, Guillain-Barre syndrome, Lyme disease, AIDS, infectious mononucleosis and autoimmune diseases.

SEQUELAE/COMPLICATIONS OF FACIAL NERVE PALSY

Peripheral facial paralysis may result in following complications:
- **Incomplete recovery:** It can result in facial asymmetry, epiphora (due to inability to close eye), drooling of saliva and difficulty in chewing food (due to weak oral sphincter). Drooling during chewing and drinking and impairment of speech may result in social problems.
- **Exposure keratitis:** Evaporation of tears from the opened eye results in dryness that leads to keratitis and corneal ulcer. The condition becomes worse when lesion is above the geniculate ganglion. The findings of corneal irritation are redness, itching, foreign body sensation and visual blurring.
- **Synkinesis (mass movement):** While closing the eye corner of mouth twitches. It may happen vice versa. It occurs due to cross innervation of fibers.
- **Tics and spasms:** Involuntary movements of the facial muscles occur, which are due to the faulty regeneration of fibers.
- **Contractures:** The fixed contraction or fibrosis of atrophied muscles affects movements of face. The facial symmetry is maintained at rest.
- **Crocodile tears (gustatory lacrimation):** The condition is characterized by the lacrimation during the mastication. The faulty regeneration of parasympathetic fibers occurs and they supply lacrimal gland instead of the salivary glands. Treatment consists of the section of greater superficial petrosal nerve or tympanic neurectomy.
- **Frey's syndrome (gustatory sweating):** This condition is characterized by the sweating and flushing of skin over the parotid during mastication. It happens in some cases of parotid surgery.
- **Psychological and social problems.**

BELL'S PALSY

Bell's palsy is an idiopathic demyelinating disease. It is characterized by an acute isolated unilateral lower motor neuron facial paralysis.
- It accounts for over 50% of acute facial palsies.
- Both sexes are equally affected.
- There is no age bar, but incidence rises with increasing age.
- Risk factors include diabetes (angiopathy) and pregnancy (retention of fluid).

Etiology

- **Viral infection:** Many reports suggest viral infections due to herpes simplex, herpes zoster and Epstein-Barr virus. Some consider Bell's palsy a part of the

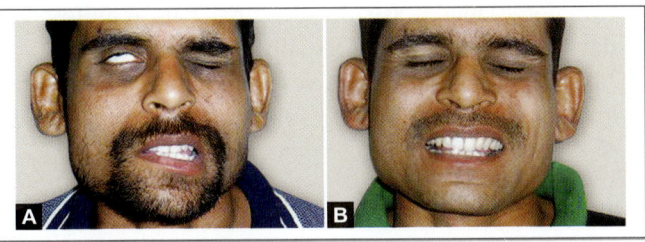

Figs 18.9A and B: Right Bell's facial palsy. (A) Note the inability to close the eye and move the angle of mouth, and upward rolling of eye ball (Bell's phenomenon); (B) Recovery of facial palsy

polyneuropathy. Other cranial nerves may also be involved.
- *Vascular ischemia:* Primary ischemia may be induced by cold or emotional stress. It causes increased capillary permeability that leads to exudation of fluid, edema and compression of microcirculation of the nerve (secondary ischemia).
- *Hereditary:* About 10% of patients give positive family history. The narrow Fallopian canal (hereditary predisposition) can make the nerve susceptible to early compression at the slightest edema.
- *Autoimmunity:* T-lymphocyte changes have been seen.

Clinical Features

This sudden onset of complete or incomplete isolated unilateral lower motor neuron facial palsy present (Fig. 18.9) with following features:
- Inability to close eye
- Bell's phenomenon (when patient tries to close the eye, eyeball turns up) (Fig. 18.9A).
- Dribbling of saliva from the angle of mouth
- Asymmetrical face
- Epiphora (tears flowing down from the eye)
- Earache may precede or accompany the facial palsy
- Hyperacusis (sensitivity to loud sounds due to stapedial palsy)
- Diminished taste sensation: It may occur due to the involvement of chorda tympani
- Bell's palsy is recurrent either ipsilateral or contralateral in 12% of patient.

Diagnosis

Diagnosis of Bell's palsy is usually clinical and by exclusion. Patient requires careful history and examination to exclude other known causes of facial paralysis.
- *Laboratory tests:* Some patients need radiological studies, complete blood count (CBC), peripheral blood smear, sedimentation rate, blood sugar and serology.
- *Nerve excitability tests:* They are done daily or on alternate days to monitor nerve degeneration.
- *Topodiagnostic tests:* They help in establishing the site of lesion.

Differential Diagnoses

The presence of any of the cause (Box 18.1) will rule out the diagnosis of Bell's palsy.

Treatment

Regular electrophysiological assessment is important to know the extent of nerve damage and determine the need of surgical decompression.

General Measures

- *Reassurance.*
- *Analgesics:* For the relief of ear pain.
- *Eye care:* Eye must be protected against exposure keratitis. The preventive measures include:
  - Artificial tears (methylcellulose drops) every 1–2 hours and 4–5 times per day
  - Eye ointment followed by patching or taping the eye
  - Cover for the eye in night
  - Protecting the eye from wind, foreign bodies and drying with glasses and moisture chambers
  - Temporary tarsorrhaphy (may be needed in some cases).
- *Physiotherapy:* The facial muscles massage though does not influence recovery, gives psychological support. Active facial movements should be encouraged.

Medical Treatment

- *Steroids:* Though their utility has been doubtful they are used by many, if patient reports within 1 week. Steroids have been reported to prevent incidence of synkinesis and crocodile tears and shorten the recovery time. Prednisolone (1 mg/kg/day) divided into morning and evening doses for 5–10 days depending upon whether the paralysis is incomplete or is recovering. Thereafter the doses are tapered in next 5–10 days.

> **Contraindications:** Pregnancy, diabetes, hypertension, peptic ulcer, pulmonary tuberculosis and glaucoma.

- *Acyclovir:* Steroids are generally combined with acyclovir.
- *Other drugs:* Vasodilators, vitamins, mast cell inhibitors and antihistaminics are of no avail.

Surgical Facial Nerve Decompression

It relieves pressure on the nerve fibers and improves their microcirculation. Both the vertical and tympanic segments of nerve are decompressed. Some favor decompression of the whole Fallopian canal including labyrinthine segment. The approaches include postaural and middle fossa.

Prognosis

- Majority of the patients (85–90%) recover fully.
- Ninety five percent patients of incomplete Bell's palsy recover completely.
- The chances of complete recovery are better when clinical recovery begins within 3 weeks of onset.
- Some of the patients (10–15%) do not recover completely and some stigmata of regeneration remains.
- Recurrent facial palsy may not recover fully.

RECURRENT FACIAL PALSY

- In 3–10% cases of Bell's palsy, recurrent episodes of facial palsy occur.
- In cases of unilateral recurrent facial palsy, facial nerve neuroma should be ruled out.
- Other causes include Melkersson's syndrome, diabetes, sarcoidosis and tumors.

MELKERSSON'S SYNDROME

- This idiopathic disorder has a triad of facial paralysis, swelling of lips and fissured tongue.
- Patients get recurrent attacks of facial palsy.
- Treatment is similar to Bell's palsy.

RAMSAY HUNT SYNDROME OR HERPES ZOSTER OTICUS (VARICELLA-ZOSTER VIRUS)

The disease is caused by varicella-zoster virus (VZV) that starts replicating first in geniculate ganglia and then travels down and affect, facial nerve, inner ear and spiral and vestibular ganglia. Ganglia of trigeminal and CN VIII have also been implicated (Figs 18.10A and B).

Clinical Features

- Painful vesicles with erythematous base appear in the canal and concha, behind pinna and or soft palate. Later vesicles rupture and form crusts.

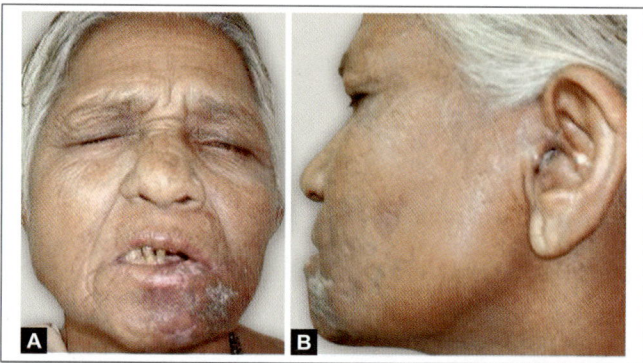

Figs 18.10A and B: Recovering facial palsy and herpes lesions. (A) Front view is showing left facial paresis and healing herpes lesions; (B) Lateral view showing herpes lesions of left external ear

- Unilateral facial palsy and deep ear pain manifest 1–2 days later. Facial paresis usually recovers over weeks.
- About 25% patients have vertigo, nystagmus, tinnitus and hearing loss.

Treatment

- Tab. acyclovir 800 mg 5 times a day or famcyclovir seen 500 mg TDS or valacyclovir 1 gm TDS for 7 days.
- Tab. prednisone tapering dose 6 days course beginning usually with 1 mg/kg.
- Topical antibiotic/steroid ear drops.
- Eye care.

TEMPORAL BONE FRACTURE

Facial nerve palsy is due to intraneural hematoma, compression by a bony spicule or transection of nerve. Traditionally, temporal bone fractures are divided into three categories:

1. Transverse
2. Longitudinal
3. Oblique/mixed

The differences between longitudinal and transverse temporal bone fractures are enumerated in Table 18.2.

> *Temporal bone fracture:* Clinical features include hearing loss, dizziness, facial weakness, ear bleeding, hemotympanum, raccoon eyes, and/or bruising over the mastoid cortex (Battle's sign).
> - *Radiological investigation:* The best radiologic examination is a fine cut, axial and coronal, temporal bone CT scan.
> - *Indications for surgical exploration of the facial nerve:*
>   - Immediate onset of complete facial paralysis.
>   - Delayed onset of complete facial paralysis associated with:
>   - Radiologic evidence of a fracture through the Fallopian canal of facial nerve.
>   - Poor prognostic testing with electroneuronography or electromyography.

IATROGENIC OR SURGICAL TRAUMA

Facial nerve may be damaged accidentally during stapedectomy, tympanoplasty or mastoid surgery. The paralysis may be immediate (needs earliest surgical decompression and repair) or delayed (treated conservatively). The exposed nerve may be pressed by the pressure on ear packing. This just needs removal of ear pack.

Surprisingly, even if the facial nerve is surgically removed secondary to a parotid tumor, facial nerve functions can spontaneously return. The precise mechanism of this rare occurrence is not known.

Table 18.2: Differences between longitudinal and transverse temporal bone fractures

Characteristics	Longitudinal	Transverse
Frequency	More common (80%)	Less common (20%)
Site of blow	Parietal	Occipital
Otic capsule	Usually otic capsule sparing	Usually disrupting
Fracture line	From squamous part of temporal bone to foramen lacerum, parallel to long axis of petrous pyramid	From foramen magnum to foramen spinosum through jugular foramen, across the petrous pyramid
Injury to external and middle ear	Common	Absent
Ear bleeding	Common	Absent because tympanic membrane is intact
Hemotympanum	Absent	Common
CSF otorrhea	Present	Absent (CSF may pass through Eustachian tube)
Labyrinth or CN VIII injury	Uncommon	Common
Hearing loss	Usually conductive	Usually sensorineural
Vertigo	Uncommon (may be present due to concussion)	Generally severe due to labyrinth or CN VIII injuries
Facial paralysis	Uncommon (20%)	Common (50%)
Onset of facial palsy	Usually delayed	Usually immediate
Site of facial nerve injury	Horizontal tympanic segment	Meatal or labyrinthine segment geniculate ganglion

Abbreviation: CSF—cerebrospinal fluid; CN—cranial nerve

Prophylaxis

Thorough anatomical knowledge and temporal bone dissection under good quality operative microscope trains the surgeon and avoids facial nerve injuries during the ear surgeries. Other tips, which help in avoiding damage to the nerve, are as follows:

- Always work along the course of facial nerve and never across the nerve.
- Constant irrigation during the drilling avoids thermal injury to the facial nerve.
- Diamond burr must be used when working near the nerve.
- If nerve is exposed, do not get scared. Just handle the nerve gently. Avoid unnecessary handling and instrumentations.
- Do not remove those granulations which penetrate facial nerve.

HYPERKINETIC DISORDERS OF FACIAL NERVE

The involuntary twitching of facial muscles on one or both sides occurs in cases of hemifacial spasm and blepharospasm.

Hemifacial Spasm

There occurs involuntary unilateral repeated twitching of facial muscles. There are two types of hemifacial spasms idiopathic and secondary:

1. ***Essential or idiopathic:*** Cause is not known.
   Treatment consists of the following:
   - Selective section of the branches of facial nerve in the parotid.
   - Puncturing the facial nerve with a needle in its tympanic segment.
   - Injection of botulinum blocks the neuromuscular junction by preventing release of acetylcholine in the affected muscle.
2. ***Secondary:*** The irritation of facial nerve can be caused by following cerebellopontine angle disorders:
   - Acoustic neuroma
   - Congenital cholesteatoma
   - Glomus tumor
   - Vascular loop at the cerebellopontine angle: It is treated by microvascular decompression through posterior fossa craniotomy.

Blepharospasm

Twitching and spasms of the orbicularis oculi muscles on both sides results in closure of both the eyes causing functional blindness.

- The cause, which is yet not certain, perhaps lies in the basal ganglia.
- Treatment includes:
  - Selective section of nerves supplying muscles around the eye on both sides.
  - Injection botulinum A into the peripheral muscles gives relief for 3–6 months. It can be repeated if required.

SURGICAL TREATMENT OF FACIAL NERVE PALSY

- **Suppurative otitis media (SOM):** In addition to the aggressive antibiotic therapy following surgical measures are taken in cases of SOM:
    - *Myringotomy:* It is indicated in cases of acute otitis media (AOM) and coalescent mastoiditis.
    - *Tympanomastoid surgery:* In cases of coalescent mastoiditis and cholesteatoma.
- **Decompression:** The facial nerve is compressed by intraneural edema, hematoma and a fractured bone in the Fallopian canal. The compressed nerve is exposed in surgical decompression. The facial nerve sheath is slit to relieve pressure.

    When electrical tests indicate progressive nerve weakness (> 90%) facial nerve decompression should be done at the earliest in cases of Bell's palsy, Ramsay Hunt syndrome and longitudinal temporal bone fracture.
- **End-to-end anastomosis:** It is a suitable procedure for extratemporal part of facial nerve. The gap between the severed ends of nerves are few millimeters. The two ends should be approximated without any tension. A 9/0 or 10/0 monofilament suture is used to tie the nerve ends.
- **Nerve graft (cable graft):** It is indicated when the gap between severed ends is more and cannot be closed without tension by end-to-end anastomosis. Nerve graft is usually taken from greater auricular nerve, lateral cutaneous nerve of thigh or the sural nerve. In the Fallopian canal, graft may not need any suturing.
- **Hypoglossal-facial anastomosis:** It is indicated when proximal facial nerve stump cannot be identified. Anastomosis of hypoglossal nerve to the severed peripheral end of the facial nerve improves the muscle tone and permits some movements of facial muscles. It leads to unilateral atrophy of tongue muscles. However, patient adjusts to the difficulty in chewing and articulation within few weeks.
- **Plastic procedures:** The procedures such as facial slings, face lift operation, slings of masseter and temporalis muscle, improve cosmetic appearance in cases where nerve grafting is not possible or has failed. The slings of masseter and temporalis muscle provide not only the facial symmetry but also some movement to face.

Self-evaluation Exercises

1. Which of the following is the shortest and most narrow segment of facial canal?
    a. Labyrinthine segment
    b. Tympanic segment
    c. Mastoid segment
    d. Meatal segment
2. Which of the following is the longest segment of facial nerve?
    a. Labyrinthine segment
    b. Tympanic segment
    c. Mastoid segment
    d. Meatal segment
    e. Intracranial and parotid
3. During superficial parotidectomy which is said to be the most reliable landmark to identify main trunk of facial nerve?
    a. Tympanomastoid suture
    B. Mastoid tip
    c. Styloid process
    d. Auricular cartilage
4. Which of the following statement are not true for the facial nerve and middle ear relations?
    a. Landmark used for identification of geniculate ganglion of facial nerve is processus cochleariformis
    b. Tympanic segment of facial nerve lies above the oval window and below the horizontal semicircular canal
    c. Mastoid segment of facial nerve always lies behind the tympanomastoid suture and can be located 6–8 mm deeper to tympanomastoid fissure
    d. A patient with lesion between geniculate ganglion and nerve to stapedius will have phonophobia and loss of stapedial reflex and taste sensation
    e. None of the above
5. Which of the following statements are related with the upper motor neuron facial palsy?
    a. Patient can shut both eyes with equal power and can wrinkle his forehead scalp bilaterally
    b. Upper face has a bilateral corticobulbar innervations
    c. Lesions of corticobulbar fibers (in brainstem and genu of internal capsule) result in upper motor neuron facial palsy such as in pseudobulbar palsy
    d. Blink reflex remains intact bilaterally and liquid drips out from the corner of mouth
    e. All of the above

Contd...

Contd…

6. Which of the following is not the cause of recurrent facial paralysis?
    a. Facial nerve neuroma
    b. Diabetes
    c. Melkersson-Rosenthal syndrome
    d. Sarcoidosis
    e. None of the above
7. Which of the following is not the feature of Melkersson-Rosenthal syndrome?
    a. Recurrent upper motor neuron facial paralysis
    b. Fissured tongue
    c. Circumoral edema
    d. None of the above
8. Which of the following statements are not true for Ramsay-Hunt syndrome?
    a. Herpes-zoster virus infection
    b. Involves geniculate ganglion of facial nerve
    c. Vesicular eruptions are seen in concha, posteromedial surface of pinna and soft palate
    d. None of the above

Filling the Blanks

9. In the nerves _____ helps promote regeneration of severed axons. It is produced mainly by Schwann cells and forms a sleeve for regenerating axons.
10. In the upper part at the lateral end (fundus) of internal auditory canal, a vertical crest called _____, separates facial nerve canal from the superior vestibular nerve canal.
11. _____ fracture of temporal bone occur due to a blow from the side of head and has less chances of facial palsy. Patient will have conductive hearing loss.
12. Ecchymosis seen over the mastoid in cases of temporal bone fracture is called _____ sign.
13. _____ fractures of temporal bone result from occipital blow to head and are more likely to cause injury to labyrinth and facial nerve.

True (T)/False (F)

14. Facial nerve supplies to all the muscles derived from first branchial arch.
15. Chorda tympanic nerve, a branch of facial nerve carries afferent postganglionic parasympathetic secretomotor fibers to submandibular and sublingual salivary glands after joining lingual nerve in infratemporal fossa.
16. Greater petrosal nerve, a facial nerve branch from geniculate ganglion carries preganglionic secretomotor fibers for lacrimation, so the tearing is lost in suprageniculate or transgeniculate lesions of facial nerve.
17. Facial nerve exits anterior to digastric ridge and lies above the posterior belly of digastric.
18. The corticobulbar fibers bilaterally innervate the facial motor neurons to the lower face.
19. Bell's palsy is an idiopathic isolated upper motor neuron facial palsy. In Bell's palsy, hyperacusis is due to the paralysis of stapedius muscle.
20. In cases of lower motor neuron facial nerve paralysis, eyeball turns up and out while closing the eyes and this is called Bell's phenomenon.
21. Facial paralysis during pregnancy can occur in cases of preeclampsia.
22. Facial nerve palsy is common in cases of longitudinal temporal bone fracture.
23. Transverse fractures of temporal bone are less common than longitudinal fractures.
24. The most common cause of high frequency SNHL in cases of head injury is labyrinthine concussion.
25. Mastoidectomy is the most common cause of iatrogenic facial nerve palsy.

Answers

1. a	2. e	3. a	4. e	5. e
6. e	7. a	8. d	9. Endoneurium	10. Bill's bar
11. Longitudinal	12. Battle's	13. Transverse	14. F	15. F
16. T	17. T	18. F	19. F	20. T
21. T	22. F	23. T	24. T	25. T

Chapter 19

Tumors of the Ear and Cerebellopontine Angle

⊙ Specific Learning Objectives

After going through the chapter, you should be able to answer the following questions:
- Describe some common tumors of the external ear and their management.
- Describe the clinical features and management of glomus tumors of middle ear.
- Which is the most common cancer of middle ear? Describe its clinical features and management.
- Describe the clinical features and management of acoustic neuroma.

BENIGN TUMORS OF EXTERNAL EAR

Osteomas/exostoses are the most common benign tumors of external auditory canal (EAC) and usually need no treatment. Ear polyps, which are usually not true neoplasms, are (see Chapter 'Otologic Symptoms and Examination') commonly associated with chronic suppurative otitis media (CSOM). Congenital disorders of external ear such as preauricular sinus and cyst are discussed in Chapter 'Diseases of External Ear'.

Osteoma

- This single, smooth, bony, hard, pedunculated tumor arises from the cancellous bone of EAC.
- It usually arises from the posterior meatal wall near the osteocartilaginous junction.
- Surgical removal is done either by fracturing its pedicle or by a drill.

Exostoses

- *Types:* Exostoses arise from compact bone. They are multiple and bilateral.
- *Occupations:* It is common in divers and swimmers, as their ear canals are frequently exposed to cold water.
- *Sex:* Males are affected more than females (3:1).
- *Clinical features:* They present as smooth, sessile, bony swellings in the deeper part of the bony meatus near the tympanic membrane.
- *Treatment:* They need surgical removal only if they impair hearing or cause retention of wax. They are removed with high speed drill. The deep exostoses lie close to facial canal. Therefore, the gouge and hammer are not used.

Cysts

- *Sebaceous cyst:* The most common site for sebaceous cyst is postauricular sulcus below and behind the lobule.
- *Sebaceous adenoma:* It arises from sebaceous glands of the meatus and present as a smooth, skin-covered swelling in the outer part of EAC.
- *Dermoid cyst:* It is usually present as a rounded mass over the upper part of mastoid.
- *Treatment:* These swellings require total surgical excision.

Hemangiomas

Hemangiomas are congenital tumors seen in children and may involve other parts of face and neck.
- *Capillary hemangioma:* It is a tumor of capillaries which present as a port-wine stain and does not regress.
- *Cavernous hemangioma:* This strawberry tumor is composed of endothelial lined blood spaces and increases rapidly during the first year of childhood. After that it starts regressing and usually disappears by the fifth year of life.

Papilloma

- *Papilloma (wart)* is a viral disease. It presents as a tufted growth or flat gray plaque with rough surface. It needs surgical excision or curettage with cauterization of its base.

- ***Cutaneous horn*** is a form of papilloma with heaping up of keratin. It presents as horn-shaped tumor at the rim of helix in elderly people. Treatment consists of surgical excision.

Keratoacanthoma
- Keratoacanthoma, though a benign tumor, looks like malignant one. Patient develops a raised nodule which has a central crater.
- To begin with it grows fast, but then slowly regresses and leaves a scar.
- Treatment consists of excisional biopsy.

Neurofibroma
- The non-tender and firm swelling which patient has may be part of the von Recklinghausen's disease.
- If the tumor obstructs EAC or presents a cosmetic problem it needs surgical excision.

Ceruminoma
It is a tumor of ceruminous gland.
- ***Clinical features:*** This benign tumor presents as a smooth, firm, skin-covered polypoid swelling. It is usually attached to the posterior or inferior wall of outer part of EAC. The tumor can obstruct the EAC and results in wax collection.
- ***Treatment:*** Wide surgical excision is required to prevent recurrence. If malignancy is suspected or confirmed on biopsy, radiotherapy should be given. Malignant ceruminoma is more common than benign (2:1 ratio).

Keloid of Auricle
The common sites for keloids, which occur after trauma or piercing of the ear for ornaments, are the lobule and helix. Black races are affected more. Postauricular keloids (Fig. 19.1A) are occasionally seen after mastoid surgery.

Treatment: Surgical excision usually results in recurrence (Fig. 19.1B). Recurrence can be avoided by local injection of triamcinolone into the surgical site and pre and postoperative radiation with a total dose of 600–800 rads, which are delivered in four divided doses.

MALIGNANT TUMORS OF EXTERNAL EAR

These neoplasms are uncommon. The three most common malignant neoplasms of the auricle are as follows:
1. Basal cell carcinoma.
2. Squamous cell carcinoma.
3. Melanomas.
- ***Etiology:*** The radiation (direct sunlight) and chronic ear inflammation are the two important etiologic factors.
- ***Site:*** Most common site is auricle (85%). EAC (10%) and middle ear (5%) are rare sites of ear carcinoma.

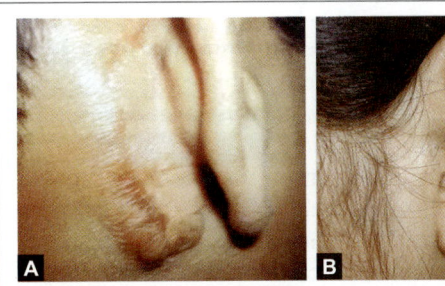
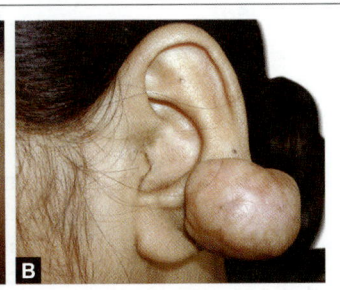

Figs 19.1A and B: (A) Keloid after postauricular mastoid surgery; (B) Recurrent keloid. Recurrence after surgery of keloid that occurred after ear piercing

Squamous Cell Carcinoma of Auricle
Clinical Features
- ***Predisposing factor:*** Prolonged exposure to direct sunlight.
- ***Age and sex:*** Common in fair-complexioned people especially in males who are in their fifties.
- ***Most common site:*** Helix.
- ***Lesion:*** A painless nodule or an ulcer with raised everted edges and indurated base.
- ***Metastases:*** Its spread to regional lymph nodes occurs very late.

Treatment
- In small lesion with no nodal metastasis, local excision with 1 cm of safety margin is sufficient.
- In large tumor coming within 1 cm of EAC with nodal metastases, total amputation of the pinna with en bloc removal of parotid gland and cervical lymph nodes is done.

Basal Cell Carcinoma of Auricle
- ***Common sites:*** They are the helix and the tragus.
- ***Age and sex:*** More common in elderly men (> 50 years).
- ***Lymphatic metastasis:*** It is rare.
- ***Clinical features:*** Nodular ulcer with raised or beaded edge and central crust, which on removal result in bleeding.
  - Lesion usually extends circumferentially into the skin but may penetrate cartilage and bone.

Treatment
- ***Superficial skin lesions:*** Radiotherapy.
- ***Lesions involving cartilage:*** Surgical excision consists of total amputation of the pinna with en bloc removal of parotid gland.

Melanoma of Auricle
- ***Predisposing factor:*** Direct exposure to sun. Common in men of light complexion.
- ***Metastases:*** It occurs in 16–50% of the cases.

Treatment

- *Early lesion:* Wedge resection and primary closure in cases of superficial melanoma which is less than 1 cm in diameter and situated over the helix.
- *Advanced lesion:* Superficial melanoma (larger than 1 cm), infiltrative melanomas, melanoma of posterior auricular surface or concha and recurrent melanomas need total amputation of the pinna with en bloc removal of parotid gland and cervical lymph nodes.

TUMORS OF MIDDLE EAR AND MASTOID

Tumors of middle ear and mastoid are divided into benign and malignant. Malignant tumors are further divided into primary and secondary (Box 19.1).

- Tumors of the ear may masquerade as chronic ear infection. While treating these chronic EAC and middle ear infections, the suspicion of neoplasm should be kept in mind.

> Glomus tumors are the most common true neoplasms of the middle ear.

- Hemangiomas, squamous cell carcinoma and rhabdomyosarcoma can also occur.

Glomus Tumors (Paragangliomas)

- This most common benign neoplasm of middle ear arises from the glomus bodies, which resemble carotid body in structure. The paraganglionic cells of the tumor are derived from the neural crest.
- Females are affected five times more than the males. It is often seen in the middle age (40-50 years). In such cases search should be made for other glomus tumors.

Pathology

- This benign non-encapsulated tumor is extremely vascular neoplasm.

Box 19.1: Tumors of the middle ear and mastoid

- **Benign**
  - *Glomus tumor*—glomus jugulare and glomus tympanicum
- **Malignant**
  - *Primary*
    - *Carcinoma*—squamous cell carcinoma, adenocarcinoma
    - *Sarcoma*—rhabdomyosarcoma, osteosarcoma, lymphoma, fibrosarcoma and chondrosarcoma
  - *Secondary*
    - *Metastatic*—carcinoma of bronchus, breast, kidney, thyroid, prostate and gastrointestinal tract
    - *From adjacent areas*—nasopharynx, external auditory canal and parotid.

- Though the tumor is locally invasive, its growth is very slow, extending over several years.
- Histology shows of masses or sheets of epithelial cells which have large nuclei and a granular cytoplasm. The thin walled blood sinusoids without any contractile muscle coat are in abundance and account for profuse bleeding.
- They carry < 3% malignancy conversion rate.
- Less than 1% tumors are associated with catecholamine secretions.

Sites

The glomus bodies are present in the dome of jugular bulb and along the course of tympanic branch of 9th cranial nerve (Jacobson's nerve) on the promontory. So there are mainly two types of glomus tumors:

1. *Glomus jugulare:* This tumor arises from the dome of jugular bulb and invades the hypotympanum and jugular foramen. It involves CN IX, X, XI and XII and may compress internal jugular vein and encroach its lumen.
2. *Glomus tympanicum:* This tumor arises from the promontory and may cause facial paralysis.

Spread

- *Local:* The tumor first fills the middle ear and then invades the tympanic membrane and present as an ear polyp, which bleeds readily. It may later on invade following structures:
  - Labyrinth, petrous pyramid and the mastoid.
  - Jugular foramen and the 9th to 12th cranial nerves.
  - Through Eustachian tube, tumor may enter into the nasopharynx.
  - Posterior and middle cranial fossa.
- *Metastatic:* Lungs and bones metastases are rare. Metastatic lymph node involvement can occur.

Clinical Features

- **Intratympanic tumor**
  - Earliest features are hearing loss and tinnitus.
    - *Hearing loss:* Conductive and slowly progressive.
    - *Tinnitus:* Pulsatile, swishing character and synchronous with pulse. It can be stopped by carotid pressure.
    - *Audible systolic bruit* over mastoid.
  - **Otoscopy**
    - *Red reflex* through intact tympanic membrane.
    - *Rising sun appearance:* When tumor arises from the floor of middle ear.
    - *Tympanic membrane* appears bluish and bulging.
    - *Pulsation sign (Brown's sign):* On increasing the ear canal pressure with Siegle's speculum, tumor pulsates vigorously and then blanches. Reverse happens with release of pressure.

- ◆ *Aquino's sign:* Otoscopy shows blenching of glomus jugulare tumor on compression of carotid artery.
- *Ear polyp*
  - *Profuse bleeding:* Either spontaneously or on attempts to clean EAC.
  - *Dizziness or vertigo*
  - *Facial paralysis*
  - *Earache* is less common than in carcinoma of the external and middle ear.
  - *Otorrhea:* It is due to secondary infection and simulates chronic suppurative otitis media polyp.
  - *Red, vascular polyp* filling the meatus, which bleeds readily and profusely on manipulation. **Biopsy is contraindicated**.
- *9th to 12th cranial nerve palsies*
  These are late features and occur several years after ear symptoms.
  - Dysphagia.
  - Dysarthria and hoarseness of voice.
  - Unilateral paralysis of soft palate, pharynx and vocal cord.
  - Weakness of trapezius and sternocleidomastoid muscles.
- *Catecholamine features:* Headache, sweating, palpitation, hypertension and anxiety.
- *Mass over the mastoid or in the nasopharynx.*

Pulsatile tinnitus: In cases of pulsatile tinnitus, always first rule out the paraganglioma (glomus tympanicum or jugulare).

Differential Diagnoses

Because of their appearance, glomus tumors may be mistaken for:
- High-riding jugular bulb or dehiscent jugular bulb.
- Aberrant carotid artery.

Jugular Foramen Syndrome

This syndrome consists of the palsies of the CN IX, X and XI, which pass through the jugular foramen. The causes include:
- Tumors
  - Glomus tumors (paraganglioma)
  - Nerve sheath tumors
  - Sarcomas
- Lymphadenopathy
- Skull fracture

Investigations

- *Catecholamines:*
  - Serum levels of catecholamines.
  - Break-down products of catecholamines in urine—vanillylmandelic acid, metanephrine, etc.
- *CT scan-head:* Bone window, 1 mm thin sections help to distinguish glomus tympanicum from the glomus jugulare. Caroticojugular spine is eroded in the glomus jugulare. The aberrant carotid artery, high or dehiscent jugular bulb can also be diagnosed.
- *MRI:* Shows soft tissue extent of the tumor.
- *Magnetic resonance angiography (MRA) and venography:* MRA and venography show invasion of jugular bulb and internal jugular vein and carotid artery.
- *Four vessel angiography:* It provides following information:
  - Extent of tumor
  - Compression of internal carotid artery
  - Finding other carotid body tumors
  - Decision for embolization of tumor
  - Brain perfusion studies and adequacy of contralateral internal carotid artery and circle of Willis.
- *Biopsy: It is contraindicated because the tumor is highly vascular and bleeds profusely.*

Phelps sign: It is seen in cases of glomus jugulare tumor and consists of destruction of bone between the carotid canal and jugular foramen.

Treatment

Treatment modalities include surgical removal, radiation, embolization and combination of these techniques.
- *Surgical removal:* Depending upon the extent of tumor it can be removed through transmeatal, transmastoid and skull base approach.
- *Radiation:* It does not cure but reduces the vascularity of the tumor and arrests its growth. Its indications are as follows:
  - Inoperable tumors
  - Residual tumors
  - Recurrences after surgery
  - Elderly patients who cannot withstand extensive skull base surgery.
- *Embolization:* Embolization reduces the vascularity of tumor before surgery. It may become the sole treatment in inoperable and irradiated patients.

Carcinoma of Middle Ear/EAC

Carcinoma of middle ear and mastoid, though the most common primary middle ear malignancy is rare tumor. It arises either primarily from middle ear or is an extension of carcinoma of deep bony meatus.

Etiology

- **Age:** Patients are in the age group of 40–60.
- **Sex:** It is slightly more common in females.
- **Chronic suppurative otitis media (CSOM):** Most patients (75%) have associated chronic ear discharge that mimics CSOM. Chronic irritation is perhaps the causative factor. Carcinoma can develop in radical mastoid cavities.
- **Radium dial painters:** Primary carcinoma of mastoid air cells is more common in these workers.

Pathology

- Types of carcinoma of EAC in order of decreasing frequency include squamous cell carcinoma, basal cell carcinoma and adenoid cystic carcinoma.
- Adenocarcinoma, which is less common, arises from the glandular elements of middle ear.

Spread

- The tumor destroys ossicles, facial canal, internal ear, jugular bulb, carotid canal, deep bony meatus and mastoid.
- Medially, it spreads toward the petrous apex. Dura is usually resistant to the spread.
- Anteriorly, it spreads and involves parotid gland, temporomandibular joint and infratemporal fossa.
- Through the Eustachian tube it can enter into the nasopharynx.
- Lymph nodes are involved at an advanced stage.

Clinical Features

Appearance of persistent and inordinate pain or blood stained discharge in chronic cases of painless mucopurulent or purulent otorrhea (CSOM or chronic otits externa) should raise the suspicion.

- Foul-smelling blood-stained discharge.
- Severe ear pain especially in night.
- An ulcerated area in the meatus or a bleeding friable polypoid mass or granulations.
- Meaty or polypoid mass in EAC (squamous cell carcinoma) (Fig. 19.2A).
- Small pimple with significant pain (adenoid cystic carcinoma).
- Serpiginous ulceration (basal cell carcinoma).
- Facial nerve palsy can occur because of local extension (Fig. 19.2B).
- Labyrinthine involvement causes SNHL and vertigo.
- **Late features:** Parotid mass, CN IX X XI and XII palsy, cervical lymphadenopathy.

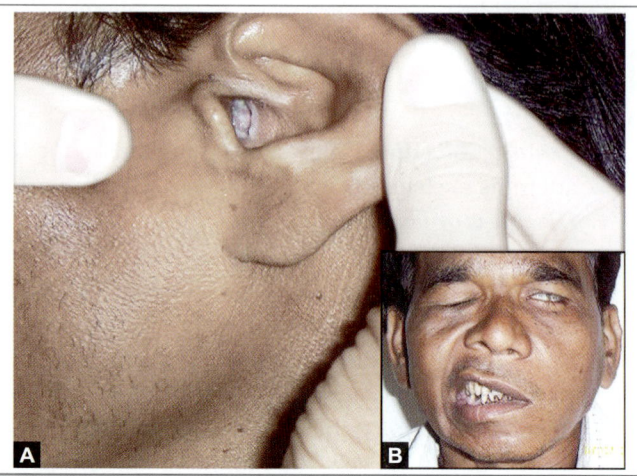

Figs 19.2A and B: (A) Carcinoma left middle ear and external auditory canal (EAC). Mass in left EAC; (B) Inset shows left facial palsy of the same patient

- Tumor may originate from nasopharynx.
- Enlargement of regional lymph nodes—preauricular, postauricular, infra-auricular and upper deep cervical.

Investigations

- **CT scan and angiography:** They show the extent of tumor and bone invasion.
- **Biopsy:** Biopsy should be taken in cases of intractable chronic otitis externa. Histopathology will confirm the nature of lesion.

Treatment

It consists of en bloc wide surgical excision with postoperative radiation. The combination of surgery and radiotherapy offers better prognosis.

- **Surgery:** Depending on the extent of tumor, it may consist of radical mastoidectomy, subtotal/total petrosectomy.
- **Radiotherapy:** Radiotherapy alone is palliative and is considered when the growth involves CN IX, X, XI and XII or spreads to the cranial cavity or nasopharynx.

Rhabdomyosarcoma

This rare tumor arises from the embryonic muscles, tissue or the pluripotential mesenchyme. It mostly affects children.

- **Early cases mimic CSOM** and have ear discharge, polyp or granulations.
- **Facial palsy** occurs early.
- **Swelling** in the surrounding region of the ear.
- **Biopsy:** It establishes the diagnosis.
- **Treatment:** A combination of radiation and chemotherapy is the best modality of treatment. Surgery is considered in selected localized tumors.
- **Prognosis:** It is poor.

INTERNAL AUDITORY CANAL (IAC) AND CEREBELLOPONTINE ANGLE (CPA)

Contents of Internal Auditory Canal

In addition to internal auditory vessels, following nerves enter the IAC (Fig 19.3):
- *Facial nerve* in anterosuperior quadrant.
- *Superior vestibular nerve* in posterosuperior quadrant.
- *Cochlear nerve* in anteroinferior quadrant.
- *Inferior vestibular nerve* in posteroinferior quadrant.

Boundaries of Cerebellopontine Angle (CPA)

CPA is a potential space in posterior cranial fossa which has following boundaries:
- *Anterior:* Petrous part of temporal bone.
- *Posterior:* Cerebellum.
- *Inferior:* Cerebellar tonsil.
- *Superior:* Pons and cerebellar peduncles.

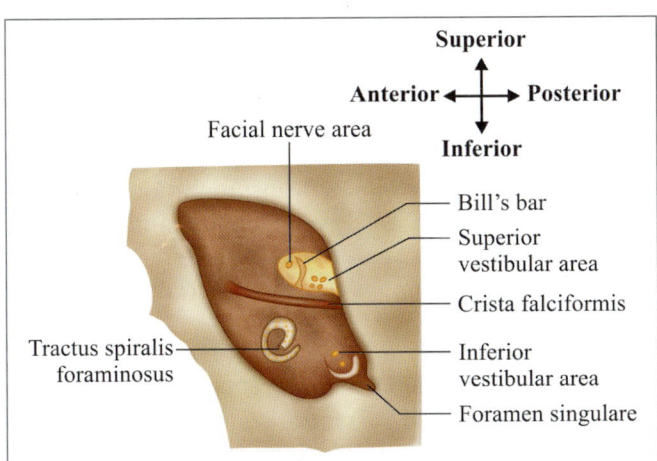

Fig. 19.3: Fundus of right internal auditory canal (IAC) as seen through the IAC

Relations of CPA (Fig. 19.4)

Facial and vestibulocochlear nerves pass superiorly and laterally through the CPA and enter into the IAC. Other cranial nerves have following relations with CPA:
- *Superior:* Trigeminal nerve.
- *Inferior:* Glossopharyngeal, vagus and accessory cranial nerves.

ACOUSTIC NEUROMA (AN)

Syn: Vestibular schwannoma or neurilemmoma

Acoustic neuroma (AN) is the most common (80%) CPA tumor and constitutes 10% of all the brain tumors.

This benign, encapsulated eighth nerve tumor is extremely slow growing. It is composed of elongated spindle cells with rod-shaped nuclei which are lying in rows or palisades. The unilateral tumors are more common. In patients of neurofibromatosis bilateral tumors are seen.

Growth

AN arises from the Schwann cells of the vestibular nerve twice as often as from the cochlear nerve. It reaches the CPA (Figs 19.4A to D) after eroding and widening IAC. Anterosuperiorly it involves the CN V and inferiorly involves the CN IX, X and XI, which lie in jugular foramen. The big AN can displace brainstem and put pressure on cerebellum and raise intracranial tension. Seventy percent of ANs grow slowly over years and 30% remain stable.

Genetic Association and Von Recklinghausen Disease

Five percent of AN patients have neurofibromatosis (NF), which is also called *von Recklinghausen's disease*. The NF associated tumors are not capsulated and may be multiple or bilateral. These AN tumors are more aggressive. Though rarely, they can undergo malignant change.

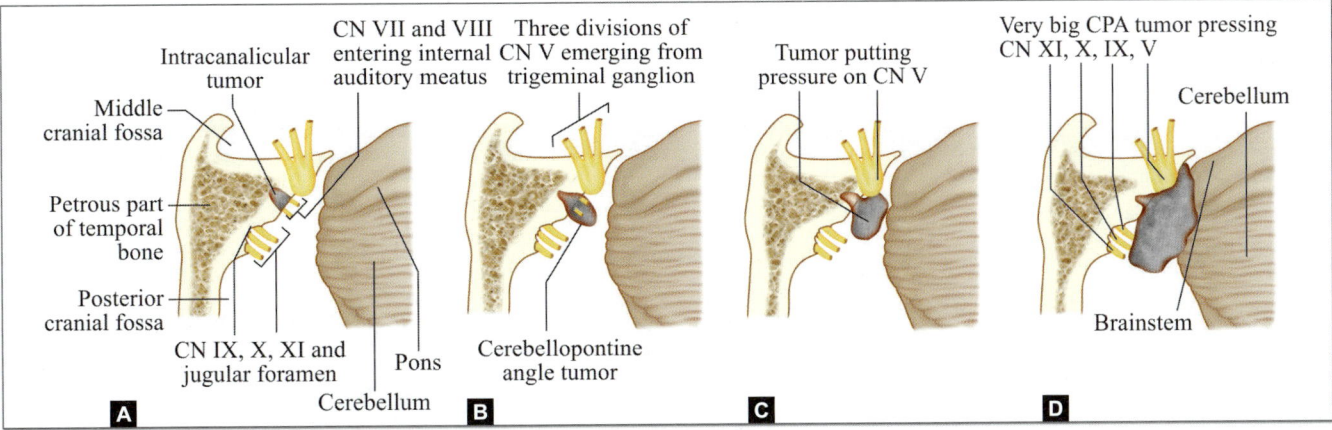

Figs 19.4A to D: Acoustic neuroma. (A) Intracanalicular tumor; (B) Cerebellopontine angle tumor; (C) Tumor pressing trigeminal nerve; (D) Tumor pressing glossopharyngeal, vagus, and accessory nerves, brainstem and cerebellum

Clinical Features

Acoustic neuroma: Asymptomatic AN occurs in about 2% of the population.

> The cases of progressive unilateral sensorineural hearing loss (SNHL) and unilateral tinnitus must be investigated to rule out AN.

- ***Onset:*** The growth of AN is extremely slow and patient's history may extend over several years.
- ***Age and sex:*** Patients are usually in age group of 40–60 years. Female to male ratio is 3:2.
- ***Intracanalicular tumor:*** It is limited to IAC and can put pressure on cochlear and vestibular nerves and internal auditory artery. Progressive unilateral SNHL, which is often accompanied by tinnitus, is the most common presenting symptom.
    - ***Hearing loss:*** Progressive unilateral SNHL. Difficulty in understanding speech is out of proportion to the pure tone hearing loss. Some patients present with sudden SNHL.
    - ***Tinnitus***
    - ***Vestibular symptoms:*** Imbalance or unsteadiness occurs in 50% of patients. Sudden-onset rotatory vertigo is rare because slow growth of tumor results in vestibular compensation.
- ***Facial nerve:*** Sensory fibers are more sensitive and affected early. Motor fibers are more resistant so are affected late.
    - ***Histeliberger's sign:*** Numbness of posterior aspect of concha, which is supplied by the sensory fibers of the facial nerve.
    - ***Electrogustometry:*** Loss of taste from anterior 2/3 tongue.
    - ***Schirmer's test:*** Reduced lacrimation.
    - ***Blink reflex:*** It is delayed.
- ***CN V:*** The first extracanalicular nerve to be involved is trigeminal. The tumor is in CPA and of about 2.5 cm size.
    - Reduced corneal sensitivity.
    - Numbness or paresthesia of face.
- ***CN IX and X***
    - Dysphagia, hoarseness of voice and nasal regurgitation of fluid.
    - Palatal, pharyngeal and laryngeal paralysis.
- ***CN XI, XII, III, IV and VI:*** They are involved when tumor is very large.
- ***Brainstem:*** Long motor and sensory tracts are involved.
    - Weakness and numbness of the arms and legs with exaggerated tendon reflexes.
- ***Cerebellum:*** Finger-nose test, knee-heel test, dysdiadochokinesia, ataxic gait, inability to walk along a straight line with tendency to fall to the affected side.
- ***Raised intracranial tension***
    - Blurring of vision, headache, nausea, vomiting, and diplopia (CN VI involvement).
    - ***Fundus examination:*** Papilloedema (blurring of disk margins).

Audiometry

Retrocochlear hearing loss occurs. The differences between the cochlear and retrocochlear hearing losses are given in Table 19.1:
- Hearing loss is more marked in high frequencies.
- Poor speech discrimination disproportionate to pure tone hearing loss. Roll over phenomenon (reduction of discrimination score when loudness is increased beyond a particular limit) is commonly observed.
- Recruitment absent.
- Threshold tone decay test is positive.
- ***Impedance:*** Stapedial reflex absent.
- ***Brainstem evoked response audiometry:*** A delay of >0.2 m/sec in wave V between two ears is significant. Wave V may be absent or prolonged.

Caloric Test

Diminished or absent response in 96% of patients.

Table 19.1: Differences between cochlear and retrocochlear hearing losses

Hearing tests	Cochlear hearing loss	Retrocochlear hearing loss
Speech discrimination score	< 90%	Very poor
Roll over phenomenon	Absent	Present
Recruitment	Present	Absent
SISI score	> 70%	< 20%
Tone decay	Absent	Present
Stapedial reflex	Present	Absent
Stapedial reflex decay	Normal	Abnormal
BERA	Interval between wave I and V normal	Wave V delayed or absent

Abbreviations: SISI—short increment sensitivity index; BERA—brainstem evoked response audiometry

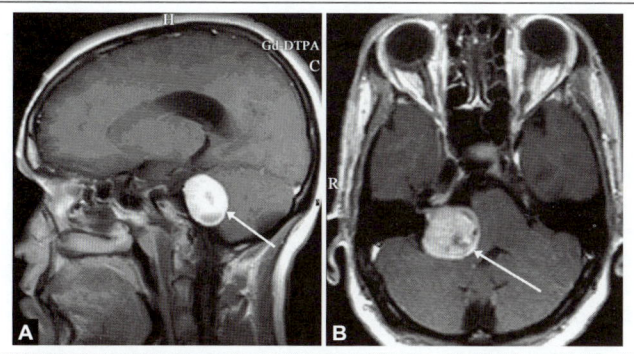

Figs 19.5A and B: MRI of brain with gadolinium contrast in a case of CPA tumor. (A) Sagittal section; (B) Axial section (arrows showing)
Source: Dr Ritesh Prajapati, Consultant Radiologist, Anand, Gujarat

Gadolinium-enhanced MRI

Thin section gadolinium-enhanced MRI (Figs 19.5A and B) is the gold standard for diagnosis of AN and is superior to CT scan. Intracanalicular tumor of a few millimeters size can be diagnosed. On the basis of size AN is classified into four groups:
1. Intracanalicular (limited to IAC).
2. Small size (up to 1.5 cm).
3. Medium size (1.5-4 cm).
4. Large size (over 4 cm).

Vertebral Angiography

It is helpful in differentiating acoustic neuroma from other CPA tumors.

Differential Diagnoses

AN is the most common CPA tumor. It should be differentiated from the following CPA tumors that are listed in order of descending frequency:
- Meningioma
- Lipomas
- Epidermoid
- Cholesterol granulomas
- Cholesteatoma
- Arachnoidal cyst
- Aneurysm
- Metastasis
- Schwannoma of other cranial nerves such as CN V, VII, IX, X, and XI.

AN should be differentiated from other common causes of dizziness (Table in Chapter 'Peripheral Vestibular Disorders').

Treatment

The treatment of first choice is surgical removal. The second choice is gamma knife surgery. Conventional external radiotherapy (low tolerance of the central nervous system to radiation) and chemotherapy do not have any role in the treatment.
- **Surgery:** The surgical approach depends upon the size and extent of the tumor. The following approaches are employed:
  - Middle cranial fossa and transtemporal supralabyrinthine.
  - Translabyrinthine.
  - Retrolabyrinthine.
  - Suboccipital/retrosigmoid.
- **Gamma knife surgery:** This stereotactic gamma-irradiation therapy or linear accelerator (LINAC) delivers high dose of ionizing radiation to the tumor and minimizes its effect on the surrounding neural tissue. It facilitates arrest of the tumor growth and reduction in its size. It can be used in following patients:
  - Patient is not willing for surgery.
  - Tumor < 3 cm.
  - Contraindications to surgery.
  - Residual tumor after surgery.
- **Conservative approach:** Patients who are elderly or have serious medical problems may be kept under wait and watch policy because ANs are slow growing.

Self-evaluation Exercises

1. The features of carcinoma of middle ear does not include:
   a. Elderly persons
   b. Chronic ear discharge
   c. CN III palsy
   d. Pain in the ear
   e. Friable ear polyp with tendency to bleed
2. Which of the following is not true for glomus tumors (paraganglioma)?
   a. Tumors grow very slowly and are multicentric in origin
   b. Common sites are carotid bifurcation, jugular foramen and promontory of middle ear
   c. Diagnostic biopsy should be done
   d. None of the above

Contd...

Section 2 • Ear

Contd…

3. Which of the following is not true for glomus jugulare?
   a. Rising sun appearance
   b. Aquino's sign; B. Brown's sign
   c. Phelps sign
   d. Management includes preoperative embolization, surgery and radiotherapy
   e. None of the above
4. Which of the following are not the clinical features of acoustic neuroma?
   a. Unilateral tinnitus and sensorineural hearing loss are the earliest features
   b. Facial palsy is a late feature
   c. The earliest extracanalicular cranial nerve to be involved is abducent
   d. None of the above
5. Differential diagnoses of acoustic neuroma include:
   a. Endolymphatic hydrops
   b. Cerebellopontine angle meningioma
   c. Congenital choleseatoma
   d. All of the above

True (T)/False (F)

6. A patient with glomus jugulare can have ear bleeding, pain, tinnitus and progressive deafness and a red swelling behind the intact tympanic membrane which blanches on pressure with pneumatic speculum.
7. Exostoses of external auditory canal present as multiple bony swellings and are common in swimmers.
8. Osteoma of external auditory canal is usually single and occurs at tympanomastoid suture line.
9. In Aquino's sign otoscopy shows blenching of glomus jugulare tumor on compression of carotid artery.
10. Phelps sign is seen in cases of glomus jugulare tumor and consists of destruction of bone between the carotid canal and jugular foramen.
11. Brown's sign (Pulsation sign) is seen in glomus jugulare tumor. During otoscopy with pneumatic speculum, on raising the pressure red mass behind the drum pulsates vigorously while reverse occurs on releasing the pressure.
12. Treatment of choice if the glomus tympanicum is restricted to promontory is radiotherapy.
13. The most common site of origin of acoustic neuroma is inferior vestibular nerve.
14. Hitzelberger sign is numbness in the posterosuperior wall of external auditory canal (supplied by CN VII) in cases of glomus jugulare.
15. Audiogram in a patient with acoustic neuroma can have any type of asymmetrical sensorineural hearing loss that may be high frequency, low frequency, flat, and sudden hearing loss. Difficulty in understanding speech is out of proportion to the hearing loss.
16. MRI scan with Gadolinium is the most sensitive diagnostic modality for acoustic neuroma.

Answers

1. c	2. c	3. e	4. c	5. d	6. T
7. T	8. T	9. T	10. T	11. T	12. F
13. F	14. F	15. T	16. T		

Problem-oriented Cases (Spot Diagnosis)

1. A 30-year-old female has been suffering from bilateral hearing loss for 5 years. She does not give any past history of ear discharge. She says that her hearing loss increased during her pregnancy.[1]
2. A patient comes to you with ear bleeding, pain, tinnitus and progressive deafness. On examination, you see a red swelling behind the intact tympanic membrane which blanches on pressure with pneumatic speculum.[2]
3. A 10-year-child develops torticollis, a tender swelling behind the angle of mandible and fever. He has been suffering from chronic foul smelling ear discharge for 5 years. Ear examination shows purulent putrid discharge with granulations in the ear canal.[3]
4. A child with an acute suppurative otitis media was being treated with antibiotic ear drops, oral antibiotics and analgesics. Two weeks later the child develops a swelling over the mastoid, pain in the ear, fever and pulsatile ear discharge.[4]
5. An adult lady develops hearing loss during pregnancy. Her mother had similar problem. Hearing loss is bilateral and slowly progressive. She feels that her hearing improves in noisy background. Pure tone audiometry shows conductive hearing loss. Bone conduction dips at 2000 Hz.[5]
6. An elderly man, who has been suffering from chronic ear discharge for many years, develops facial palsy and pain in the ear which is worse at night. Otoscopy shows a friable ear polyp which has a tendency to bleed.[6]

---

[1]Otosclerosis, [2]Glomus jugulare, [3]Bezold's abscess, [4]Coalescent mastoiditis, [5]Otosclerosis, [6]Carcinoma of middle ear

Section 3: Nose and Paranasal Sinuses

Chapter 20

Anatomy and Physiology of Nose and Paranasal Sinuses

Specific Learning Objectives

After going through the chapter, you should be able to answer the following questions:
- Describe the anatomy of nasal septum including its blood and nerve supply.
- Describe the anatomy of lateral wall of nasal cavity including its blood and nerve supply.
- Describe in detail the structures of middle meatus and ostiomeatal complex.
- Describe the maxillary sinus and its various relations.
- Describe the various groups and types of ethmoidal sinuses including their variations.
- What do you know about: (1) Osteocartilaginous frame work of nose; (2) Frontal sinus; (3) Sphenoid sinus; (4) Olfaction and its pathway; (5) Mucociliary mechanism and factors affecting them?

INTRODUCTION

The nasal cavity and paranasal air sinuses are lined by mucosa, which warm, moisten and filter inspired air. The nasal cavity begins at the external nares and posteriorly opens through the choanae into the nasopharynx. The two nasal cavities are separated from each other by midline nasal septum and bounded laterally by three shelf-like bones, the conchae (turbinates). All the four paranasal air sinuses drain into meatuses between the conchae on the lateral nasal wall and are named after the bones that contain them (maxillary, ethmoid, frontal and sphenoid). The ophthalmic (CN V_1) and maxillary (CN V_2) divisions of the trigeminal nerve (CN V) provide the sensory innervation of nose and paranasal sinuses. The olfactory nerves carry smell information from the upper part of the nasal cavity. The glands of mucosa are supplied by the postganglionic fibers from the pterygopalatine ganglion, which receive preganglionic fibers from the greater petrosal branch of facial nerve. CT anatomy is described in Chapter 'Diagnostic Imaging'.

ANATOMY OF NOSE

EXTERNAL NOSE

The external nose has important cosmetic value and enhances personality and beauty of an individual.

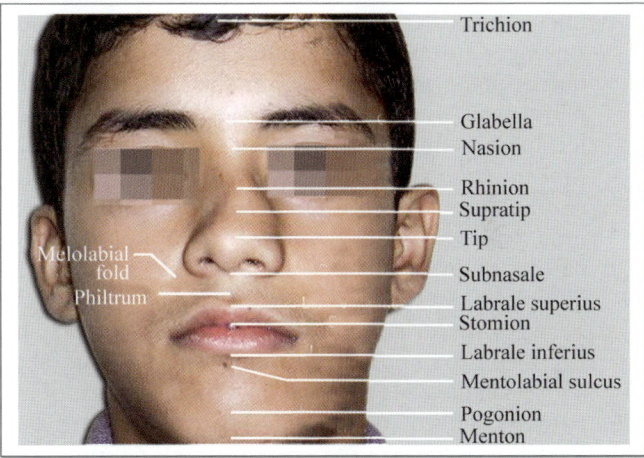

Fig. 20.1: Crooked nose ('C' shaped). Note soft tissue anatomic landmarks (reference points)

Figure 20.1 shows a crooked nose with 'C' shaped deformity and soft tissue anatomic landmarks (reference points). This pyramidal structure is made up of osteocartilaginous framework, which is covered by muscles and skin.

Osteocartilaginous Framework of Nose

The upper one-third of external nose is bony (nasal bones) and forms bridge (root) of the nose while lower two-third is cartilaginous and forms dorsum of the nose (Figs 20.2 and 20.3).

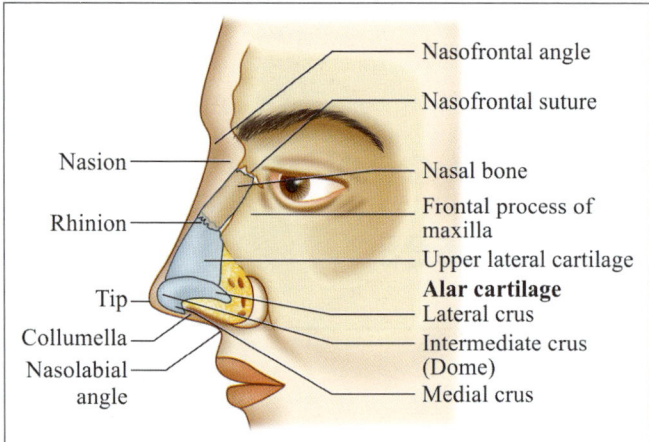

Fig. 20.2: External nose structure—lateral view

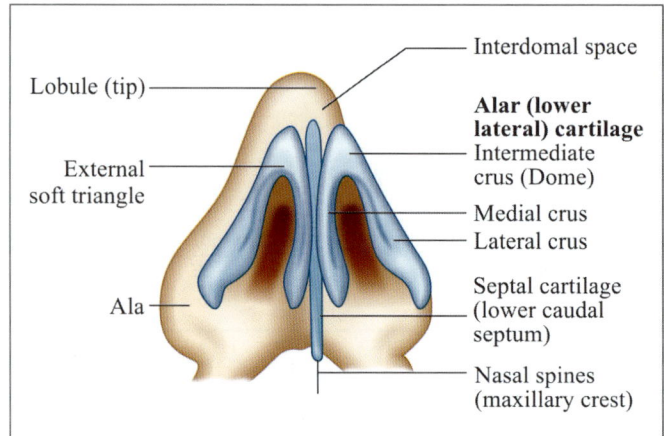

Fig. 20.3: External nose structure—basal view

- **Bony Part:** The two nasal bones meet in the midline and rest on the nasal process of the frontal bone. They are held between the frontal processes of the maxillae.
- **Cartilaginous Part:** It is made up of mainly upper and lower lateral cartilages and septal cartilages. These cartilages are connected with one another and with the adjoining bones by perichondrium and periosteum.
    - **Upper lateral cartilages:** They are attached to the under surface of the nasal bones above and extend up to the lower lateral cartilages below. Both side cartilages fuse with each other and with the upper border of the septal cartilage and form dorsal surface of the nose. The lower free margin, which can be seen intranasally, forms limen vestibuli or nasal valve.
    - **Lower lateral cartilages:** This U-shaped alar cartilage has two crura lateral and medial. The lateral crus, which overlaps lower margin of upper lateral cartilage, forms the ala while medial crus lies in columella.
    - **Lesser alar (or sesamoid) cartilages:** They may be two or more in number and lie above and lateral to alar cartilages. Most of the lower free margin of ala consists of fibrofatty tissue and not the alar cartilage.
    - **Septal cartilage:** The anterosuperior border of septal cartilage, which supports the dorsum of the nose, extends from under surface of nasal bones to the nasal tip. It is discussed in detail in other Section of this Chapter.

Supratip depression deformity of nose: It occurs due to loss of septal cartilage support such as in cases of septal abscess and excessive removal of septal cartilage during submucosal resection of septum.

Nasal Musculature

The facial muscles, which bring about movements of the nose, include procerus, nasalis (transverse and alar parts), levator labii superioris alaeque nasi (muscle with the longest name) and depressor septi.

Nasal Skin

The skin, which covers nasal bones and upper lateral cartilages, is thin and freely mobile. But skin covering the alar cartilages is thick and adherent and contains many sebaceous glands.

Rhinophyma: Hypertrophy of sebaceous glands of external nose skin results in this lobulated tumor (*see* Chapter 'Diseases of External').

Dangerous Area of Face (Danger Triangle Area)

This triangular area, venous drainage of which goes intracranially, extends from nasion to angles of mouth and includes external nose and upper lip. The inferior ophthalmic vein, which receives angular vein, drains into cavernous sinus. The infection of this area has the potential to cause cavernous sinus thrombosis.

Development

Above the roof of stomodeum, the mesenchymal frontonasal process grows downward and merges with the maxillary processes, which arise from first branchial arch. The ectodermal thickening of olfactory placode invaginates as a pit between the frontonasal process and lateral nasal process. The frontonasal process forms median nasal process and upper lip philtrum. The lateral nasal process forms the lower lateral cartilage and lobule of the lateral portion of nose. The olfactory placode invaginates internally to rest high in the nasal cavity and forms olfactory epithelium.

Chapter 20 • Anatomy and Physiology of Nose and Paranasal Sinuses

Congenital cleft lip deformity occurs due to the failure of the fusion of medial frontonasal process and lateral maxillary process.

INTERNAL NOSE

The nasal septum divides the internal nose into two halves right and left nasal cavities. The nasal cavities communicate with the exterior through anterior nares (nostrils) and with the nasopharynx through posterior nasal choanae. The anterior and inferior skin-lined portion of internal nose is called vestibule and posterior mucosa-lined portion makes nasal cavity proper. Each nasal cavity has four boundaries lateral and medial walls, roof and floor.

- *Lateral wall of nasal cavity:*
  - *Bones:* The lateral wall is formed by following bones:
    - *Nasal bone*
    - *Maxilla:* Frontal process and medial surface maxilla and medial wall of maxillary sinus
    - *Lacrimal bone*
    - *Inferior turbinate*
    - *Ethmoid:* Lateral mass of ethmoidal bone
    - *Palatine bone:* Perpendicular plate
    - *Sphenoid:* Medial pterygoid plate
  - *Turbinates:* Three scroll-like bony projections, inferior, middle and superior turbinates (conchae) are seen over the lateral wall. Sometimes, a fourth turbinate, concha suprema is also seen (Figs 20.4 and 20.5).
    - *Inferior turbinate:* This is the largest turbinate and is a separate bone.
    - *Middle turbinate:* This is the part of ethmoidal bone and is described in other Section of this Chapter.
    - *Superior turbinate:* This is the smallest turbinate and a part of ethmoidal bone and may get pneumatized by one or more ethmoidal air cells. It

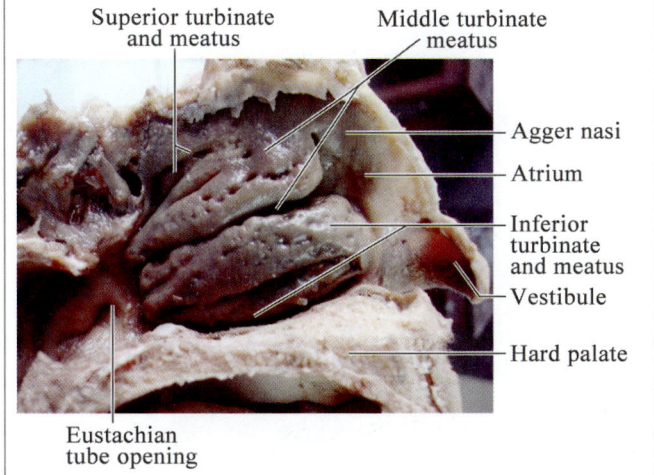

Fig. 20.5: Lateral wall of nasal cavity of cadaver showing turbinates and meatuses

is situated posteriorly and superior to the middle turbinate and is not visible on anterior rhinoscopy examination.
- *Supreme turbinate:* It may be seen lying above the superior turbinate in some cases.
- *Meatuses:* The three corresponding spaces present below and lateral to each turbinate are inferior, middle and superior meatus (Figs 20.6 to 20.8).
  - *Inferior meatus:* It is present along the whole length of the lateral wall. Nasolacrimal duct opens in the anterior part of inferior meatus. The opening of nasolacrimal duct is guarded by Hasner's mucosal valve.
  - *Middle meatus:* It lies below the middle turbinate and is described in other Section of this Chapter.
  - *Superior meatus:* It is present only in the posterior third of lateral wall of nose. Posterior ethmoidal sinuses open in this space.

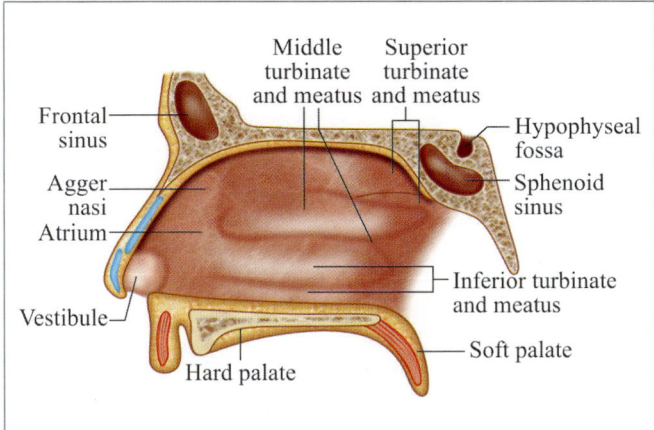

Fig. 20.4: Lateral wall of nasal cavity showing turbinates and meatuses

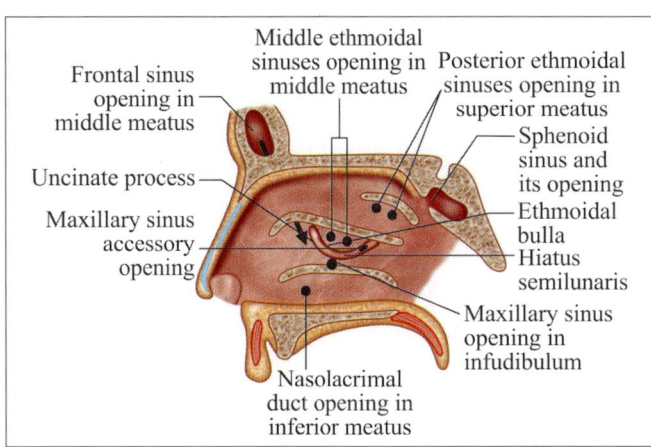

Fig. 20.6: Openings of paranasal sinuses. Lateral wall of nose after removal of turbinates

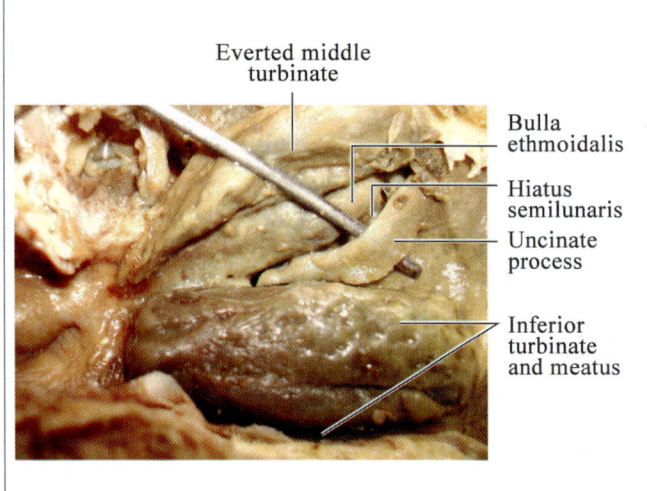

Fig. 20.7: Cadaveric dissection of osteomeatal complex. Middle turbinate is reflected upward. Probe lies in the ethmoidal infundibulum and is coming out through the lower attachment of uncinate process

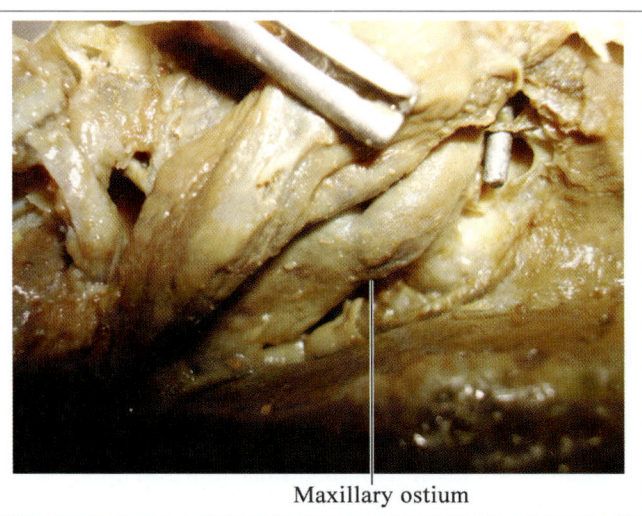

Fig. 20.8: Cadaveric dissection of osteomeatal complex. Middle turbinate is reflected upward. Uncinate process is removed and the ethmoidal infundibulum is opened. The probe is showing the frontal sinus opening. Note the maxillary ostium

- **Sphenoethmoidal recess:** It lies above the superior turbinate. The sphenoid sinus opens into this recess medial to the superior turbinate about 1 cm above the upper margin of posterior choana close to the posterior border of septum.
- **Atrium:** This shallow depression lies in front of the middle meatus and above the vestibule.
- **Medial wall:** It is formed by the nasal septum, which has been described in other Section of this Chapter.
- **Roof:** It has three parts—anterior sloping part (nasal bones), middle horizontal part (cribriform plate of ethmoid through which olfactory nerves pass) and posterior sloping part (body of sphenoid bone).
- **Floor:** Floor of the nose makes roof (hard palate) of the oral cavity. It is made up of two bones—palatine process of the maxilla (anterior three-fourth) and horizontal plate of the palatine bone (posterior one-fourth).

Vestibule of Nose

This anteroinferior portion of nasal cavity is lined by skin, which contains sebaceous glands, hair follicles and the hair (vibrissae). For the internal and external nasal valves see Chapter 'Nasal Septum'.

- **Limen nasi (nasal valve):** This area is the greatest constriction of respiratory tract. Its boundaries include:
  - **Floor:** Floor of the nose.
  - **Superior and lateral:** The caudal margin of upper lateral cartilage.
  - **Medial:** Columella and lower part of the nasal septum up to mucocutaneous junction.

Rhinoplasty: Injudicious resection of lateral nasal cartilage during rhinoplasty can produce collapse of nose during inspiration.

Nasal Septum

Nasal septum (Fig. 20.9) can be divided into three parts—columellar septum, membranous septum and septum proper. The columellar and membranous parts can be moved from side to side.

1. **Columellar septum:** It is covered on either side by skin. The columella contains medial crura of lower lateral cartilages, which are joined together with fibrous tissue.

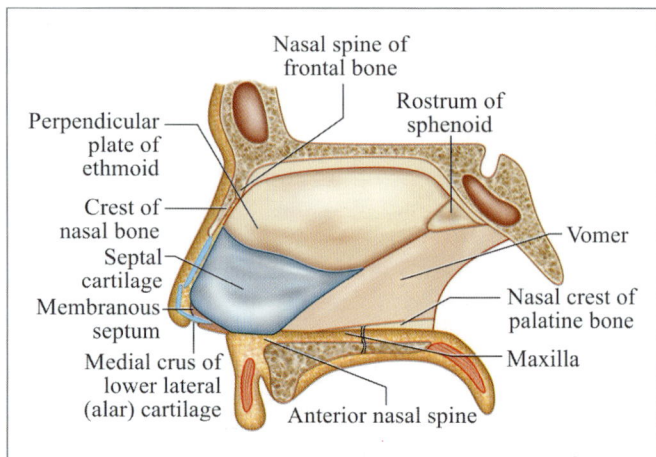

Fig. 20.9: Structure of the nasal septum lateral view. Bony and cartilaginous part seen after removing the mucosa. Posterior triangular segment of cartilaginous septum generally overlaps the bony septum

2. ***Membranous septum:*** It lies between the columella and the caudal border of septal cartilage and consists of only double layer of skin. There is no bony or cartilaginous support in membranous septum.
3. ***Septum proper:*** It is covered with mucous membrane and consists of osteocartilaginous framework. The principal constituent of septum proper is large quadrilateral septal cartilage. Other major constituents are the perpendicular plate of ethmoid and vomer. Other bones, which make very small contributions, include crest of nasal bones, nasal spine of frontal bone, rostrum of sphenoid, crests of palatine and maxilla including the anterior nasal spine of maxilla.

- ***Septal cartilage:*** This large quadrilateral septal cartilage is wedged between vomer and ethmoid plate.
  - ***Inferior margin:*** It lies in a groove of vomer and rests anteriorly on anterior nasal spine.
  - ***Caudal septal deviation:*** It occurs due to dislocation of inferior margin of septal cartilage from anterior nasal spine.
  - ***Septal spur:*** It is the result of dislocation of the inferior margin of septal cartilage from the vomerine groove.
  - ***Superior margin:*** Septal cartilage fuses with the upper lateral cartilages of external nose. *Therefore septal deviation may be associated with deviation of dorsum of nose.*

> **Depression of nasal dorsum:** Septal cartilage also provides support to the tip and dorsum of cartilaginous part of external nose. Septal cartilage destruction, which can be caused due to septal abscess, injuries, tuberculosis or excessive removal during septal surgery, results in depression of dorsum of nose and drooping of the nasal tip.

Middle Meatus and Osteomeatal Complex (Figs 20.7, 20.8 and 20.10)

Middle meatus space lies below the middle turbinate. It is present in the posterior half of the lateral wall. The osteomeatal complex includes middle turbinate, bulla ethmoidalis, uncinate process and ethmoidal infundibulum. It is important as ostium of frontal, maxillary and anterior ethmoidal sinuses are present in this area.

> **Functional endoscopic sinus surgery (FESS):** Any mucosal swelling and congenital anomaly of osteomeatal unit can cause obstruction, stasis and repeated infections of the upstream sinuses. FESS puts stress on this complex, which needs normal restoration to enhance sinus drainage.

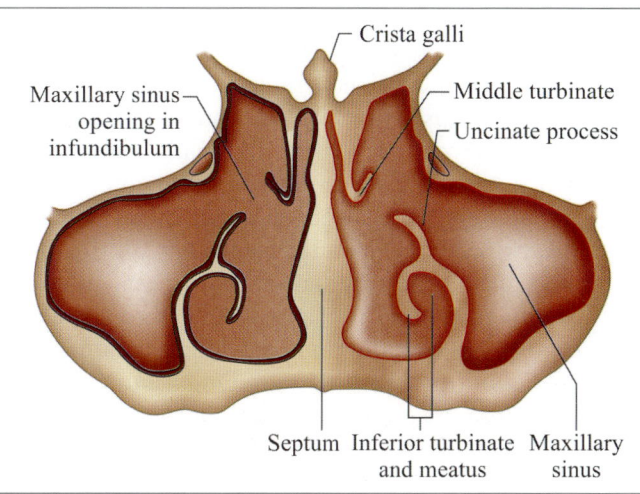

Fig. 20.10: Osteomeatal complex. Coronal section of nose and paranasal sinuses at the level of osteomeatal complex. The uncinate process is in sagittal plane bounding the infundibulum in which opens the ostium of maxillary sinus

- ***Middle turbinate:*** This lower ethmoidal turbinate is attached to the lateral wall through the ground basal lamella. Its anterior one-third lies in sagittal plane and is attached to the lateral edge of cribriform plate, (floor of anterior cranial fossa). Its middle one-third lies in frontal plane and is attached to lamina papyracea (medial wall of orbit). Its posterior one-third, runs horizontally and is attached to lamina papyracea and medial wall of maxillary sinus.

> - **CSF rhinorrhea and anosmia:** They can be caused by the damage to cribriform plate due to the fracture of middle turbinate.
> - **Paradoxical middle turbinate:** In some cases lateral surface of middle turbinate is convex. It can cause narrowing of the middle meatus. It can affect ventilation and mucociliary clearance in osteomeatal unit.
> - **Concha bullosa:** It is pneumatization of the middle turbinate. It is present in 30% of the population and is usually asymptomatic. It drains into the frontal recess directly or through agger nasi cells. The enlarged middle turbinate can affect ventilation and mucociliary clearance in osteomeatal unit. The obstruction to the drainage system of concha bullosa results in symptoms. It requires endoscopic sinus surgery (removal of medial wall of concha or entire concha bullosa).

- ***Bulla ethmoidalis:*** Middle ethmoidal air cells form this rounded bulge and they open on or above it. As the bulla ethmoidalis lies anterior to the ground lamella of middle turbinate, these air cells are considered part of anterior group of ethmoidal cells. If not pneumatized,

bulla ethmoidalis may remain like a solid bony prominence. It may extend superiorly to base of skull and posteriorly to ground lamella of middle turbinate.
- *Lateral sinus of Grunwald:* Sometimes there are spaces above or behind the bulla ethmoidalis, which are called suprabullar or retrobullar recesses respectively and together form lateral sinus of Grunwald. It is bounded superiorly by the base of skull, laterally by lamina papyracea, inferiorly by the bulla, and medially opens (through hiatus semilunaris superior) in to the middle meatus.
- *Hiatus semilunaris:* This two-dimensional gap lies between the posterosuperior free border of uncinate process and bulla. It opens laterally into a three-dimensional funnel-shaped space called ethmoidal infundibulum.
- *Uncinate process:* This small thin lamina of ethmoid bone forms floor and medial wall of the ethmoidal infundibulum. This sickle shape bone runs from anterosuperior to posteroinferior direction.
  - *Two borders:* The free posterosuperior border is sharp and runs parallel to surface of bulla ethmoidalis. The anteroinferior border is attached to the lateral wall of nose.
  - *Two ends:* Posteroinferior end is attached to inferior turbinate and divides the lower membranous part of middle meatus into anterior and posterior fontanelle, which are devoid of bone. If perforated they open into the maxillary sinus. The anterosuperior end may be inserted laterally on the lamina papyracea, upwards into the base of skull or medially into the middle turbinate and accounts for the variations in the drainage of frontal sinus.
- *Ethmoidal infundibulum:* Frontal sinus opens into the anterosuperior part of infundibulum just posterior to posterior wall (opening) of agger nasi cells (curved ridge running downwards and forwards above the atrium). Anterior ethmoidal air cells open into the infundibulum. Maxillary sinus, which may have accessory openings, opens into posterior part of the infundibulum.
  - *Boundaries:*
    - *Medial:* Uncinate process and frontal process of maxilla and sometimes lacrimal bone.
    - *Lateral:* Lamina papyracea.
- *Agger Nasi:* It is an elevation that lies just anterior to the attachment of middle turbinate and if pneumatized contains agger nasi cells, which communicate with frontal recess.

Large agger nasi cells can constrict the frontal recess and can impair the frontal sinus drainage.

Linings of Internal Nose

- *Skin of nasal vestibule:* Vestibule is lined by skin (stratified squamous epithelium), which contains hair, hair follicles and sebaceous glands.
- *Olfactory epithelium:* The olfactory epithelium that is paler in color lines the olfactory region, which includes roof of nasal cavity and area above superior concha.
- *Respiratory mucosa:* The respiratory mucous membrane, which covers the lower two-third of the nasal cavity, shows variable thickness. It is thickest over nasal conchae especially at their ends. It is thick over the nasal septum and thin in the meatuses and floor of the nose. This respiratory mucous membrane is pseudostratified ciliated columnar epithelium and contain plenty of goblet cells. It is highly vascular and contains erectile tissue. The submucosal layer contains both racemose and tubular glands that secrete serous and mucous secretions for the surface mucous blanket.

Blood Supply of Nose

Branches of both external and internal carotid arteries supply the nose (Box 20.1). Sphenopalatine and greater palatine branches of internal maxillary artery (branch of external carotid artery) supply posterior inferior part of internal nose. Branches of facial artery (branch of external carotid artery) supply anterior inferior nasal cavity. Anterior and posterior ethmoidal branches of ophthalmic artery (branch of internal carotid artery) supply superior part of nasal cavity (Figs 20.11 and 20.12). For the retrocolumellar vein see Chapter 'Diseases of External Nose and Epistaxis'.

Little's area or Kiesselbach's plexus in the anteroinferior part of nasal septum just above the vestibule is the vascular area, where anterior ethmoidal, sphenopalatine, greater palatine and septal branch of superior labial arteries and their corresponding veins form an anastomosis. This is the most common site for epistaxis and the bleeding polyp (fibroangioma) of septum.

Box 20.1: Blood supply of nose

Internal Carotid System
- *Ophthalmic artery*
  - Anterior ethmoidal artery
  - Posterior ethmoidal artery

External Carotid System
- *Maxillary artery*
  - *Sphenopalatine artery:* Nasopalatine, posterior nasal septal branches and posterior lateral nasal branches.
  - *Greater palatine artery*
  - *Infraorbital artery:* Nasal branch of anterior superior dental artery.
- *Facial artery:* Superior labial artery

Chapter 20 • Anatomy and Physiology of Nose and Paranasal Sinuses

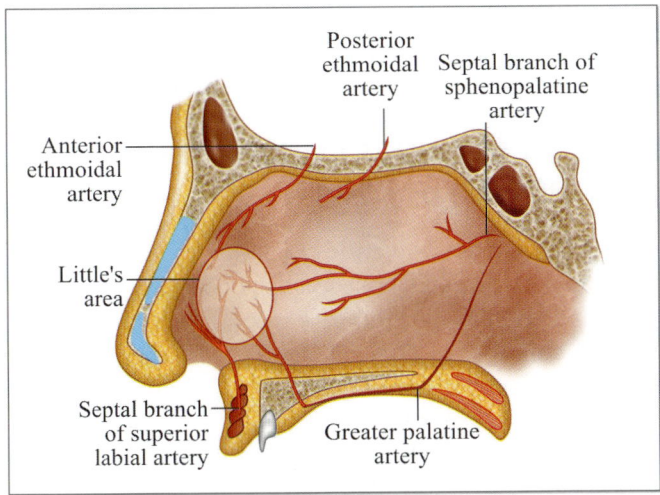

Fig. 20.11: Blood supply of nasal septum

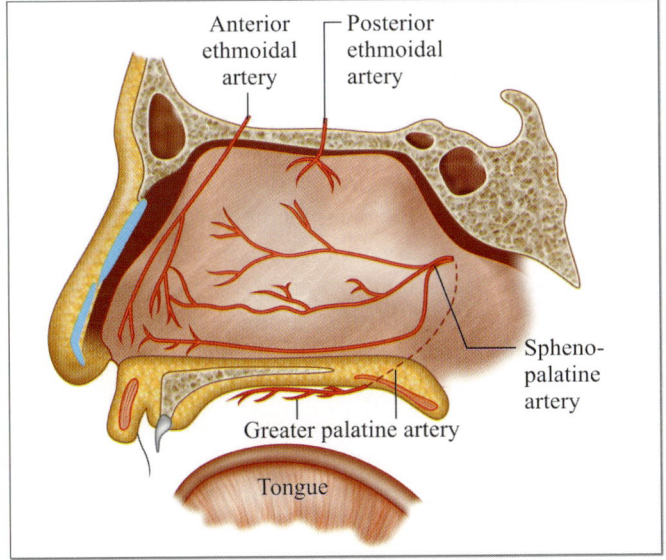

Fig. 20.12: Blood supply of lateral wall of nose

Submucosal Vascular Plexus

The submucosal venous plexus of respiratory mucosa of nose, which consists of arterioles, capillaries, vascular sinusoids, venous plexuses and venules, resembles erectile tissue of genitalia. This deeper specialized vascular plexus is present in the erectile tissue of inferior turbinate and adjacent septum and posterior part of middle turbinate. It is under the control of autonomic nervous system. Stimulation of sympathetic vasomotor nerves causes vasoconstriction (noradrenaline secretion), while parasympathetic stimulation causes vasodilation (acetylcholine secretion) and watery nasal discharge (secretomotor). Stronger mechanical or chemical stimulation of internal nose may cause apnea and bradycardia.

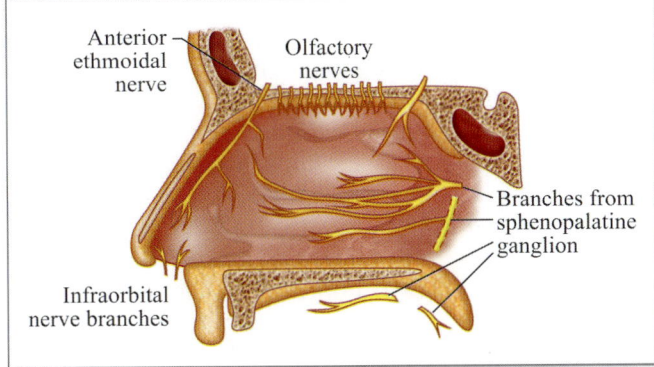

Fig. 20.13: Nerve supply of lateral wall of nose

Nerve Supply of Nasal Cavity (Fig. 20.13)

- ***Olfactory nerves:*** These central filaments of the olfactory cells, which are arranged into 12–20 nerves, carry sense of smell from the olfactory region of nose. They pass through the cribriform plate and end in the olfactory bulb.

> *Injury of olfactory nerves:* Olfactory nerves carry meningeal sheaths of dura, arachnoid and pia mater and because of this injury to these nerves can result in CSF rhinorrhea and meningitis.

- ***Trigeminal nerve:*** The ophthalmic division (anterior ethmoidal nerve) and maxillary division (sphenopalatine and infraorbital branches) carry common sensation (such as touch and irritation from acrid odors). Both these divisions supply to the skin of external nose.
  - Branches of infraorbital nerve supply vestibule of nose.
  - The posterior two-third of nasal cavity (septum and lateral wall) is supplied by branches of sphenopalatine ganglion, which pass through the sphenopalatine foramen situated near the posterior end of middle turbinate, where it can be blocked by placing a pledget of cotton of 4% xylocaine.
  - Anterosuperior part of the nasal cavity (lateral wall and septum) is supplied by anterior ethmoidal nerve, which can be blocked by placing the cotton pledget impregnated in 4% xylocaine high up inside of nasal bones.
- ***Autonomic nervous system***
  - ***Parasympathetic:*** These nerve fibers are secretomotor and supply the nasal glands. The greater superficial petrosal nerve, which carry preganglionic fibers from the parasympathetic nucleus situated in brainstem, joins deep petrosal nerve (postganglionic vasomotor sympathetic

fibers) and forms nerve to pterygoid canal (vidian nerve), which reaches to the sphenopalatine ganglion where only parasympathetic fibers relay. The branches of sphenopalatine ganglion pass through sphenopalatine foramen and supply nasal cavity. Parasympathetic fibers, which supply to nasal blood vessels, cause vasodilation.

- *Sympathetic:* The preganglionic sympathetic nerve fibers come from upper two thoracic segments of spinal cord (origin from hypothalamus) and relay in superior cervical ganglion. The postganglionic fibers form a plexus around internal carotid artery, from which deep petrosal nerve arises that joins the preganglionic parasympathetic fibers of greater petrosal nerve to form the nerve to pterygoid canal (vidian nerve). These postganglionic sympathetic vasomotor fibers reach the nasal cavity without relaying in the sphenopalatine ganglion and cause vasoconstriction of nasal vessels (decongestion of nasal cavity).

> *Vidian neurectomy:* Some surgeons are of opinion that excessive rhinorrhea (vasomotor and allergic rhinitis) can be controlled by section of the vidian nerve.

- *Facial nerve:* It supplies to the muscles of the external nose.

Lymphatic Drainage

- *Submandibular lymph nodes:* The external nose and anterior part of nasal cavity drain into submandibular lymph nodes.
- *Retropharyngeal and upper jugular nodes:* Posterior part of nasal cavity drains into upper jugular nodes either directly of through the retropharyngeal nodes.
- *Perineural intracranial spread:* The perineural intracranial spread of cancer is possible through the lymphatics of the upper nasal cavity, which communicate with subarachnoid space along the olfactory nerves.

ANATOMY OF PARANASAL SINUSES

On each side there are four paranasal air sinuses in four cranial bones—frontal, maxilla, ethmoid and sphenoid. They are divided into two groups:

1. *Anterior group:* The sinuses, which open anterior to basal lamella of middle turbinate in the middle meatus, form anterior group of paranasal sinuses. They are maxillary, frontal and anterior ethmoid sinuses.
2. *Posterior group:* The sinuses, which open posterior and superior to basal lamella of middle turbinate, form posterior group of paranasal sinuses. They are posterior ethmoid and sphenoid sinuses. The posterior ethmoidal sinuses open in the superior meatus and sphenoid sinuses open in sphenoethmoidal recess.

MAXILLARY SINUS (ANTRUM OF HIGHMORE) (Fig. 20.14)

It is the first to develop and is largest paranasal sinus (15 ml capacity in adult). It occupies the body of maxilla and is pyramidal in shape. The base faces towards lateral wall of nose and apex is directed laterally into the zygomatic process.

- *Boundaries*
  - *Anterior wall:* The anterior facial surface of maxilla (canine fossa) is related to cheek.
  - *Posterior wall:* It is in relation with the infratemporal and pterygopalatine fossa.
  - *Medial wall:* It is thin and membranous at places and faces middle and inferior meatuses.
  - *Floor:* It is situated about 1 cm below the level of floor of nose in adults. Until 3 years of age, sinus floor is 4–5 mm above the nasal floor. It is formed by alveolar process of the maxilla. The roots of all the molars, second premolar and sometimes first premolar (depending on the extent of pneumatization and age of the person), are situated in the floor of maxillary sinuses. These teeth roots are separated from the sinus mucosa by a thin lamina of bone, which may be dehiscent. The chances of oroantral fistulae are high after the extraction of these teeth. Infection of these teeth can result in maxillary sinusitis.
  - *Roof:* The roof of the maxillary sinus is the floor of the orbit and is traversed by infraorbital nerve and vessels.

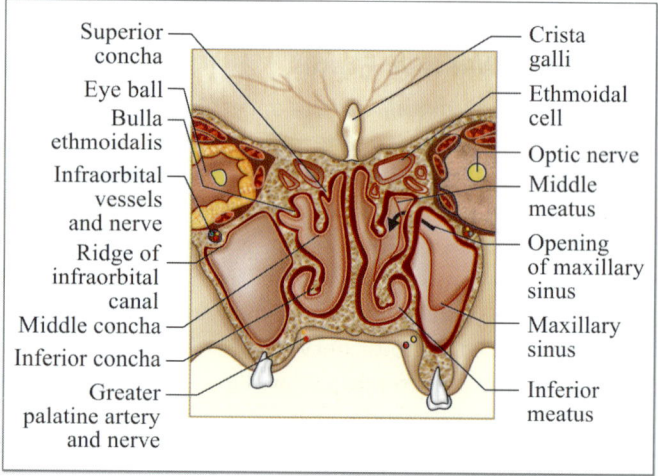

Fig. 20.14: Coronal section of nose and paranasal sinuses seen from behind

- **Ostium of maxillary sinus:** It is situated higher in medial wall and opens in the posterior part of ethmoidal infundibulum.
- **Accessory ostium:** In 30% of population, an accessory ostium, which may be quite large, is seen behind and in front of the natural main ostium. The maxillary sinus does not drain through accessory ostium and is bypassed by the mucus blanket.

> **Functional endoscopic sinus surgery (FESS):** During FESS, accessory maxillary ostium is joined with the natural maxillary ostium to prevent recirculation of the mucopus into the maxillary sinus.

Frontal Sinus

The frontal sinus is situated above and deep to the supraorbital ridge. It lies between the inner and outer tables of the lower part of frontal bone. The shape and size of this loculated sinus vary (very large to absent). The bilateral frontal sinuses are often asymmetric. The intervening bony septum, which is thin and often obliquely placed, may be deficient in some cases. A very large sinus may extend into the roof of the orbit.

- **Relations:**
  - **Anterior wall** of the sinus is related to the forehead skin.
  - **Floor** is in relation with orbit.
  - **Posterior wall** relations are meninges and frontal lobe of brain.
- **Ostium** of frontal sinus is situated in its floor and opens into the frontal recess, which depending upon the attachment of uncinate process opens either in the infundibulum or medial to the uncinate process into the middle meatus.

Ethmoidal Sinuses (Fig. 20.15)

Ethmoidal sinuses are thin walled air cavities in lateral masses of ethmoid bone. They vary in number (3–18) and lie between upper third of lateral nasal wall and the medial wall of orbit. Clinically they are divided into two groups—anterior and posterior. Anterior ethmoid group opens into the middle meatus. Posterior ethmoid group opens into the superior meatus and some in sphenoethmoidal recess.

- **Boundaries**
  - **Roof:** It is closed by the frontal bone, which forms the floor of anterior cranial fossa.
  - **Lateral wall:** Lamina papyracea separates it laterally from the orbit.

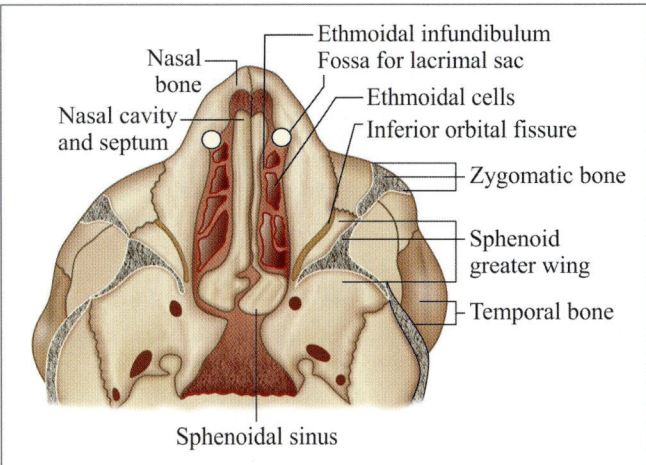

Fig. 20.15: Axial section of nose and paranasal sinuses in the upper part showing ethmoidal and sphenoidal sinuses

> **FESS:** Lamina papyracea is paper thin and can be easily damaged during intranasal surgery and destroyed by ethmoidal infections. Optic nerve, which is at risk during posterior ethmoid surgery, is in close relationship with posterior group of ethmoidal air cells.

- **Agger nasi cells:** These are most anterior of anterior ethmoid cells and lie in close proximity of frontal recess. They are situated at the agger ridge, which is present just anterior to anterosuperior attachment of middle turbinate.
- **Grand (basal) lamella:** This bony insertion of middle turbinate into the skull base and lateral nasal wall separates anterior from posterior ethmoid cells. Grand lamella can be divided into three parts. Anterior one-third inserts into lamina cribrosa, middle one-third (oblique anterosuperior to posteroinferior course) into lamina papyracea and posterior one-third horizontal part inserts into lateral nasal wall.

> - **Big agger nasi cells** can obstruct drainage of frontal sinus and their removal provides better view of nasofrontal duct during endoscopic sinus surgery.
> - **Frontoethmoid cells:** In frontal recess encroaching frontal sinus.
> - **Haller cells:** These ethmoid cells extend into the roof of maxillary sinus in the region of maxillary sinus ostium. These cells may remain asymptomatic or affect maxillary sinus ventilation and drainage resulting in recurrent or chronic maxillary sinusitis. They are present in 10% of population.

Contd...

Contd…

- **Onodi cells:** These are posterior ethmoid cells and extend either laterally or superiorly along the sphenoid sinus. The optic nerve can lie within them. Onodi cells must be recognized during the endoscopic sinus surgery on posterior ethmoid to avoid optic nerve injury.

Sphenoid Sinus (Figs 20.16 and 2.17)

The two sphenoid sinuses, one on each side are rarely symmetrical. They occupy body of sphenoid bone and are separated by a thin bony septum, which is usually obliquely situated and may even be deficient. The ostium, which is situated in the upper part of anterior wall, drains into sphenoethmoidal recess.

The anterior wall of sphenoid sinus is 7 cm away from anterior nasal spine at 30° angle.

- **Relations:** The relations are important during the endoscopic sinus surgery and transsphenoidal hypophysectomy. The extent and relations of sphenoid sinus depend upon the degree of pneumatization, which may extend into the wings of sphenoid, pterygoid plates and clivus.
    - *Anterior part:* The superior relations are olfactory tract, optic chiasma and frontal lobe. The lateral wall relations are optic nerve, internal carotid artery and maxillary nerve. These structures may be dehiscent in the lateral wall of sinus.
    - *Posterior part:* Roof of sinus is floor of sella turcica (pituitary gland fossa). Lateral wall is related to cavernous sinus, which contains internal carotid artery and CN III, IV and ophthalmic and maxillary divisions of trigeminal (CN V_1 and V_2).

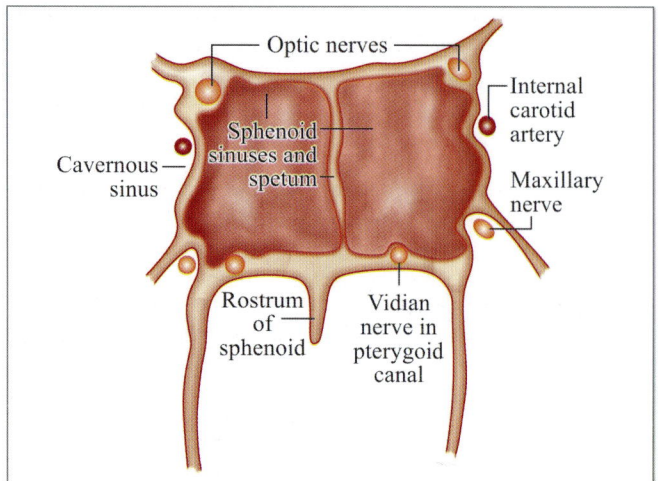

Fig. 20.16: Sphenoidal sinuses coronal section showing important structures situated in relation with sphenoid sinus walls

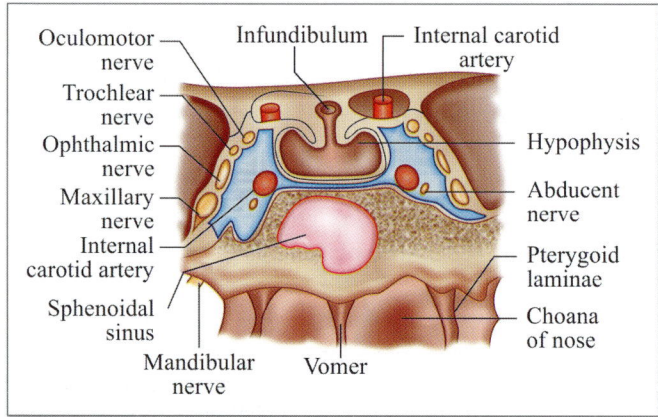

Fig. 20.17: Relations of sphenoid sinus with cavernous sinus and pituitary fossa and gland

Mucous Membrane of Paranasal Sinuses

The mucous membrane of paranasal sinuses is thinner and less vascular and is continuous with that of the nasal cavity through the sinuses openings. It is ciliated pseudostratified columnar epithelium with numerous mucoserous glands and goblet cells. They produce mucus blanket which has two layers—inner thin serous layer or sol phase and outer viscous mucus layer or gel phase. Cilia, which help in drainage of mucus, are more marked near the ostia.

Mucus Drainage of Sinuses

Mucus secretions of paranasal sinuses travel to their ostium in a spiral manner. The cilia propel mucus through the ostium into their respective meatuses.

The mucus from anterior groups of sinuses passes along the lateral pharyngeal gutter. Hypertrophy of lateral pharyngeal lymphoid occurs in infection of anterior sinuses. The mucus from posterior group of sinuses spreads over the posterior pharyngeal wall.

- *Maxillary sinus:* In the maxillary sinus, secretion transports (stellate pattern) begin from floor and along all the four walls (anterior, posterior, medial and lateral) and roof and converge at the natural ostium.
- *Frontal sinus:* Its secretions flow in both directions along medial aspect of ostium. They flow out of sinus along floor and inferior parts of anterior and posterior walls. From the medial aspect of ostium, secretions flow superiorly and then laterally along the roof of frontal sinus.

CT vs plain X-ray: The plain CT scan without contrast is the first line of screening study of the nose and paranasal sinuses. The plain PNS X-rays do not offer adequate views of osteomeatal complex, sphenoid and ethmoid sinuses due to the overlapping of structures.

Lymphatic Drainage

The lymphatic of sinuses form a capillary network in mucosa. They drain into upper deep cervical nodes, either directly or through lateral retropharyngeal nodes.

Blood Supply

The paranasal sinuses are supplied by the branches of both external carotid artery (facial artery and sphenopalatine branch of maxillary artery) and internal carotid artery (anterior and posterior ethmoidal branches of ophthalmic artery) (Table 20.1). Sphenopalatine artery, which divides into two main branches, enters the nasal cavity through sphenopalatine foramen (posterior to middle turbinate).

Endoscopic sinus surgery (ESS): The septal branch of sphenopalatine artery passes across the inferior aspect of anterior surface of sphenoid sinus and can be damaged during ESS sphenoidectomy.

Nerve Supply

Paranasal sinuses are mainly supplied by branches of trigeminal nerve (CN V) (Table 20.1).
- The supraorbital, supratrochlear and anterior and posterior ethmoidal nerves are branches of ophthalmic division of trigeminal nerve (CN V_1).
- The greater palatine, posterolateral nasal and superior nasal branches of the infraorbital nerve are branches of maxillary division of trigeminal nerve (CN V_2) and supply maxillary sinus.
- The sphenopalatine nerve, which also carries parasympathetic secretomotor fibers, is also the branch of maxillary division (CN V_2).

Development of Paranasal Sinuses

The paranasal sinuses, which develop as out-pouchings from the mucous membrane of nose, continue to grow during childhood and early adult life (Table 20.2). At the time of birth, only the maxillary and ethmoidal sinuses are present. Radiologically, maxillary sinus is distinguished at 4–5 months, ethmoid at 1 year and sphenoid at 4 years and frontal at 6 years of age.

Pediatric rhinosinusitis: At birth, both frontal as well as sphenoid sinuses are absent and therefore not clinically significant in young children.

PHYSIOLOGY OF NOSE

The functions of the nose include olfaction, respiration, air conditioning of inspired air, protection of lower airway, vocal resonance and nasal reflex.

RESPIRATION

Humans are natural nose breathers. A newborn with bilateral choanal atresia may asphyxiate to death if immediate airway management is not done. Mouth breathing is learned later in life. The nose allows breathing during eating.

Inspiratory and expiratory air currents during quite respiration pass between the turbinates and nasal septum (Figs 20.18A and B). Little air passes below (i.e. inferior meatus) and above the level of turbinates (i.e. olfactory region). Sniffing helps weak odorous substances reaching olfactory area.

Table 20.1: Blood and nerve supplies of paranasal sinuses

Sinuses	Arteries	Nerves
Frontal	Supraorbital, supratrochlear	Supraorbital, supratrochlear
Maxillary	Maxillary (main) and facial	Maxillary
Anterior ethmoidal	Anterior ethmoidal	Anterior ethmoidal
Posterior ethmoidal	Posterior ethmoid and sphenopalatine	Posterior ethmoid and sphenopalatine
Sphenoidal	Posterior ethmoid and sphenopalatine	Posterior ethmoid and sphenopalatine

Table 20.2: Development and growth of paranasal sinuses

Sinus	At birth	Adult size	Growth	Radiological appearance (age)
Maxillary	Present	15 years	Biphasic growth: Birth–3 years, 7–12 years	4–5 months
Ethmoid	Present	12 years	Size increases upto 12 years	1 year
Frontal	Absent	13–18 years	Invades frontal bone (2–4 years), size increases until teens	6 years
Sphenoid	Absent	12–15 years	Reaches sella turcica (7 years), dorsum sellae (late teens), basisphenoid (adult)	4 years

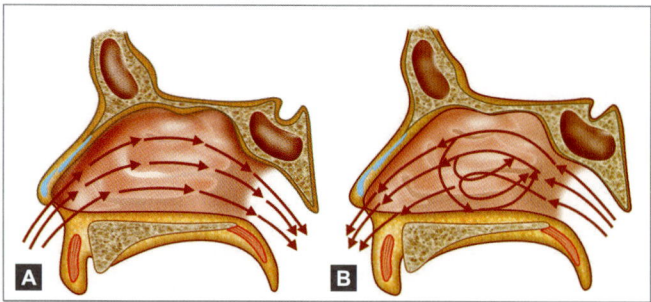

Figs 20.18A and B: Nasal airflow. (A) Inspiratory air flow. 50% of the total airflow passes through middle part of nose. 35% air passes through inferior meatus and only 15% through olfactory region; (B) Expiration. Limen nasi converts the expiratory air current into eddies under the cover of inferior and middle turbinates and ventilates sinuses

During expiration, friction offered at nasal valve converts air currents into eddies under cover of inferior and middle turbinates. These eddies ventilate the sinuses through their openings in the nose. Anterior end of inferior turbinate increases and decreases in size and thus regulates inflow of air.

Nasal Cycle

The alternate opening and closing of each side of nose is called nasal cycle. It varies every few hours and is characteristic of an individual. Kayser first described it in 1895. Nasal cycle, which is observed in up to 80% of normal subjects, has also been studied with the help of rhinomanometry. There occur rhythmic cyclical congestion and decongestion of nasal mucosa (perhaps under the control of autonomic innervation), which control the airflow through nasal cavity. Most of the people are not conscious about this alteration in airflow because the total resistance of nasal airflow remains constant.

AIR-CONDITIONING OF INSPIRED AIR

Nose acts as an 'air-conditioner' and filters, purifies, moistens and warms the inspired air for lungs. In 24 hours we breathe 500 cubic feet of air. Air is efficiently filtered, humidified, adjusted to proper temperature and cleared of all the dust, bacteria and viruses by the nose.

- *Filtration and purification:* Nasal vibrissae filter coarse particles (up to 3 mm). Finer particles of 0.5-0.3 mm (such as dust, pollen and bacteria) adhere to the mucus (electrostatic attraction with the nasal mucus blanket), which is secreted by mucous glands and spread all over the nasal mucous membrane. But particles <0.5 mm pass through the nose into lower airways.
- *Temperature control:* The turbinates double the surface area of nasal mucosa. The large surface of nasal mucosa is structurally adapted (highly vascular with cavernous venous spaces or sinusoids) to regulate temperature of the inspired air. The mucous membrane of middle and inferior turbinates and adjacent part of the septum controls the blood flow that regulates the size of turbinates. This 'radiator' mechanism warms up the inspired cold air (which may be < 0°C) to near body temperature (37°C). Hot air is cooled to the body temperature.
- *Humidification:* The serous glands of nasal mucous membrane regulate the relative humidity (75-100%) of the inspired air, which is dry in winter and humid in summer. Approximately 1 liter of water is evaporated from nasal mucosa in 24 hours. During expiration, nose removes water (maintaining hydration) and heat (preventing hypothermia) from expired air.

Humidity and ciliary function: Moisture facilitates the function of the ciliary epithelium. Fifty percent relative humidity (dry air) can stop ciliary function in 8–10 minutes, which predisposes to infections of the respiratory tract and affects gas exchange.
Nasal obstruction and sleep apnea: Nasal obstruction affects gaseous exchange in the lungs, which results in pO_2 fall and pCO_2 rise that causes apnea spells during sleep.

PROTECTION OF AIRWAY

- *Enzymes and immunoglobulins:* Enzymes and immunoglobulins are present in nasal secretions. Muramidase (lysozyme) kills bacteria and viruses. Immunoglobulins (IgA and IgE) and interferon provide immunity against upper respiratory tract infections.
- *Sneezing:* Foreign particles, irritating nasal mucosa are expelled by this protective reflex. Copious flow of nasal secretions (due to irritation) washes noxious substance out.

Mucociliary Mechanism

Nasal mucosa is rich in mucous and serous secretory glands (600-700 ml of nasal secretions in 24 hours), which form a mucus blanket that spread over the mucosa. Mucus blanket consists of two layers superficial mucus layer and deep serous layer and floats (5-10 mm/minute) on the cilia. Cilia beat constantly (10-20 times per second at room temperature) like a "conveyer belt" towards the nasopharynx. The complete sheet of mucus blanket reaches into the pharynx in 10-20 minutes. This viscous mucus blanket entraps bacteria, viruses and dust particles from the inspired air and carries them into pharynx and gets swallowed into stomach and digested.

- *Ciliary biphasic beats:* The ciliary biphasic beats have two strokes rapid effective stroke (extended cilia reach superficial mucus layer) and slow recovery stroke, in which cilia bend (reach deep thin serous layer) and travel slowly in the reverse direction. The effective strokes move the mucus blanket in one direction.

- **Factors affecting ciliary beating:** The ciliary movements can be affected by:
  - Environmental pollution
  - Humidity
  - Drying
  - Drugs such as adrenaline
  - Excessive heat and cold
  - Hypertonic and hypotonic solutions
  - Smoking (nicotine)
  - Infections—viral and bacterial
  - Parasympathetic system
  - Airborne external irritants—SO_2 and CO_2
  - The cilia and lysozyme act best at nasal secretion pH 7, the alteration of which (due to infections and certain nasal drops) can affect the functions of cilia and lysozyme.

Kartagener's syndrome: In this **immotile cilia syndrome** cilia are defective and cannot beat effectively and lead to stagnation of mucus. There is absence of dynein arm on the peripheral ciliary microtubules. Patient presents with triad of—
- Chronic rhinosinusitis (mucus accumulation in nose),
- Bronchiectasis and
- Situs inversus

VOCAL RESONANCE

Nose acts as a resonating chamber for the speech. For phonating nasal consonants (M/N/NG), sound passes via nasopharynx and nose. When either nose or nasopharynx is blocked (rhinolalia clausa), speech becomes denasal and M/N/Ng are pronounced as B/D/G respectively. Reverse happens in velopharyngeal insufficiency (rhinolalia aperta).

NASAL REFLEXES

- **Sneezing:** Irritation of nasal mucosa causes sneezing. If a finger is pressed under the columella it may abort sneezing.
- **Cardiopulmonary responses:** Strong nasal stimuli result in profound cardiopulmonary responses such as breathing cessation and bradycardia. It is relevant to sleep apnea syndrome.
- **Appetite:** Good smell of food results in reflex secretion of saliva and gastric juice.
- **Nasobronchial and nasopulmonary reflexes:** They affect pulmonary functions.

Pulmonary resistance: Nasal obstruction increases pulmonary resistance, which can be reversed by treating nasal obstruction.
- Nasal packing lowers pO_2, which becomes normal after removal of pack.
- Chronic nasal obstruction (tonsil and adenoid hypertrophy) in children causes pulmonary hypertension and cor pulmonale, which can be reversed after their surgical treatment.

OLFACTION

Olfactory system is highly developed in animals and is important for their communication and survival and gives warnings of the environmental dangers. In humans it is comparatively less developed but plays an important role in enjoying delicious and sumptuous food.

Olfaction and ammonia: Vapors of ammonia cause irritation and stimulate fibers of the trigeminal nerve (not olfactory). The olfaction is affected in patients of nose block and food tastes bland and unpalatable.

Olfactory Pathways

Olfactory system is an important constituent of limbic system.

- **Olfactory receptor cells:** Olfactory epithelium in the olfactory region of nose contains millions of olfactory receptor cells, peripheral processes of which reach the mucosal surface and expand into a ventricle that have several cilia and receive odorous substances.
- **Olfactory nerves:** Central processes of the olfactory cells make olfactory nerves.
- **Olfactory bulb:** Olfactory nerves pass through the cribriform plate of ethmoid and end in the mitral cells of the olfactory bulb.
- **Olfactory tract:** Axons of mitral cells traverse in olfactory tract.
- **Cerebrum:** Olfactory tract carries smell to the prepiriform cortex and the amygdaloid nucleus.
- **Disorders of smell:** See Chapter 'Nasal symptoms and examination'.

Olfactory receptor cells: Primary olfactory receptor cells are able to regenerate entirely while other special sensory primary neurons cannot.

Vomeronasal Organ of Jacobson

This accessory olfactory tissue is present in 1–3 mm tubule with an oval orifice. It is situated 1 cm behind the caudal end of septum and 3 mm above the nasal floor. The color of mucosa in this area is pale yellowish. Though electrovomerogram has been recorded in response to odorants yet its function in humans remain uncertain.

PHYSIOLOGY OF PARANASAL SINUSES

FUNCTIONS

The functions of the paranasal sinuses, which are not well proved, include:
- Air-conditioning of the inspired air (humidification and warming)
- Keep the nasal chambers moist
- Resonance to voice
- Protect the delicate structures in the orbit (eye) and the cranium (brain)
- Lighten the skull bones
- Rapid growth of face
- Absorption of shock to the face and skull
- Increasing the area of olfactory membrane
- Regulation of intranasal pressure.

VENTILATION OF SINUSES

Ventilation of paranasal sinuses takes place through their ostia. It is paradoxical and reverse to lungs. Sinuses get emptied of air during inspiration and filled with air during expiration. Inspiration causes negative pressure (–6 mm to –200 mm of H_2O) in the nose. Expiration causes positive pressure in the nose and sets up eddies that ventilate the sinuses.

Self-evaluation Exercises

1. The major constituent of nasal septum is quadrangular septal cartilage.   **T/F**
2. Nasal septum is composed of following components:
    a. Major constituent quadrangular septal cartilage
    b. Important contribution from perpendicular plate of ethmoid and vomer
    c. Minor contributions come from sphenoid rostrum, frontal nasal spine, anterior nasal spine, crests of maxilla, palatine and nasal bones
    d. All of the above
3. Which of the following is not true for vomeronasal organ?
    a. Vestigial structure
    b. Said to be related with olfaction
    c. Seen as a pit on the posterosuperior part of nasal septum
    d. None of the above
4. Which of the following are true for respiratory cilia?
    a. Length about 5–7 micron
    b. Rate of ciliary beat about 10–20 times per second at room temperature
    c. Ratio of effective phase and recovery phase of ciliary beat 1:3
    d. Nasal cilia are approximately 0.3 micron thick
    e. All of the above
5. Which of the following is true for ethmoidal infundibulum?
    a. Situated in lateral wall of nose
    b. Communicates with nasal cavity through hiatus semilunaris
    c. Opening of the maxillary sinus is situated near its floor
    d. All of the above
6. Which of the following are not true for sphenopalatine ganglion?
    a. Innervates nose, palate and lacrimal gland (associated with lacrimation)
    b. Anesthetized by injecting xylocaine just above and behind the posterior end of middle turbinate and into the greater palatine foramen and canal
    c. Preganglionic secretomotor fibers from greater petrosal nerve relay here
    d. All of the above
7. Which of the following is not true for sphenoid sinus?
    a. In an adult the distance between its opening and anterior nasal spine is about 7 cm
    b. Its cavity may show indentations of internal carotid artery, optic nerve, vidian nerve and maxillary division of trigeminal nerve
    c. Drains into sphenoethmoidal recess
    d. None of the above

Contd...

Contd...

8. Sinuses draining anterior to basal lamella:
   a. Maxillary sinus
   b. Frontal sinus
   c. Anterior ethmoidal sinuses including agger nasi cells
   d. All of the above

True (T)/False (F)
9. Direction of nasolacrimal duct is downwards, forward and medially.
10. Nasolacrimal duct courses anterior to maxillary ostium and opens into inferior meatus.
11. Uncinate process of ethmoidal bone forms lateral wall of ethmoidal infundibulum, which lies in the lateral wall of nose.
12. Hiatus semilunaris, a two-dimensional door like space lies between bulla ethmoidalis and uncinate process.
13. Posterior fontanelle is situated in the lateral wall of middle meatus.
14. Schneiderian membrane (mucosa) is the pseudostratified ciliated columnar respiratory mucosa of nose.
15. The pH of 'mucous blanket' of nose is 7.
16. Normal nasal temperature is 32°C. All nasal ciliary activity ceases at 7–10°C.
17. Main current of nasal airflow during inspiration is through the upper part of the nasal cavity (medial to superior turbinate and meatus) in a parabolic curve.

Answers

1. T	2. d	3. c	4. e	5. d	6. d
7. d	8. d	9. F	10. T	11. F	12. T
13. T	14. T	15. T	16. T	17. F	

Chapter 21

Nasal Symptoms and Examination

Specific Learning Objectives

After going through the chapter, you should be able to answer the following questions:
- What are the nasal symptoms and how will you take history and perform examination in these patients?
- What are the abnormalities that you can see during your anterior rhinoscopy examination and their causes?
- How will you perform the examination of paranasal sinuses and what will you look for during the examination?
- What are the different types of smell disorders and their causes?
- What are the different causes of unilateral nasal obstruction and how they are different from the causes of bilateral nasal obstruction?
- What do you know about the causes of proptosis?
- Which are the common sites of epistaxis and the vessels involved in the bleeding from those sites?
- Enumerate the causes of epistaxis and explain some of the common causes. How will you evaluate a case of epistaxis?
- How would you manage a case of anterior epistaxis? What is the procedure and complications of posterior nasal packing?

INTRODUCTION

External nose does not need any special instrument for examination. Anterior rhinoscopy allows assessment of nasal cavity, septum and inferior middle turbinate and meatus. A child's nose can be examined with a wide speculum otoscope. For general scheme of case taking and general set up of Bull's eye lamp light source and head mirror *see* Chapter 'History and Examination'.

HISTORY TAKING

History must include the details of all the complaints mentioned in the chief complaints (Table 21.1). It begins with the appearance of first symptom and extend up to the time of consultation. It usually consists of the mode of onset (sudden/gradual), preceding events causing onset, course of symptoms (progressive/constant/fluctuant and continuous/intermittent), factors aggravating/relieving, other accompanying complaints and the treatment taken. In cases of unilateral disorder, note the side and site of affliction. If both the sides of nose are affected, then it should be mentioned which is worst affected. Many a time, negative answers are equally important in arriving at a diagnosis. Inquiries are made for any systemic diseases, which patient might be suffering from such as diabetes, hypertension, tuberculosis, HIV/AIDS and coronary, liver, kidney and bleeding disorders.

Table 21.1: Common complaints of nose and paranasal sinuses

Main complaints	Associated complaints
• Nasal stuffiness/obstruction	• Headache
• Nasal discharge—anterior/postnasal drip	• Vomiting
• Sneezing	• Fever
• Itching	• Facial fullness/pain
• Nose bleed (epistaxis)	• Exophthalmos
• Nasal crusting	• Change in voice (hypernasal/hyponasal)
• Disturb smell	• Snoring/obstructive sleep apnea (OSA)
• Emitting foul smell to others	• Cough
• Swelling nose and paranasal sinuses	• Epiphora
• Nose deformities—congenital or acquired	• Hearing loss (conductive)
• Injury/foreign body (FB)	

Unilateral purulent blood stained nasal discharge in children: It is usually due to foreign body nose unnoticed by parents.

EXAMINATION

Box 21.1 shows the general format of examination of nose and paranasal sinuses and causes of common findings.

Chapter 21 • Nasal Symptoms and Examination

> **Box 21.1: Examination of nose and paranasal sinuses—findings and their causes**
>
> **Physical Examination of Nose**
> - **External nose:**
>   - *Swelling:* Furuncle, septal abscess, dermoid, glioma, sebaceous cyst
>   - *Scars:* Operation, trauma
>   - *Sinus:* Congenital dermoid
>   - *Ulcer/neoplasm:* Rhinophyma, basal cell/squamous cell carcinoma or melanoma, herpes simplex/zoster
>   - *Deformity:* Deviated or twisted nose, hump, depressed bridge, bifid or pointed tip, destruction of nose (trauma, syphilis, and cancer), and longer nose appearance in aged persons due to drooping of the nasal tip
>   - *Palpation:* Raised temperature, tenderness, fluctuation, fixity of skin, thickening of soft tissues, crepitation (fracture)
>   - *Enlargement of bony skeleton:* Paget's disease or fibro-osseous dysplasia
>   - *Cartilaginous enlargement:* Chondroma or chondrosarcoma
> - **Vestibule:** Furuncle, fissure (chronic rhinitis), crusting, dislocated caudal end of the septum and tumors (cyst, papilloma, carcinoma or melanoma).
> - **Anterior rhinoscopy**
>   - *Nasal cavity:* Narrow (septal deviation or hypertrophy turbinates, polyp, growth), wide (atrophic rhinitis); discharge (mucoid, mucopurulent, purulent, blood); crusting; foreign body.
>   - *Septum:* Deviation, spur, ulcer, perforation, swelling (hematoma or abscess), growth (rhinosporidiosis, hemangioma, fibroangioma), bony destruction (syphilis), or cartilaginous destruction (lupus vulgaris).
>   - *Floor of nose:* Defect (cleft palate or fistula), swelling (dental cyst), neoplasm (hemangioma), or granulations (foreign body or osteitis).
>   - *Inferior and middle turbinates:* Enlarged and swollen (hypertrophic rhinitis, concha bullosa), small and rudimentary (atrophic rhinitis). Congested in inflammation and pale in allergy.
>   - *Inferior and middle meatuses:* Discharge/polyps in the middle meatus (infection of maxillary, frontal or anterior ethmoidal sinuses) and between the middle turbinate and the septum (posterior group of ethmoid sinuses).
>   - *Mass:* Polyp, rhinosporidiosis, carcinoma
>   - *Probing:* Site of attachment, consistency, mobility and sensitiveness of the mass, bleeding on touch.
> - **Posterior rhinoscopy**
>   - *Posterior choanae:* Atresia, polyp
>   - *Posterior ends of inferior turbinates:* Hypertrophy
>   - *Discharge:* In middle meatus (infection of maxillary, frontal or anterior ethmoidal sinuses); above middle turbinate (infection of the posterior ethmoid or the sphenoid sinuses).
>   - *Nasopharynx:* See Chapters 'Pharyngeal Symptoms and Examinations and Tumors of Nasopharynx'.
>
> **Functional Examination of Nose**
> - **Patency of nose:** Spatula test/cotton-wool test
> - **Sense of smell:** Clove oil, peppermint, coffee, and essence of rose.
>
> **Examination of Paranasal Sinuses**
> - **Inspection and palpation**
>   - *Swelling or fullness:* Cheek, upper lip, lower and upper eyelids and the malar region, forehead and root of nose.
>   - *Orbit and eyeball:* Margins, swelling, proptosis, eye movements, vision (acuity and field), convergence, pupil reactions, fundus, redness, and displacement of eye ball.
>   - *Vestibule of mouth:* Obliteration/fullness/swelling in gingivolabial/gingivobuccal sulcus
>   - *Upper alveolus and palate:* Swelling, ulcer, loose teeth, or carries teeth
>   - *Swelling and tenderness:* Maxillary/canine fossa/frontal/between nose and eye (anterior ethmoid)
> - **Transillumination:** For maxillary, frontal and ethmoidal sinuses

EXTERNAL NOSE

The external nose needs proper inspection as well as palpation for the skin lesions and the osteocartilaginous framework deformities (Box 21.1).

Swelling and cysts:
- ***Dermoids:*** They occur over nasal bones and columella.
  - **Dermoid cyst:** It can present as a discharging sinus over the osteocartilaginous junction of nasal bridge.
- ***Furuncle (Figs 21.1A and B):*** It presents as a tender red swelling near the tip of nose.
- ***Dental cysts/abscess:*** They present as swelling near the nasal alae.
- ***Rhinophyma:*** It presents as enlargement of the lower part of nose.
- ***Rodent ulcer:*** Basal cell carcinoma (Fig. 21.2A)
- ***Nasolabial cyst (Fig. 21.2B):*** It obliterates alar facial fold and cause smooth swelling in the floor of nasal vestibule and upper part of upper lip.

Palpation of external nose differentiates between bony, cartilaginous and soft tissue swelling and diagnose deformity, fracture (crepitus) and other lesions.

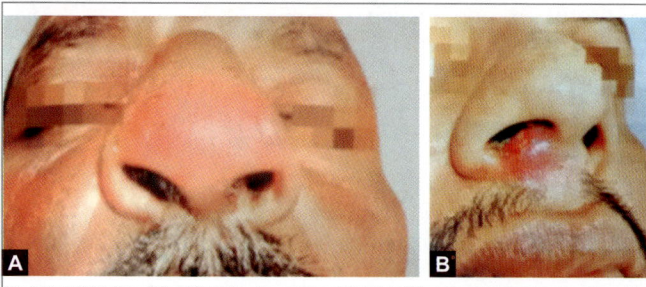

Figs 21.1A and B: Nasal furuncle. (A) External nose swelling; (B) Furuncle in the vestibule

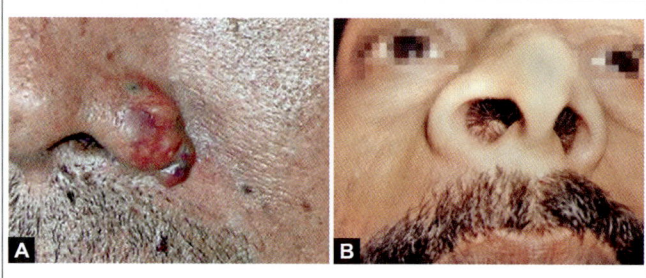

Figs 21.2A and B: (A) An early rodent ulcer (basal cell carcinoma) of nasomaxillary skin; (B) Nasolabial cyst

Vestibule is an anterior skin lined part of nasal cavity having vibrissae (hairs in nasal vestibule). It can be easily evaluated by lifting the tip of nose. For further details, refer to Chapter 'Diseases of External Nose'.

ANTERIOR RHINOSCOPY (EXAMINATION OF NASAL CAVITY)

Thudicum Nasal Speculum

A Thudicum or Vienna type of nasal speculum, which is held in the left hand, assists in widening the vestibule (Figs 21.3A and B). The blades of speculum are inserted into the less sensitive skin lined vestibule and should not touch the septal mucosa which is very sensitive and vascular. The nasal speculum is closed while introducing and opened during examination and remains partially open when removing from the nose (avoid picking vibrissae). The size of the nasal speculum should be chosen according to the age of patient and size of the nose.

Examination

Patient's head needs to be tilted in different directions to examine different sites in the nose—septum, inferior turbinate and meatus, middle turbinate and meatus and floor of the nose (Box 21.1).
- *Posture test:* Drainage of purulent discharge from various sinuses depends upon the posture of patient.

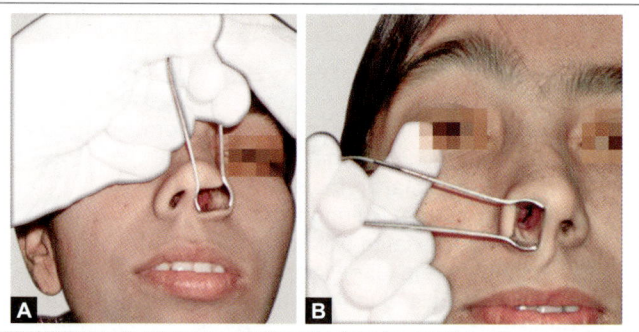

Figs 21.3A and B: Anterior rhinoscopy. Two ways of holding and introducing of the nasal speculum

After wiping out the purulent discharge from the middle meatus, note the following points:
- *Frontal sinus:* Pus reappears immediately if the patient is sitting in upright position (head forward chin down position).
- *Ethmoidal sinus:* Pus reappears after some time (10–15 minutes) if the patient is sitting in upright position.
- *Maxillary sinus:* Pus reappears if the head is so bent that the affected maxillary sinus is in upward position.

POSTERIOR RHINOSCOPY

It consists of examining the nasopharynx and posterior part of nasal cavity by the postnasal mirror (Fig. 21.4A). The patient opens his mouth and breathes quietly. Postnasal mirror is warmed but should not be hot. It is always better to test on the back of hand before introducing. The examiner depresses the patient's tongue with a tongue depressor that is held in left hand and introduces posterior rhinoscopic mirror (postnasal mirror). The mirror should be held in right hand like a pen and carried towards posterior pharyngeal wall, along the tongue but without touching the posterior third of tongue (to avoid gag reflex). The reflected light from the head mirror illuminates the area of nasopharynx and the examiner sees the reflected

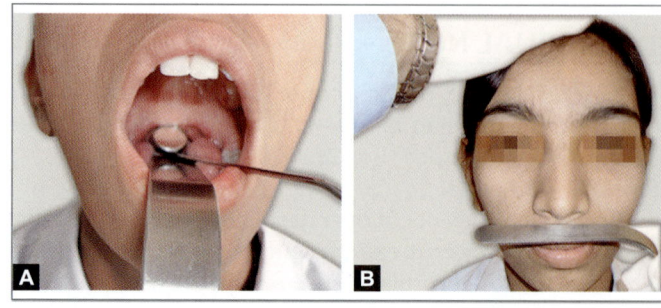

Figs 21.4A and B: Nasal examination. (A) Posterior rhinoscopy; (B) Spatula test for patency of nose

image of the postnasal space in the postnasal mirror. If the patient is quiet and relaxed, then usually soft palate does not contract and hide the view. This procedure especially needs concentration, patience and practice. For the structures seen during this procedure *see* Box 21.1.

PATENCY OF NASAL CAVITIES

- *Spatula test* (Fig. 21.4B): A clean cold stainless steel tongue depressor is held below the nose while patient exhales. Each area of mist formation on either side is compared.
- *Cotton-wool test:* A fluff of cotton is held below each nostril and its movements indicate the nasal blow of air while the patient inhales or exhales.
- *Alae nasi movements:* In cases of inspiratory obstruction, alae nasi collapse onto the septum.
- *Cottle test: See* Section of 'Nasal Valves Disorders'.

SENSE OF SMELL

See Section 'Smell' of this Chapter.

Ammonia: It stimulates the fibers of trigeminal nerve and is not used for testing smell.

PARANASAL SINUSES

They are examined by inspection, palpation and transillumination. The anterior group of sinuses (maxillary, frontal and anterior ethmoid) drains in middle meatus. The posterior ethmoid drains into superior meatus. The sphenoid sinus opens into sphenoethmoidal recess.

All the structures, which are adjacent to the different walls of these sinuses, need attention of the examiner. Sphenoid sinus, which opens in the sphenoethmoidal recess, lies deep and cannot be examined directly. Frontal sinus has three walls—anterior, posterior and floor but only the anterior wall can be examined externally. For the methods and findings of examination of paranasal sinuses *see* Box 21.1.

Tenderness

Tenderness of the sinuses can be elicited by pressure or percussion with a finger on their walls (Fig. 21.5).
- *Frontal sinus:* Anterior wall and floor above the medial part of eyebrow and above the medial canthus.
- *Maxillary sinus:* Anterior wall over the cheek lateral to nose (Fig. 21.5B).
- *Anterior ethmoids:* Medial wall of orbit just behind the root of nose.

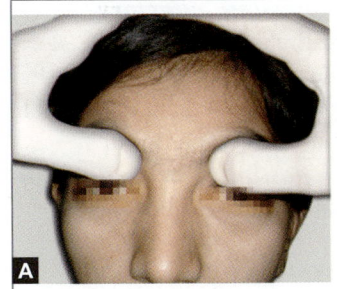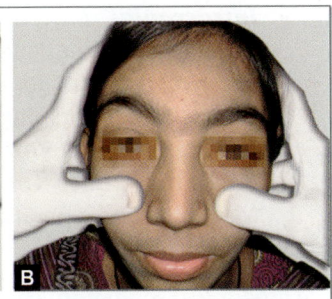

Figs 21.5A and B: Tenderness of the sinuses elicited by pressure with finger on their walls. (A) Frontal sinuses; (B) Maxillary sinuses

Transillumination

- *Maxillary sinus:* A specially made light source is placed in the mouth that is closed. Normally, a crescent of light in the inferior fornix and glow in the pupil, which are equally bright on either side can be seen. The affected side maxillary sinus will not transmit light if there is pus, thickened mucosa or a neoplasm.
- *Frontal sinus:* A small light source is placed in the superomedial angle of the orbit. The transmission of light from the anterior wall of the both side frontal sinuses is compared.

Endoscopic Examination

See Chapter 'Operations of Nose and Paranasal Sinuses'.

SPECIAL INVESTIGATIONS

SMELL

The odorous substance should be volatile and reach the olfactory area. Any lesion anywhere in the olfactory pathway (olfactory mucosa, olfactory nerves, olfactory bulbs and tract and the cortical center of olfaction) will affect smelling power of the person.

Physiological Factors Affecting Olfaction

They include age, satiety, gender, adaptation and habituation and odor mixtures.

Causes of Olfactory Disorders

- *Loss of smell (anosmia and hyposmia):* It can result from—
  - *Nasal obstruction* due to nasal polyps, enlarged turbinates, edema of mucous membrane as in common cold, allergic and vasomotor rhinitis.
  - *Atrophic rhinitis*
  - *Peripheral neuritis:* Toxic or influenzal
  - *Injury to olfactory nerves and olfactory bulb:* Fractures of anterior cranial fossa.

- *Intracranial lesions pressing olfactory tracts:* Abscess, tumor and meningitis
- **Parosmia:** It refers to perversion of smell. Patient interprets the odors incorrectly, which are usually disgusting. The causes of parosmia include:
  - *Recovery phase of postinfluenzal anosmia:* Misdirected regeneration of nerve fibers.
  - *Intracranial tumor*.

> **Three most common causes of anosmia:** They are sinonasal disease, post-upper respiratory tract infection and trauma (injury to olfactory nerves at cribriform plate or brain injury).

Tests for Smell

In routine testing, patient is asked to close eyes and smell common odors such as lemon, peppermint, rose, garlic, coffee, and cloves. Each side of the nose is tested separately. Quantitative estimation (quantitative olfactometry) needs special equipment.
- **Electro-olfactogram (EOG):** Electrode is placed on the olfactory epithelium. It records a slow, negative and monophasic potential in response to odorants. EOG represents a 'generator potential'.

> **Kallmann syndrome:** It consists of anosmia, congenital hypogonadism and amenorrhea in females.

NASAL OBSTRUCTION

Causes of Nasal Obstruction
- **Unilateral nasal obstruction**
  - *Infectious:* Furuncle, hypertrophic turbinate, concha bullosa, antrochoanal polyp and unilateral sinusitis.
  - *Congenital:* Atresia and stenosis of nares, unilateral choanal atresia, nasoalveolar cyst.
  - *Traumatic:* Foreign body, rhinolith, deviated nasal septum (DNS) and synechia
  - *Neoplasms:* Papilloma, bleeding polyp of septum, benign and malignant tumors of nose and paranasal sinuses, and nasopharynx.
- **Bilateral nasal obstruction**
  - *Infectious:* Bilateral vestibulitis, rhinosinusitis (infectious, allergic and others), bilateral nasal polyps, atrophic rhinitis, septal abscess and large choanal polyp.
  - *Congenital:* Congenital atresia of nares, bilateral choanal atresia and Thornwald's cyst.
  - *Structural:* Collapsing nasal alae, stenosis of nares, DNS, adhesions between soft palate and posterior pharyngeal wall.
  - *Traumatic:* Septal hematoma.
  - *Neoplasms:* Large benign and malignant tumors.
  - *Miscellaneous:* Hypertrophic turbinates and big adenoids.

Differential Diagnosis (Flow chart 21.1)

Observe the nose during normal and exaggerated nasal breathing and watch for the collapse of internal and external nasal valves. The site and causes of nasal obstruction include:
- **Vestibule:** Caudal septal dislocation, synechia or stenosis
- **Nasal valve:** Post-rhinoplasty synechia
- **High septal deviation:** Examine the upper part of nasal septum.
- **Turbinates:** Hypertrophic turbinates or concha bullosa
- **Choanal:** Choanal atresia, choanal polyp
  - *Unilateral choanal atresia:* This pediatric disease is usually asymptomatic and usually missed.
  - *Choanal polyp:* It is usually not visible on the anterior rhinoscopy but can be seen easily with posterior rhinoscopy and nasal endoscopy examination.
- **Polyps and septal hematoma and abscess**
- **Tip ptosis:** It contributes to decreased nasal airflow.

NASAL VALVES DISORDERS (FIG. 21.6A)

- **Internal nasal valve:** It is the narrowest area of airway. It is bounded by septum, lower margin of upper lateral cartilage (ULC) and anterior aspect of inferior turbinate. The septal deformities and loss of ULC support can lead to nasal obstruction. The ULC may be thickened, twisted and concave or absent because of prior surgery.
- **External nasal valve:** It is at the level of caudal septum. This laterally based space is bounded by bony pyriform nasal aperture, lateral margin of ULC and lateral crura of lower lateral cartilage (LLC). The causes of external valve compromise includes rhinoplasty, aging and caudal septal dislocation or trauma.
- **Cottle test (Fig. 21.6B):** This test is done for the abnormality of the nasal valve. The cheek is drawn laterally and the patient breathes quietly. If there is subjective improvement in nasal airway, the test is positive, which indicates nasal valve compromise. The test also can be performed by lateralizing the ULC with a cotton-tipped applicator.

PROPTOSIS (EXOPHTHALMOS)

Proptosis (G. *proptosis*, a falling forward) refers to protrusion of the eyeball. It can be congenital (familial) or acquired and unilateral or bilateral. Unilateral is caused by tumors of nasopharynx, paranasal sinuses and retro-orbital region and bilateral is caused by hyperthyroidism.

Chapter 21 • Nasal Symptoms and Examination

Flow chart 21.1: Showing anterior rhinoscopy findings of various causes of nasal obstruction

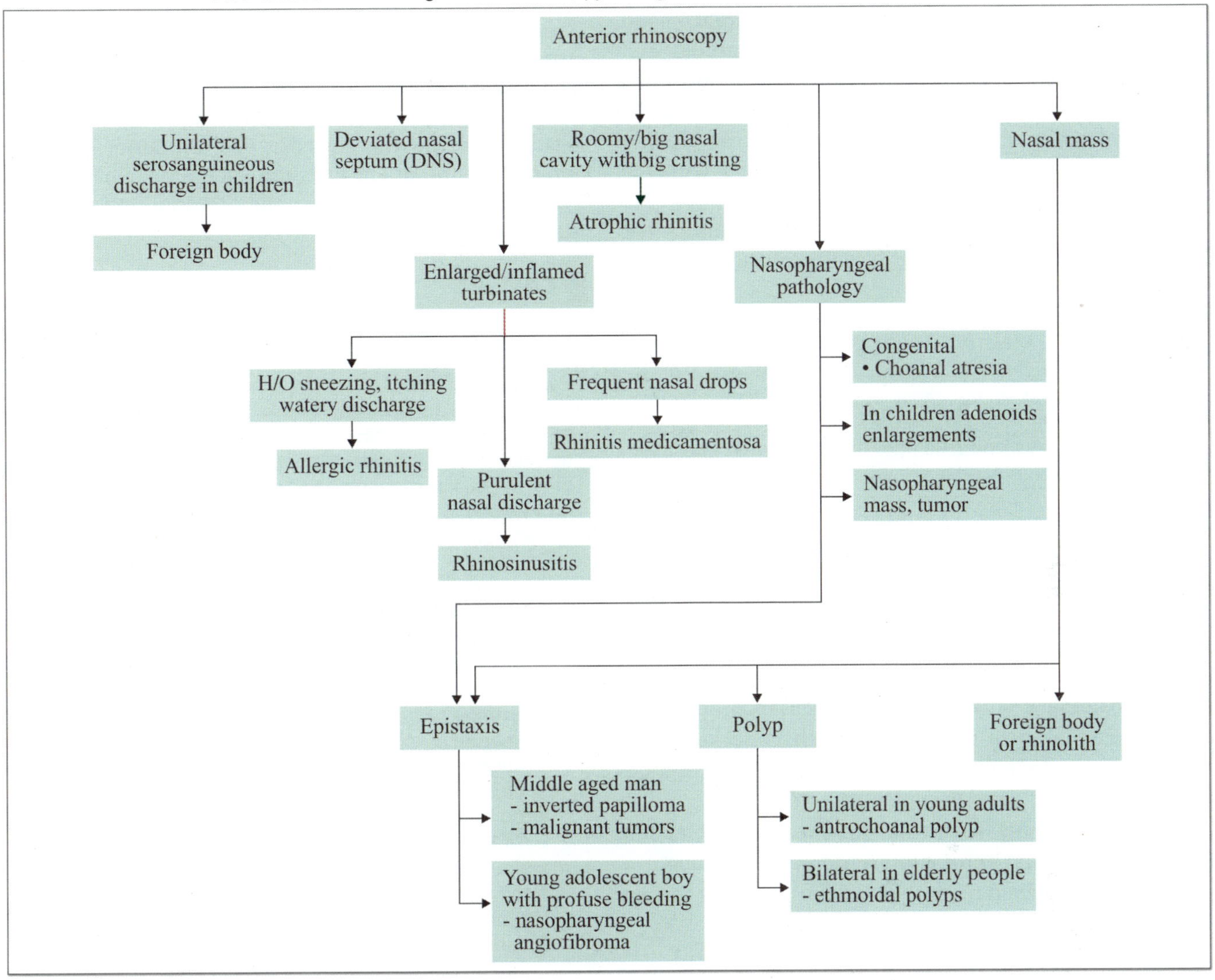

```
                            Anterior rhinoscopy
    ┌──────────┬──────────────┬──────────────┬──────────────┐
Unilateral   Deviated nasal  Roomy/big nasal              Nasal mass
serosanguineous septum (DNS) cavity with big crusting
discharge in children              │
    │                        Atrophic rhinitis
Foreign body                       │
                         Enlarged/inflamed       Nasopharyngeal
                            turbinates              pathology
                     ┌────────┴────────┐        ┌──────┴────────┐
              H/O sneezing, itching  Frequent nasal drops   Congenital
              watery discharge           │                  • Choanal atresia
                     │              Rhinitis medicamentosa
              Allergic rhinitis    Purulent                In children adenoids
                                   nasal discharge         enlargements
                                         │
                                   Rhinosinusitis          Nasopharyngeal
                                                           mass, tumor

              Epistaxis              Polyp            Foreign body
                                                      or rhinolith
         Middle aged man         Unilateral in young adults
         - inverted papilloma    - antrochoanal polyp
         - malignant tumors
                                 Bilateral in elderly people
         Young adolescent boy    - ethmoidal polyps
         with profuse bleeding
         - nasopharyngeal
         angiofibroma
```

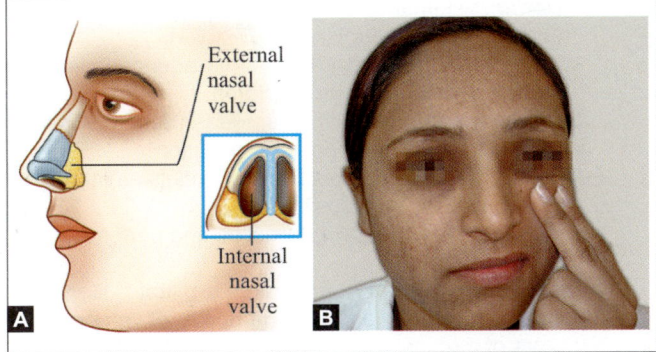

Figs 21.6A and B: Nasal valves. (A) External nasal valve (inset shows internal nasal valve); (B) Cottle test

- **Pertinent anatomy:** The orbit is related to frontal sinus (superiorly), maxillary sinus (inferiorly), ethmoid sinus (medially) and sphenoid sinus (posteromedially).
- **Causes:** ENT causes include
  - *Congenital and familial*
  - *Trauma:* Maxillofacial injuries, orbital hemorrhage after endoscopic sinus surgery.
  - *Infection:* Complications of rhinosinusitis such as subperiosteal abscess, orbital cellulitis and cavernous sinus thrombosis, fungal rhinosinusitis, Wegener's garnulomatosis.
  - *Cysts:* Mucocele of frontoethmoid sinus.
  - *Benign tumors:* Inverted papilloma, osteoma, ethmoidal polyps and fungus, juvenile nasopharyngeal angiofibroma and fibrous dysplasia.
  - *Malignant tumors:* Carcinoma and sarcomas of nose, paranasal sinuses and nasopharynx.
- Other causes are as follows:
  - *Vascular:* Cavernous hemangioma, carotid cavernous fistula (pulsatile proptosis).
  - *Endocrine:* Grave's disease (*see* Chapter 'Disorders of Thyroid').

- **Orbital:** Pseudotumor of orbit, orbital cellulitis and abscess, inflammations of lacrimal gland, tumors of orbital contents such as dermoid cyst, cavernous and capillary hemangioma, schwanoma, glioma, retinoblastoma, histiocytosis X, orbital menangioma, pleomorphic adenoma of lacrimal gland, rhabdomyosarcoma, lymphoma, leukemic deposits, melanoma of choroid.
- *Management:* Clinical features, imaging studies and biopsy will confirm the diagnosis. The cause of proptosis should be treated.

- **Dermoid cyst** is the most common pediatric benign tumor of orbit.
- **Rhabdomyosarcoma** is the most common pediatric malignant tumor of orbit.

EPISTAXIS (NOSEBLEED)

Bleeding from the nose is called epistaxis (synonym: nosebleed). Epistaxis is a symptom and one should try to find its local and systemic causes.
- Approximately 50% population experience nosebleed in their life but it is serious enough to seek medical consultation in less than 10%. Some patients present as an emergency. There is no age bar.
- Children usually have mild anterior nasal bleeding while elderly have profuse posterior nose bleeding.
- Males are affected more than females but after the age of 50 years both the sexes are affected equally.

PERTINENT ANATOMY

Little's Area/Kiesselbach's Plexus

Little's area is situated in the anteroinferior part of nasal septum and is supplied by branches of both external and internal carotid arteries. For the further details of blood supply of nose, see Chapter 'Anatomy and Physiology of Nose and Paranasal Sinuses'.

The four arteries which anastomose richly and form a vascular plexus (Kiesselbach's plexus) in this region, are:
1. Anterior ethmoidal.
2. Septal branch of superior labial.
3. Septal branch of sphenopalatine.
4. Greater palatine.

This vascular area is the most common site of nosebleed in children and young adults. It gets dried due to the effect of inspiratory current and easily traumatized due to frequent picking (fingering) of nose.

Retrocolumellar Vein

It runs vertically downward just behind the columella and crosses the floor of nose. It is a common source of venous bleeding in young people.

Woodruff's plexus: This source of posterior epistaxis is situated below the posterior end of inferior turbinate. Sphenopalatine artery exits the sphenoplataine foramen 1 cm inferior and anterior to the posterior end of middle turbinate.

CAUSES

Causes of epistaxis can be divided into local and general (Box 21.2).

Common causes of epistaxis: The most common cause of nosebleed in children is repeated fingernail trauma to Little's area. In elderly people, most common cause is atherosclerotic changes and hypertension. In many cases, no obvious cause is ascertained (idiopathic). In vicarious menstruation, nosebleed occurs at the time of menstruation.

Box 21.2: Causes of epistaxis

- **Local causes** (nose, paranasal sinuses and nasopharynx)
  - **Trauma:** Finger nail trauma (obsessive compulsive disorder), injuries of nose (accidental, homicidal, surgery), maxillofacial trauma, head injuries, nasal intubation, foreign bodies, rhinolith, blowing of nose too hard and violent sneezing.
  - **Infections:** Rhinosinusitis, nasal vestibulitis, sinusitis, adenoiditis, diphtheria, pyogenic granuloma, rhinosporidiosis, granulomatous lesions (tuberculosis, syphilis, sarcoidosis, Wegener's granuloma), atrophic rhinitis, rhinitis sicca, maggots, leeches and neglected foreign body.
  - **Neoplasms**
    - **Benign:** Hemangioma, inverted papilloma, juvenile angiofibroma, aneurysms.
    - **Malignant:** Epidermoid carcinoma, adenocarcinoma, sarcoma, esthesioneuroblastoma.
  - **Environmental:** High altitudes, sudden decompression (Caisson's disease), chemicals, pollution.
  - **Drugs:** Nasal sprays and drops of antihistaminics and steroids, sniffing of cocaine, snuff.
  - **Miscellaneous:** Septal deformities and perforation.
- **General causes**
  - **Cardiovascular:** Hypertension, mitral stenosis, congestive heart failure, eclampsia of pregnancy, tumors of mediastinum (raised venous pressure).
  - **Hemopoietic:** Aplastic anemia, leukemia, thrombocytopenic and vascular purpura, coagulopathies (congenital and acquired), hemophilia, Christmas disease, polycythemia vera, multiple myeloma.
  - **Nutritional:** Malnutrition, scurvy, alcohol abuse, vitamin A, D, C, E and K deficiencies and high doses of vitamin E.

Contd…

Contd…

> - ***Blood vessels:*** Arteriosclerosis, collagen diseases and hereditary hemorrhagic telangiectasia (HHT).
> - ***Liver disease:*** Hepatic cirrhosis (deficiency of factor 2, 7, 9 and 10).
> - ***Kidney disease:*** Chronic nephritis and renal failure.
> - ***Drugs:*** Aspirin, nonsteroidal anti-inflammatory drugs (NSAIDs) (ibuprofen and diclofenac) and anticoagulant therapy (heparin and coumadin).
> - ***Acute infections:*** Influenza, measles, chickenpox, whooping cough, rheumatic fever, infectious mononucleosis, typhoid, pneumonia, malaria, dengue fever.

EVALUATION

The initial evaluation of nosebleed patients includes assessment of hemodynamic stability, airway compromise and vital parameters.

History

Complete history includes following questions:
- Side of bleeding; worst side if bleeding is bilateral.
- Symptoms of posterior nasal bleeding such as expectoration of blood and hematemesis.
- Precipitating events such as trauma, acute infection, nasal drops and sprays and surgery.
- Duration and amount of bleeding.
- Syncopal or near syncopal attacks.
- Risk factors such as hypertension, leukemia, hemophilia, purpura, congestive heart failure, renal failure and liver dysfunction and their medications.
- Drugs such as aspirin, NSAIDs (ibuprofen), heparin, antiplatelet drugs, high doses of vitamin E.
- Past history of bleeding and its treatment.
- Family history of bleeding tendencies such as hemophilia.

Examination

- Examination should include vital parameters, complete ear, nose and throat examination, general features and systemic examination.
- The examination is often treatment oriented and should try to locate the cause and site of bleeding. Patient needs reassurance.

SITES OF EPISTAXIS

- ***Little's area:*** The most common site of bleeding in children and young people is Little's area.
- ***Above middle turbinate:*** Area supplied by anterior and posterior ethmoidal branches of ophthalmic artery (branch of internal carotid artery).
- ***Below middle turbinate:*** Area supplied by sphenopalatine branch of internal maxillary artery (branch of external carotid artery).
- Sometimes, the bleeding site may be hidden by middle and inferior turbinates.

Local decongestant helps in localization of the bleeding site and packing of the nose.

- ***Posterior nasal cavity and nasopharynx:*** Pateint will have posterior epistaxis and blood will come in throat and swallowed and spitted out.
- ***Diffuse epistaxis:*** In general systemic disorders, there occurs diffuse bleeding from septum and lateral nasal wall.

Anterior Epistaxis

- In anterior epistaxis, blood flows from anterior nasal opening (Table 21.2).
- It is more common than posterior nasal bleeding. The common sites are Little's area and anterior part of lateral nasal wall.
- It is usually mild and may be controlled by local pressure (pinching of nose) or anterior packing.
- It mostly affects children and young adults and the most common cause is trauma.

Posterior Epistaxis

- Posterior nasal bleeding is less common but more severe and occurs spontaneously. Most of the patients are more than 40 years of age. Bleeding is so severe that most patients require hospitalization and postnasal packing (Table 21.2).

Table 21.2: Differences between anterior and posterior epistaxis

	Anterior nasal bleeding	Posterior nasal bleeding
Incidence	More common	Less common
Common sites	Little's area	Posterosuperior part of nasal cavity
Localization	Easy	Difficult
Common age	Children and young people	Elderly people, more than 40 years
Common cause	Trauma (fingernail, frequent picking of nose)	Arteriosclerosis and hypertension
Nasal endoscope	Not required	Required
Severity	Mild bleeding	Profuse bleeding
Management	Comparatively easy and in OPD	Difficult and in operation theater
Anesthesia	Usually local	Usually general

- The blood can be seen in the pharynx. It is swallowed by the patient and then later on vomited out as a coffee colored vomitus. The latter may wrongly be considered as hematemesis.
- The bleeding site is difficult to localize. It is mostly in posterosuperior part of nasal cavity.
- The most common cause is hypertension and arteriosclerosis.

INVESTIGATIONS

Recurrent and profuse nosebleed cases need following investigations, which are ordered as per the suspected cause:
- *Complete blood count:* Anemia, leukemia and thrombocytopenia.
- Bleeding time, clotting time, prothrombin time, partial thromboplastin time.
- *Radiological:* X-ray chest, CT, MRI and angiography.

TREATMENT

The treatment includes general measures, nasal cautery, anterior and posterior nasal packing, arterial embolization, ligation and surgery.

A. General Measures

The following general measures are taken in cases of epistaxis:
- Home care (Box 21.3).
- Reassurance and mild sedation.

Box 21.3: Home care of epistaxis patients

Patients and their relatives are given following instructions if bleeding occurs at home:
- **Prevention**
  - Avoid frequent cleaning (obsessive-compulsive tendencies) of nose with tissue paper or finger.
  - Maintain proper nasal hydration with saline, gels and ointment.
  - Increase ambient humidity with a bedroom humidifier.
- **Treatment**
  - Pinch the nose with thumb and index finger for about 5 minutes. It usually stops the bleeding from the Little's area, which is the most common site of bleeding.
  - Place a small piece of cotton soaked in decongestant nasal drops.
  - Lean back no further than 45°.
  - In **Trotter's method**, patient sits and leans little forward over a basin to spit any blood. Patient breathes quietly from the mouth.
  - Cold compresses over the nose results in reflex vasoconstriction. Drops of ice-cold water directly in the nose.
  - Report to doctor if bleeding does not stop.

- *Position of the patient:* Sitting with a backrest.
- *Recording of blood loss:* Direct and through spitting and vomiting.
- *Monitoring of vital parameters:* Pulse, temperature, blood pressure and respiration, hemodynamic stability (blood transfusion if needed) and airway compromise.
- *Intermittent oxygen:* Bilateral nasal packing increases pulmonary resistance due to nasopulmonary reflex.
- *Antibiotics* in cases of infection and nasal packing.
- *Investigation and treatment of the cause.*

B. Nasal Cautery

Light anterior nasal packing should be done after cauterization.
- *Chemical cautery* with a bead of silver nitrate is helpful in cases of mild bleeding.
- *Electrocautery (monopolar, bipolar or suction cautery):* It is employed in cases of failure and severe bleeding.
  - *Topical anesthesia* with 4% xylocaine and then local infiltration with xylocaine adrenaline are used before cauterization.
  - *Endoscopic nasal cautery:* Posterior bleeding points are seen and cauterized better under endoscopic vision. With the help of suction cautery, the procedure may be done successfully under local anesthesia and sedation.
  - *Complication:* Avoid deep and bilateral cautery as it can cause septal perforation.

C. Anterior Nasal Packing (Fig. 21.7)

- *Indications:* Anterior nasal packing is done in cases of active anterior epistaxis. Cauterization of the bleeding

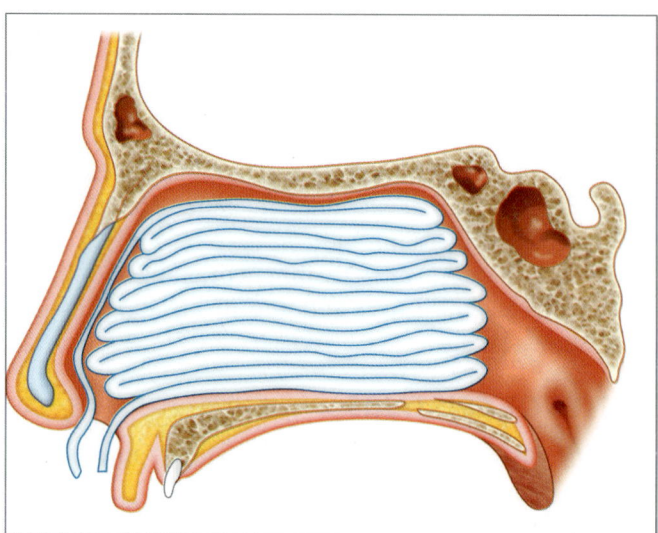

Fig. 21.7: Anterior nasal packing in horizontal layers with nonresorbable vaseline gauze strip

area is tried first. But if bleeding is profuse and the site of bleeding cannot be localized, anterior nasal packing is done.
- **Method:** Nose must be cleared of blood clots by suction and forceps. One meter long ribbon gauze (width 2.5 cm in adults and 12 mm in children), which is soaked in liquid paraffin, is packed tightly in each nasal cavity by layering the gauze from floor to the roof and from before backwards. The initial few centimeters of ribbon gauze are folded upon it and introduced along the floor. Some consultants prefer vertical layers of ribbon gauze from back to the front. If bleeding starts from another nose then posterior nasal bleeding must be suspected. Either one or both nasal cavities may be packed.
- **Removal:** Pack can be removed after 24 hours or after 2–3 days.
- **Packing materials:** In addition to ribbon gauze, other packing materials include Merocel Pope or Kennedy nasal sponges, prefashioned anterior nasal balloons, gelfoam, and oxidized cellulose (Surgicel).
- **Systemic antibiotics** are started to prevent infection and toxic shock syndrome.

D. Posterior Nasal Packing

Postnasal packing usually requires general anesthesia and patient needs hospitalization.
- **Indications:** Posterior nasal packing is done when cauterization fails and posterior bleeding site cannot be determined.
- **Methods:**
  - *Gauze:* A piece of gauze is rolled into the shape of a cone. Then three silk ties are tied to this cone-shaped gauze (Figs 21.8A and B). A rubber catheter is passed through the nose. Its pharyngeal end is brought out from the mouth and the silk threads of postnasal pack are tied to it. The catheter along with the silk threads is gradually withdrawn from nose and postnasal pack tied with silk threads is guided into the nasopharynx with the index finger. Anterior nasal cavity is now also packed. The silk threads are tied over a dental roll. The third silk thread, which is cut short, hangs in the oropharynx and helps in easy removal of the postnasal packing.
  - *Foley's catheter (Fig. 21.9):* Some ENT surgeons use Foley's catheter, the bulb of which is inflated with saline. The catheter is pulled out and choana is blocked by the inflated bulb. Then anterior nasal packing is done.
  - *Nasal balloon (Fig. 21.10):* The current variety of nasal balloon has two bulbs, one lies in postnasal space while another remains in nasal cavity.

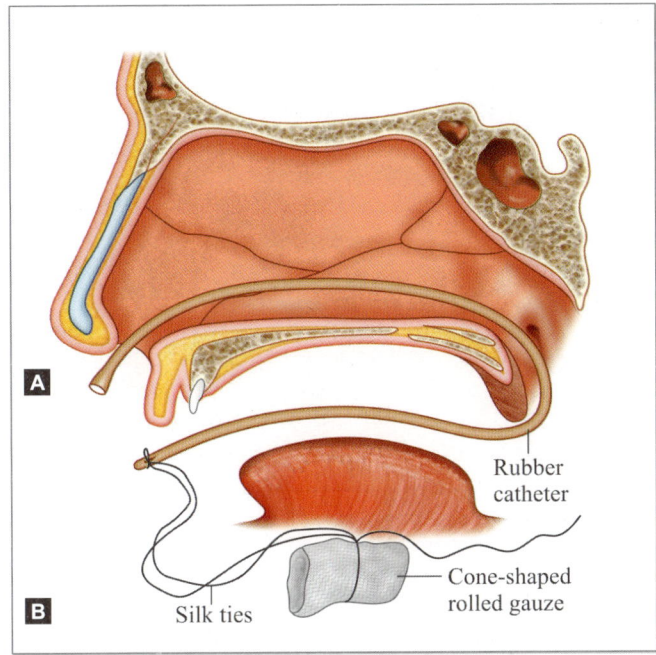

Figs 21.8A and B: Posterior nasal packing. (A) Procedure; (B) Postnasal pack

Posterior epistaxis: One to two percent of patients die within 1 year.

E. Arterial Embolization

Arterial embolization is done in refractory cases of epistaxis. It is an invasive process and performed in angiography suite by an experienced neuroradiologist.
- **Method:** First diagnostic angiography of bilateral carotid system is done. Then in ideal cases, catheter is

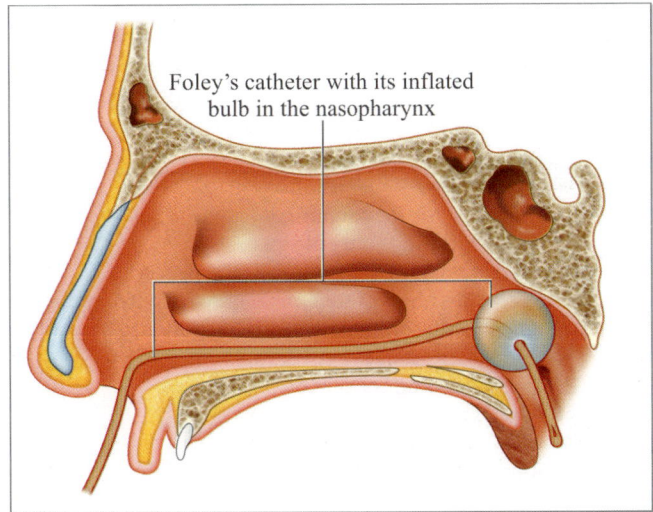

Fig. 21.9: Posterior nasal packing with Foley's catheter

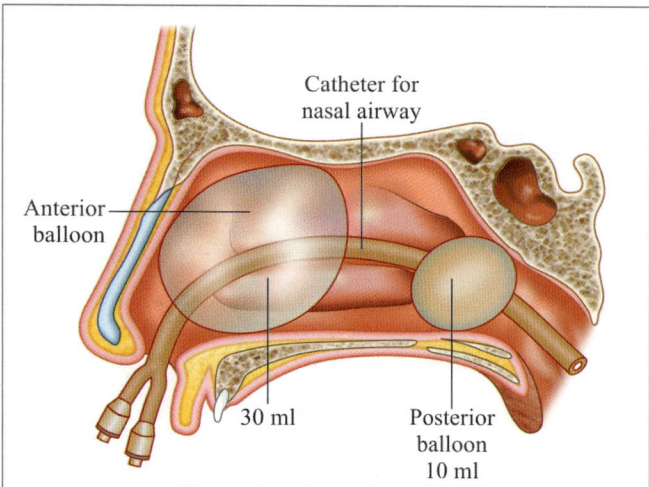

Fig. 21.10: Epistaxis balloon. Smaller (10 ml) posterior balloon and bigger (30 ml) anterior balloon are inflated. Channel of catheter provides airway for nasal breathing

guided into internal maxillary artery. Gelfoam and/or polyvinyl alcohol particles are used for embolization.
- *Contraindications:* It is contraindicated in cases of severe atherosclerotic disease, anomalous anastomosis and allergy to contrast.

F. Arterial Ligation

- *External carotid artery:* Ligation of external carotid artery above the origin of its first branch (superior thyroid artery) is done, when the area of profuse bleeding (supplied by external carotid system) is not controlled by packing and cauterization. The facilities of embolization and ligation of its more peripheral branches have obviated its need.
- *Maxillary artery:* The internal maxillary artery can be approached in various ways. It is ligated in cases of uncontrollable posterior epistaxis.
    - *Transantral:* In Caldwell-Luc approach, posterior wall of maxillary sinus is removed and clips are applied to the maxillary artery or its branches. In pterygopalatine fossa, the maxillary artery is usually anteroinferior to the maxillary and vidian nerves.
    - *Endoscopic ligation* of the maxillary artery can also be done through nose.
- *Ethmoidal arteries:* The bleeding area above the level of middle turbinate if not controlled by cautery and packing is managed by ligation of anterior and posterior ethmoidal arteries. They are exposed in the medial wall of the orbit. The foramina of anterior and posterior ethmoidal arteries are about 18 mm and 28 mm respectively away from anterior lacrimal fossa crest. They are situated in frontoethmoid suture. The external ethmoid incision is employed.
- *Endoscopic ligation of sphenopalatine artery (SPA):* It can be done under local anesthesia but some prefer general anesthesia. SPA is identified and ligated with a clip as it enters the nose through sphenopalatine foramen near the posterior end of middle turbinale. The mucosal flap is reflected in the posterior part of lateral nasal wall.

G. Surgical Treatment

- *Persistent nasal septal bleeding:* The elevation of mucoperichondrial flap from the nasal septum results in fibrosis and constriction of blood vessels. Submucous resection operation with removal of septal spur also achieves the same end result.
- *Hereditary hemorrhagic telangiectasia or Osler-Weber-Rendu Disease:* Hereditary hemorrhagic telangiectasia involves the anterior part of nasal septum and causes recurrent episodes of profuse bleeding.
    - *Laser:* Lesion can be managed by Argon, potassium titanyl phosphate (KTP) and neodymium-doped yttrium aluminium garnet (Nd: YAG) lasers. The recurrence, which is well known in the surrounding mucosa, needs repeated application of lasers.
    - *Septodermoplasty:* The anterior part of septal mucosa is excised and a split skin graft is used.

Self-evaluation Exercises

1. Which are not true for ammonia?
    a. Used for testing sense of smell
    b. Used in nose for testing reflex lacrimation
    c. Stimulates fibers of trigeminal nerve supplying the nasal mucosa
    d. Patient with complete anosmia responds to inhalation of ammonia
    e. None of the above
2. Kallmann syndrome consists of:
    a. Anosmia
    b. Congenital hypogonadism
    c. Amenorrhea in females
    d. All of the above

Contd...

Contd…

> 3. Arteries which participate in the formation of Kiesselbach's plexus include:
>   a. Anterior ethmoidal
>   b. Greater palatine
>   c. Superior labial
>   d. All of the above
>
> **True (T)/False (F)**
> 4. Transillumination test was commonly performed to diagnose maxillary and frontal sinusitis.
> 5. Little's area is the anteroinferior part of nasal septum and is the most common site of epistaxis. It constitutes about 10% cases of nosebleed.
> 6. Woodruff's plexus of veins is situated inferior to the posterior end of inferior turbinate and is a site of posterior epistaxis in adults.
> 7. Anterior and posterior ethmoidal arteries are the branches of ophthalmic artery, which is a branch of internal carotid artery.
>
> **Answers**
>
> | 1. a | 2. d | 3. d | 4. T | 5. F |
> |------|------|------|------|------|
> | 6. T | 7. T | | | |

Chapter 22

Diseases of External Nose and Vestibule

⊙ Specific Learning Objectives
After going through the chapter, you should be able to answer the following questions:
- Describe common infections of external nose and vestibule and their management.
- Describe common tumors of external nose and vestibule and their management.
- What do you know about: (1) Dermoid cyst of nose; (2) Rhinophyma; (3) Saddle nose deformity?

INFECTIONS

People usually rub their nasal vestibule and surrounding skin. Minor abrasions and hair follicles are common sites of both acute and chronic infections. Coagulase-positive staphylococci are the most common pathogens. Nose is free of pathogens in majority of normal people.

Cellulitis of Nose
- *Etiology:* The causative organisms are streptococci and staphylococci. The infection may be an extension from the nasal vestibule.
- *Clinical features:* A red, swollen and tender nose.
- *Treatment:* Systemic antibacterial, hot fomentation and analgesics.

Furuncle or Boil of Nose
- *Etiology:* Infection of hair follicle by *Staphylococcus aureus*.
- *Predisposing factors:* These are:
  - Picking of the nose
  - Plucking the nasal vibrissae
- *Clinical features:* A small, red, exquisitely painful and tender swelling, which spread to the tip and dorsum of nose and rupture spontaneously in the nasal vestibule (Fig. 22.1).
- *Treatment:* Medical treatment includes warm compresses, analgesic and topical and systemic antibiotics.
  - The incision and drainage is done if fluctuation appears.
  - Furuncle should not be squeezed or prematurely incised because infection can spread to cavernous sinus.

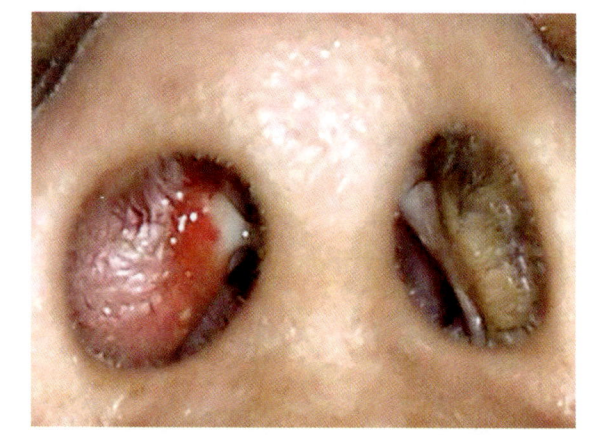

Fig. 22.1: Furuncle right nasal vestibule

- *Complications:*
  - Cellulitis of the upper lip
  - Septal abscess
  - Cavernous sinus thrombosis

Nasal Vestibulitis
- *Etiology:* This diffuse dermatitis is caused by *S. aureus*.
- *Predisposing factors:* They are:
  - Nasal discharge due to rhinosinusitis and allergy.
  - Frequent picking or wiping of nose with handkerchief.
- *Clinical features:* It has two types—acute and chronic.
  - *Acute:* Acute red, painful and tender swelling.
  - *Chronic:* Crusts, scales, painful fissure, erosion and excoriation (Fig. 22.2).
  - The infection may involve upper lip.

Chapter 22 • Diseases of External Nose and Vestibule

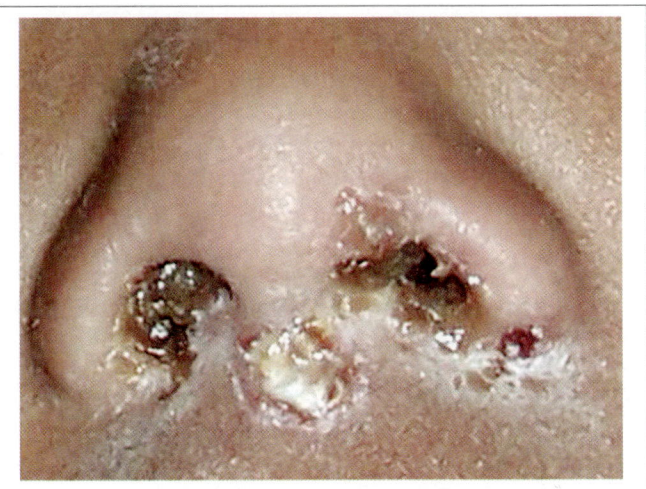

Fig. 22.2: Nasal vestibulitis

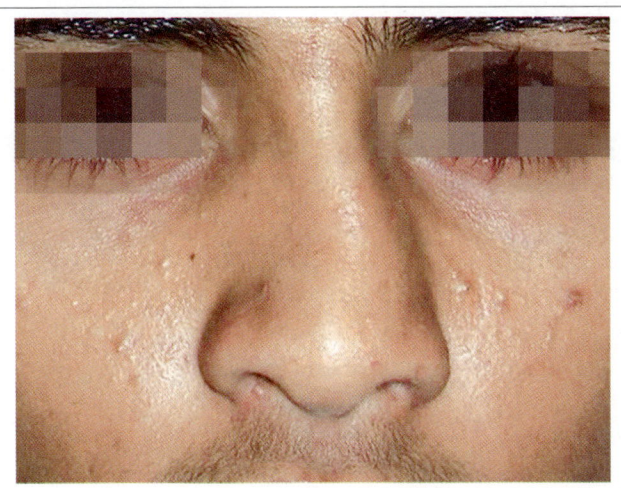

Fig. 22.3: Crooked nose 'S' shaped

- *Treatment:*
  - Treat the cause of nasal discharge.
  - Clean all the crusts and scales and apply antibiotic-steroid ointment. Treatment is continued for few days after the apparent cure to prevent likely relapse.
  - A chronic fissure is cauterized with silver nitrate.

DEFORMITIES OF EXTERNAL NOSE

The appearance of the external nose is frequently the subject of concern. These nasal deformities can be either congenital or acquired. The acquired defects are usually due to injuries. Plastic surgery (rhinoplasty) is required for the restoration of appearance. The most common deformity is the familial hump nose.

Hump Nose

- Hump may involve bone, cartilage or both.
- *Treatment:* Reduction rhinoplasty.

Saddle Nose Deformity (Depressed Nasal Dorsum)

It may be bony, cartilaginous or both.
- *Etiology:*
  - Depressed nasal fracture is the most common cause.
  - Excessive removal of septum in submucous resection.
  - Septal hematoma.
  - Septal abscess.
  - Granulomatous lesions of nose: Leprosy, tuberculosis and syphilis.
- *Treatment:* Augmentation rhinoplasty fills the dorsum of nose with cartilage, bone or a synthetic implant. Autografts are usually preferred over allografts. The chances of extrusion are more with synthetic implants, (silicone and teflon).

- In cases of cartilaginous depression, septal or auricle cartilage is laid in a single or multiple layers.
- In case of both cartilaginous and bony deformity, cancellous bone from the iliac crest is used as graft.

Crooked and Deviated Nose

In crooked nose, the dorsum of the nose (from frontonasal angle to the tip) is curved in either C or S-shaped (Fig. 22.3). In deviated nose, dorsum of the nose (from frontonasal angle to the tip) is deviated to one side.
- *Etiology:* Trauma is the most common cause. As the nose grows, injuries, which may be sustained during birth, neonatal period or childhood, can manifest into these deformities.
- *Treatment:* Rhinoplasty or septorhinoplasty corrects deformity and nasal obstruction.

Stenosis and Atresia of Nares

- *Etiology*
  - Web formation and stenosis may occur after trauma or surgery of nasal tip or vestibule. In Young's operation, which is done in atrophic rhinitis, nares are deliberately closed with vestibular skin flaps.
  - Destructive inflammatory lesions of nose.
  - Congenital atresia due to noncanalization of epithelial plug. It is rare.
- *Treatment:* Reconstructive plastic surgery.

TUMORS OF EXTERNAL NOSE

They can be divided into three categories—congenital, benign and malignant (Table 22.1). For intranasal tumors see Chapter 'Tumors of Nose, Paranasal Sinuses and Jaws'.

Table 22.1: Classification of swellings of external nose and vestibule. For the similar name intranasal tumors see Chapter 'Tumors of Nose, Paranasal Sinuses and Jaws'

Congenital	Benign	Malignant
Dermoid	Rhinophyma or potato tumor	Basal cell carcinoma (rodent ulcer)
Encephalocele or meningoencephalocele	Papilloma	
	Hemangioma	Squamous cell carcinoma (epithelioma)
Glioma	Pigmented nevus	
Nasoalveolar cyst	Seborrheic keratosis	Melanoma
	Neurofibroma	
	Tumors of sweat glands	

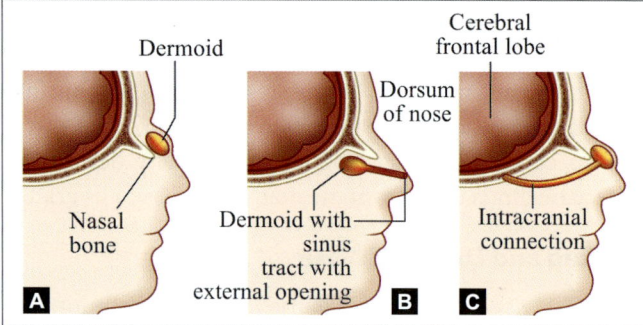

Figs 22.4A to C: Nasal dermoid. (A) Simple dermoid lies superficial to nasal bones; (B) Dermoid with sinus. Dermoid situated deep to nasal bones and sinus tract has an external pit in the midline of dorsum of nose; (C) Dermoid with intracranial connection

Dermoid Cyst of Nose

- **Types:** It is of two types (Figs 22.4A to C).
  - **Simple dermoid:** It presents as a midline swelling over the nasal bones and does not have any external opening.
  - **Dermoid cyst with sinus:**
    - **External pit:** Infants and children present with a pit or a sinus over the dorsum of nose. Hair may be protruding out from the sinus.
    - **Intracranial connection:** The sinus track communicate intracranially. Dermoid cyst lies between nasal bones and upper part of septum.
- **Treatment:** Surgery consists of splitting of the nasal bones and removal of cyst along with its extension in the upper part of the nasal septum. Intracranial extension needs associated neurosurgical approach.

Extranasal Encephalocele or Meningoencephalocele

Herniation of brain tissue with meninges occurs through a congenital bony defect, which may be intranasal or extranasal.

- **Clinical features:** An extranasal meningoencephalocele presents with pulsatile swelling. This cystic swelling is reducible and shows cough impulse. Swelling may be present in the following sites:
  - Root of nose (nasofrontal variety).
  - Side of nose (nasoethmoidal variety).
  - Anteromedial aspect of the orbit (naso-orbital variety).
- **Treatment:** It needs neurosurgery, which includes severing the stalk from the brain and repairing the bony defect.

Extranasal Glioma

Most of the gliomas, which are nipped off portions of encephalocele (during embryonic development), are extranasal (60%). Other types include intranasal (30%) and both intra and extranasal (10%).

- **Clinical feature:** Firm subcutaneous swellings may be seen on nasal bridge, side of nose or near the inner canthus.
- **Treatment:** Glioma is removed by external nasal approach.

Rhinophyma or Potato Tumor

This slow growing benign tumor occurs due to the hypertrophy of sebaceous glands in the region of nasal tip. Most of the patients are elderly male.

- **Clinical features:** It is usually seen in long-standing cases of acne rosacea.
  - Patient presents with pink and lobulated mass over the nose with superficial vascular dilation, which gives unsightly appearance to the face.
  - The big tumors can cause nasal obstruction and obstructed vision.
- **Treatment:** Paring down of the mass is done with knife or laser. The raw area is allowed to re-epithelialize. The complete excision of tumor is usually followed by skin grafting.

Basal Cell Carcinoma (Rodent Ulcer) of External Nose

This is the most common malignant tumor of external nose (87%). It equally affects either sex and occurs in the age of 40–60 years.

- **Clinical features:**
  - Common sites are tip and ala of nose (Fig. 21.2A).
  - This slow growing lesion may present as a cyst, pearly papule, nodule or an ulcer with rolled edges.
  - The lesion, which remains confined to the skin for a long time, may invade underlying cartilage or bone.
  - Lymph node metastasis is extremely rare.
- **Treatment:** The extent of surgery depends on the size, location and depth of the tumor.

- **Early lesion:** It may be treated with cryosurgery, irradiation or surgical excision. The latter includes 3–5 mm of normal skin around the tumor mass.
- **Recurrent and extensive lesions:** The wide resection of recurrent and extensive lesions involve cartilage and bone. The large surgical defect is closed by plastic surgery (local or distant flaps or a prosthesis).

Squamous Cell Carcinoma (Epithelioma) of External Nose

This is the second most common malignant tumor of external nose (11%). It equally affects either sexes and occurs in the age group of 40–60 years.

- **Clinical features:**
  - It presents as an infiltrating nodule and an ulcer with rolled out edges.
  - The common sites are lateral wall of the vestibule and columella. It may extend into nasal floor and upper lip.
  - Nodal metastases to the parotid and submandibular nodes are seen in 20% cases.
- **Treatment:**
  - **Early lesion:** It responds well to radiotherapy.
  - **Advanced lesions:** Advanced lesions, which involve bone or cartilage, need wide surgical excision and plastic repair of the defect.
  - **Metastatic cervical lymph nodes:** They require neck dissection.

Melanoma Nose

- **Clinical features:** This slow growing, rare lesion may present as superficially spreading type or nodular invasive type.
- **Treatment:** It is treated with surgical excision.

Self-evaluation Exercises

True (T)/False (F)
1. Nasal tip deformity is corrected by augmentation rhinoplasty.
2. Rhinophyma, hypertrophy of sweat glands of nasal tip is associated with acne rosacea.

Answers
1. T   2. F

Chapter 23

Infectious Rhinosinusitis

⊙ Specific Learning Objectives

After going through the chapter, you should be able to answer the following questions:
- How will you differentiate acute bacterial rhinosinusitis from acute viral rhinosinusitis and how would you manage them?
- What are the etiological and predisposing factors of chronic rhinosinusitis and how would you manage this condition?
- Enumerate the complications of rhinosinusitis and their alarming sign and symptoms.
- What do you know about the: (1) Mucocele of paranasal sinuses; (2) Samter's triad; (3) Pathophysiology of sinusitis?
- How will you differentiate the cavernous sinus thrombosis from orbital cellulitis and how would you manage them?
- Describe different types of nasal polypi, their differentiating features and management.

INTRODUCTION

Rhinosinusitis (RS) is an inflammation of the nose and paranasal air sinuses. Its common causes include viral, bacterial and allergic. RS in children is a multifactorial disease and the importance of predisposing factors changes with increasing age.

There is almost always involvement of nose in all the inflammatory sinus condition. Therefore, Task Force of the Rhinology and Paranasal Sinus Committee in 1997 suggested the term rhinosinusitis (RS), instead of sinusitis. Formerly, sinusitis and rhinitis were described separately.

CLASSIFICATION

The RS can be divided into different types on the basis of duration. Patients whose symptoms never disappear completely for more than 12 weeks are termed chronic rhinosinusitis (CRS). Patients who have complete recovery between the episodes of RS, which lasts for more than 7 days, are considered to have recurrent rhinosinusitis.
- Acute rhinosinusitis (< 4 weeks duration)
    - Viral rhinosinusitis (VRS)
    - Acute bacterial rhinosinusitis (ABRS)
- Subacute rhinosinusitis (4–12 weeks duration)
- Chronic rhinosinusitis (> 12 weeks duration)
    - With polyps
    - Without polyps
- Recurrent acute rhinosinusitis (3 episodes in 6 months or 4 or > 4 episodes of acute RS in 1 year).

Sinusitis

In the anatomical classification, the sinusitis can be maxillary, ethmoidal, frontal, sphenoidal, multisinusitis (involvement of >1 sinus), unilateral, bilateral and pansinusitis (involvement of all the sinuses). The commonly involved sinuses are maxillary and ethmoid. A sinusitis is termed open if pus can drain through its natural ostium while it is not possible in close type. The latter causes more severe symptoms and can cause complications.

Acute rhinosinusitis: It is primarily an infectious disease that can range from acute viral rhinosinusitis (the common cold) to acute bacterial rhinosinusitis.

VIRAL RHINOSINUSITIS (COMMON COLD)

The average attacks of viral rhinosinusitis (VRS) in a year in an adult can be two to four. Approximately 20–30% cases of acute rhinosinusitis are viral.

Etiology
- The common viruses are—rhinovirus (most common in adults) and parainfluenza viruses.
- Other viruses are adenovirus, picornavirus and its subgroups such as rhinovirus, coxsackie and echo viruses.
- Respiratory syncytial virus (RSV) and influenza virus are more destructive to respiratory cilia. These have

many serotypes, which vary in potency and severity of infection.
- The infection is usually contracted through airborne droplets.
- Incubation period is 1–4 days and illness lasts for 2–3 weeks.

Clinical Features

VRS and ABRS have many common clinical presentations.
- Usually VRS begins with sore throat, which lasts for 1 or 2 days and then followed by cough and nasal discharge.
- In beginning there may be burning sensation at the back of nose, nasal stuffiness, rhinorrhea and sneezing.
- Patient has chill and low-grade fever.
- Nasal watery discharge is profuse and may become mucopurulent due to secondary bacterial invasion (*Streptococcus haemolyticus, pneumococci, staphylococcus, Haemophilus influenzae, Klebsiella pneumoniae* and *Morexella catarrhalis*).

Treatment

There is no approved treatment. The following ancillary therapies though prescribed traditionally, have little supporting data.
- *Efficient in symptom control:* Decongestants, anticholinergics, and first generation antihistamines (diphenhydramine, chlorpheniramine, clemastine).
  - *Antihistamines:* Symptoms can be easily controlled with antihistaminics and nasal decongestants. Antihistamines may impair psychomotor performance often without sedation and other noticeable symptoms. Patients should not drive and operate heavy machinery. In elderly patients (> 65–70 years of age) they are avoided as the risks of delirium and cognitive decline are high. As the rhinorrhea is diminished due to anticholinergic property newer less sedating antihistamine are less effective.
  - *Oral decongestants:* They may cause insomnia and agitation. Use with caution in cases of hypertension, ischemic heart disease, glaucoma, prostatic hypertrophy, diabetes mellitus and geriatric patients. They are contraindicated in patients using MAO inhibitors or having uncontrolled hypertension or severe coronary artery disease.
  - *Ipratropium bromide nasal spray:* It reduces rhinorrhea.
  - *Topical decongestants:* Use is limited to 3 days.
- *Possible efficacy:* Zinc gluconate lozenges, vitamin C (2–3 g/day in divided doses), *Echinacea* extract and saline irrigation are helpful in some cases.
- *No significant benefit:* Guaifenesin, saline spray, steam, "nonsedating" antihistamines (loratidine, fexofenadine, cetrizine) are not of much help.
- *Analgesics:* Non-aspirin containing analgesics are preferred as aspirin causes increased shedding of viruses.
- *Others:* Chicken soup.
- *Antibiotics have no role in VRS.*
- *General:* Bed rest and plenty of fluids are encouraged.

Course

- The VRS resolves within 3 weeks in most of the adults regardless of bacterial colonization (*Streptococcus pneumoniae, M. catarrhalis* and *H. influenzae*), which are significantly more symptomatic.
- Less than 2% in adults and 30% in children, VRS progress to ABRS.

Complications

- Complications are occasional and include sinusitis, pharyngitis, tonsillitis, bronchitis, pneumonia and otitis media.
- In *influenzal rhinitis* (influenza viruses A, B or C) complications due to bacterial invasion are common.
- In *rhinitis associated with exanthemas* (measles, rubella, chickenpox) secondary infection and complications are more frequent and severe.

ACUTE BACTERIAL RHINOSINUSITIS (ABRS)

Distinguishing a VRS from ABRS though not easy is important. In ABRS, symptoms of VRS after several days suddenly start worsening instead of slowly improving.

Microbiology

- *Most common bacteria:* In adults as well as in children they are *S. pneumoniae, H. influenzae* and *M. catarrhalis*.
- *Other:* They include anaerobes, *Streptococcal* species and *Staphylococcus aureus*.
- *Anaerobic organisms and mixed infections:* They are seen in maxillary sinusitis of dental origin.

Predisposing Factors

They are following:
- Viral rhinosinusitis
- Allergic rhinosinusitis
- Trauma—maxillofacial injuries
- Physical stigmata such as deviated nasal septum (DNS)

- Swimming and diving: Infected water enters the sinuses through the ostia. High content of chlorine gas in swimming pools causes chemical inflammation.
- Barotraumas.
- Dental infections and extraction of upper molars and premolars. They involve maxillary sinus.
  - Periapical dental abscess may burst into the sinus.
  - The root of a tooth, during extraction, may be pushed into maxillary sinus.

All the etiologic factors mentioned in chronic rhinosinusitis (CRS) can also contribute in inciting ABRS.

Pathology

- Acute inflammation of mucosa leads to congestion and increased activity of serous and mucous glands. Exudation of fluid and outpouring of polymorphonuclear cells occur.
- The exudate, which is serous in beginning, becomes mucopurulent and causes destruction of mucosal lining. Failure of ostium to drain pus results in empyema of the sinus with destruction of its bony walls. Dental infections are very fulminating.
- The progress of disease depends on the:
  - Virulence of organisms
  - Defense system of the host
  - Structural features of osteomeatal complex

Clinical Features

Fewer than 5 in 1,000 colds are followed by ABRS. Symptoms of upper respiratory tract infection which last for more than 10 days or worsen after 5 to 7 days indicate ABRS.
- Predictors of ABRS
  - Best predictors of ABRS, which differentiate it from VRS, include:
    - Maxillary toothache
    - Poor response to decongestants
    - Colored/purulent nasal discharge
    - Abnormal transillumination
  - Other predictors include unilateral facial pain, pain with bending and mildly elevated ESR.
  - Findings having little predictive value include headache, difficulty in sleeping, sore throat, sneezing, malaise, itchy eyes, fever or sweats and painful chewing.
  - Severe symptoms include both high-grade fever and purulent nasal discharge for 3–4 consecutive days.
- Rhinorrhea may be thick, thin, clear or purulent.
- Cough may remain throughout the day and may be more at night.
- Headache usually comes up on waking, gradually increases and reaches its peak at about mid-day and then starts subsiding (office headache).
- Ethmoidal pain, which may be aggravated by movements of the eyeball, is localized over the bridge of the nose, medial and deep to the eye.
- Halitosis, periorbital edema and nasal congestion may be present.
- Additional adult features may be facial pain, headache and dental and gum pain (especially in maxillary sinus involvement). Pain may be aggravated by stooping, coughing or chewing.
- Nasal examination shows edema, hyperemia and purulent debris. The most specific feature is purulent exudates in middle meatus. Nonspecific features are facial tenderness on palpation over sinuses and the maxillary teeth.
- Postural test is done if no frank pus is seen in the middle meatus. *Method:* Middle meatus is decongested with a pledget of cotton soaked in topical decongestant. The patient is instructed to sit with the affected sinus turned up. Purulence in the middle meatus may be seen after 10–15 minutes.

Investigations

- ***Transillumination test:*** The affected sinus is found opaque. It is performed in a darkroom using a bright light. For more detail see Chapter 'Nasal Symptoms and Examination'. Frontal sinuses often develop asymmetrically. Interpretations:
  - ***Normal:*** Typical light transmission
  - ***Dull:*** Reduced light transmission
  - ***Opaque:*** No light transmission
- ***Nasal endoscopy examination:*** See Chapter 'Operations of Nose and Paranasal Sinuses'.
- ***CT imaging:*** Indications include refractory and recurrent cases of ABRS and in suspected cases of complications to determine extent of orbital, bony and CNS involvement. CT is done after the completion of antibiotic course. The findings may include obstruction of osteomeatal complex, polypoid changes and bony abnormalities.
  - Plain sinus X-ray (Fig. 23.1A) is now not recommended.
  - A limited sinus CT scan (coronal sections only) provides excellent imaging detail (Fig 23.1B). It cuts 50% of radiation exposure.
  - New low dose CT scanners have only 10–15% of radiation exposure.
  - Red flag findings are unilateral disease, sinus expansion and bony erosion.
  - Abnormal findings are sinus opacification, air-fluid level, marked mucosal thickening and polyps.
  - Findings not generally concerning are small retention cysts, concha bullosa, minimal mucosal thickening.
- ***Antral puncture:*** Aspiration of fluid from sinus is done for the identification of infecting organism. Gram's

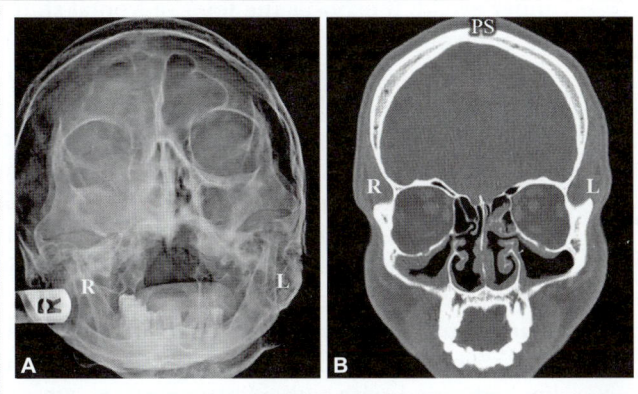

Figs 23.1: (A) X-ray paranasal sinus Water's view showing right side haziness in frontal, ethmoidal and maxillary sinuses (pansinusitis); (B) Plain CT scan paranasal sinuses coronal section. Mucosal thickening in left ethmoidal sinus. Circumferential mucosal thickening and polyp formation in bilateral maxillary sinuses

staining, culture and sensitivity are done especially in refractory cases and complications. The recovery of bacteria in a density of at least 104 colony-forming units/ml is considered significant.

Plain radiographs and ARBS: In the present era of CT the role of plain radiographs are debatable. Radiographs show presence of fluid or clouding of the sinuses (Fig. 23.1A). Completely opaque sinuses usually (about 85%) have pus in them, while 50% sinuses that show thickened mucous membrane with central aeration have pus in them.

Course

- The following causes are considered in patients who fail to respond to appropriate antibiotics. Tumors, granulomatous diseases, allergic rhinitis and invasive fungus (immunocompromised patients) and allergic fungal sinusitis. CT imaging and biopsy will confirm the diagnosis.
- Patients with recurrent ABRS are evaluated for predisposing factors, which include anatomical abnormalities especially of osteomeatal complex, immunodeficiency, allergies, irritants and cystic fibrosis. Recurrent ABRS cases need endoscopy and culture and sensitivity of the sinus/nasal fluid.

Differential Diagnosis

- *Mucocele and neoplasms of the sphenoid sinus:* They clinically mimic acute sphenoiditis. They should always be excluded in any case of isolated sphenoid sinus involvement though that is rare.
- *Diphtheritic rhinitis:* Diphtheria, which is rare these days, may be primary or secondary to faucial diphtheria. A grayish tenacious membrane, removal of which causes bleeding, covers the inferior turbinate and the floor of nose. Excoriation of anterior nares and upper lip are present in some cases. Treatment consists of isolation of the patient, systemic penicillin and diphtheria antitoxin.
- *Irritative rhinitis:* It is caused by exposure to dust, smoke, irritating gases (ammonia, formalin, acid fumes), foreign body and intranasal manipulation. Patient develops an immediate catarrhal reaction with sneezing, rhinorrhea and nasal congestion, which usually pass off rapidly with removal of the offending agents. The symptoms may persist if nasal epithelium has been damaged and the infection supervenes.

Treatment

The reasonable strategy for many patients is to treat symptomatically and recommend antibiotics only if symptoms do not begin to improve. The incidence of severe complications and progression from acute to chronic rhinosinusitis is extremely low. If the symptoms are severe or worsening and clinical suspicion of ABRS is high include antibiotics in the treatment regime.

- *Antibiotics:* They have not been shown to decrease the risk of complication or progression to CRS. Expensive antibiotics are unneccessarily prescribed when equally effective and less expensive alternatives are available.
  - *First line of antibiotics* in uncomplicated ABRS, are amoxicillin and trimethoprim-sulfamethoxazole for 10–14 days. The course may be extended to 3 weeks in cases of partial improvement.
    - Amoxicillin (40 mg/kg daily) 500 mg 8 hourly or 875 mg 12 hourly.
    - Trimethoprim-sulfamethoxazole 160 mg/800 mg 12 hourly.
  - *First line alternatives* (only for patients allergic to both first line antibiotics) are doxycycline and azithromycin.
    - Doxycycline hyclate 100 mg 12 hourly.
    - Azithromycin 500 mg daily for 3 days.
    - Cefuroxime axetil 250–500 mg 12 hourly.
    - Cefdinir 300 mg 12 hourly or 600 mg daily.
    - *Others:* Loracarbef, clarithromycin and cefprozil.
  - *Second line of antibiotics* in cases of first line failure (or severe symptoms, suspected complications and resistance). Combination of amoxicillin and clavulanate, cefpodoxime and cefuroxime (have activity against beta-lactamase-producing bacteria and resistant *S. pneumoniae*). In adults fluoroquinolones are also recommended.
    - Amoxicillin high dose 875–1,000 mg 8 hourly.
    - Amoxicillin/clavulanate potassium 875/125 to 2,000/125 12 hourly.

- Levofloxacin 500 mg daily (increased risks of tendon rupture in those over age 60, in kidney, heart and lung transplant patients and with use of simultaneous corticosteroid).
  - **Intravenous antibiotics** in cases of complications: For suspected penicillin-resistant pneumococci: Cefotaxime (50–75 mg/kg per day in 4 divided doses), with or without vancomycin (40 mg/kg/day in 4 divided doses). Then antibiotic based on the report of culture and sensitivity of aspirated fluid from sinus must be started. If needed surgical drainage must be considered.
  - **Metronidazole:** In cases of anaerobic organisms seen in sinusitis of dental origin.
- **Adjunctive therapy:** They are not well proved but do give symptomatic relief (see treatment of VRS) and include:
  - **Nasal steroid spray:** For recurrent acute RS or acute RS superimposed on CRS addition of following high dose nasal corticosteroids for 3 weeks may decrease duration of symptoms and improve rate of clinical success.
    - Flunisolide 25 mcg/spray—8 sprays (200 mcg) each nostril 12 hourly.
    - Mometasone furoate or Fluticasone 50 mcg/spray—4 sprays (200 mcg) each nostril 12 hourly.
  - **Oral and topical decongestant:** Nasal decongestant drops (1% ephedrine, 0.1% xylo-or oxymetazoline) not for > 5 days because of the potential for rebound congestion and development of rhinitis medicamentosa.
  - **Steam inhalation** alone or medicated with menthol or Tincture Benzoin Co. is done 15–20 minutes after nasal decongestion.
  - **Hot fomentation and analgesics.**
- **Surgery:** The surgery is reserved for patients with threatened intraorbital and intracranial complications. The reported success of endoscopic sinus surgery (ESS) is about 80–90%. It is indicated in following conditions:
  - **Persistent disease** despite medical therapy.
  - **Recurrent RS** with identifiable and related anatomical or acute pathological abnormalities in the osteomeatal complex.
  - **Empyemas**, which do not respond to antibiotics, need surgical drainage. ESS are successfully employed in managing empyema of paranasal sinuses. Following procedures may be considered if facilities of functional endoscopic sinus surgery (FESS) are not available.
    - *Antrum puncture in maxillary sinus empyema:* It is rarely required in the era of FESS. Details of antrum puncture and FESS can be seen in Chapter 'Operations of Nose and Paranasal Sinuses'.
    - *Trephining for empyema of frontal sinus:* It is done through an incision on the medial part of upper eyelid. It exposes the floor of frontal sinus, the bone of which is removed with a cutting drill. The pus is collected for culture and sensitivity and sinus is irrigated. A plastic catheter is inserted and fixed and sinus is irrigated with normal saline two or three times daily. The patency of frontonasal duct can be determined by adding a few drops of methylene blue to the irrigating fluid and its exit can be confirmed in the nose. Drainage tube is removed when frontonasal duct becomes patent.
    - *Empyema of ethmoid or sphenoid sinuses:* This also needs surgical drainage, which can be performed with either intranasal or external approach (sphenoethmoidectomy).

> *Antibiotic resistance patterns in ABRS:* Penicillin resistant *S. pneumoniae* (25–40%), beta lactamase producing *H. influenzae* (30–40%) and beta lactamase producing *M. catarrhalis* (92%).

CHRONIC RHINOSINUSITIS (CRS)

The noninfectious factors important in the pathogenesis of RS are patency of sinus ostia, nasal airflow, mucociliary activity, immunocompetence and the nature and quantity of secretions.

Bacterial Causes

The microbial pathogens present in CRS include *S. aureus*, coagulase-negative *Staphylococcus*, anaerobic and Gram-negative bacteria.

Etiologic and Predisposing Factors

Many CRS patients do not have bacterial cause but have hyperplastic mucosal disease such as nasal polyposis. There occurs hyperemia and edema of mucous membrane with hypertrophy of seromucinous glands and increase in goblet cells. Blood sinusoids especially over the turbinates are distended.

The underlying etiological and predisposing factors and associated conditions of CRS are following:
- **Infections:** Viral, bacterial, fungal and parasitic infections of neighboring organs such as pharynx (tonsils and adenoids) and upper teeth.
- **Traumatic:** Maxillofacial injuries, foreign bodies, surgery and nasal packing.
- **Hypersensitivity:** Allergy IgE mediated and non IgE mediated hypersensitivities, aspirin hypersensitivity with asthma and polyps and vasomotor factors.
- **Environmental:** Cold and wet climate and overcrowding.
- **Immunodeficiency:** Congenital and acquired (AIDS).

- ***Endocrinal:*** Diabetes, pregnancy and hypothyroidism.
- ***Mucociliary abnormalities:*** Cystic fibrosis and primary ciliary dysmotility.
- ***Mass:*** Neoplasms of nose, sinuses and nasopharynx (benign and malignant), retention cysts, antrochoanal and ethmoidal polyps.
- ***Autoimmune or idiopathic:*** Granulomatous (sarcoid and Wegener's), vasculitis (systemic lupus erythematosus (SLE) and Churg Straus Syndrome) and pemphigoid.
- ***Pollution:*** Chronic irritation from dust, smoke, cigarette smoking and snuff.
- ***Structural defects:*** DNS, synechia, choanal atresia and osteomeatal complex abnormalities.
- ***Lifestyle:*** Excessive intake of carbohydrates and lack of exercise.

Clinical Features

The following sign and symptoms may be divided into two types—major and minor. The presence of two or more major factors or one major factor and two minor factors (Table 23.1) or purulent nasal discharge make the diagnosis of CRS.

- ***Duration:*** Chronic rhinosinusitis is diagnosed if patients have symptoms for more than 12 weeks.
- ***Predisposing factors:*** The features of predisposing factors must be sought for.
- ***Nasal obstruction:*** It may worsen on lying and affects the dependent side of nose.
- ***Nasal discharge and post-nasal drip:*** It may be mucoid or mucopurulent, thick and viscid. Patient can have a constant desire to blow the nose and clear the throat.
- ***Headache:*** The swollen turbinates especially middle impinging on the nasal septum results in headache.
- ***Anterior rhinoscopy:*** It reveals dull red nasal mucosa and swollen turbinates, which pit on pressure and shrink with topical decongestants (compared from hypertrophied inferior turbinate).
- ***Sinuscopy:*** Nasal endoscopy may show allergic or cobble stoned mucosa (sarcoid), presence and location of purulent discharge and polyps.

Table 23.1: Major and minor factors in chronic rhinosinusitis

Major factors	Minor factors
• Facial pain/pressure	• Headache
• Facial congestion/fullness	• Fever
• Nasal obstruction/blockage	• Halitosis
• Nasal discharge/purulence	• Fatigue
• Discolored postnasal discharge	• Maxillary dental pain
• Hyposmia	• Cough
• Purulent nasal discharge	• Ear pain/pressure/fullness

Samter's triad (aspirin triad syndrome): Nasal polyps in adults are associated with asthma that is aspirin-sensitive.

Investigations

- ***Nasal endoscopy***
- ***Culture and sensitivity:*** Aspiration of purulent discharge near the ostium (not from nasal floor) under endoscopic guidance with a sinus secretion aspirator is done. For culture calginite swabs are good but discharge may not easily adhere to the swab.
- ***CT scan:*** It shows the extent of disease, complicating anatomy, asymmetry of skull base and orbital blowout fracture. CT scan is done before surgery and in cases of antibiotic failure. The presence of just only sinus mucosal abnormalities does not mean much and is not an indication for surgery as these findings may be incidental in asymptomatic patients also.
  - If CT scan suggests no inflammatory disease that means patient is not having RS. The alternative diagnoses include allergic rhinitis, atypical facial pain, migraine or tension headache, nasal drying, gastroesophageal reflux disease (GERD), atrophic rhinitis, temporomandibular joint (TMJ) and dental pain.
- ***Allergy evaluation:*** It is almost mandatory before the consideration of surgery as approximately 60% patients have evidence of allergy.

Differential Diagnoses

- ***Cystic fibrosis or primary ciliary dyskinesia:*** If the polyps are present in children then cystic fibrosis or primary ciliary dyskinesia syndrome must be ruled out.
- ***Fungal infection:*** In cases of very sticky, rubbery, yellow, tan or green mucus, special stains for fungus should be performed.
- ***Systemic diseases:*** In cases of failure of antibiotic and surgical treatment, systemic diseases (sarcoid, Wegener's granulomatosis) and mucosal and ciliary abnormalities should be considered.
- ***Gastroesophageal reflux disease:*** If the presenting complaint is postnasal discharge then patient must be evaluated for GERD.

Chronic hyperplastic rhinosinusitis: Eosinophilic infiltration is the hallmark in most of the patients and about 50% of patients have asthma.

- ***Hypertrophic rhinitis:*** It is discussed with hypertrophied turbinates in Chapter 'Nasal Septum Disorders'.

Medical Treatment

Treat the cause with particular attention to tonsils, adenoids, allergy, personal habits (smoking or alcohol indulgence), environment and work situation (smoky and dusty surroundings).

- Broad-spectrum antibiotics and steroids are usually started immediately and then changed as per the report of culture and sensitivity. A 28-day antibiotic course is used along with a nasal steroid spray (NSS). It may be combined with short course of tapering oral steroids, before the case is considered for surgery. The NSS is tapered and started again if symptoms recur.
    - Culture directed topical antibiotic:
        - Mupirocin, 5 g in 45 ml saline, as nasal irrigation in cases of *S. aureus*.
        - Gentamicin, 80 mg in 500 ml saline, as nasal irrigation, in cases of *Pseudomonas*.
- Saline nasal douching daily before NSS helps in some refractory cases. One to three tablespoons of saline (1–2 teaspoons of salt and 1 teaspoon of baking soda per 1 quart of water) should be used per sitting. This helps to keep the nose free from viscid secretions and also remove superficial infection.
- Allergy, if present must be managed.
    - Topical antihistamines
    - Anticholinergics (ipratropium)
    - Leukotriene modifier (montelukast, zafirlukast and zileuton) may be helpful in some cases.
    - In cases of associated allergic fungal sinusitis, desensitization and antifungal agents may be helpful.
- Nasal decongestants relieve nasal obstruction and improve sinus ventilation. Excessive and longtime use is avoided because it may lead to rhinitis medicamentosa and affect mucociliary clearance.

Surgical Treatment

- ***Endoscopic sinus surgery (ESS)***
    - In antibiotic failures when CT scan is positive, ESS is considered. Massive polyps are usually not cured with antibiotics and recurrence usually occurs after surgery. Long term NSS and oral steroids (especially perioperative) do prevent and delay recurrence after the removal. Noninclusion of sinus ostium, postoperative scarring and systemic diseases (sarcoid, Wegener's granulomatosis), mucosal and ciliary abnormalities can result in failure.
    - For ESS and other operations, *see* Chapter 'Operations of Nose and Paranasal Sinuses'. Following procedures may be considered if facilities for ESS are not available or fails.
- ***Maxillary sinus***
    - Antral puncture and irrigation.
    - Intranasal antrostomy is done if antral puncture and sinus irrigations fail. An inferior meatus antrostomy is made that provides aeration and free drainage to maxillary sinus.
    - Caldwell-Luc operation: The antrum is approached through the anterior wall with sublabial incision. After removing the irreversible diseases, another window is created between the antrum and inferior meatus (inferior meatus antrostomy).
- ***Frontal sinus***
    - Intranasal drainage procedures facilitate free drainage through the frontonasal duct and include correction of deviated septum, removal of polyps or anterior part of middle turbinate, intranasal ethmoidectomy and treatment of maxillary sinusitis.
    - Trephination of frontal sinus.
    - External frontoethmoidectomy (Howarth's or Lynch operation): The frontal sinus is approached through the floor. A curvilinear incision is made around the inner margin of the orbit. Diseased mucosa and ethmoid cells are removed and a new frontonasal duct is created.
    - Osteoplastic flap operation (unilateral or bilateral): Through a coronal or a brow incision, the anterior wall of frontal sinus is elevated as an osteoplastic flap, which is based inferiorly. The diseased mucosa and purulent material are removed and the sinus drained through a new frontonasal duct. In some cases it is desirable to obliterate the sinus after removing all diseased and normal mucosa of the sinus.
- ***Ethmoid sinuses***
    - ***Intranasal ethmoidectomy:*** It is done for ethmoid infection and polyps, which are removed between the middle turbinate and the medial wall of orbit (lamina papyracea). The frontal and sphenoid sinuses are also drained by this approach. ESS is better technique.
    - ***External ethmoidectomy:*** Ethmoid sinuses can be removed through medial orbital incision.
    - ***Frontosphenoethmoidectomy:*** This surgery also provides access to sphenoid and frontal sinuses.
- ***Sphenoid sinus:*** It is approached after removing its anterior wall. It can be done by external ethmoidectomy, trans-septal approach and ESS.

COMPLICATIONS OF RHINOSINUSITIS

The complications of sinusitis (Box 23.1) can broadly be divided into acute and chronic and local and distant. The acute local complications such as orbital, intracranial and bony are more common.

> **Box 23.1: Complications of rhinosinusitis**
>
> *Acute*
> - Orbital
>   - Inflammatory edema
>   - Orbital cellulitis
>   - Subperiosteal abscess
>   - Orbital abscess
>   - Cavernous sinus thrombosis
> - Intracranial
>   - Abscess: Extradural, subdural, cerebral
>   - Meningitis
>   - Encephalitis
>   - Cavernous and superior sagittal sinus thrombosis
> - Bony
>   - Osteitis and osteomyelitis (Pott's puffy tumor)
> - Dental
> - Toxic shock syndrome
>
> *Chronic*
> - Mucocele/pyocele
>
> *Associated diseases*
> - Otitis media
> - Adenotonsillitis
> - Bronchiectasis

> The alarming signs and symptoms for intracranial and intraorbital extension of rhinosinusitis include:
> - High fever
> - Severe pain
> - Worsening headache
> - Meningeal signs
> - Infraorbital hypesthesia
> - Altered mental status
> - Significant facial swelling
> - Diplopia
> - Ptosis
> - Chemosis
> - Proptosis
> - Abnormal pupillary or extraocular movements

MUCOCELE AND PYOCELE

Mucocele, the chronic cysts of sinuses are lined with pseudostratified or low-columnar epithelium containing few goblet cells. These round or oval cysts grow concentrically and expand very slowly over 10 years or more.

Pyocele is similar to mucocele but its contents are purulent. It can result from infection of a mucocele.

Etiology

The suggested etiologies are:
- Obstruction of sinus ostium.
- Obstruction of minor salivary gland duct present within the mucosal lining of sinuses.

Maxillary Mucocele

- It is an incidental finding on radiographs and rarely requires specific treatment.
- If needed, it can be aspirated through puncture of either inferior meatus or canine fossa.

Frontoethmoidal Mucocele

This is the ***most common*** type of mucocele.
- ***Clinical features:*** It presents with frontal headache, proptosis, deep nasal and periorbital pain and diplopia. The latter is caused due to inferior and lateral displacement of eyeball.
  - The swelling is cystic and non-tender; eggshell crackling may be elicited.
- ***Imaging:*** It shows clouding of sinus with sclerosis of surrounding skull and loss of scalloped outline of frontal sinus.
- ***Treatment:*** It requires surgical removal (fronto-ethmoidectomy) or endoscopic marsupialization into the nasal cavity.
  - Ethmoidal mucocele causes a bulge in the middle meatus of nose and can be drained by uncapping the ethmoidal bulge (or with external ethmoid operation) and establishing free drainage.

Sphenoethmoidal Mucocele

- ***Clinical features:*** They present with headache (occipital and vertex), deep nasal pain, diplopia, visual field disturbance and eyeball displacement.
  - ***Exophthalmos*** is always present and the pain is localized to the orbit and forehead.
  - ***Superior orbital fissure syndrome:*** There occurs involvement of CN III, IV, VI and ophthalmic division of CN V.
  - ***Orbital apex syndrome:*** Involvement of CN II, III, IV, V_1, V_2, VI.
- ***Imaging:*** Radiographic findings confirm the diagnosis. The slow expansion leads to destruction of sphenoid and posterior ethmoid sinuses.
- ***Treatment:*** It includes opening the mucocele widely into the nasal cavity.
  - ***Endoscopic sinus surgery:*** Anterior wall of the sphenoid sinus is removed, cyst wall uncapped and its fluid contents evacuated.
  - ***External:*** Ethmoidectomy with sphenoidotomy is performed.

ORBITAL COMPLICATIONS

Purulent frontal and ethmoidal sinusitis may result in orbital complications (Table 23.2). The infection can travel into the orbit through thin lamina papyracea and thrombophlebitis.

Clinical Features

- ***Inflammatory edema of eyelids:*** It is the first indication of orbital involvement and progresses to cellulitis, erythema, proptosis and fever (101°F).

Table 23.2: Chandler classification of orbital involvement

Inflammatory edema	Lid edema with normal visual acuity and extraocular movements
Orbital cellulitis	Diffuse edema of orbital contents but no discrete abscess formation
Subperiosteal abscess	Pus collection along lamina papyracea; inferior and lateral eyeball shift
Orbital abscess	Pus within orbit, proptosis, chemosis, ophthalmoplegia, dim vision
Cavernous sinus thrombosis	Bilateral involvement of eyes, toxic look and findings of meningismus

- *Orbital cellulitis:* Later on chemosis increases, ophthalmoplegia occurs and fundus shows mild vascular congestion (Table 23.2).
- *Subperiosteal abscess:* Fever may increase to 102°F–104°F and an abscess may form along medial wall of orbit and within periorbita.
- *Superior orbital fissure syndrome:* It presents with deep orbital pain, frontal headache and progressive paralysis of CN VI, III and IV.
- *Orbital apex syndrome:* It consists of features of superior orbital fissure syndrome and involvement of the optic nerve and maxillary division of the trigeminal.

Diagnosis

CT scan and ultrasound will confirm the abscess formation.

Treatment

- Orbital inflammation and cellulitis need sinus drainage and intravenous antibiotics.
- An abscess needs surgical drainage. The failure to drain the abscess can lead to permanent orbital sequelae and intracranial complications.

OSTEOMYELITIS AND OSTEITIS

Osteomyelitis is an infection of bone marrow while the osteitis means infection of the compact bone. Osteomyelitis can be of either the maxilla or the frontal bone.

Osteomyelitis of Maxilla

It is more common in infants and children than adults because of the spongy bone in the anterior wall of the maxilla. Infection usually starts in the dental sac and spreads to the maxilla. The primary infection of the maxillary sinus rarely causes osteomyelitis.

- *Clinical features:* They include erythema, swelling of cheek, edema of lower lid, purulent nasal discharge and fever. Subperiosteal abscess and fistulae form in infraorbital region, alveolus or palate, or in zygoma. Sequestration of bone can occur.
- *Treatment:* It includes large doses of antibiotics, drainage of abscess and removal of the sequestra.
- *Complications:* Damage to temporary and permanent tooth-buds, maldevelopment of maxilla, oroantral fistula, persistently draining sinus and epiphora.

Osteomyelitis Frontal Bone

It is more common in adults because frontal sinus is not developed in infants and children.

- *Etiology:* It usually results from acute infection of frontal sinus, which may be direct or through thrombophlebitis. Other causes are trauma and surgery.
- *Pott's puffy tumor:* A subperiosteal abscess develops over anterior surface of frontal sinus and results in the swelling of overlying soft tissue.
- *Extradural abscess:* Pus may form internally as an extradural abscess.
- *Treatment:* It consists of large doses of antibiotics, drainage of abscess and trephining of frontal sinus through its floor.
  - It may require removal of sequestra and necrotic bone with osteoplastic flap.

CAVERNOUS SINUS THROMBOSIS

The infection of paranasal sinuses especially ethmoid and sphenoid (less commonly the frontal) and orbit can cause thrombophlebitis of the cavernous sinuses (Fig. 23.2).

- *Clinical features:* The clinical features include bilateral orbital involvement, rapidly progressive chemosis and ophthalmoplegia, retinal congestion, high fever (105°F) and prostration (Table 23.3).
  - The condition progresses so rapidly that even immediate aggressive treatment usually cannot save vision and patient's life.
- *Diagnosis:* CT scan confirms the diagnosis.

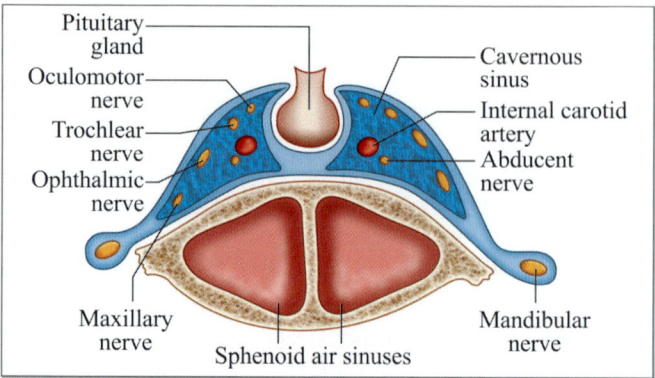

Fig. 23.2: Cavernous sinus relations and contents

Table 23.3: Differences between orbital cellulitis and cavernous sinus thrombosis

	Orbital cellulitis	Cavernous sinus thrombosis
Source	Commonly ethmoid sinuses	Nose, sinuses, orbit, ear and pharynx
Onset and progress	Slow	Abrupt
Cranial nerve involvement	Involved concurrently with complete ophthalmoplegia	Involved individually and progressively
Side	Usually involve affected side eye	Involves both eyes
Toxemia	Absent	Present
Fever	Present	High temperature with chills
Mortality	Less	Very high

- *Treatment:* It includes intravenous antibiotics, drainage of abscess and orbital decompression. Heparinization slows progression of thrombosis.

INTRACRANIAL COMPLICATIONS

Frontal, ethmoid and sphenoid sinuses form floor of the anterior cranial fossa and infection from these can cause following intracranial complications:
- Meningitis
- Encephalitis
- Extradural abscess
- Subdural abscess
- Brain abscess
- Cavernous sinus thrombosis.

The infection spreads either directly through the defect in posterior wall of frontal sinus or through diploic frontal vessels (subdural abscess).
- *Clinical features:* Thrombosis of dural vessels results in focal cerebral abscess, seizures and neurologic deficits.
  - Neck rigidity is an alarming sign in cases of sinusitis.
  - Other features of raised CSF pressure include headache, intractable vomiting and deterioration in consciousness.
- *Management:* It needs close collaboration with neurosurgeon. Treatment usually consists of intravenous antibiotics and proper drainage of involved sinus.

HYPERTROPHIED TURBINATES

See Chapter 'Nasal Septum Disorders'.

NASAL POLYPS

Nasal polyps are traditionally divided into antrochoanal polyp and bilateral ethmoidal polyps. They are non-neoplastic masses of edematous sinonasal mucosa.

Etiology

The exact etiology of nasal polyps is not well understood. They are usually manifestations of:
- *Rhinosinusitis:* Allergic, non-allergic and non-allergic rhinitis with eosinophilia (NARE) syndrome.
- *Cystic fibrosis:* Disorders of ciliary motility and abnormal composition of nasal mucus.
- *Allergic fungal sinusitis.*
- *Samter's triad:* It is the triad of nasal polyps, asthma and aspirin intolerance.
- *Kartagener's syndrome:* Bronchiectasis, sinusitis, situs inversus and ciliary dyskinesis.
- *Young's syndrome:* Sinopulmonary disease and azoospermia.
- *Churg-Strauss syndrome:* Asthma, fever, eosinophilia, vasculitis and granuloma.
- *Nasal mastocytosis:* Nasal mucosa is infiltrated with mast cells with few eosinophils. Skin tests for allergy and IgE levels are normal.
- *Neoplasms:* Simple nasal polyp may be associated with malignancy, which is common in people above 40 years and should be excluded by histological examination.

Pathology

- There occurs collection of extracellular fluid and edema of nasal mucosa (polypoidal change), especially of middle meatus and middle turbinate. The polyps are sessile in the beginning and later become pedunculated due to the effect of gravity and the excessive sneezing.
- The polyps are usually lined with ciliated columnar epithelium, which on exposure to atmospheric irritation may undergo metaplastic change to transitional and squamous type. Submucosa contains large intercellular spaces filled with eosinophils and round cells.

Clinical Features

- Nasal polyps can occur at any age.
- They usually present with nasal stuffiness/obstruction.
- Patients may have partial or total anosmia (loss of sense of smell) and headache.
- Paroxysmal sneezing, watery nasal discharge and itching indicate allergy.
- Nasal purulence indicates associated infective cause.
- Nasal polyps can be sessile or pedunculated, solitary or multiple, unilateral or bilateral.
  - Polyps usually appear as pale, smooth, glistening, grape-like masses.
  - They do not bleed on touch while infective or neoplastic lesions may bleed.
  - They are insensitive to probing. This feature differentiates solitary polyp from hypertrophy of the turbinate or cystic middle turbinate.
  - Big polyps, which protrude out from the nostril (Fig. 23.3A), appear pink and vascular (simulating neoplasm).

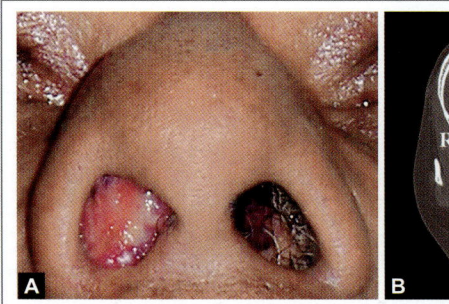
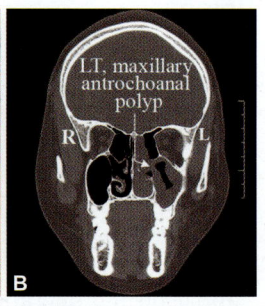

Figs 23.3A and B: (A) Big nasal polyp protruding out from right nostril; (B) Plain CT scan paranasal sinuses coronal section. A case of left antrochoanal polyp obliterating left nasal cavity and showing mucosal thickening in left maxillary sinus

- Their gradual progression may result in broadening of nose and increased intercanthal distance.

Staging

Polyps can be staged as following according to their size.
- *Stage I:* Limited to the extent of middle turbinate.
- *Stage II:* Extending beyond the limit of middle turbinate.
- *Stage III:* Approaching to inferior turbinate.
- *Stage IV:* Going up to the floor of nose.

Ethmoidal polyps (Table 23.4): Their common sites of origin are uncinate process, bulla ethmoidalis, ostia of sinuses and medial surface and edge of middle turbinate. Nasal polyps usually never arise from the septum or the floor of nose.

Antrochoanal Polyp

- *Origin:* It arises from the maxillary antrum near its accessory ostium and comes out and grows towards posterior choana and anterior nasal cavity (Table 23.4).
- *Parts:* It consists of three parts:
  1. *Antral:* A thin stalk.
  2. *Choanal:* Round and globular.
  3. *Nasal:* Flat from side to side.
- It is usually single and unilateral and is seen in children and young adults.
- Unilateral nasal obstruction may become bilateral, when polyp grows into the nasopharynx and obstructs both sides choanae.
- Voice becomes thick and dull (hyponasality).
- Mucoid nasal discharge may be unilateral or bilateral.
- A soft, smooth, grayish and mobile mass covered with nasal discharge may be seen through both anterior and posterior rhinoscopy.
- A large antrochoanal polyp may be seen hanging down in the oropharynx and/or protruding out from the nostril, which look pink and congested.

Table 23.4: Differences between antrochoanal and ethmoidal polyp

	Antrochoanal polyp	Ethmoidal polyps
Age	Common in children	Common in middle age
Etiology	Usually infection	Allergy or multifactorial
Number	Solitary	Multiple
Side	Unilateral	Bilateral
Origin	Maxillary sinus	Ethmoidal sinuses
Growth	Grows towards posterior choana	Grow towards anterior nares
Lobes	Two (dumbbell) or three (trilobed)	Multiple small and grape-like masses
Obstruction	Usually unilateral	Usually bilateral
History	Relatively short	Relatively long
Recurrence	Uncommon	Common
Treatment	Usually surgical	Usually medical

- If an antrochoanal polyp grows only posterior, it may be missed on anterior rhinoscopy.
- Table 23.4 shows the differences between antrochoanal and ethmoidal polyps.

Differential Diagnoses

- *Blob of mucus:* It may look like a polyp but disappears on blowing the nose.
- *Hypertrophied middle turbinate:* It is pink in color and hard like bone and can be easily differentiated from polyp with probe testing.
- *Angiofibroma:* It occurs exclusively in adolescent males and present with profuse recurrent episodes of epistaxis. If suspected, it should not be probed because that can cause brisk bleeding.
- *Malignancy:* They are fleshy pink in appearance, friable in nature and have tendency to bleed on touch. A red and fleshy, friable and granular mass presenting with epistaxis and orbital complications can be due to malignancy. Some time a polyp masquerade a malignancy, so all polyps are subjected to histology.
- *Pediatric masses:* Mucoviscidosis, gliomas and encephalocele. From encephalocele, on FNAC, CSF can be aspirated. It presents like a polyp.
- *Other causes of nasal obstructions:* The causes of unilateral and bilateral nasal obstructions are covered in detail in Chapter 'Nasal Symptoms and Examination'.

Polyps in children: Glioma, encephalocele, meningoencephalocele present as polyps in children. So the polyp in children must be aspirated before surgery and tested for CSF. Direct removal can lead to CSF leak and intracranial complications such as meningitis.

Investigations

- CT scan of paranasal sinuses (Fig. 23.3B) shows not only the extent and nature of lesion but also helps to plan surgery. They have replaced plain X-rays.
- X-ray of paranasal sinuses show opacity of the involved antrum.
- X-ray lateral view soft tissue nasopharynx shows globular swelling of antrochoanal polyp, which is differentiated from angiofibroma by the presence of a column of air behind the polyp.

Treatment

- *Medical:* Early polypoidal changes usually revert to normal with antihistaminics, control of allergy and infection and steroids (local and systemic).
    - Steroids also prevent recurrence after surgery. Contraindications for steroids include hypertension, peptic ulcer, diabetes, pregnancy and tuberculosis.
- *Surgical:* Currently almost all the polyps, which do not respond to medical treatment, are managed by ESS.
    - *Snare:* Solitary pedunculated polyp can be removed with snare.
        - Krause's nasal snare is used for removal of nasal polyps and partial turbinectomy. The polyp mass is engaged in the wire loop and avulsed.
    - *Intranasal ethmoidectomy:* Multiple ethmoidal polyps need uncapping of the ethmoidal air cells through intranasal route. It is best performed with functional endoscopic sinus surgery (FESS), which facilitates drainage and ventilation to the other involved sinuses such as maxillary, sphenoidal or frontal.
    - *External ethmoidectomy:* It is done through the medial wall of the orbit by an external incision, which lies medial to medial canthus. This external approach is considered in cases of recurrence, when surgical landmarks are distorted and ill-defined.
    - *Transantral ethmoidectomy (Caldwell-Luc approach):* It is indicated when maxillary antrum is also involved. The maxillary antrum is opened and the ethmoid air cells are exenterated through the medial wall of the antrum. This procedure can be avoided with the use of angled sinuscopes.
    - *An antrochoanal polyp* can be avulsed either through the nasal or oral route. Recurrence, which is uncommon after complete removal, may need Caldwell-Luc operation.

FUNGAL SINUSITIS

See Chapter 'Nasal Manifestation of Systemic Diseases'.

ATROPHIC RHINITIS (OZENA)

See Chapter 'Nasal Manifestation of Systemic Diseases'.

Self-evaluation Exercises

1. Which of the following are true for acute bacterial rhinosinusitis?
    a. Most common causative organisms include *Streptococcus pneumoniae* followed by *Haemophilus influenza*
    b. First line of antibiotic treatment is amoxicillin for 10 days
    c. The second line of antibiotic in refractory cases is amoxicillin with clavulanic acid
    d. All of the above
2. The cystic fibrosis does not include:
    a. Chronic sinusitis and multiple nasal polyps
    b. Recurrent chest infections
    c. Malabsorption syndrome
    d. Sweat chloride test confirms the diagnosis
    e. None of the above
3. Which of the following are not true for Kartagener's syndrome?
    a. Caused by deficiency of ATPase motor protein dynein
    b. Characterized by respiratory infections and sterility
    c. Immotile cilia syndrome
    d. Electron microscope shows absence of dye inside the arms in A-tubules
    e. None of the above
4. Clinical features of Kartagener's syndrome include:
    a. Recurrent/chronic sinusitis
    b. Bronchiectasis
    c. Sterility
    d. Situs inversus
    e. All of the above.
5. The cranial nerves which pass through the cavernous sinus are:
    a. III   b. IV
    c. VI   d. V (ophthalmic and maxillary divisions)
    e. All of the above
6. Which of the following is not the feature of cavernous sinus thrombophlebitis/infection?
    a. Unable to move eye in any direction (ophthalmoplegia)
    b. Ptosis and dilated pupil (loss of pupillary light reflex)
    c. Altered skin sensation over the maxilla and frontal bones
    d. Loss of corneal blink reflex
    e. None of the above
7. The clinical features of Sluder's neuralgia do not include:
    a. Rhinorrhea
    b. Increased lacrimation
    c. Nasal stuffiness
    d. None of the above

Contd...

Section 3 • Nose and Paranasal Sinuses

Contd...

8. Which of the following are not the features of antrochoanal polyp?
   a. Arises from maxillary sinus
   b. Grows anteriorly
   c. Often bilateral
   d. Treatment of choice functional endoscopic sinus surgery (FESS)
9. Which of the following are not the features of ethmoidal polyp?
   a. Usually bilateral
   b. Multiple in number
   c. Middle aged patients
   d. Arise from uncinate process and middle turbinate
   e. None of the above
10. Samter's triad consists of:
    a. Nasal polyps
    b. Bronchial asthma
    c. Aspirin sensitivity
    d. All of the above
11. The common causes of nasal polyps are:
    a. Aspirin intolerance
    b. Fungal sinusitis
    c. Chronic rhinosinusitis of allergic and nonallergic origin
    d. All of the above
12. The common causes of Rhinolalia clausa include:
    a. Allergic rhinitis
    b. Adenoids
    c. Nasal polyps
    d. All of the above
13. Syndromes with infertility and sinopulmonary disease include:
    a. Cystic fibrosis
    b. Kartagener's syndrome
    c. Young's syndrome
    d. All of the above

True (T)/False (F)

14. Caldwell-Luc operation is considered in cases of recurrence of antrochoanal polyp.
15. Topical steroid is the most effective medical treatment of nasal polyps. The next line of treatment is functional endoscopic sinus surgery.
16. Ethmoidal polyps are often associated with bronchial asthma and allergy is an etiological factor.
17. Common cold is most often caused by rhinovirus.
18. Anaerobic and mixed infections occur in sinusitis of dental origin.
19. The cavernous sinus is situated lateral to the body of sphenoid bone in the floor of anterior cranial fossa.
20. In cavernous sinus thrombophlebitis/infection, the abducent is the first cranial nerve to be affected resulting in medially deviated eyeball.
21. Pott's puffy tumor develops due to the pyogenic infection of frontal sinus (osteomyelitis).

Answers

1. d	2. e	3. e	4. e	5. e	6. e
7. d	8. b, c	9. e	10. d	11. d	12. d
13. d	14. T	15. T	16. T	17. T	18. T
19. F	20. T	21. T			

Chapter 24

Nasal Manifestation of Systemic Diseases

> **Specific Learning Objectives**
>
> After going through the chapter, you should be able to answer the following questions:
> - What are the differences between Wegener's granulomatosis and peripheral T-cell neoplasms and how will you manage them?
> - What are the etiological factors and clinical features of atrophic rhinitis and how will you manage such patient?
> - What are the etiological factors and clinical features of rhinoscleroma and how will you manage such patient?
> - What do you know about rhinosporidiosis?
> - Describe different types of fungal sinusitis and their diagnoses.

INTRODUCTION

Formerly several granulomatous lesions were called lethal midline granuloma. Various systemic diseases involving the nose, which are discussed in this Chapter, can be classified into four major groups—vasculitides, bacterial infection, fungal infections and lymphomas (Table 24.1).

These lesions are usually the manifestations of systemic diseases, which always have other systemic features that help in making the diagnosis. Biopsy from nasal lesions not only establishes the correct diagnosis but also excludes a neoplasm. Many of these diseases simulate neoplasms.

WEGENER'S GRANULOMATOSIS (WG)

In addition to respiratory tract, WG also involves kidneys and skin. It should be differentiated from peripheral T-Cell neoplasm (*see* Table 24.2) and in cases of large septal perforation from drug abuse (cocaine).

Table 24.1: Systemic diseases involving nose

Group	Diseases
Vasculitides	Wegener's granulomatosis, sarcoidosis and Churg-Strauss syndrome
Bacterial	Rhinoscleroma, syphilis, tuberculosis, lupus and leprosy
Fungal	Rhinosporidiosis, aspergillosis, mucormycosis, histoplasmosis and blastomycosis
Lymphoma	Peripheral T-cell neoplasm (non-healing midline granuloma)

Clinical Features

There are three main types of WG—Types 1, 2 and 3.
1. ***Type 1 limited form:*** Patient presents with clear, purulent or blood stained nasal discharge (chronic rhinosinusitis), which does not respond to medical treatment. Other nasal findings include severe pain over dorsum of nose, very large nasal crusts and granulations and later on septal perforation and saddle nose deformity (Figs 24.1A and B). The general symptoms of systemic vasculitis are weakness, malaise, fatigue, night sweats and migratory arthralgias.
2. ***Type 2 with pulmonary involvement:*** Cough, hemoptysis and single or multiple cavity lesions in X-ray chest.

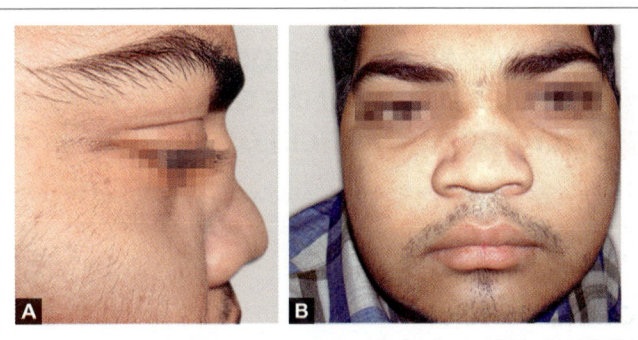

Figs 24.1A and B: Saddle nose deformity due to Wegener's granulomatosis. The puffiness of face is due to steroid therapy. (A) Lateral view; (B) Front view

3. ***Type 3 with wide dissemination:*** Involvement of multiple organs such as airway, lungs, renal and skin. Destruction can involve eyes, ear, orbit, palate, oral cavity or oropharynx.
    - ***Otological findings:*** Unilateral or bilateral serous otitis media and profound sensorineural hearing loss.
    - ***Oral cavity:*** Diffuse gingival lesions, minor salivary gland involvement and oral ulcers.
    - ***Subglottic involvement:*** In a case of very short segment of upper tracheal stenosis, WG should be ruled out.
    - ***Kidneys:*** Renal failure is usually the cause of death.

Diagnosis

- ***CBC:*** Anemia and raised ESR.
- ***Urine:*** Red cells, casts and albumin in urine and raised serum creatinine levels.
- ***X-ray chest:*** Single or multiple cavity lesions.
- ***Biopsy:*** It is diagnostic. WG shows necrosis and ulceration of mucosa, epithelioid granuloma and necrotizing vasculitis, which may involve small arteries and veins such as arterioles, capillaries and venules.
- ***Cytoplasmic antineutrophilic cytoplasmic antibody (c-ANCA):*** It is so specific for WG that it may preclude the need for biopsy such as in subglottic stenosis. But a negative c-ANCA does not rule out WG. The raised titer of c-ANCA is an ominous sign.

Treatment

- ***Immunosuppressive therapy:*** Oral cyclophosphamide (2 mg/kg/day for 6 months to 1 year and then after the disappearance of symptoms tapered gradually) and prednisone (1 mg/kg/day for 1 month and then gradually tapered following 2 months). In cases of relapse this standard protocol is started again.
- ***Trimethoprim-sulfamethoxazole (Bactrim/Septran):*** It cures the early limited type 1 WG. It may be continued indefinitely after the discontinuation of standard protocol because it may prevent relapse.

PERIPHERAL T-CELL NEOPLASM (NONHEALING MIDLINE GRANULOMA, POLYMORPHIC RETICULOSIS)

This destructive disease of the nose and midfacial region is differentiated from WG by the absence of pulmonary and renal involvement (Table 24.2).

Clinical Features

- Unilateral lesions in nose extending to soft tissue of nose, upper lip, oral cavity, maxillary sinus and orbit.
- Lesions are explosive and rapidly progressive.

Table 24.2: Comparison of Wegener's granulomatosis and peripheral T-cell neoplasms

	Wegener's granulomatosis	Peripheral T-cell neoplasm
Distribution of lesion	Focal and localized Bilateral	Diffuse Unilateral
Onset	Gradual	Explosive
Progress	Gradual	Rapid
Ear, tracheal, and renal	Involvement common	Involvement very uncommon
Histology	Vasculitis	Polymorphic lymphoid infiltrate
c-ANCA	Diagnostic	Negative
EBV-RNA	Absent	Detected
Immuno-histochemical study	No role	Diagnostic
Treatment	Immunosuppression	Radiotherapy

Abbreviations: c-ANCA, cytoplasmic antineutrophilic cytoplasmic antibody; EBV-RNA, Epstein-Barr virus-ribonucleic acid

- Secondary infection of lesions by gram-negative and anaerobic organisms.

Diagnosis

- ***Biopsy:*** It will show mixed population of cells (mature lymphocytes, plasma cells and large lymphoreticular cells), which resembles picture of lymphoma.
- ***Immunohistochemical studies:*** By using antibodies to leukocytes-common antigen CD45RB, B-cell lineage markers CD20, T-cell lineage markers CD3, CD43, CD45RO and natural killer marker CD57.
- ***EBV-RNA:*** Detected by *in situ* hybridization.

Treatment

- ***Localized lesion:*** Curative radiotherapy followed by surgical debridement and a nasal prosthesis.
- ***Multiorgan disease:*** Standard leukemia protocol.

ATROPHIC RHINITIS (OZENA)

This chronic inflammation of nose is characterized by the roomy nasal cavities and foul-smelling large crusts in posterior nasal cavity. There occurs atrophy of nasal mucosa and turbinate bones.

Atrophic rhinitis is of two types: primary and secondary. The primary atrophic rhinitis is more common and will be described in more detail.

Etiology

The exact cause of primary atrophic rhinitis is not known but various theories and predisposing factors, which have been proposed, are following:

- **Hereditary:** More than one family member can be affected.
- **Hormonal:** It usually starts at puberty. Females are affected more than males. Spontaneous regression of symptoms occurs after menopause.
- **Racial:** White and yellow races are more affected.
- **Dietary:** Deficiency of vitamin A, D or iron are seen. Patients are usually from low socioeconomic level.
- **Infective:** The various organisms cultured from nose are *Klebsiella ozaenae (Perez bacillus), diphtheroids, Proteus vulgaris, Escherichia coli, Staphylococci* and *Streptococci*. They are not considered primary causative organisms but are said to be secondary invaders, which are responsible for foul smell.
- **Autoimmune:** Some unspecified agents are said to trigger antigenicity of nasal mucosa that leads to production of antibodies which destroy nasal mucosa.

Pathology

The respiratory ciliated columnar epithelium of the nasal cavity is replaced by stratified squamous type. There occur atrophy of seromucinous glands, venous blood sinusoids and nerve elements. Obliterative endarteritis, which causes resorption of turbinates and widening of nasal chambers, can be seen in the mucosa, periosteum and bone. The disease persists for years and usually recovers spontaneously in middle age.

Clinical Features

- Patients are usually females around puberty. They emit foul smell from the nose, which make them social outcast. Patients themselves are not aware of this foul smell because of marked anosmia (merciful anosmia).
- Nasal obstruction due to large crusts filling the nose is present in spite of unduly wide nasal chambers.
- Epistaxis usually occurs when the crusts are removed.
- Greenish or grayish black color big dry crusts are seen.
- Roomy nasal cavities and atrophy of turbinates allow easy visibility of posterior wall of nasopharynx and ostium of sinuses.
- Nasal mucosa looks pale.
- Septal perforation and saddle nose deformity are not uncommon.
- Atrophic pharyngitis: Atrophic changes occur in the pharyngeal mucosa, which looks dry and glazed with crusts.
- Obstruction to Eustachian tube may result in middle ear effusion, which present with deafness.
- Atrophic laryngitis: Patient has cough and hoarseness of voice.
- X-ray of paranasal sinuses: Sinuses become small, underdeveloped and thick walled and appear opaque. The development of sinuses get arrested. Antral puncture becomes difficult due to thick sinus walls.

Treatment

Complete cure is not yet possible. Treatment consists of both medical and surgical management.

- **Medical:** It aims at maintaining nasal hygiene and removal of crusts to take care of putrefying smell and further crust formation.
  - **Warm normal saline or alkaline nasal irrigation:** It facilitates removal of crusts. One teaspoonful of alkaline powder (sodium bicarbonate 1 part, sodium biborate 1 part, and sodium chloride 2 parts) is dissolved in 280 ml of water. It is used for irrigating the nasal cavities 2 to 3 times a day. Later on just once every 2 to 3 days is sufficient. The alkaline solution loosens the crusts and removes thick tenacious discharge. Hard crusts need to be removed with forceps or suction.
  - **25% glucose in glycerin:** Application of this paint, after the removal of crusts, inhibits the growth of proteolytic organisms responsible for foul smelling.
  - **Antibiotics:** Spraying and painting of antibiotics may eliminate secondary infection.
    - Kemicetine antiozaena solution, which contains Chloromycetin, estradiol and vitamin D2, has been found useful.
    - Systemic use of streptomycin (effective against Klebsiella), 1 g/day for 10 days, has shown to reduce crusting and bad odor.
  - **Estradiol nasal spray:** It is said to increase vascularity of nasal mucosa and regenerate seromucinous glands.
  - **Placental extract:** The submucosal intranasal injection provides symptomatic relief.
  - **Potassium iodide:** This oral preparation has been shown to promote and liquefy nasal secretions.
- **Surgical**
  - **Young's operation:** In this plastic surgery both the nostrils are completely closed within the nasal vestibule with flaps. Nasal mucosa may revert to normal and crusting is reduced. The nostrils are opened again after about 6 months or later.
  - **Modified Young's operation:** The nostrils are partially closed that avoids the discomfort of nasal obstruction.
  - **Narrowing the nasal cavities:** Narrowing of the nasal airway helps in decreasing the crusting. The techniques include:
    - Submucosal intranasal injection of teflon paste.
    - Fat, cartilage and bone, etc. under the mucoperiostium of floor and lateral wall of nose and septum.
    - Medial displacement of lateral nasal wall.

Secondary Atrophic Rhinitis

- Syphilis, lupus, leprosy and rhinoscleroma cause atrophic changes and destruction of the nasal structures.

- The long-standing purulent rhinosinusitis, radiotherapy and excessive surgical removal of turbinates can result in atrophic rhinitis.
- Unilateral atrophic changes on the wider side nasal cavity are seen sometimes in cases of marked deviation of nasal septum.

RHINITIS SICCA

The respiratory ciliated columnar epithelium of anterior part of nose undergoes squamous metaplasia with atrophy of seromucinous glands.
- *Clinical features:* This crust-forming lesion of anterior third of nose (especially nasal septum) is seen in workers (bakers, iron and goldsmiths), who work in hot, dry and dusty surroundings.
  - The removal of crusts from the anterior part of septum causes ulceration, nosebleed and later on even septal perforation.
- *Treatment:* Patient is instructed to correct the occupational surroundings and use masks and filters. Following measures help immensely:
  - Application of bland or antibiotic-steroid ointments.
  - Avoidance of frequent nose pricking and removal of crusts.
  - Nasal saline douche.

RHINITIS CASEOSA

In this uncommon condition, granulomatous sinus mucosa destroys bony walls of sinus.
- *Clinical features:* It usually involves one side of nose and mostly affects males.
  - Examination reveals offensive purulent discharge and inspissated cheesy material, which is possibly the result of chronic rhinosinusitis.
  - This condition needs differentiation from malignancy.
- *Treatment:* It consists of removal of debris and granulation tissue, which restore free drainage of the affected sinus.
- *Prognosis:* It is usually good.

SARCOIDOSIS

This granulomatous disease resembles tuberculosis. There is absence of caseation. Although the cause is not known, sarcoidosis is associated with abnormalities of cell-mediated and humoral immunity.

Clinical Features

There occurs involvement of lungs, lymph nodes, skin, eyes (episcleritis), salivary glands (parotid swelling), oropharynx (tonsillar hypertrophy), larynx (epiglottic swelling and subglottic swelling) and neuropathy (sudden deafness and unilateral or bilateral facial nerve palsy).
- *External nose:* Raised papular lesions may coalesce and form bluish-red swellings. These firm and elastic lesions extend deeply and involve entire dermis.
- *Lupus pernio:* This nasal sarcoidosis presents with chronic violaceous cutaneous lesions over nose, cheeks, ears and fingers.
- *Nasal symptoms:* Nasal obstruction, pain and sometimes epistaxis.
- *Nasal findings:* Crusting and diffuse mucosal swelling involving septum, inferior turbinate, nasal vestibule and skin of face.

Diagnosis

In addition to the positive findings of X-ray chest and biopsy, it is necessary (before labeling the case as sarcoidosis) to exclude other causes of granulomatous lesions.

Treatment

Systemic and topical steroids.

RHINOSCLEROMA

Von Hebra coined the term rhinoscleroma in 1870. Rhinoscleroma is endemic in several parts of the world. In India, northern parts are affected more than the southern states. There is no age and sex bar.

Etiopathology

The causative microorganism, *Klebsiella rhinoscleromatis* (Frisch bacillus), is a Gram-negative bacillus. Mode of infection is not clear. The disease begins in the nose but extends to nasopharynx, oropharynx, larynx (mostly subglottic region), trachea and bronchi.

Clinical Features

There are four stages of this disease: catarrhal, atrophic, granulomatous and cicatricial.
1. *Catarrhal:* Foul smelling purulent nasal discharge for weeks to months.
2. *Atrophic stage:* This stage presents with crusting, which resembles atrophic rhinitis.
3. *Granulomatous stage:* Multiple granulomatous nodules, which enlarge and coalesce, are seen in nasal mucosa. Subdermal infiltration of lower part of external nose and upper lip gives "woody" feel. These painless nodules are non-ulcerative and can be found in pharynx, larynx, trachea and bronchi.
4. *Cicatricial stage:* Fibrosis leads to stenosis of nares, distortion of upper lip and adhesions in the nose, nasopharynx, oropharynx and larynx. The subglottic stenosis manifests as respiratory distress.

Diagnosis

- **Biopsy:** Submucosa is infiltrated with plasma cells, lymphocytes, eosinophils, Mikulicz cells and Russell bodies. ***The vacuolated Mikulicz cells (almost diagnostic) are large foamy histiocytes***. The central nucleus stains well with hematoxylin and eosin. Cytoplasm contains causative bacilli. Russell bodies are homogeneous eosinophilic inclusion bodies (accumulation of immunoglobulins secreted by the plasma cells). They are found in the plasma cells.
- **Culture of infected tissue:** The causative organisms are cultured and that is diagnostic.

Treatment

- **Antibiotics:** Both streptomycin (1 g/day) and tetracycline (2 g/day) for 4–6 weeks. Repeat if necessary after 1 month. Treatment is stopped when two consecutive cultures are negative.
- **Steroids:** They reduce fibrosis.
- **Surgery:** In fourth stage of fibrosis and stenosis, surgery is required to establish the airway and correct nasal deformity. A silastic stent facilitates re-epithelialization.
- **Radiotherapy:** It is not effective.

TUBERCULOSIS

- Tuberculosis of nose secondary to lung tuberculosis is more common than primary tuberculosis of nose.
- Anterior part of nasal septum and anterior end of inferior turbinate are the common sites of involvement.
- Nodular infiltration is usually followed by ulceration and perforation of cartilaginous part of nasal septum.
- **Diagnosis:** Biopsy and special staining of sections for acid-fast bacilli, culture of organisms confirm the diagnosis.
- **Treatment:** Antitubercular therapy.

LUPUS VULGARIS

This low-grade tuberculous infection affects nasal vestibule and the skin of nose and face.
- **Skin lesions:** Brown and gelatinous (apple-jelly) nodules.
- **Nasal vestibule:** Chronic vestibulitis and perforation in the cartilaginous part of nasal septum.
- **Diagnosis:** Biopsy confirms the diagnosis. It is difficult to isolate tubercle bacilli by culture and animal inoculation in lupus vulgaris.
- **Treatment:** Antitubercular therapy.

LEPROSY

Leprosy is common in the tropics and caused by *Mycobacterium leprae*. It is widely prevalent in India. The nose is involved more commonly in lepromatous type in comparison to tuberculoid or dimorphous forms of leprosy. Common sites of involvement are anterior part of nasal septum and anterior end of inferior turbinate.

Clinical Features

- It presents initially with excessive nasal discharge with red and swollen mucosa.
- Crusting and bleeding occurs later.
- Nodular lesions on the septum ulcerate and cause perforation of cartilaginous part of septum.
- **Late sequelae:** Atrophic rhinitis, depression of nasal bridge (saddle nose deformity), destruction of anterior nasal spine with retrusion of the columella.

Diagnosis

Scrapings of nasal mucosa and biopsy: Acid fast lepra bacilli are present in the foamy appearing histiocytes called lepra cells.

Treatment

- **Antibiotics:** Dapsone, rifampicin and isoniazid.
- **Reconstruction procedures:** They are performed when disease is inactive.

SYPHILIS

Syphilis is usually classified into two types: acquired and congenital (*see* Section 'Syphilis' of Chapter 'Sensorineural Hearing Loss').

Acquired Syphilis

It is further divided into three types—primary, secondary and tertiary.
1. **Primary:** Primary chancre of the vestibule is rare.
2. **Secondary:** Present in nose with simple rhinitis with crusting and fissuring in the nasal vestibule. The presence of mucous patches in the pharynx, skin rash, fever and generalized lymphadenitis suggest the diagnosis.
3. **Tertiary:** Nasal septum gumma destroys both bony and cartilaginous parts of nasal septum. Other findings include offensive nasal discharge with crusts, bony and cartilaginous sequestra, saddle nose deformity and perforation of the hard palate.

Congenital Syphilis

It has two forms—early and late.
1. **Early form:** (First 3 months of life), it manifests as "snuffles" and subsequently other findings appear such as purulent nasal discharge, fissuring and excoriations of nasal vestibule and skin of upper lip.

2. ***Late form:*** In puberty, clinical features of tertiary syphilis manifest such as gumma and perforation of nasal septum. Other stigmata of syphilis (corneal opacities, deafness and Hutchinson's teeth) are also present.

Complications

They include vestibular stenosis, perforations of nasal septum and hard palate, secondary atrophic rhinitis and saddle nose deformity.

Diagnosis

- ***Serological tests:*** VDRL
- ***Biopsy of the tissue:*** Special stains demonstrate *Trepenoma pallidum*.

Treatment

- ***Penicillin:*** Benzathine penicillin 2.4 million units IM every week for 3 weeks with a total dose of 7.2 million units.
  - Nasal alkaline wash
  - Removal of nasal crusts
- ***Surgery:*** Removal of bony and cartilaginous sequestra and correction of deformities are done when disease becomes inactive.

RHINOSPORIDIOSIS

This fungal granuloma is caused by *Rhinosporidium seeberi*. It is seen in southern states of India, Pakistan and Sri Lanka. This fungus is acquired through contaminated water of ponds frequented by animals. It usually involves nose, nasopharynx, lip, palate, conjunctiva, epiglottis, larynx, trachea, bronchi, skin, vulva and vagina. Yet it is not possible to culture the fungus and transfer the disease to experimental animals.

Lifecycle: The three stages of life cycle of *Rhinosporidium seeberi* are trophic stage (endopores increase in size and their nucleus and cytoplasm divides and form trophocyte filled with young endospores), development of sporangium (trophocyte and its endospores mature and form sporangium) and production of endospores (sporangium rupture and release endospores).

Clinical Features

- ***Symptoms:*** Blood-tinged nasal discharge, nasal stuffiness and frank epistaxis.
- ***Nose findings:*** A leafy, pink to purple color polypoidal mass attached to nasal septum or lateral wall may extend into the nasopharynx and hang behind the soft palate. The surface of the mass is studded with white dots (sporangia of fungus). The mass is very vascular and bleeds easily on touch.

Diagnosis

Biopsy: Sporangia, oval and round in shape are filled with spores which are bursting through its chitinous wall.

Treatment

- ***Surgery:*** Complete excision of the mass and cauterization of its base. Recurrence is not uncommon.
- ***Medical:*** No drugs are effective. Dapsone has shown some success.

FUNGAL SINUSITIS

- ***Types:*** Fungal rhinosinusitis has five distinct forms:
  - ***Invasive:***
    - Acute invasive fungal sinusitis
    - Chronic invasive fungal sinusitis
  - ***Noninvasive:***
    - Fungus balls
    - Saprophytic fungal infection
    - Allergic fungal rhinosinusitis
- ***Immunology:*** The evaluation of the immunologic status of the patient is very important because fungal sinusitis is related to host immunocompetency.
- ***Clinical features:*** The chronic symptoms in noninvasive fungus include facial pain, nasal obstruction, cacosmia, nasal polyps, proptosis and allergic mucin casts.

Acute Invasive Fungal Sinusitis

- ***Etiology:*** The most common fungi are aspergillus species and mucorales (mucormycosis).
  - ***Aspergillus:*** This species have narrow hyphae with regular septations and 45° branching.
  - ***Mucormycosis:*** It is more common in diabetics. Fungal elements are broad, ribbon-like (10–15 mm), irregular and rarely septated.
- ***Clinical features:*** The immunocompromised patients (diabetic, transplant, leukemia, and AIDS) are most at risk for invasive fungus. These cases need quick evaluation and aggressive management. Steroids administration may be one of the precipitating factors.
  - ***Acute clinical picture:*** It includes palatal erosion, impairment of vision, limitations in extraocular movements, fever, nasal and facial anesthesia and nasal necrosis.
  - ***Mucopurulence:*** It is variable depending on the neutropenia of the host.
- ***Investigations:*** The investigations are as follows:
  - ***CBC:*** Immunosuppressed patients may show neutropenia and evidence of left shift.
  - ***Coagulation profile:*** Platelets, bleeding time, prothrombin time and partial thromboplastin time.
  - ***Blood sugar:*** It is found raised in invasive fungus especially mucormycosis.

- **Culture:** An endoscopic aspirate culture is done with immediate fungal stains.
- **Biopsy:** If fungal stains are negative and suspicion is strong then biopsy with immediate frozen section and fungal stains are done. Coagulation abnormalities if any are corrected before biopsy.
- **CT scan:** A coronal CT scan is the minimum requirement of any fungal sinus surgery.
  - Axial scans provide additional information for the funguses of frontal and sphenoidal sinuses. Contrast studies are ordered if invasive fungus shows bony erosion, intracranial and orbital extension.
- **Treatment:** Attempts must be made to reverse the immunocompromised status by controlling its cause.
  - **Antifungal agents:** The systemic and topical antifungal agents appropriate for the cultured fungus must be started immediately.
  - **Conservative debridement:** Repeated conservative debridement (removal of necrotic tissue) may be needed in operative candidates, whose immunocompromised state can be reversed. Orbital exenteration should be avoided, when patient is not blind, even if there is involvement of the orbit. In cases of bone marrow transplant, when ingraft fails, immunocompromised state cannot be reversed and heroic surgeries are futile and must not be done.
    - *Intravenous amphotericin B* is usually started while awaiting fungal report.
    - *Ketoconazole and itraconazole:* If *Pseudallescheria boydii* grows on culture.
- **Prevention:** The use of high-efficiency particulate air filter systems and elimination of potted plants can reduce fungal infection in high-risk neutropenic patients.

Chronic Invasive Fungal Sinusitis

- **Causative fungi:** *A. flavus* (most common), *A. fumigatus*, *Alternaria*, *P. boydii*, *Sporothrix schenckii*.
- **Types:** There are two types of chronic indolent invasive fungal sinusitis and both progress over weeks to months to years.
  - **Granulomatous:** It infects immunocompetent patients.
  - **Nongranulomatous:** It occurs in immunocompromised patients.
- **Diagnosis:** Fungal culture and biopsy with special fungus stains confirm the diagnosis.
- **Treatment:** It consists of—
  - Repeated courses of antifungal therapy.
  - Surgical debridement.
  - Attempts to control the cause of immunocompromise.

Fungus Balls

- **Causative fungal species:** The fungi presenting with balls are *A. flavus*, *A. fumigatus*, *Alternaria* and *Mucor*.
- **Sites:** Maxillary sinus is most commonly involved followed in descending frequency by sphenoid, ethmoid and the frontal.
- **Clinical features:** This noninvasive fungus may remain asymptomatic for months to years but may become invasive if the patient becomes immunocompromised.
  - It may present with facial pain and cacosmia.
- **CT scan:** Fungus balls show total or partial sinus opacification (hyperdense area) and rarely bony erosion.
- **Diagnosis:** It is usually diagnosed at surgery and suspected on CT scans.
  - Culture may be negative but fungus can be seen with special stains.
- **Treatment:** Usually no antifungal therapy is required. The recurrence after surgical removal is uncommon.

Saprophytic Fungal Infection

- **Clinical:** The fungus grows on mucocrusts, seen after endoscopic sinus surgery (ESS).
- **Treatment:** It includes removal of crusts.
- **Prevention:** The patient is instructed to irrigate the nose weekly with sterile saline and wear a mask in moldy environments.

Allergic Fungal Rhinosinusitis (AFRS)

The manifestations of this noninvasive fungus occur because of a hypersensitivity response by the patient to the fungus. It responds to systemic steroids.

- **Etiology:** Dematiaceous (darkly pigmented) fungal species include *Alternaria*, *Bipolaris*, and *Curvularia*.
- **Clinical features:** Allergic fungal rhinosinusitis (AFRS) is found in cases of allergy, polyps and allergic mucin nasal casts.
- **Laboratory:**
  - Eosinophilia.
  - Total immunoglobulin IgE is raised along with fungus-specific IgE and IgG, which are difficult to evaluate as many fungi cause AFRS.
  - In quiescent AFRS, total IgE may be normal.
- **CT scan:** Imaging shows heterogeneity of tissue densities within the sinuses. Post contrast MRI shows fungal growth with changes of sinusitis (Fig. 24.2).
- **Histopathology:** Hyphae are seen in eosinophil-rich mucin without any evidence of tissue invasion. So the pathologist should assess the mucin not the polyp.
  - An allergic mucin contains necrotic inflammatory cells, eosinophils and Charcot-Leyden crystals (byproduct of eosinophil degranulation).
- **Treatment:** It includes surgery, steroids, immunotherapy and antifungal agents.

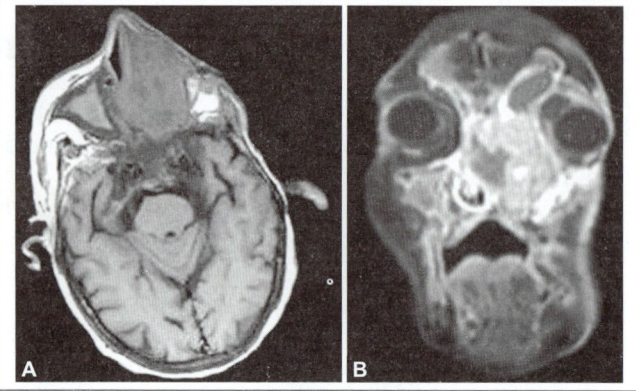

Figs 24.2A and B: Post-contrast coronal MRI showing fungal growth with changes of sinusitis. Moderate contrast enhancement in left nasal cavity mass

- **Surgery:** Surgical removal of all allergic mucin.
- **Steroids:** If it is difficult to remove allergic mucin completely, then remission is achieved with systemic steroids. In cases of recurrence, repeated surgical removal of mucin combined with perioperative steroids (prednisone 60 mg for several days and tapered off over 2 to 4 weeks) is beneficial.
- **Immunotherapy:** It contains fungal agents, started within 4–8 weeks of surgery, and prevents recurrence.
- **Oral antifungal agents:** Their role is controversial. A long course of oral itraconazole (400 mg daily for 1 month and tapered over 3 months) needs regular monitoring of liver functions. It has shown good results.

Self-evaluation exercises

1. Which of the following are not correct for rhinoscleroma?
   a. Gram-negative coccobacillus (*Klebsiella rhinoscleromatis*) infection
   b. Stages—catarrhal, granulomatous and cicatricial
   c. Woody infiltration of the upper lip
   d. Usually the patients are adults
   e. Nasal obstruction and crusting of nose
   f. None of the above
2. Which of the following are correct for rhinoscleroma?
   a. Broadening of nasal dorsum
   b. Involvement of subglottic region and trachea leads to airway obstruction
   c. Mikulicz' cells and Russell bodies are characteristic features seen on histology
   d. Drugs used include streptomycin, ciprofloxacin and tetracycline
   e. All of the above
3. The features of congenital syphilis include:
   a. Perforation of nasal septum
   b. Saddle nose deformity
   c. Snuffles in newborn
   d. Atrophic rhinitis
   e. All of the above
4. The acute fulminant fungal sinusitis is commonly seen in:
   a. Immunosuppressed patients
   b. Diabetes
   c. HIV
   d. Transplant and chemotherapy
   e. All of the above
5. Management of acute fulminant fungal sinusitis includes:
   a. Treatment of the incriminating factors
   b. Aggressive surgical debridement
   c. Amphotericin-B
   d. All of the above
6. Which of the following statements are true for the acute invasive fungal infection (mucormycosis) of nose and sinuses?
   a. Lateral nasal walls and turbinates involvement
   b. Quickly spreads to orbit, palate, face and cranium
   c. Fungal hyphae invade blood vessels and cause ischemic necrosis
   d. Treatment includes surgical debridement and amphotericin-B
   e. All of the above

Contd...

Contd...

True (T)/False (F)

7. Russell bodies are seen in plasma cells and contain rounded eosinophilic structures.
8. Syphilis involves nasal bones while tuberculosis affects nasal cartilage.
9. The fungal infection of nose rhinosporidiosis presents as nasal polyp.
10. Patients of atrophic rhinitis suffers more because they perceive offensive smell emanating from their own noses.
11. In patients of atrophic rhinitis degenerative changes in olfactory mucosa results in anosmia.
12. Alkaline nasal douche mixture contains sodium chloride (2 parts), sodium bicarbonate (1 part) and sodium borate (1 part).
13. Alkaline nasal douche is prepared in glucose water.
14. Noninvasive fungal sinusitis include fungal ball and fungal allergic sinusitis (presenting with polyps) and do not require antifungal treatment.
15. *Aspergillus* species is rare etiological agent in nose and paranasal sinus mycoses.

Answers

1. f	2. e	3. e	4. e	5. d	6. e
7. T	8. T	9. T	10. F	11. T	12. T
13. F	14. T	15. F			

Pearls and Nuggets (Refresh your knowledge)

- **Sluder's neuralgia:** This neuralgia of sphenopalatine ganglion presents with neuralgic pain in lower-half of face, nasal congestion, rhinorrhea and increased lacrimation.
- **Facial plastic surgery:** Good results depend on two factors: 1) Reasonable patient expectations and 2) proper surgical capability.
  - **Rhinoplasty:** The success depends mainly on the aesthetic liking of the patient.
  - **Blepharoplasty:** Preoperative basic ophthalmologic examination is must including visual acuity, visual fields and dry eyes.
  - **Rhytidectomy:** It can correct wrinkling in only the lower two-thirds of the face and the neckline.
- **Asthmatic bronchitis:** Asthmatic patients, frequently, have allergy to aspirin (acetylsalicylic acid).
- **Antibiotic resistance patterns in acute bacterial rhinosinusitis:** Penicillin resistant *S. pneumoniae* (25–40%), beta lactamase producing *H. influenzae* (30–40%) and beta lactamase producing *M. catarrhalis* (92%).
- **Chronic hyperplastic rhinosinusitis:** Eosinophilic infiltration is the hallmark in most of the patients and about 50% of patients have asthma.
- **Life-threatening injuries:** Most of them can be identified during the primary survey.
- **Cervical spine immobilization in trauma patients:** It is vital to maintain cervical spine immobilization while managing the airway.
- **Blood loss:** Young healthy patients can lose up to 30% of blood volume with minimal symptoms.
- **Intubation:** It is required if the patient has Glasgow Coma Scale/Score of 8 or less.
- **Facial trauma:** Thin cut (1–3 mm) facial CT with coronal reformatting is the ideal imaging study.
- **Mandibular fractures:** Open reduction and internal fixation (ORIF) with bone plates and lag screws is the most accepted treatment. It provides stable rigidity and early patient function.
- **Condylar fractures:** Severe fractures are problematic even with the open reduction and internal fixation.

Chapter 25

Allergic and Nonallergic (Vasomotor) Rhinitis

⊙ Specific Learning Objectives

After going through the chapter, you should be able to answer the following questions:
- What are the different types of allergic response in allergic rhinitis?
- What are the clinical features of allergic rhinitis (AR) and how will you evaluate these patients? What are the complications of AR?
- Which are the different treatment modalities of patients with allergic rhinitis? Describe their indications, merits and demerits.
- Describe different types of nonallergic rhinitis. What do you know about: (1) Rhinitis medicamentosa; (2) Vasomotor rhinitis; (3) Nonallergic rhinitis with eosinophilia (NARE)?

ALLERGIC RHINITIS (AR)

Definition: *A symptomatic disorder of nose induced by an IgE mediated inflammation after allergen exposure (ARIA).*

Rhinitis is the most common chronic disease of human beings. One in six people suffer from rhinitis. Allergic rhinitis (AR) constitutes more than 50% of all allergies in India, and its incidence is steadily increasing worldwide.

Surprisingly, it is more common in developed countries where the pollution is lesser in comparison to developing countries. Allergic rhinitis and asthma frequently coexist; in fact AR appears first in about 45% of patients.

The essential symptoms of this IgE-mediated atopic allergic disease are: nasal pruritus, congestion, rhinorrhea and paroxysms of sneezing. Demonstration of allergic hypersensitivity by in vivo or in vitro testing of specific-IgE antibody to aeroallergens is mandatory for confirming the diagnosis of AR.

PATHOGENESIS

IgE is produced by plasma cells which are regulated by T suppressor lymphocytes and T helper cells. In genetically predisposed persons, allergens produce specific IgE antibodies which are 'Y' shaped, and have Fc and Fab portions. Fc end of IgE becomes fixed to tissue mast cells and blood basophils. On subsequent exposure, allergen combines with Fab end of IgE antibodies which are already fixed to mast cells. Two such IgE antibodies, which bridge the allergen and mast cell, activate the mast cell. The disruption of mast cells leads to the release of chemical mediators which are of two types—preformed and newly synthesized (Table 25.1). Histamine, leukotrienes, prostaglandins and others stimulate H_1 receptors in the nasal mucosa and blood vessels, and produce rhinorrhea and mucosal edema. Itching and sneezing are produced by the stimulation of nerve endings.

Types of Allergic Response

There are two types of clinical allergic response—immediate and delayed. The clinical manifestations of early and late phases are overlapping in cases of recurrent and continuous exposure of allergens.

Table 25.1: Mediators released by sensitized mast cells and their effects

Name of mediator	Effects
Preformed	
Histamine	Vasodilatation and bronchospasm
Eosinophilic chemotactic factor for anaphylaxis	Attracts eosinophils
Neutrophil chemotactic factor	Attracts neutrophils
Heparin	Enhances phagocytosis
Newly formed	
Prostaglandins	Vasoactive and bronchospastic
Leukotriene	Vasoactive and bronchospastic
Platelets aggregating factor	Platelets released histamine and serotonin
Thromboxane A	Spasmogenic
Tumor necrosis factor	Attracts neutrophils and eosinophils

1. *Immediate (early phase):* It occurs within 5–30 minutes of exposure and leads to release of vasoactive amines, such as histamine, which clinically manifest as sneezing, discharge, blockage and bronchospasm. The stimulated mast cells secrete chemical mediators (histamine, prostaglandins and leukotrienes).
2. *Late (delayed phase):* The late phase, which occurs 2–8 hours after exposure, is due to infiltration of eosinophils, neutrophils, basophils, monocytes and CD4$^+$ T cells at the site of allergen deposition. This delayed phase clinically manifests as swelling, congestion and thick secretion, which subside slowly.

CLASSIFICATION

There are two clinical types of AR—seasonal (hay fever) and perennial. Patients of AR who have a decreased resistance to acute rhinitis, upper respiratory tract infection (URI), sinusitis and otitis media, may develop asthma.

- *Seasonal allergic rhinitis:* Hay fever and summer colds are common terms for seasonal AR which produce stuffy/runny nose, paroxysm of sneezing and itchy nose/eyes/throat and excess mucus in nose/throat. The condition may be a mere nuisance, or interferes with work and recreation. Pollens of common trees often cause early springtime hay fever while late springtime pollens come from the grasses.
  - *Hay fever:* It is a misnomer because neither it is caused by hay nor it produces fever.
  - *Summer cold:* It should not be confused with acute rhinitis (coryza); that is caused by virus and not by allergens.
  - *Rose fever:* It is also a misnomer because colorful or fragrant flowering plants rarely cause allergy, as their pollens are too heavy to be airborne.
- *Perennial allergic rhinitis:* Perennial rhinitis is caused by allergens that are present through all seasons, and they include animal dander (cats, dogs, horses and other pets, wool and feathers), cosmetics, molds, foods and house dust. Allergies that become worse in wintertime, when the hot air furnaces are turned on, are due to house dust. Molds spoil bread, rot fruit and mildew clothing. These fungi also grow on dead leaves, grass, hay, straw, grains and houseplants and in the soil. Mold spores may be in the outside air all year except in mountain area when snow covers the ground. Damp places, such as basements and laundry rooms, are ideal places for the fungal growths. Molds can also be found in cheeses and fermented alcoholic beverages.

Angioedema: Deficiency of C1 esterase inhibitor, an inherited condition causes angioedema. The increased production of C1 esterase leads to anaphylatoxins that causes capillary permeability and edema.

CLINICAL FEATURES

Diagnostic symptoms: They include:
- *Nasal pruritus:* Itching may also involve eyes, palate, and pharynx.
- *Paroxysms of sneezing:* Some patients have a 'tickling' sensation without sneezing while others are exhausted with sneezing.
- *Rhinorrhea:* This is a clear watery discharge, which may be extraordinarily profuse. A postnasal 'drip' may occur, though less often than in infective rhinitis.

Symptoms

- *Bilateral nasal stuffiness:* It is due to venous stasis of the inferior turbinates and mucosal edema. Obstruction from polyps tends to be constant. It occurs more commonly in vasomotor rhinitis than AR. Some patients complain of anosmia intermittently or continuously, even in the absence of obstruction.
- *Severity:* Symptoms vary in severity from day to day, or even from hour to hour. The severity of symptoms is more in seasonal AR in comparison to perennial AR.
- *Age:* Though there is no age and sex bar, AR usually affects school going children. A common sequence is eczema in infancy, then rhinitis followed by asthma. Nasal allergy is less common after 50 years of age.
- *Associated symptoms:* Allergic rhinitis may be associated with—
  - *Lower respiratory symptoms:* Cough, wheezing, chest tightness and dyspnea.
  - *Eye:* Eye irritation.
  - *Skin:* Pruritus and eczematous dermatitis.
- *Allergens:* The history must include a survey of allergen exposure associated with home, work, hobbies, and habits as well as medications.

Examination

- *Allergy salute:* The external nose examination may show a transverse nasal crease across the middle of nasal dorsum (Dennie-Morgan line), which occurs due to repeated upward rubbing of nose simulating a salute.
- *Inferior turbinate:* Examination reveals edematous and inflamed submucosa but in severe conditions, mucosa may look pale, boggy or blue-tinged due to vascular engorgement and venous congestion. Vascular dilatation and stasis lead to a purplish discoloration of inferior turbinates. Anterior and posterior ends of inferior turbinates may become much enlarged. There occurs intercellular transudation of tissue fluid (edema) due to damage to capillary endothelium and loosening of cellular cement.

- ***Thin watery discharge:*** It occurs from increased activity of the seromucinous glands.
- ***Polyps:*** They are pedunculated portions of edematous mucosa and may be single or multiple. They usually develop in the ethmoidal sinuses and from the middle turbinate or antral lining.
- ***Superadded infection:*** It is not uncommon. The mucosa becomes reddish in color and the secretions become more viscid (jelly-like) and purulent.

Complications/Associated Conditions

- ***Sinuses:*** The common findings are generalized thickening of the lining mucosa, development of polyps (single or multiple) and effusion into the sinuses. The fluid is sterile and clear, but may become thick and gum-like in some chronic cases.
- ***Eyes:*** Ocular features include edema of lids, congestion, cobblestone conjunctiva, and allergic shiners (dark circles under the eyes).
- ***Ears:*** Serous otitis media due to Eustachian tube block manifests with retracted tympanic membrane and fluctuating and conductive hearing loss.
- ***Pharynx:*** Hyperplasia of submucosal lymphoid tissue manifests as granular pharyngitis. Persistent AR in children can result in 'adenoid faces' and orthodontic problems.
- ***Larynx:*** Edema of vocal cords present with hoarseness of voice.
- ***Bronchial tree:*** AR patients have fourfold risk of developing bronchial asthma.

INVESTIGATIONS

- ***Complete blood count:*** The eosinophil count of the blood is raised, especially in the morning, and always in the presence of an extrinsic allergen.
- ***Nasal smear:*** Eosinophils may be found in great numbers in the nasal secretions and on microscopic examination of the nasal mucosa and polyps.
- ***Intranasal provocation test:*** It is a crude method, which is occasionally used these days. A drop of test solution can induce rhinorrhea, and sometimes lacrimation.
- ***Elimination tests:*** It can occasionally be helpful, especially in suspected food allergies.

Specific-IgE Antibody Tests

Allergy tests reveal an immune response to either one or more allergens. These positive test results must be correlated with the history before concluding the incriminating allergen(s). IgE antibodies are detected by *in vivo* (skin tests) or *in vitro* methods.

Skin Tests

Prick and intradermal skin tests generate a localized pruritic wheal (induration) and flare (erythema) which is maximal at 15–20 minutes. It is a very useful tool for the diagnosis of allergic respiratory disease (rhinitis and asthma). The negative and positive (histamine) controls are important for valid results and accurate interpretation.
- It is more sensitive, specific, and rapid than in vitro radioallergosorbent testing (RAST).
- *Precautions*
    - Antihistamines (H_1 antagonists, tricyclic antidepressants, phenothiazines) must be withdrawn prior to skin testing.
    - There is very small risk of inducing a systemic reaction in prick type of testing.
- The selected intradermal tests to suspected allergens can be performed.

In Vitro Tests of IgE Antibody

Allergen-specific IgE antibodies are detected in serum by ***radioallergosorbent test (RAST)*** or ***enzyme-linked immunosorbent assay (ELISA)***. A negative response of allergen-specific IgE is sufficient to rule out significant inhalant allergy.
- *Advantages*
    - No risk of a systemic reaction, and test results are not affected by antihistaminics.
    - Serial measurement of total IgE is useful in allergic fungal sinusitis.
- *Disadvantages*
    - In vitro tests are less sensitive than skin tests because they estimate circulating IgE. Atopic allergy is caused by IgE antibodies bound to mast cells. It can give false-positive results in patients with high total serum IgE levels.
    - The test results are not immediately available.

TREATMENT

The main treatment modalities of allergy rhinitis are avoidance of the allergen, pharmacotherapy, immunotherapy and local surgical interventions.

Avoidance Therapy

Though it may not reduce the underlying immunologic sensitivity, avoidance of allergen exposure cures the clinical manifestations. So if it is possible, then it should always be considered in addition to other modalities of treatment. Accurate diagnosis of the causative allergens is mandatory for the success of avoidance therapy.
- ***Pollens:*** Closing windows and remaining in air-conditioned environments can significantly decrease pollen exposure.

- **Animal dander:** The patient may benefit from keeping away from their pet animals.
- **House dust mites:** The mattress and pillows should be encased in dust-proof material. The bedroom should not have carpets, upholstered furniture and stuffed animals. Control the relative humidity (< 50%). The room should be cleaned frequently.
- **Mold spores:** Gardening and fanning should be avoided. Indoor mold spores can be avoided by repairing leaks and cleaning mold buildup in sinks, shower curtains and pipes.

Drug Therapy

Antihistamines

Though not in all the cases, antihistamine therapy is helpful in allergic rhinitis and in urticaria. Antihistamines rarely alleviate symptoms of asthma but they are not contraindicated in treating associated rhinitis or pruritus.
- *First-generation (chlorpheniramine, brompheniramine, diphenhydramine, clemastine, hydroxyzine):* Their use is limited due to sedation and dry mucous membranes, seizures and tachyarrhythmias.
- *Second-generation (loratidine, cetrizine, acrivastine):* They do not readily cross blood-brain barrier and are non-sedating H_1 receptor-blocking drugs.
- *Third-generation (fexofenadine, desloratadine, levocetrizine, tecastemizole):* Rupatadine is a new selective histamine H_1 receptor and platelet activating factor antagonist.
- *Topical (azelastine, levocabastine):* They are used intranasally and avoid the systemic side effects.

Sympathomimetic Drugs (Nasal Decongestants)

Alpha-adrenergic agonists (vasoconstricting) are used orally and topically as nasal decongestants.
- *Oral (pseudoephedrine and phenylephrine):* The common side effects of oral decongestants are insomnia, tremor and tachycardia. Though freely available and widely used in India, phenylpropanolamine (PPA) has been removed from USA market due to the reports of hemorrhagic strokes.
- *Topical (phenylephrine, naphazoline, oxymetazoline and xylometazoline):* Daily use of topical nasal decongestants can lead to rhinitis medicamentosa due to the rapid development of rebound vasodilation.

Corticosteroids

- *Systemic:* Short-term systemic burst therapy is indicated for treatment of severe AR. While using steroids, due attention must be paid to their side effects and toxicity, such as hypothalamic-pituitary-adrenal suppression.
- *Topical (steroid nasal spray):* Long-term topical corticosteroid (flunisolide, beclomethasone, mometasone, budesonide, fluticasone and triamcinolone) nasal therapy is an effective, comparatively safe and an essential aspect of management of the inflammatory phase of the AR.
  - Their potential side effects are epistaxis, nasal irritation, crusting and nasal septal perforation and potential risk of growth inhibition in children. It is desirable to break their use for 1–2 weeks every 2–3 months.
  - All commercially available steroids' nasal sprays are more or less similar in their efficacy, often requiring only a single daily dose after an initial period of therapy with four doses daily for 1 week.

Mast Cell Stabilizers (Cromolyn and Nedocromil)

These drugs help in prophylaxis and prevent the response to allergen by stabilizing the mast cell.

Sodium chromoglycate, 2% solution, is available as nasal drops and spray and as an aerosol powder.

Anticholinergic Agents (Nasal Topical Ipratropium Bromide)

Ipratropium is preferred as adjunctive treatment of allergic as well as nonallergic rhinitis because it does not cause rhinitis medicamentosa. Though ipratropium does not alleviate sneezing, pruritus, or nasal congestion, it is useful for treatment of postnasal drip and rhinorrhea.

Leukotriene Modifiers

They (zileuton, zafirlukast, montelukast) act by inhibiting formation of leukotrienes or blocking their effect. Combination therapy (montelukast 10 mg and levocetrizine 5 mg) is reported to be a more effective strategy than monotherapy, in cases of moderate-to-severe symptoms of persistent AR.

Anti-IgE Antibody Therapy

Studies have shown omalizumab efficacy in allergic rhinitis but the use is limited due to its high cost and parenteral administration.

Immunotherapy

Treatment of AR by the repeated long-term injection of allergen has been shown to be an effective method for reducing or eliminating clinical manifestations.
- *Indications:* The best candidates for immunotherapy are the cases of severe allergic rhinitis who respond poorly to drug and avoidance therapy, or when allergens are unavoidable.
- *Immunologic effects:* Immunotherapy produces IgG blocking antibody.
- *Clinical effects:* While on immunotherapy, there is significant decrease in symptoms and medication usage.

Some patients become completely asymptomatic. The beneficial effect may persist even after the cessation of treatment.

Procedure

A sterile aqueous solution of incriminating allergen(s) is administered by subcutaneous injection in gradually increasing doses once or twice a week until a maintenance dose is reached. Then the interval is increased to every 4 weeks. The maintenance dose is usually 1–10,000 times the starting dose. Gradually increasing doses minimize the risk of systemic allergic reactions during immunotherapy. Three to five years is the usual course of therapy. *Now sublingual and nasal routes of administrations are also available but the doses are 20-100 times more than the subcutaneous injections.*

> **Surgical treatment of allergic rhinitis:** In some of the refractory and selective cases following surgical procedures may be considered—radiofrequency ablation, laser ablation or surgical removal of the inferior turbinate.

Step Care Approach of Allergic Rhinitis and Its Impact on Asthma (ARIA)

ARIA classification and guidelines are given in Fig 25.1 and Table 25.2.

NONALLERGIC RHINITIS (VASOMOTOR RHINITIS)

Approximately, 10% of the population suffers from chronic or recurrent nasal symptoms. The prevalence of nonallergic rhinitis (NAR) in otolaryngology practice is high (about 40%). In many cases, it is difficult to differentiate NAR from AR. AR is more common than NAR. Quite commonly, patients have mixed features of both NAR and AR. Both conditions have similar presentations, manifestations,

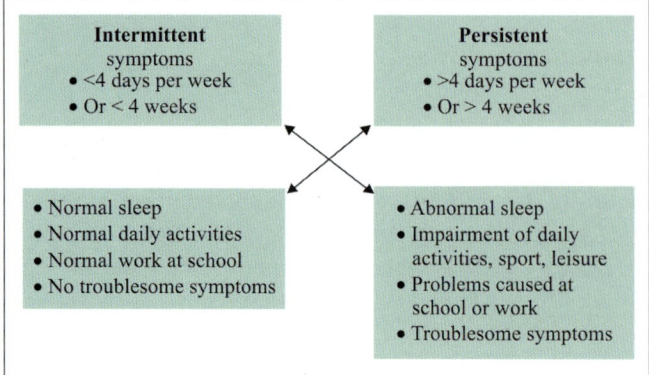

Fig. 25.1: Classification of allergic rhinitis ARIA (Allergic rhinitis and its impact on asthma)

Table 25.2: Step care approach of allergic rhinitis and its impact on asthma (ARIA)

Symptoms and disease	Recommendations
Mild intermittent disease	Oral antihistamines or intranasal cromolyn sodium
Moderate severity or persistent disease	Intranasal corticosteroids
Severe symptoms	Oral nonsedating antihistamines and intranasal corticosteroids
Severe and persistent symptoms	A short course of oral steroids and immunotherapy
Persistent nasal obstruction	Short course of intranasal decongestant or oral decongestant and antihistamines
General instructions to all patients	Avoid allergens, irritants and nonspecific stimuli

and treatment. Nonallergic rhinitis presents with all the symptoms of AR (such as rhinorrhea, congestion and sneezing) but these patients have negative allergic history, skin testing and nasal cytology. Nasal itching and paroxysmal sneezing are usually lesser with NAR in comparison to AR. Other common terms used for NAR are vasomotor rhinitis and perennial rhinitis.

PATHOPHYSIOLOGY

The rich blood supply of nasal mucosa is similar to the erectile tissues that have venous sinusoids or 'lakes' surrounded by smooth muscle fibers. These smooth muscle fibers act as sphincters and control the filling and emptying of sinusoids. Sympathetic stimulation causes vasoconstriction and decongestion of nose, while parasympathetic stimulation causes not only excessive secretion from the nasal glands (rhinorrhea) but also vasodilation and engorgement (congestion of nose).

Autonomic nervous system, which supplies the nasal mucosa, is under the control of hypothalamus and emotions play a significant role in NAR. Autonomic nervous system is not stable in cases of NAR. Nasal mucosa becomes hyperreactive and responds unduly to change in temperature, humidity, blasts of air, dust or smoke.

TYPES OF NONALLERGIC RHINITIS (NAR)

The symptoms of NAR include rhinorrhea, congestion and sneezing. Some of these conditions have been given specific terms, which are categorized under the NAR (vasomotor rhinitis).

Nonallergic Rhinitis with Eosinophilia (NARE)

Patients have perennial symptoms with episodes of watery discharge, itching, sneezing and epiphora. They have negative and irrelevant reports by skin and *in vitro* allergy testing. The specific allergy triggers are absent, but aggravating factors usually include weather changes and exposure to chemical irritants. Nasal smear shows marked eosinophilia.

Drug-Induced Rhinitis

- Several anti-hypertensive drugs, such as beta-blockers, alpha-blockers, angiotensin-converting enzyme (ACE) inhibitors and vasodilators can result in nasal congestion and stuffiness.
- The anticholinesterase drug (neostigmine) used in myasthenia gravis have acetylcholine like action, which lead to nasal stuffiness.
- Aspirin and NSAID are well known to cause sinusitis and asthma.
- Contraceptive pills (estrogen) can cause nasal obstruction.

Rhinitis Medicamentosa

The long-term use of cocaine and topical nasal decongestants causes rebound congestion and leads to rhinitis medicamentosa.

Treatment: It consists of withdrawal of topical decongestant, oral and/or topical steroid therapy, and surgical reduction of hypertrophied turbinates are usually effective.

Honeymoon Rhinitis

Too much sexual activity can lead to nasal congestion and rhinorrhea.

Emotional Rhinitis

Nose mucosa may react to several emotional conditions, such as anxiety, tension, hostility, humiliation, resentment and grief.

Treatment: It includes counseling for emotional adjustment. Imipramine like antidepressants have anticholinergic effect.

Hormone-Related Rhinitis

- *Hypothyroidism:* Due to the hypoactivity of sympathetic and predominance of parasympathetic system there occurs nasal congestion and discharge. These patients need supplement thyroid hormone.
- *Menstruation:* Fluctuating levels of hormones during menstruation can cause nasal symptoms.
- *Puberty:* The changing hormone concentrations during puberty can result in rhinitis.
- *Pregnancy:* Pregnant women may develop edema of the nasal mucosa due to hormonal changes. The common nasal symptoms are watery discharge and stuffiness. The severity of these nasal symptoms parallels blood estrogen levels. Nasal symptoms decrease towards term

because the blood is shunted away from nose towards the growing uterus. The persistent congestion may lead to secondary infection and rhinosinusitis.

Treatment: Usually, these women respond to limited local measures, such as saline drops and topical steroids. Limited surgery (cryosurgery) to hypertrophied turbinate is done in refractory cases.

Gustatory Rhinitis

The ingestion of hot and spicy food leads to mucoid or watery nasal discharge. The onset is immediate and lasts for as long as the food is ingested. Stimulation of afferent sensory nerves activates the parasympathetic nerves, which lead to nasal gland secretion, sweating and epiphora.

Non Airflow Rhinitis

In laryngectomy and tracheostomy cases, there is no nasal airflow. The turbinates are swollen due to loss of vasomotor control. Similar changes also occur in cases of choanal atresia and adenoid hypertrophy. Stagnation of discharge in the nasal cavity can lead to infection.

Idiopathic or Vasomotor Rhinitis (VMR)

When no cause of NAR is found, the condition is termed VMR which is usually said to be due to imbalance of autonomic nerve fibers that supply to nasal mucosa. It can be either increased parasympathetic, or decreased sympathetic activity.

CLINICAL FEATURES

It is important to note the pattern and timing of symptoms, exacerbating and relieving factors, and environmental triggers. Exclusion of systemic diseases and hormonal imbalances must be done.

Symptoms

- *Paroxysmal sneezing:* Especially in morning while getting out of the bed.
- *Excessive rhinorrhea:* In some cases, profuse and watery discharge is the presenting and only symptom. The nose may start dripping when the patient bends forward. This should be distinguished from CSF rhinorrhea.
- *Nasal obstruction:* The bilateral nasal stuffiness usually alternates from one side to other. This is generally more marked at night, when the dependent side of nose is often blocked.
- *Postnasal drip:* Though uncommons it can be the only symptom.

Examination

- *Nose:* The mucosa is usually boggy and edematous with clear mucoid secretions. The turbinates are usually congested and hypertrophic.

- **Pharynx:** Mucosal injection and lymphoid hyperplasia involving tonsils, adenoids, and base of tongue may be seen.
- **Complications:** Nonallergic rhinitis cases may subsequently develop polyps, turbinate hypertrophy and sinusitis.

INVESTIGATIONS

- Absolute eosinophil count
- Nasal smear
- Skin and in vitro allergy tests to rule out allergic rhinitis
- Acoustic rhinometry for measuring nasal patency
- Smell testing
- CT scan in cases of sinus disease
- MRI in cases of mass lesions

TREATMENT

Medical

- *Avoidance of inciting factors* such as coming in and going out of AC room, too much humidity, blasts of air, dust and smoke.
- *Antihistaminics and oral decongestants:* Relieve nasal obstruction, sneezing and rhinorrhea.
- *Steroid nasal spray*
- *Systemic steroids* are reserved for complicated and refractory cases.
- *Psychological counseling* for emotional adjustment.
- *Exercise* is an important adjunct to treatment.
- *Tranquilizers* help in some patients.

Surgical

It is more or less similar to allergic rhinitis.
- Reduction of hypertrophied turbinates.
- Correction of deviated nasal septum.
- Removal of polyps.
- Sectioning of the parasympathetic secretomotor fibers to nose (vidian neurectomy) for controlling refractory excessive rhinorrhea.

Self-evaluation Exercises

1. In some of the refractory and selective cases, surgical treatment of allergic rhinitis targeting inferior turbinate includes:
    a. Radiofrequency ablation
    b. Laser ablation
    c. Surgical removal
    D. All of the above

True (T)/False (F)

2. Deficiency of C1 esterase inhibitor, an inherited condition causes angioedema.
3. The increased production of C1 esterase leads to anaphylatoxins that causes capillary permeability and edema.
4. Cromolyn sodium provides protection against nasal allergy when used just after the exposure to allergen.
5. Vidian nerve section has been used in cases of vasomotor rhinitis with excessive watery rhinorrhea.
6. Nasal smear shows decreased number of eosinophils in nonallergic eosinophilic rhinitis.
7. The topical use of xylometazoline cannot cause rhinitis medicamentosa.

Answers

1. d   2. T   3. T   4. F   5. T   6. F   7. F

Chapter 26

Nasal Septum Disorders

Specific Learning Objectives

After going through the chapter, you should be able to answer the following questions:
- What are the different presentations and types of nasal septal fracture and their management?
- Describe the etiology, types, clinical features and treatment of deviated nasal septum.
- How will you differentiate and manage septal hematoma and septal abscess?
- What do you know about: (1) Septal perforation; (2) Hypertrophied inferior turbinate; (3) Choanal atresia; (4) Nasal synechia

For the pertinent anatomy and blood supply of nasal septum refer to Chapter 'Anatomy and Physiology of Nose and Paranasal Sinuses'.

FRACTURE OF NASAL SEPTUM

Facial trauma can result in fracture of nasal septum. It may be inflicted on the nose from the front, side or below. The nasal septum can get buckled and fractured vertically and horizontally (Figs 26.1A and B). For nasal bone fracture, see Chapter 'Maxillofacial Trauma'.

Features

- ***Multiple pieces of fracture:*** In a smashed nose, septum is crushed to pieces, which may overlap each other or project into the nasal cavity.
- ***A crushing blow from the front*** may cause buckling, twisting, fractures and duplication of nasal septum with telescoping of its fragments.
- ***Caudal dislocation of septal cartilage:*** Trauma to the lower nose can cause fracture of the septal cartilage and its dislocation from the vomerine groove without associated fractures of nasal bones.
- ***Epistaxis:*** Patient can have profuse epistaxis.
- ***Septal hematoma:*** If the septal mucosa is intact, septal trauma can cause septal hematoma, which should be drained early to prevent resorption of the septal cartilage and saddle nose deformity.

Types

- **"Jarjavay" fracture (Fig. 26.1A):** This horizontal fracture starts just above the anterior nasal spine and

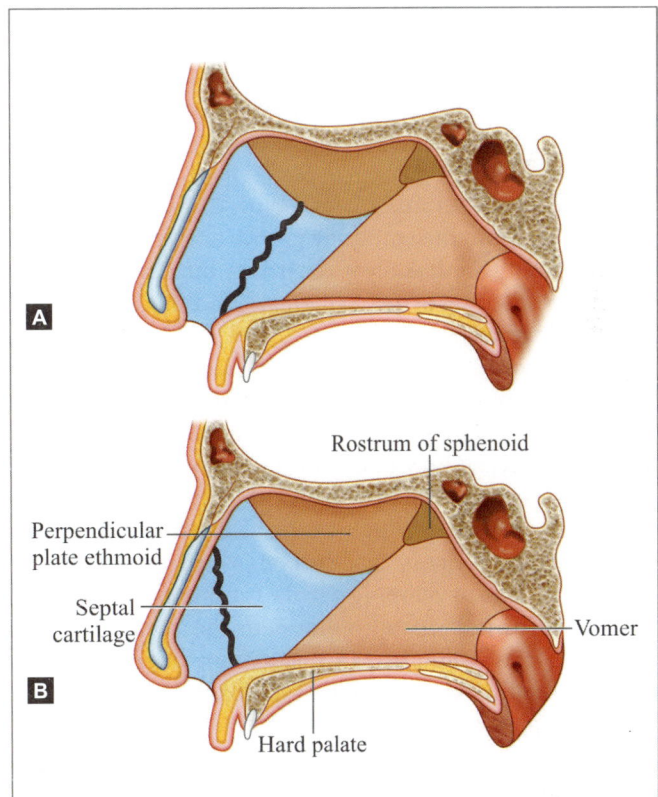

Figs 26.1A and B: Types of nasal septum fractures. (A) Jarjavay horizontal fracture; (B) Chevallet vertical fracture

runs backwards parallel and above the junction of septal cartilage with the vomer. It results from blows from the front.

- "Chevallet" fracture (Fig. 26.1B). This vertical fracture starts from anterior nasal spine and runs upwards towards the junction of bony and cartilaginous dorsum of nose. It results from blows from below.

Treatment
They need early treatment.
- Hematoma is drained at the earliest.
- Dislocated septal cartilage and fractured segments of septum are repositioned and supported between mucoperichondrial flaps. The mattress sutures are taken and nasal packing is done.
- Associated fractures of nasal pyramid are treated.

Complications
- Deviation of the cartilaginous nose.
- Asymmetry of nasal tip, columella and the nostril.
- Septal hematoma and nasal synechia.

DEVIATED NASAL SEPTUM (DNS)

DNS is a common condition. Patient usually presents with nasal obstruction. There is no age and sex bar but usually males are affected more than females. DNS is more common in Caucasians in comparison to the native Americans. In some hereditary cases, it runs in families.

Etiological Factors
- *Accidental trauma:* A lateral blow displaces the septal cartilage from the vomerine groove and maxillary crest. A crushing frontal blow results in buckling, fractures and telescoping of its fragments. Childhood injuries are often forgotten.
- *Natal trauma:* Trauma inflicted to the fetus at difficult delivery (forceps) should be immediately attended. They can lead to septal deviation in later life.
- *Antenatal:* Abnormal intrauterine postures can compress nose and upper jaw.
- *Developmental:* Nasal septum develops from the tectoseptal process that descends and meets the two halves of the developing palate. The latter descends and widens further to accommodate the teeth. Buckling of the nasal septum can result from unequal growth between the palate and the skull base. If septum starts growing at a more rapid rate than face, it becomes buckled.
- *Mouth breathers:* Buckling of nasal septum in children can result from highly arched palate, which occurs in mouth breathers such as in adenoid hypertrophy.
- *Cleft lip and palate:* They may be associated with dental abnormalities.
- *Mass in nose:* Tumors and polyps of nose can result in deviation of the nasal septum to opposite side.

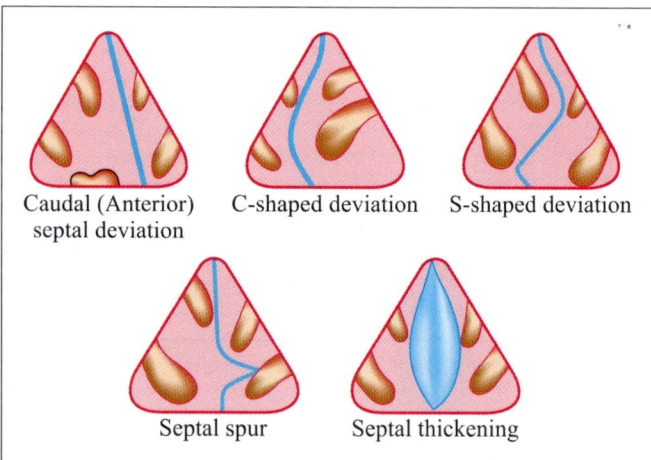

Fig. 26.2: Types of deviated nasal septum

Types
Deviation may be bony/cartilaginous, anterior/posterior, horizontal/vertical and superior/inferior (Fig. 26.2).
- *Anterior dislocation (caudal septal deviation):* Septal cartilage dislocates from anterior nasal spine into one of the nasal cavity (Figs 26.3A and B). It is better seen at the base of nose (Fig. 26.4).
- *C-shaped deformity:* The nasal septum becomes like an arc. On the concave side, nasal cavity is wider that can lead to compensatory hypertrophy of turbinates or atrophic changes. The septal blood vessels get stretched on the convex surface of DNS.
- *S-shaped deformity:* It can be either in vertical or anteroposterior plane and may cause bilateral nasal obstruction.
- *Spurs:* Spur is a shelf-like projection of cartilage, bone or both, which may press on the lateral wall of nose. It is usually found at the junction of vomer bone and cartilage. A spur can give rise to headache and predispose the patient to repeated epistaxis.

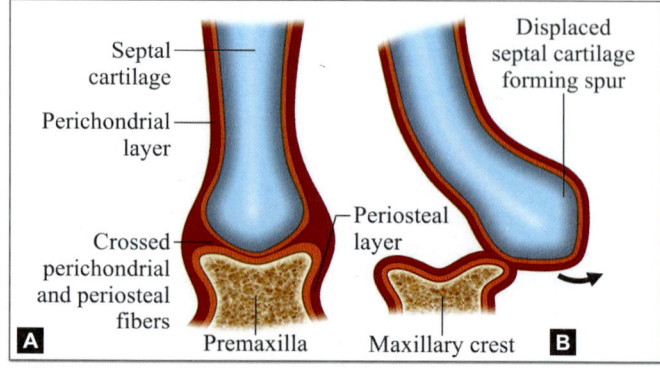

Figs 26.3A and B: Inferior aspect of septum and maxillary crest. (A) Normal; (B) Displaced septal cartilage shifted from the crest and forming spur

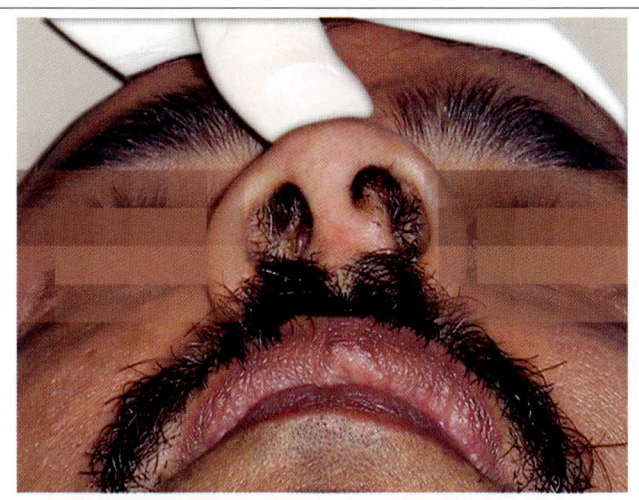

Fig. 26.4: Caudal septal deviation better seen at base of nose

- *Thickening:* It occurs due to organization of hematoma, overriding of fractured and dislocated septal fragments.

Clinical Features

Surprisingly, many patients who have gross DNS do not have any complaint whereas some patients with minor DNS complain the most.
- *Nasal Obstruction:* It may be unilateral or bilateral and is the most common symptom of DNS. High septal deviation causes more nasal obstruction than lower ones because respiratory currents pass through upper part of nasal chamber.
- *Headache:* A spur, pressing on the lateral wall of nose, can present with neuralgic headache. Sinusitis and negative pressure in sinuses can also cause headache. It can result from improper working of sinus ostium due to DNS.
- *External deformity:* Septal deflections may be associated with external nasal deformities (cartilaginous, bony or both) and deformities of the nasal tip and columella.
- *Epistaxis:* Mucosa over the convex part of DNS gets exposed to the dry air currents that causes crust formation. The removal of these crusts can cause bleeding.
- *Hyposmia/anosmia:* Severe DNS may not allow the inspired air to reach the olfactory region.

Complications

- *Mouth breathing:* It can lead to recurrent infection of pharynx, larynx and lungs.
- *Sleep apnea*
- *Recurrent and chronic rhinosinusitis:* Obstruction of sinus ostia due to marked DNS, can result into poor ventilation and drainage of the sinuses.
- *Middle ear infection:* DNS can affect the Eustachian tube and predisposes patients to middle ear infection.
- *Atrophic rhinitis:* Atrophic changes may occur on the concave side.
- *Asthma:* DNS may act as a trigger for bronchospasm.

Treatment

The treatment is surgical correction that can be done with or without endoscopic vision under general or local anesthesia. Surgery is considered when DNS produces nasal obstruction and other clinical features and complications. For details of the septal surgery, see Chapter 'Operations of Nose and Paranasal Sinuses'.

Submucous Resection (SMR)

The mucoperichondrial and mucoperiosteal flaps on either side of the septum are elevated. The deflected parts of the bony and cartilaginous septum are removed.

Septoplasty

It is a conservative septal surgery. Only the most deviated part of nasal septum is removed. Remaining septal framework is corrected and repositioned. The flaps are raised only on one side of the septum. Septoplasty is replacing SMR operation.
- *Septal surgery in children:* It can interfere with the growth of nasal skeleton and is usually avoided. But in severe DNS causing marked nasal obstruction a very limited septoplasty can be considered.

SEPTAL HEMATOMA

It refers to collection of blood under the mucoperichondrium and mucoperiosteum of the nasal septum.

Etiology

- Nasal trauma
- Septal surgery
- Spontaneous in bleeding disorders.

Clinical Features

- Bilateral nasal obstruction occurs.
- Frontal headache with a pressure feeling on the nasal bridge.
- Bilateral septal swelling, which is soft, fluctuant, smooth and round.

Treatment

- *Aspiration:* Small hematoma is aspirated with a wide bore needle.
- *Incision and drainage:* Larger hematoma needs incision and drainage. It is done through a small horizontal incision that is parallel to the nasal floor.

A small piece of mucosa is excised, which facilitates drainage.
- Nasal cavities are packed to prevent reaccumulation of blood.
- *Systemic antibiotics* prevent septal abscess.

Complications

- *Thickened septum:* Organization of hematoma into fibrous tissue.
- *Septal abscess:* It leads to necrosis of cartilage and depression of nasal dorsum.

SEPTAL ABSCESS

Etiology

- Secondary infection of septal hematoma.
- Furuncle and upper lip.
- Acute infection such as typhoid and measles.
- Diabetic patients are at high risk.

Clinical Features

- Bilateral nasal obstruction.
- Pain and tenderness over the bridge of nose.
- Fever with chills.
- Frontal headache.
- Red and swollen skin over the nose.
- Smooth bilateral swelling of the nasal septum with fluctuation and congestion of septal mucosa.
- Enlarged and tender submandibular lymph nodes.

Treatment

Incision and Drainage

It is performed at the earliest. Pus should be sent for culture and sensitivity examination. The preferred site of incision is dependent part of the abscess. Small piece of septal mucosa is excised, which facilitates drainage. Necrotic pieces of septal cartilage must be removed. In some cases, incision needs to be reopened daily for 2–3 days for draining pus and removal of necrotic pieces of septal cartilage.

Systemic Antibiotics

They may need to be changed as per the report of culture and sensitivity and continued for a period of 10 days.

Complications

- *Saddle nose deformity:* The necrosis of septal cartilage causes depression of the nasal dorsum in the supratip area. It needs augmentation rhinoplasty, which is performed after 2–3 months.
- *Septal perforation* due to necrosis of septal flaps.
- *Meningitis*
- *Cavernous sinus thrombosis.*

PERFORATION OF NASAL SEPTUM

Etiology

- *Trauma:* Habitual nose picking and perforation of septum for putting ornaments.
- *Septal surgery:* SMR and cauterization of septum (chemicals and galvanocautery).
- *Septal abscess:* Infected hematoma.
- *Nasal myiasis:* Maggots nose.
- *Foreign body:* Rhinolith and neglected foreign body.

Chronic granulomatous conditions: Lupus, tuberculosis and leprosy cause perforation in the cartilaginous part of septum. Syphilis leads to perforation in the bony part.

- *Wegener's granuloma:* This midline destructive lesion may cause total septal destruction.
- *Occupational:* Chrome platters and painters.
- *Drug induced:* Snuff and cocaine addicts and long-term use of topical corticosteroids.
- *Idiopathic.*

Clinical Features

- Whistling sound during inspiration and expiration in small anterior perforations.
- Nasal obstruction due to crust formation.
- Epistaxis occurs when crusts are removed.

Diagnosis

- Biopsy in cases of granulomatous lesions will reveal the exact nature of disease.
- Hemogram and serological tests help in diagnosing systemic diseases.

Treatment

- *Medical:* Treatment of the cause of perforation.
- *Small perforations:* Surgically closed with plastic flaps.
- *Larger perforations:* Difficult to close surgically. Alkaline nasal douches and application of a bland ointment keep the nose crust-free. A thin silastic button, which can be worn by the patients, relieves the symptoms.

Polychondritis: Seventy to eighty percent patients have involvement of the nasal septum.

HYPERTROPHIED TURBINATES

In hypertrophic rhinosinusitis, there occurs thickening of mucosa, submucosa, seromucinous glands, periosteum and bone. The causes and predisposing factors are similar to chronic rhinosinusitis which is well covered in Chapter 'Infectious Rhinisinusitis'.

Clinical Features

- Nasal obstruction is the presenting symptom.
- Turbinal mucosa is thick and does not pit on pressure. No occurs shrinkage with topical decongestant due to presence of underlying fibrosis.
- The inferior turbinate is hypertrophied (mulberry appearance) in its entirety including anterior end, posterior end and inferior border.

Anterior ethmoidal neuralgia: Concha bullosa of middle turbinate pressing on the nasal septum can result into anterior ethmoidal neuralgia.

Treatment

Priority should be given to the treatment of etiological and predisposing factors of the disease. In the refractory cases surgery is considered. Surgical reduction of inferior turbinates can be achieved with following methods:

- Linear cauterization
- Submucosal diathermy
- Cryosurgery of turbinates
- Submucous resection of turbinate bone
- Laser, microdebrider and radiofrequency
- Total and partial turbinectomy (partially removed at its anterior end, inferior border or posterior end).
  - *Turbinectomy scissors:* These long and blunt tipped scissors are bent at an obtuse angle. They are used for turbinectomy and cutting the nasal septal cartilage.
- Hypertrophied middle turbinate can be removed partially or totally.
- *Caution:* Excessive removal of turbinates can result in persistent crusting and atrophic changes.

Compensatory Hypertrophic Rhinitis

In marked deviation of septum, the roomier side of the nose shows hypertrophy of inferior and middle turbinates to reduce the wide space (to avoid drying and crusting). Hypertrophic changes require reduction of turbinates.

NASAL SYNECHIA

Etiology

Injury to opposing surfaces of nasal mucosa between the nasal septum and turbinates can result in adhesion formation by scar tissue. The common causes include intranasal surgical procedures such as:

- Septal surgery
- Polypectomy
- Removal of foreign bodies
- Reduction of nasal fractures
- Endoscopic sinus surgery
- Anterior nasal packing
- Infective ulcerative lesions.

Clinical Features

- Nasal synechia can impede drainage from the sinuses and cause recurrent sinusitis.
- Patient presents with nasal obstruction, headache and nasal discharge.
- Minor synechia may remain asymptomatic.

Treatment

It consists of cutting of synechia and prevention of their recurrence by placing a thin silastic, plastic, and cellophane sheets or gelatin sponge.

Prevention of nasal synechia: To prevent synechia formation after nasal surgery, packing of ribbon gauze with liquid paraffin is helpful.

CHOANAL ATRESIA

It refers to closure of posterior nasal choana. This congenital anomaly is caused by persistence of primitive bucconasal membrane.

Clinical Features

Choanal atresia can be classified as unilateral and bilateral; complete and incomplete; bony (90%) and membranous (10%).

Unilateral

It is more common but remains undiagnosed till adult life.
- Ipsilateral mucoid discharge without any air bubbles.

Bilateral

Newborns are natural nose breather and bilateral choanal atresia causes respiratory obstruction, which if not managed immediately, can prove fatal.

- Asphyxia endangers newborn's life.
- *Cyclic asphyxia:* Newborn breathes intermittently through mouth.
- *Difficulty in suckling:* Bilateral nose block makes suckling difficult.

Diagnosis

- Catheter cannot be passed from nose to pharynx.
- Drops of methylene blue into the nose do not come into the pharynx.
- X-ray lateral view after putting radio-opaque dye into the nose will show the atresia.
- CT scan shows extent and nature of atresia.

Choanal atresia: It is usually unilateral and more common in females (2:1). It is usually seen on the right side. The bony atresia is more common than membranous (9:1).

Treatment

- ***Tracheostomy or endotracheal intubation:*** Emergency management for airway is required in bilateral choanal atresia.
- ***McGovern's technique:*** A nipple with a large hole can obviate the need for tracheostomy. It provides a good oral airway.
- ***Correction of atresia (recanalization)/endoscopic atresioplasty:*** With the endoscopic approach choana can be created by drilling out the atresia.

Self-evaluation Exercises

1. Patients with deviated nasal septum can present with:
   a. Recurrent sinusitis
   b. Compensatory hypertrophy of turbinate
   c. Nasal stuffiness
   d. Epistaxis
   e. All of the above
2. Complications of septal abscess include:
   a. Depression of nasal bridge
   b. Meningitis
   c. Cavernous sinus thrombophlebitis
   d. All of the above
3. Which of the following are not true for choanal atresia?
   a. Usually unilateral
   b. More common in females (2:1)
   c. Usually seen on the right side
   d. Bony atresia more common than membranous (9:1)
   e. None from above

True (T)/False (F)

4. Concha bullosa of middle turbinate pressing on the nasal septum can result into anterior ethmoidal neuralgia.
5. To prevent synechia formation after nasal surgery, packing of ribbon gauze with liquid paraffin is helpful.

Answers

1. e   2. d   3. e   4. T   5. T

Pearls and Nuggets (Refresh your knowledge)

- **Septal hematoma:** Before reducing the nasal bone fractures, a septal hematoma must be ruled out because failure to drain it may result in a septal abscess, septal perforation and/or saddle nose deformity.
- **Polychondritis:** Seventy to eighty percent patients have involvement of the nasal septum.

Chapter 27

Maxillofacial Trauma

⊙ Specific Learning Objectives

After going through the chapter, you should be able to answer the following questions:
- How will you classify the maxillofacial injuries and evaluate them?
- How will you manage different types of nasal bone fractures?
- What are the etiological factors and clinical features of tripod (zygoma) fracture and how will you manage it?
- What are the characteristic features of orbital blow out fractures and how will you manage them?
- Describe the LeForte classification of nasomaxillary fractures and their clinical features and management.
- Describe different types of mandibular fractures and their management?
- What do you know about: (1) Oroantral fistula; (2) CSF rhinorrhea; (3) Rhinolith; (4) Maggots nose (nasal myiasis)?

INTRODUCTION

Injuries of the maxillofacial region involve both soft tissues and bones. In this era of fast life and expressways the incidence of automobile accidents are significantly increasing. The management of facial trauma is usually preceded by general management, which includes maintenance of airway and management of hemorrhage and associated injuries.

ETIOLOGY

The maxillofacial trauma can be caused by:
- Motor vehicle accidents
- Industrial injuries
- Sports injuries
- Altercations—fistfights
- Gunshot and other penetrating injuries
- Animal bites
- Burns

CLASSIFICATION

For the sake of description and management, the injuries of maxillofacial region can be divided into following:
- Soft tissue injuries of face
- Maxillofacial fractures
- Orbital fractures
- Fractures of the mandible
- Maxillofacial trauma in children

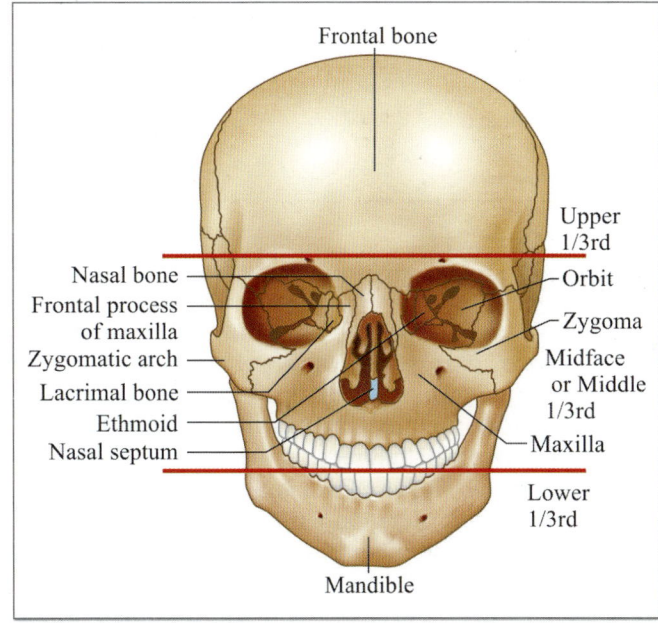

Fig. 27.1: Norma frontalis showing three maxillofacial regions and common fracture sites

The maxillofacial region (Fig. 27.1) can be divided into three parts—upper, middle and lower one-third (Box 27.1). The upper third lies above the supraorbital ridge while lower third consists of mandible and lower teeth. The middle third lies between the supraorbital ridge and angle of mouth.

> **Box 27.1: Classification of fractures of maxillofacial region**
>
> - **Upper third of the face**
>   - Frontal sinuses
>   * Anterior wall
>   * Posterior wall
>   * Floor
>   * Frontonasal duct
>   - Supra-orbital ridge
>   - Frontal bone
> - **Middle third of the face**
>   - Nasal bones and septum
>   * Depressed
>   * Angulated
>   - Naso-orbital Ethmoid (NOE)
>   - Zygomatic arch
>   - Orbit (blow-out fracture)
>   * Floor
>   * Medial wall
>   - Maxillary and malar region
>   * Central (naso-maxillary complex)
>   – Le Fort I
>   – Le Fort II
>   – Le Fort III
>   * Lateral (malar-maxillary complex)
> - **Lower third of the face**
>   - Temporomandibular joint
>   - Mandible
>   * Symphyseal or parasymphyseal
>   * Body
>   * Angle
>   * Ramus
>   * Coronoid
>   * Condylar
>   * Alveolar

GENERAL PRINCIPLES

- *Trimodal distribution of death after trauma:* It consists of deaths within seconds to minutes (overwhelming head and brain injury), from minutes to hours (golden hour for trauma care) and days to weeks (progressive organ failure and infection).
- *Airway, breathing and circulation (ABC):* They need immediate consideration and action. Resuscitation measures start simultaneously along with the initial survey (such as pupil size and reactivity and level of consciousness) and consists of intravenous fluids, nasogastric tube (not in fractures of cribriform plate and midface), cardiac monitors, urinary catheter (not in urethral injury), radiological and laboratory investigations. Injection tetanus toxoid 0.5 mL is given to patients, who are not recently immunized.
- *Associated injuries:* In blunt trauma cases X-ray chest posteroanterior (PA) view, lateral cervical spines and anteroposterior (AP) pelvis are usually ordered. The secondary survey includes head-to-toe examination of completely undressed patient. The respective specialists should attend the associated injuries of head, cervical spines, neck, larynx, chest, abdomen and limbs. The eyeball injuries are managed by ophthalmologists.

> *Life-threatening injuries*: Most of them can be identified during the primary survey.

EVALUATION

Evaluation of maxillofacial trauma includes history, physical examination, imaging and laboratory investigations.

RADIOLOGY

The radiological investigations include:
- *Plain radiographs:* Open-mouthed Towne's and lateral oblique (for mandible).
- CT scan axial and coronal 3 mm cuts.
- Panorex.

The wide availability of spiral high-resolution CT scanners has replaced plain X-rays for the assessment of craniomaxillofacial injuries. The exception is an isolated nasal bone fracture. The axial cuts are best for frontal, naso-orbital-ethmoid (NOE), zygomatic arch and vertical orbital wall fractures, while coronal sections are good for orbital roof and floor and pterygoid plates. For mandible most surgeons prefer plain X-rays and panoramic tomography.

> *CT and facial trauma:* Thin cut (1–3 mm) facial CT with coronal reformatting is the ideal imaging study. Three-dimensional reconstruction (of < 1.5 mm slices) displays overall facial architecture.

SOFT TISSUE INJURIES

Facial Lacerations

Facial lacerations are thoroughly cleaned of any dirt and foreign materials and are closed layer by layer.

Parotid Gland

The exposed parotid tissue needs suturing. Both ends of the injured parotid duct (Stensen's) should be identified and sutured with fine suture over a polyethylene tube, which is left for 3 days to 2 weeks.

Facial Nerve

The cut ends of the nerve are identified (needs superficial parotidectomy) and sutured with 8-0 or 10-0 silk.

FRONTAL SINUS

The fractures of frontal sinus can be linear horizontal, linear vertical and comminuted of anterior and posterior walls.

Anterior Wall Fractures

They may be depressed (cosmetic defect) and comminuted. In these fractures, frontal sinus is approached either through an existing external skin wound or a brow incision. While elevating the bone fragments do not strip them from the periosteum. The frontal sinus is inspected to rule out posterior wall fracture.

Posterior Wall Fractures

These fractures are associated with dural tears, brain injury and cerebrospinal fluid (CSF) rhinorrhea and require neurosurgical management. Dural tears are repaired with temporalis fascia and small frontal sinuses are obliterated with fat.

Frontonasal Duct

The chances of obstruction to sinus drainage are high and that may result in a mucocele. To avoid this complication, a large communication between the sinus and the nose is created. Small frontal sinuses need complete removal of the sinus mucosa and obliteration with fat.

SUPRAORBITAL RIDGE

Clinical Features

Supraorbital ridge fractures present with following sign and symptoms:
- Periorbital ecchymosis (purplish patch caused by extravasation of blood into the skin).
- Flattening of the eyebrow.
- Proptosis or downward displacement of eye.
- Impacted bone fragment in the orbit.

Treatment

These fractures require open reduction through an incision either in the brow or in transverse skin line of the forehead.

FRONTAL BONE

Frontal bone fractures, which usually involve the orbit, can be depressed and linear. Brain injury and cerebral edema require neurosurgical management.

NASAL BONES AND SEPTUM

Because of the projection of nose on the face, nasal bone fracture is the most common fracture of maxillofacial region. Nasal bone fractures are the third most common fractures of the body (first clavicle and second wrist).

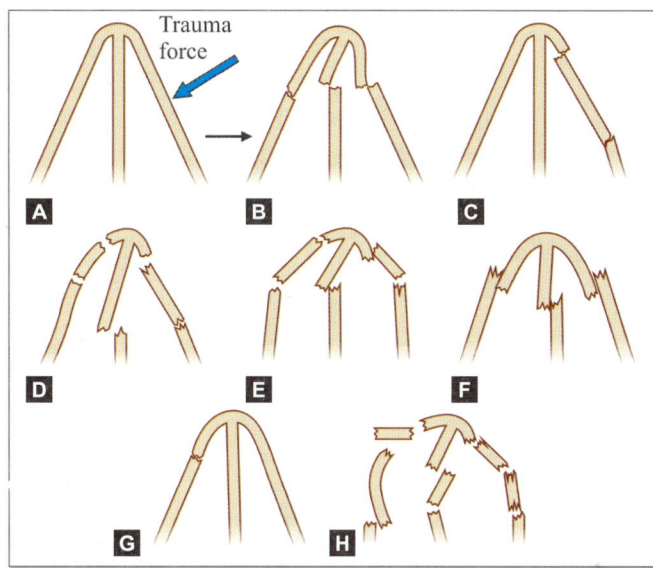

Figs 27.2A to H: Nasal fracture patterns. (A) Traumatic force from lateral side of nasal bone; (B) Fracture of perpendicular plate of ethmoid; (C) Unilateral fracture of nasal bone; (D) Bilateral fracture of nasal bones; (E) Open book-splayed; (F) Impacted fracture; (G) Greenstick and (H) Comminuted fracture

Nasal fractures often involve nasal septum which may be buckled, dislocated or fractured into several pieces (Figs 27.2A to H). Septal hematoma can occur. For the nasal septal fracture *see* Chapter 'Nasal Septum Disorders'.

Types

Magnitude and direction (front or side) of traumatic force determine the depth and type of injury. There are two types of nasal fractures—depressed (frontal blow) and angulated (lateral blow).
- *Depressed:* The lower parts of nasal bones are thinner and easily fractured. A frontal blow can cause an open book fracture, where nasal septum collapses and nasal bones splay out. Greater force can result in comminuted fractures of not only nasal bones but also frontal processes of maxillae, which flatten and widen the nasal dorsum.
- *Angulated:* A lateral blow can cause either unilateral depression of nasal bone on the side of injury or fracture of both the nasal bones and the septum. It results in deviation of nasal bridge (Fig. 27.3A).

Clinical Features

- Pain.
- Swelling appears within few hours and hides defect.
- Nasal obstruction.
- Bleeding from nose and external wound.
- Nasal deformity (depressed from the front or side) and nasal pyramid deviation.

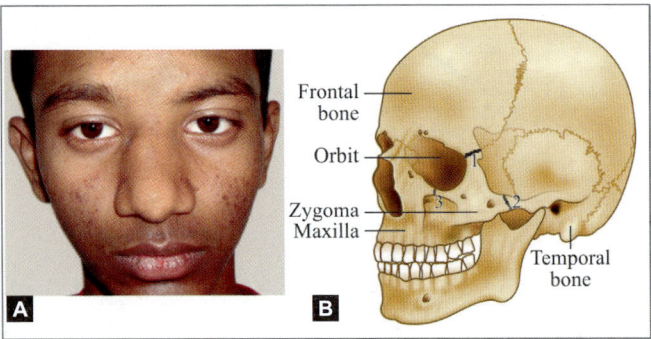

Figs 27.3A and B: (A) Nasal bone fracture. Note right side displacement of bridge of nose. (B) Left zygoma (tripod) fracture showing three sites of fracture. (1) Zygomaticofrontal; (2) Zygomaticotemporal; (3) Infraorbital

- Periorbital ecchymosis (purplish patch caused by extravasation of blood into the skin).
- External lacerations, exposure of nasal bones and cartilage in compound fractures.
- Tenderness, crepitus and mobility of fractured fragments.
- Septal deviation/hematoma.

Diagnosis
- *Clinical:* Diagnosis is usually clinical.
- *X-rays:* Waters', right and left lateral and occlusal views which though usually do not change the line of management, are important for documentation and medicolegal matter.

Treatment
The active treatment is needed only in cases of deformity and septal deviation. It consists mainly of closed and open reduction. The presence of swelling not only hides deformity but also interferes with accurate reduction. The best time for reduction is either immediate (before the appearance of edema) or when swelling has subsided (after 5–7 days). The reduction should be done within 2 weeks otherwise fracture heals. The healing is faster in children.
- *Closed reduction:* Depressed fractures can be reduced by a straight blunt elevator along with outside digital manipulation. Laterally displaced nasal bridge can be reduced only with external firm finger pressure. Impacted fracture fragments require disimpaction, which is performed with the help of Walsham and Asche's forceps (*see* Chapter on 'Instruments'). Septal hematoma is drained. Though simple fractures do not need intranasal packing, unstable fractures need both intranasal packing as well as external splint.
  - *Walsham's forceps:* They are used for the disimpaction and reduction of the fractures of nasal bones.
  - *Asch's septum forceps:* They are used for reducing fractures of nasal septum by lifting the nasal septum forwards.
- *Open reduction:* It is required occasionally when closed methods fail and in some cases of septal injuries deformities.
- *Rhinoplasty and septorhinoplasty:* Healed nasal deformities are corrected by rhinoplasty and septorhinoplasty.

Septal hematoma: Before reducing the nasal bone fractures, a septal hematoma must be ruled out because failure to drain it may result in a septal abscess, septal perforation and saddle nose deformity.

NASO-ORBITAL ETHMOID (NOE)
The fractures of NOE region occur when the force directly hits over the nasion. The fractures can involve nasal bones, perpendicular plate of ethmoid, ethmoidal air cells and medial orbital wall. They get displaced posteriorly. Medial canthal ligament can be avulsed. Injury can extend to cribriform plate, frontal sinus, frontonasal duct, extraocular muscles, eyeball and the lacrimal apparatus.

Clinical Features
- *Signs of medial canthal tendon disruption:* They are:
  - *Telecanthus:* The widening (>35 mm) of the intercanthal distance (normal is half of the interpupillary distance) occurs due to lateral displacement of medial orbital wall.
  - *Narrowing of palpebral fissure:* The distance between the medial and lateral canthus decreases.
  - *Epiphora:* There occurs overflow of tears upon cheek.
- *Pug nose:* There occur depression of nasal bridge and elevation of nose tip.
- *Periorbital ecchymosis:* It is the purplish patch caused by extravasation of blood into the skin of periorbital region.
- *Orbital hematoma:* It occurs due to bleeding from anterior and posterior ethmoidal arteries.
- *CSF leakage:* It can occur due to fracture of cribriform plate and dura.
- *Displacement of eyeball.*

Diagnosis
CT scan evaluates naso-orbital ethmoid (NOE) region.

Treatment

- *Closed reduction:* It is indicated in uncomplicated cases. After the reduction it is stabilized with wires tied over the lead plates.
- *Open reduction:* It is indicated in extensive comminuted nasal and orbital bones fracture and injuries to lacrimal apparatus, medial canthal ligaments and frontal sinus.
  - *Method:* An H-type incision, is employed and if necessary extended to the eyebrows for accessing frontal sinuses. The repair of medial canthal ligaments and lacrimal apparatus is done first. Medial canthal ligaments are repaired with a wire. The fractures of nasal bones and medial orbital walls are reduced and nasal bridge height is achieved. Intranasal packing helps in restoring the contour.

ZYGOMA (TRIPOD FRACTURE)

- Zygoma fracture (caused by direct trauma) is the second most common fracture (after nasal bones) of maxillofacial region.
- Fracture line involves zygomaticofrontal suture, orbital floor, infraorbital margin and foramen, anterior wall of maxillary sinus and the zygomaticotemporal suture (Fig. 27.3B).
- The flattening of the malar prominence and a step-deformity of infraorbital margin results from the inferior and posterior displacement of the lower segment of zygoma, which is separated from its three processes (tripod fracture).
- Orbital contents may get herniated into the maxillary sinus.

Clinical Features

- Ecchymosis of periorbital region (including conjunctiva and maxillary buccal sulcus) within 2 hours of injury is pathognomonic.
- Flattening of malar eminence with step-deformity of inferior and lateral margins of orbit.
- Hypesthesia or anesthesia over anterior portion of face occurs due to injury of infraorbital nerve.
- Trismus (difficulty in opening mouth) occurs due to impaction of fractured zygoma fragment and coronoid process of mandible.
- Oblique slant of palpebral fissure occurs due to inferior displacement of lateral palpebral ligament (lateral canthal tendon).
- Lateral canthus and pupil of eye are at lower level in comparison to the normal eye.
- Diplopia (double vision) and restricted upward ocular movements (entrapment of inferior rectus muscle).
- Periorbital emphysema may occur due to leak of air from the maxillary sinus on nose blowing.

Diagnosis

- Waters' and exaggerated Waters' views show the fracture and displacement and clouding of maxillary sinus (presence of blood).
- CT scan shows comminuted fractures and depression of orbital floor and herniation of orbital contents.

Treatment

Open reduction and internal wire fixation is indicated in displaced fractures.

- The frontozygomatic suture is approached through lateral brow incision.
- Displaced fracture is reduced by passing an elevator behind the zygoma.
- A separate incision in the lower lid exposes infraorbital margin. The fracture of orbital floor can also be repaired through this incision.
- Transantral approach: The antrum is exposed as in Caldwell-Luc operation. Maxillary sinus blood is aspirated and then fracture is reduced. Antral packing helps in stabilizing the reduced fracture and removed after 10 days.

ZYGOMATIC ARCH

- The two fractured fragments of zygomatic arch fracture have three fracture lines. There occurs impingement of fragments on the condyle or coronoid process.
- *Clinical features:* Characteristic depression is seen in the area of zygomatic arch.
  - *Local pain and tenderness:* They are aggravated during talking and chewing and limit the movements of mandible.
- *Diagnosis:* Submentovertical view of the skull shows zygomatic arch fracture. Waters' view is also helpful. CT scan is replacing plain X-rays.
- *Treatment:* Open reduction.
- *Method:* A vertical incision above and in front of the ear is used. Temporal fascia is incised and an elevator is passed deep to it. The elevator is passed under the depressed arch fragments and elevated. Fragments remain stable even without fixation.

ORBIT (BLOWOUT FRACTURE)

There are two types of blowout fractures—pure and impure.

1. *Pure blowout fracture:* It is an isolated fracture of orbital floor and occurs when a non-penetrating blunt object (ball, fist, hockey puck and cork) strikes the globe. The increased intraorbital pressure results in blowing out of thin walls (especially floor) of orbit. The orbital contents get herniated into maxillary antrum. There is no damage to orbital rim.

- **Clinical features:** The patient may present with:
  - *Pain* confined to orbit.
  - *Ecchymosis* of lid, conjunctiva and sclera.
  - *Enophthalmos:* It is a good indicator.
  - *Inferior displacement of the eyeball.*
  - *Diplopia:* The entrapment of inferior rectus and inferior oblique muscles result in restricted up and down movement of the eyeball.
  - *Hypoesthesia or anesthesia* over anterior portion of face (infraorbital nerve injury).
  - *Forced duction test* is done after topical conjunctival anesthesia. The episcleral tissue in the region of inferior oblique insertion is grasped with fine-toothed forceps. By passively rotating, restrictions of the eyeball movements are checked. The complete restriction of passive movements indicates entrapment of muscle. This test is done in operation room after the reduction of blow out fracture. The free passive movements of eyeball indicate success of surgery.

> **Forced duction test:** It detects extraocular muscle entrapment.

2. **Impure blowout fracture (rim fracture):** In contrast to pure blowout fracture orbital rim gets involved along with the floor of the orbit. The zygomatic and Le Fort II maxillary fractures are usually accompanied by fractures of orbital floor. The repair of zygomatic component of injury may unmask undiagnosed impure blowout fracture by revealing enophthalmos.
   - **Diagnosis:**
     - Waters' view shows a teardrop shaped opacity (herniating orbital fat) hanging from the roof of maxillary antrum (teardrop sign) and loss of double cortical lines (orbital rim and floor).
     - CT scan is replacing plain Waters' view.
   - **Treatment:**
     - *Indications for surgery* are enophthalmos, diplopia and entrapment of inferior rectus and oblique muscles.
     - *Transantral approach:* Through this approach, orbital floor fracture is easily reduced with a finger after opening the maxillary antrum. The packing kept in the antrum supports the reduced fragments.
     - *Infraorbital approach:* It can be used either alone or in combination with transantral approach. An incision in a skin crease of the lower eyelid is made. In badly comminuted fractures of orbital floor, an autogenous bone graft (iliac crest, nasal septum, outer table of calvarium and anterior wall of antrum) or cartilage (septal and conchal) is used for reconstruction of the floor of the orbit.

Inorganic implants such as gelfilm, silicon and teflon sheets, Marlex mesh and titanium mesh, have also been used.

NASO-MAXILLARY COMPLEX

Types

In 1901, the French surgeon Rene Le Fort described three typical patterns of the fractures of naso-maxillary complex (in fresh cadavers after using low-velocity impact forces), which are now called Le Fort I, II and III (Fig. 27.4). These Le Fort fractures, which are usually bilateral, may be mixed.

1. **Le Fort I fracture (Transverse):** The fracture line runs above and parallel to the palate and crosses lower part of nasal septum, maxillary antra and the pterygoid plates.
2. **Le Fort II fracture (Pyramidal):** The fracture line runs through the root of nose, lacrimal bone, floor of orbit, upper part of maxillary sinus and pterygoid plates. It has some clinical features of zygomatic fractures.
3. **Le Fort III fracture (Craniofacial disjunction):** There occurs complete separation of facial bones from the cranial bones. The fracture line runs through the root of nose, ethmofrontal junction, superior orbital fissure, lateral wall of orbit, frontozygomatic and temporozygomatic sutures and the upper part of pterygoid plates.

Clinical Features

- **Mobile palate:** *It is a pathognomonic sign of Le Fort fracture.* After stabilizing the forehead with one hand,

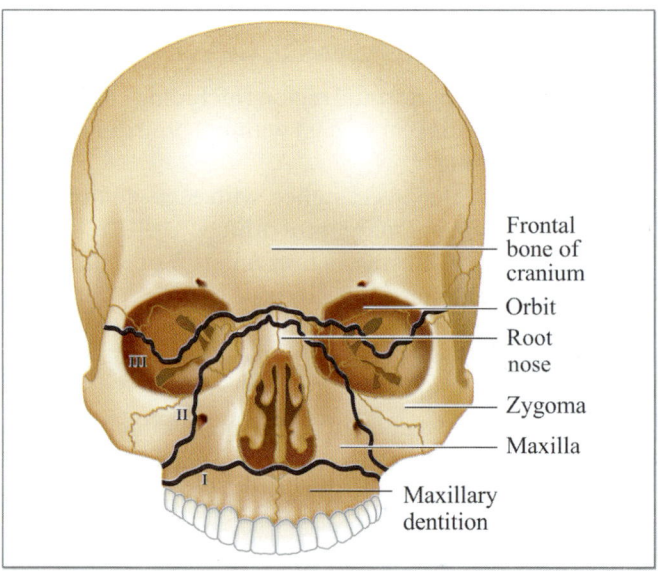

Fig. 27.4: Le Fort classification of fractures of naso-maxillary complex crossing nasal septum and pterygoid plates. (I) Transverse (separating maxillary dentition); (II) Pyramidal (fracture of root of nose, medial wall and floor of orbit and maxilla), (III) Craniofacial disjunction (separating face from the cranium)

examiner tries to see the mobility of palate and upper teeth with other hand.
- Facial edema and ecchymosis.
- Malocclusion of teeth with anterior open bite.
- Elongation or compression of midface.
- Epistaxis.
- Step-offs or movement of facial skeleton at fracture site.
- CSF rhinorrhea, blindness and airway obstruction in Le Fort II and Le Fort III fractures.

Diagnosis

CT scans better delineate fracture lines and the displacement of fragments and is replacing plain X-rays.

Treatment

Airway restoration and control of severe hemorrhage (maxillary artery and its branches) are the first priorities. Good cosmetic and functional results need early treatment. But associated intracranial and cervical spine injuries may delay reduction and fixation. Surgery includes:
- Open reduction and interosseous wirings.
- Interdental and intermaxillary wiring using arch bars.
- Wire slings from frontal bone, zygoma or infraorbital rim to the teeth or arch bars.

MANDIBLE

Classification

Figure 27.5 shows Dingman's classification of mandible fractures according to their location. The incidences of multiple and single fractures are almost equal. Angle's classification also refers to fracture of the mandible.
1. Condylar fractures are the most common and others in descending frequency are fractures of the angle, body and symphysis.
2. Fractures of the ramus, coronoid and alveolar processes are uncommon.

Factors Affecting Displacement

Factors affecting the displacement of mandibular fractures are:
- Pull of mandible muscles on the fragments.
- Direction of fracture line.
- Bevel of the fracture.

Mode of Injury

Though condylar fractures are caused by indirect trauma to the chin and opposite side of the mandible body, the most common cause of other mandibular fractures is direct trauma.

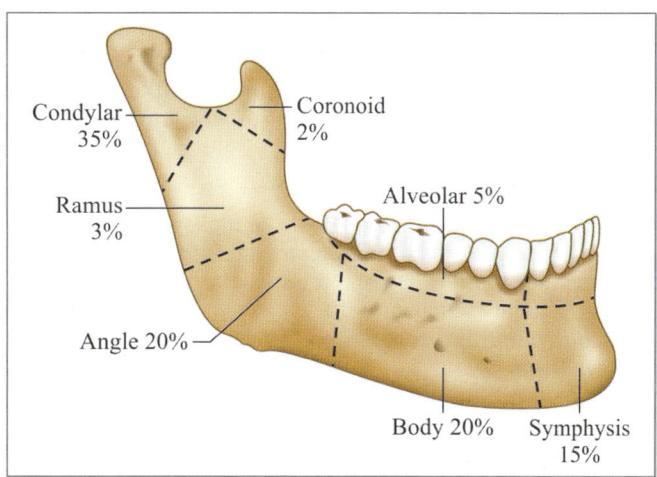

Fig. 27.5: Dingman's classification of mandible fractures. In descending order common fractures are condylar, angle, body, and symphysis (CABS)

Clinical Features

- *Fractures of condyle:* Pain, trismus, tenderness at fracture site, malocclusion of teeth and deviation of jaw to the opposite side on opening the mouth (due to displacement of fragments).
- *Fractures of angle, body and symphysis:* The intraoral and extraoral inspection and palpation reveal malocclusion of teeth, ecchymosis of oral mucosa, and step-deformity, tenderness and crepitus at fracture site.

Diagnosis

- X-rays PA view of the skull for condyle.
- Right and left oblique views of mandible are helpful.
- *Panorex view is gold standard.*
- CT scan is indicated in severely comminuted and displaced condylar fractures.

Treatment

Both closed as well as open methods can be employed for reduction and fixation.
- *Closed methods:* They include interdental wiring and intermaxillary fixation and external pin fixation. In condylar fractures, intermaxillary fixation with arch bars and rubber bands is done. The intermaxillary wires are usually removed in three weeks and jaw exercises encouraged. Immobilization beyond three weeks in condylar fractures can result in ankylosis of temporomandibular joints. The intermaxillary wires may be reapplied for another week if occlusion is not good. The process may need repetition till the bite and jaw movements are satisfactory.
- *Open methods:* After exposing the fracture site, fragments are fixed by direct interosseous wiring, which is strengthened by a figure of eight wire tie. Compression

plates, which avoids prolong immobilization and intermaxillary fixation, are widely used to fix the fragments. The indications include edentulous patients with bilateral condylar fractures and children.

- *Mandibular fractures*: Open reduction and internal fixation (ORIF) with bone plates and lag screws is the most accepted treatment. It provides stable rigidity and early patient function.
- *Condylar fractures*: Severe fractures are problematic even with ORIF.

OROANTRAL FISTULA

Oroantral fistula is situated on the upper alveolus or gingivolabial sulcus. It is a communicating track between the maxillary antrum and oral cavity. *First molar is most commonly incriminated tooth.*

Etiology

- *Extraction of the upper second premolar and molars* is the most common cause because the roots of these teeth are closely related to the cavity of maxillary antrum. Apical tooth abscess is also important predisposing factor.
- *Postoperative complications of Caldwell-Luc operation:* Sublabial incision may fail to heal.
- *Carcinoma of maxilla:* Erosion of the floor of maxillary antrum.
- *Penetrating injuries and fractures of maxilla.*
- *Infection of maxilla:* Osteitis and syphilis.

Clinical Features

- *Nasal regurgitation:* Semisolid food and liquids pass through fistula and come into antrum and then to nose.
- *Foul smelling discharge from fistula and nose:* It occurs due to infection of maxillary antrum.
- *Inability to create positive and negative pressures in the oral cavity:* Patient finds it difficult to blow musical instruments and suck through a straw as air gets leaked through the oroantral fistula.
- *Probe test:* A probe can be passed through the fistulous track from oral cavity into the antrum.

Treatment

- *Recent fistula:* Immediately after tooth extraction, make sure that there is no infection and retained tooth piece in the antrum. Conservative treatment includes suturing of gum margins and a course of antibiotics.
- *Chronic or large fistula:* After treating maxillary sinusitis with antibiotics and repeated antral irrigations, the surgical repair is done with a palatal or a buccal flap. The fistulous track lined by squamous epithelium is excised and bony edges of fistula are drilled and prepared for the flaps.
- *Caldwell-Luc operation:* It provides a nasoantral window for free drainage. It helps in removing a retained tooth root, foreign body (FB) and diseased mucosa.
- *Cancer maxilla:* In these cases fistula is closed by a dental obturator. Whenever required antrum can be examined.

CEREBROSPINAL FLUID RHINORRHEA

As the name suggests, CSF rhinorrhea means CSF leaks come out through nasal cavity.

The most common site of CSF rhinorrhea is cribriform plate. Next common site is ethmoidal sinuses.

Etiology

- *Idiopathic.*
- *Traumatic (immediate and delayed):*
  - Head injuries, temporal bone fracture and maxillofacial traumas.
  - Surgeries of frontal, ethmoid and sphenoid sinus, hypophysectomy and endoscopic sinus surgery.
- *Tumors:* Intracranial neoplasms such as tumors of the pituitary and olfactory bulb, large osteomas of frontoethmoid region and skull base neoplasms such as sinonasal and nasopharyngeal cancers.
- *Congenital defects:* Encephalocele.
- *Hydrocephalus and benign intracranial hypertension.*
- *Infection:* Sinus mucocele and osteomyelitis.

Sites and Pathways

- *Anterior cranial fossa:* CSF reaches the nose through the cribriform plate, ethmoid air cells or frontal sinus.
- *Middle cranial fossa:* CSF reaches the nose through sphenoid sinus.
- *Otorhinorrhea:* In transverse temporal bone fracture CSF enters into the middle ear and then comes to nasopharynx and nose through the Eustachian tube.

Diagnosis

Patient presents with dribbling of clear fluid from the nose on bending and straining. CSF rhinorrhea should be differentiated from the usual nasal discharge of rhinitis and sinusitis (Table 27.1).

- *Physical:* CSF remains clear when stand in a test tube, whereas nasal discharge leaves a sediment because of mucus and other proteins.

Table 27.1: Differences between CSF rhinorrhea and nasal secretions

	CSF rhinorrhea	Nasal secretions
History	Surgery, injury and tumor	Sneezing, stuffiness, itching
Discharge flow	Few drops or a stream of fluid	Continuous
Aggravation	Straining and forward bending	Allergy, infection, crying
Sniffing back	Impossible	Possible
Character	Thin, watery and clear	Mucus, mucopurulent, tears
Taste	Sweet	Salty
Sugar content	Normally more than 30 mg/dl	Less than 10 mg/dl
β 2 transferrin	Present	Absent

- *Reservoir sign:* CSF collected in the sinus especially sphenoid during the night sleep comes out through nose in the morning when patient flexes his head.
- *Nasal discharge stiffens the handkerchief* while CSF does not.
- *Glucose content:* Oxidase-peroxidase paper strip or biochemical tests will show the glucose content of CSF. Compare with sugar in CSF obtained from lumbar puncture as sugar is reduced in cases of meningitis.

> β 2 transferrin: It is specific for CSF and confirms the diagnosis of CSF leak.

- *Electronic nose:* This novel strategy can distinguish between CSF and serum.
- *Otorhinorrhea:* Middle ear may show fluid and conductive hearing loss.
- *Double ring sign or target sign:* In traumatic cases, when CSF is mixed with blood, double ring sign (or target sign) helps in diagnosis. Discharge is placed on a piece of filter paper, which shows a central spot of blood and peripheral halo of CSF that spreads more and faster than blood.

Complications

- Meningitis and intracranial infections.
- Pneumocephalus and secondary brain compression.

Localization of CSF Leak (CSF Tracers)

Site of leak can be seen in high resolution CT (thin coronal cuts with bone window). HRCT shows the area of bony defect. Intrathecal agents, which are used for localizing the site of CSF leaks are visible dyes, radionuclide markers and radiopaque dyes (Table 27.2).

Table 27.2: CSF tracers

Visible dyes	Fluorescein
Radionuclide markers	Radioactive iodine (I^{131}) serum albumin (RISA), technetium (99mTc)-labeled serum albumin and diethylene-triamterene-penta-acetic acid (DTPA) and Indium (In^{111})-labeled DTPA
Radiopaque dyes	Metrizamide

- *Intrathecal fluorescein:* Injection fluorescein 10% 0.1 mL diluted in patient own CSF is infused slowly over 30 minutes. Nasal endoscopy identifies the characteristic green color of the fluorescein in nose and sinuses at the site of CSF leak.
- *Radionuclide cisternography:* Radionuclide is injected intrathecally and pledgets of cotton are placed close to the suspected sites of CSF leak such as olfactory slit (cribriform plate), middle meatus (frontal and ethmoidal sinuses), sphenoethmoidal recess (sphenoid sinus) and Eustachian tube (temporal bone). Monitoring of the distribution of tracer is done with a scintillation camera. These pledgets are assayed for tracer 12–24 hours later with a gamma counter.
- *CT cisternography:* CT is done after intrathecal administration of radiopaque contrast (metrizamide), which shows the presence of CSF leak.
- *MRI cisternography:* It is a non-invasive and non-ionizing technique. Heavily T2 weighted image with fat suppression and video reversal provides a means to image CSF.

Treatment

The cause of CSF rhinorrhea needs early treatment.
- *Early traumatic CSF rhinorrhea:* These are managed conservatively by:
  - Placing the patient in strict bed rest and head elevation (semi-sitting position).
  - Patient is advised to avoid nose blowing, sneezing, coughing and straining.
  - Stool softeners.
  - Prophylactic antibiotics prevent meningitis.
  - If needed subarachnoid drainage through a lumbar catheter.
  - Acetazolamide and mannitol decrease intracranial pressure.
  - Nasal packing and drops are not used.
- *Persistent CSF rhinorrhea:* These patients need surgery. The repair can be:
  - *Intracranial approach:* Done by neurosurgeons.
  - *Nasal endoscopic approach:* It is usually preferred in leaks from the frontal sinus, cribriform plate, ethmoid and sphenoid sinuses.

Following are the main steps:
- Identification of the site of CSF leak.
- Preparing the site for the graft that is usually fascia (or fat from thigh or abdomen).
- Insinuating the fascia in extradural space.
- Repairing the bony defect (if >2 cm size) with conchal or septal cartilage.
- Putting back the nasal mucosa over the leaking site.
- Putting surgicele, gelfoam and merocele for further strengthening.
- Betadine/Betnovate-N impregnated nasal packing.
- Lumbar drain when CSF pressure is high.

FOREIGN BODY NOSE

Foreign bodies (FBs) are often seen in children. They may be living (maggots) and non-living. Non-living consists of organic (seeds and grams) and inorganic such as piece of paper, chalk, button, pebbles, beads and cell-battery. Iatrogenic FBs include sponges, cotton swabs and gauze packing.

Food and vomiting material can enter the nose through the incompetent nasopharyngeal sphincter. Bullets enter directly through penetrating wound. Sequestration of bone *in situ* can also occur.

Clinical Features

- Patient or the parents of children come with clear history of FB in nose.
- Sneezing, nose block and bleeding are common symptoms.
- Many children do not tell or simply forget to report to their parents. These children present with unilateral foul smelling nasal discharge with or without blood staining.
- **On examination:** FB is visible (Figs 27.6A and B).

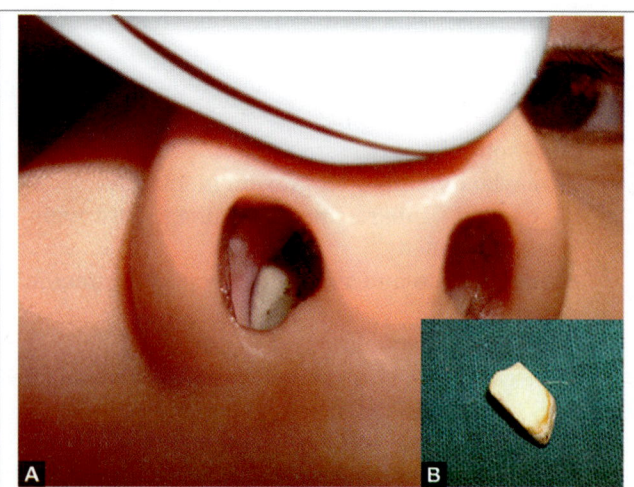

Figs 27.6A and B: (A) Foreign body (chalk writing stick) in right nose; (B) Removed piece of chalk writing stick

Foreign body nose in children: A unilateral foul smelling purulent nasal discharge in a child is mostly due to forgotten foreign body nose.

Complications

A FB nose if not removed can result in:
- Nasal infection and sinusitis.
- Rhinolith formation.
- Swallowing and sticking in esophagus.
- Inhalation into the tracheobronchial tree.

Treatment

FBs need removal:
- ***Paper piece and cotton swab:*** They are removed with a pair of forceps.
- ***Solid and rounded foreign bodies:*** A blunt hook or Eustachian catheter is passed beyond the limit of FB. Then the FB is dragged out along the nasal floor.
- ***Children and apprehensive patients:*** General anesthesia with cuffed endotracheal tube should be used. Patient should be kept in Rose's position and nasopharynx is packed.
- ***Nasal endoscopes:*** They facilitate the removal of FB lodged far posterior in the nose, which may need to be pushed into nasopharynx.

Causes of unilateral blood stained mucopurulent discharge:
- Forgotten FB nose in children.
- Rhinolith and sequestra.
- Nasal diphtheria in children.
- Nasal myiasis (maggots).
- Acute and chronic unilateral sinusitis.
- Malignancy of nose and paranasal sinuses in elderly patients.

RHINOLITH

Rhinolith refers to nasal calculus or concretions (single or multiple) that forms around FB, blood clot or inspissated secretion in nose. Deposition of carbonates and phosphates of calcium and magnesium occurs gradually but progressively. It grows into a large irregular mass (hard or friable), which may result in pressure necrosis of septum and lateral wall of nose.

Clinical Features

Rhinoliths are seen in adults. Patients present with:
- Unilateral nasal obstruction and foul-smelling discharge which may be blood-stained.

- The mucosal ulceration and granulations can cause epistaxis and neuralgic pain.
- A grey brown/greenish-black mass, which feels stony hard on probing, is seen in the nose. It may look white also.

Treatment

- Rhinolith should be removed under general anesthesia.
- While manipulating it may break off because it is usually brittle and friable.
- Large rhinolith usually needs lateral rhinotomy and removed in broken pieces.

NASAL MYIASIS (MAGGOTS NOSE)

This condition is not uncommon in India and mostly seen in months of August, September and October.

Etiopathology

- Maggots are larvae of flies (Genus *Chrysomya*). They can infest nose, nasopharynx and paranasal sinuses and cause extensive destruction.
- Foul smelling nasal discharge attracts flies, which lay their eggs (about 200) that hatch into larvae within 24 hours. Later on secondary infection occurs.
- The common causes of foul smelling nasal discharge include atrophic rhinitis, syphilis and leprosy. These diseases are characterized by nasal crusting and loss of nasal sensation. Poor hygiene is an important contributing factor.

Clinical Features

- Initially patients may have irritation, sneezing and lacrimation and later on headache.
- Patient presents with epistaxis (thin blood-stained nasal discharge), puffy eyelids and lips, fever, toxemia and cellulitis of nose and face.
- Later on the maggots start crawling out of the nose.
- Patient emits foul smell.
- Maggots lead to destruction of nose and paranasal sinuses, soft tissue of face, palate (perforation) and even eyeball.
- Fistulae may form around the nose.
- Intracranial complications can kill the patient.

Treatment

- ***Removal of the maggots by forceps:*** While removing, maggots go away from light into darker cavities.
- ***Topical liquid paraffin, diluted chloroform or ether and turpentine oil nasal drops:*** They are used to irritate and stupefy the maggots so they come out of the nose. Maggots of nose are best treated by chloroform diluted with water.
- ***Nasal douche with warm saline:*** It facilitates removal of slough, crusts and dead maggots.
- ***Antibiotics:*** They take care of secondary infection.
- ***Personal hygiene:*** It should be observed to prevent the recurrence.

Self-evaluation Exercises

1. Which of the following does not apply for mandibular fracture?
   a. The posterior part of mandible displaced superiorly by the contraction of masseter muscle
   b. Inability to close the mouth
   c. Bloodstained saliva from mouth
   d. Intense pain in the ipsilateral jaw
   e. None from above

True (T)/False (F)

2. Le Fort's classification is of fractures of mandible.
3. Mandibular fracture can cause anesthesia of chin or ipsilateral lower lip because of the laceration of the inferior alveolar nerve of mandibular division of trigeminal nerve.
4. Angle's classification refers to fracture of the mandible.
5. First premolar is most commonly incriminated tooth in cases of oroantral (orodental) fistula.
6. The most common site of CSF rhinorrhea is frontal bone and the next common site is sphenoid sinuses.
7. Beta-2 transferrin is the diagnostic test for CSF rhinorrhea.
8. Maggots nose are best treated by nasal saline drops.

Answers

1. e 2. F 3. T 4. T 5. F 6. F 7. T
8. F

Chapter 28

Tumors of Nose and Paranasal Sinuses

⊙ Specific Learning Objectives

After going through the chapter, you should be able to answer the following questions:
- What do you know about: (1) Fibrous dysplasia; (2) Inverted papilloma?
- What are the etiological factors and clinical features of maxillary carcinoma?
- How will you evaluate, classify and stage a patient with carcinoma of maxilla?
- How will you manage a case of carcinoma of maxillary sinus?

INTRODUCTION

Both benign and malignant tumors of the nose and paranasal sinuses are uncommon. The malignant neoplasms of this region are more common than benign. The separation of nasal tumors from tumors of paranasal sinuses is difficult except in early stages. In addition to primary tumors, these areas can be encroached with growths of nasopharynx, cranial and oral cavity.

> **Most common malignant tumor of nose and paranasal sinuses**: Squamous cell carcinoma is most common and constitutes about 80% of the malignant tumors of nose and paranasal sinuses.

Benign tumors are smooth and localized while the malignant masses are friable and with a granular surface that bleed on touch. Tumors of nose and paranasal sinuses can be divided into three categories—benign, intermediate and malignant (Table 28.1).

ANGIOFIBROMA

This tumor arises in the posterior part of nasal cavity near the sphenopalatine foramen and is discussed in detail in the Chapter of 'Tumors of Nasopharynx'.

INTRANASAL MENINGOENCEPHALOCELE

Meningoencephalocele is usually seen in infants and young children. Herniation of brain tissues and meninges occur through foramen cecum or cribriform plate.

Table 28.1: Classification of tumors of nose and paranasal sinuses

Benign	Intermediate	Malignant
Squamous papilloma	Inverted papilloma	Squamous cell carcinoma
Encephalocele*	Meningioma	Adenocarcinoma
Glioma*	Hemangioma	Adenoid cystic carcinoma
Dermoid*	Hemangiopericytoma	Malignant melanoma
Neurofibroma	Ameloblastoma	Olfactory neuroblastoma
Schwannoma	Plasmacytoma	Lymphoma
Angiofibroma*		Osteogenic sarcoma
Osteoma		Chondrosarcoma
Chondroma		Fibrosarcoma
Ossifying fibroma		Rhabdomyosarcoma*
Cementoma		
Fibrous dysplasia*		
Odontogenic tumor*		

*These tumors are seen in children

- **Clinical:** A smooth polyp like mass in the upper part of nose between the septum and middle turbinate that increases in size on crying and straining.
- **Differential diagnosis:** It can be easily misdiagnosed as a polyp, which if avulsed results in CSF rhinorrhea and meningitis.
- **Biopsy:** *It is contraindicated.*

- **CT scan:** It demonstrates the defect in the base of skull.
- **Treatment:** Frontal craniotomy with severing of the stalk from the brain is done along with the repair of dural and bony defect by neurosurgeon. Later on, intranasal mass is removed by ENT surgeon.
- **Extranasal meningoencephalocele:** See Chapter on 'Diseases of External Nose'.

GLIOMAS

- Thirty percent gliomas are intranasal and 10% both intra and extranasal.
- Gliomas arise from interstitial tissue of CNS.
- Patients are infants and children.
- It presents as a firm polyp and may be seen protruding at the anterior nares.
- **Extranasal Glioma:** See Chapter 'Diseases of External Nose'.

Most common congenital tumor of the nose in children: It is the glioma.

NASAL DERMOID

- Widening of upper part of nasal septum with splaying of nasal bones and hypertelorism.
- A pit or a sinus in the midline of nasal dorsum with hair protruding in some cases may be seen.
For more detail *see* Chapter 'Diseases of External Nose'.

MONOSTOTIC FIBROUS DYSPLASIA

In this disease, bone is replaced by fibrous tissue.
- **Site:** The most common site is maxilla (Fig. 28.1) followed by ethmoid and frontal sinuses.
- **Clinical features:** Patient develops disfigurement of face, nasal obstruction and displacement of the eye.
- **Treatment:** Wide removal (surgical resculpturing) provides good cosmetic and functional results.

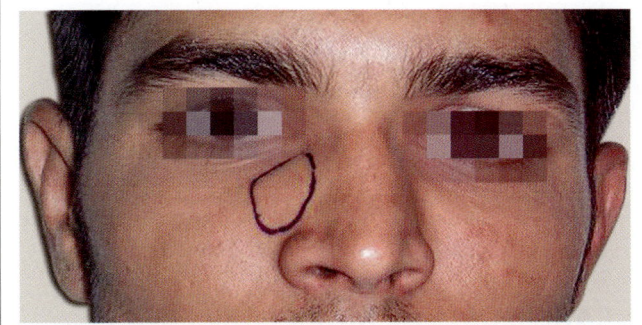

Fig. 28.1: Fibrous dysplasia. Disfigurement of face due to the fullness on the right side of nose

SQUAMOUS PAPILLOMA

- Verrucous growth like warts in the vestibule and lower part of nasal septum.
- Single or multiple and pedunculated or sessile.
- **Treatment:** Local excision (even with cryosurgery and laser) is done. The cauterization of the base prevents recurrence.

OSTEOMAS

Osteoma is formed of mature lamellar bone.
- **Most common site:** Frontal sinus followed by ethmoid and maxillary.
- Asymptomatic and seen incidentally on X-rays.
- The obstruction to the sinus ostium can lead to mucocele and pressure symptoms in the orbit, nose and cranium.
- **Treatment:** Symptomatic osteoma needs surgical removal.

PLEOMORPHIC ADENOMA

This rare tumor, which usually arises from the nasal septum, needs wide surgical excision.

CHONDROMA

In addition to pure chondroma there are mixed types such as fibro, osteo and angiochondromas. Histological differentiation between benign and malignant tumors is not completely defined.
- **Common sites:** Nasal cavity and nasal septum.
- Pure chondroma is smooth, firm and lobulated growth.
- **Treatment:** Wide excision is required as they can undergo malignant transformation.

SCHWANNOMA AND NEUROFIBROMA

These indolent inactive, sluggish, painless tumors have slow progressive growth and become symptomatic by obstructing sinus ostium. This rare tumor can present as yellow, firm round mass with blood vessels on its surface causing pressure necrosis of surrounding bones. They arise from components of peripheral nerve.
- **Schwannoma:** It is an isolated encapsulated tumor.
- **Neurofibroma:** It is woven into the nerve and may be multiple.
- **CT scan and MRI:** Neuroma and neurilemmoma show irregular patchy appearance.
- **Treatment:** These tumors need conservative local excision. Malignant change can occur in cases with multiple neurofibromatosis (von Recklinghausen's disease).

OSSIFYING FIBROMA AND CEMENTOMA

- *Ossifying fibroma:* Histologically it looks similar to fibrous dysplasia.
  - *Age:* It is seen in young adults.
  - *Radiology:* The sclerotic bony margin can be seen.
  - *Treatment:* It can be shelled out easily.
- *Cementoma:* It is a variant of ossifying fibroma and needs local excision.

AMELOBLASTOMA (ADAMANTINOMA) AND CALCIFYING EPITHELIAL TUMOR OF PINDBORG

These rare tumors account for only 1% of all jaw tumors.
- Locally aggressive tumors arise from the odontogenic tissue and usually involve maxillary sinus.
- *Treatment:* Surgical excision.

INVERTED PAPILLOMA

(Transitional cell papilloma or Ringertz tumor or Schneiderian papilloma)

The neoplastic epithelium of this papilloma grows towards underlying stroma rather than on the surface therefore is called inverted papilloma. *It is thought to be caused by human papilloma virus (HPV).*

- *Clinical features:* It is mostly seen in males between 40–70 years of age.
  - This is unilateral (nasal obstruction and discharge) and arises from the middle meatus. Epistaxis is not uncommon.
  - It presents as red or grey masses, which may be translucent, edematous and simulate nasal polyps. It can invade paranasal sinuses and orbit (proptosis, diplopia and epiphora).
  - *CT and MRI:* Show site and extent of tumor
  - *Biopsy:* It will confirm the diagnosis.
- *Treatment:* It is wide surgical excision. Inadequate removal results in recurrence.
  - *Lateral rhinotomy:* Medial maxillectomy and en bloc ethmoidectomy.
  - *Endoscopic sinus surgery (ESS):* Some surgeons have obtained good results with ESS.
- *Prognosis:* Inverted papillomas are known for their recurrence.
  - In 10–15% cases they convert into squamous cell carcinoma.

Inverted papilloma: The excision should be aggressive because this aggressive nasal benign tumor has frequent coexisting carcinoma.

MENINGIOMAS

Benign and encapsulated tumors of arachnoidal origin.
- *Intracranial meningioma:* It can invade sinuses.
  - *Radiology:* Hyperostosis of ethmoidal region.
  - *Treatment:* It needs surgical excision. Radiotherapy is able to stabilize inoperable tumors.
- *Extracranial meningioma:* It arises from ectopic arachnoid tissue and needs electron microscopy for identification.

HEMANGIOMAS

- *Capillary hemangioma (bleeding polyp of nasal septum):* It occurs on the anteroinferior part of nasal septum as a soft, dark red and pedunculated/sessile tumor.
  - It presents with recurrent epistaxis and nasal obstruction.
  - This smooth growth may become ulcerated.
  - *Treatment:* Local excision with surrounding mucoperichondrium.
- *Cavernous hemangioma:* It arises from the turbinates.
  - *Treatment:* Surgical excision with cryotherapy. Extensive disease needs combination of radiotherapy and surgical excision.

HEMANGIOPERICYTOMA

This rare vascular tumor arises from the pericytes, which surround the capillaries. It is common in nose but may also involve sinuses.
- *Clinical features:* Most of the patients are in the age group of 60–70 years and present with epistaxis.
  - Tumor may be slowly enlarging but aggressively infiltrating and have varying appearance.
- *Biopsy:* Brisk bleeding occurs on biopsy. The nature of the tumor, whether benign or malignant, cannot be distinguished histologically.
- *Treatment:* It consists of wide surgical excision. Delayed recurrence is likely.
  - Radiotherapy is indicated for inoperable and recurrent lesions.

PLASMACYTOMA

- Solitary plasmacytoma of nose predominantly affects males over 40 years.
- *Treatment:* If total regression does not occur with radiotherapy, surgery is done.
- *Prognosis:* Patients need long term follow-up as there are chances of developing multiple myeloma.

CARCINOMA OF MAXILLARY SINUS

- *Incidence:* Malignancy of paranasal sinuses accounts for 15% of all upper respiratory tract neoplasms.

- **Sites:** *The most common site of carcinoma is the maxillary sinus followed in descending order by ethmoids, frontal and sphenoid.*
  - In nose, squamous cell carcinoma may arise from the vestibule, anterior part of nasal septum (Nose-picker's cancer) and the lateral wall of nasal cavity.

Histology: More than 80% of the malignant tumors of nose and paranasal sinuses are squamous cell carcinomas. Other in descending order, are adenoid cystic carcinoma and adenocarcinoma. Melanoma and sarcomas are rare.

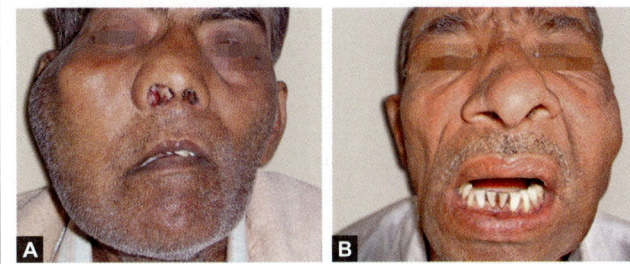

Figs 28.2A and B: Malignancy maxillary sinus. (A) Note swelling of face and infratemporal fossa region and mass in right nasal cavity; (B) Trismus indicating retromolar extension

Etiology

The exact cause of sinus malignancy is not yet clear but following are some predisposing factors:
- ***Industrial workers:*** Workers of hardwood furniture industry, nickel refining, leather work and mustard gas manufacturing have higher incidence of sinonasal cancer.
  - Adenocarcinoma of the ethmoids and upper nasal cavity is more common in workers of furniture industry.
  - Workers of nickel refining are more prone to develop squamous cell and anaplastic carcinoma.
- ***Geographical:*** Bantus of South Africa who use locally made snuff, which is rich in nickel and chromium, have higher incidence of sinonasal cancer.
- ***Aflatoxin:*** It is found in certain foods and dust.
- ***Polycyclic hydrocarbons***
- ***Mesothorium (thorotrast):*** It is a radiopaque dye used in antrum.

Clinical Features (Fig. 28.2A and B)

- ***Early:*** Facial pain, nasal obstruction and epistaxis. The lesion arises from the sinus mucosa and may remain silent for a long period, during which patient has vague symptoms of rhinosinusitis such as nasal stuffiness, blood stained nasal discharge, facial paresthesia or pain and epiphora.
- ***Eye and Orbit:***
  - ***Diplopia*** and squint due to involvement of oculomotor nerves and extraocular muscles.
  - ***Loss of vision*** due to the involvement of optic.
  - ***Proptosis*** due to tumor compression of periorbita.
  - ***Epiphora*** due to involvement of lacrimal duct.
- ***Facial numbness*** due to involvement of branches of infraorbital nerve (CNV_2).
- ***Facial swelling*** due to involvement of facial soft tissue.
- ***Malocclusion,*** widening of upper alveolus, loose and nonvital teeth due to involvement of upper alveolus.
- ***Trismus*** due to involvement of pterygoid muscles.
- ***Neck swelling*** due to involvement of jugular chain lymph nodes.
- ***Deafness:*** Serous otitis media due to involvement of nasopharynx.
- ***Mass:*** Necrotic intranasal mass and/or alveolar/palatal mass or ulceration.
- ***Cranial nerves involvement:*** CN II, III, IV, V_1 and V_2, VI.

Late features of carcinoma maxillary sinus: Following features appear when tumor spreads and destroys the bony confines and involves surrounding structures.
- *Medial spread towards nasal cavity:* Nasal obstruction, discharge and epistaxis.
- *Anterior spread towards face:* Swelling of the cheek (Fig. 28.2A) and later invasion of the facial skin.
- *Inferior spread towards alveolus:* Expansion of alveolus, dental pain, loosening of teeth, poor fitting of dentures, ulceration of gingiva, swelling of hard palate.
- *Superior spread towards orbit:* Facial paresthesia/anesthesia, proptosis, diplopia, ocular pain and epiphora.
- *Posterior spread into pterygomaxillary and infratemporal fossa:* Trismus due to involvement of pterygoid plates and the muscles (Fig. 28.2B).
  - Spread to nasopharynx, sphenoid sinus, skull base.
- *Intracranial spread:* Through ethmoids, cribriform plate and foramen lacerum.
- *Lymphatic spread:* Neck swelling (cervical node metastases of submandibular and upper jugular nodes) is uncommon and occurs in the advanced stages.
  - Maxillary and ethmoid sinuses drain primarily into retropharyngeal nodes (inaccessible to palpation).
- *Distant metastases:* Though rare they mostly occur in lungs and occasionally in bones.

Diagnosis

- ***Radiographs:*** CT scan has replaced plain X-rays, which show opacity of sinus with expansion and destruction of the bony walls.
- ***CT scan and MRI (Fig 28.3):*** Axial and coronal planes show bony (CT) and soft tissue (MRI) extent of tumor and help in the staging of disease.

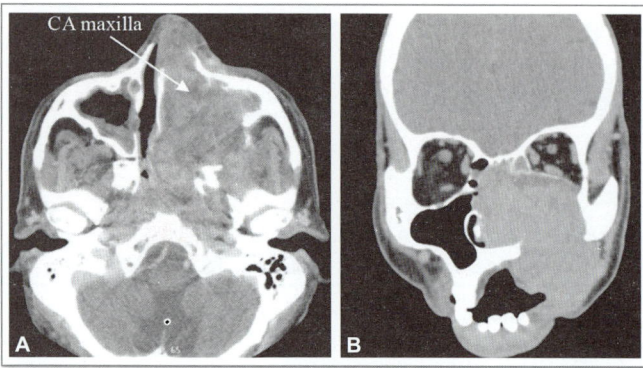
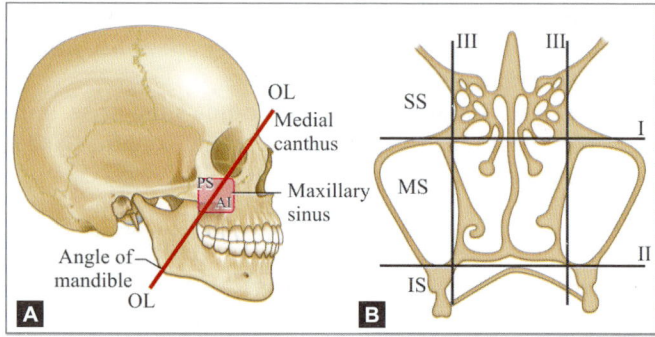

Figs 28.3A and B: (A) Contrast CT scan of nose and paranasal sinuses axial section. A large growth of left maxillary sinus. It is destructing the medial wall of maxillary sinus and extending into the left nasal cavity. It is destructing the posterolateral wall of maxillary sinus and pterygoid plates and extending into pterygopalatine fossa and pterygomaxillary fissure and involves lateral pterygoid muscle. Posteriorly the mass is extending into the nasopharynx through the choana with complete obliteration of nasopharyngeal lumen; (B) CT scan coronal section Ca Maxilla with infraorbital extension. Note tumor is reaching up to skull base

Figs 28.4A and B: Classifications of maxillary carcinoma. (A) Ohngren's classification. OL, Ohngren's line; AL, anteroinferior region; PS, posterosuperior region; (B) Lederman's classification. I, II, III, two horizontal and one vertical lines of Sebileau; SS, suprastructure; MS, mesostructure; IS, infrastructure

- **Endoscopy:** Endoscopy of the nose and maxillary sinus facilitates examination and an accurate biopsy.
- **Biopsy:** Biopsy is taken from the growth in the nose or mouth. In early suspected cases, sinus may be explored through Caldwell-Luc operation but preferred approach is endoscopic intranasal. Direct visualization of the tumor site helps in staging.

Classification and Staging

Classifications provide valuable insight in planning the treatment and predicting the prognosis.
- **Ohngren's classification:** An imaginary line, which extends between medial canthus and the angle of mandible, divides the maxilla into two regions: anteroinferior and posterosuperior (Fig. 28.4A). Anteroinferior growths are easy to manage and have better prognosis than posterosuperior tumors.
- **Lederman's classification:** Two horizontal lines of Sebileau, one passing through the orbit floors and other through antral floors, divide the area into three regions (Fig. 28.4B):
  - **Suprastructure:** Ethmoid, sphenoid and frontal sinuses and the olfactory area of nose.
  - **Mesostructure:** Maxillary sinus and the respiratory part of nose.
  - **Infrastructure:** Containing alveolar process.
  The vertical line at the plane of medial wall of orbit separates ethmoid sinuses and nasal fossa from the maxillary sinuses. Suprastructure and infrastructure of Lederman's classification is not similar to Ohngren's classification.
- **TNM classification:** According to American Joint Committee on Cancer (AJCC), TNM classification is for squamous cell carcinoma (Tables 28.2 and 28.3). The CT scan and MRI are usually required for staging these tumors.
- **Histopathological classification:** In addition to the location and extent of tumor, histological nature of malignancy is also important in deciding the line of treatment.
  - Grades of squamous cell carcinoma:
    - Well differentiated
    - Moderately differentiated
    - Poorly differentiated
  - Cell types—They include:
    - Squamous cell carcinoma
    - Undifferentiated carcinoma
    - Transitional cell carcinoma
    - Carcinoma with inverted papilloma
  - **Vascular or perineural invasion:** Their presence or absence should be noted.

Most antral malignancies are anterior ethmoidal because they usually invade anterior and posterior ethmoid sinuses.

> **Superior orbital fissure:** In cases of tumor compressing the structures traversing the superior orbital fissure, patient experiences pain and altered sensation on the skin of the anterior scalp and dorsum of the nose. Branches of the ophthalmic division of trigeminal nerve (CN V_1), which carry general sensation from frontal region and dorsum of the nose, traverse through superior orbital fissure. Tumor of the maxillary sinus, which lies inferior to the orbit, erodes the superior orbital fissure through the floor of the orbit.

Treatment

- **Surgery:** It is the mainstay therapy. Complete radical maxillectomy includes removal of maxilla along with the nasal bone, the ethmoid sinus, and in some cases pterygoid plates. It is adequate when tumor is confined to maxilla, or extends to facial soft tissues, palate, or

Table 28.2: Primary tumor (T) staging (American Joint Committee on Cancer (AJCC)) of carcinoma nasal cavity, maxillary and ethmoid sinuses

Maxillary sinus	
T_1	Tumor limited to maxillary sinus mucosa with no involvement of bone
T_2	Tumor involving bone of hard palate and/or middle meatus. No extension to posterior wall of maxillary sinus and pterygoid plates
T_3	Tumor involving bone of the posterior wall of maxillary sinus, floor or medial wall of orbit; ethmoid sinuses, subcutaneous tissues
T_{4a}	Tumor involving any of the following: anterior orbital contents, skin of cheek, pterygoid plates, infratemporal fossa, cribriform plate, sphenoid or frontal sinuses
T_{4b}	Tumor involving any of the following: Orbital apex, dura mater, brain, middle cranial fossa, cranial nerves (other than maxillary division of trigeminal nerve), nasopharynx, or clivus
Nasal cavity and ethmoid sinus	
T_1	Tumor restricted to any one subsite
T_2	Tumor involving two subsites in a single region or extending to involve an adjacent region within the nasoethmoidal complex
T_3	Tumor involving medial wall or floor of the orbit, maxillary sinus, palate, or cribriform plate
T_{4a}	Tumor involving any of the following: Anterior orbital contents, skin of nose or cheek, minimal extension to anterior cranial fossa, pterygoid plates, sphenoid or frontal sinuses
T_{4b}	Tumor invades any of the following: Orbital apex, dura, brain, middle cranial fossa, cranial nerves (other than maxillary division of trigeminal nerve), nasopharynx, or clivus

Note: For the regional lymphadenopathy (N) *see* Chapter 'Neoplasms of the Oral Cavity'

Table 28.3: Staging of cancer of nose and paranasal sinuses

Stage 1	$T_1 N_0 M_0$
Stage 2	$T_2 N_0 M_0$
Stage 3	$T_3 N_0 M_0$; $T_{1-3} N_1 M_0$
Stage 4 A	$T_4 N_{0-1} M_0$
Stage 4 B	$T_{1-4} N_{2-3} M_0$
Stage 4 C	$T_{1-4} N_{1-3} M_1$

anterior orbit but without invasion of the ethmoidal roof, posterior orbit, or pterygoid region. Figure 28.5A shows Weber-Ferguson incision.

- **Radiotherapy:** It is given either before or after surgery. Curative radiotherapy or chemoradiation may make the inoperable tumors operable. Neutron beam irradiation is most suited to adenoid cystic carcinomas.
  - *Preoperative radiotherapy:* A full course of preoperative radiotherapy is followed 4–6 weeks later by total or extended maxillectomy.
  - Indications of postoperative radiotherapy
    - Large tumors
    - Positive margins
    - Perineural or perivascular invasion
    - Lymph node metastasis
  - Adverse affects of radiotherapy
    - **5,800 rad:** Severe panophthalmopathy with severe corneal ulceration in 100% cases.
    - **2,800–5,400 rad:** Cataracts and visual disturbances in 86% cases.

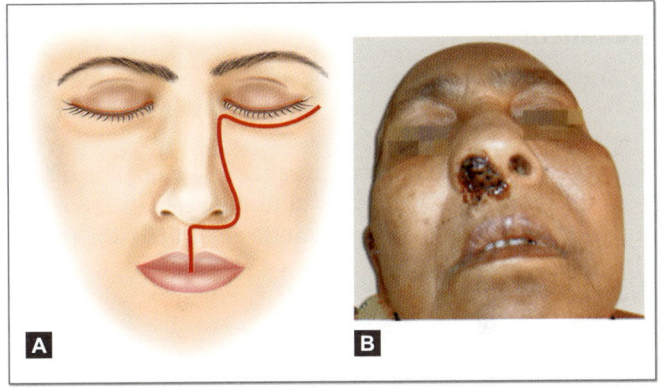

Figs 28.5A and B: (A) Weber-Ferguson's incision for maxillectomy starts at the upper lip philtrum on the operative side and goes up to the columella. It continues round the margin of the ala and up the lateral border of the nose. Near the medial canthus of eye it turns laterally in a rounded fashion to go 5 mm below the lower lid margin; (B) Dark brown colored polypoidal mass covered with clotted blood coming out of right side nose. Biopsy: Small cell undifferentiated carcinoma/neuroblastoma. Immunohistochemistry advised to confirm the origin

- **Eye ball:** Some surgeons prefer to spare the eye whereas others intentionally include the eye during surgery and irradiation. Orbital exenteration in patients with ethmoid tumor has been reported to increase survival.

- **T_1 and T_2 tumors:** They may be treated by maxillectomy or radiotherapy.
- **T_3 and T_4 tumors:** Usually a combination of radiotherapy and surgery is employed.

Prognosis

Overall, 5-year survival is about 30%. The multimodal treatment, which is combination of chemotherapy, radiation and surgery, improve the results.

MALIGNANCY OF ETHMOID SINUS

Ethmoid sinuses are usually involved from extension of maxillary sinus growths.

Clinical Features

- *Early features:* Nasal obstruction, blood stained nasal discharge and retro-orbital pain.
- *Late features:* Broadening of the nasal root, lateral displacement of eyeball and diplopia.
  - *Intracranial:* Meningitis due to invasion of cribriform plate.
  - *Cervical lymph node involvement:* Rare.

Imaging

- *CT scan:* It shows the extent of disease.
- *MRI:* It reveals intracranial spread.

Treatment

- *Early cases:* Preoperative radiotherapy, followed by total ethmoidectomy through lateral rhinotomy approach.
- *Late stages:* Craniofacial resection (when cribriform plate is involved) exposes anterior cranial fossa and facilitates total exenteration of the growth in one piece.

Prognosis

Five years survival is about 30%.

MALIGNANCY OF FRONTAL SINUS

It is uncommon and usually seen in middle aged males. Male female ratio is 5:1.
- *Presenting features:* Pain, swelling of the frontal region and swelling above the medial canthus (erosion of floor of frontal sinus).
  - *Orbital features:* When growth extends to ethmoids.
  - *Involvement of dura of anterior cranial fossa:* Growth invades the posterior wall of the sinus.
- *Treatment:* Preoperative radiation followed by surgery, which includes removal of frontal and ethmoid sinuses and orbital exenteration. This neurosurgical approach resects the dura of anterior cranial fossa.

MALIGNANCY OF SPHENOID SINUS

- Very rare
- Clinical features similar to the inflammatory lesions of sphenoid sinus

- CT and MRI scan show the extent of disease and biopsy through sphenoidectomy confirm the diagnosis.
- *Treatment:* Radiotherapy is the mainstay of treatment.

ADENOCARCINOMA

- *Common sites:* It is usually seen in upper nasal cavity and ethmoid.
- *Occupations:* It is common in persons who are associated with woodworking, furniture making and leather work.
- *Treatment:* They have aggressive local progression and need aggressive surgical en bloc resection.

ADENOID CYSTIC CARCINOMA

- *Spread:* These tumors, which are usually seen in antrum, spread to skull base along the neural sheath.
  - Distant metastases are more common than regional metastasis.
- *Treatment:* It usually includes surgical resection with irradiation (preferably neutron beam).
  - *Three modality therapy:* Some recommend combination of chemotherapy (regional infusion with 5-fluorouracil), surgery (maxillary resection) and irradiation.

Perineural invasion: It is most commonly seen in adenoid cystic carcinoma.

MALIGNANT MELANOMA

- Patients are of 50 years of age and of either sex.
- Immunological defenses play an important role in the control of this tumor.

Clinical Features

- *Black colored nasal mass and discharge:* A slaty-grey or bluish-black polypoid mass and black nasal discharge.
  - Amelanotic varieties are non-pigmented.
- *Sites:* Common site is anterior part of nasal septum followed by middle and inferior turbinate.
- *Metastases:* Regional (cervical lymph node) metastases and distant (blood stream) metastases are common.

Treatment

- *Wide surgical excision:* A five-year survival rate after surgical excision is about 30%.
- *Radiotherapy and chemotherapy:* They suppress the immune processes.

OLFACTORY NEUROBLASTOMA

- *Origin:* Tumor of olfactory placode.
- *Sex and age:* Seen in either sex and in any age group.
- *Clinical:* A cherry red, polypoidal mass in the upper third of the nasal cavity (Fig. 28.5B).
- *Biopsy:* Very vascular and bleeds profusely on biopsy.
- *Spread:* Lymph node and systemic metastases can occur.
- *Treatment:* Though moderately radiosensitive it is treated with radiation.
    - Some favor surgical excision followed by radiation.
    - Craniofacial resection is suggested for the tumors of cribriform plate.

SARCOMAS

- *Osteogenic sarcomas and chondrosarcoma:* They have relentless local progression and are more common in mandible than maxilla.
- *Treatment* includes en bloc resection and/or irradiation (preferably neutron beam).
    - Some prefer induction chemotherapy.

RHABDOMYOSARCOMA

Rhabdomyosarcoma is the most common pediatric malignancy of upper respiratory tract.

- This aggressive tumor shows rapid progression and dissemination.
- *Histological subtypes:* They include alveolar, botryoid and embryonal.
- *Treatment:* It is usually multimodality and includes clear surgical margins supplemented by irradiation and chemotherapy.

Self-evaluation Exercises

1. Which of the following is not true for the inverted papilloma (Ringertz tumor)?
    a. Unilateral nasal papilloma arising from the lateral wall of nose
    b. Polypoidal masses may resemble allergic nasal polyps
    c. Inward growth of squamous or transitional cell epithelium towards fibrovascular stroma lends the name of inverted papilloma to it
    d. It is well-known for its recurrence and malignant change (squamous cell carcinoma in 10–15% of patients)
    e. None of the above
2. Which of the following are true for malignancy paranasal sinuses?
    a. Nearly 80% are squamous cell carcinoma
    b. Maxillary sinus is the most common site
    c. Other sites in decreasing order are nasal cavity, ethmoid sinuses, frontal and sphenoid sinus
    d. All of the above
3. Risk factors for squamous cell carcinoma of paranasal sinuses include:
    a. Smoking
    b. Nickel and chromium plating industry
    c. Leather industry
    d. Polycyclic volatile hydrocarbons, mustard gas, and isopropyl oil
    e. All of the above
4. Which of the following are not true for ethmoidal cancer?
    a. Most of the ethmoidal cancers are extensions of carcinoma maxilla
    b. Patients die of meningitis
    c. Patients with adenocarcinoma of ethmoid usually give history of wood-dust exposure
    d. None from above

True (T)/False (F)

5. The most common site of fibrous dysplasia is frontal sinus.
6. The most common site of osteoma is maxillary sinus.
7. Bleeding polyp of the nose is the hemangioma/fibroangioma of nasal septum.
8. Glioma is the most common congenital tumor of the nose in children.
9. Perineural invasion is most commonly seen in adenocarcinoma.
10. Wood workers are at greater risk factor for adenocarcinoma of sinonasal tract.
11. Ohngren's line is useful in assessing the prognosis of carcinoma of frontal sinus.
12. In cases of tumor compressing the structures traversing the superior orbital fissure, patient experiences pain and altered sensation on the skin of the anterior scalp and dorsum of the nose.

Contd…

Contd…

13. Branches of the ophthalmic division of trigeminal nerve (CN V), which carry general sensation from frontal region and dorsum of the nose, traverse through inferior orbital fissure.
14. Tumor of the maxillary sinus, which lies inferior to the orbit, erodes the superior orbital fissure through the floor of the orbit.
15. Treatment of $T_3N_0M_0$ squamous cell carcinoma of maxilla consists of maxillectomy and radiotherapy.

Answers

1. e	2. d	3. e	4. d	5. F	6. F
7. T	8. T	9. F	10. T	11. F	12. T
13. F	14. T	15. T			

Problem-oriented Cases (Spot Diagnosis)

1. A child aged 2 years has severe bilateral sensorineural hearing loss. Hearing aids were used but with no benefit. What for will you further evaluate the child?[1]
2. A 20-year-old female from Uttar Pradesh is having nasal obstruction and crusting of nose. Your examination of patient reveals an infiltrating lesion that involves nasal vestibule and upper lip with broadening of nasal dorsum.[2]
3. A biopsy taken from a granulomatous lesion of nose shows Mikulicz's cells and eosinophilic structures in the cytoplasm of the plasma cells.[3]
4. A 10-year-old boy presents with chronic sinusitis and multiple nasal polyps, recurrent chest infections and malabsorption syndrome. Sweat chloride test confirms the diagnosis.[4]
5. A 4-year-old child presents with chronic right side serosanguinous (purulent blood tinged) nasal discharge, which is not getting cured with medical treatment.[5]
6. A 3-year-old child presents with a unilateral single nasal polyp, which dose not bleed on touch. Which condition you would like to rule out or confirm?[6]
7. An elderly diabetic patient develops left-sided orbital cellulitis. CT scan shows evidence of left-sided maxillary sinusitis. Gram-stained smear of orbital exudates reveals irregularly branching septate hyphae.[7]
8. An immunocompromised patient with severe aspergillosis is hospitalized. He is suffering from invasive fungal sinusitis. He has been administered NSAIDs, antihistamines, and adrenal corticoids. Now which parenteral antifungal agent you would like to start?[8]

---

[1]Cochlear implant, [2]Rhinoscleroma, [3]Rhinoscleroma, [4]Cystic fibrosis, [5]Foreign body nose, [6]Intranasal meningocele, [7]Aspergillus maxillary sinusitis, [8]Amphotericin B

Section 4: Oral Cavity and Salivary Glands

Chapter 29

Anatomy of Oral Cavity

⊙ Specific Learning Objectives
After going through the chapter, you should be able to answer the following question:
- Describe the subsites of cancer in oral cavity and their lymphatic drainage.

ORAL CAVITY

It extends from the lips to the junction of hard and soft palate and circumvallate papillae (Figs 29.1 and 29.2). The subsites of oral cavity categorized by the American Joint Committee on Cancer Staging (AJCC) are shown in Table 29.1.
- Hard palate is included in the oral cavity whereas soft palate is the part of oropharynx. The anterior two-third of tongue is the part of oral cavity while the posterior one-third of tongue is included in oropharynx.

LIPS

Lips form the anterior boundary of the oral cavity.

- **Parts:** The two surfaces of lip, skin and mucosal, become continuous with one another round its red margin, which is called vermilion.
- **Vermilion border:** The site along which the two lips meet with one another is marked by a line that indicates transition from a dry vermilion to a moist vermilion.

- An ulcerative squamous cell carcinoma lesion fixes the skin early to the deep substance of lip because of the 2 mm distance between the epithelium and muscle.
- **Commissure of mouth:** As far as possible, it should be spared during the surgery because it is very delicate and difficult to reconstruct.

Lymphatic Drainage
- **Lower lip:** Medial part of lower lip drains into submental (level Ia) while lateral part to submandibular nodes (level Ib).

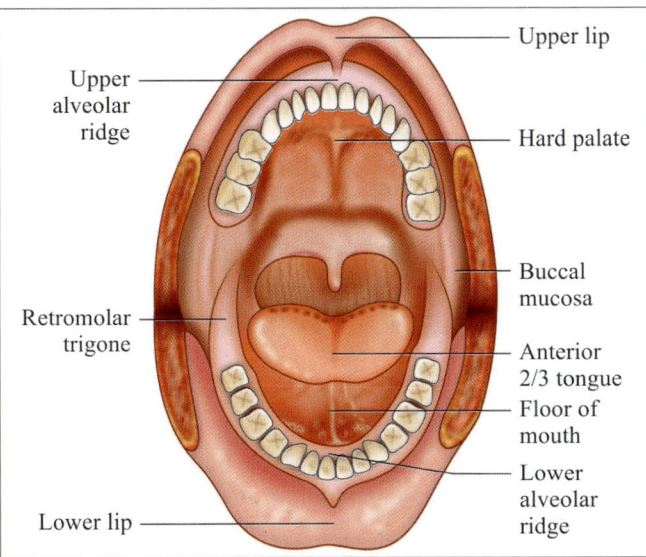

Fig. 29.1: Oral cavity overview

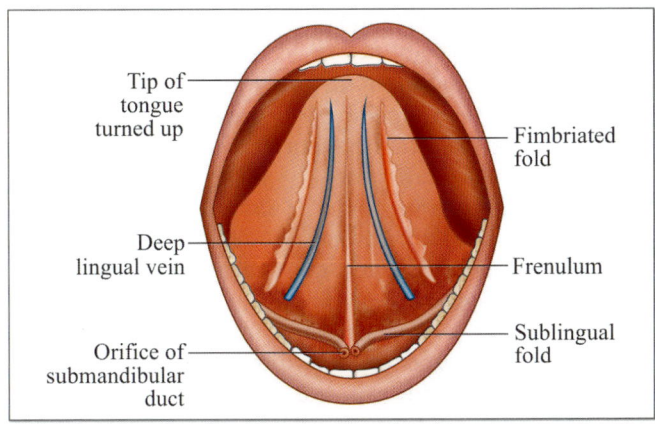

Fig. 29.2: Inferior surface of tongue and floor of mouth

Table 29.1: Subsites of cancer in oral cavity

- *Lip (vermilion surface)*
    - Upper lip
    - Lower lip
    - Commissures
- *Buccal mucosa* (includes mucosa of cheek and inner surface of lips up to line of contact of opposing lip)—mucosal surfaces of:
    - Upper and lower lips
    - Cheeks
    - Retromolar area
    - Upper and lower buccoalveolar sulci
- *Anterior two-third of tongue* (anterior to circumvallate papillae)
    - Dorsal and ventral surfaces
    - Lateral borders
    - Tip
- *Hard palate*
- *Lower alveolar ridge* (alveolus and gingiva)
- *Upper alveolar ridge* (alveolus and gingiva)
- *Floor of mouth*
- *Retromolar trigone*

Source: AJCC 1997

- *Upper lip:* It drains into preauricular, infraparotid and submandibular nodes.

ALVEOLI AND GINGIVAE

Gums (gingivae) surround the teeth and cover the upper and lower alveolar ridges.
- *Lymphatic drainage:*
    - *Upper alveolus:*
        - Buccal aspect drains to submandibular nodes
        - Lingual aspect drains either directly to upper deep cervical or through the lateral retropharyngeal nodes.
    - *Lower alveolus:* The central part of both buccal and lingual surfaces of mucosa drains to submental whereas lateral parts drain to submandibular nodes.

FLOOR OF MOUTH (FIG. 29.2)

Floor of mouth is a crescent-shaped area that lies between the gingivae and ventral surface of tongue. There are few minor salivary glands in the floor of mouth.
- *Examination:*
    - *Anterior portion of the floor* (frenulum, sublingual papillae with openings of submandibular ducts) is examined when patient raises the tip of tongue towards the hard palate.
    - *Lateral portion of the U-shaped floor of mouth* is examined by displacing the tongue in medial direction with the help of a tongue depressor.
- *Lymphatic drainage:*
    - *Anterior portion of floor of mouth* drains into submental and submandibular nodes (level I). Lymphatics here cross the midline.
    - *Posterior portion* drains into upper deep cervical nodes (level II and III).

BUCCAL MUCOSA

It is covered with non-keratinizing stratified squamous epithelium. Buccal mucosa lines the inner surface of cheeks and lips and extends between the superior and inferior gingivobuccal sulcus. It extends posteriorly up to pterygomandibular raphe and anteriorly to the meeting line of lips. It covers parotid duct, minor salivary glands, buccinator muscle and upper and lower alveoli.

Lymphatic Drainage

Buccal mucosa drains into submental and submandibular nodes and from there to the deep cervical lymph nodes.

> Carcinoma of buccal mucosa is the second most common cancer of oral cavity after the tongue.

Retromolar Trigone

Retromolar trigone is a triangular area of mucosa that covers anterior border of the ascending ramus of mandible. It lies behind the third molar, where the pterygomandibular raphe is attached to the mandible. Its base lies posterior to the last molar and its apex is towards the maxillary tuberosity. The pterygomandibular raphe provides origin to superior constrictor and buccinator muscles.

HARD PALATE

Hard palate forms the roof of the oral cavity and floor of the nasal cavity. It contains high number of minor salivary glands.

> In hard palate, minor salivary glands tumors (such as adenoid cystic, mucoepidermoid and adenocarcinoma) are more common than squamous cell carcinoma. Most of the squamous cell carcinoma of upper alveolus and hard palate arises from maxillary antrum.

Lymphatic Drainage

- Anterior part of palate drains to submandibular nodes
- Posterior part drains either directly to the upper deep cervical or via lateral retropharyngeal nodes.

TONGUE

Anterior two-third of tongue is the content of the oral cavity (Fig. 29.3). Posterior one-third (base of tongue) is situated behind the circumvallate papillae and forms anterior wall oropharynx.
- *Parts:* Oral tongue has the tip, lateral borders and dorsum and ventral surfaces of the tongue.

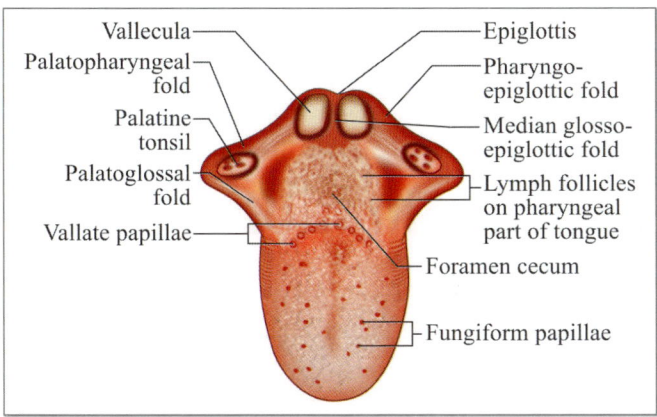

Fig. 29.3: Dorsum of the tongue and oropharynx

- Carcinoma of tongue is the most common cancer of oral cavity.
- The interlacing tongue muscle fibers and constant movement of tongue (speech and chewing) facilitate spread and wide dissemination of tongue cancer.
- During the surgery, palpation of tongue tumors and excision of cancer lesion with 2 cm safe margin are of paramount importance.

Lymphatic Drainage

- Tip drains to submental and deep jugular cervical chain.
- Ventral surface drains to the submandibular nodes.
- The rest of the anterior two-third of tongue drains to the deep jugular chain of lymph nodes. These level III nodes are situated between digastric and omohyoid muscles.
- Central portion and base drain into deep cervical nodes of both sides.

Lymphatics from anterior portion of mouth can sometimes drain directly to lower jugular chain (levels III and IV).

The patients with cancer of lateral border of anterior two-third can have enlargement only of jugulodigastric and jugulomohyoid lymph nodes.

Pre-Facial and Post-Facial Lymph Nodes

These lymph nodes are present near the anteroinferior angle of masseter muscle where facial artery crosses the inferior margin of mandible. Prefacial and post-facial lymph nodes are often affected in cancer of mouth patients and should be removed along with the radical or modified radical neck dissection.

TASTE BUDS

They are in highest number (250) in circumvallate papillae and least (1–18) in fungiform papillae. There are practically no buds in filiform papillae. Foliate papillae have second highest number (100) of taste buds.

Self-evaluation Exercises

1. Which are the two most common cancer of oral cavity?
   a. Buccal mucosa
   b. Tongue
   c. Lip
   d. Alveolus
2. Which is the most common site for minor salivary gland tumor?
   a. Lips
   b. Floor of mouth
   c. Hard palate
   d. Tongue
3. Which of the following statements are not true for taste buds?
   a. Highest number (250) in circumvallate papillae
   b. Least (1–18) in fungiform papillae
   c. Practically no buds in filiform papillae
   d. Foliate papillae have second highest number (100) of taste buds
   e. None of the above

True (T)/False (F)

4. The interlacing tongue muscle fibers and constant movement of tongue (speech and chewing) check the spread and wide dissemination of tongue cancer.
5. The patients with cancer of lateral border of anterior two-third can have enlargement only of jugulodigastric and jugulomohyoid lymph nodes.
6. Posterior part of hard palate drains either directly to the upper deep cervical or via lateral retropharyngeal nodes.
7. Vertical midline sulcus of upper lip extending from nasal columella to vermilion border is called philtrum.

Answers
1. a, b   2. c   3. e   4. F   5. T   6. T   7. T

Chapter 30

Oral Symptoms and Examination

⦿ Specific Learning Objectives

After going through the chapter, you should be able to answer the following questions:
- What are the different oral symptoms and how will you conduct the examination of oral cavity?
- What are the different findings you seek during examination of oral cavity and their causes?
- How will you evaluate a case of cancer of oral cavity?

For general scheme of case taking and general set up of Bull's eye lamp light source and head-mirror *see* Chapter 'History and Examination'.

ORAL CAVITY

Symptoms

Patients may come to doctor after observing some findings in their mouth, such as an abnormal growth, coating of tongue, cleft lip, cleft palate and oroantral fistula. Patient may see their circumvallate papillae of tongue in the mirror or feel by finger and develop cancer phobia.

- *Pain:* May be referred to the ear. It can occur in any part of the oral cavity.
- *Xerostomia:** Dryness of mouth can be caused by mouth breathing, radiotherapy and generalized lesions of the salivary glands. 1,000–1,500 mL of saliva is secreted in 24 hours. Major amount of saliva, when salivary glands are not stimulated is secreted by submandibular glands.
- *Excessive salivation:* The common causes of excessive salivation are—ulcers of mouth and pharynx, poor orodental hygiene, ill fitting denture and iodide therapy.
- *Dysgeusia:*** Patient can have unilateral or bilateral perverted, diminished and loss of taste. It may be associated with lesions, such as heavily coated tongue, injury to chorda tympani or the facial nerve. Taste buds on the anterior two-third of tongue appreciate sweet, sour and salt tastes.

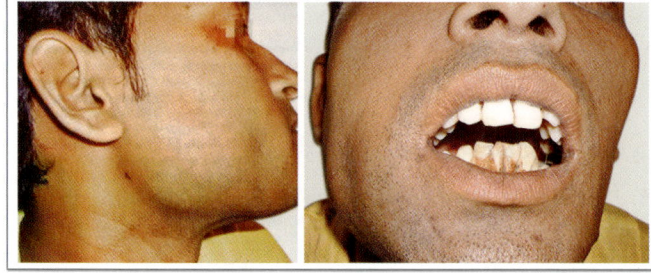

Fig. 30.1: Trismus in a patient of masticator space abscess

- *Trismus:**** The common causes of difficulty in opening the mouth, which are related to the local oral cavity are oral submucous fibrosis, ulcerative lesions, dental abscess (Fig. 30.1), trauma to mandible and maxilla, and malignant lesions of buccal mucosa and retromolar trigone.
- *Other:* Other oral cavity complaints include ulcers, swelling, ankyloglossia, cleft lip, cleft palate, injury, halitosis, toothache and gums swelling and bleeding.

- **Sense of taste:** It is highly redundant due to its rich innervation. It is nearly impossible to lose all sense of taste.
- **Taste and flavor:** They are usually confused with each other. The taste includes only the ability to sense sweet, salty, bitter and sour tastes. Flavor includes both taste and smell (80%). Patients with taste problems may be having flavor and a smell disorders.

---
*G. xeros, dry + G. stoma, mouth
**Dys, bad, difficult + G. geusis, taste
***L. fr. G. trismus, a creaking, rasping

Chapter 30 • Oral Symptoms and Examination

Table 30.1: Findings on examination of oral cavity

- **Lips (upper and lower):** Swellings, growths, vesicles, ulcers, crusts, scars, unilateral and bilateral clefts.
- **Buccal mucosa:** Change in color, ulceration, vesicles, bullae (pemphigus), white stria (lichen planus), blanched appearance with submucosal fibrous bands (submucous fibrosis), leukoplakia, erythroplakia, pigmentation, atrophic change in mucosa, swelling or growth.
- **Opening of parotid duct:** Red, swollen, secretions (viral and suppurative parotitis).
- **Gums of upper and lower jaws:** Red and swollen gums (gingivitis), ulcerated gums covered with membrane (viral ulcers and Vincent's infection), hyperplasia (pregnancy and dilantin therapy), growths (benign or malignant neoplasms of maxilla or mandible), periodontitis.
- **Teeth:** Number, tartar, loose teeth, carious, malocclusion (fractures of mandible and maxilla, abnormalities of temporomandibular joint), impacted last molar.
- **Hard palate:** Cleft palate, oronasal fistula (trauma and syphilis), high arched palate (mouth breathing in adenoids), swelling (tumors of palate and nose), bony growth in midline of hard palate (torus palatinus), ulcers/growths (benign and malignant).
- **Tongue:** Macroglossia (hemangioma, lymphangioma, cretinism, edema and abscess), ankyloglossia (congenital tongue tie, cancer tongue and floor of mouth, painful ulcer, abscess), deviation on protrusion (hypoglossal paralysis on the side of deviation), bald and smooth tongue (iron deficiency anemia, median rhomboid glossitis, geographical tongue), fissures (Melkersson's syndrome, syphilis), ulcers (aphthous, traumatic due to jagged tooth and denture, malignant, syphilitic and tubercular), red/white lesions (leukoplakia, erythroplakia), proliferative growth (malignancy).
- **Floor of mouth:** Short frenulum (tongue-tie), scar (trauma and corrosive burn), ulcer (trauma, erosion of submandibular duct stone, aphthous ulcer, malignancy), swelling (ranula, sublingual dermoid, calculus of submandibular duct, benign and malignant tumors, Ludwig's angina).
- **Opening of submandibular duct:** Red, swollen, secretions.

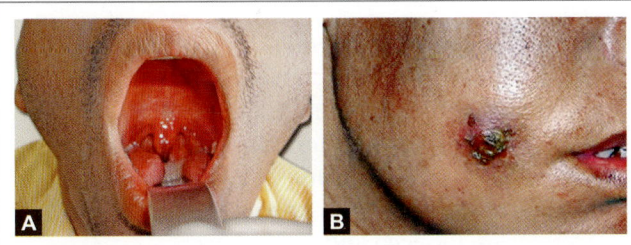

Figs 30.2A and B: (A) Tongue depressor used in the examination of oral cavity and oropharynx; Note submucosal cleft palate with bifid uvula; (B) Skin involvement in buccal mucosa carcinoma

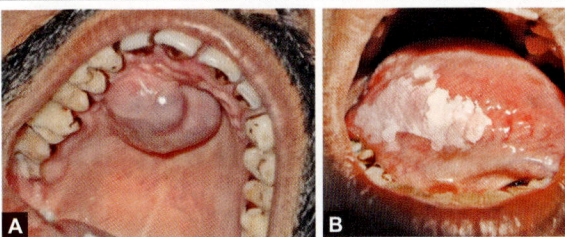

Figs 30.3A and B: (A) Hard palate hemangioma; (B) Hairy leukoplakia tongue
Source: (A) Dr Amit Goyal, AIIMS, Jodhpur

Examination

Examine all the different parts of oral cavity by both inspection, as well as palpation (Table 30.1). Tongue depressors (Fig. 30.2A) are used in the examination of oral cavity and oropharynx and are available in different sizes for children and adults.

- **Lips:** They have an outer (cutaneous), an inner (mucosal) surface and a vermilion border.
- **Buccal mucosa:** It is examined by asking the patient to open the mouth and then retracting the cheek with a tongue depressor.
  - Look for not only the change in color but also change in surface appearance. Parotid duct opening can be seen opposite the crown of upper second molar tooth. Examine the skin of the cheek because carcinoma of buccal mucosa can invade the same (Fig. 30.2B).
- **Teeth and gums:** Examine gums and teeth of both upper and lower jaws. Cheeks and lips are retracted with the help of tongue depressor for examining the outer surface of gums while tongue is pushed away for examining the inner surface of gums.
- **Hard palate:** See for any swelling (Fig. 30.3A), ulcer and cleft.
- **Anterior two-third tongue:** Tongue should be examined in its natural position and then patient is asked to protrude it and move it in different directions (Figs 30.3B to 30.5).
- **Floor of mouth:** The floor of mouth consists of the area that lies under the tongue and two lateral gutters (Fig. 30.5B). The latter are examined by two tongue depressors that retract tongue and cheek. The submandibular duct opens on the summit of raised papilla on either side of the tongue frenulum. The swellings in the floor of mouth are examined by bimanual palpation, which help in differentiating between submandibular salivary gland and submandibular lymph nodes (Fig. 30.6A).

Tongue Depressor

One blade of Lack's tongue depressor is slightly bent at the end. The bent end is used for holding the depressor and supports the little finger of the examiner. The other blade

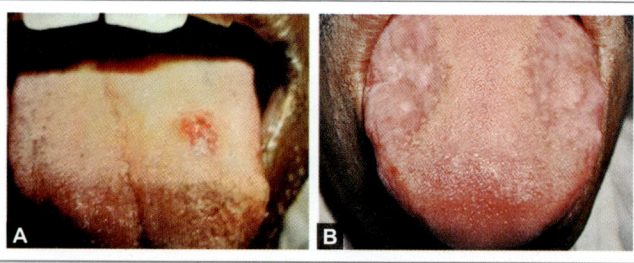

Fig. 30.4A and B: (A) Tongue bite during chewing food; (B) Glossitis involving bilateral margins of the tongue. A 38-year-old male patient with complaints of burning sensations on the margins of tongue for 5 days

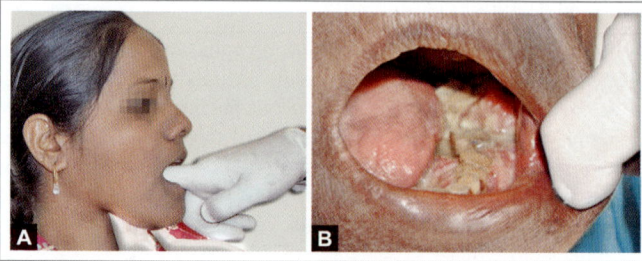

Figs 30.6A and B: (A) Bimanual palpation of floor of mouth and submandibular region; (B) Carcinoma left lower alveolus (premolar to retromolar region) extending to buccal mucosa, floor of mouth and cheek skin

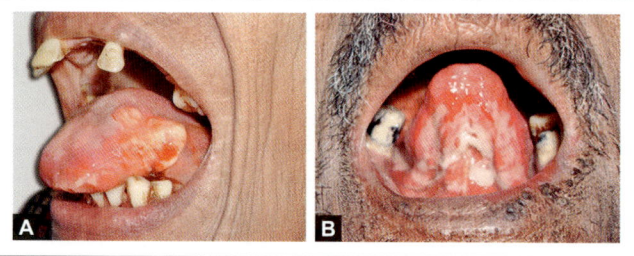

Figs 30.5A and B: (A) Carcinoma anterior two-third tongue left lateral margin. Note two separate infiltrative lesions involving tip and middle one-third tongue; (B) Ulcerative lesions involving under surface of tongue and floor of mouth. Note that the tip of tongue is touching the hard palate

depresses the tongue and is used like a lever to depress anterior two-thirds of the tongue with the fulcrum over the lower teeth.

Caution: Touching of the posterior one-third of the tongue with the tongue depressor must be avoided as it usually leads to the gag reflex and not tolerated by the patient.

- *Uses:* It is used for examining the oral cavity and the pharynx. In addition to the depressing of tongue it can also be used for:
  - Squeezing the tonsil
  - Retraction of cheek laterally and tongue medially
  - Test for gag reflex
  - Checking nasal air blast (cold spatula test)
  - Spatula test for suspected case of tetanus.

Sialography: It is used to diagnose stones, chronic inflammation and tumors in parotid and submandibular glands. It is contraindicated in acute inflammation and acute sialectasis.

EVALUATION OF ORAL CANCER PATIENTS

The diagnosis of oral cancer is primarily clinical and confirmed by histopathology. A detailed history, physical examination including palpation (Fig. 30.6A) and investigations should include the following elements:

- *History:*
  - *Symptoms:* They include changes in the size of existing denture, otalgia, oral-dental pain, odynophagia, facial numbness, trismus, dysarthria, dysphagia, bleeding, halitosis and weight loss.
  - *Personal and past history:* Patient is inquired about medications, allergies, medical illnesses, previous surgeries, tobacco and alcohol use.
- *Examination:*
  - *Local lesion:* Dimension and extension including crossing midline, adjacent structures involved; fixation to underlying periosteum of mandible (Fig. 30.6B) and maxilla, regional lymphatic spread.
  - *Need for reconstruction:* Explore need for reconstruction and their options, and available free and pedicled flap.
  - *Dental evaluation:* Before radiation treatment, prosthodontic evaluation for surgical obturator in cases of maxillectomy.
  - *Speech and swallowing:* Consultation and counseling with speech and swallowing pathologist.
- *Investigations:*
  - *Routine:* ECG, X-ray chest (preferably both postero-anterior and lateral views) and basic laboratory profile, liver profile in alcoholics.
  - *Biopsy:* Punch/incisional biopsy from the periphery of the tumor including some normal adjacent mucosa confirms the tissue diagnosis. Areas of necrosis and infection should be avoided as this tissue may confuse the pathologist.
  - *Fine needle aspiration cytology (FNAC):* It is indicated in cases of suspicious nodes in the presence of known primary carcinoma.

- **Synchronous second primary cancer:** Search for synchronous upper aerodigestive tract cancers. About 15% patients of the oral cavity cancer have multiple primary cancers, which are present in the upper aerodigestive tract. Risk factors (such as smoking and alcohol) are common for all these cancer sites.
- **Panendoscopy:** It includes bronchoscopy, esophagoscopy and direct laryngoscopy, and has been advocated by many in all head and neck cancer patients.
- **Imaging:** They help in knowing the extent of primary tumor and regional lymphadenopathy.
- **Computerized tomography:** CT is best for demonstrating cortical bone erosion and lymph node metastases.
- **Magnetic resonance imaging:** MRI is best for seeing soft tissue invasion by tumor and extension into medullary bone.
- **Orthopantogram:** In patients with suspected mandibular invasion, panorex or orthopantogram facilitates dental evaluation.
- **Ultrasound:** Abdominal ultrasound detects liver metastasis.
- **Positron emission tomography (PET) and single-photon emission computed tomography (SPECT):** In stage IV patients, PET and SPECT identify occult distant metastasis.

Self-evaluation Exercises

1. Some of the causes of excessive salivation are:
    a. Oral iodides
    b. Poorly fitting denture
    c. Ulcers in oral cavity
    d. Peritonsillitis
    e. All of the above
2. Sialography is used to diagnose which lesions of parotid and submandibular glands:
    a. Stones
    b. Chronic inflammation
    c. Tumors
    d. All of the above

True (T)/False (F)

3. About 500 mL of saliva is secreted in 24 hours.
4. Major amount of saliva, when salivary glands are not stimulated is secreted by parotid glands.
5. Sialography is contraindicated in acute inflammation of salivary glands and acute sialectasis.

Answers

1. e   2. d   3. F   4. F   5. T

Pearls and Nuggets (Refresh your knowledge)

- **Peutz-Jeghers syndrome:** The benign intestinal polyps are associated with perinasal, perioral and buccal mucosal pigmentation.
- **Psammoma bodies:** They are seen in the papillary carcinoma of thyroid gland.
- **HIV/AIDS:** Biopsy of new oral lesions must be done early to rule out malignancy.
- **Oral thrush in adults:** The common risk factors are corticosteroid and broad spectrum antibiotics, pregnancy, diabetes mellitus, nutritional deficiency and human immunodeficiency virus.
- **Viral sialadenitis:** Mumps is the most common parotid viral infection. Less common viral infections are Cytomegalovirus, Coxsackie and Epstein-Barr viruses.
- **Bacterial sialadenitis:** It is usually caused coagulase positive S. aureus. S. pneumoniae, E. coli, H. influenzae and oral anaerobe infections may also occur.
- **Sjogren's syndrome:** A positive ANA, RF, SS-a, SS-b and an elevated ESR are indicative of Sjogren's syndrome. Biopsy from lip confirms the diagnosis and shows atrophy of minor salivary glands with an abundance of lymphocytes and histiocytes.
- **Malignancy of salivary glands:** Their presentation may be similar to benign tumors and can lead to delay in diagnosis.
- **Cleft and craniofacial anomalies:** The care of these patients needs many medical and surgical subspecialties and requires a team management.
    - **Initial management:** The children need a secure airway and adequate nutrition.
- **Cleft lip:** Maxillary prominence fails to fuse with intermaxillary segment.
- **Cleft palate:** Eustachian tube dysfunction can cause persistent otitis media with effusion and recurrent acute otitis media.
- **Tongue:** All the intrinsic and extrinsic muscles of tongue are supplied by the hypoglossal nerve except the palatoglossal, which is innervated by vagal accessory nerve.

Chapter 31

Oral Mucosal Lesions

Specific Learning Objectives

After going through the chapter, you should be able to answer the following questions:
- Describe the etiopathogenesis, clinical features and management of oral submucous fibrosis.
- Describe the various clinical forms of oral leukoplakia and their management. How will you differentiate it from erythroplakia?
- What are the different clinical forms of lichen planus and their management?
- How will you differentiate between the two forms of candidiasis and manage them?
- What do you know about: (1) Pemphigus vulgaris; (2) Mucous membrane pemphigoid; (3) Erythema multiforme; (4) Acute necrotizing ulcerative gingivitis; (5) Premalignant lesions of oral cavity?
- What are the differences between primary and secondary herpes simplex infection and how will you manage them?
- Describe the predisposing factors, clinical forms and management of recurrent aphthous stomatitis.

INTRODUCTION

Impairment to oral health can lead to malnutrition, infection, impaired communication, pain and an impaired quality of life. The various oral mucosal lesions are enumerated in the Box 31.1. The purpose of this chapter is to provide an overview of some of the common oral mucosal disorders.

RED/WHITE LESIONS

ORAL SUBMUCOUS FIBROSIS (OSMF)

It is an insidious painless oral cavity disease, which is characterized by juxta epithelial deposition of fibrous tissue that sometimes even extends to the pharynx. Joshi in 1953 first described this condition in India. The disease is prevalent (2–5 per 1,000) throughout the Indian subcontinent.

Etiopathogenesis

Several factors operate together and cause this disorder. Exact etiology of this condition is not known but the following factors have been incriminated:
- *Prolonged local irritation:*
  - *Chewing of betel, areca nut and tobacco:* Most of these patients have habit of chewing *paan* (a specially prepared leaf), betel nut (*sopari*) and

> **Box 31.1: Oral mucosal lesions**
> - *Red/white lesions*: Oral submucous fibrosis, oral leukoplakia, oral hairy leukoplakia, oral lichen planus, chronic discoid lupus erythematosus, candidiasis, fordyce spots, nicotine stomatitis.
> - *Vesiculobullous/ulcerative lesions*: Pemphigus vulgaris, mucous membrane (cicatricial) pemphigoid, primary herpes simplex infection, recurrent herpes simplex infection, herpes simplex infection, hand foot and mouth disease, herpangina, acute necrotizing ulcerative gingivitis, recurrent aphthous stomatitis, Behcet's syndrome, erythema multiforme, traumatic (eosinophilic) granuloma, traumatic ulcers, radiation mucositis, blood disorders, drug-induced oral lesions.
> - *Pigmented lesions*: Melanotic macules, melanoma, amalgam tattoo.
> - *Systemic diseases*: Cardiovascular, endocrine, gastroenterology, neurological, renal, hematological (leukemia, agranulocytosis, pancytopenia, cyclic neutropenia, sickle cell anemia).
> - *Collagen-vascular and granulomatous disorders*: Sjögren's syndrome, systemic lupus erythematosus, scleroderma, dermatomyositis-polymyositis, sarcoidosis, Wegener's granulomatosis.
> - *Lesions of tongue*: Geographical tongue, hairy tongue, fissured tongue, tongue tie.

tobacco. The hard and rough surface of betel nut causes mechanical irritation. *Alkaloids* in betel nut (such as *arecoline*) cause chemical irritation and

stimulate collagen synthesis and the proliferation of buccal mucosa fibroblasts. *Tannins* in betel nut stabilize the collagen fibrils and render them resistant to degradation by the collagenase.
  - *Smoking* of cigarettes/*bidies* also leads to local irritation.
  - *Alcohol:* Consumption of too much alcohol has been linked with premaligant and malignant conditions.
  - *Excessive amount of chilies and spices* in the daily food may also be an additional factor.
- *Dietary deficiency:* As there occurs recurrent vesicle formation and ulceration of the oral mucosa a dietary deficiency of iron, vitamins B-complex and A has been proposed. With vitamin A, zinc and antioxidants patients feel improvement. Lack of fruits and vegetables in diet has been linked with leukoplakia, erythroplakia and submucous fibrosis.
- *Socioeconomic status:* People of lower socioeconomic status have been seen to be at higher risk of developing leukoplakia, erythroplakia and submucous fibrosis.
- *Cell-mediated immune process:* Some consider it a cell-mediated immune reaction to arecoline. Arecanut chewing causes collection of activated T-lymphocytes and macrophages in subepithelial layers of oral mucosa, which result in reduced production of antifibrotic cytokines (less collagenase) and increased production of fibrinogenic cytokines (act on mesenchymal cells and proliferate fibroblasts). These lead to increased production of collagen.
- *Localized collagen disease:* As the histopathological changes seen in submucous fibrosis are similar to the collagen diseases such as rheumatoid arthritis and scleroderma, some scientists think it to be a localized collagen disorder.
- *Racial:* Disease usually affects Indians or people of Indian origin living abroad. Sporadic cases are also seen in Nepal, Thailand, South Vietnam and Sri Lanka.
- *Genetic:* As the disease usually affects Indians and not all the people who chew *paan, sopari* and tobacco, some authorities strongly feel it to be genetic disorder.

Pathology

- Early cases show polymorphonuclear leukocytes, eosinophils and few lymphocytes while lymphocytes and plasma cells appear in advanced cases. The higher population of activated T-lymphocytes mainly T-helper/inducer lymphocytes (minor population of B-cells), macrophages and high $CD4_+$ and $CD8_+$ lymphocyte ratio in subepithelial tissue suggest main role of cellular immune response and minor role of humoral immunity.
- The cytokines produced by macrophages and T-lymphocytes lead to synthesis of collagen and fibrosis.
- There occurs a fibroelastotic transformation of connective tissues in lamina propria associated with epithelial atrophy, which is sometime preceded by vesicle formation.
- Juxta-epithelial fibrosis occurs with atrophy or hyperplasia of overlying epithelium, which shows areas of epithelial dysplasia. The process of fibrosis and loss of vascularity can extend deeper into the muscles.

Potential for Malignant Change

- Leukoplakia and squamous cell carcinoma are some time associated with this condition as the predisposing factors for all these disorders are common
- The malignant transformation (Fig. 31.1A) has been observed in 3–7.6% of cases.

Clinical Features

- *Age and sex:* Though there is no age and sex bar, the disease mostly affects male patients of 20–40 years.
- *Habits:* History of chewing of *paan, sopari* or tobacco is almost always present.
- *Trismus:* The majority of the patients present with gradually progressive painless difficulty in opening the mouth. (Fig. 31.1B).
- *Ankyloglossia:* The disease may advance and cause difficulty in protruding out the tongue.
- *Soreness and burning mouth:* Some patients have soreness of mouth with constant burning sensation, which worsens during meals especially of pungent spicy type. In later stages, patient develops insidious, painless and progressive trismus and ankyloglossia.
- *Vesicles/Ulcers:* Few patients complain of repeated vesicular eruption on the palate and pillars. Initially there occurs patchy redness of mucous membrane with formation of vesicles, which rupture and form superficial ulcers.
- *Fibrous bands:* The most common sites of white fibrotic bands (Fig. 31.2A) are soft palate, faucial pillars, retromolar area and buccal mucosa. In later stages, fibrosis develops in the submucosal layers along with the blanching of mucosa with loss of suppleness. Fibrosis and scarring, which can be seen and felt has

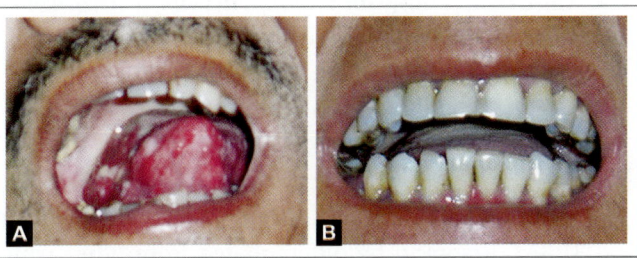

Figs 31.1A and B: Oral submocous fibrosis (OSMF). (A) Malignancy of tongue right lateral margin in case of OSMF; (B) OSMF. Severe trismus with 0.73 cm mouth opening

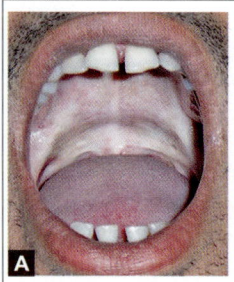 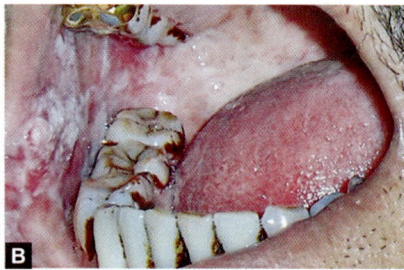

Figs 31.2A and B: (A) Oral submucous fibrosis. White fibrous bands involving soft palate, faucial pillars and retromolar area; (B) Leukoplakia of buccal mucosa. Opaque elevated thickened and leathery lesion

Box 31.2: Grafts and flaps tried for reconstruction in the management of oral submucous fibrosis
- Bilateral tongue flap
- Nasolabial flaps
- Island palatal mucoperiosteal flap
- Bilateral radial forearm free flap
- Buccal pad of fat graft
- Temporalis fascia graft
- Split skin graft

also been demonstrated in the underlying muscle that lead to further restrictive mobility of soft palate, tongue and jaw.

Treatment

- *Medical*
    - *Local steroids/hylase:* Topical injection of steroids, which may be combined with hylase, into the area of fibrous bands (injection dexamethasone 4 mg and hylase 1500 IU in one mL intraoral submucosal biweekly at different sites for 8–10 weeks) is more effective than their systemic use. This brings significant improvement in symptoms and relieves trismus.
    - *Avoidance of irritant factors* (areca nuts, *pan*, tobacco, pungent foods) is of paramount importance.
    - *Vitamins and minerals:* Treat anemia and vitamin deficiencies. Vitamin A, zinc and antioxidants therapy has shown some beneficial effect.
    - *Jaw opening exercises:* They are encouraged.
- *Surgical:* Number of surgical procedures have been reported.
    - *Surgical incision of fibrous bands:* Severe trismus associated with marked fibrous bands can be treated by surgical excision and grafting. It gives immediate dramatic improvement in opening of the mouth but usually results in rebound trismus.
    - *Lasers* have also been used to cut the fibrous bands.
    - *Coronoidectomy and temporal muscle myotomy*.
    - *Reconstruction:* Several types of grafts and flaps have been tried after cutting the fibrous bands (Box 31.2).

ORAL LEUKOPLAKIA

Leukoplakia clinically present as a white patch (Fig. 31.2B and 31.3A). It should be differentiated from other white lesions of oral mucosa such as lichen planus, discoid lupus erythematosus, white spongy nevus and candidiasis.

Risk Factors

The exact cause is not known but the risk factors include:
- *The incriminating factors,* which are seen along with this lesion, are:
    - *Tobacco smoking*
    - *Smokeless tobacco:* Tobacco chewing
    - *Alcohol abuse:* It is especially harmful if combined with smoking
    - *Areca nut and betel*
- *Associated diseases:* The lesion is some time associated with:
    - Submucous fibrosis
    - Hyperplastic candidiasis
    - Plummer-Vinson syndrome.
- *Sex:* Males are affected two to three times more often than females.
- *Age:* Mostly it is seen in the fourth decade of life.

Clinical Features

- *Site:* Though the most common sites are buccal mucosa (especially in India) and oral commissures, it may also be seen over floor of mouth, tongue, gingivobuccal sulcus and lip.
- *Lesion:* Widely variable clinical lesions include homogeneous and smooth, focal, diffuse, heterogeneous and multifocal with variable texture.
    - The white, yellowish or gray surface alteration with ill-defined margins. Plaques may be small circumscribed or extensive and soft, thicker or feel crusty.
    - Surface texture can be finely granular, slightly papillary, ulcerative, erosive, nodular, or verrucous.
- *Induration:* Induration indicates malignant change and immediate biopsy should be taken.

Clinical Forms

There are different clinical types of leukoplakia. Nodular and erosive types have higher incidence of malignant transformation.

- *Homogenous leukoplakia (thin leukoplakia):* This smooth or wrinkled white patch is less associated with malignancy. Macular lesion may gradually progress to more opaque elevated thickened, furrowed, leathery

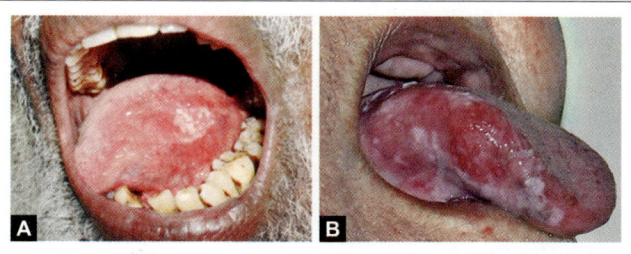

Figs 31.3A and B: (A) Leukoplakia tongue anterior two-third lateral margin without induration. Note nodular white patches with erythematous base; (B) Erythroplakia tongue. Bright red velvety patch on the lateral margin of tongue

or wrinkled appearance. Some lesions may disappear over time.
- *Nodular (speckled) leukoplakia:* There occur nodular white patches with erythematous base (Fig. 31.3A).
- *Erosive leukoplakia (erythroleukoplakia)* presents white patches, which has erosions and fissures and is interspersed with red patches (erythroplakia).

Erythroplakia
- Erythroplakia presents as a bright red velvety red patch (Fig. 31.3B) or plaque usually over lower alveolar mucosa, gingivobuccal sulcus and the floor of the mouth.
- The lesion is irregular and clearly demarcated from adjacent normal epithelium.
- Red vascular connective tissue of the submucosa shines through the mucosa due to decreased keratinization of mucosal epithelium.
- Clinically lesion may look like granular and/or interspersed with areas of leukoplakia, which is usually indistinguishable from erythroleukoplakia type of leukoplakia.
- Most of the erythroplakia lesions show severe dysplasia, carcinoma *in situ* and frank invasive carcinoma. The malignant potential is 17 times higher than in leukoplakia.
- Treatment of this lesion needs excision biopsy either surgically or with CO_2 laser and regular follow-up.

- *Proliferative verrucous leukoplakia:* This uncommon variant of leukoplakia is multifocal and persistent and occurs more often in women. A thin flat white patch progresses to leathery thickened and papillary to verrucous quality. Recurrence rate is high and 70% cases develop squamous cell carcinoma.

Histopathology
- It ranges from hyperkeratosis and acanthosis to dysplasia (disordered cell growth and architectural distortion) and carcinoma *in situ* to invasive squamous cell carcinoma. The dysplasia is traditionally graded as mild, moderate and severe.
- About 25% of leukoplakias show epithelial dysplasia that may be from mild to severe grades. Higher grade of dysplasia indicates increased chances of malignant change.
- A clinical shift from homogeneous to heterogeneous, speckled and nodular form is an indication for rebiopsy.

Potential for Malignant Change
- Leukoplakia is the most common premalignant oral mucosal lesion.
- The chances of malignant change are from 1–17.5% (average 5%).
  - *Age and duration:* More the age and duration of the lesion greater are the chances of malignant change.
  - *Site:* Leukoplakia of floor of the mouth and ventral surface of tongue have higher incidence of malignant change.

Management
- *Biopsy:* An incisional biopsy (multiple biopsies in extensive lesions) must be taken from suspicious areas (such as erythematous, granular, ulcerated and indurated) to know the grades of dysplasia and rule out malignancy.
- *Benign or minimal dysplasia:* Observation or excision. Spontaneous regression is not uncommon in homogenous variety if incriminating factors are removed.
- *Premalignant lesions of moderate to severe dysplasia:* Excision
  - *Methods of complete removal:* Scalpel excision, laser ablation, electrocautery and cryoablation.
- *Chemoprevention:* It is indicated in treated cases and mild dysplasia. The agents include retinoids, antioxidants, cyclooxygenase (COX)-2 inhibitors.

ORAL LICHEN PLANUS
Clinical Features
- Oral lesions may be associated with skin lesions, which consist of pruritic, purple, polygonal papules that are seen on the forearms and medial side of thigh.
- The multifocal and bilateral nature of lesion differentiates lichen planus from other oral mucosal disorders. Wickham's striae is a feature of lichen planus.

Clinical Forms
In cases of erosive lichen planus and atrophic lichen planus, there is risk of malignant change.
- *Reticular lichen planus:* Symmetrical bilateral asymptomatic buccal lesions often in lower mucobuccal folds are seen in middle-aged population. White keratotic striae form lace-like pattern over a normal or erythematous mucosa. No active treatment except reassurance is required.

- *Erosive lichen planus:* It is characterized by painful ulcer on the buccal mucosa, gingivae and lateral tongue, which is surrounded by a keratotic periphery. Treatment consists of topical steroids.
- *Atrophic or erythematous lichen planus:* Thinned edematous glossy reddened mucosa with loss of surface keratinization dominates faint white striae.
- *Bullous lichen planus:* In this rare variant, the bullae size ranges from few millimeters to over 1 cm. They rupture and result in painful ulceration.

Treatment

- *Corticosteroids:* Topical intralesional injections and systemic.
- *Other alternatives:* Hydroxychloroquine, azathioprine and retinoids.

CHRONIC DISCOID LUPUS ERYTHEMATOSUS

- Oral lesions are similar to those of erosive form of lichen planus. They are always associated with skin lesions.
- Malignant change usually occurs in labial lesion near vermilion border in males. These patients should avoid bright sunlight by the application of ultraviolet barrier cream to the lips.

CANDIDIASIS (MONILIASIS)

This infection is caused by *Candida albicans* and has two forms—thrush and chronic hypertrophic candidiasis.

Acute Pseudomembranous Candidiasis (Thrush)

- *Age:* This condition can be seen in infants, children and adults.
- *Lesion:* Thrush presents as white/gray patches on the oral mucosa and tongue, which when wiped off, leave an erythematous mucosa.
- *Predisposing conditions:* Adults are usually affected when they are immunocompromised, dehydrated and suffering from diabetes, AIDS, some systemic malignancy and taking broad spectrum antibiotics, cytotoxic drugs, steroids and radiation.
- *Treatment includes:*
    - Topical application of nystatin and clotrimazole.
    - Systemic antifungal agents are fluconazole, itraconazole and ketoconazole.
    - Management of predisposing condition.

Chronic Hypertrophic (Hyperplastic) Candidiasis or Candidal Leukoplakia

This invasive *C. albicans* infection has high incidence of malignant change.

- *Most common site:* The lesion mostly affects anterior buccal mucosa often placed posterior to labial commissure along the occlusal line. A triangular pattern is seen with its apex directed posteriorly.
- *Appearance:* The dense chalky plaques of keratin cannot be wiped off. They are thicker and more opaque than noncandidal leukoplakia.
- *Treatment*
    - *Surgery:* This condition usually requires excisional surgery.
    - *Antifungal:* Long-term (many months) antifungal (such as nystatin, amphotericin or miconazole) therapy eliminates candidal infection and reduces the risk of malignant transformation.

Median Rhomboid Glossitis

- The exact cause of this condition is not well understood. Some believe it to be a persistence of tuberculum impar. Recent studies have revealed chronic candida infection.
- As the name suggests a red rhomboid area, devoid of papillae is seen on the dorsum of tongue in front of foramen cecum.
- The condition is asymptomatic and an incidental finding and does not need treatment.

Oral thrush in adults: The common risk factors are corticosteroid and broad spectrum antibiotics, pregnancy, diabetes mellitus, nutritional deficiency and human immunodeficiency virus.

FORDYCE'S SPOTS

- The aberrant sebaceous glands may be seen as yellowish or yellow-brown spots, which shine through the buccal or labial mucosa.
- They are seen equally in both the sexes and are considered normal.

NICOTINE STOMATITIS

- The condition is a misnomer as nicotine is not the cause of this disease.
- In smokers (especially reverse smoking) palatal mucosa shows pin point red spots in the center of umbilicated papular lesions, which are due to inflammation of the minor salivary glands. The openings of the ducts of minor salivary glands react to the heat of the smoke
- *Treatment:* Patients are advised to give up the habit of smoking.

VESICULOBULLOUS/ULCERATIVE LESIONS

PEMPHIGUS VULGARIS

This autoimmune mucocutaneous life threatening disorder is characterized by intraepithelial cleavage and affects older age group of 50–70 years.

Clinical Features

Upper aerodigestive tract lesions precede skin lesions by months to years in more than 70% of the patients.
- *Lesions:* The initial vesiculobullous lesions produce erosions, blisters, ulcers and pain that tend to run a chronic course. In contrast to pemphigoid, pemphigus ulcers heal faster and without scarring. Healing is followed by formation of new lesions.
- *Sites:* Predominantly oropharynx, soft palate and buccal and labial mucosa. Erythematous and friable gingival marginal lesions bleed easily on slightest provocation. They extend to alveolar mucosa.

Treatment

Treatment includes systemic steroids and cytotoxic drugs.

MUCOUS MEMBRANE PEMPHIGOID OR CICATRICIAL PEMPHIGOID

This is a heterogeneous cluster of autoimmune subepithelial disorder.

Clinical Features

- *Head and neck sites:* Oral mucosa is most commonly involved followed by ocular (conjunctiva), nasal, nasopharyngeal, laryngeal and esophageal areas. Keratinized tissue of palatal and gingival area is more commonly affected than buccal.
- *Lesions:* Patchy distribution of vesicles and bullae and erythematous features. Bulla filled with clear or hemorrhagic fluid ruptures to form superficial ulceration, which are covered with shaggy collapsed mucosa. Skin lesions may be absent.

Treatment

Similar to pemphigus treatment consists of steroids.

HERPES SIMPLEX VIRUS: HERPETIC GINGIVOSTOMATITIS OR OROLABIAL HERPES

The herpes simplex virus infection has two types of clinical presentation—primary and secondary.

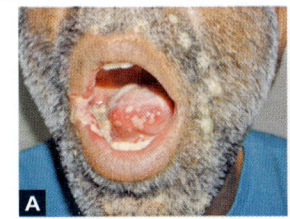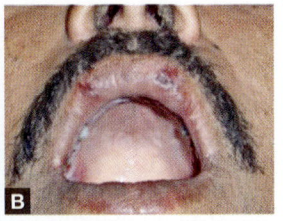

Figs 31.4A and B: (A) Herpetic gingivostomatitis involving perioral skin; (B) Herpes labialis

Primary Herpes Simplex Infection

- *Prevalence:* Affects 60–90% of population. Common in children and less common in adults.
- *Lesion:* Group of thin-walled, delicate and short-lived clusters of multiple small vesicles which like herpangina rupture and form ulcers surrounded by inflammation.
- *Site:* Any part of the oral cavity both keratinized and non-keratinized can be involved (Fig. 31.4A).

Treatment

Symptomatic and supportive.

Secondary Herpes Simplex Infection or Recurrent Herpes Simplex Infection

In recurrent human herpes simplex virus (HHV-1) infection, virus lies dormant in the trigeminal ganglion. Once reactivated, they travel along peripheral sensory nerves and involve oral cavity mucosa.

Clinical Features

- *Age:* It usually affects adults and is milder in form as adults develop some immunity to herpes virus.
- *Provocations:* Some of the common precipitating factors are emotional stress, fatigue, fever, pregnancy and immune deficiency states.
- *Prodrome:* Painful, tingling and burning with subsequent vesicles at the site.
- *Lesions:* Pinhead size clustered vesicles occur over erythematous and edematous background. After 1–2 days vesicles rupture and form tender ulcers and ultimately crusting. Crusting phase is of 5–7 days. Ulcers heal without scarring. In immunosuppressed patients ulcers are big and scarring occurs.
- *Herpes labialis:* This is the most common clinical form of recurrent herpes (Fig. 31.4B). The frequency ranges from 5–23%. The site of affection is the vermilion border of the lip, skin vermilion junction and adjacent skin. The site remains same in repetitive episodes.

Treatment

- *Topical:* Topical docosanol cream and penciclovir cream for herpes labialis.

- **Systemic:** Immunocompetent adults usually do not require the specific treatment. Antiviral acyclovir, 200 mg, five times in a day for 5 days helps in cutting down the course of recurrent herpes labialis.

HAND, FOOT AND MOUTH DISEASE

In this viral infection, which usually affects children, vesicles occur not only in oral cavity (palate, tongue and buccal mucosa) but also on the skin of hands, feet and sometimes even buttocks.

HERPANGINA

- *Causatives organism:* Coxsackie viral infection.
- *Age:* It mostly affects children.
- *Lesion:* There occurs multiple, small vesicles which rupture to form small ulcers. These ulcers are usually 2–4 mm in size and have a yellow base and red areola around them.
- *Most common sites:* Movable mucosa of the faucial pillars, tonsils, soft palate and uvula.
- *Treatment:* No special treatment is needed. Ulcers usually heal by themselves within a week time.

ACUTE NECROTIZING ULCERATIVE GINGIVITIS

- *Causative microorganisms:* Vincent's infection, anaerobic fusiform bacilli and spirochete (Borelia vincenti).
- *Age:* Usually affects young adults and middle-aged persons.
- *Lesions:* It starts at the interdental papillae and then spreads to free margins of the gingivae. Gingivae become red and edematous.
- *Vincent's angina:* Ulcers, which get covered with necrotic slough, can be seen over the gingivae and on the tonsils.
- Diagnosis can be confirmed by smear from the affected area.
- *Treatment:* It includes
    - Systemic antibiotics which also cover the anaerobes (penicillin, erythromycin and metronidazole).
    - Frequent mouth washes with sodium bicarbonate solution.
    - Attention to dental hygiene.

RECURRENT APHTHOUS STOMATITIS

This most common non-traumatic form of oral ulcerative disease chiefly affects oral and oropharyngeal mucosa.

Etiology

The exact etiology is not well understood. The multifactorial etiology may have following factors:

- *Autoimmune disease:* Both T-cell mediated and antibody-mediated processes.
- *Predisposing factors*
    - Local physical trauma
    - Ultraviolet light
    - Psychological stress
    - Hormonal influences
    - Professional groups
    - Higher socioeconomic status
    - Non-smokers and non-users of smokeless tobacco.
    - Food hypersensitivity: Nuts (walnuts, hazelnuts, Brazil nuts), spices, tomatoes, and chocolate
    - HIV
    - Nutritional: Hematinic and other deficiency states such as vitamin B_{12}, folic acid and iron.

Clinical Features

- *Lesions and their sites:* It is characterized by recurrent, painful and superficial ulcers on the movable mucosa of oral cavity (lips, cheeks, tongue and floor of mouth) and oropharynx (soft palate and tonsillar pillars). It spares fixed mucosa of the hard palate and gingivae.

Herpes vs aphthous: Absence of vesicles and blistering and involvement of only non-keratinized mucosa differentiate aphthous from herpes infection.

- *Clinical forms:* The clinical forms are divided into three classes—minor, major and herpetiform aphthous ulcers.
    - *Minor:* Most common form. Small multiple ulcers occur in anterior mouth (Figs 31.5A and B).
    - *Major:* Major ulcers are deeply crated, very big (2–4 cm) and sharply marginated (Fig. 31.6A). In immunocompromised patients, these major ulcers are more severe, deeper and painful and last for longer than 6 weeks time and may serve as a marker for HIV progression.

Herpetiform aphthous stomatitis: The disproportionate pain, adult onset and absence of vesicles differentiate herpetiform ulcers from herpes ulcerations (Fig. 31.6B).

Treatment

- *Mild and infrequent episodes:* Symptomatic treatment.
    - Lignocaine viscous helps in relieving local pain.
    - Topical application of steroids and cauterization with 10% silver nitrate help many patients.
    - Tetracycline (250 mg) dissolved in 50 mL of water four times a day as mouth rinse and then to be swallowed.
- *Severe and continuous episodes:* Short-term systemic steroids.
- *Major ulcers:* Intralesional steroids.

Chapter 31 • Oral Mucosal Lesions

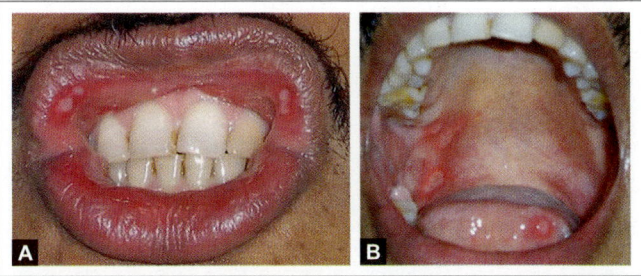

Figs 31.5A and B: (A) Minor aphthous ulcers on non-keratinized labial mucosa of anterior oral cavity; (B) Minor aphthous ulcers on non-keratinized mucosa of tongue, anterior tonsillar pillar and soft palate

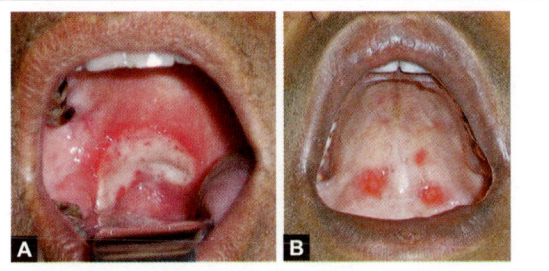

Figs 31.6A and B: (A) A major aphthous ulcer. Deeply crated very big ulcer with sharp margins involving right anterior tonsillar pillar and soft palate; (B) Herpetiform aphthous ulcers (very small and multiple) on non-keratinized mucosa of soft palate and absence of vesicles

> *HIV:* Oral manifestations include oral candidiasis, hairy leukoplakia and recurrent aphthous ulcers.

BEHÇET'S SYNDROME (OCULO-ORO-GENITAL SYNDROME)

It is a triad of:
- Aphthous-like ulcers (with punched out edge). The edge of the ulcer is characteristically punched out.
- Genital ulcerations.
- Uveitis.

The syndrome can also involve other systems of the body such as skin, joints and central nervous system.

ERYTHEMA MULTIFORME

Erythema multiforme (EM) is a self-limiting, mucocutaneous disease of unknown etiology. It is usually associated with either herpes simplex infection or drug ingestion (antiseizures and sulphonamides).

Clinical Features

It has rapid onset and involves skin and/or mucous membranes. About 25% of patients have only oral lesions. Mucosal and cutaneous bullae and ulceration occur in symmetrical distribution.

- *Oral mucosal lesions*
  - *Lesions:* Oral mucosal vesicles or bullae soon rupture and form irregular size and shape ulcers, which are covered with pseudomembrane (fibrinous plaque) and bleed easily.
  - *Site:* Any part of oral mucosa can be involved but the common sites are lips, buccal mucosa and tongue.

> *Diagnostic feature of erythema multiforme:* Hemorrhagic crusts on the vermilion portion of lips with edema and severe tenderness are the distinctive feature.

  - *Oral and oropharyngeal dysfunctions:* Sialorrhea, pain, odynophagia, dysarthria, inability to chew and swallow.
- *Skin lesions*
  - *Target or iris lesions* (concentric erythematous to pigmented patches) on the palms, soles and extensor surfaces of the extremities can be seen if the skin is involved.

Treatment

- *Specific* treatment is controversial.
- *Symptomatic treatment:* Analgesics, oral hygiene, bland mouth rinses, topical steroids, antifungal, and anesthetics.
- *Short-course of corticosteroids:* In EM minor cases as the disease is self-limiting.
- *Antivirals:* In cases of prior HHV-1 infection.

RADIATION MUCOSITIS

- Radiation therapy can affect the oral and pharynx mucosa. The mucosa initially becomes red and later on forms spotty areas of mucositis which coalesce to form large ulcerated areas that are covered by slough.
- Mucositis of cancer chemotherapy (such as methotrexate, 5-fluorouracil and bleomycin) has erythema, edema and ulceration.

BLOOD DISORDERS

- *Acute leukemia:* Acute lymphoblastic leukemia occurs in young children while acute myeloid leukemia affects middle aged and elderly people. It can cause hypertrophy of gums with ulceration and bleeding.
- *Agranulocytosis:* It may present as ulcerations in throat with severe neutropenia.
- *Cyclical neutropenia (periodic falls in neutrophil count):* Patients are prone to infections and oral ulceration.
- *Pancytopenia:* There occurs a drop in RBC count, white cell count and platelets. CBC and peripheral blood films

usually indicate the diagnosis, which further needs the study of bone marrow aspiration.

Leukemia: Oral findings include pale mucous membrane, gingival hypertrophy and petechial hemorrhages.

DRUG-INDUCED ORAL LESIONS

- Drugs like penicillin, tetracycline, sulfa drugs, barbiturates and phenytoin can cause erosive, vesicular and bullous lesions in mouth.
- Contact stomatitis (erythema, vesicles and bullae) can occur due to local reaction of mouth washes, lozenges, chewing gum, tooth paste or to prosthetic dental materials.

LESIONS OF TONGUE

GEOGRAPHICAL TONGUE OR MIGRATORY GLOSSITIS

- This asymptomatic condition is characterized by erythematous area, which is devoid of papillae and surrounded by an irregular keratotic white outline (Fig. 31.7A).
- The shape of lesions keeps on changing.
- It does not require any treatment.

HAIRY TONGUE

- *Clinical features:* The excessive formation of keratin causes elongation of the filiform papillae on the dorsum of the tongue. Due to chromogenic bacteria, they look like brown or black color hair.

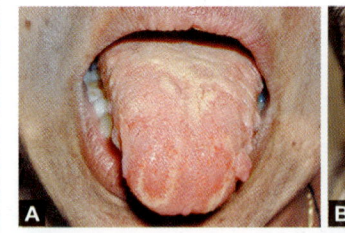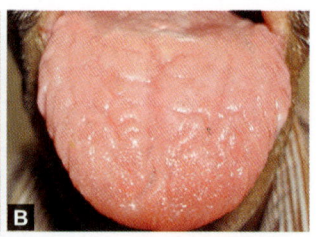

Figs 31.7 and B: (A) Geographical tongue. Note the erythematous area that is devoid of papillae and surrounded by an irregular keratotic white outline; (B) Fissured tongue

- *Smoking:* It could be one of the factors.
- *Treatment:*
  - Scraping of the lesions with a tongue cleaner.
  - Application of half strength hydrogen peroxide.
  - Vitamins.
  - Smoking is prohibited.

FISSURED TONGUE (FIG. 31.7B)

It may be congenital or acquired.
- *Acquired:* It may be due to syphilis, deficiency of vitamin B complex or anemia.
- *Congenital:* In Melkersson Rosenthal syndrome, congenital fissuring of tongue (scrotal tongue) is associated with recurrent attacks of facial palsy.

TONGUE TIE (ANKYLOGLOSSIA)

A mobile tongue helps not only in speech but also in maintaining orodental hygiene. It cleans the debris and prevents dental plaques. Symptomatic tongue tie is not common.
- Once the tongue is protruded beyond the lower incisors it can not cause speech problems.
- *Treatment:* Thick significant tongue tie needs transverse surgical release with vertical closure. Thin mucosal fold is simply incised.

Self-evaluation Exercises

1. Precancerous oral lesions having malignant potential are:
   a. Erythroplakia (erythroplasia)
   b. Leukoplakia
   c. Lichen planus
   d. Submucous fibrosis
   e. All of the above
2. Wickham's striae is a feature of lichen planus.   T/F
3. Oral findings of leukemia include:
   a. Pale mucous membrane
   b. Gingival hypertrophy
   c. Petechial hemorrhages
   d. All of the above
4. Oral manifestations of HIV include:
   a. Oral candidiasis
   b. Hairy leukoplakia
   c. Recurrent aphthous ulcers
   d. All of the above

True (T)/False (F)

5. Fordyce's spots represent normal variants of ectopic sweat glands.
6. Fordyce's spot are present as granules in oral cavity.
7. Hand, foot and mouth disease is caused by Herpes zosters virus.

Answers

1. e   2. T   3. d   4. d   5. F   6. T   7. F

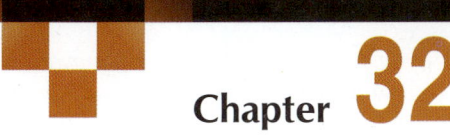

Disorders of Salivary Glands

⊙ Specific Learning Objectives

After going through the chapter, you should be able to answer the following questions:
- What are the predisposing factors, clinical features and complications of the acute suppurative parotitis and how will you manage it?
- What do you know about: (1) Recurrent parotitis of childhood; (2) Sialolithiasis; (3) Pleomorphic adenoma; (4) Mucoepidermoid carcinoma; (5) Sjogren's syndrome; (6) Frey's syndrome?

INTRODUCTION

Salivary gland disorders can be broadly divided into following categories:
- Congenital
- Inflammatory
- Obstruction and trauma
- Neoplasms
- Degenerative conditions.

Congenital disorders, which include aplasia/agenesis, ductal atresia, fistula and ectopic salivary tissue, are rare.

INFLAMMATORY DISORDERS

MUMPS

Mumps is an acute viral parotitis, which is caused by the paramyxovirus (RNA virus).

Mumps is the most common cause of nonsuppurative acute sialadenitis. It mostly affects children.

Epidemiology

- Mumps is highly contagious.
- The peak incidence occurs in the spring in temperate climates (little variation in tropics).
- The paramyxovirus is endemic in the community. It is disseminated by means of airborne droplets from salivary, nasal and urinary secretions.
- This paramyxovirus enters through the upper respiratory tract and then localizes in glandular and central nervous system tissue.
- It has an incubation period of 2–3 weeks.
- Viral infection of salivary glands may be locally asymptomatic.

Clinical Features

- Viral prodome: Low-grade fever, headache, myalgia, anorexia, arthralgia and malaise just before parotid swelling
- Mumps is characterized by localized pain, which is exacerbated on chewing.
- Parotid gland swelling is tense and firm.
- Painful swelling of the gland causes displacement of the pinna, otalgia, trismus and dysphagia.
- There is bilateral parotid gland swelling in 75% of cases but submandibular gland might be affected in rare cases. Usually one side parotid will swell first followed by enlargement of the other gland in 1–5 days.
- The overlying parotid skin is stretched with a glazed appearance, but there is usually no erythema or warmth.

Investigation

- Viral serology: Complement fixing soluble (S) antibodies against the nucleoprotein core of the virus is associated with active infection and their levels peak at 10 days to 2 weeks and disappear within 8–9 months. A fourfold increase in antibody titer is diagnostic for acute infection. Complement fixing viral (V) antibodies against outer surface hemagglutinin appear later than S antibodies and persist at low levels for many years.
- A leukocyte count may show leukopenia.
- There is an elevation in the serum salivary type amylase.

Treatment

Supportive measures include:
- Bed rest
- Oral hygiene
- Hydration
- Dietary modifications to minimize glandular secretory activity.

Fever usually subsides before the resolution of glandular edema, which may take several weeks.

Complications

They include orchitis, aseptic meningitis, pancreatitis, nephritis and sensorineural hearing loss.

Prevention

Subcutaneous injection of vaccination (live attenuated Jerry Lynn vaccine), usually in combination with measles and rubella vaccines is given after 12 months of age. The antibodies produced by vaccine, persist for at least 5 years. The vaccine is contraindicated in pregnancy, immunocompromised states and allergies to neomycin.

ACUTE SUPPURATIVE SIALADENITIS

> The parotid is most commonly involved salivary gland.

The parotid gland's serous saliva, unlike mucinous saliva of other salivary glands, is deficient in lysosomes, IgA antibodies and sialic acid, which have antimicrobial properties. The saliva from other glands (submandibular and sublingual glands) contains high molecular weight glycoproteins that competitively inhibit bacterial attachment to the epithelial cells of the salivary ducts.

Predisposing Factors

- **Age:** It usually affects 50 and 60 years old people (equal incidence among men and women).
- **Debilitating conditions:** Malignant lesion and pre-existing infection.
- **Postoperative period:** Major abdominal and hip repair surgery. It occurs within the first two postoperative weeks.
- **Local:** Stenosis and sialolithiasis.
- **Systemic diseases:** Diabetes mellitus, hypothyroidism, renal failure and Sjögren's syndrome.
- **Dehydration and significant hemorrhage:** The retrograde bacterial contamination of the salivary ducts from the oral cavity occurs due to the stasis of salivary flow.
- **Medications**.

Causative Microorganisms

- Penicillin resistant *Staphylococcus aureus* in hospitalized patients.
- *Streptococcus pyogenes*, *Streptococcus viridans*, *Streptococcus pneumoniae* and *Haemophilus influenzae* (community-acquired cases).
- **Anaerobic bacteria:** *Peptostreptococcus*, *Bacteroides* species and *Fusobacterium*.

Clinical Features

- It usually presents with rapid onset of pain and swelling over the affected salivary gland, fever, chills and malaise.
- Dehydration with dry mucous membranes and local tenderness, warmth and induration.
- Bimanual palpation results in suppurative discharge from the duct orifice.

Investigations

- Leukocytosis with neutrophilia and normal serum amylase.
- Computed tomography (CT) and ultrasound (US) is indicated to look for abscess formation if patient does not respond to medical treatment (Fig. 32.1A).
- Cultures of purulent drainage from the duct orifice. Percutaneous needle aspiration limits the amount of contamination.

Treatment

It begins with aggressive medical treatment and includes:
- Prompt fluid and electrolyte replacement, oral hygiene, reversal of salivary stasis and antimicrobial therapy.
- Salivary flow should be stimulated by sialogogues such as lemon drops and orange juice.
- Regular external and bimanual massage, starting from the distal bed of the gland and working in the direction of duct drainage helps greatly in drainage.
- Analgesics and local heat application alleviate discomfort.
- Antimicrobial therapy, which might need change after the culture results, should be continued for 1 week after

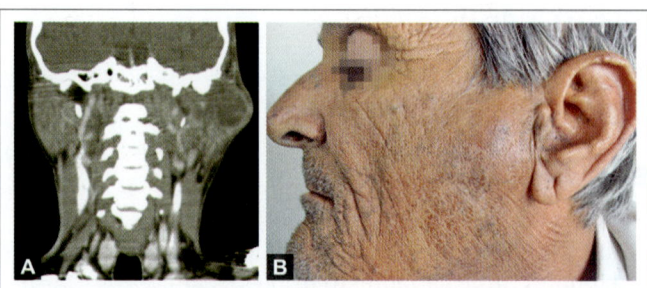

Figs 32.1A and B: (A) Contrast CT scan shows left parotid abscess. Coronal image show peripherally enhancing hypodense lesion in left parotid gland; (B) Left side parotid abscess. 57 year-old-male diabetic irradiated patient of right side carcinoma tonsil. Patient had painful swelling that reduced in size with antibiotics and abscess got localized
Source: Dr Swati Shah, Professor, Radiodiagnosis, GCR Medical College, Ahmedabad

resolution of symptoms. Antibiotics include augmented penicillin (Beta-lactamase producing bacteria in 75% cases), antistaphylococcal penicillin, a first-generation cephalosporin, vancomycin or linezolid (for methicillin-resistant *S. aureus* infection) and metronidazole (for anaerobes).
- Surgical drainage of a loculated abscess is done if conservative measures fail.

PAROTID ABSCESS

- Multiple small abscesses may coalesce and form large abscess in an advanced case of suppurative parotitis (Fig. 32.1B).

> US examination of the swelling will reveal the abscess. The usual fluctuation may not be elicited due to the dense fibrous capsule (derived from investing layer of deep cervical fascia) of the parotid gland.

Treatment

Incision and drainage: In addition to medical treatment, acute parotitis abscess needs incision and drainage. It is done under the cover of antibiotics.

RECURRENT PAROTITIS OF CHILDHOOD

Boys are affected more than girls. This disease of unknown etiology is characterized by periodic episodes of swelling and pain.

> Recurrent parotitis of childhood is the second most common inflammatory salivary gland disease of childhood (8 months to 16 years) after mumps.

Clinical Features (Figs 32.2A and B)

- Recurrent episodes of acute or subacute unilateral parotid gland swelling along with fever, malaise and pain after a meal.
- Exacerbations occur every 3–4 months and last for days to weeks.

- ***Sialography:*** Sialectasis appears as numerous scattered punctate pools of contrast.
- ***Ultrasound:*** An enlarged gland with multiple small hypoechoic areas.
- ***MR sialography:*** This noninvasive study may be used during acute episodes.
- ***Culture and sensitivity:*** Pus must be sent for culture.

Treatment

Treatment includes:
- Adequate hydration
- Gland massage
- Local heat
- Sialagogues
- Appropriate intravenous penicillinase-resistant antistaphylococcal antibiotics.

Most cases resolve spontaneously in late adolescence.

TUBERCULOUS MYCOBACTERIAL DISEASE

> The most common manifestation of *Mycobacterium tuberculosis* infection in the head and neck is cervical lymphadenopathy. Older children and adults are affected more.

Clinical Features

Constitutional signs: They include fever and night sweats. Weight loss might be absent.
Clinically, there are two different forms.
1. ***An acute inflammatory lesion with diffuse glandular edema:*** It may be confused with an acute sialadenitis or an abscess.
2. ***A chronic tumorous lesion:*** It is seen as a discrete slow growing mass that mimics a neoplasm.

Treatment

- ***Multiple drugs AKT***
- ***Complete surgical excision:*** When diagnosis is uncertain and the lesion is resistant to medical therapy, complete surgical excision is both diagnostic and curative.

ACTINOMYCOSIS

The most common type of actinomycosis infection is cervicofacial (55%). Isolated parotid involvement can occur by means of retrograde ductal migration and direct spread of an invasive cervicofacial infection.

Clinical Features

- Painless, indurated enlargement of the involved salivary gland. It might mimic a neoplasm.
- Multiple draining cutaneous fistulas: It is quite common. A chronic purulent drainage might occur with

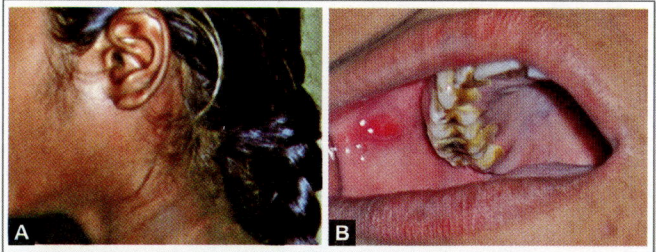

Figs 32.2A and B: (A) Left side acute parotid gland swelling in a 10-year-old girl; (B) Stensen's duct opening of right side parotid gland is congested

granulomatous involvement and spread to adjacent tissue. The periphery of the lesion is densely fibrotic and avascular.
- A history of recent dental disease and manipulation is common.

Diagnosis

Smears and stains for sulfur granules and the organisms: Needle aspiration of the mass or a fistula swab. Sulfur granules have also been described for nocardiosis

Treatment

- Penicillin six weeks parenteral course followed by an additional six months of oral course completely eradicates the organism.
- Other acceptable alternatives include clindamycin, doxycycline and erythromycin.
- Surgical excision is necessary to remove extensive fibrosis and sinus tracts, when antibiotics fail. It also helps in diagnosis.

OBSTRUCTIVE DISORDERS

SIALOLITHIASIS

The formation of stones in the salivary ductal system is called **sialolithiasis**. Parotid stones are mostly located at the hilum or parenchyma, while in the submandibular gland, they tend to develop in the duct.

Etiology

Exact etiology is uncertain. Salivary stasis and ductal inflammation and injury are important contributing factors. Elderly people are more affected than children. Most of the patients are male.

Eighty to ninety percent of calculi develop in Wharton's duct of submandibular gland. The reasons are the following:
- Wharton's duct is longer and has a larger caliber. It is angulated against gravity as it courses around the mylohyoid muscle.
- Submandibular secretions are more viscous and have a higher calcium and phosphorus concentration.

Composition

They are composed mainly of calcium phosphate and carbonate in combination with an organic matrix of glycolproteins and mucopolysaccharides and small amounts of other salts such as magnesium, potassium and ammonium.

Clinical Features

- Recurrent episodes of postprandial salivary colic pain and swelling.
- Past history of recurrent attacks of acute suppurative sialadenitis might be present.
- Bimanual palpation reveals the presence of a stone in most cases.
- Parotid stones might be seen just at the orifice of Stensen's duct or along the course of the duct.

Investigations

- ***Plain radiographs*** (intraoral and occlusal views) identify radiopaque stones and in the submandibular gland 80% of stones are radio-opaque.
- ***Ultrasound:*** It detects 90% of stones if they are > 2 mm.
- ***CT scanning*** with fine cuts is very accurate at detecting salivary stones.

Treatment

- ***Nonsurgical management:*** It consists of the use of:
  - Sialogogues
  - Local heat
  - Hydration
  - Massaging of the involved gland
  - Antibiotic coverage is started in cases of infection.
  - ***Manually milking out:*** Submandibular stones nearer the duct orifice may be manually milked out through the duct opening (Figs 32.3A to C).
- ***Surgical management:*** It consists of:
  - ***Incision of duct:*** Submandibular stones, which are no more than 2 cm from the duct orifice, may be either manually milked out through the duct opening or the duct is incised directly over the stone. There is no need for closure of Wharton's duct after the procedure.
  - ***Sialadenectomy:*** Submandibular stones located more proximal and near gland will require

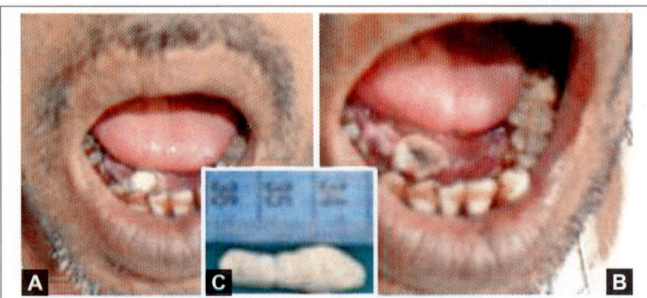

Figs 32.3A to C: Wharton's duct calculus. This patient had right submandibular abscess. (A) Right side Wharton's duct calculus coming out from its opening; (B) Appearance of Wharton's duct opening (too much dilated) after the milking out of calculus. The submandibular abscess drained through this opening; (C) Gross appearance and measurement of the removed Wharton's duct calculus

sialadenectomy, which may be performed either through transcervical or transoral approach. Parotid stones are more difficult to manage because of the anatomy of Stensen's duct.
- **Recent advances:** Use of various combination of baskets, graspers and intracorporeal lithotripsy have been employed to treat sialolithiasis in both the parotid and submandibular glands.
  - ***Extracorporeal shock wave lithotripsy (ESWL):*** It reduces stones to small fragments, which are then flushed out of the duct with spontaneous salivation or the use of a secretagogue. ESWL is breaking up of calculi by focussed ultrasound arising from the machine outside of body.
  - ***Sialoendoscopy:*** Rigid endoscopes are used to visualize and remove salivary duct stones.

NEOPLASMS OF SALIVARY GLANDS

Seventy percent of the salivary gland tumors arise in the parotid gland (Fig. 32.4A).
- The chances of a tumor being benign are more in major salivary glands (80% of parotid and 50–60% of submandibular) while less in minor salivary glands (25%). Therefore, majority of the minor salivary glands tumors are malignant.

The sign and symptoms of malignancy are rapid growth, restricted mobility, fixity of overlying skin, pain and facial nerve involvement.

- The tumors of salivary glands are either of epithelial or mesenchymal origin and can be benign and malignant (Table 32.1).

Most common salivary gland tumors: Pleomorphic adenoma is the most common salivary gland tumor and the number two is mucoepidermoid carcinoma.

- Other tumors in series of common frequency are adenoid cystic carcinoma, adenocarcinoma, malignant mixed tumor and Warthin's tumor (second most common benign tumor).

Table 32.1: Tumors of salivary glands

Benign	Malignant
Epithelial (adenomas)	*Epithelial*
• Pleomorphic adenoma	• Mucoepidermoid carcinoma
• Adenolymphoma (Warthin's tumor)	• Adenoid cystic carcinoma (cylindroma)
• Oncocytoma	• Acinic cell carcinoma
• Monomorphic adenoma	• Adenocarcinoma
	• Malignant mixed tumor
	• Squamous cell carcinoma
	• Undifferentiated carcinoma
Mesenchymal	*Mesenchymal*
• Vascular: Hemangioma	• Lymphoma
• Lymphatic: Lymphangioma	• Sarcoma
• Lipoma	
• Neurofibroma	
• Benign cyst	

- The pleomorphic adenoma of the parotid gland needs surgical excision that provides both definitive diagnosis and adequate treatment.
- Management of other types of salivary neoplasms is challenging because of their relative infrequency and variable biologic behavior.

- ***Nonneoplastic and noninflammatory parotid swellings:*** The common causes are obesity, hypothyroidism, diabetes mellitus, and malnutrition.
- ***Most common parotid tumor in children:*** It is lymphoma.

PLEOMORPHIC ADENOMA

- **Site:** This most common benign slow growing tumor of salivary glands, usually arise from the tail of parotid (Fig. 32.4B) and submandibular glands. It can also arise from minor salivary glands and deep lobe of the parotid, which presents as a parapharyngeal tumor in the oropharynx.
- **Clinical feature:** The tumor may be quite large at first presentation. It is usually seen in the third and fourth decade and has propensity for females.
- **Histopathology:** These 'mixed tumors' have both epithelial and mesenchymal elements in variable amount. The stroma may be mucoid, fibroid, vascular, myxochondroid or chondroid.
- **Treatment:** This encapsulated tumor sends pseudopods into the surrounding glands, therefore it is essential that surgical excision of the tumor should include surrounding normal gland tissue. These pseudopods may be left behind if the tumor is simply 'shelled out'. Superficial parotidectomy is done for superficial parotid tumor.

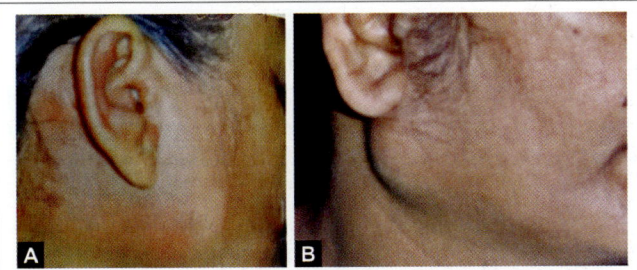

Figs 32.4A and B: (A) Swelling of the parotid gland; (B) Tail of parotid gland

WARTHIN'S TUMOR OR ADENOLYMPHOMA (PAPILLARY CYSTADENOMA LYMPHOMATOSUM)

- *Age and sex:* Warthin's tumor is commonly seen between fifth and seventh decade with male preponderance (5:1).
- *Site:* The most common site is the tail of the parotid and is bilateral in 10% cases. They may be multiple.
- *Gross pathology:* It is a rounded encapsulated tumor, which may be at times cystic with mucoid or brownish fluid.
- *Histopathology* shows its epithelial and lymphoid elements.
- *Treatment:* Usually superficial parotidectomy is performed. However, they can be enucleated without danger of recurrence.

ONCOCYTOMA

- It comprises less than 1% of all salivary gland tumor and usually does not grow more than 5 cm in size.
- It is mostly seen in the superficial parotid lobe of the elderly people.
- This oxyphil adenoma arises from acidophilic cells (oncocytes).
- Oncocytoma shows increased uptake of technetium-99. It may be malignant, benign or cystic in nature.
- Treatment is superficial parotidectomy.

HEMANGIOMAS

- Hemangiomas are the most common benign parotid tumors in children and predominantly affect females.
- Congenital hemangioma grows rapidly in the neonatal period and then involutes spontaneously. Cutaneous hemangioma coexists in 50% of the cases.
- Characteristically, they are soft and painless and increase in size with crying or straining. The overlying skin shows bluish discoloration.
- Treatment is surgical excision if they do not regress.

LYMPHANGIOMAS

- These less common tumors feel soft and cystic and involve parotid and submandibular glands.
- They do not regress in size spontaneously and need surgical excision.

MUCOEPIDERMOID CARCINOMA

- This slow growing malignant tumor of parotid can metastasize and involve facial nerve. Mucoepidermoid tumors of minor salivary glands are more aggressive while in major salivary glands they behave like pleomorphic adenoma.
- The mucoepidermoid tumor has both the areas of mucin producing cells as well as squamous cells.
- The tumors have been classified as low grade and high grade. The tumors, which have greater epidermoid element, are more malignant.
  - Low grade tumors are more common in children. They have good prognosis and 90% 5 years survival rates.
  - High grade tumors are more aggressive. They have poor prognosis and 30% 5 years survival rate.

Treatment

- Low grade parotid tumors are managed by superficial or total parotidectomy. Surgery depends upon the location and extent of the tumor. Facial nerve is preserved.
- The aggressive high grade tumors need total parotidectomy and facial nerve is sacrificed if invaded by tumor. Facial nerve is grafted in same sitting.
- If needed radical neck dissection is also combined.

ADENOID CYSTIC CARCINOMA (CYLINDROMA)

- This is a slow growing tumor, which infiltrates widely into the tissue planes and muscles. It is the most common malignant tumor of the submandibular salivary gland.
- It spreads through perineural spaces and lymphatics and causes pain and facial nerve palsy.
- Distant metastases can occur in lungs, brain and bones.

Treatment

- Treatment is by radical parotidectomy, which includes large surrounding normal tissue.
- Radical neck dissection is done if nodal metastases are present.
- Postoperative radiation is given if the margins of the tumor are not clear.
- Local recurrences after surgical excision, which may be as late as 10–20 years, are common.

ACINIC CELL CARCINOMA

Among the malignancies of parotid gland, this has the best prognosis. This low grade tumor appears similar to a benign mixed tumor. It presents as a small, firm, movable and encapsulated tumor. Bilateral tumors are also seen. Metastases are rare.

Treatment is superficial or total parotidectomy.

SQUAMOUS CELL CARCINOMA

This rapidly growing painful tumor infiltrates and ulcerates through the skin, and metastasizes to neck nodes.

Treatment is by radical parotidectomy, which includes surrounding part of muscle, mandible, temporal bone and the involved skin. Radical neck is combined if nodal metastases are present. Postoperative radiotherapy is given.

MALIGNANT MIXED TUMOR

This tumor can develop in pre-existing benign mixed tumor. Rapid growth and appearance of pain in a slow growing benign tumor indicates malignant change. A 'de novo' tumor has much shorter history.
Treatment is radical parotidectomy.

ADENOCARCINOMA

This highly aggressive tumor mostly arises in minor salivary glands and sends distant metastases.

LYMPHOEPITHELIAL CARCINOMA OR UNDIFFERENTIATED CARCINOMA

This rare aggressive painful tumor has a tendency to spread rapidly. It becomes fixed to skin and ulcerates. It causes facial paralysis and cervical nodal metastasis. Treatment is wide excision combined with radical neck dissection and postoperative radiotherapy.

- *Malignancy of salivary glands:* Their presentation may be similar to benign tumors and can lead to delay in diagnosis.
- *Superficial parotidectomy:* This surgical treatment is adequate in cases of oncocytoma, pleomorphic adenoma, basal cell adenoma, and acinic cell carcinoma of parotid gland. Because of the section of greater auricular nerve, it is followed by anesthesia of the lower part of pinna.

XEROSTOMIA

Xerostomia refers to dryness of mouth resulting from diminished or arrested salivary secretion. Xerostomia causes difficulty in chewing, swallowing and phonation, adherence of food to the buccal mucosa and multiple dental caries.
- Diabetes and cystic fibrosis should be assessed.
- Sedatives, antipsychotics, antidepressants, antihistamines and diuretics are most often associated with oral dryness.
- Salivary gland exposure to therapeutic irradiation > 4,000 cGy will result in severe and permanent secretory hypofunction.

Mikulicz's disease and Sjogren's syndrome: Mikulicz's disease consists of xerostomia and xero-ophthalmia and is the most common presentation of Sjogren's s syndrome.

SJÖGREN'S SYNDROME

Sjögren's syndrome is a chronic autoimmune disorder of the exocrine glands. The salivary and lacrimal glands are primarily affected. The lymphocytic infiltration results in glandular hypofunction leading to dryness of the mouth and eyes. The disease might even evolve into a malignant lymphoid process.

Types

There are two types of Sjogren's syndromes:
1. *Primary Sjögren's syndrome:* This type of Sjögren's syndrome is confined to the exocrine glands.
2. *Secondary Sjögren's syndrome:* Patients have the characteristic signs and symptoms of primary Sjögren's syndrome associated with features of other autoimmune disease.

Secondary Sjögren's syndrome is the triad of keratoconjunctivitis sicca (involvement of lacrimal gland), xerostomia (involvement of salivary glands and mucous glands of the oral cavity) and autoimmune connective tissue disorders such as rheumatoid arthritis.

Epidemiology

- The estimated prevalence of Sjögren's syndrome is believed to be 1–3%.
- The disease is most commonly seen in patients during their fourth to fifth decade of life.
- More than 90% of patients are women.

Clinical Features

- Predominant clinical presentation: Dryness of the mouth and eyes.
- Salivary gland enlargement is most common in the parotid glands and occurs in 25–66% of patients. The bilateral enlargement may be recurrent and episodic or chronic and fixed.
- Patients with persistent unilateral or bilateral parotid gland enlargement are at higher risk for the development of lymphoma.
- Xerostomia causes difficulty in chewing, swallowing and phonation, adherence of food to the buccal mucosa and multiple dental caries.
- *Most common ocular complaint:* Foreign body sensation in the eye ('gritty' or 'sandy' feeling).

- **Schirmer's test:** For tear secretion rate assessment (*see* Chapter 'Facial Nerve Disorders').
- Staining of damaged corneal and conjunctival epithelia by rose Bengal dye is specific for keratoconjunctivitis sicca.

Laboratory Investigations

Laboratory investigations show raised erythrocyte sedimentation rate, positive rheumatoid factor and positive antinuclear antibodies. Biopsy from the lower lip shows evidence of involvement of minor salivary glands.

Treatment

The treatment consists of symptomatic therapy and prevention of irreversible damage to the teeth and eyes.

- **Sjögren's syndrome:** A positive ANA, RF, SS-a, SS-b and an elevated ESR are indicative of Sjögren's syndrome. Biopsy from lower lip confirms the diagnosis and shows atrophy of minor salivary glands with an abundance of lymphocytes and histiocytes.
- **Mikulicz disease:**
  - It consists of xerostomia and xerophthalmia.
  - Treatment of choice is steroid therapy.

Sarcoidosis: The clinical features include parotid swelling, facial paralysis, cervical lymphadenopathy, and diabetes insipidus.

FREY'S SYNDROME (GUSTATORY SWEATING)

- **Gustatory sweating** manifests several months after the parotidectomy operation. It is characterized by sweating and flushing of the preauricular skin during mastication.
- This condition is the result of aberrant innervation of sweat glands by parasympathetic secretomotor fibers which were destined for the parotid. Thus, these postganglionic fibers from the otic ganglion carried by auriculotemporal nerve, instead of causing salivary secretion cause secretion from the sweat glands.
- The placement of a sheet of fascia lata between the skin and the underlying fat may prevent secretomotor fibers reaching the sweat glands.

Treatment

- Usually no treatment other than reassurance is required.
- In cases of significant nuisance and social embarrassment, the condition is treated by tympanic neurectomy of Jacobson's nerve, which carries preganglionic parasympathetic secretomotor fibers from the inferior salivary nucleus through the glossopharyngeal nerve.

Self-evaluation Exercises

1. Complications of mumps do not include:
   a. Unilateral sensorineural hearing loss
   b. Thyroiditis
   c. Pancreatitis
   d. Orchitis
   e. None of the above
2. The clinical features of sarcoidosis include:
   a. Parotid swelling
   b. Facial paralysis
   c. Cervical lymphadenopathy
   d. Diabetes insipidus
   e. All of the above
3. The common causes of nonneoplastic and noninflammatory parotid swellings are:
   a. Obesity
   b. Hypothyroidism
   c. Diabetes mellitus
   d. Malnutrition
   e. All of the above

Contd...

Contd...

4. Which of the following is related with Sjogren's syndrome?
    a. Autoimmune disease associated with collagen disorder
    b. Predominantly seen in women (9:1)
    c. Between the ages of 40 and 60 years
    d. Dryness of the eyes and dry mouth are the most common features
    e. All of the above
5. Which of the following is not true for Sjogren's syndrome?
    a. Parotid enlargement may be chronic or relapsing
    b. Parotid enlargement develops in one-third of patients
    c. Three to ten percent patients develop lymphoma
    d. None of the above
6. Which of the following is not true for Mikulicz is disease?
    a. Xerostomia
    b. Xerophthalmia
    c. Rheumatoid arthritis
    d. Treatment of choice is steroid therapy
    e. None of the above
7. Which of the following is not true for Frey's syndrome?
    a. Flushing and sweating of skin of parotid region during eating in parotidectomy patients
    b. Sympathetic postganglionic nerve fibers supplying the parotid gland are misdirected
    c. Sectioning of the Jacobson's nerve (tympanic branch of glossopharyngeal nerve carrying preganglionic secretomotor fibers for parotid gland) on the promontory of middle ear (tympanic neurectomy) alleviate the symptoms
    d. None of the above
8. Superficial parotidectomy is adequate in cases of:
    a. Oncocytoma
    b. Pleomorphic adenoma
    c. Basal cell adenoma
    d. Acinic cell carcinoma
    e. All of the above
9. Some of the causes of xerostomia are:
    a. Antihistamines
    b. Uremia
    c. Sjögren's syndrome
    d. Mouth breathing
    e. All of the above

True (T)/False (F)
10. Because of the section of greater auricular nerve, superficial parotidectomy is followed by anesthesia of the lower part of pinna.
11. Eighty percent of salivary calculi are seen in parotid gland.
12. Twenty percent of submandibular gland calculi are radiolucent.
13. Most common parotid tumor in children is lymphoma.
14. Submandibular gland is the most common site of pleomorphic adenoma.
15. Hemangioma is present in neonates with an isolated unilateral parotid swelling with bluish overlying skin.
16. Hemangioma swelling does not increase when child cries.
17. Adenoid cystic carcinoma is the most common malignant tumor of the submandibular salivary gland.
18. Adenoid cystic carcinoma has no tendency for perineural invasion.
19. Among the malignancies of parotid gland, acinous cell carcinoma has the best prognosis.

Answers

1. e	2. e	3. e	4. e	5. d	6. c
7. b	8. e	9. e	10. T	11. F	12. T
13. T	14. F	15. T	16. F	17. T	18. F
19. T					

Chapter 33

Neoplasms of Oral Cavity

Specific Learning Objectives

After going through the chapter, you should be able to answer the following questions:
- Which are the etiological and risk factors of oral carcinoma?
- What are the subsites and TNM staging of oral cancer?
- How will you evaluate and manage a patient with oral tongue cancer?
- What are the clinical features of buccal carcinoma and how will you manage such patients?

INTRODUCTION

The tumors of oral cavity can be classified into two major categories—benign and malignant. Benign tumors and tumor-like lesions can be further divided into two groups—solid and cystic. Tori and dermoid cysts are congenital lesions. Malignant tumors have two histopathological types—carcinoma and sarcoma (Table 33.1).

BENIGN TUMORS OF ORAL CAVITY

PAPILLOMA

- Squamous papilloma is usually associated with human papillomavirus (HPV)-6 and HPV-11 virus subtypes. It is one of the most frequently occurring conditions.
- *Age:* Peak incidence in third to fifth decades of life.
- *Most common sites:* Soft and hard palate, uvula, tongue, lips and buccal mucosa.
- *Clinical features:* Pedunculated and white in color and less than 1 cm in size mass. Surface usually wart like but may be smooth.
- *Treatment:* Surgical excision or ablation with CO_2 laser.

PLEOMORPHIC ADENOMA

- Most common benign neoplasm of minor salivary gland.
- *Common sites:* Soft and hard palate.
- *Clinical features:* Painless progressive submucosal tumor.

Table 33.1: Tumors of the oral cavity

Benign
• Solid
▪ Papilloma
▪ Pleomorphic adenoma
▪ Hemangioma
▪ Lymphangioma
▪ Granular cell tumor
▪ Ameloblastoma
▪ Torus (congenital)
◆ Torus palatinus
◆ Torus mandibularis
▪ Inflammatory
◆ Pyogenic granuloma
◆ Irritation fibroma
• Cystic
▪ Mucocele
▪ Ranula
◆ Simple
◆ Plunging
▪ Dermoid cysts (congenital)
◆ Sublingual
◆ Submental
Malignant
• Carcinoma
▪ Squamous cell carcinoma
▪ Nonsquamous cell carcinoma
◆ Minor salivary gland tumors
◆ Melanoma
◆ Lymphoma
• Sarcoma
▪ Kaposi's sarcoma

- *Treatment:* Wide surgical excision.
- *Prognosis:* High recurrence rate.

HEMANGIOMA

- Oral hemangiomas (Fig. 33.1A) constitute 14% of all hemangiomas
- *Age:* Mostly seen in children.
- *Most common site:* Lip
- *Clinical feature:* Soft, painless, red or blue mass of usually < 2 cm size. Large tumors can encroach any part of oral cavity and oropharynx.
- *Differential diagnosis:* Pyogenic granuloma
- *Treatment:* Spontaneous regression occurs in congenital hemangioma. Large and persistent hemangiomas need surgical excision after microemboloization. Sclerotherapy, cryosurgery and laser have been tried.
- *Phlebectasias:* Dilated veins on oral and tongue mucosa in 40–50 years old patients.

LYMPHANGIOMA

- *Most common site:* Anterior two-thirds of tongue.
- *Clinical features:* Diffuse (macroglossia) or localized compressible soft swelling.
- *Treatment:* Small tumors totally excised. In large diffuse swellings partial excision reduces the bulk.

GRANULAR CELL TUMOR

- *Origin:* From Schwann cells (formerly thought to arise from the muscle and called myoblastoma).
- *Most common site:* Tongue (other: soft palate, uvula and labial mucosa).
- *Clinical features:* Firm, painless, sessile submucosal nodule of less than 1.5 cm size.
- *Congenital epulis:* Involves gums of future incisors in female infants.
- *Treatment:* Excision biopsy.
- *Prognosis:* Recurrence less than 10%.

AMELOBLASTOMA

- Most common odontogenic neoplasm.
- *Origin:* From rests of primitive dental lamina related to the enamel organ in alveolar bone.

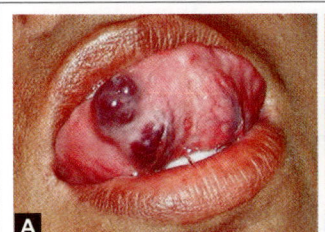 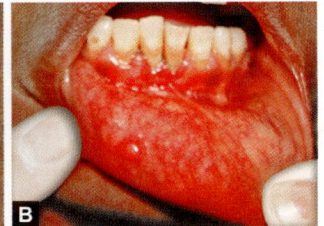

Figs 33.1A and B: (A) Hemangioma tongue; (B) Mucous retention cyst of lower lip

- *Age:* Third decade of life.
- *Most common site:* Molar/ramus area of mandible.
- *CT scan:* Shows unilocular or multilocular radiolucency with cortical bone expansion.
- *Treatment:* En bloc resection with at least 1 cm margins of normal appearing tissue.
- *Recurrence rate:* 22%.
- *Malignant transformation:* Rare.

TORUS

Torus is a frequently observed developmental anomaly. It presents as a bony outgrowths in the second decade of life. It continues to grow slowly throughout the life.

Clinical Features

- Tori are more common in females.
- These pedunculated or multilobulated broadly based smooth bony masses are usually asymptomatic.
- In later life, they may interfere with denture placement and get repeatedly injured while eating.
- Torus palatinus is found in the midline of hard palate.
- Torus mandibularis is found on the lingual surface of mandible in the premolar region.

Treatment

Removal from the underlying cortex with osteotomes or cutting burrs.

PYOGENIC GRANULOMA

- *Pathology:* Reactive granuloma in response to trauma and chronic irritation.
- *Most common sites:* Anterior gingivae (other: tongue, buccal mucosa and lips).
- *Clinical features:* Soft smooth reddish (purple) raised or pedunculated mass. Bleeds on touch.
- *Pregnancy granuloma or epulis gravidarum:* Starts in first trimester of pregnancy and regresses after delivery. Not removed during pregnancy.
- *Epulis granulomatosa:* Occurs after tooth extraction.
- *Treatment:* Excisional biopsy with removal of predisposing factor.
- *Recurrence:* Uncommon. Common in pregnancy.

IRRITATION FIBROMA

- This common tumor-like condition of oral cavity is found in 1.2% of adults.
- It usually becomes apparent during and after fourth decade.
- Asymptomatic solitary sessile or pedunculated firm mass which is seldom larger than 1.5 cm.
- Sites are buccal, labial and tongue mucosa.

- History of chronic irritation is present.
- **Treatment:** Conservative excisional biopsy.

MUCOCELE

- This is a soft cystic bluish color retention cyst of minor salivary gland.
- Though it can occur anywhere in oral cavity, its most common site is the lower lip (Fig. 33.1B).
- **Treatment:** Surgical excision.

RANULA

- Ranula, a cystic grayish translucent swelling, occurs in the lateral part of the floor of mouth and pushes the tongue up.
- Ranula is the result of obstruction of the ducts of sublingual salivary gland.
- *Plunging ranula* is quite big and extends into the neck.

Treatment

- *Excision:* Small ranula may be completely excised.
- *Marsupialization:* Large ranula needs marsupialization. It is difficult to excise the ranula completely because of its thin wall and ramifications.

DERMOID CYSTS

- Dermoid cysts are lined by keratinized squamous epithelium. They are formed from epithelial rests that are found along embryonic fusion lines. They contain elements of epidermal appendages such as hair follicles, sweat glands and connective tissue.
- Head and neck accounts for about 7% of total dermoid cysts; of this, 6.5–23% are found in floor of the mouth.
- As they enlarge, difficulties in deglutition, speech and respiration occur.
- There are two types of dermoids in this region: sublingual and submental:
  i. *Sublingual dermoid* is situated above the mylohyoid.
     - It can be either median or lateral
     - It shines as a white mass through the mucosa.
  ii. *Submental dermoid* develops below the mylohyoid muscle.
     - It presents as a submental swelling.
- **Treatment:** Complete excision of the cyst.

CARCINOMA OF ORAL CAVITY

Epidemiology

In Indian males, mouth/oropharynx are the most common sites of cancer while in females they are on number four. This preventable disease is caused by tobacco, alcohol, *paan*, reverse smoking, areca nut and betel quid.

In Banglore cancer registry, mouth cancer was found the fifth leading sites of cancer for females. In Barshi, it was found fourth leading cancer for both males and females. In Ahmedabad, tongue and mouth were seen the top leading sites of cancer in males.

Risk Factors

The risk factors, which are associated with the development of oral cavity cancers, include several 'Ss' such as smoking, spirit, *sopari* (areca nut), sharp and septic tooth, syphilitic glossitis and syndrome Plummer-Vinson. Tobacco and alcohol are the most common preventable factors.

- *Smoking:* Incidence of oral cancer is six times more in smokers. Reverse smoking, where burning end of the 'churat' (rolled tobacco leaf) is put in the mouth, is the cause of higher incidence of cancer of the hard palate. Pipe smoking has been associated with lip cancer. Forty percent of patients who continue smoking after definitive treatment develop recurrence or second head and neck malignancy.
- *Alcohol:* Cancer of upper aerodigestive tract occurs six times more in heavy drinkers. Individuals who both smoke and drink have 35 times more risk. Alcoholic mouthwashes have also been implicated.
- *Chewing of paan, sopari and tobacco: Paan* (specially prepared leaf), *sopari* (betel nut, product of Areca catechu tree), quid (powdered tobacco mixed with lime) are chewed in the mouth and carcinoma develops at the site of their lodgment. This bad habit is largely responsible for oral cancer in Indians. Betel nut is a mild stimulant similar to that of coffee.
- *Avitaminosis and malnutrition:* Riboflavin deficiency is proposed to be responsible for cancer in alcoholics. Plummer-Vinson syndrome (iron deficiency anemia and dysphagia in females) is related with cancer of oral cavity and postcricoid region.
- *Dental caries, sharp jagged teeth and ill fitting dentures:* They cause chronic irritation, which may result in malignant change.
- *Human papillomavirus:* The role of HPV has been reported in a subset of head and neck squamous cell carcinoma.
- *Environmental ultraviolet light exposure:* It has been associated with lip cancer.
- *Long-term immunosuppression:* There is 30 fold increased risk in patients with renal transplant.
- *HIV infection:* Kaposi's sarcoma can occur in oral cavity.
- *Other carcinogenic factors proposed in the etiology are following:*
  - Hot spicy food
  - Xeroderma pigmentosa
  - Chronic glossitis
  - Cirrhosis.

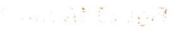

Subsites of Oral Cavity

The oral cavity extends from the lips to the level of anterior tonsillar pillar. For the subsites of cancer in oral cavity (AJCC, 2002) *see* Fig. 29.1, Table 29.1 in Chapter 29 'Anatomy of Oral Cavity'.

Clinical Evaluation and Investigations

For history taking, clinical evaluation, investigation and imaging studies, *see* Chapter 'Oral Symptoms and Examination' in the Section of 'Oral Cavity and Salivary Glands'.

> *Premaligant conditions of oral cavity:* They include leukoplakia, eryhthroplakia, lichen planus, chronic discoid lupus erythematosis, and oral submucous fibrosis. See Chapter 'Oral Mucosal Lesions'.

Staging

Table 33.2 shows AJCC staging and TNM classification.

CARCINOMA LIPS

Clinical Features

- *Sex:* Males in the age group of 40–70 years.
- *Lesion:* Exophytic and ulcerative types.
- *Most common site:* Between the midline and commissure of the lower lip.
- *Local spread:* Initially tumor spreads laterally and later infiltrates deeply and spread into anterior triangle of neck and invade mandible.
- *Regional lymphatic metastasis:* It is late and involves submental and submandibular nodes. At later stage, deep cervical nodes may get involved.
- *Histopathology:* Mostly squamous cell carcinoma.

Table 33.2: AJCC cancer staging and UICC TNM classification of oral cancer

Primary tumor (T)	
T_x	Unable to assess primary tumor
T_0	No evidence of primary tumor
T_{is}	Carcinoma *in situ*
T_1	Tumor is < 2 cm in greatest dimension
T_2	Tumor > 2 cm and < 4 cm in greatest dimension
T_3	Tumor > 4 cm in greatest dimension
T_4 (lip)	Primary tumor invading cortical bone, inferior alveolar nerve, floor of mouth, or skin of nose or chin
T_{4a} (oral)	Tumor invades adjacent structures (e.g. cortical bone, into deep tongue musculature, maxillary sinus) or skin of face
T_{4b} (oral)	Tumor invades masticator space, pterygoid plates, or skull base or encases the internal carotid artery
Regional lymphadenopathy (N)	
N_x	Unable to assess regional lymph nodes
N_0	No evidence of regional metastasis
N_1	Metastasis in a single ipsilateral lymph node, <= 3 cm in greatest dimension
N_{2a}	Metastasis in single ipsilateral lymph node, > 3 cm and < 6 cm
N_{2b}	Metastasis in multiple ipsilateral lymph nodes, all nodes < 6 cm
N_{2c}	Metastasis in bilateral or contralateral lymph nodes, all nodes < 6 cm
N_3	Metastasis in a lymph node > 6 cm in greatest dimension
Distant metastases (M)	
M_x	Unable to assess for distant metastases
M_0	No distant metastases
M_1	Distant metastases
TNM staging	
Stage 0	$T_{is}\ N_0\ M_0$
Stage I	$T_1\ N_0\ M_0$
Stage II	$T_2\ N_0\ M_0$
Stage III	$T_3\ N_0\ M_0$; $T_{1-3}\ N_1\ M_0$
Stage IVA	$T_{4a}\ N_{0-1}\ M_0$; $T_{1-4a}\ N_2\ M_0$
Stage IVB	$T_{4b}\ N_{0-2}\ M_0$; $T_{1-4b}\ N_3\ M_0$
Stage IVC	$T_{1-4b}\ N_{1-3}\ M_1$

Source: American Joint Committee on Cancer (AJCC) Staging Manual, 6th edition. Chicago; 2002

Treatment

Either radiation therapy or surgery for stage I tumors gives cure rates greater than 85%. Surgery for large tumors consists of excision with adequate safety margin and repair. Block dissection is done if lymph nodes are involved. Postoperative radiotherapy to chin and neck region is planned in high-risk advanced stage tumors.

Abbe-Estlander flap: It is used to reconstruct defects in cases of carcinoma of lip involving angle of mouth (commissure). Such defects require partial commissure reconstruction.

CARCINOMA GINGIVA/ALVEOLAR RIDGE

- *Common features:* Failure of socket healing after tooth extraction; sudden difficulty in wearing denture; superficial ulceration or proliferative tissue at the gingival margin.
- *Most common site* is the lower jaw in the premolar region and just behind the first molar (Figs 33.2A and B).
- *Local spread:* To cheek, floor of mouth, retromolar trigone and hard palate. After invading underlying bone, it spreads rapidly along the neurovascular bundle.
- *Nodal metastases:* The enlargement of submandibular and upper jugular nodes is common at the time of presentation.

Treatment

Surgery is preferred over radiotherapy. Radiations lead to radio-osteonecrosis.
- Early lesion on the lower alveolus is excised (marginal resection of the mandible).
- Extensive tumor of lower alveolus requires segmental or hemimandibulectomy. Access is achieved via lip split approach. Block dissection is needed when lymph nodes are involved.
- Tumors confined to hard palate, upper alveolus and floor of maxillary antrum needs partial maxillectomy with block dissection if nodes are enlarged.
- Upper alveolar tumor involving inferior structure of maxilla requires total maxillectomy followed by postoperative radiotherapy.
- Primary reconstruction should always be undertaken.

CARCINOMA ORAL TONGUE

Gross Pathology

- *Pre-existing lesions:* Some patients have pre-existing leukoplakia, dental ulcer and syphilitic glossitis.
- *Common site:* Middle third of the lateral border. Figures 33.3 and 33.4 show different types of lesions. The lesion extends early on to the ventral surface of the tongue and floor of mouth. The tip and dorsum are uncommon sites.
- *Local spread:* Deeply into the musculature (causes ankyloglossia), inferiorly into the floor of mouth and laterally into alveolus and mandible.
- *Lymph node metastases:* Bilateral and contralateral lymph node involvements can occur.
- *Histopathology:* Squamous cell carcinoma is most common.

Clinical Features

- This is commonly seen in 50–70 years of men.
- Early lesions are painless and may remain asymptomatic. Lesion arises in an atrophic depapillated area with an erythroplakia patch with peripheral streaks and areas of leukoplakia.

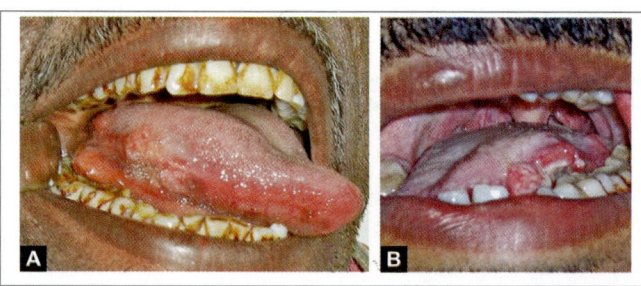

Figs 33.3A and B: (A) Carcinoma tongue right lateral margin. Nodular lesion with induration of the surrounding tissue; (B) Carcinoma tongue right lateral margin. Ulcerative lesion with rolled edges and grayish white shaggy base with induration

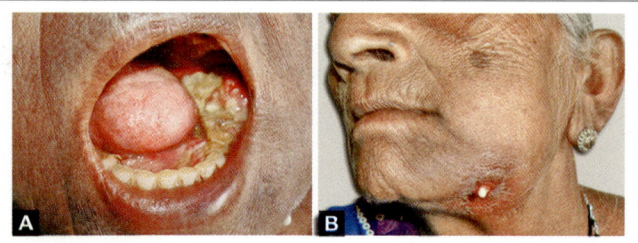

Figs 33.2A and B: (A) Carcinoma left lower alveolus (premolar to retromolar region) extending to buccal mucosa, floor of mouth and cheek skin; (B) Note the lower jaw swelling and pus from skin lesion

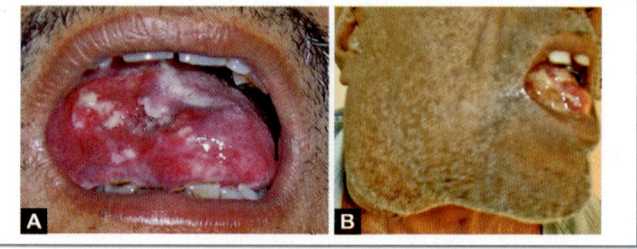

Figs 33.4A and B: (A) Malignancy tongue. Nonhealing ulcer with infiltration; (B) An advanced case (Stage IV: $T_4 N_3$) of right side carcinoma tongue (tumor invades into deep tongue musculature) with secondary neck nodes (lymph node > 6 cm in greatest dimension)

- Painful ulcer/growth/lump is a late feature.
- Referred earache occurs due to common nerve supply (branches of mandibular division of trigeminal) of the tongue (lingual nerve) and ear (auriculotemporal).
- Enlarged lymph node presents as mass in the neck (Fig. 33.4B). About 50% patients have palpable nodes at the time of presentation. About 12% of the patients present with only lump in neck.
- *Late features:* Dysphagia, odynophagia (leads to drooling of saliva), ankyloglossia, slurred speech, bleeding and cachexia.
- *Lesion:* Often it is exophytic with areas of ulceration.
  - *Exophytic:* An exophytic lesion like a papilloma.
  - *Ulcerative:* A nonhealing ulcer with rolled edges (Fig. 33.3B) and grayish white shaggy base with induration. The ulcer may be present superficially or in depths of a fissure infiltrating underlying muscle (Fig. 33.4A).
  - A submucous nodule with induration of the surrounding tissue.
  - The lesion may be associated with leukoplakia.

Treatment

The main modalities of treatment, which depends on the staging of the cancer (Table 33.2), are surgery and radiotherapy. One should try to preserve function of the tongue along with the total eradication of cancer.
- *Stage I ($T_1 N_0$):* Equal results with radiotherapy and surgery. Simple intraoral excision is preferred. Formal reconstruction is not required if less than one-third of the tongue is excised.
- *Stage II ($T_2 N_0$):* Treated by radiotherapy (including tumors and regional lymph nodes) or by surgical excision (hemiglossectomy) with prophylactic neck dissection.
- *Stage III or IV:* Hemiglossectomy (depending on the extent of the tongue lesion) combined with marginal, segmental or hemimandibulectomy (depending upon the extent of involvement of mandible) and radical neck dissection of lymph nodes (commando operation) followed by postoperative radiotherapy. This strategy gives better results than either surgery or radiotherapy alone. A rim mandibular resection is advised when lesion reaches but does not invade alveolus (Fig. 33.5A).

CARCINOMA FLOOR OF MOUTH

Clinical Features

- *Male/female ratio:* It is 4:1.
- *Early features:* Lesion may remain asymptomatic or cause soreness and irregularity in the floor of mouth.
- *Submandibular swelling:* It may be due to enlarged submandibular salivary gland and node metastases.
- *Lesion:* Ulcerative and infiltrative lesions.

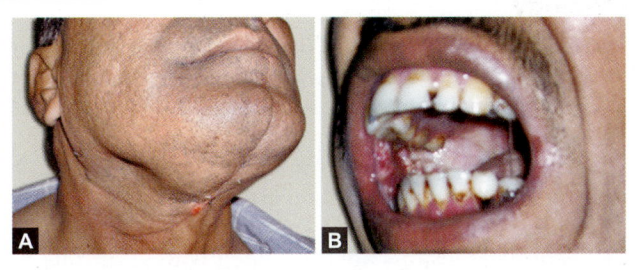

Figs 33.5: (A) External neck incision of Commando operation; (B) Malignancy buccal mucosa right side with trismus

- *Leukoplakia:* It is more common in the floor of mouth than at other sites.
- *Common site:* Begins anteriorly near the opening of submandibular duct that get obstructed and leads to enlargement of submandibular gland.
- *Local spreads:* Ventral aspect of the tongue, lingual gingiva, mandibular periosteum and deeply into the floor of mouth and submental space.
- *Lymphatic metastases:* Submandibular and jugulodigastric nodes and may be bilateral.
- *Histopathology:* Usually squamous cell carcinoma.

Treatment

- *Stage I:* If there is no involvement of tongue, lingual gingiva and nodes than small lesions are treated with wide excision or radiotherapy. Both offer equal results.
- *Stage II:* Prophylactic neck dissection or irradiation is done for stage II cancer because there is high incidence of micrometastases (40%).
- *Stage III and IV:* These patients need surgery and radiotherapy. Large tumor with involvement of tongue, gingiva, mandible and nodes require hemiglossectomy, marginal or segmental mandibular resection, and radical neck dissection. Resultant defect is reconstructed with either a local or distant flap.

CARCINOMA BUCCAL MUCOSA

Buccal mucosa lines the inner surface of cheeks and lips and extends between the superior and inferior gingivobuccal sulcus. It extends posteriorly up to pterygomandibular raphe and anteriorly up to the meeting line of lips. Buccal mucosa drains into submental and submandibular nodes.

Most common cancers of oral cavity: Carcinoma of tongue is the most common cancer of oral cavity and the second most common site is the buccal mucosa.

Pathology

- *Most common sites (Figs 33.5B and 33.6A):* Angle of mouth and the plane of occlusion to retromolar region. Gingivobuccal sulcus where *paan* and tobacco quid is kept.
- *Multicentric:* Buccal mucosa cancer may be multicentric as the entire buccal mucosa is 'condemned'.
- *Lesion:*
  - Exophytic lesions are associated with erythroleukoplakia.
  - Ulceroinfiltrative lesions may infiltrate deeply.
  - Verrucous carcinoma.
- *Local spread:*
  - The ulcer may spread deeply and involves different layers of cheek such as submucosa, muscle, subcutaneous fat and skin.
  - Patient develops trismus if buccinator, masseter, or medial pterygoid muscle is involved.
  - If the lesion spreads radially, it involves angle of the mouth and lip anteriorly; retromolar trigone and medial pterygoid muscle posteriorly; upper gingivobuccal sulcus and maxilla superiorly; and lower gingivobuccal sulcus and alveolar ridge and gums inferiorly.
- *Lymphatic spread:* Submandibular, submental, and parotid nodes. Later on upper jugular nodes are affected. In some cases, there occurs direct involvement of upper jugular nodes skipping the submandibular group. Nodal involvement develops in about 50% cases.
- *Histopathology:* Squamous cell carcinoma is most common but salivary gland tumors are also seen.

Clinical Features

- Early lesions are asymptomatic
- Pain and bleeding
- *Trismus:* Involvement of buccinator, masseter or pterygoid muscles leads to trismus (Fig. 33.5B).
- *Late feature:* Fungating foul smelling bleeding mass over the cheek or in the oral cavity.

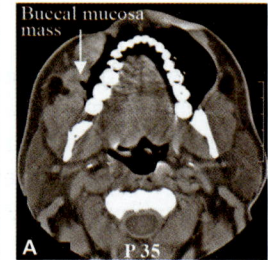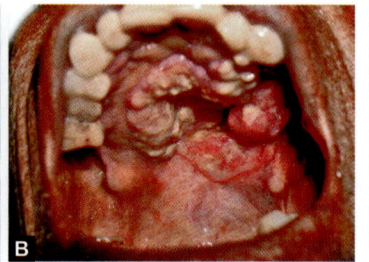

Figs 33.6A and B: (A) Carcinoma buccal mucosa. Contrast CT scan neck axial section. Enhancing thickening of right buccal mucosa (12–14 mm thickness) with mild stranding of adjacent buccal planes; (B) Carcinoma left side hard palate crossing midline and extending to alveolus and floor of nasal cavity

Verrucous Carcinoma

Verrucous carcinoma appears as soft white velvety area of superficial proliferative exophytic lesion (like a white papillary growth), which has considerable keratinization. The deep invasion and induration are minimal. The tumor behaves like a low-grade squamous cell carcinoma. The lymph node metastasis is late.

Treatment

- *Stage I (T_1N_0):* Wide excision with safety margin including underlying buccinator muscle followed by quilted split-skin graft.
- *Stage II (T_2N_0):* Radiotherapy to the primary lesion and regional lymph nodes if bone is spared. If bone (maxilla and mandible) is involved or growth infiltrates the muscle, excision of the growth combined with marginal or segmental mandibulectomy or partial maxillectomy along with the reconstruction is done.
- *Stage III and IV:* Surgical resection combined with neck dissection and reconstruction and postoperative radiotherapy.
- *Reconstruction:*
  - Free radial forearm flap: Lesion extending to retromolar area, maxillary tuberosity or tonsillar fossa.
  - Buccal fat pad with or without temporalis muscle flap: For reconstruction of maxillary defects, hard and soft palate defects, and cheek and retromolar defects.

CARCINOMA HARD PALATE

It is common in India as some people have the bad habit of reverse smoking (keeping the burning end of *bidi* or cigar in the mouth).

Hard palate contains high number of minor salivary glands. Minor salivary glands tumors (adenoid cystic, mucoepidermoid and adenocarcinoma) are more common than squamous cell carcinoma. Most of the squamous cell carcinoma of upper alveolus and hard palate arises from maxillary antrum.

Clinical Features

- *Lesion:* Superficial ulcer with rolled out edges, which may be felt by tongue as painless irregularity on the palate.
- *Local spread:* To gingiva, lip, soft palate. The invasion of hard palate can involve floor of the nasal cavity and the maxillary antrum (Fig. 33.6B). This condition should be differentiated from cancer of maxillary antrum and nose, which could spread to and involve hard palate.
- *Lymphatic metastasis:* It is late and involves submandibular and upper jugular nodes and indicates poor prognosis.

Treatment

- Small tumors are excised along with the hard palate.
- Tumors confined to hard palate, upper alveolus and floor of maxillary antrum needs partial maxillectomy with block dissection if nodes are enlarged.
- Surgical defect in the palate needs closure or a suitable prosthesis.

CARCINOMA RETROMOLAR TRIGONE

- It may be either primary or secondary (extension of growths from the gingiva, floor of mouth, buccal mucosa or the palate).
- Depending on the extent of lesion, wide surgical excision with block dissection is done.

Concurrent multiple primary cancers: About 15% oral cancer patients have multiple primary cancers of the upper aerodigestive tract as the risk factors (smoking and drinking) are common. That is why these patients need panendoscopy to rule out second primary.

MINOR SALIVARY GLAND TUMORS

Minor salivary gland tumors are mostly malignant (adenoid cystic carcinoma 40%, adenocarcinoma 30% and mucoepidermoid carcinoma 20%).

- Most common site is palate. Other sites are tongue, cheek, lip, gums and floor of mouth.
- *Treatment:* Wide surgical excision along with block dissection, if nodes are involved.

MELANOMA

- Very rare in oral cavity.
- *Most common sites:* Hard palate (50%) and upper gingiva (25%).
- *Sex:* Males female ratio 2:1.
- *Age:* Most patients are in sixth decade.
- *Clinical features:* Initial raised, nodular and flat lesions remain asymptomatic.
  - *Lesion:* Area of higher pigmentation (black to brown) after many years ulcerates, bleeds and becomes painful. Rare in amelanotic (nonpigmented) area.
  - *Rapid growth:* Destruction of underlying bone.
- *Metastasis:* Both the regional lymph node and distant metastases. Fifty percent patients come with metastasis at the time of presentation.

Treatment

Wide surgical excision followed by radiotherapy.

Prognosis

- Recurrence is quite common.
- Prognosis is very poor (5-year survival only 5%). Indicators of poor outcome are following:
  - Main guide to prognosis: Histological tumor thickness (Breslow) in mm from the granular cell layer to the deepest identifiable melanocyte.
  - Malignant melanocytes in blood vessels.
  - Multiple or atypical mitoses.
  - Destruction of underlying bone.
  - Presence of metastases.

KAPOSI'S SARCOMA

- This vascular tumor is seen in acquired immune deficiency syndrome (AIDS) patients.
- It is multifocal in origin and primarily affects skin but may also be seen in the oral cavity.
- It presents as a reddish purple nodule or a plaque mostly on the palate.
- The tumor consists of spindle cells with hemorrhagic cleft-like spaces.
- Chemotherapy is advised when they do not respond to antiretroviral therapy.

Self-evaluation Exercises

1. Which of the following is not true for cancer tongue?
   a. Tip is the most common site for carcinoma of oral tongue
   b. Patient develops referred earache because the anterior two-third tongue receive its somatosensory innervation from the vagus nerve
   c. The best treatment for stage III carcinoma of oral tongue is wide excision
   d. All of the above

True (T)/False (F)

2. The most common site of minor salivary gland tumor is the floor of mouth.
3. The best treatment for stage III $T_2 N_1 M_0$ carcinoma of buccal mucosa will be surgical excision of growth with supraomohyoid neck dissection and postoperative radiotherapy.
4. Abbe-Estlander flap is used to reconstruct defects in cases of carcinoma of lip involving angle of mouth (commissure). Such defects require partial commissure reconstruction.
5. Soft palate and lower gingiva are the most common sites of melanoma in the oral cavity.

Answers

1. d   2. F   3. T   4. T   5. F

Section 5: Pharynx and Esophagus

Chapter 34

Anatomy and Physiology of Pharynx and Esophagus

⊙ Specific Learning Objectives

After going through the chapter, you should be able to answer the following questions:
- What are the components of Waldeyer's ring and their functions and lymphatic drainage?
- What are the differences between adenoids and palatine tonsils?
- Describe the blood supply of tonsil and its bed.
- Name the three divisions of pharynx and their different subsites and lymphatic drainage.
- Describe various normal constrictions and sphincters of the esophagus.
- Describe the different stages of swallowing.

PHARYNX

Pharynx is a 12–14 cm long conical tube which forms upper part of the air and food passages. It extends from basiocciput and basisphenoid to the lower border of cricoid cartilage. Inferiorly, it becomes continuous with the esophagus through pharyngo-esophageal junction (1.5 cm width), which is the narrowest part of gastrointestinal tract apart from the appendix. The width of pharynx base, which faces towards skull base, is 3.5 cm. Pharynx is traditionally divided into three parts—nasopharynx, oropharynx and hypopharynx (Fig. 34.1).

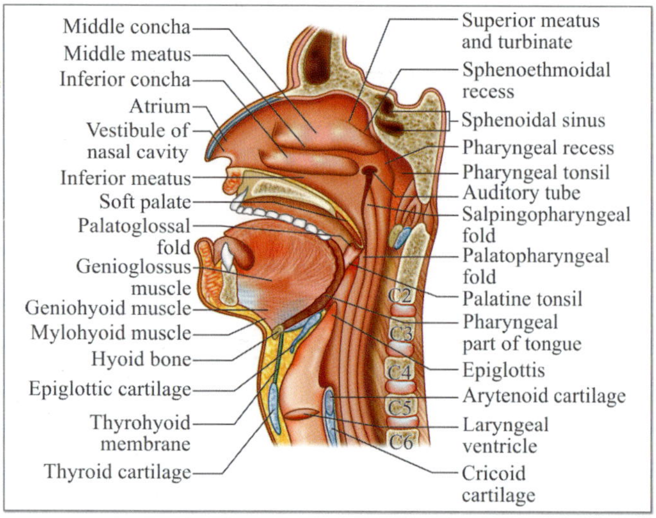

◼ PHARYNGEAL WALL (FIG. 34.2)

From within outwards it is composed of four layers—mucous membrane, pharyngeal aponeurosis (pharyngobasilar fascia), muscular coat and buccopharyngeal fascia.

1. *Mucous membrane:* The pharyngeal mucosa is ciliated columnar in the nasopharynx and stratified squamous elsewhere. It is continuous with mucous membrane of Eustachian tubes, nasal cavities, mouth, larynx and esophagus. There are numerous mucous glands.

Fig. 34.1: Sagittal section of nose, mouth, pharynx and larynx

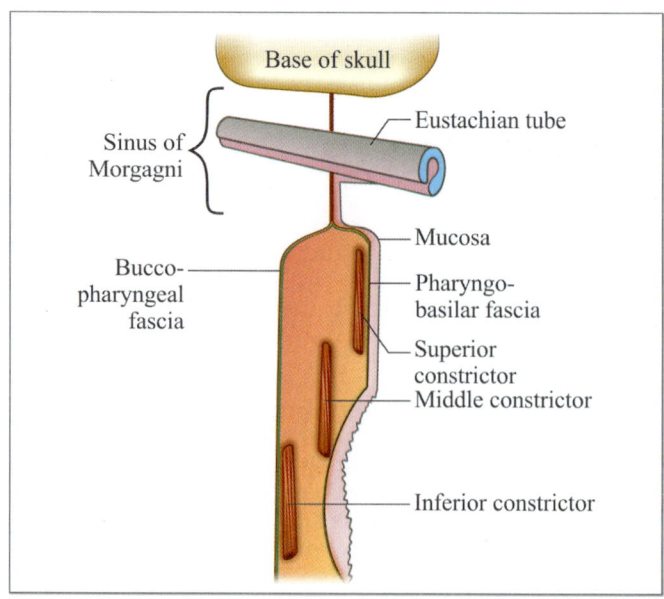

Fig. 34.2: Pharyngeal wall. Coronal section

2. ***Pharyngeal aponeurosis (pharyngobasilar fascia):*** This fibrous layer lines the muscular coat and fills up the gap left in the muscular layer especially near skull base. It is thick between the superior border of superior constrictor muscle and base of skull and becomes thin and indistinct inferiorly.
3. ***Muscular coat:*** It consists of two layers of muscles—external and internal
    i. ***External layer:*** It consists of three horizontal circular muscles—superior, middle and inferior constrictor muscles.
    ii. ***Internal layer:*** It consists of three vertical muscles stylopharyngeus, salpingopharyngeus and palatopharyngeus muscles.
4. ***Buccopharyngeal fascia:*** This fascial layer covers outer surface of the constrictor muscles. In the upper part, it extends anteriorly and covers the buccinator muscle. Above the superior constrictor, it merges with pharyngeal aponeurosis.

PHARYNGEAL SPACES

The pharyngeal spaces where abscesses can form include retropharyngeal and parapharyngeal spaces (*see* Chapter 'Deep Space Neck Infections').

Killian's Dehiscence

This potential gap lies between the two parts of inferior constrictor muscle: oblique fibers of thyropharyngeus and transverse fibers of cricopharyngeus. This weak area is common site for following:
- ***Perforation:*** Perforation during esophagoscopy. This gap is also called 'gateway of tears'.
- ***Herniation:*** Herniation of pharyngeal mucosa in cases of Zenker's diverticulum (pharyngeal pouch).

> **Hypopharyngeal diverticulum:** Incoordination between contraction of thyropharyngeal muscles and relaxation of cricopharyngeal sphincter at the upper end of esophagus can lead to hypopharyngeal diverticulum. The cricopharyngeal sphincter fails to relax when thyropharyngeal muscles is contracting.
> - **Structures passing between superior and middle constrictors:** Glossopharyngeal nerve and stylopharyngeus muscle.
> - **Structure passing between middle and inferior constrictor muscles:** Superior laryngeal artery and vein and internal laryngeal branch of superior laryngeal nerve.

WALDEYER'S RING (FIG. 34.3)

Mucosa associated lymphoid tissue (MALT) in subepithelial layer of pharynx is aggregated at the entrance of

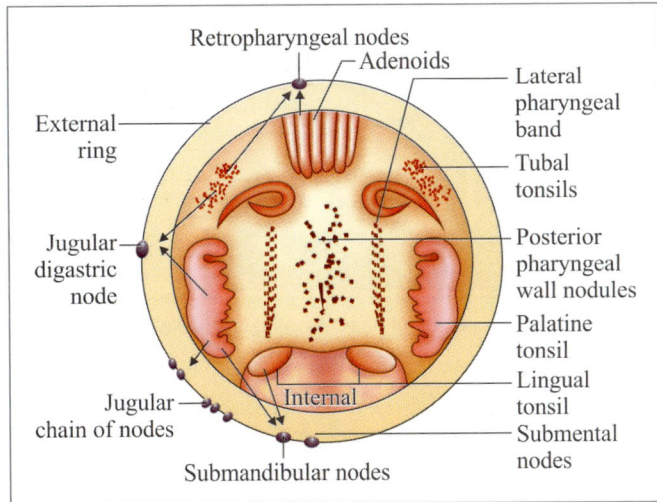

Fig. 34.3: Waldeyer's ring

aerodigestive tract and are collectively called Waldeyer's ring. Waldeyer's ring consists of:
- Adenoids or nasopharyngeal tonsil
- Tubal tonsils (fossa of Rosenmuller)
- Lateral pharyngeal bands
- Palatine tonsils
- Nodules (posterior pharyngeal wall)
- Lingual tonsils

Functions of Tonsils and Adenoids
- ***Immunology and host defenses:*** T-lymphocytes in parafollicular region provide cell-mediated immunity against viruses, bacteria and fungi. Once the pathogens enter into these lymphoid aggregations they are taken care of by IgM and IgG antibodies, which are produced by plasma cells.
- ***Sentinels at the portal of aerodigestive tract:*** Tonsils and adenoids act as protective sentinels against harmful intruders into the air and food passages. The crypts in tonsils increase the surface area for contact with foreign substances.
- ***Antibody production especially secretory IgA:*** B-lymphocytes in the germinal centers of these lymphoid follicles make antibodies IgA.

NASOPHARYNX

Nasopharynx is the uppermost part of the pharynx and lies behind the nasal cavities (Fig. 34.4).
- ***Extension:*** It extends from the base of skull to the soft palate (level of hard palate and atlas).
- ***Epithelium:*** Functionally, nasopharynx is the posterior extension of nasal cavity and is lined with pseudostratified ciliated columnar epithelium.
- ***Communications:*** It communicates with nasal cavity, middle ear cavity and oropharynx.

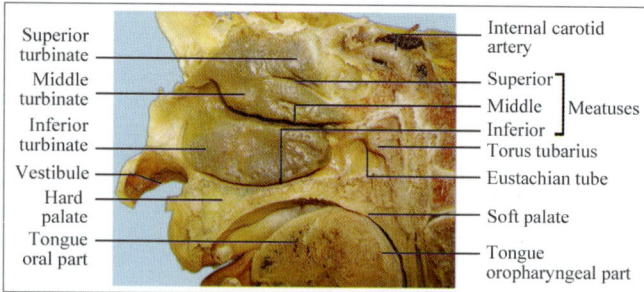

Fig. 34.4: Sagittal section of head showing lateral wall of nasal cavity and nasopharynx

Boundaries

- ***Roof and the posterior wall:*** They imperceptibly merge with each other. Roof is formed by basisphenoid and basiocciput. Posterior wall is formed by the arch of the atlas vertebra that articulates with dense of axis and covered by prevertebral muscles and fascia.
    - ***Nasopharyngeal tonsil (adenoids):*** Adenoids are present at the junction of roof and posterior wall of nasopharynx and throw the overlying mucous membrane into radiating folds. They increase in size up to the age of 6 years and after that gradually atrophies.
    - ***Nasopharyngeal bursa:*** This epithelial lined median recess, which is seen within the adenoid mass, extends from pharyngeal mucosa to periosteum of basiocciput. It represents the embryonic site of attachment of notochord to the pharyngeal endoderm.
    - ***Rathke's pouch:*** This dimple above the adenoids (junction of nasal septum and roof of nasopharynx) is the reminiscent of the buccal mucosal invagination, which forms the anterior lobe of pituitary.
- ***Floor:*** Anteriorly soft palate; posteriorly communicates with the oropharynx through nasopharyngeal isthmus. Floor of nasopharynx is the roof of oropharynx.
- ***Anterior:*** It communicates with nasal cavities through posterior nasal apertures (choanae). Posterior ends of nasal turbinates and meatuses can be seen through posterior choanae.
- ***Lateral wall:*** Structures seen on lateral wall are following:
    - ***Pharyngeal opening of Eustachian tube:*** It is situated 1.25 cm behind the posterior end of inferior turbinate.
    - ***Torus tubarius:*** It is an elevation, which is raised by the cartilage of Eustachian tube and bounds the Eustachian tube above and behind.
    - ***Tubal tonsil:*** This collection of subepithelial lymphoid tissue is continuous with adenoid tissue and forms a part of the Waldeyer's ring. It is situated at the tubal elevation.
    - ***Fossa of Rosenmuller:*** It is a recess that is situated above and behind the tubal elevation.
    - ***Salpingopharyngeal fold:*** It is raised by the salpingopharyngeus muscle and extends from the lower end of the torus tubarius to the lateral pharyngeal wall.

Sinus of Morgagni

This is a space which lies between the base of the skull and upper free border of superior constrictor muscle. Following structures pass through this space:
- Eustachian tube
- Levator veli palatini muscle, and
- Ascending palatine artery, which is a branch of the facial artery.

Passavant's Ridge

This mucosal ridge, which encircles the posterior and lateral walls of nasopharyngeal isthmus, is raised by fibers of palatopharyngeus muscle. When soft palate contracts during deglutition or speech, it makes firm contact with Passavant's ridge and cut off nasopharynx from the oropharynx.

Lymphatic Drainage

Lymphatics of the nasopharynx and the structures present on its boundaries drain into:
- Retropharyngeal and parapharyngeal lymph nodes.
- Upper deep cervical nodes either directly or through retropharyngeal and parapharyngeal lymph nodes.
- Spinal accessory chain of nodes: They are present in the posterior triangle of the neck.
- Contralateral cervical lymph nodes: Nasopharyngeal lymphatic crosses midline.

Functions of Nasopharynx

- ***Airway:*** A conduit for air to its way to the larynx.
- ***Middle ear ventilation:*** Eustachian tube ventilates and drains the middle ear. Dysfunctions of Eustachian tube can affect middle ear.
- ***Resonance:*** It is a part of resonating chamber for voice production. Nasopharyngeal obstruction (rhinolalia closa) and velopharyngeal incompetence (rhinolalia aperta) produce changes in voice.
- ***Drainage:*** It is a drainage channel for middle ear cleft, nasal and nasopharyngeal mucus secretions.
- ***Nasopharyngeal isthmus:*** It cuts off nasopharynx from oropharynx during swallowing, vomiting, gagging and speech.

- **Tornwald's disease:** This is an abscess that develops in nasopharyngeal bursa. Infected bursa usually presents with persistent postnasal discharge or crusting.
- **Craniopharyngioma:** It arises from Rathke's pouch.
- **Eustachian tube functioning:** Enlarged or infected tubal tonsils can affect Eustachian tube.
- **Nasopharyngeal carcinoma:** Fossa of Rosenmuller is a common site for the nasopharyngeal carcinoma.
- **Passavant's ridge:** It represents superior interdigitation of the superior constrictor and palatopharyngeal muscles.
- **Rouviere's node:** This most superior node of the lateral group of retropharyngeal lymph nodes is common site of lymphatic metastasis from the nasopharynx.

ADENOIDS

These nasopharyngeal tonsils, which are covered with ciliated columnar epithelium, are situated at the junction of the roof and posterior wall of the nasopharynx. Adenoids are composed of vertical ridges of lymphoid tissue, which are separated by deep clefts. Adenoids have no crypts and capsule whereas palatine tonsils have both capsule and crypts (Table 34.1). Adenoid tissue shows physiological enlargement during the first 6 years of life and then tends to regress and almost completely disappears by 20 years of age.

Blood Supply

Branches of external carotid artery supply to adenoids:
- Ascending palatine branch of facial artery.
- Ascending pharyngeal artery.
- Pharyngeal branch of the third part of maxillary artery.

Lymphatic Drainage

Adenoids drain into upper deep jugular nodes directly or through retropharyngeal and parapharyngeal nodes.

OROPHARYNX

This middle part of pharynx lies behind the oral cavity. It extends from the plane of hard palate above to the plane of hyoid bone below.

Table 34.1: Differences between palatine tonsils and adenoids

	Adenoids	Palatine Tonsils
Number	Single	One on each side
Site	Nasopharynx	Tonsillar fossa in oropharynx
Crypts or furrows	Only furrows	Only crypts
Capsule	Absent	Present
Epithelium	Ciliated columnar	Squamous stratified
In adults after 20 years of age	Absent	Present

Communications

- *Anterior:* It communicates with oral cavity through oropharyngeal isthmus.
- *Superior:* It communicates with nasopharynx through nasopharyngeal isthmus.
- *Inferior:* It communicates with laryngopharynx.

Boundaries

- *Posterior wall:* Retropharyngeal space that lies opposite the axis and upper part of the third cervical vertebra.
- *Anterior wall:* The upper part of anterior wall communicates with oral cavity through oropharyngeal isthmus. The structures present in the lower part are: base of tongue, lingual tonsils and valleculae.
  - *Oropharyngeal isthmus:* It is bounded by following structures:
    - *Above:* Soft palate
    - *Inferior:* Dorsal surface of tongue
    - *Lateral:* Palatoglossal arch (anterior tonsillar pillars).
  - *Base of tongue:* It lies posterior to circumvallate papillae and insertion of palatoglossal muscle.
  - *Lingual tonsils:* Situated in the base of tongue.
  - *Valleculae:* These cup-shaped spaces, one on each side, lie between the base of tongue and anterior surface of epiglottis. The median glossoepiglottic fold separates the two valleculae. Laterally they are bounded by the pharyngoepiglottic fold that is the upper limit of pyriform sinus of laryngopharynx.
- *Lateral wall:* Both anterior and posterior tonsillar pillars emerge from the soft palate and enclose tonsillar fossa, in which is situated the palatine tonsil. So the structures present in the lateral wall include:
  - Palatine or faucial tonsil.
  - *Anterior pillar or palatoglossal arch:* The palatoglossus muscle is present in this fold.
  - *Posterior pillar or palatopharyngeal arch:* The palatopharyngeus muscle lies in this fold.
- *Superior:* Anteriorly soft palate makes the roof of oropharynx. Posteriorly it communicates with nasopharynx through nasopharyngeal isthmus at the plane of hard palate and atlas vertebra.
- *Inferior:* It communicates with laryngopharynx at the plane of upper border of epiglottis and the pharyngoepiglottic folds and third cervical vertebra.

Lymphatic Drainage

Oropharynx drains in the following lymph nodes:
- Upper jugular chain particularly the jugulodigastric (tonsillar) node.
- Retropharyngeal and parapharyngeal nodes: Soft palate, lateral and posterior pharyngeal walls and the base of tongue.
- Posterior cervical group.

Functions of Oropharynx

- A common conduit for the passage of both air and food.
- Oropharyngeal phase of deglutition.
- Vocal tract for certain speech sounds.
- Taste: The base of tongue, soft palate, anterior pillars and posterior pharyngeal wall contain taste buds.
- Local defense and immunity.

- **Infection or compensatory enlargement of lingual tonsils** may occur after tonsillectomy.
- **Retention cysts:** Valleculae are common sites for retention cysts.
- **Carcinoma of base of tongue:** Lymphatics of base of tongue cross mid-line and drain bilaterally therefore cancer of this area can cause secondary neck nodes on both the sides.

PALATINE (FAUCIAL) TONSILS

Site and Extension

Palatine tonsil is an ovoid mass of lymphoid tissue. It is situated in the lateral wall of oropharynx (tonsillar fossa) between the anterior (mucosal fold of palatoglossal muscle) and posterior tonsillar pillars (mucosal fold of palatopharyngeal muscle). It extends superiorly into the soft palate, inferiorly into the tongue base and anteriorly into palatoglossal arch (formed by palatoglossal muscle).

Surfaces and Poles

A tonsil has two surfaces medial and lateral and two poles upper and lower. Surface epithelium of tonsil is continuous with the epithelium of oropharynx. Tonsillar crypts are tube like invaginations from the surface epithelium. Infections of tonsil can involve any of these components.

- **Supratonsillar fossa:** The medial surface of tonsillar upper pole has a semilunar fold between anterior and posterior pillars. This fold encloses a potential space called supratonsillar fossa.
- **Anterior tonsillar space:** The lower pole is attached to the tongue. Here a triangular fold of mucous membrane extends from anterior pillar to the anteroinferior part of tonsil. This fold encloses a anterior tonsillar space.

Tonsillar Crypts

The nonkeratinizing stratified squamous epithelium on medial surface of tonsil dips into the tonsillar mass and forms crypts (12–15). Openings of crypts can be seen on the medial surface of the tonsil (Figs 34.5 and 34.6).

- **Crypta magna or intratonsillar cleft:** It is situated near the upper part of tonsil. It is very large and deep and represents the ventral part of second pharyngeal pouch.

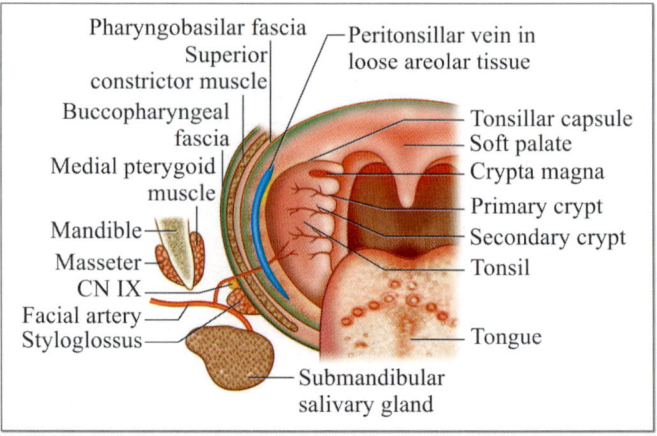

Fig. 34.5: Bed of tonsil

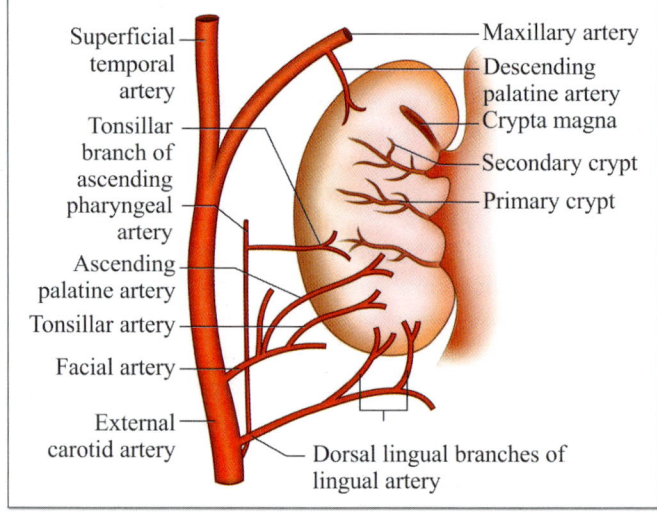

Fig. 34.6: Blood supply and crypts of tonsil

- **Secondary crypts:** They arise from the main crypts within the substance of tonsil.
- **Content:** Crypts may be filled with cheesy material, which consists of epithelial cells, bacteria and food debris and can be expressed out with pressure over the anterior tonsillar pillar.

Capsule

Lateral surface of tonsil is covered by a well-defined fibrous capsule, which is separated from the bed of tonsil by loose areolar tissue that allows easy dissection during tonsillectomy. In this same plane occurs the peritonsillar abscess. Some fibers of palatoglossus and palatopharyngeus muscles are attached to tonsillar capsule.

Bed of the Tonsil (Fig. 34.5)

The superior constrictor, glossopharyngeal nerve and styloglossus muscle form the bed of tonsil. Lateral to the superior constrictor muscles lies facial artery, submandibular gland, posterior belly of digastric, medial pterygoid muscle and the angle of mandible.

Blood Supply (Fig. 34.6)

- *Arterial supply:* The main artery of tonsil is tonsillar branch of facial artery. Other branches of external carotid artery that supply the tonsil are:
  - Ascending pharyngeal artery from external carotid.
  - Ascending palatine, a branch of facial artery.
  - Dorsal lingual branch of lingual artery.
  - Descending palatine branch of maxillary artery.

> *Bleeding after tonsillectomy*: The ascending pharyngeal, facial, lingual and maxillary arteries are all branches of external carotid artery that may need to be ligated in cases of refractory bleeding after tonsillectomy.

- *Venous drainage:* Veins from the tonsils drain into paratonsillar veins, which are present on lateral surface of tonsil and drain into the common facial vein and pharyngeal venous plexus.

Lymphatic Drainage

Palatine tonsils drain into the jugulodigastric (tonsillar) nodes of upper deep cervical group, which are situated below the angle of mandible.

Nerve Supply

The sensory nerve supply to tonsil is from:
- Maxillary division of trigeminal nerve (CN V_2): Lesser palatine branches from sphenopalatine ganglion.
- Glossopharyngeal nerve (CN IX).

> - *Tonsillolingual sulcus:* It separates the tonsil from tongue and is a common site for carcinoma.
> - *Tonsillectomy:* Tonsils may be larger in childhood and usually regress in size near puberty. If they become the seat of disease, they may be removed.
> - *Styloid process:* The styloid process when enlarged may be palpated intraorally in the lower part of tonsillar fossa. The glossopharyngeal nerve and styloid process can be approached through the tonsil bed after tonsillectomy.
> - *Bleeding after tonsillectomy:* External carotid artery may need to be ligated in cases of refractory bleeding after tonsillectomy as its branches (ascending pharyngeal, facial, lingual and maxillary arteries) supply the tonsils.
> - *Second pharyngeal pouch:* Palatine tonsil develops in the second pharyngeal pouch.

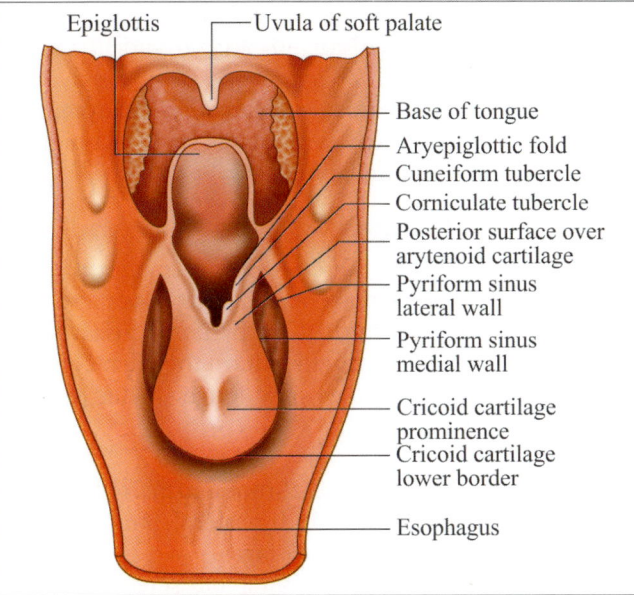

Fig. 34.7: Structures of hypopharynx. Posterior view of laryngopharynx

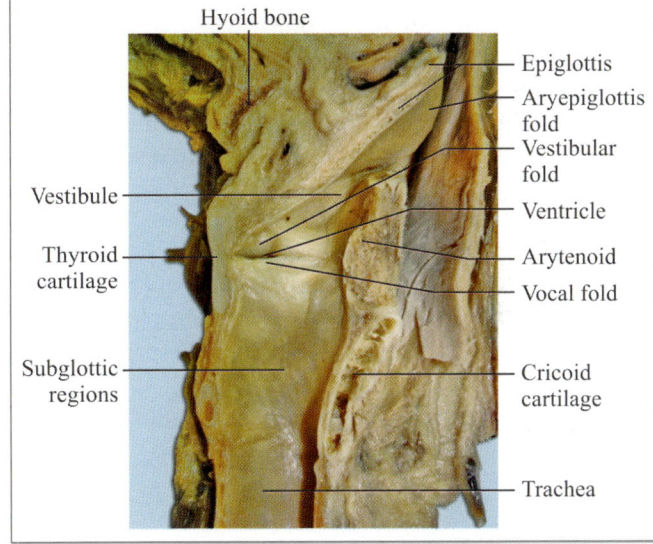

Fig. 34.8: Sagittal section of larynx and laryngopharynx

HYPOPHARYNX (LARYNGOPHARYNX)

Hypopharynx, which is the lowest part of the pharynx, lies behind and partly lateral to the larynx (Figs 34.7 and 34.8). It extends superiorly from the plane of hyoid bone to the lower border of cricoid cartilage. Posteriorly, it lies on the 3rd, 4th, 5th, 6th cervical vertebrae.

Communications

- *Superior:* It is continuous with oropharynx at the level of hyoid bone.

- **Inferior:** It becomes continuous with esophagus at the level of lower border of cricoid cartilage and 6th cervical vertebra.
- **Anterior:** It communicates with larynx through the laryngeal inlet, which is bounded by the epiglottis, aryepiglottic folds and arytenoids.

Hypopharynx Subsites

It is subdivided into three regions—pyriform sinus, postcricoid region and posterior pharyngeal wall.

1. *Pyriform sinus (fossa):* Each pyriform fossa lies on either side of the larynx. They form the lateral channel for food. Foreign bodies may lodge in the pyriform fossa.
   Boundaries:
   - *Lateral:* Thyrohyoid membrane and thyroid cartilage.
   - *Medial:* Aryepiglottic fold, posterolateral surface of arytenoid and cricoid cartilages.
   - *Superior:* Pharyngoepiglottic fold separates it from vallecula.
   - *Inferior:* It opens into the esophagus at the level of lower border of cricoid cartilage.
2. *Postcricoid region:* This anterior wall of laryngopharynx (pharyngoesophageal junction) extends between the level of arytenoids and lower border of cricoid lamina.
3. *Posterior pharyngeal wall:* It extends from the level of hyoid bone to the level of inferior border of cricoid cartilage between the apices of pyriform fosse.

Lymphatic Drainage

- *Pyriform sinus:* It drains into the upper jugular chain through the thyrohyoid membrane.
- *Posterior pharyngeal wall:* Lateral retropharyngeal or parapharyngeal nodes and then to deep cervical lymph nodes.
- *Postcricoid region:* Parapharyngeal nodes and nodes of supraclavicular and paratracheal chain.

Functions

- Common pathway for air and food.
- Provides a vocal tract for resonance of certain words.
- Helps in deglutition.

> - **Internal laryngeal nerve** runs submucosally in the lateral wall of pyriform fossa. It causes referred earache in cases of carcinoma pyriform fossa. It is accessed here for local anesthesia.
> - **Postcricoid carcinoma:** It is a common site for carcinoma, which usually develops from Plummer-Vinson syndrome especially in females.
> - **Cancer of Pyriform fossa:** Pyriform fosse have rich lymphatic network and carcinoma of this region has high frequency of nodal metastases.

ESOPHAGUS (FIG. 34.9)

Esophagus is a 25 cm long muscular tube that begins from the lower end of hypopharynx at the level of lower border of cricoid cartilage (C6) to the cardiac end of stomach (T11). Cervical esophagus inclines to the left from its origin to thoracic inlet. Thoracic esophagus also inclines to the left from T7 to the esophageal opening in the diaphragm.

CONSTRICTIONS

Esophagus shows four normal constrictions, which can be seen in esophagogram as well as during esophagoscopy. These constrictions, where foreign bodies can be held up, are at the following approximate levels:

1. Pharyngoesophageal junction (C6)-15 cm from the upper incisors.
2. Arch of aorta (T4)-22 cm from upper incisors.
3. Left main bronchus (T5)-25 cm from upper incisors.
4. Diaphragm (T10)-40 cm from upper incisors.

Structure

The esophageal wall consists of following four layers from within outwards:

1. *Mucosa:* It is stratified squamous epithelium.
2. *Submucosa*
3. *Muscular layer:* It has two layers—inner circular and outer longitudinal fibers. Circular fibers at the lower end get modified and form cardiac sphincter. The muscle fibers are striated in upper third, smooth in the lower third and both striated and smooth in the middle third of esophagus.
4. *Fibrous layer:* It loosely covers the esophagus.

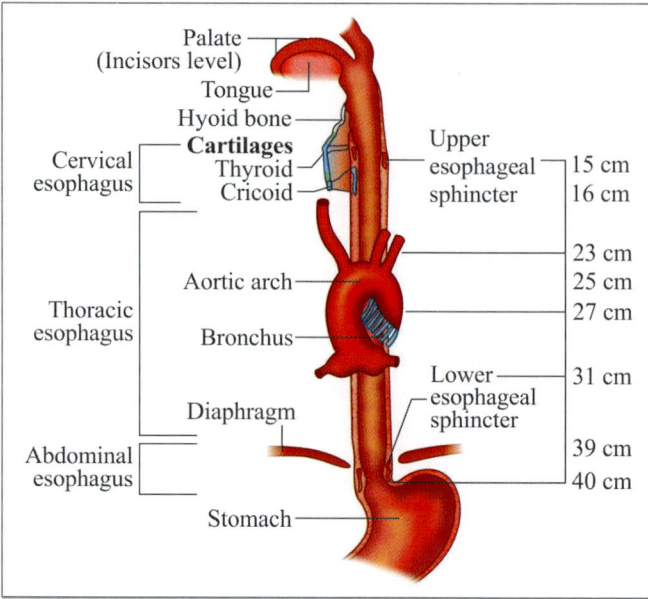

Fig. 34.9: Esophagus and its relations

Nerve Supply

- *Parasympathetic:* It is mediated by branches of vagus nerve (CN X) that has synaptic connections to myenteric (Auerbach's) plexus. Meissner's submucosal plexus is sparse in esophagus.
- *Sympathetic:* Sympathetic trunk.

Lymphatic Drainage

- *Cervical esophagus:* Deep cervical group of nodes.
- *Thoracic esophagus:* Posterior mediastinal nodes.
- *Abdominal esophagus:* Gastric lymph nodes.

ESOPHAGEAL SPHINCTERS

Esophageal manometry shows two high-pressure zones, which form the physiological sphincters of esophagus. The middle portion of esophagus shows active peristalsis that is weaker in the upper part and becomes gradually stronger towards the lower part of esophagus.

- *Upper esophageal sphincter (UES):* Upper esophageal sphincter is about 3–5 cm long and functions during the act of swallowing. It begins from the upper border of esophagus. This functional unit correlates anatomically with junction of the thyropharyngeus and cricopharyngeus, which are powerful striated muscles. UES is closed at rest and protects respiratory passage from regurgitation of esophageal contents. It does not allow air to enter into the esophagus except during swallowing.
- *Lower esophageal sphincter (LES):* LES is also about 3–5 cm long. This relatively high pressure zone prevents gastric contents reflux into the esophagus. LES has a pressure of 10–25 mm Hg. It is situated at lower portion of esophagus just above the esophagogastric junction. It is more subtle and created by the asymmetrical arrangement of smooth muscle fibers in the distal esophageal wall. It opens in response to primary peristalsis and vomiting and allows air to escape from the stomach.
  - *Factors affecting LES tone:* They include the following: food, gastric distension, gastrointestinal hormones, drugs and smoking.

PHYSIOLOGY OF SWALLOWING

The process of swallowing is usually divided into three phases: oral (buccal), pharyngeal and esophageal. The swallowing center in medulla integrates functions of cranial nerves V, VII, IX, X and XII. Various mechanical and neuromuscular conditions can disrupt this process.

- *Oral phase:* The food is chewed, lubricated (with saliva) and converted into a bolus. The tongue is elevated against the palate and food is propelled into oropharynx. It is a voluntary phase.
- *Pharyngeal phase:* Once the bolus of food comes into oropharynx, a series of reflex actions occurs, which do not allow the food to go into nasopharynx, oral cavity and larynx and facilitate carrying the food past oropharynx and laryngopharynx into the esophagus.
  - *Nasopharynx:* Closure of nasopharynx occurs when soft palate contracts against the Passavant's ridge. Nasopharyngeal isthmus shuts the nasopharynx from oropharynx.
  - *Oropharynx:* Closure of oropharyngeal isthmus, which occurs due to the sphincteric action of palatoglossal muscles when tongue contracts against palate, prevents the entry of food back into oral cavity.
  - *Larynx:* Closure of laryngeal inlet by contraction of aryepiglottic folds and closure of false and true cords prevent aspiration of food material into the larynx. There occurs temporary cessation of respiration and rising of larynx under the base of tongue. The function of epiglottis is not clear but is seen deflecting backwards while food passes into the pyriform fossa.
  - *Hypopharynx:* When pharyngeal muscles contract cricopharyngeus muscles relax and food passes from pharynx into the esophagus. These actions are well timed and synchronous.
- *Esophageal phase:* Once the food enters into the esophagus, cricopharyngeal sphincter closes and primary peristalsis of esophagus takes the food bolus down into the stomach. Gastroesophageal sphincter (GES) relaxes well before the arrival of peristaltic wave. Bolus of food is taken into the stomach with the peristaltic waves and then gastroesophageal sphincter closes.

Gastroesophageal Reflux

Reflux of food (gastric content) into esophagus is prevented with the following:

- Functioning gastroesophageal sphincter.
- Negative intrathoracic pressure and slight positive intra-abdominal pressure.
- Pinch-cock effect of diaphragm.
- Mucosal folds.
- Esophagogastric angle.

> **Heartburn (pyrosis)** refers to the feeling of substernal burning that is highly specific of gastroesophageal reflux disease (GERD).

> - *Killian-Jamieson's space:* It lies between cricopharyngeus and circular fibers of the esophagus.
> - *Lamier Hackemann's space:* It lies between circular and longitudinal fibers of the esophagus.

Section 5 • Pharynx and Esophagus

Self-evaluation Exercises

1. Which of the followings are not correct for adenoids?
   a. Situated in the roof and posterior wall of nasopharynx
   b. Have a capsule on external surface
   c. Have crypts
   d. Present at birth but disappears by puberty
   e. All of the above
2. Structures passing between superior and middle constrictors:
   a. Glossopharyngeal nerve
   b. Eustachian tube
   c. Superior laryngeal nerve
   d. Stylopharyngeus muscle
3. Structure passing between middle and inferior constrictor muscles:
   a. Glossopharyngeal nerve
   b. Superior laryngeal artery and vein
   c. Recurrent laryngeal nerve
   d. Internal laryngeal branch of superior laryngeal nerve
4. Structures passing between upper border of superior constrictor muscle and base of skull are:
   a. Levator veli palatine
   b. Eustachian tube
   c. Ascending palatine artery
   d. All of the above

True (T)/False (F)

5. Waldeyer's ring of lymphoid tissue is situated in both nasopharynx and oropharynx.
6. Palatine tonsil develops in the first pharyngeal pouch.
7. Main blood supply to tonsil is from the tonsillar branch of lingual artery.
8. Passavant's ridge represents superior interdigitation of the superior constrictor and palatopharyngeal muscles.
9. Killian-Jamieson's space lies between cricopharyngeus and circular fibers of the esophagus.
10. Killian dehiscence is found between the middle constrictor and thyropharyngeus.
11. Rouviere's node, the most superior node of the lateral group of retropharyngeal lymph nodes is common site of lymphatic metastasis from the nasopharynx.
12. Lamier-Hackemann's space lies between circular and longitudinal fibers of the esophagus.

Answers

1. b, c	2. a, d	3. b, d	4. d	5. T	6. F
7. F	8. T	9. T	10. F	11. T	12. T

Pearls and Nuggets (Refresh your knowledge)

- **Adenohypophysis:** This anterior lobe of pituitary gland is derived from an outgrowth of oral ectoderm called Rathke's pouch.
- **Palatal muscles:** All the muscles of palate are supplied by the vagal accessory nerve except the tensor palati, which is innervated by mandibular division of trigeminal nerve.
- **Styloid process:** All the three muscles arising form the styloid process have different nerve supplies. Stylohyoid by facial nerve; styloglossus by hypoglossal nerve; and stylopharyngeus by glossopharyngeal nerve.
- **Submucous cleft palate:** The clinical features include bifid uvula, notch in posterior border of hard palate, and deficient palatal muscles.
- **Third aortic arch:** It gives rise to the common carotid arteries.
- **Nucleus solitarius in medulla:** Most visceral sensation other than pain such as taste sensations, chemoreceptor and baroreceptor information from carotid sinus and carotid body go to this nucleus through facial, glossopharyngeal and vagus nerves. Lesions of carotid body and carotid sinus result in problems in self regulating blood pressure. The nuclei found throughout the length of the medulla are solitary nucleus and spinal nucleus of CN V.

Chapter 35

Pharyngeal Symptoms and Examination

> **Specific Learning Objectives**
>
> After going through the chapter, you should be able to answer the following questions:
> - What will be the symptoms of the patients of nasopharyngeal diseases and the findings you will be looking for during your examination?
> - What are the symptoms of oropharyngeal disorders and their findings you will be seeking during examination?
> - What are the different causes of dysphagia and their characteristic features?
> - How will you evaluate a patient with dysphagia?

EVALUATION OF PHARYNX

For general scheme of case taking and general set-up of bull's eye lamp, light source and head mirror, *see* Chapter 'History and Examination'. Pharyngeal symptoms include sore throat, ulcers, growth, pain, odynophagia (painful swallowing), stridor, voice change, nasal voice, dysphagia (difficulty in swallowing), snoring, cough, sputum, injury and foreign body. The associated complaints include fever, headache, earache, conductive hearing loss, vomiting, nasal regurgitation, loss of weight and anorexia. History of the symptoms must be taken in detail such as duration, mode of onset, severity, progression and factors aggravating and relieving, etc. Patient must be inquired about the habits of chewing *paan*, sopari and tobacco, smoking and alcohol.

NASOPHARYNX

Symptoms

Symptoms of nasopharyngeal disorders are:
- Nasal obstruction
- Nasal discharge anterior or posterior
- Epistaxis
- Hearing loss: Conductive
- Symptoms of cranial nerve palsies
- Neck swelling: Metastatic neck nodes.

Examination

Box 35.1 shows the protocol of examination, nasopharyngeal structures, pathological findings seen during examination and their causes. Examination of cranial nerves and regional lymph nodes is important. The tumors of nasopharynx can involve any of the cranial nerve often CN IX, X and XI and cervical lymph nodes (upper internal jugular and along accessory nerve).

- **Anterior rhinoscopy:** Some part of the nasopharynx can be seen in decongested nose (with vasoconstrictors) even on anterior rhinoscopy.
- **Posterior rhinoscopy:** It provides fragmented view of nasopharynx, which is mentally reconstituted by the examiner. The examiner has to tilt the mirror in different directions to visualize the structures present on different walls of the nasopharynx. For the detail method *see* Chapter 'Nasal Symptoms and Examination'. (*see* also Nasopharynx Section in Chapter 'Pharyngeal Symptoms and Examination') next to 'Posterior Rhinoscopy' in Table 21.1 of Chapter 21.
  - *Retraction of soft palate with catheters:* It facilitates postnasal mirror examination in some difficult cases and requires good local or general anesthesia. In this method, a soft rubber catheter is passed through the nostril and then taken out from the mouth through the oropharynx. Both ends of catheter are held together, and pulled forward. Retraction of soft palate makes the mirror examination easy. This method is becoming obsolete with the advent of sinuscope and flexible nasopharyngolaryngoscopy.
- **Digital examination:** Though uncomfortable for the patient, it is a simple method to palpate the nasopharynx. Examiner, standing behind and right to the patient invaginates patient's cheek between the teeth with his

> **Box 35.1: Examination of nasopharynx: Methods of examination, nasopharyngeal structures, pathological findings and their causes**
>
> - *Methods:*
>   - *Anterior rhinoscopy*
>   - *Posterior rhinoscopy*
>   - Retraction of soft palate with catheters
>   - *Digital examination*
>   - *Endoscopy:* Sinuscope, flexible nasopharyngolaryngoscope
>   - *Examination of cranial nerves*
>   - *Examination of neck nodes*
> - *Nasopharyngeal structures:*
>   - *Anterior:* Posterior border of nasal septum, choanae, posterior ends of turbinates and meatuses
>   - *Lateral:* Opening of Eustachian tube (ET), torus tubarius and pharyngeal recess (fossa of Rosenmuller)
>   - *Floor:* Upper surface of soft palate
>   - *Roof and posterior wall:* Adenoids, median recess of nasopharyngeal bursa within the adenoid mass, Rathke's pouch dimple above the adenoids (junction of nasal septum and roof of nasopharynx)
> - *Pathological findings and their causes:*
>   - *Discharge:* Middle meatus (infections of anterior group of sinuses), superior meatus (infections of posterior group of sinuses)
>   - *Crusting:* Atrophic rhinitis and nasopharyngitis
>   - *Mass:*
>   - Smooth pale mass (antrochoanal polyp)
>   - Pink lobulated mass (angiofibroma)
>   - Irregular bleeding mass (carcinoma)
>   - Smooth swelling in the roof (Thornwald's cyst and abscess)
>   - Irregular mass with radiating folds (adenoids)
>   - Mulberry irregular mass filling the lower part of choana (hypertrophy of inferior turbinate)
>   - *Bleeding* (nasopharyngeal angiofibroma and carcinoma)

left finger and introduces right index finger behind and above the soft palate into the nasopharynx. This method is not employed in cases of angiofibroma.

- *Endoscopy:* It gives a bright and magnified view of the nose and nasopharyngeal structures. It can be performed by rigid and flexible fiber-optic scopes.
  - *Rigid nasal endoscope (sinuscope or rhinoscope):* They are available in different sizes and angles and introduced through the nose after instilling and spraying local anesthetic and decongestant. *See* Chapter 'Operations of Nose and Paranasal Sinuses'.
  - *Flexible nasopharyngolaryngoscope:* It offers views of nose, pharynx and larynx. *See* Chapter 'Laryngeal Symptoms and Examination'.

OROPHARYNX

Oropharynx lies behind the oral cavity, and includes tonsils and their pillars, soft palate, base of tongue, and posterior pharyngeal wall (Fig. 35.1). Oropharynx lies behind the anterior tonsillar pillars, hard palate and V-shaped row of lingual circumvallate papillae.

Symptoms

The lesions of oropharynx can disturb swallowing, phonation, respiration and hearing. The common symptoms and their causes are mentioned in Box 35.2.

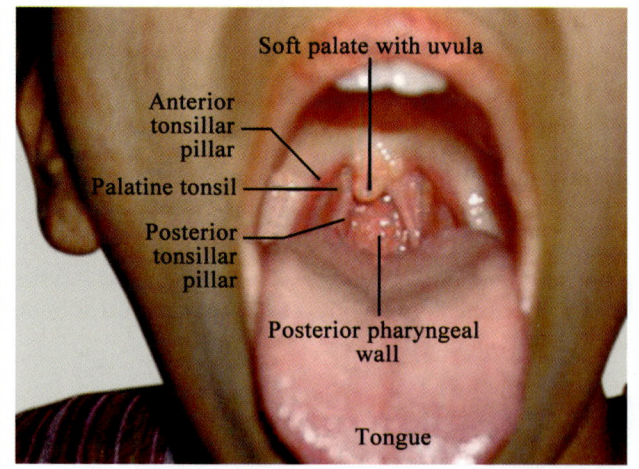

Fig. 35.1: Oropharyngeal structures seen through opened mouth

- *Middle ear symptoms:* A conductive hearing loss can occur due to Eustachian tube malfunction, which may result from enlarged tonsils (interfere movements of soft palate), cleft palate and palatal paralysis. The infections of pharyngitis and tonsillitis can travel to the middle ear through Eustachian tube.
- *Cancer phobia:* Some structures in the oropharynx may be noticed by certain patients during their self examination. Hypertrophic circumvallate and foliate

Box 35.2: Oropharyngeal symptoms and their causes

- **Sore throat and/or odynophagia:** Tonsillitis, pharyngitis, aphthous ulcers, abscesses (peritonsillar, parapharyngeal, retropharyngeal) and lingual tonsillitis
- **Dysphagia:** Tonsillar enlargements, benign and malignant tumors of tonsils, base of tongue, posterior pharyngeal wall and parapharyngeal region
- **Nasal regurgitation of fluid:** Paralysis of soft palate, cleft palate and palatal perforation
- **Change in voice:** Hypernasality (paralysis of palate), muffled or hot potato voice (space occupying lesions of the oropharynx)
- **Referred earache:** Ulcers, tumor, infection of the base of tongue, tonsil, pillars and palate
- **Snoring and obstructive sleep apnea (OSA):** Large tonsils, soft palate and tongue
- **Halitosis (bad smell from the mouth):** Infected tonsils and malignant tumors

papillae can generate cancer fear in these patients who need reassurance.

Examination

The examination begins by asking the patient to open the mouth widely. Tongue depressor is used to examine tonsillolingual sulcus and to express contents of tonsillar crypts. The base of tongue is examined by laryngeal mirror. The structures of oropharynx and their common lesions are mentioned in Box 35.3.

- **Tonsils and pillars:** For expressing the material from tonsil crypts, pressure on the anterior pillar is applied with the edge of tongue depressor. Palpation should always be performed with a gloved finger to know the consistency of the mass. There is uniform congestion of the pillars, tonsils and pharyngeal mucosa in acute tonsillitis; however, congestion of only anterior pillars indicates chronic tonsillitis. Ulcer and proliferative growth may extend to or from the tonsil, base of tongue, and the retromolar trigone.
- **Soft palate:** In cases of peritonsillar abscess, uvula becomes edematous and displaced to the opposite side. To note the movement of soft palate, patient is asked to say 'AA'. Deviation of the uvula and soft palate occurs to the healthy side in cases of vagus palsy, which may be associated with paralysis of posterior pharyngeal wall that manifests as a 'curtain effect' (the paralyzed side of palate moves like a sliding curtain). In cases of submucous cleft palate, in addition to bifid uvula, a notch can be palpated in the midline of the posterior part of hard palate.
- **Base of tongue and valleculae:** Posterior one-third of tongue is best examined by indirect laryngoscopy and finger palpation. It lies between the V-shaped row of circumvallate papillae and the valleculae. Valleculae are two shallow depressions that lie between the base of tongue and the epiglottis.
- **Palpation:** Palpation of oropharynx including base of tongue is very important as it helps in locating the infiltrative growth and its extension which is usually missed during inspection. If the patient fails to relax, and does not cooperate even after 4% xylocaine spray, palpation must be conducted under general anesthesia.

Box 35.3: Findings of oropharyngeal examination and their causes

- **Tonsils:** Present/absent
    - **Size:** Large and obstructive; small and embedded
    - **Symmetry:** Unilateral or bilateral enlargement
    - **Crypts:** White or yellow spots at the openings (follicular tonsillitis); white excrescences which are not easily wiped off (keratosis); expression of cheesy material (normal) and frank pus (septic tonsil)
    - **Membrane:** Membranous tonsillitis (diphtheria and Vincent's angina)
    - **Ulcer:** Malignant, aphthous, Vincent's angina, tuberculosis and ulcerating tonsillolith
    - **Mass:** Cystic (retention cyst), pedunculated or sessile solid mass (papilloma, fibroma), proliferative growth (cancer)
    - **Bulge:** Peritonsillitis and abscess, parapharyngeal abscess and tumor
    - **Palpation:** Hard (malignancy or tonsillolith), pulsation (internal carotid artery aneurysm) and bony (an elongated styloid process)
    - **Tonsillar pillars:** Congestion, ulcer and proliferative growth
- **Soft palate:** Redness, bulge or swelling (peritonsillitis), fibrous band (submucous fibrosis), vesicles, cleft palate, notch in the midline on posterior part of hard palate (submucous cleft palate), paralysis, ulcers/growths (benign and malignant)
    - **Uvula:** Edematous, displaced to the opposite side (peritonsillar abscess, palatal palsy), bifid uvula, 'curtain effect' (paralysis of posterior pharyngeal wall)
- **Posterior pharyngeal wall:** Lymphoid nodules (granular pharyngitis), postnasal purulent drip (chronic sinusitis), thin glazed mucosa and crusting (atrophic pharyngitis), ulcers/growths (benign and malignant)
- **Base of tongue and valleculae:** (Indirect laryngoscopy and palpation): Color of mucosa (normal or congested); prominent veins, varicosities at the base of tongue, lingual thyroid, ulceration (malignancy, tuberculosis, syphilis), solid swelling (lingual thyroid, lymphoma, carcinoma base of tongue), cystic swelling (vallecular cyst, dermoid and thyroglossal cyst)

The examiner must insert his/her finger in patient's cheek (especially in children) between the upper and lower teeth to prevent biting on the examiner's finger.

LARYNGOPHARYNX

For the evaluation (symptoms and examination) of laryngopharynx, kindly *see* Chapter 'Laryngeal Symptoms and Examination'.

EVALUATION OF ESOPHAGUS

The symptoms of heartburn, dysphagia and odynophagia almost always suggest a primary esophageal disease.
- *Heartburn (pyrosis):* This is sensation of substernal burning that often radiates to the neck. It is highly indicative of gastroesophageal reflux disease (GERD). It is the reflux of acidic (rarely alkali) material into the esophagus, and discussed in detail in Chapter 'Disorders of Esophagus'.
- *Odynophagia:* It is sharp retrosternal pain on swallowing indicative of esophagitis due to candida, herpes viruses, cytomegalovirus (CMV), especially in immunocompromised patients. The traumatic causes include caustic ingestions and pill-induced ulcers (*see* Chapter 'Disorders of Esophagus').
- *Dysphagia:* The difficulty in swallowing is discussed in detail in other Section of this Chapter.

BARIUM ESOPHAGOGRAPHY

Barium evaluation is gold standard for swallowing disorders and esophageal function. It allows evaluation of tongue movement, soft palate elevation, epiglottic tilt, laryngeal closure and peristalsis of pharyngoesophageal segment (Figs 35.2A and B). It differentiates between mechanical lesions and motility disorders.
- *Contraindications:* Barium swallow is not used in cases of aspiration. Other contraindications include perforation of pharynx and esophagus.
- *Indications and findings (Figs 35.3A to C):*
  - *Malignant lesions:* They show irregular narrowing of lumen along with mucosal destruction, ulceration and shouldering effect. The length of tumor is important for its staging.
  - *Benign strictures:* Smooth narrowing (may be at multiple sites) of a short or long part of esophagus.
  - *Cardiac achalasia (cardiospasm):* Markedly dilated, elongated, and tortuous esophagus (megaesophagus) having fluid level in lumen.
  - *Esophageal varices:* Irregular filling defects (like a string of pearls) in lower portion of esophagus.

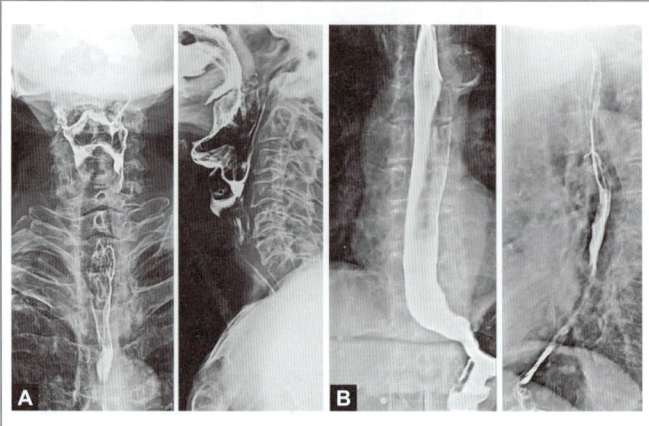

Figs 35.2A and B: Normal barium swallow. (A) Upper esophagus; (B) Lower esophagus
Source: Dr Swati Shah, Professor, Radiodiagnosis, GCRI Medical College, Ahmedabad

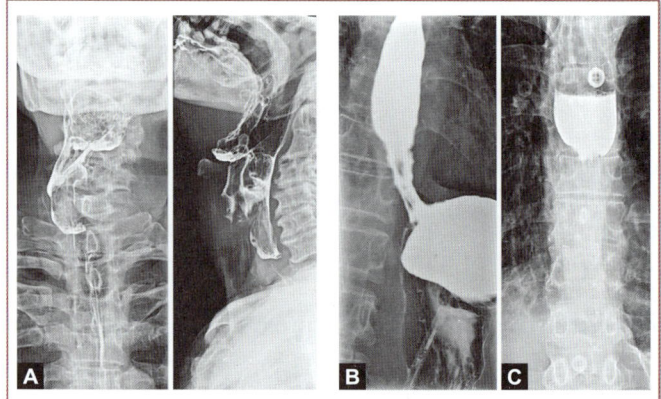

Figs 35.3A to C: Barium swallow. (A) Filling defect in left pyriform fossa; (B) Mucosal irregularity in lower third of esophagus and esophageal-gastric junction; (C) Abrupt obstruction at mid-esophageal level
Source: Dr Swati Shah, Professor, Radiodiagnosis, GCRI Medical College, Ahmedabad

 Barium swallow vs esophagoscopy: Many clinicians prefer flexible endoscopy if they strongly suspect mechanical lesions. In motility disorders, barium swallow is done first as it provides more physiologic examination.

ESOPHAGOSCOPY

See Chapter 'Endoscopies'.

DYSPHAGIA

It refers to difficulty in swallowing. It can be divided into two types: oropharyngeal (difficulty in transferring food bolus from oropharynx to upper esophagus) and esophageal (difficulty in transporting bolus through the body of esophagus).

CAUSES

The cause of dysphagia may lie in oral cavity, pharynx or esophagus (Box 35.4).

EVALUATION

History

- *Sudden onset:* Foreign body and impaction of food on a stricture and malignancy, and neurological lesions.
- *Gradually progressive:* Malignancy (short history with weight loss) and peptic strictures (long history with heartburn).
- *Chronic but not progressive:* Benign stricture.
- *Intermittent:* Spasmodic episodes.
- *Liquids/solids:* More with liquids (paralytic lesions), more with solids and progressing to liquids (malignancy).
- *Intolerance to acid food and fruit juices:* Ulcerative lesions.
- *Associated complaints:*
  - *Regurgitation and heartburn:* Hiatus hernia.
  - *Regurgitation of undigested food* in lying down and coughing in night: Hypopharyngeal diverticulum.
  - *Nasal regurgitation:* Palatal paralysis.
  - *Aspiration into lungs:* Laryngeal paralysis.

Physical Examination

The physical examination should include oral cavity, oropharynx, hypopharynx, larynx, neck, chest and nervous system including cranial nerves. The lesions of oral cavity and pharynx can be seen during physical examination whereas esophageal causes require investigations such as barium swallow and esophagoscopy.

Investigations

Upper endoscopy, barium swallow, manometry and pH recording are the mainstay of dysphagia evaluation.

- *Hemogram:* Iron deficiency anemia in Plummer-Vinson syndrome.
- *X-ray chest:* For advanced esophageal lesions, cardiovascular, pulmonary and mediastinal diseases and pneumomediastinum.
- *X-ray neck lateral and frontal projections:* For cervical osteophytes, lesions of postcricoid and retropharyngeal region.
  - Useful in children.

Box 35.4: Causes of dysphagia

- **Oral causes:** They include disorders of following functions and structures
  - **Chewing:** Trismus, fractures of mandible and maxilla, cancer of the upper and lower jaw and temporomandibular joints disorders
  - **Lubrication:** Causes of xerostomia such as radiotherapy and Mikulicz disease
  - **Tongue:** Paralysis, swelling, painful ulcers, carcinoma, abscess and total glossectomy
  - **Palate:** Cleft palate, palatal palsy, oroantral and oronasal fistula, carcinoma palate
  - **Floor of mouth:** Cancer and Ludwig's angina
- **Pharyngeal causes:**
  - **Tumors:** Tonsil, soft palate, pharynx, base of tongue, supraglottic larynx, or even obstructive hypertrophic tonsils
  - **Inflammatory:** Acute tonsillitis, peritonsillar abscess, retropharyngeal abscess, parapharyngeal abscess, acute epiglottitis and edema of larynx
  - **Spasmodic:** Tetanus and rabies
  - **Paralytic:** Palatal palsy, which present with nasal regurgitation, may be caused by diphtheria, bulbar palsy, or cerebrovascular accidents. Lesions of vagus and bilateral superior laryngeal nerves can lead to aspiration
- **Esophageal causes:** The lesions may lie in the lumen, on the wall, or outside the wall of esophagus
  - **Lumen obstruction:** Atresia, foreign body, strictures and benign and malignant tumors
  - **Mucosal inflammation:** Acute and chronic esophagitis
  - **Motility disorders:**
    - **Hypomotility:** Achalasia, scleroderma and amyotrophic lateral sclerosis
    - **Hypermotility:** Cricopharyngeal spasm and diffuse esophageal spasm
  - **External pressure:**
    - **Hypopharyngeal diverticulum**
    - **Hiatus hernia**
    - **Cervical spines:** Osteophytes
    - **Thyroid:** Enlargement, tumors and thyroiditis
    - **Mediastinal:** Tumor, lymph node enlargement, aortic aneurysm and cardiac enlargement
    - **Vascular rings:** Dysphagia lusoria (Fig. 35.4)

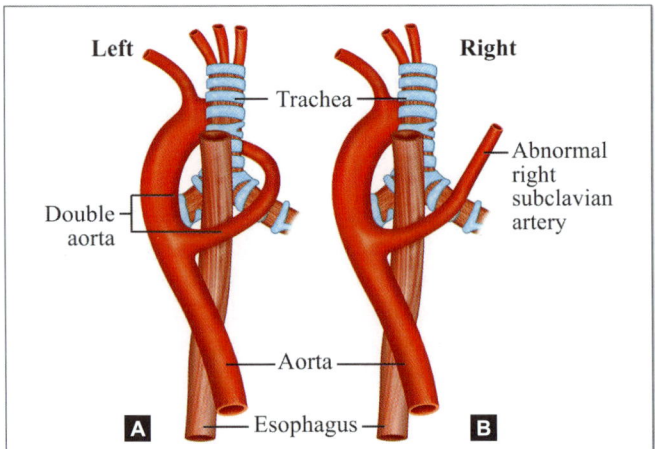

Fig. 35.4: Dysphagia lusoria: Pressure on thoracic esophagus from abnormal great vessels as seen from behind. (A) Double aorta; (B) Abnormal right subclavian artery

- Shows radiopaque foreign bodies.
- Saying 'e' during exposure brings the tongue anterior, and shows oropharynx better.
- Blowing through closed mouth distends hypopharynx.
- **Computed radiography and digital radiography:** In this filmless technique, image is captured on an array of digital elements, and is read directly into a computer.
  Advantages:
  - **Soft tissue differences:** It can emphasize subtle soft tissue differences even if the image is suboptimally exposed.
  - **Invert image:** Radiodense elements appear whiter than radiolucent elements on traditional films but computer technology can invert the image and some aspects of anatomy, and pathology can be visualized better.
- **Barium swallow:** For malignancy, cardiac achalasia, strictures, diverticulum, hiatus hernia and esophageal spasms.
- **Cineradiography:** For motility disorders of esophageal wall and sphincters.
- **Ultrasound:** Transesophageal echosonography can evaluate the depth of malignant ulcer, which helps in staging the disease.
- **Manometry and pH studies:** For motility disorders, gastroesophageal reflux and esophageal spasm (spontaneous or acid induced). A pressure transducer along with a pH electrode and an open-tipped catheter measure the pressures of esophageal wall and sphincters. Gastroesophageal reflux disease is measured by pH electrode, which also measures the effectiveness of esophagus to clear the acid load.
- **Esophagoscopy (flexible and rigid):** For direct examination of esophageal mucosa and biopsy (*see* Chapter 'Endoscopies').
- **Associated investigations:** They vary from case to case such as bronchoscopy for bronchial carcinoma, cardiac catheterization for vascular anomalies and thyroid scan for malignant thyroid.

Self-evaluation Exercises

Filling the blanks:
1. _____ is caused by the compression of esophagus by an abnormal right subclavian artery, which abnormally arise directly from the aorta and passes anterior or posterior to esophagus.

Match the following clinical features with their causes:

2. Regurgitation and heartburn	a. Palatal paralysis
3. Regurgitation of undigested food in lying down	b. Hiatus hernia
4. Nasal regurgitation	c. Laryngeal paralysis
5. Aspiration into lungs	d. Hypopharyngeal diverticulum

Match the following barium swallow findings with their causes:

6. Malignant lesions	a. String of pearls appearance
7. Benign strictures	b. Irregular narrowing of lumen and shouldering
8. Cardiac achalasia (cardiospasm)	c. Smooth narrowing
9. Esophageal varices	d. Megaesophagus

True (T)/False (F)
10. Many clinicians prefer flexible endoscopy if they strongly suspect mechanical lesions.
11. In motility disorders, barium swallow is done first as it provides more physiologic examination.

Answers
1. Dysphagia lusoria 2. b 3. d 4. a 5. c
6. b 7. c 8. d 9. a 10. T
11. T

Pharyngitis and Adenotonsillar Disease

> **Specific Learning Objectives**
> After going through the chapter, you should be able to answer the following questions:
> - What do you know about: (1) Infectious mononucleosis; (2) Keratosis pharyngitis; (3) Tonsilloliths?
> - Describe in detail the differential diagnoses, complications and management of streptococcal tonsillitis/pharyngitis.
> - What are the differentiating features between acute follicular tonsillitis and diphtheritic tonsillitis?
> - Describe the etiological and predisposing factors, clinical features and complications of chronic adenotonsillar hypertrophy.

INTRODUCTION

Infections of pharynx, tonsil and adenoids account for a significant proportion of childhood illnesses. They often lead to two of the most common pediatric surgeries—tonsillectomy and adenoidectomy. The predominant symptom of oropharyngeal infection is sore throat. Sore throat is one of the most common chief complaints with which patients consult to physicians.

PHARYNGITIS

Pharyngitis refers to inflammation of the pharynx mainly oropharynx. Acute catarrhal or superficial tonsillitis is a part of generalized pharyngitis, and is mostly seen in viral infections. In parenchymatous tonsillitis, which affects tonsil substance, tonsil is uniformly enlarged and red. Pharyngitis is common in adults while tonsillitis is mainly a disease of children. Majority of pharyngeal infections in adults are viral. The *Streptococcus pyogenes* only accounts for 5–10% in adults.

Irritative Pharyngitis

The causes of this common condition include:
- Postnasal drip
- Laryngopharyngeal reflux
- Occupational and environmental exposures.

Bacterial Pharyngitis

- In children, bacterial pharyngitis accounts for 30–40% of cases while in adults, it accounts for only 5–10%.
- Most cases of bacterial pharyngitis are caused by group A β-hemolytic *Streptococcus pyogenes* (GABHS).
- Hoarseness and cough are not suggestive of pharyngitis.
- It is important to confirm the diagnosis of GABHS because majority of acute pharyngitis cases do not have streptococcal infection.
- *See* the Section 'Streptococcal Tonsillitis-Pharyngitis' of this Chapter.

Viral Pharyngitis

- ***Coxsackievirus infections***
  - ***Herpangina:*** It mostly affects children. Child presents with fever, sore throat, and vesicular eruption surrounded by a zone of erythema on the soft palate and pillars (*see* Chapter 'Oral Mucosal Lesions').
  - ***Acute lymphonodular pharyngitis:*** It presents with fever, malaise and sore throat. White yellow, solid nodules on the posterior pharyngeal wall may be seen on examination.
- ***Cytomegalovirus:*** It affects immunosuppressed transplant patients. The infection mimics infectious mononucleosis but heterophil antibody test is negative.
- ***Pharyngoconjunctival fever:*** It is caused by adenovirus, and presents with sore throat, fever and conjunctivitis. Pain in abdomen mimics appendicitis.
- ***Measles:*** It is characterized by Koplik's spots (white spots surrounded by red areola) on the buccal mucosa opposite the molar teeth 3–4 days before the rash.
- ***Common cold (Rhinovirus, Coronavirus, Parainfluenza virus):*** It may affect tonsils and pharynx, and present with sore throat, dysphagia and fever. Tonsils may be enlarged but there is no exudate.

- ***Herpes simplex virus:*** It may cause exudative or nonexudative pharyngitis, which may be associated with gingivostomatitis (*see* Chapter 'Oral Mucosal Lesions').

Treatment
- Treatment of viral infection is nonspecific and symptomatic.
- Antibiotics are used for secondary bacterial colonization. Gram-negative and *S. aureus* infections increase by about 50% in these viral diseases.

INFECTIOUS MONONUCLEOSIS

Infectious mononucleosis is caused by Epstein-Barr virus.

Clinical Features
- Often affects older children and young adults.
- Fever, sore throat and exudative pharyngitis.
- Both tonsils are enlarged, congested and covered with membrane.
- Marked local discomfort.
- Lymphadenopathy: Lymph nodes are enlarged in the posterior triangle of neck.
- Hepatosplenomegaly.

Diagnosis
- ***Characteristic feature:*** Petechiae at the junction of hard and soft palate.
- ***Complete blood count:*** Fifty percent lymphocytes, of which 10% are atypical. White cell count is normal in first week and rises in second week.
- ***Serological tests:*** Monospot and Paul Bunnell or ox-cell hemolysis test shows high titers of heterophil antibody.

Treatment
- ***Symptomatic*** and recovery may take weeks.
- ***Antibiotics:*** No role except in secondary bacterial infection. Ampicillin causes skin rash in this condition and should be avoided.
- ***Management of upper airway obstruction:*** Airway obstruction can occur due to significantly enlarged tonsils. It is managed with:
  - Nasopharyngeal airway
  - High dose steroids
  - Tonsillectomy or tracheostomy.

> ***Infectious mononucleosis:*** Amoxicillin and ampicillin can cause a salmon-colored rash.

STREPTOCOCCAL TONSILLITIS-PHARYNGITIS

Infection spreads into the crypts which become filled with purulent material. The openings of crypts present yellowish spots of pus (acute follicular tonsillitis) which may coalesce, and form a membrane on the surface of tonsil (acute membranous tonsillitis).

Etiology
- ***GABHS*** is a precursor of two serious conditions acute rheumatic fever and poststreptococcal glomerulonephritis. It is the most common cause of acute bacterial tonsillitis-pharyngitis. Epidemic forms are seen in recruit camps and daycare facilities. GABHS are Gram-positive cocci that grow in chain.
  - ***Natural reservoir:*** Skin, nasopharynx and oropharynx.
  - ***Spread:*** Mostly through aerosolized microdroplets; less commonly by direct contact, and rarely through ingestion of contaminated non-pasteurized milk and foods.
  - ***Seasons:*** Autumn and winter.
- ***Non-group A beta-hemolytic streptococcal infection*** is clinically similar to GABHS. It is comparatively less common.
- ***The other bacteria*** may primarily infect the tonsil or may be secondary to a viral infection and mimic GABHS infection. They include *staphylococci, pneumococci* and *H. influenzae*.

Clinical Features

The disease often affects school going children (peak 5–6 years), but may affect infants and individuals above 50 years of age.

Symptoms
- ***Throat pain:*** Dry throat, fullness in throat or sore throat.
- ***Dysphagia:*** Difficulty in swallowing or odynophagia.
- ***Fever:*** Temperature (38–40°C) may be associated with chills and rigors. The child may present as a case of pyrexia of unknown origin.
- ***Earache:*** It may be either referred or due to acute otitis media.
- ***Constitutional symptoms***v Headache, limb and back pain, malaise and constipation.
- ***Abdominal pain:*** It is due to mesenteric lymphadenitis, and simulates acute appendicitis.

Physical Findings
- ***Tongue:*** Dry and coated tongue.
- ***Breath:*** Fetid breath (halitosis).

- **Oropharynx:**
  - Hyperemia of pillars, soft palate and uvula.
  - Tonsils red and swollen with yellowish spots of pus at the opening of crypts (acute follicular tonsillitis) which may coalesce, and form a membrane on the surface of tonsil (acute membranous tonsillitis). This membrane can be easily wiped away with a swab. The enlarged tonsils may meet in midline.
  - Edema of the uvula and soft palate may be present.
- **Lymph nodes:** Enlarged and tender jugulodigastric lymph nodes.

Diagnosis

Sore throat, fever with cervical adenopathy and pharynx with exudative covering are highly suggestive of *Streptococcus pyogenes*.

- **Rapid strep tests:** Latex agglutination or enzyme-linked immunosorbent assay (ELISA) methods extract antigen (group-A streptococcal) from a swab. It is highly specific (95%), but less sensitive (60–100%) than culture.
- **Throat culture:** Swab the posterior pharynx and tonsillar area when body temperature is greater than 38.3°C, patient presents only with sore throat or rapid strep test is negative in strongly suspected cases.

Treatment

- **General:** Bed rest and plenty of fluids.
- **Symptomatic:** Analgesics and antipyretics such as aspirin and paracetamol.
- **Specific:** Antibiotics for 7–10 days reduces the chances of suppurative complications and acute rheumatic fever, but not poststreptococcal glomerulonephritis.
  - Penicillin or amoxicillin is the drug of choice. If there is no response then suspect beta-lactamase producing organisms and anaerobes, and start
    - Amoxicillin + clavulanic acid or
    - Clindamycin or
    - Erythromycin + metronidazole
- **Asymptomatic carriers:** They usually do not need any treatment except when:
  - Family member is having rheumatic fever.
  - Family members are getting recurrent streptococcal infection.

> **Group A beta-hemolytic streptococci**: It is the most common cause of acute tonsillitis and can also result in rheumatic fever and poststreptococcal glomerulonephritis.

Complications

- *Scarlet fever*
- *Rheumatic fever*
- *Acute glomerulonephritis*
- *Acute otitis media:* It may coincide with recurrent tonsillitis.
- *Subacute bacterial endocarditis (SABE):* Acute tonsillitis in cases of valvular heart disease can cause SABE, which is usually due to *streptococcus* viridans.
- *Chronic/recurrent tonsillitis* due to incomplete resolution of tonsil infection, which may persist in lymphoid follicles of the tonsil like microabscesses.
- *Peritonsillar abscess*
- *Parapharyngeal abscess*
- *Retropharyngeal space infection*
- *Cervical abscess:* Suppuration of jugulodigastric nodes.

Differential Diagnosis of Membranous Pharyngitis-Tonsillitis

In membranous tonsillitis an exudative membrane forms over the medial surface of the tonsils. It occurs due to pyogenic organisms.

- *Agranulocytosis:*
  - Ulcerative necrotic lesions in the oropharynx.
  - Patient looks very ill.
  - *Diagnosis:*
    - Total leukocyte count: 50–2000/cumm
    - Polymorph neutrophil 5% or less.
- *Leukemia:* In children, acute lymphoblastic leukemia is more common (75%) than acute and chronic myelogenous (25%) leukemia. In adults, 80% are nonlymphocytic and 20% are acute lymphocytic leukemia.
  - TLC: Greater than 100,000/cumm.
  - Progressive anemia.
  - Bone marrow examination: Blasts cells are seen.
- *Aphthous ulcers:* Small/large, single/multiple painful ulcers on any part of oral cavity or oropharynx. Solitary big ulcer may involve the tonsil and pillars (*see* Chapter 'Oral Mucosal Lesions').
- *Malignancy tonsil:* See Chapter 'Tumors of Oropharynx'.
- *Traumatic ulcer:* Any injury to oropharynx. It may be accidental due to a toothbrush, a pencil or finger. It heals by formation of a membrane which appears within 24 hours.
- *Diphtheria:* See following Section and Table 36.1.
- *Infectious mononucleosis:* See previous Section.
- *Vincent's angina:* See Chapter 'Oral Mucosal Lesions'.
  - *Causative organism:* Fusiform bacilli and spirochetes.
  - *Clinical features:* It has insidious onset with mild fever and discomfort in throat. It presents with membrane, which usually involves one tonsil. This pseudomembrane can be easily removed, and reveal an irregular ulcer.
  - *Diagnosis:* Throat swab shows the causative organisms.

Differential Diagnoses of White Patches on Tonsils

In addition to the above-mentioned causes of membranous pharyngitis-tonsillitis, following conditions can present with white lesions on the tonsils: candidiasis, herpes ulcers, tuberculosis, syphilis, papilloma, cyst, keratosis and tonsillolith.

FAUCIAL DIPHTHERIA

The increasing coverage of child population by diphtheria immunization [combined (DPT, DT) and single vaccines] has significantly reduced the incidence of diphtheria. The disease was quite common and feared of. It is now fortunately seen uncommonly. However, it should be kept in mind whenever any membrane is seen on the tonsils of a child (Table 36.1).

- ***Causative organisms:*** Gram-positive bacilli *Corynebacterium diphtheriae.*
- ***Spread:*** It spreads by droplet infection. Diphtheria carriers harbor organisms in their throat.
- ***Incubation period:*** 2–6 days.

Clinical Features

- Children are affected more.
- Diphtheria has slow onset of local discomfort.
- Fever seldom rises above 38°C.
- The dirty gray tenacious membrane extends beyond the tonsils on to the soft palate and posterior pharyngeal wall and after removal, leaves a raw bleeding surface.
- Larynx and nasal cavity can also be affected.
- Cervical lymph nodes (jugulodigastric) get enlarged and tender, and may present as 'bull-neck' appearance.
- The child looks ill and toxemic.

Diagnosis

Diphtheria is usually a clinical diagnosis and in cases of doubt, the child should be treated on the line of diphtheria without wasting much time.

- Urine may show albumin.
- Smear and culture of throat swab will reveal *Corynebacterium diphtheriae.*

Complications

Diphtheria exotoxin is toxic to heart and nerves.

- ***Heart:*** Myocarditis, cardiac arrhythmia and acute circulatory failure.
- ***Neurological:*** Paralysis of palate, diaphragm and ocular muscles.
- ***Larynx:*** Airway obstruction.

Treatment

- ***Antidiphtheric serum:*** Antidiphtheric serum (ADS) is started immediately on clinical suspicion to neutralize the free diphtheria exotoxin. Dose depends on the site, duration and severity of disease.
    - ***20,000 to 40,000 units:*** History of less than 48 hours, or membrane is limited to tonsils only.
    - ***80,000 to 120,000 units:*** History of more than 48 hours, or membrane extends beyond tonsils.
    - ***Mode of administration:*** Intravenous infusion in saline in about 60 minutes.

Table 36.1: Distinguishing features of acute follicular (streptococcal) tonsillitis and diphtheria

Features	Acute follicular tonsillitis	Diphtheria
Past history	Recurrent sore throat with fever	Contact with diphtheria patient
Diphtheria vaccination	Taken	Not taken
Age	No age bar	Children
Onset	Acute	Insidious
Throat pain	Severe	Mild
Fever	High grade	Low grade
Hoarseness of voice and respiratory distress	Never	Present in advanced disease
Bull neck due to cervical lymphadenopathy	Absent	Not uncommon
Pulse rate	In proportion to fever	Out of proportion to fever and weak
Toxemia	Absent	Present in advanced disease
Tonsillar membrane	Limited to tonsil and easily removed	May extend to adjacent structures, and difficult to remove, and leaves raw bleeding area
Throat swab	Streptococci	*Corynebacterium diphtheriae*
Urine	No albumin	Albumin often present
First line of treatment	Antibiotics	Antidiphtheric serum
Mortality	Nil	High

- **Sensitivity test:** Horse serum is tested by conjunctival or intracutaneous test with diluted antitoxin. Adrenaline must be kept ready for any hypersensitivity reaction.
- **Desensitization:** Desensitization is required if patient is hypersensitive to ADS.
- Antibiotics:
  - Benzyl penicillin 600 mg 6 hourly for 7 days.
  - Erythromycin 500 mg 6 hourly orally in penicillin sensitive individuals.

TONSILLAR CONCRETIONS/TONSILLOLITHS

Tonsillolith (calculus of the tonsil) may be seen in chronic tonsillitis. The blocked tonsillar crypt causes retention of debris, which consists of inorganic salts of calcium and magnesium (formation of stone).

Clinical Features

- The affected crypt gradually enlarges, and may ulcerate on medial surface of tonsil.
- Retained material may have bacterial growth and then presents with halitosis and sore throat.
- Whitish foul-tasting and foul-smelling cheesy material can be expressed from tonsils.
- Tonsilloliths are usually seen in adults. Patient presents with local discomfort and foreign body sensation. They are diagnosed by palpation and probing.

Treatment

- **Conservative:** Expression of concretions/cheesy material and chemical cauterization of crypts with topical silver nitrate application.
- **Tonsillectomy:** In cases of persistent pain, halitosis and foreign body sensation.

INTRATONSILLAR ABSCESS

Accumulation of pus within the blocked tonsillar crypt can occur in cases of acute follicular tonsillitis.

- *Clinical Features*
  - Marked local pain and dysphagia.
  - Tonsil swollen and red.
- *Treatment*
  - Antibiotics
  - Drainage of the abscess
  - Tonsillectomy

TONSILLAR CYST

Blocked tonsillar crypt may present as a yellowish swelling over the tonsil.
- Usually they are asymptomatic.
- If symptomatic, it is drained.

KERATOSIS PHARYNGITIS

- White or yellowish dots or horny excrescences on the surface of tonsils, pharyngeal wall and lingual tonsils are characteristics of this benign condition. These excrescences are firmly adherent and cannot be wiped off. They are the result of hypertrophy and keratinization of epithelium.
- Patient does not have features of acute follicular tonsillitis such as sore throat, fever, cervical nodes and exudates. Patients just notice them during their self throat examination and get concerned.
- *Treatment:*
  - The spontaneous regression does occur so, no specific treatment is required.
  - The concerned patients need reassurance.

DISEASES OF LINGUAL TONSILS

Hypertrophy, infection and abscess can occur in lingual tonsil. Compensatory hypertrophy of lymphoid tissue may occur in response to repeated infections especially in tonsillectomy patients.

Clinical Features

- Discomfort on swallowing
- Feeling of lump in the throat
- Dry cough
- Thick voice
- Lingual tonsil are enlarged, congested or studded with follicles
- Cervical lymph nodes are enlarged

Treatment

- Antibiotics
- Diathermy coagulation or excision of lingual tonsils (by conventional or laser surgery).

Lingual Tonsillar Abscess

- *Clinical features:*
  - Severe unilateral dysphagia and excessive salivation.
  - Pain in the tongue
  - Enlarged and tender jugulodigastric nodes.
- *Complications:* Laryngeal edema.
- *Treatment:* Antibiotics, analgesics, proper hydration and incision and drainage of the abscess.

CHRONIC ADENOTONSILLAR HYPERTROPHY

Chronic adenotonsillar hypertrophy (Fig. 36.1) can cause obstructive sleep apnea (OSA) and affect craniofacial growth and microbiologic flora of tonsils and adenoids.

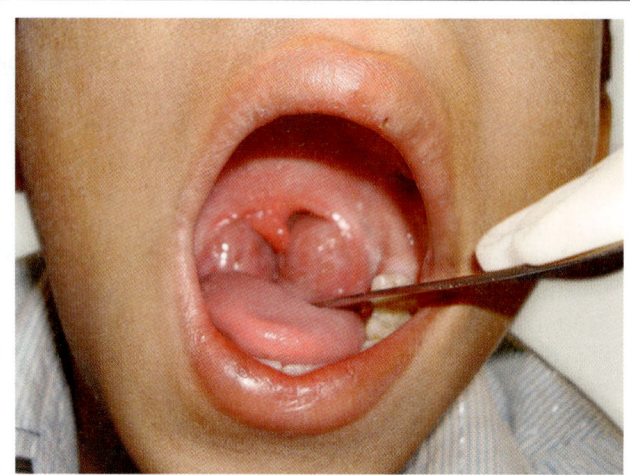

Fig. 36.1: Kissing tonsils

Etiology

- ***Physiological:*** There occur physiological enlargement of adenoids and tonsils (associated with generalized lymphoid hyperplasia) in the first to the fourth year of life. It is due to increased immunologic activity.
- ***Infection:*** β-lactamase producer pathogenic bacteria.
- ***Recurrent rhinitis and sinusitis.***
- ***Allergy*** of upper respiratory tract.
- ***Irritation:*** Second hand smoke exposure.

Clinical Features

The size of the adenoid mass (relative to the available space in the nasopharynx) and infection are important in causing the nasal, aural and general symptoms such as aprosexia (lack of concentration).

- ***Nasal:***
  - ***Nasal obstruction:*** Mouth breathing is one of the most common symptoms. It interferes with feeding and suckling (respiration and feeding cannot take place simultaneously). The child may fail to thrive.
  - ***Nasal discharge:*** The choanal obstruction and associated chronic rhinosinusitis may present with wet bubbly nose.
  - ***Epistaxis:*** Not common.
  - ***Rhinolalia clausa:*** Voice becomes toneless and loses nasal quality.
- ***Ear:*** Eustachian tube obstruction and infection may result in following features:
  - ***Conductive hearing*** loss and retracted tympanic membrane.
  - ***Recurrent acute otitis media.***
  - ***Chronic suppurative otitis media.***
  - ***Serous otitis media.***

Adenoid Facies and Craniofacial Growth Abnormalities

The characteristic facial appearance called 'adenoid facies' and craniofacial growth abnormalities are caused due to chronic nasal obstruction and mouth breathing. The features, some of which are reversed after adenotonsillectomy, include:

- An elongated face
- Retrognathic mandible
- Dull expression
- Dark circles under the eyes
- Open mouth
- Pinched nose due to disuse atrophy of alae nasi
- Hitched up upper lip
- Open bite, protrusive maxilla and buccal posterior crossbite
- Prominent and crowded upper teeth
- High arched hard palate because of the absence of moulding action of the tongue.

> ***Orthodontic procedures:*** The children with adenotonsillar hypertrophy, which are considered for orthodontic procedures for malocclusion, should have an ENT evaluation.

Airway Obstruction

- ***Excessive loud snoring at night.***
- ***Cor pulmonale and pulmonary hypertension:*** Chronic upper airway obstruction due to chronic adenotonsillar hypertrophy leads to pulmonary ventilation-perfusion abnormality and chronic alveolar hypoventilation. The chronic hypercapnia and hypoxia result in respiratory acidemia, pulmonary artery vasoconstriction, and right ventricular dilation and then eventually cardiac failure.
- ***Obstructive sleep apnea.***

Diagnostic Assessment of Tonsils and Adenoids

- ***Clinical:*** Confirm the features of adenotonsillar hypertrophy mentioned above.
- ***Postnasal mirror examination:*** An adenoid mass can be seen.
- ***X-ray soft tissue nasopharynx lateral view:*** Reveal size of adenoids, and extent of nasopharyngeal air space compromise (Fig. 36.2).
- ***Sinuscope and flexible nasopharyngoscope under topical anesthesia:*** Shows details of the nasopharynx.
- ***Nasal obstruction:*** Evaluate for other causes of nasal obstruction such as turbinate hypertrophy.

Chapter 36 • Pharyngitis and Adenotonsillar Disease

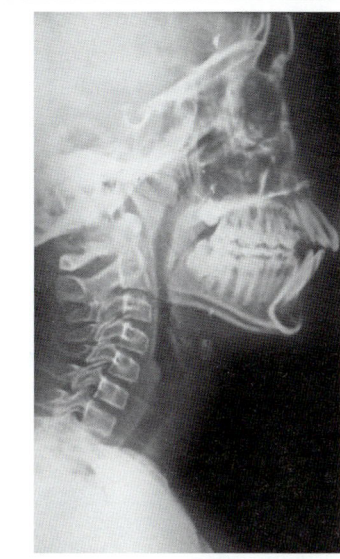

Fig. 36.2: Soft tissue opacity in nasopharynx

1-4+ Grading of tonsillar hypertrophy: It is based on the percentage projection of tonsil medially from the anterior tonsillar pillar.
- **1+:** up to 25% projection
- **2+:** 25-50% projection
- **3+:** 50-75% projection
- **4+:** 75-100% projection such as kissing tonsils

Treatment

- **Medical:** Following measures may cure early disease without resort to surgery:
  - Breathing exercises
  - Decongested, saline or steroid nasal drops
  - Antihistaminics
  - Antibiotics
  - Management of any associated nasal allergy
- **Surgical:** Adenotonsillectomy
  - For indications, contraindications, preoperative assessment, surgical techniques, postoperative care and complications see Chapter 'Adenotonsillectomy'.

Submucous cleft of palate: See for bifid uvula and translucent line through the mid soft palate, and palpate for notching of posterior part of hard palate. It is important before adenotonsillectomy.

OBSTRUCTIVE SLEEP APNEA (OSA) IN CHILDREN

In children, adenotonsillar hypertrophy is the most common cause of sleep apnea.

Clinical Features

The sleep disturbances may have following consequences:
- Episodes of apnea
- Too much loud snoring
- Chronic mouth breathing
- Interrupted sleep with frequent awakening and nightmares
- Hypersomnolence
- Poor school/work performance
- Dysphagia
- Hyponasal speech (rhinolalia clausa)
- **Failure to thrive:** OSA in children may disrupt growth hormone during REM sleep.
- **Enuresis:** Children with secondary enuresis (develop later in childhood) associated with significant airway obstruction due to adenotonsillar hypertrophy usually respond to adenotonsillectomy. Primary enuresis, which is congenitally present, does not respond to this surgery.
- **Obesity:** Like adults (classic obesity-related pickwickian syndrome), obesity is not a factor in pediatric OSA due to adenotonsillar hypertrophy.

Diagnosis

- **Polysomnography:** This expensive testing is not must in pediatric OSA, which is associated with confirmed adenotonsillar hypertrophy. But it is required in children where OSA is not associated with adenotonsillar hypertrophy.
- **Sleep sonography:** Tape recording of night sleep patterns at patient's home reliably detects evidence of OSA. It is an easy and most economical method of diagnosing OSA.
- **X-ray chest and ECG** should be taken preoperatively.

Common causes of rhinolalia clausa: They are allergic rhinitis, hypertrophy of adenoids and nasal polyps.

Self-evaluation Exercises

1. The common causes of rhinolalia clausa include:
    a. Allergic rhinitis
    b. Adenoids
    c. Nasal polyps
    d. All of the above
2. Which are not true for pharyngoconjunctival fever:
    a. Epidemics
    b. Follicular conjunctivitis
    c. Acute pharyngitis
    d. Fever
    e. None of the above
3. Which are true for herpangina:
    a. Self limiting infection
    b. Children
    c. Sore throat
    d. Fever
    e. All of the above
4. Which are not true for infectious mononucleosis:
    a. Sore throat and fever
    b. Generalized lymphadenopathy
    c. Splenomegaly
    d. Atypical lymphocytes in peripheral smear
    e. None of the above
5. The clinical features of Vincent's angina do not include:
    a. Gingivitis
    b. Stomatitis
    c. Ulceration of tonsils
    d. None of the above
6. Some of the causes of gray white membrane on the tonsils are:
    a. Infectious mononucleosis
    b. Streptococcal tonsillitis
    c. Diphtheria
    d. All of the above
7. In children with adenoid hyperplasia, adenoid facies show:
    a. Crowded teeth
    b. High-arched palate
    c. Open mouth
    d. Under slung lower jaw and underdeveloped/pinched nostrils
    e. All of the above
8. Nasopharyngeal obstruction due to adenoid hypertrophy cannot cause:
    a. Sinusitis
    b. Serous otitis media
    c. Cor pulmonale
    d. None of the above

True (T)/False (F)

9. Faucial diphtheria can cause palatal palsy.
10. Cor pulmonale cannot occur in children with chronic obstruction of upper respiratory tract due to enlarged tonsils and adenoids.
11. Management of adenoid hypertrophy with conductive hearing loss due to otitis media with effusion (OME) is adenoidectomy with grommet insertion.

Filling the blanks

12. In _____, yellow spots over the tonsil are not easy to wipe off.
13. Most common causative microorganism of acute tonsillitis is _____ .

Answers

1. d 2. e 3. e 4. e 5. d 6. d
7. e 8. d 9. T 10. F 11. T
12. Keratosis pharyngitis
13. *Streptococcus haemolyticus* (Group A beta-hemolytic *Streptococcus pyogenes*)

Chapter 37

Obstructive Sleep Apnea

Specific Learning Objectives
After going through the chapter, you should be able to answer the following questions:
- How will you classify the sleep disordered breathing? What are the differences between snoring and obstructive sleep apnea?
- What are the causes and pathophysiological factors of snoring and obstructive sleep apnea?
- How will you evaluate patients of snoring and obstructive sleep apnea?
- How will you manage the patients of snoring and obstructive sleep apnea?

INTRODUCTION

Sleep disordered breathing (SDB) is a type of intrinsic sleep disorder (dyssomnia). It encompasses primary snoring, upper airway resistance syndrome (UARS), obstructive sleep apnea syndrome and obesity-hypoventilation syndrome (Pickwickian syndrome). SDB (apnea-hypopnea index of 5 or more per hour of sleep) occurs in about 9% women and 24% men between the ages of 30 and 60 years. Among the women SDB is more common in postmenopausal age. About 70% SDB patients are obese.

About 25% of adults snore and the prevalence rises with increasing age. About 60% of males over 60 years of age have snoring. Though snoring does indicate some obstruction in upper airway most snorers have no obstructive sleep apnea (OSA). Although OSA patients are typically loud snorers, not all people who snore have OSA. Snoring and OSA probably represent a continuum of a similar pathology. There is difference between the noise of snoring and stridor.

- **Sleep apnea:** Cessation of breathing for 10 s or more during sleep. The airflow is usually measured at the nose and lips.
- **Apnea index:** Number of episodes of apnea during one hour of sleep.
- **Hypopnea:** Drop of 50% airflow associated with EEG defined arousal or 4% drop in O_2 saturation.
- **Respiratory disturbance index (RDI) or apnea hypopnea index:** Number of apnea and hypopnea episodes during one hour sleep.
- **Arousal:** Transient awakening from sleep.
- **Arousal index:** Number of arousal during one hour sleep, < 4 is normal.

CLASSIFICATION

- **Snoring:** In this noisy breathing, a rough, rattling inspiratory noise is produced by vibration of pendulous soft palate or occasionally of vocal cords, during sleep.
  - **Primary snoring:** In these snorers, an apnea-hypopnea index is less than 5.
  - **Upper airway resistance syndrome:** These patients have an apnea-hypopnea index of less than 5 but have an elevated arousal index (more than 5).
- **Sleep apnea:** There are three classes of sleep apnea—central, obstructive and mixed.
  i. **Obstructive sleep apnea syndrome (OSAS):** In OSAS transient upper airway obstruction results in intermittent cessation of airflow and breathing though there is normal respiratory effort. This is the most common type of sleep apnea and is managed by ENT surgeons. An apnea-hypopnea index is more than 5. During the episodes, oxyhemoglobin desaturation becomes less than 90%.
  ii. **Central sleep apnea:** Intermittent failure in the respiratory drive centers in central nervous system (CNS) results in cessation in airflow and breathing. The phrenic nerve and diaphragm become temporarily inactive. There is no obstruction in upper respiratory tract. This class of sleep apnea is managed by neurologists and sleep specialists.
  iii. **Mixed sleep apnea:** This variant of OSA has components of both central and obstructive sleep apnea.
- **Pickwickian syndrome:** This syndrome is characterized by obesity and hypersomnolence. It was described

by Charles Dickens in 'The Pickwick Papers'. In obese persons, weight of neck, redundant soft palate and thick base of tongue contribute to OSA.

PATHOPHYSIOLOGY OF OBSTRUCTIVE SLEEP APNEA (OSA)

An obstruction at any level of upper respiratory tract (URT) (i.e. from nose to the true vocal cords) can result in OSA. During inspiration there occurs a negative pressure within URT. Muscle relaxation of whole body (including muscles of URT) occurs during the deeper stages of sleep (Stages III, IV and REM). These two factors (muscle relaxation and negative pressure) result in collapse and obstruction of the airway in the patients, who have redundant tissue or narrow airway. Obstruction of airway leads to oxyhemoglobin desaturation that results in arousal and brings the patient to a lighter level of sleep. The upper respiratory airway is established again with the loud snorting breathing.

Sleep Patterns in OSA

During the deep stages of sleep (Stages III, IV and REM) most obstructive events occur as the muscles are most relaxed. So the OSA patients mainly have less deep sleep of Stages I and II. Due to these restless sleep patterns, these patients are deprived of deep sleep and have daytime somnolence. So the OSA patients have quick onset of sleep and multiple arousals. The successful treatment of OSA results in increase in REM sleep.

Factors Aggravating OSA

Certain factors are known to exacerbate OSA episodes. Most snoring is not pathologic and may be prevented by life style changes by managing factors mentioned in Box 37.1.

DIAGNOSIS AND EVALUATION OF OSA

History

Though not found totally reliable, history of sleep apnea is elicited from the spouse. The symptoms are listed in Box 37.2. Though not pathognomonic the typical symptoms

---

Box 37.1: Factors aggravating OSA

- Alcohol
- Sedatives including antihistamines and cough suppressants
- Allergic rhinitis
- Upper respiratory infections (URI)
- Weigh gain
- Supine position

Box 37.2: Symptoms of obstructive sleep apnea

- Snoring
  - Family members complain about patient's loud snoring
- Daytime somnolence
  - Drowsiness at work
  - Fall asleep at work, while driving and on telephone
- Morning headache and fatigue
- Restless sleep
  - Patient does not feel rested after night sleep
- Periods of apnea (cessation of breathing) resulting in frequent arousals at night
  - Sudden awakening and gasping for air
- Decreased libido and impotence
- Indigestion and gastroesophageal reflux disease
- Hypertension
- Decreased cognitive function including memory loss
- Personality changes, depression and psychosis
- Nocturnal headache, sweating and enuresis

---

are snoring, day time somnolence, morning headache and restless sleep. Periods of apnea result in frequent arousals at night. The neurobehavioral symptoms affect school and work performance.

Physical Examination

- **ENT head and neck examination:** Patients with OSA need complete ENT, head and neck examination and measurement of blood pressure, neck circumference and body mass index. The common findings, which constitute even the etiological factors, are mentioned in Box 37.3. In children OSA is generally due to tonsil and adenoid hypertrophy. For pediatric OSA *see* Chapter 'Pharyngitis and Adenotonsillar Diseases'.

Box 37.3: Etiological findings on physical examination in patients with OSA

- **Nose:** Deviated septum, hypertrophic turbinates, allergic rhinitis, nasal valve collapse, polyps/tumors
- **Oral cavity:** Macroglossia, retrognathia, micrognathia, large mandibular tori
- **Oropharynx:** Large tonsils, redundant or large soft palate, large uvula and lateral pharyngeal wall, fullness in base of tongue, lingual tonsillar hypertrophy, banding of posterior pharyngeal wall
- **Laryngopharynx:** Lateral pharyngeal wall collapse, omega-shaped epiglottis, tumor
- **Larynx:** Vocal cord palsy and tumor
- **Neck:** Full and thick neck (Pickwickian syndrome)
- **Children:** Tonsil and adenoid hypertrophy, nasopharyngeal cyst, encephalocele, choanal atresia, deviated nasal septum and craniofacial or orthodontic malformations
- **General:** Obesity, achondroplasia, chest wall deformity, Marfan's syndrome.

- **Body mass index:** The body weight in kilogram is divided by the height in square meters.
  - *Normal:* 18.5 to 24.9
  - *Over weight:* 25 to 29
  - *Obesity:* 30 to 34.9
- **Collar size:** Neck circumference at the level of cricothyroid membrane should not exceed 42 cm in male and 37.5 cm in females.
- **Systemic examination:** Further examination is needed in patients with cor pulmonale and hypertension.

Flexible Nasopharyngolaryngoscopy

This endoscopy examination offers a view of entire nasopharynx, laryngopharynx and larynx.
- **Muller's maneuver:** This test is done before the uvulopalatopharyngoplasty (UPPP) to know whether the patient will benefit from this surgery or not. It is performed to find the level and degree of obstruction in cases of obstructive sleep apnea. After passing the scope, examiner pinches the patient's nostrils and patient attempts to inhale with closed mouth. The base of tongue, lateral pharyngeal wall and palate are examined for collapsibility. If the laryngopharynx and/or larynx collapse, it means test is positive. It indicates that obstruction is below the level of soft palate. These patients will not benefit from UPPP and may need tracheostomy. The severity is rated from 0 (minimal collapse) to 4+ (complete collapse).

Radiography

Imaging studies may involve lateral cephalometric X-rays, fluoroscopy, CT scan or MRI.

Standard lateral cephalometric tracings identifies soft-tissue and skeletal obstruction in upper airway. Though limited by two dimensions this simple and cost-effective method measures posterior airway space and evaluates maxillary and mandibular development.

Polysomnography

This is the gold standard test in the evaluation of OSA. It differentiates snoring without OSA, with OSA and central sleep apnea. It also identifies the severity of the apnea. This expensive test can be done in a sleep lab or in a patient's home. It requires the patient to spend a night.
- **Parameters:** This highly sensitive and specific test measures following elements:
  - Electroencephalogram (EEG) shows brain activity.
  - Electromyogram (EMG) shows chin and leg muscle (anterior tibialis) movements.
  - Electrocardiogram (ECG) shows cardiac rhythm.
  - Electrooculogram (EOG) shows eye movements.
  - Pulse oximetry shows blood oxygen saturation.
  - Respiratory effort monitoring of chest and abdomen.
  - Air movement at nose and mouth.
  - Monitoring of body positions.
  - **Optional:** End-tidal CO_2 monitor, esophageal manometer, nasal CPAP/bilevel positive airway pressure.
- **Indications:** Not everyone who snores need sleep study. The snorers, who have following elements, need sleep study.
  - Hypersomnolence, morning headache and restless sleep.
  - Socially disruptive loud snoring.
  - Prior to any surgery for sleep apnea or snoring.

Home Sleep Studies

These measures are economical. They are not as sensitive or specific as a formal sleep lab polysomnography. Some studies measure only pulse oximetry while others have multichannel recording devices.

Multiple Sleep Latency Test

This test is done during the day in a sleep laboratory. The patient is allowed to take several naps. This test measures the time that patient takes to fall asleep. An average sleep onset of less than 5 minutes indicates excessive daytime sleepiness, which is considered pathologic.

SEVERITY OF OSA

- **Respiratory disturbance index:** Respiratory disturbance index (RDI) is the sum of apneas and hypopneas. On the basis of RDI, OSA can be classified into three groups:
  - Mild (10–30)
  - Moderate (30–50)
  - Severe (>50)
- **Degree of oxyhemoglobin desaturation (SaO_2):** It is less than 85% in moderate OSA and less than 60% in severe OSA.
- **Epworth Sleepiness Scale:** It assesses the daytime sleepiness (Table 37.1). Patients answer the questions on the scale from 0 to 3.

COMPLICATIONS OF OSA

The chronic OSA patients if not treated can develop significant morbidity and mortality due to following conditions, which can be reversed to normal with the successful treatment of OSA.
- Cardiac arrhythmias
- Cerebrovascular accidents
- Angina and myocardial infarction
- Congestive heart failure
- Cor pulmonale and chronic heart failure
- Hypertension: Systemic and pulmonary
- Peripheral edema

Table 37.1: Epworth sleepiness scale

Answer the chances of dozing/sleeping in the following situations on the scale 0 to 3*	
Situation	Score* (0-3)
Reading	
Watching TV	
Theater/meeting place	
At traffic light while driving vehicle	
Sitting in passenger seat of a car for 1 hour	
Rest after lunch without alcohol	
On lying down to rest	
**Total Score	

*Score/scale: 0, never doze; 1, slight chance of dozing; 2, Moderate chance of dozing; 3, High chance of dozing.
**Total score less than 8 is normal.

- Polycythemia
- Excessive day time somnolence can result in
  - Accidents during driving vehicle or operating dangerous machines.
  - Less exercise and more weight gain and more severe sleep apnea.

Road accidents and OSA: The decrease psychomotor vigilance results in seven fold increase in the risk of motor vehicle accidents in OSA patients.

NONSURGICAL TREATMENT

Flow chart 37.1 shows the management of snoring both with and without OSA. Discomfort and poor compliance are major stumbling blocks in the nonsurgical measures in managing snoring and OSA.

Lifestyle Modifications

Behavioral modifications (Box 37.4) though may reduce snoring and OSA especially in mild cases, patients' compliance is usually a problem.

Positional therapy: The patient is advised to sleep sideway rather than on the back. A rubber ball tied to the back of pajama prevents the patient to adopt supine position, which aggravates the symptoms.

Nasal Continuous Positive Airway Pressure (CPAP)

This ventilator type machine is the most effective mean in the nonsurgical management of OSA. Continuous positive airway pressure (CPAP) provides a sort of pneumatic splint to airway and increases its caliber. Though it is 100% effective in treating OSA, patient's compliance is not very good and about 30% patients eventually stop using this. In CPAP, an airtight mask is kept over the patient's nose with the help of a strap wrapped around the head. The optimum pressure for opening the airway, which is determined during sleep study, is usually kept at 5–20 cm of H_2O.

Bilevel positive airway pressure and auto-titrating PAP: They have little better patient compliance. Bilevel positive airway pressure (BiPAP) delivers positive pressure at two fixed levels—a higher inspiratory and a lower expiratory pressure. Auto-titrating PAP (APAP) continuously adjusts the pressure.

Box 37.4: Lifestyle modifications for the management of snoring and OSA

- Adopt an athletic lifestyle and exercise daily
- Lose weight
- Avoid sedatives (tranquilizers, sleeping pills, antihistaminics and cough suppressants) at bed time
- Avoid alcoholic drinks within 4 hours of retiring to bed
- Avoid heavy dinner within 3 hours of going to bed
- Avoid getting overtired
- Establish regular sleeping patterns
- Sleep sideway rather than on the back
- Raise the head end of the bed about 4" by placing bricks under the bedposts
- Nonsnorer partner should go to sleep first.

Intraoral Devices

Tongue-retaining device (TRD) and mandible advancement device (MAD) hold the tongue and/or mandible forward during the sleep and keep the airway open. Similar to CPAP, discomfort and poor compliance are major concerns.

SURGICAL TREATMENT OF OSA

The surgeries are planned according to the location of the obstruction.

Uvulopalatopharyngoplasty

This technically easy operation is the most common surgery performed for OSA. The oropharyngeal airway is enlarged in an anterior-superior and lateral dimensions. It is a type of radical tonsillectomy. The tonsils and uvula are removed along with the posterior edge of the soft palate. The anterior and posterior faucial pillars are sutured together. Similarly, the nasal and oral side mucosas of the cut edge of soft palate are sutured together. Patients usually stay for 1 to 2 days in the hospital.

- *Results:* UPPP is very effective in treating snoring but significant improvement (50% or more reduction in RDI) in OSA occurs in about 50% of patients. UPPP alone does not reduce the mortality of OSA. The tracheostomy and CPAP have shown dramatic improvement in

Flow chart 37.1: Management of snoring both with and without OSA

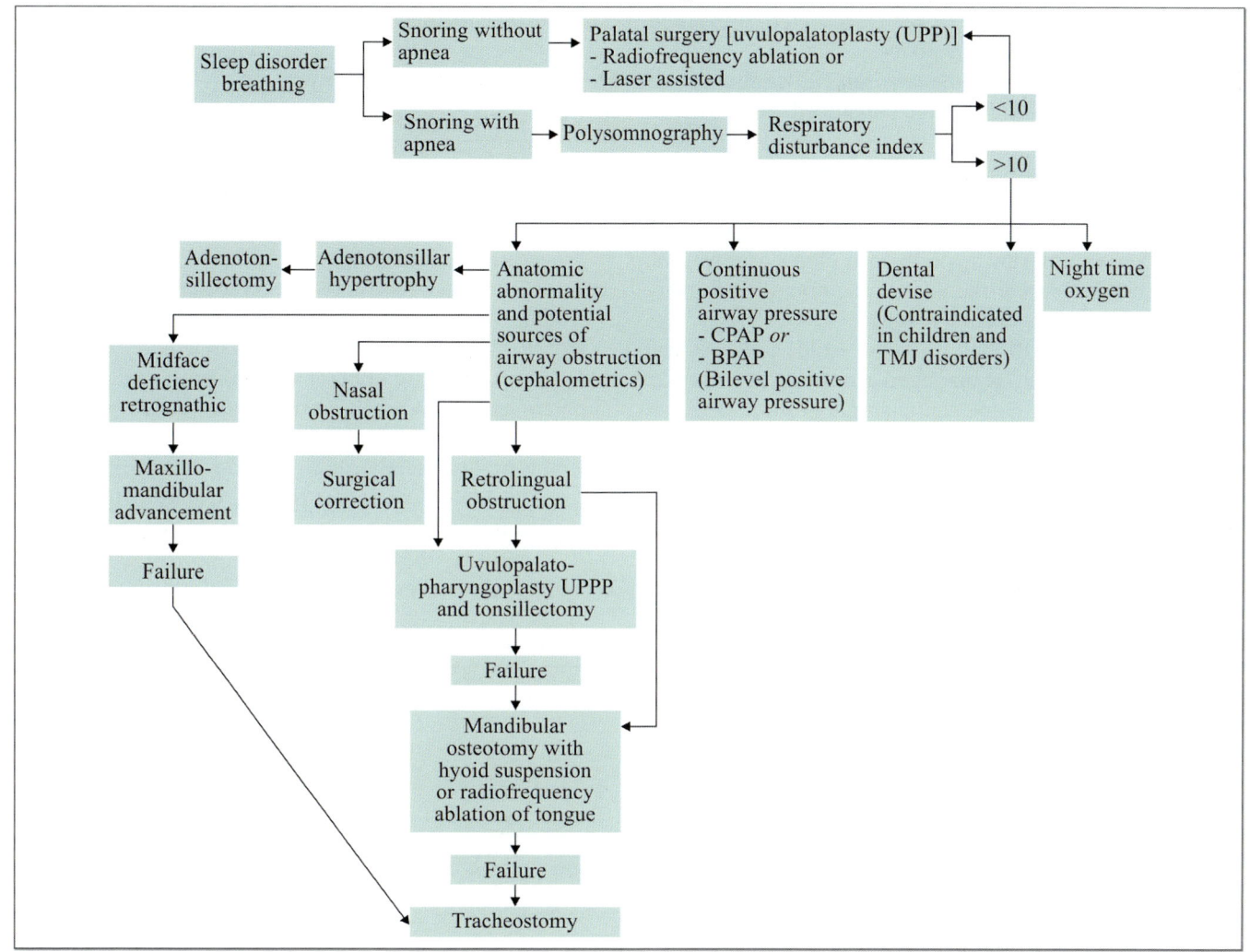

OSA mortality. Therefore patient should be told that additional procedures may be required if UPPP fails.
- **Complications:** They are similar to tonsillectomy and includes bleeding (most common), temporary velopharyngeal incompetence (in 5–10% of patients) and nasopharyngeal stenosis (rare). Other minor postoperative complaints, which are temporary, include dry mouth, throat tightness, increased gag reflex and alteration in taste.

Other Surgical Procedures

- **Hypopharyngeal and base of tongue procedures:** The findings, which suggest hypopharyngeal obstruction, include:
  - **Morbid obesity:** Body mass index greater than 31 kg/m^2
  - **Mandibular skeletal deficiency**
  - **Lateral cephalometric radiogram:** PAS less than 11 mm
  - **Flexible laryngoscopy:** Narrow retrolingual space
    - **Muller's maneuver:** Lateral pharyngeal wall collapse
  - **Apnea-hypopnea index:** Greater than 30
- **Procedures for advancing base of tongue:** They can be performed in presence of fullness in the base of the tongue.
  - **Partial midline glossectomy:** This can be performed with the help of either a laser or Bovie cautery.
  - **Tongue base radiofrequency:** Radiofrequency (RF) needle is inserted submucosally which coagulates tissue and causes scarring. RF can be used in five to six sittings to reduce the size of tongue.
  - **Advancement genioplasty with hyoid suspension:** In cases of obstruction at the level of base of tongue, retrognathia and micrognathia, the airway is enlarged by advancing genial tubercle of mandible (origin of genioglossus muscle) anteriorly and suspending hyoid bone from mandible by permanent sutures

or wire. A rectangular chin portion of mandible including genial tubercles is resected and then rotated 90° and fixed by plates.

- **Hyoid myotomy and suspension:** The midline hyoid bone is isolated and then advanced over thyroid cartilage.

- *Mandibular and maxillary advancement:* This procedure is more major than UPPP. It employs sagittal split and LeFort I osteotomies. These osteotomies are then fixed in anterior position with plates and screws. They effectively treat the anatomic anomalies causing OSA and offer long-lasting results.
- *Nasal surgery:* Though rarely a sole cause, nasal obstruction should be managed according to its cause. The procedures include septal surgery and removal of polyps and tumors.
- *Tracheostomy:* Though neither preferred by surgeon nor liked by the patient this gold standard treatment of OSA is almost 100% effective. Tracheostomy bypasses the upper airway entirely but needs daily care throughout the life, which is a major stumbling block. It is probably the first line of surgery in very severe OSA or in those who are significantly obese or debilitated.

SURGICAL TREATMENT OF SNORING WITHOUT OSA

- *Uvulopalatoplasty:* Laser-assisted uvulopalatoplasty (LAUP) or Bovie-assisted uvulopalatoplasty (BAUP) can be performed under local anesthesia as an OPD procedure. In this procedure uvula is amputated and 1 cm trenches are created in the soft palate on either side of the uvula. The soft palate elevates and stiffens after healing. It may be performed in two to four stages, each separated by about 1 month. In this way the soft palate resection is titrated to treat snoring without velopharyngeal incompetence.
  - It is highly effective and resolution of snoring occurs in 85–90% of patients. Though it may help in mild or moderate OSA, generally it is contraindicated in cases of OSA.
- UPPP is also very effective in treating snoring.

Self-evaluation Exercises

1. Which of the following conditions cannot cause snoring?
    a. Nasopharyngeal angiofibroma
    b. Tonsillar enlargement
    c. Antrochoanal polyp
    d. Adenoid hypertrophy
    e. None of the above
2. Which of the following are related with Muller's maneuver?
    a. Performed with flexible nasopharyngolaryngoscopy
    b. Find the level and degree of obstruction in cases of obstructive sleep apnea
    c. Patient makes maximal inspiratory effort with nose and mouth closed
    d. Base of tongue, lateral pharyngeal wall and palate are examined for collapsibility
    e. All of the above
3. Which of the following operations are done for obstructive sleep apnea?
    a. Tracheostomy
    b. Adenotonsillectomy
    c. Uvulopalatopharyngoplasty
    d. All of the above

True (T)/False (F)

4. The degree of obstruction with Muller's maneuver in cases of obstructive sleep apnea is rated from 0 (minimal collapse) to 4+ (complete collapse).
5. Although obstructive sleep apnea (OSA) patients are typically loud snorers, not all people who snore have OSA.
6. Snoring and obstructive sleep apnea (OSA) probably represent a continuum of a similar pathology.
7. Polysomnography is the gold standard test in the evaluation of snoring and obstructive sleep apnea (OSA).

Answers
1. E   2. E   3. D   4. T   5. T   6. T
7. T

Chapter 38

Tumors of Nasopharynx

Specific Learning Objectives

After going through the chapter, you should be able to answer the following questions:
- What are the characteristic clinical features of nasopharyngeal angiofibroma?
- How will you evaluate and manage a case of nasopharyngeal angiofibroma?
- How the nasopharyngeal carcinoma spreads and manifests its clinical features?
- How will you evaluate and manage a case of nasopharyngeal carcinoma?
- What do you know about Thornwaldt's disease?

INTRODUCTION

Primary tumors of nasopharynx are relatively rare. The most common benign tumor juvenile nasopharyngeal angiofibroma (JNA), malignant tumor nasopharyngeal carcinoma (NPC) and Thornwaldt's disease will be discussed in this chapter.

Benign Tumors of Nasopharynx

Majority of the nonepithelial benign tumors in nasopharynx are vascular. JNA, though rare is the most common benign tumor of nasopharynx. Other benign tumors, which are very rare and arise from the roof and lateral wall of nasopharynx, include.
- *Teratoma:* It is congenital tumor. True teratomas have tissues which are derived from all the three germinal layers. Other congenital tumors include hairy polyp (dermoid with skin appendages) and epignathi (well developed fetal parts). Congenital tumors have female preponderance (6:1).
- *Pleomorphic adenoma:* From minor salivary glands.
- *Chordoma:* From the notochord.
- *Hamartoma:* A focal malformed normal tissue that resembles neoplasm such as hemangioma.
- *Choristoma:* Tissues at an abnormal site.
- *Chraniopharyngioma:* From Rathke's pouch.
- *Paraganglioma*
- *Squamous papilloma*

Rathke's pouch: It may persist as craniopharyngeal canal in nasopharynx. It forms anterior pituitary.

Malignant Tumors of Nasopharynx

Cancer of the nasopharynx was found uniformly high in six of the eight North East registry areas in India (ICMR 2006). Carcinoma is the most common variety of nasopharyngeal malignancy but other rare types include:
- **Lymphomas:** Non-Hodgkin's type of lymphoma is more common than Hodgkin's. Almost all are B-cell type.
- **Rhabdomyosarcoma in children:** Embryonal rhabdomyosarcoma presents as a polyp in the nasopharynx.
- **Plasmacytoma:** Solitary or part of generalized multiple myelomatosis.
- **Chordoma:** From remnant of notochord.
- **Adenoid cystic carcinoma:** From minor salivary glands.
- **Hemangiopericytoma**
- **Melanoma**

- *Most common malignant tumor of nasopharynx in children:* It is rhabdomyosarcoma.
- *Most common site of rhabdomyosarcoma in the head and neck region:* It is orbit.

JUVENILE NASOPHARYNGEAL ANGIOFIBROMA (JNA)

JNA is the most common benign tumor of nasopharynx.

Etiology

The exact cause is yet not known.

- A primary aberration of pituitary-gonadal axis is suggested but not proved.
- The tumor is almost exclusively seen in adolescent males in the second decade of life. So it is considered to be testosterone dependent.
- A hamartomatous nidus of vascular tissue in the nasopharynx is said to be activated when male sex hormone appears.

Pathology

Angiofibroma consists of varying amount of vascular and fibrous tissues. Vessels do not have muscle coat and are just endothelium lined. It results into severe bleeding, which cannot be controlled by application of adrenaline. The tumor is covered with nasopharyngeal mucosa and clinically may appear deceptively avascular.

Site of Origin

The site of origin is a matter of dispute. Currently it is believed to arise close to the superior margin of sphenopalatine foramen (bounded by palatine bone, horizontal ala of vomer and root of pterygoid process). In past it was said to arise from the roof of nasopharynx or the anterior wall of sphenoid bone.

Growth and Extensions

Nasopharyngeal fibroma is a locally invasive benign tumor. It destroys the adjoining structures and grows in the following directions and regions:
- ***Anteriorly*** into the nasal cavity and produce nasal obstruction, epistaxis and nasal discharge.
- ***Posteriorly*** into nasopharynx.
- ***Laterally*** into the pterygopalatine fossa (pushing posterior wall of maxillary sinus), pterygomaxillary fissure and thence to infratemporal fossa and cheek (*see* Fig. 38.1A).
- ***Superiorly*** the tumor invades floor of middle cranial fossa anterior to foramen lacerum and lies lateral to carotid artery and cavernous sinus. Tumor may go into sella turcica through sphenoid sinus and lies medial to carotid artery. Anterior cranial fossa can be invaded through ethmoid roof and cribriform plate.
- ***Orbit:*** It enters into the orbit through the inferior orbital fissure. It invades apex of the orbit. It may enter the orbit through superior orbital fissure. It produces proptosis and 'frog-face deformity'.
- ***Paranasal sinuses:*** Maxillary, sphenoid and ethmoid.

Clinical Features

Most common presentation:
- Profuse and recurrent episodes of epistaxis and unilateral nasal obstruction occur in more than 80% of cases.
- It occurs exclusively in males of 10–25 years of age.
- Patient is usually markedly anemic.
- Denasal speech.

- ***Ear:*** Conductive hearing loss and serous otitis media occur due to obstruction of Eustachian tube.
- ***Local findings:*** Pink or purplish nasopharyngeal mass, which is sessile, lobulated or smooth and obstructs one or both choanae. Consistency is firm but digital palpation is never done because it can result in profuse bleeding.
- ***Clinical features of advanced tumor (frog-face deformity):***
  - Broadening of nasal bridge.
  - Proptosis and superior orbital fissure syndrome.
  - Swelling of cheek and infratemporal fossa.
  - Involvement of 2nd, 3rd, 4th, 5th cranial nerves: Diplopia and visual field defects.

Spot diagnosis: In an adolescent male, profuse recurrent episodes of nosebleed suggest juvenile nasopharyngeal angiofibroma until proven otherwise.

Diagnostic Radiology

- ***Computed tomography (CT) scan with contrast enhancement axial and coronal sections (Fig. 38.1A):*** CT is gold standard for JNA and has replaced conventional radiographs. The extent of tumor, bony destruction and displacements can be seen.
  - ***Antral sign (Holman-Miller sign):*** Anterior bowing of posterior wall of maxillary sinus (anterior wall of pterygopalatine fossa) is characteristic of JNA.
- ***Magnetic resonance imaging (MRI):*** It is indicated when soft tissue extensions are present in following regions:
  - Intracranial
  - Infratemporal fossa
  - Orbit
  - Surveillance of residual and recurrent tumor.
- ***Carotid angiography:*** Extension and vascularity of the tumor and its feeding vessels can be seen. It is done for embolization therapy.

Chapter 38 • Tumors of Nasopharynx

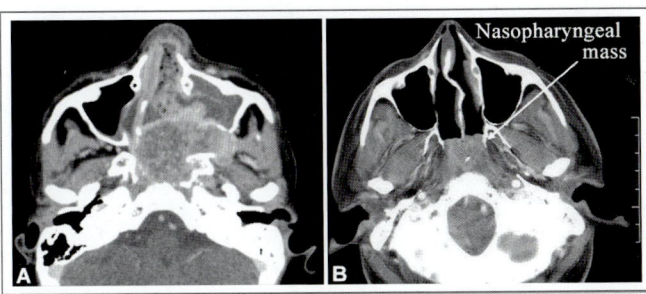

Figs 38.1A and B: Contrast CT scan (A) Juvenile nasopharyngeal angiofibroma. Note the pterygopalatine fossa and infratemporal fossa extension; (B) Nasopharyngeal mass axial section. Large soft tissue density mass causing complete obliteration of nasopharyngeal lumen. Laterally it is obliterating lateral recesses and openings of Eustachian tubes. It is also extending into both posterior choanae. Mass shows foci of calcification
Source: (A) Dr Amit Goyal, AIIMS, Jodhpur; (B) Dr Ritesh Prajapati, Consultant Radiologist, Anand, Gujarat

Staging

Sessions's classification, modified by Radkowski reflects the clinical behavior of JNA (Table 38.1).

> **Diagnosis**
> In most cases, clinical features and CT scan findings will confirm the diagnosis. Biopsy is contraindicated because it results in the profuse bleeding.

Treatment

Open surgical excision is the treatment of choice.
- **Surgical approaches:** Depending upon the origin and extensions of angiofibroma, following approaches may be employed. Occasionally combined approaches are employed especially in significant extension into infratemporal fossa, middle cranial fossa and cavernous sinus (Table 38.1). Autologous transfusion preoperatively if the patient status permits should be considered.
    - **Transpalatine:** Tumors confined to nasopharynx, nasal cavity and sphenoid sinus.
    - **Le Fort 1 osteotomy approach:** For extension to paranasal sinuses, pterygopalatine fossa and infratemporal fossa.
    - **Medial maxillectomy:** It provides access to orbit, ethmoid and sphenoid sinuses and anterior skull base.
    - **Sardana's approach:** Transpalatine + Sublabial.
    - **Extended lateral rhinotomy:** It gives wide exposure.
        - Via facial incision
        - Via degloving approach
    - Extended Denker's approach
    - Intracranial-extracranial
    - Infratemporal fossa
- **Measures to reduce the vascularity of tumor:** The intraoperative blood loss may be significant (about 2 liters). Following preoperative measures can reduce the vascularity of tumor.
    - **Embolization of the feeding vessels:** After carotid angiography, feeding vessels from external carotid artery can be embolized. It reduces the size of tumor and operative bleeding. Surgery must be performed within 24–48 hours of embolization as later on collateral develops and vascularization occurs from opposite side.
    - **Estrogen therapy:** Stilboestrol 2.5 mg three times a day for 3 weeks. Not preferred currently.
    - **Preoperative radiation:** Generally not favored.
    - **Cryotherapy.**
- **Endoscopic resection:** For early tumors limited to nose, nasopharynx, ethmoid and sphenoid. Preoperative embolization of feeding vessels and early control of internal maxillary artery facilitate tumor mobilization.
- **Radiation therapy (3000 to 3500 cGy in 15-18 fractions in 3–3.5 weeks):** It is debatable and may be considered for more advanced tumor with significant intracranial extension. The mass regresses slowly over 1–3 years.

Complications: Though less with current intensity modulated radiation therapy (IMRT), the feared complications in these young patients are following:

Table 38.1: Radkowski classification of juvenile nasopharyngeal angiofibroma (JNA) and suggested surgical approach

Stage*	Tumor extent*	Surgical approach
IA	Tumor limited to nose and nasopharyngeal vault	Transpalatal or endoscopic
IB	Extension to paranasal sinuses	Medial maxillectomy by lateral rhinotomy or endoscopic
IIA	Minimal extension to pterygomaxillary fissure (PMF)	Extended lateral rhinotomy or Le Forte 1
IIB	Full extension to PMF and/or erosion of orbital bones	Extended lateral rhinotomy and removing anterior wall of maxillary sinus and along with part of nasal pyriform aperture
IIC	Extension to infratemporal fossa and/or cheek or posterior to pterygoid plates	Infratemporal fossa approach or maxillary swing approach (facial translocation)
IIIA	Erosion of skull base: minimal intracranial	Combined intracranial and/or extracranial
IIIB	Extensive intracranial and/or cavernous sinus extension	Neurosurgery/radiation

*Radkowski D and others; Arch Otoalryngol Head and Neck 122:122, 1996

- Secondary malignancy
- Abnormal craniofacial development
- Cataracts
- Optic atrophy
- Osteoradionecrosis.
- **Chemotherapy:** Doxorubicin, vincristine and decarbazine have been tried in combination in very aggressive recurrent tumors.

Recurrence

Recurrence of tumor after surgical removal is not uncommon and ranges from 30–50%. Revision surgery and radiotherapy are the options which may be considered.

Though well-documented, spontaneous regression with advancement of age is uncommon.

NASOPHARYNGEAL CARCINOMA (NPC)

NPC is most common in southern states of China, Taiwan and Indonesia. In Guangdong Province of Southern China, NPC is the third most common malignancy among men. Here the people are predominantly of Mongoloid origin. In India, nasopharyngeal cancer constitutes only 0.5% of all body cancers (common in north east states).

Etiology

The exact etiology is yet unknown. NPC is a multifactorial disease. The various factors include genetic susceptibility, environmental factors, dietary and personal habits.
- **Genetic:** Chinese, whether they live in China or elsewhere, have a higher genetic susceptibility to NPC.
  - **EBV:** Gains on chromosome 12 and allelic losses on 11q, 13q, and 16q causes invasive carcinoma.
- **Viral:** Epstein-Barr virus (EBV) is usually associated with NPC. Specific viral markers are used to screen people in high-risk areas. IgA against both EA and VCA are done for screening of NPC.
- **Environmental:** Air pollution, smoke from burning of incense and wood (polycyclic hydrocarbon).
- **Smoking:** Tobacco and opium.
- **Dietary:**
  - Nitrosamines in dry salted fish and preserved foods.
  - Diet deficient in vitamin C, fresh fruits, carotene and fibers. Vitamin C blocks nitrosification of amines.

Pathology

- Squamous cell carcinoma (SCC) has various grades of its differentiation or variants such as transitional cell carcinoma and lymphoepithelioma. SCC is most common (85%).
- On the basis of histology, WHO has reclassified epithelial growths into three types (Table 38.2). Type I keratinizing squamous cell carcinoma can be graded into well, moderately and poorly differentiated.
- Lymphomas are 10% and the rest 5% include rhabdomyosarcoma, malignant mixed salivary tumor and malignant chordoma.

Table 38.2: WHO classification of epithelial carcinoma based on histopathology

Type 1 (25%)	Keratinizing squamous cell carcinoma, EBV –ve, 10% survival
Type 2 (12%)	Nonkeratinizing carcinoma, EBV +ve, 50% survival Without lymphoid stroma With lymphoid stroma
Type 3 (63%)	Undifferentiated carcinoma, EBV +ve, 50% survival Without lymphoid stroma With lymphoid stroma

%, % of NPC; EBV, Epstein-Barr Virus; Survival, 5-year survival

Spread

- **Most common site of origin:** Fossa of Rosenmuller
- **Local spread:**
  - **Anterior:** Choana, nasal cavity and orbit
  - **Posterior:** Retropharyngeal space
  - **Inferior:** Oropharynx and laryngopharynx
  - **Lateral:** Eustachian tube, parapharyngeal space, pterygoid muscles and infratemporal fossa (via sinus of Morgagani).
  - **Superior:** Middle cranial fossa (via foramen lacerum and ovale), jugular foramen, hypoglossal canal, posterior cranial fossa.
- **Lymph node** (ipsilateral, contralateral and bilateral) involvement is common and early feature because nasopharynx has rich lymphatic network. Metastasis to cervical nodes can be either direct or through the retropharyngeal and parapharyngeal nodes.
- **Distant metastasis:** Lungs, bone and liver.

Clinical Features

- **Age and sex:** It is mostly seen in 4th and 5th decades of life. Incidence starts rising from 2nd decade of life. Males are three times more prone than females.
- *The most common presenting feature* of NPC is **cervical lymphadenopathy** (60–90%) followed in descending order by:
  - Conductive hearing loss
  - Nasal obstruction
  - Epistaxis
  - Cranial nerve palsies (CN VI most common and the first cranial nerve to be affected)
  - Headache
  - Earache
  - Neck pain (involvement of retropharyngeal nodes causes neck stiffness and torticollis)
  - Weight loss

- **Types of tumor:** Three forms:
  I. **Proliferative:** Polypoid tumor fills the nasopharynx and causes nasal obstruction.
  II. **Ulcerative:** Epistaxis is common.
  III. **Infiltrative:** Growth infiltrates submucosally.
- **Clinical features of spread:**
  - **Nose:** Unilateral nasal obstruction and blood stained discharge, denasal speech (rhinolalia clausa).
  - **Ear:** Unilateral conductive hearing loss, otalgia, serous or suppurative otitis media, tinnitus and dizziness. Tumor may enter into the middle ear through the Eustachian tube.
  - **Ophthalmoneurologic:** Squint and diplopia due to involvement of CN VI, ophthalmoplegia (CN III, IV and VI), facial pain and reduced corneal reflex (invasion of CN V through foramen lacerum), exophthalmos and blindness (invasion of CN II at orbital apex).
  - **Jugular foramen syndrome:** Involvement of IX, X and XI cranial nerves (Fig. 38.2) due to enlargement of lateral retropharyngeal lymph nodes.
  - **Collet-Sicard syndrome:** Involvement of IX, X, XI and XII cranial nerves. CN XII may be involved due to extension of growth to hypoglossal canal.
  - **Horner's syndrome:** Due to involvement of cervical sympathetic chain.
  - **Cervical nodal metastases:** Patient may present with only cervical lump. It is usually seen between the angle of jaw and the mastoid. Other nodes are spinal accessory in the posterior triangle of neck and supraclavicular nodes. Nodal metastases during first consultation are seen in 75% and about half of them have bilateral nodes. First echelon nodes, the retropharyngeal nodes of Rouviere may be detected on CT.
  - **Distant metastases:** Bone (thoracolumbar vertebrae, pelvis and femoral heads), lung and liver.

> - **Krause's nodes:** These lymph nodes are situated in the jugular foramen. Their enlargement compresses CN IX, X and XI, and produce jugular foramen syndrome.
> - **Trotter's (sinus of Morgagni) syndrome or triad:** Trotter's triad, which is seen in NPC, consists of conductive hearing loss (due to Eustachian tube obstruction), immobility of soft palate and temporoparietal neuralgia in the distribution of mandibular division of trigeminal nerve. The associated trismus and preauricular fullness may be seen in some cases.
> - **Unilateral serous otitis media in elderly person:** Must rule out NPC.

Endoscopy and Biopsy

- **Endoscopy:** Flexible and rigid endoscopes are employed.
- **Biopsy:** It is essential to show the exact histology of the malignancy. Submucosal disease may need deep biopsies. Submucosal spread, beneath a normal mucosa, is quite common.

> **Occult primary:** Nasopharynx is a common site for occult primaries. Nasopharyngeal curettage must be performed in cases of strong suspicion. A strip of mucosa and submucosa from the region of fossa of Rosenmuller is taken for histology.

- **Fine-needle aspiration cytology (FNAC):** FNAC of cervical node will confirm secondary metastasis.

Serology

- **Anti-EBV IgA (anti-VCA and anti-EA) anti viral capsid antigen and anti early antigen titers:** High IgA anti-VCA titer is very sensitive and high IgA anti-EA titer is very specific for detecting early occult disease. EBV titers may be used for surveillance after treatment.
- **EBV DNA titers (anti-EBV-specific DNase)** correlate with stage, treatment response, relapse and survival. They may be used for predicting prognosis.

Radiology

- **MRI with gadolinium and fat suppression:** It is the diagnostic imaging modality of choice. Coronal views assess petroclinoid fissure, foramina (lacerum, ovale, rotundum and spinosum) and cavernous sinus. Axial views evaluate retropharyngeal, paranasopharyngeal, pterygomaxillary space and infratemporal fossa.
- **Contrast CT (Fig. 38.1B):** Evaluate bone involvement, skull base erosion and cervical lymphadenopathy particularly in presence of extracapsular spread.
- **Positron emission tomography:** For distant metastasis and residual and recurrent disease after treatment.

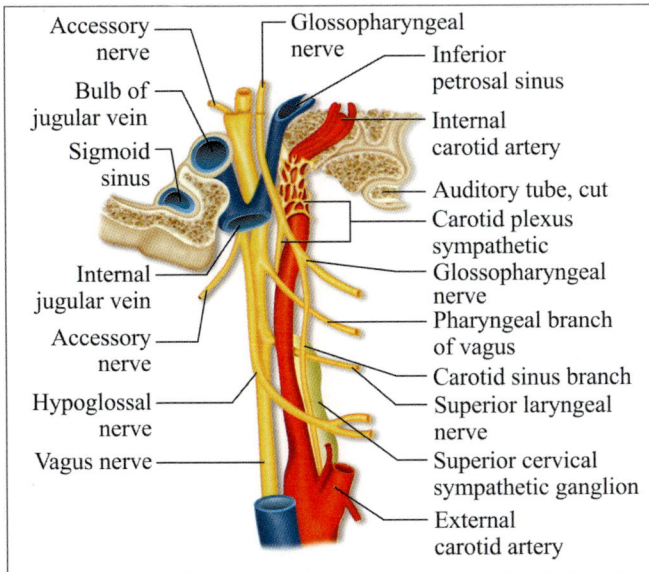

Fig. 38.2: Right jugular foramen and structures passing through it

TNM Classification

In nasopharynx carcinoma, node (N) classification is different from other mucosal carcinoma of head and neck region (Table 38.3). Less weight is given to Level 1 and 2 nodes (even 6 cm nodes are considered N_1 category). Node enlargement (irrespective of the size) of supraclavicular fossa or Ho's triangle (triangle between medial and lateral ends of clavicle and the point where neck meets the shoulder) is considered N_3 category.

Table 38.3: AJCC Cancer Staging (2002) and UICC TNM classification of malignant tumors of nasopharynx

Primary tumor (T)	
T_X	Cannot be assessed
T_0	No tumor
T_{is}	Carcinoma in situ
T_1	Tumor is confined to nasopharynx
T_2	Tumor extends to soft tissues of oropharynx or nasal fossa
T_{2a}	No parapharyngeal extension
T_{2b}	With parapharyngeal extension
T_3	Tumor invades bones and/or paranasal sinuses
T_4	Intracranial extension, involvement of cranial nerves, infratemporal fossa, hypopharynx, orbit, or masticator space
Regional lymph nodes (N); size in greatest dimension	
N_X	Cannot be assessed
N_0	No nodal metastases
N_1	Single ipsilateral node except supraclavicular fossa <= 6 cm
N_2	Bilateral or contralateral nodes except supraclavicular fossa <= 6 cm
N_{3a}	Any node > 6 cm
N_{3b}	Supraclavicular node of any size
Distant metastasis (M)	
M_X	Cannot be assessed
M_0	No distant metastasis
M_1	Distant metastasis
Stage grouping	
Stage 0	$T_{is}\ N_0\ M_0$
Satge I	$T_1\ N_0\ M_0$
Stage IIA	$T_{2a}\ N_0\ M_0$
Stage IIB	$T_{2b}\ N_0\ M_0$ or $T_{1-2b}\ N_1\ M_0$
Stage III	$T_3\ N_0\ M_0$ or $T_{1-3}\ N_{1-2}\ M_0$
Stage IVA	$T_4\ N_{0-2}\ M_0$
Stage IVB	$T_{1-4}\ N_3\ M_0$
Stage IVC	$T_{1-4}\ N_{0-3}\ M_1$

Treatment

- **Irradiation:** It is the primary treatment of choice. External radiation or intracavitary implants (brachytherapy) or both are used.
    - External beam radiotherapy is most commonly used. Opposing lateral fields include primary tumor, upper neck and third anterior matched field irradiate lower cervical and supraclavicular nodes. A tumor dose of 6000–7000 radiations is given. The stereotactic radiosurgery, three-dimensional conformal (3DCRT) and IMRT are safer and more precise.
    - Overall survival is in the range of 50–80%.
- **Systemic chemotherapy:** It may be used as palliation for distant metastases or in radiation failures. Single and combination chemotherapy (cisplatinum/5-flurouracil) have been used as an adjunct to radiation. Induction, adjuvant, concomitant or their combinations have shown improvement in survival.
- **Radical neck dissection:** It may be done for persistent nodes when primary has been controlled.

Recurrent Disease

Recurrent or residual tumor may be managed with second course of radiation (tele or Gold 198 brachytherapy), nasopharyngectomy, or skull base surgery in selected cases.

Prognosis

The prognosis of NPC is relatively better in keratinizing squamous cell carcinoma.

THORNWALDT'S DISEASE (PHARYNGEAL BURSITIS)

The pharyngeal bursa represents attachment of notochord to endoderm. It is a median recess that is located in the posterior wall of the nasopharynx in the adenoid mass.

Clinical Features

The infection of pharyngeal bursa (Thornwaldt's Disease) may present with:
- Persistent postnasal discharge and crusting in the nasopharynx.
- Nasal obstruction due nasopharyngeal swelling.
- Serous otitis media due to Eustachian tube obstruction.
- Dull occipital headache.
- Recurrent sore throat.
- Low-grade fever.
- A cystic and fluctuant swelling in the posterior wall of nasopharynx.

Treatment

- Antibiotics for infection.
- Marsupialization of the cystic swelling with removal of the lining membrane.

> **Luschka pouch:** Persistence of this invagination pouch causes Thornwaldt's cyst which may get infected and form an abscess in the nasopharynx. Notochord, which is attached to the endoderm in the area of nasopharynx, produces this invagination pouch. Pharyngeal bursa is a site for Thornwaldt's cyst.

Self-evaluation Exercises

1. Trotter's (sinus of Morgagni) syndrome is the triad of:
   a. Conductive hearing loss (due to Eustachian tube obstruction)
   b. Immobility of soft palate
   c. Neuralgic pain in the distribution of mandibular division of trigeminal nerve
   d. All of the above
2. Clinical features of nasopharyngeal angiofibroma include:
   a. Exclusively in young adolescent boys
   b. Episodes of profuse nosebleed
   c. Nasal obstruction
   d. All of the above
3. Nasopharyngeal cancer can involve:
   a. Nasal cavity
   b. Oropharynx
   c. Tympanic cavity
   d. Orbit
   e. All of the above
4. The modalities of treatment of nasopharyngeal angiofibroma include:
   a. If the mass is arising from the lateral wall of nose extending only into the nasopharynx, transpalatal approach is used
   b. Hormones
   c. Intensity modulated radiotherapy
   d. All of the above
5. The most common presentation of carcinoma of nasopharynx is:
   a. Metastatic cervical lymphadenopathy
   b. Unilateral serous otitis media
   c. Facial pain
   d. All of the above

True (T)/False (F)

6. Radiotherapy is the treatment of choice in angiofibroma of nasopharynx.
7. Carcinoma of nasopharynx is related to herpes zoster virus infection.
8. The basal cell carcinoma is the most common histological variety of carcinoma of nasopharynx.
9. Surgery is usually the first line of treatment for carcinoma of nasopharynx.
10. Patient of carcinoma of nasopharynx can present with squint, facial pain, blindness and mass in the neck.
11. Chances of metastases are highest in cancer of nasopharynx.
12. Rhabdomyosarcoma is the most common malignant tumor of nasopharynx in children.
13. Orbit is the most common site of rhabdomyosarcoma in the head and neck region.
14. Persistence of Luschka pouch (an invagination pouch) causes Thornwaldt's cyst which may get infected and form an abscess in the nasopharynx.
15. The benign tumor nasopharyngeal angiofibroma erodes bone and is known for its recurrence on incomplete removal and can spread intracranially.
16. Biopsy is contraindicated in nasopharyngeal angiofibroma.
17. Histological diagnosis of angiofibroma of nasopharynx is made by excisional biopsy.
18. In nasopharyngeal carcinoma prognosis is relatively better in keratinizing squamous cell carcinoma.
19. The associated trismus and preauricular fullness may be seen in some cases of Trotter's (sinus of Morgagni) syndrome or triad.

Filling the blanks

20. The most common site of carcinoma of nasopharynx is _____.
21. Type of voice in nasopharyngeal fibroma is _____.
22. _____ lymph nodes are situated in the jugular foramen.

Contd...

Contd…

23. The enlargement of Krause's lymph nodes compresses CN IX, X and XI, and produce _____.
24. Antral (Holman-Miller) sign is a feature of _____.
25. Trotter's triad is seen in _____.
26. Nasopharyngeal chordoma originates from the _____.
27. Most common site of origin of nasopharyngeal angiofibroma is _____.
28. Notochord, which is attached to the endoderm in the area of nasopharynx, produces _____.
29. Pharyngeal bursa is a site for _____ cyst.
30. _____ pouch may persist as craniopharyngeal canal in the nasopharynx. It forms anterior pituitary.

Answers

1. d
2. d
3. e
4. d
5. d
6. F
7. F
8. F
9. F
10. T
11. T
12. T
13. T
14. T
15. T
16. T
17. T
18. T
19. T
20. fossa of Rosenmuller (pharyngeal recess)
21. rhinolalia clausa
22. Krause's
23. jugular foramen syndrome
24. Nasopharyngeal angiofibroma
25. nasopharyngeal carcinoma
26. notochord
27. sphenopalatine foramen
28. Luschka pouch
29. Thornwaldt's
30. Rathke's

Pearls and Nuggets (Refresh your knowledge)

- **Chordoma:** It arises from the remnants of notochord. Characteristic histological features include physaliferous cells (foamy cells with compressed nuclei).
- **Contraindications for biopsy:** They include nasopharyngeal angiofibroma, glomus tumor of the middle ear, carotid body tumor of the neck and benign parapharyngeal tumors.
- **DiGeorge sequence:** The absence of thymus (few T-cells in the paracortex of lymph nodes) and parathyroid glands (hypocalcemia) results from the improper development of the third and fourth pharyngeal pouches. Young girls get repeated episodes of viral and fungal infections.
- **Muller's muscles:** These extraocular smooth muscles of eye lids are supplied by sympathetic fibers. Its paralysis in Horner syndrome causes partial ptosis.
- **Nasogastric feeding:** About 2000 K calories can be given without any untoward side effect by nasogastric feeding.
- **Jugular foramen syndrome:** It is caused by a tumor, which compresses contents that are passing through the jugular foramen. It consists of paralysis of CN IX, X and XI, which pass through the jugular foramen along with the internal jugular vein. It can be seen in patients of malignancy nasopharynx, glomus jugular, large acoustic neuroma or thrombophlebitis of jugular bulb. The syndrome consists of following features:
  - Reduction in the parotid gland secretion is the autonomic deficit.
  - Axonal lesions result in retrograde chromatolysis (changes in the neuronal cell bodies) in the nucleus ambiguus.
  - Loss of gag reflex.
  - Uvula deviated towards the opposite side of the lesion.

Chapter 39

Tumors of Oropharynx

Specific Learning Objectives

After going through the chapter, you should be able to answer the following questions:
- What are the etiological factors, pathological types and prophylactic measures of oropharyngeal carcinoma?
- How will you evaluate and manage a case of oropharyngeal carcinoma?
- Describe carcinoma of base of tongue.
- Describe malignancy of tonsil.
- What do you know about: (1) Parapharyngeal tumors; (2) Stylalgia (Eagle's syndrome); (3) Carcinoma of soft palate?

MALIGNANT TUMORS

INTRODUCTION

The high and increasing incidence of oropharyngeal cancer is becoming a serious health problem. The management of these tumors needs a multidisciplinary team, which consists of head and neck cancer surgeon, reconstructive surgeon, speech and swallowing therapist, prosthodontist, dentist and radiation and medical oncologist. **Benign tumors are far less common than the malignant ones.**

For the purpose of description of malignant tumors, oropharynx is divided into four different subsites:
1. Posterior one-third (or base) of tongue
2. Palatine tonsillar area including fossa and pillars
3. Soft palate
4. Posterior pharyngeal wall.

HISTOPATHOLOGY

The tissue of origin for most of the oropharyngeal carcinomas are stratified squamous epithelium, minor salivary glands and lymphoepithelium of Waldeyer's ring. Squamous cell carcinoma (SCC) accounts for 90% of all oropharyngeal malignancies. Some of the varieties are listed below:
- **Squamous cell carcinoma (SCC):** It is the most common variety of carcinoma. It shows various grades—well, moderately and poorly differentiated.
    - Keratinizing SCC
    - Nonkeratinizing SCC
    - Basaloid SCC
    - Verrucous carcinoma
    - Spindle cell carcinoma
    - **Lymphoepithelial carcinoma:** This is a poorly differentiated variant of SCC and shows admixture of lymphocytes. The common sites of this include tonsil, base of tongue and vallecula.
- **Minor salivary gland tumors:** Minor salivary gland malignancy is mostly seen on the palate and fauces.
    - Adenoid cystic carcinoma
    - Mucoepidermoid carcinoma.
- **Lymphomas:** Hodgkin and non-Hodgkin arise from the tonsil and base of tongue in young adults and children. Cervical nodes get enlarged.
- **Sarcomas.**

Grading

The current WHO grading system is largely based on classic broders classification. It describes following three grades:
1. Grade 1: Well differentiated.
2. Grade 2: Moderately differentiated.
3. Grade 3: Poorly differentiated.

RISK FACTORS

- Tobacco-smoking
- Alcohol
- Chewing of betel nut and tobacco
- Human papilloma virus (HPV) type 16 for SCC of tonsil: Tumor specific vaccines for HPV-positive disease are under investigation.

INCIDENCE

- **Geography:** The incidence is high in South Central Asia, South Africa and Europe. In Indian males, mouth/oropharynx are the most common sites of cancer while in females they are on number four.
- **Age:** The incidence and mortality increases with age.
- **Gender:** These tumors are three times more common in men than women (12.48 males and 5.52 females in 100,000 Indian population).
- **Racial-ethnic:** Among men, highest rate is in blacks followed in descending order by whites (non-Hispanic), Vietnamese and native Hawaiians.

PREVENTION

- **Bad habits:** Stop smoking and chewing of betel nut and tobacco.
- **Diet:** Fresh fruits and vegetables may reduce the relative risk of cancer of upper aerodigestive tract.

EVALUATION

Clinical Features

- **Early:** Throat irritation, burning sensation with acidic food, neck swelling and odynophagia.
- Referred unilateral earache is common.
- **Late:** Dysphagia, dysarthria or hot potato voice, trismus, obstructive airway symptoms, hearing loss (serous otitis media due to Eustachian tube obstruction), and weight loss.
- Hemoptysis and oral bleeding in tonsil cancer.

Types of Lesion

Three types of lesions are:
1. **Exophytic:** Superficially spreading and exophytic types are usually seen in the palatine arch. Metastases are rare.
2. **Ulcerative:** Ulcerative and infiltrative types deeply invade the adjoining structures. They are usually seen in base of tongue and tonsil.
3. **Submucosal.**

> **Prognosis:** Because of marked tendency for regional metastasis, prognosis is poor in ulcerative lesions than exophytic type of growth.

Imaging Studies

- **Computed tomography (CT) with contrast:** CT shows bony involvement (such as cortical mandibular invasion, cervical spines and skull base) and secondary neck nodes.
- **Magnetic resonance imaging (MRI):** Coronal, transverse and sagittal planes T1W and T1W with gadolinium-diethylene pentaacetate (Gd-DTPA) contrast and fat suppression. MRI shows soft tissue infiltration such as tongue base, parapharyngeal and pre-epiglottic and bone marrow involvement.
- **X-ray chest posteroanterior (PA) and lateral views:**
  - Acute or chronic diseases (e.g. Tuberculosis).
  - Pulmonary metastasis.
  - Synchronous pulmonary primary carcinoma.
- **Positron emission tomography (PET):** Indications.
  - High tumor grade and large tumor volume.
  - Recurrent tumor.
  - Neck metastasis of unknown origin.
  - Post-treatment surveillance.
- **Fusion PET-CT:** Provide improved anatomic localization of tumors and metastasis.

Biopsy

- Usually under local anesthesia with cup forceps but general anesthesia is preferred for base of tongue tumor. Panendoscopy should be performed.
- Fine needle aspiration cytology (FNAC) from neck mass may be done if primary and secondary are clinically evident.

STAGING

The Union for International Cancer Control (UICC) tumor nodes and metastasis (TNM) classification and American Joint Committee on Cancer (AJCC) cancer staging are shown in Table 39.1.

TREATMENT

The treatment modalities and protocols vary from center to center. They depend upon the site and extent of disease (Table 39.1), patient's general condition, surgeon's experience and philosophy, and facilities available. The treatment modalities include:
- Surgery
- Radiotherapy
- Chemotherapy
- Combination of surgery and radiotherapy
- Chemotherapy as an adjunct to surgery or radiotherapy
- Palliative therapy

CARCINOMA BASE OF TONGUE

This is very common in India.

Clinical Features

- **Neck swelling:** Mostly patient presents with metastases in cervical nodes.
- **Early symptoms:** They are mostly ignored by the patient for a long time and include sore throat, feeling of lump in the throat and slight discomfort on swallowing.

Table 39.1: AJCC cancer staging (2002) and UICC TNM classification of malignant tumors of oropharynx

Primary tumor (T) tumor size in greatest dimension	
T_X	Cannot be assessed
T_0	No tumor
T_{is}	Carcinoma in situ
T_1	Tumor <= 2 cm
T_2	Tumor > 2 cm but <= 4 cm
T_3	Tumor > 4 cm
T_{4a}	Tumor invades any of the following: larynx, deep or extrinsic muscles of tongue, medial pterygoid muscle, hard palate or mandible
T_{4b}	Tumor invades any of the following: lateral pterygoid muscle, pterygoid plates, lateral nasopharynx, skull base or encases carotid artery
Regional lymph nodes (N) for oropharynx and hypopharynx; size in greatest dimension	
Similar to oral cancer. See Table 33.2 of Chapter 33 'Neoplasms of Oral Cavity'.	
Distant metastasis (M)	
Similar to oral cancer. See Table 33.2 of Chapter 33 'Neoplasms of Oral Cavity'.	
Stage grouping for oropharynx and hypopharynx	
Similar to oral cancer. See Table 33.2 of Chapter 33 'Neoplasms of Oral Cavity'.	

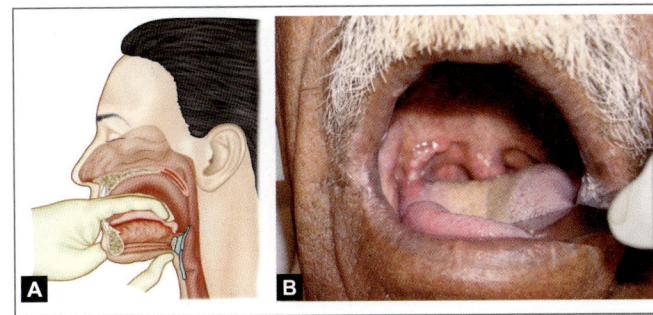

Figs 39.1A and B: (A) Bimanual palpation of oropharynx to assess tumor fixation to mandible and submucosal extent in the tongue base. Subtle mucosal abnormalities bleed after palpation; (B) Carcinoma of right tonsil involving anterior tonsillar pillar

- *Late features:* They indicate advanced disease and include referred earache, dysphagia, bleeding from the mouth, and hot potato voice.
- Deeply infiltrative ulcer with induration can be seen and palpated on base of tongue (Fig. 39.1A). The lesion may involve tongue musculature, epiglottis and pre-epiglottic space, tonsil and its pillars, and hypopharynx.

Spread
- *Local:* The deeply infiltrative ulcer involves tongue musculature, epiglottis and pre-epiglottic space, tonsil and its pillars and hypopharynx.
- *Lymphatic:* Most patients (70%) have unilateral or bilateral cervical metastases (usually jugulodigastric nodes) at the time of first consultation.
- *Distant metastases:* Bones, liver and lung.

Diagnosis
- *CT scan:* It shows tumor extension and nodal involvement.
- *Biopsy and examination under general anesthesia:* Examination and palpation under anesthesia provide better idea of the extent of lesion, which is usually far more extensive than it appears. Biopsy will confirm the diagnosis and tell the nature of malignancy.
For TNM classification and staging see Table 39.1.

Treatment
The mode of treatment varies from center to center and doctor to doctor. Tumors, which are radiosensitive (such as anaplastic carcinoma, lymphoepithelioma and lymphoma) are usually treated with radiotherapy.
- T_1 *and* T_2 *with* N_0 *or* N_1: Surgical excision with block dissection followed by radiotherapy if needed.
- T_3 *and* T_4 *lesions:* Surgical excision with mandibular resection, neck dissection and postoperative radiation.
- *T_4 lesion extending into anterior two-thirds of tongue or vallecula:* Extensive surgery consists of total glossectomy and laryngectomy in addition to the block dissection. Chemotherapy may be combined with radiotherapy and surgery in such cases.
- *Advanced cases with poor health:*
  - Palliation with radio or chemotherapy.
  - Tracheostomy and gastrostomy in terminal phases.
  - Strong analgesics for relieving pain.

CARCINOMA TONSIL (FIGS 39.1B AND 39.2A)

Spread
- *Local:* Tumor may involve soft palate and pillars, base of tongue, pharyngeal wall, parapharyngeal space, hypopharynx, pterygoid muscles and mandible.
- *Lymphatic:* Fifty percent cases show cervical node (usually jugulodigastric) involvement at the time of initial presentation.
- *Distant metastases.*

Clinical Features
- *Most common* are the persistent sore throat, difficulty in swallowing, pain in the ear and lump in the neck.
- *Late features* are bleeding from the mouth, halitosis (fetor oris), pain and trismus (due to invasion of pterygoid muscles and mandible).
- *Ulcerated lesion with necrotic base* on tonsil.

Section 5 • Pharynx and Esophagus

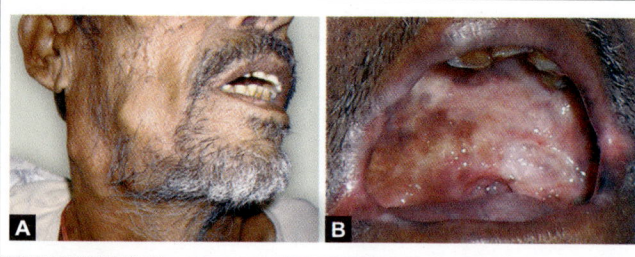

Figs 39.2A and B: (A) Malignancy of tonsil with neck node metastasis on right side; (B) Carcinoma of soft palate left side. Superficially spreading infiltrative palatal lesion involving anterior tonsillar pillar

- *Lymphomas* may simulate indolent peritonsillar abscess and present as unilateral tonsillar enlargement with or without ulceration.
- *Palpation* of tonsillar area reveals the extent of tumor and induration.

Diagnosis

Biopsy: It will reveal the histological typing.

Histopathology: Squamous cell carcinoma is the most common variety of tonsillar malignancy and second common is lymphoma.

Treatment

- *Radiotherapy:* For early and radiosensitive tumors and radiation includes cervical nodes.
- *Surgery:*
    - Excision of the tonsil for early superficial lesions.
    - Wide surgical excision with hemimandibulectomy and neck dissection (commando operation) for larger lesions and mandibular invasion.
- *Combination therapy:* Surgery with pre- or postoperative radiation.
- *Chemotherapy:* As an adjunct to surgery and radiation.

LYMPHOMA

- Lymphomas are mostly of non-Hodgkin variety.
- Most common site tonsils.
- *Lesion:* A smooth submucosal bulky mass of tonsil that may ulcerate.
- Males are affected more.
- Cervical nodes are enlarged in 40–70% of the patients.
- Treatment is radiation and/or chemotherapy.

CARCINOMA SOFT PALATE (FIG. 39.2B)

Carcinoma in faucial arch (soft palate, uvula and anterior tonsillar pillar) is often squamous cell variety (usually well-differentiated).

The superficially spreading lesions spread locally to the contiguous structures and metastasize to lymph nodes (upper deep cervical and submandibular). Nodal metastases is late.

Clinical Features

- *Most common:* Persistent sore throat, local pain and earache.
- Ulcer or growth with induration.

Treatment

- Small tumors can be easily excised.
- Large tumors involving major part of soft palate are treated with radiotherapy. Surgery is reserved for salvage as the morbidity of surgery is significant.
- Radical removal of palate and superior part of lateral pharyngeal wall through mandibulotomy (median, paramedian or lateral angular) need postoperative reconstruction.

CARCINOMA POSTERIOR PHARYNGEAL WALL

Spread

- *Local:* The submucosal spread may involve tonsil, soft palate, tongue, nasopharynx, hypopharynx, parapharyngeal space and anterior spinal ligaments.
- *Lymphatic:* Sixty percent of cases have lymph node metastases, which may be bilateral.

Clinical Features

Patient usually remains asymptomatic for a long time and present with neck swelling. X-ray soft tissue neck lateral view shows soft tissue fullness in prevertebral space (Fig. 39.3A).

Treatment

- Irradiation.
- *Surgical excision combined with block dissection and skin grafting:* Approach is usually lateral pharyngotomy with or without mandibular osteotomy.

BENIGN SWELLINGS

Some common benign lesions (papilloma, hemangioma and pleomorphic adenoma) are described here. Rare benign tumors include lipoma, fibroma and neuroma.

PAPILLOMA

- *Site:* Tonsil, soft palate and faucial pillars.
- *Lesion:* Pedunculated smooth or wart like.
- *Clinical features:* Asymptomatic noticed incidentally. Large papilloma may lead to some irritation.
- *Treatment:* Surgical excision.

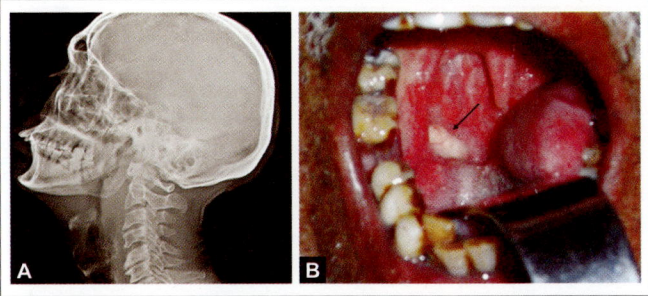

Figs 39.3A and B: (A) X-ray of soft tissue neck lateral view. Posterior pharyngeal mass. Soft tissue fullness in prevertebral space; (B) Mucous retention cyst of vallecula right side. Yellowish cystic swelling visible through the oral cavity on depressing the tongue (arrow showing)

HEMANGIOMA

- *Common sites:* Palate, tonsil, posterior and lateral pharyngeal wall.
- *Types:* Capillary and cavernous types.
- *Treatment:* Treated only if causing bleeding and dysphagia. The different modalities of treatment include:
    - Diathermy coagulation
    - Injection of sclerosing agents
    - Cryotherapy
    - Laser coagulation.

PLEOMORPHIC ADENOMA

- *Site:* Submucosal swelling on hard and soft palate.
- Potentially malignant.
- Treatment is total excision.

MUCOUS CYST

Mucous retention cysts are not uncommon.
- *Most common site:* Vallecula (Fig. 39.3B).
- Yellowish pedunculated or sessile cystic swelling.
- Usually asymptomatic and incidentally seen during examination.
- Large cysts can cause foreign body sensation in the throat.
- *Treatment:* Surgical excision of the pedunculated cyst or incision, drainage and removal of cyst wall (marsupialization).

PARAPHARYNGEAL TUMORS (FIG. 39.4A)

In parapharyngeal space (*see* Chapter 'Deep Neck Infections'), both benign and malignant tumors are seen. Commonly seen tumors include deep lobe of parotid,

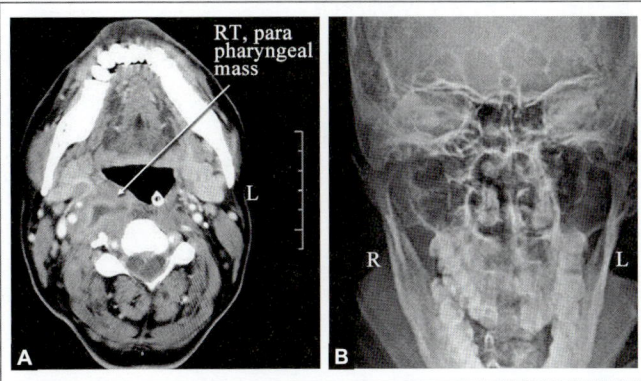

Figs 39.4A and B: (A) CT scan of parapharyngeal mass. Contrast CT scan of neck axial section. Soft tissue density mass in right parapharyngeal space, post-styloid compartment. Note the inhomogeneous enhancement with peripheral enhancing component and central nonenhancing necrotic component. Medially it involves pharyngeal mucosal space and bulges into the pharynx. Posteriorly it extends into retropharyngeal wall but not crossing midline. Laterally, loss of fat planes indicates encasing of internal and external carotid arteries and approaching internal jugular vein; (B) X-ray of skull for styloid process. Left side styloid process is thick and right side styloid process is very long

neurilemmoma, carotid body chemodectoma, lipoma and aneurysm of internal carotid artery.

They usually present with a bulge in lateral pharyngeal wall, which may distort the pillars and soft palate and look like oropharyngeal neoplasm.

- *Most common tumor of parapharyngeal space:* Neurogenic tumor
- *Internal carotid artery aneurysm:* This parapharyngeal mass displaces the tonsil and tonsillar fossa medially. Pulsations can be felt on intraoral palpation.

STYLALGIA (EAGLE'S SYNDROME)

- An elongated styloid process and calcification of stylohyoid ligament can cause pain in tonsillar fossa and upper neck. Pain radiates to the ear and gets aggravated on swallowing.
- The elongated styloid process can be palpated transorally in the tonsillar fossa.
- Many persons with elongated styloid process (an incidental and common finding on radiographs of skull) do not have any symptoms (Fig. 39.4B).
- *Diagnosis:* X-ray of skull anteroposterior or lateral view with open mouth show the elongated styloid process.

Treatment

- Symptomatic styloid process may be excised by transoral or cervical approach. Results are equivocal.

Self-evaluation Exercises

1. Which is the most common tumor of parapharyngeal space?
   a. Neurogenic tumor
   b. Deep lobe of parotid
   c. Carotid body chemodectoma
   d. Aneurysm of internal carotid artery
2. The features of internal carotid artery aneurysm include:
   a. Parapharyngeal mass
   b. Displaces the tonsil and tonsillar fossa medially
   c. Pulsations can be felt on intraoral palpation
   d. All of the above

Answers

1. a   2. d

Chapter 40

Tumors of Hypopharynx

> **Specific Learning Objectives**
>
> After going through the chapter, you should be able to answer the following questions:
> - What are the clinical features of carcinoma pyriform fossa and how will you manage it?
> - What are the risk factors of postcricoid cancer and how will you manage it?
> - What do you know about: (1) Cancer posterior pharyngeal wall; (2) Plummer-Vinson syndrome?

INTRODUCTION

Carcinoma of the hypopharynx is very common in India. Most of the tumors are squamous cell carcinoma (SCC), which have various grades of differentiation. The various subsites involved in descending order of frequency are pyriform sinus, postcricoid region and posterior pharyngeal wall.

Benign tumors of laryngopharynx are very rare and include lipoma (relatively more common), papilloma, adenoma, fibroma and leiomyoma. They usually present as smooth well-defined mass. They may be pedunculated and mobile. Treatment consists of endoscopic or open surgical excision.

Hypopharynx Subsites

It is subdivided into three regions—pyriform sinus, postcricoid region and posterior pharyngeal wall (Figs 40.1A and B). TNM classification of carcinoma laryngopharynx is given in Chapter 'Malignant Tumors of Larynx'. For the detail anatomy see Chapter 'Anatomy and Physiology of Pharynx and Esophagus'.

Risk Factors

They include following:
- Alcohol.
- Smoking.
- Chewing of betel nut and tobacco.
- Genetic predisposition.
- Plummer-Vinson or Paterson-Brown-Kelly syndrome or sideropenic anemia. It primarily affects women (85%).
- Nutritional deficiency.
- Low socioeconomic conditions.

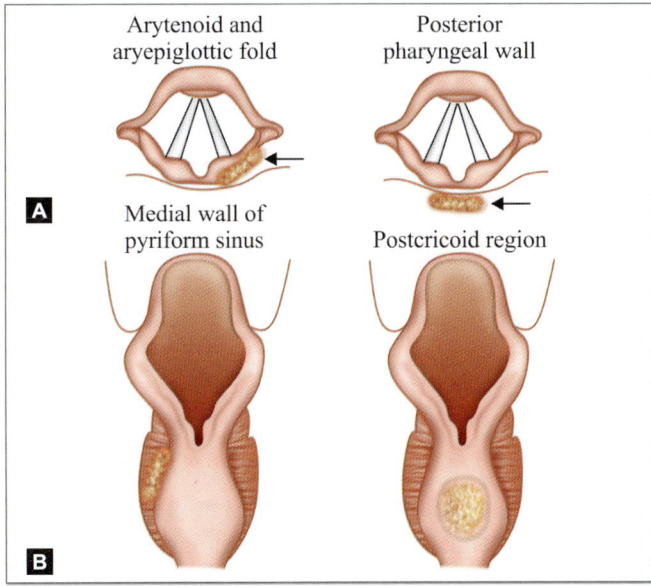

Figs 40.1A and B: Sites of hypopharyngeal cancer. (A) Indirect laryngoscopic; (B) Posterior views of laryngopharynx

CARCINOMA PYRIFORM SINUS

- It accounts for 60% of all hypopharyngeal cancers.
- Mostly affects males above 40 years of age.
- Usually patients present with metastatic neck nodes, which are very common in pyriform fossa cancer as the lymphatic metastasis is very common.

Spread

- **Locally:**
  - Superiorly to vallecula and base of tongue.
  - Inferiorly to postcricoid region.
  - Medially to aryepiglottic folds and ventricles.
  - Laterally to thyroid cartilage, thyroid gland and soft tissue mass in the neck.
- **Lymphatic:** Seventy-five percent of cases have cervical nodal metastases (upper and middle group of jugular cervical nodes, bilateral in 50% cases) at the time of first consultation. The rich lymphatic network gives rise to early lymphatic metastasis in pyriform fossa SCC. In some cases nodes appear late even after eradication of the primary.
- **Distant metastases:** It is often late and seen in lung, liver and bones.

Clinical Features

The growth usually remains asymptomatic for a long time because of the large size of the pyriform sinus.

- **Most common:** A mass of lymph nodes in the neck.
- **Early symptoms:** Sticking in the throat and 'pricking sensation' on swallowing.
- Referred otalgia or pain on swallowing.
- Increasing dysphagia.
- Hoarseness and laryngeal obstruction due to laryngeal edema and spread to larynx.
- Growth is either exophytic or ulcerative and deeply infiltrative. It can often be seen on laryngeal mirror examination. Pooling of secretions may obstruct the view.

Referred ear pain in cancer of pyriform fossa: It is through the superior laryngeal nerve which is a branch of vagus (CN X).

Diagnosis

- **Barium swallow:** Filling defect can be seen.
- **CT scan (Fig. 40.2):** Evaluate primary growth and lymph node metastasis.
- **Endoscopic examination:** It provides accurate assessment and extent of primary tumor. Panendoscopy finds any other synchronous primary.
- **Biopsy:** For histopathological diagnosis.

Treatment

- **Radiotherapy**
  - Primary treatment for early growth without nodes.
  - Planned postoperative radiotherapy usually in all cases of surgery.
- **Surgery**
  - Growth limited to pyriform fossa and larynx (vocal cord fix) and not extending to postcricoid region:

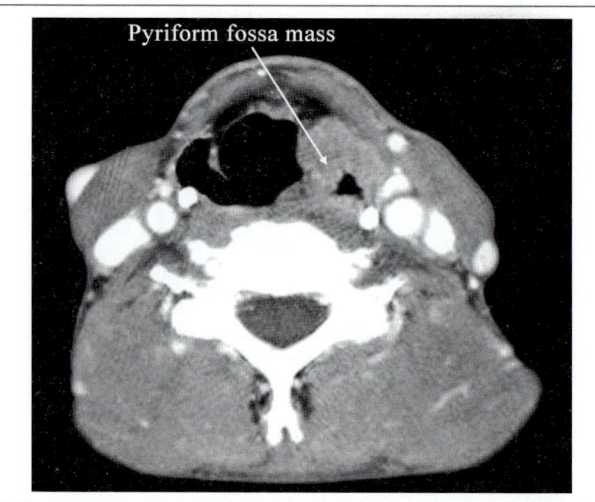

Fig. 40.2: Pyriform fossa mass. Contrast CT scan of neck axial section. Inhomogeneously enhancing mass, which is completely obliterating left pyriform fossa and involving both medial (aryepiglottic fold) and lateral wall and left side of epiglottis
Source: Dr Ritesh Prajapati, Consultant Radiologist, Anand, Gujarat

Total laryngectomy and partial pharyngectomy often combined with elective or prophylactic block dissection of lymph nodes. Pharynx is primarily closed.
  - **Growth extending to postcricoid region:** Total laryngectomy and pharyngectomy with block dissection and myocutaneous flaps or stomach pull-up for pharyngoesophageal reconstruction.
- **Curative treatment as per the staging:** (For TNM classification *see* Chapter 'Malignant Tumors of Larynx').
  - **Stage I:** Primary radiotherapy or partial pharyngectomy (PP) or partial pharyngectomy and partial laryngectomy (PPPL).
  - **Stage II:** Primary radiotherapy or chemoradiotherapy or PPPL or total laryngopharyngectomy (TLP).
  - **Stage III and IVa:** Upfront chemoradiotherapy total laryngectomy and partial pharyngectomy (TLPP) or total laryngopharyngectomy (TLP) and postoperative radiotherapy/chemoradiotherapy.

CARCINOMA POSTCRICOID

- It accounts for 30% of all laryngopharyngeal malignancies.
- One-third patients of postcricoid carcinoma suffer from an etiological factor the sideropenic anemia (Paterson-Brown-Kelly or Plummer-Vinson syndrome). It occurs in females and is characterized by hypochromic microcytic iron deficiency anemia.
- Lesion is ulcerative and infiltrative which spreads in an annular fashion and causes dysphagia.

- Patients are usually females in their twenties and thirties.

> **Plummer-Vinson syndrome:** This premalignant condition is the disease of females. It is characterized by iron deficiency anemia and dysphagia. Patients usually have koilonychia, atrophic gastritis and glossitis.

Spread

- *Local:* Cervical esophagus, arytenoids and recurrent laryngeal nerve at cricoarytenoid joint.
- *Lymphatic:* Paratracheal lymph nodes, which are bilateral and not clinically palpable.

Clinical Features

- *Most common:* Progressive dysphagia in anemic females.
- *Vocal symptoms:* Voice change and aphonia.
- Inspiratory stridor in advanced tumor occurs due to pressure on larynx and bilateral recurrent laryngeal nerves involvement.
- *General symptoms:* Malnutrition and weight loss.
- *Indirect laryngoscopy:* Edema and erythema of the postcricoid region and pooling of secretions in the hypopharynx indicates postcricoid growths.
    - *Vocal cord mobility:* Restricted vocal cord mobility due to infiltration of recurrent laryngeal nerve or posterior cricoarytenoid muscles.
- *Palpation:* Absence of laryngeal crepitus, which is felt normally while moving larynx over the cervical spine (Fig. 40.3A).

Diagnosis

- *X-ray soft tissue neck lateral view:* Shows widening of prevertebral soft tissue space.
- *Barium swallow:* Shows the lower extent of the disease (Fig. 40.3B).

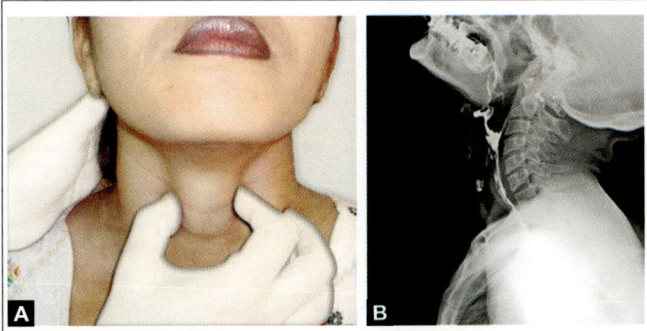

Figs 40.3A and B: (A) Post-laryngeal crepitus. On moving the larynx from side to side, normally a post-laryngeal crepitus is felt. It is absent in cases of postcricoid malignancy; (B) Barium swallow in a case of malignancy postcricoid region. Note the prevertebral soft tissue widening and irregular filling defect
Source: (B) Dr Jayesh Patel, Consultant Radiologist, Anand, Gujarat

- *Endoscopy:* It helps in assessing the extent of lesion. Panendoscopy finds other synchronous primary.
- *Biopsy:* For histopathological diagnosis.
- *CT scan (neck and thorax):* It reveals extent of disease and lymph node and lung metastasis.

Treatment

Some prefer primary surgery while others prefer initial radiotherapy.

- *Radiotherapy:* Primary radiotherapy preserves laryngeal function. Failed cases may be subjected to surgery. Some prefer planned postoperative radiotherapy.
- *Surgery:* Laryngo-pharyngo-esophagectomy with stomach pull-up or colon transposition for reconstructing pharyngoesophageal segment.
- *Curative treatment as per the staging:* (For TNM classification *see* Chapter 'Malignant Tumors of Larynx').
    - *Stage I:* Primary radiotherapy or total laryngopharyngectomy (TLP).
    - *Stage II:* Primary radiotherapy or chemoradiotherapy or TLP and postoperative radiotherapy.
    - *Stage III:* TLP or total laryngo-pharyngo-esophagectomy (TLPO) and postoperative radiotherapy/chemoradiotherapy.
    - *Stage IVa:* TLPO and gastric pull-up and postoperative radiotherapy/primary chemoradiotherapy.

Prognosis

It is poor with both irradiation and surgical treatment.

CARCINOMA POSTERIOR PHARYNGEAL WALL

This is the least common and accounts for only 10% of all laryngopharyngeal malignancy. It is mostly seen in males above 50 years of age. Growth is either exophytic (more common) or ulcerative and remains localized for long time.

Spread

- *Local:* Prevertebral fascia, muscles and vertebrae.
- *Lymphatic:* Fifty percent patients have nodal metastases (usually bilateral due to midline lesion) on their initial consultation. Retropharyngeal nodes (not clinically palpable) are also involved.

Clinical Features

They are following:
- Gradually progressive dysphagia.
- A palpable mass of nodes in the neck.
- Spitting of blood.
- *Indirect mirror examination:* Growth is either exophytic (more common) or ulcerative.

Diagnosis

- ***X-ray soft tissue neck lateral view:*** Shows vertical extent and thickness of the tumor and involvement of cervical vertebrae.
- ***CT scan*** for tumor extent and lymphatic metastasis.
- ***Endoscopy:*** It provides accurate assessment of tumor. Panendoscopy finds other synchronous primary.
- ***Biopsy:*** For histopathological diagnosis.

Treatment

- ***Radiotherapy:*** For early small lesions, particularly exophytic. It preserves function.
- ***Surgery:***
  - Early small lesions may be excised via lateral pharyngotomy and primary repair.
  - Advanced lesions may need laryngopharyngectomy and block dissection with repair of the food channel.
- ***Curative treatment as per the staging:*** (For TNM classification *see* Chapter 'Malignant Tumors of Larynx')
  - ***Stage I:*** Primary radiotherapy or Partial Pharyngectomy (PP).
  - ***Stage II:*** Primary radiotherapy or chemoradiotherapy or PP or total laryngopharyngectomy (TLP).
  - ***Stage III:*** Partial pharyngectomy or TLP and postoperative radiotherapy or chemoradiotherapy.
  - ***Stage IVa:*** Total laryngopharyngectomy and postoperative radiotherapy or chemoradiotherapy.

Prognosis

Gross 5-year cure rate is only 19%.

Self-evaluation Exercises

1. Which of the following are not true for Plummer-Vinson syndrome?
   a. Premalignant condition
   b. Disease of males
   c. Iron deficiency anemia
   d. Dysphagia
   e. None from the above
2. Patients with Plummer-Vinson syndrome usually have:
   a. Koilonychia
   b. Atrophic gastritis
   c. Glossitis
   d. All of the above
3. The referred ear pain in cancer of pyriform fossa is through superior laryngeal nerve, branch of vagus nerve. **T/F**
4. Post-laryngeal crepitus is _____ in normal persons and is _____ in patients with postcricoid malignancy.

Answers

1. b   2. d   3. T   4. present   5. absent

Chapter 41

Disorders of Esophagus

Specific Learning Objectives

After going through the chapter, you should be able to answer the following questions:
- How will you manage the patient with perforation of esophagus?
- How will you manage a patient who has consumed some corrosive substance?
- How will you treat a case of foreign body esophagus?
- What are the features of extraesophageal GERD and laryngopharyngeal reflux?
- How will you differentiate between benign and malignant strictures of esophagus and manage them?
- What do you know about: (1) Plummer-Vinson syndrome; (2) Cardiac achalasia; (3) Barret's esophagus; (4) Infectious esophagitis; (5) Zenker's diverticulum; (6) Diffuse esophageal spasm?

INTRODUCTION

The esophagus is subject to a variety of diseases (Box 41.1). The primary infections of the esophagus are rare except fungal esophagitis, which occurs in patients who are immunocompromised. Esophageal perforation is a surgical emergency. The stricture development occurs from ingestion of caustic agents. Foreign bodies (FBs) in esophagus are frequently encountered in children. The cricopharyngeal area is a frequent site. Benign tumors of the esophagus are rare. However, malignancies of the esophagus are relatively common.

Esophageal inflammatory disease like gastroesophageal reflux disease (GERD) is quite common. Peristaltic contractions of esophagus pass the food down into the stomach. The upper esophageal sphincter (UES) and lower esophageal sphincter (LES) prevent reflux of food while swallowing. Dysphagia is usually present in esophageal disorders. Odynophagia, painful swallowing indicates esophagitis.

Box 41.1: Esophageal diseases

- **Congenital:** Atresia, tracheoesophageal fistula, stenosis and dysphagia lusoria
- **Hiatus hernia:** Sliding and paraesophageal (rolling)
- **Infectious:** Monilial esophagitis, viral and granulomatous lesions
- **Inflammatory:** Gastroesophageal reflux disease (GERD) and pill-induced esophagitis
- **Injury:** Foreign bodies, drug-induced, corrosive, penetrating, and Mallory-Weiss syndrome
- **Perforation:** Spontaneous (Boerhaave's syndrome), pathological and instrumental
- **Diverticula:** Zenker's diverticulum (pharyngeal pouch), mid-esophageal diverticula, epinephric diverticula and diffuse intramural pseudodiverticulosis
- **Narrowing:** Webs, strictures and extrinsic compression
- **Motility disorders**—upper sphincter, lower sphincter and the body of esophagus
  - **Hypermotility disorder:** Cricopharyngeal spasm, diffuse esophageal spasm, nutcracker esophagus and hypertensive lower esophageal sphincter
  - **Hypomotility disorders:** Cardiac achalasia, connective tissue disease (scleroderma and amyotrophic lateral sclerosis) and hypoperistalsis—CREST syndrome
- **Neoplasms:**
  - **Benign:** Leiomyoma and others—mucosal polyps, lipomas, fibromas and hemangiomas
  - **Malignant:** Carcinoma (squamous cell carcinoma and adenocarcinoma), malignant melanoma and sarcoma
- **Miscellaneous:** Schatzki's ring, Crohn's disease, Plummer-Vinson (PV) syndrome, eosinophilic esophagitis and varices

PERFORATION OF ESOPHAGUS

Early diagnosis is essential, as mediastinitis can rapidly prove fatal. Perforation of thoracic esophagus is more serious than cervical esophagus.

Etiology

- *Instrumental trauma:* Esophagoscopy or dilatation of strictures with bougies. The most common site is just above the upper sphincter. The lower esophagus perforation near the hiatus is uncommon.
- *Spontaneous rupture:* This occurs due to vomiting and usually involves lower third esophagus. In Boerhaave's syndrome, there occurs postemetic rupture of all the layers of esophagus.
- *Pathological:* Malignancy.
- *Penetrating injuries.*

Clinical Features

- *Preceding history* of esophagoscopy, vomiting or other injury.
- *Cervical esophageal rupture*
  - Neck—Pain, local tenderness and surgical emphysema
  - Fever
  - Difficulty in swallowing.
- *Thoracic esophageal rupture*
  - Chest pain referred to the interscapular region
  - Fever 102–104°F (39–40°C)
  - Signs of shock
  - Surgical emphysema and pneumothorax
  - *Hamman's sign:* Crunching sound over the heart because of air in the mediastinum.

Diagnosis

- *X-rays of the chest and neck*
  - Widening of mediastinum and retrovisceral space
  - Surgical emphysema, pneumothorax and gas under the diaphragm
  - Pleural effusion.

> **Boerhaave's syndrome:** Patient develops severe vomiting and chest pain after drinks and heavy dinner. X-ray of chest shows hydropneumothroax.

Treatment

- *General*
  - Nil by mouth
  - Intravenous fluids for nutrition
  - Antibiotics: To combat infection
  - Management of shock.
- *Perforations of cervical esophagus:* Early cases may be managed conservatively. Drainage is required in cases of suppuration. Retrovisceral space and upper mediastinum are drained.
- *Rupture of thoracic esophagus:* Perforation is surgically repaired and pleural cavity drained within 6 hours. Repair is not possible after 6 hours but infected area needs drainage.

CORROSIVE BURNS

Etiology

Following items may be swallowed accidentally by children and by suicidal, psychotic and alcoholic adults:

- *Acids:* Various cleaners used for toilet, drain, swimming pool and metal.
- *Alkalis:* Drain and oven cleaners, dishwasher detergents and hair relaxers (conditioners).

Pathology

- *Severity:* Severity of burns depends on the nature, amount and concentration of corrosives and the duration of their contact with the tissue.
- *Extent of lesion:* Alkalis are more destructive and penetrate deep into the esophagus. Lye, a strong alkali (sodium or potassium hydroxide) burns entire esophagus and stomach. They slough and result in fatal mediastinitis and peritonitis.
- *Stages:* There are three stages of esophageal burns—(1) necrosis, (2) granulations (separation of slough) and (3) stricture. Stricture begins at 2 weeks and continues for 2 months or longer.

Clinical Features

- History of corrosive ingestion and associated burns of face, lips and oral cavity.
- Oropharyngeal, retrosternal and epigastric pain.
- Dysphagia and odynophagia.
- Hypersalivation—drooling.
- *Laryngeal*—hoarseness and stridor
- Shock.
- Mediastinitis.
- Peritonitis.
- Acid-base imbalance.

Diagnosis

- History and examination will confirm the diagnosis.
- X-rays of chest and soft tissue neck help in estimating the extent of damage.
- Esophagogastroduodenoscopy (EGD) is done within 2 days to know the extent and degree of esophageal and gastric damage for planning further treatment. Endoscope is not passed further than the first severe circumferential burn.

Grading (Table 41.1)

The grading system helps in predicting prognosis.

Chapter 41 • Disorders of Esophagus

Table 41.1: Corrosive esophageal injury

Grades	Prognosis
Grade 0	Normal
Grade 1	Mucosal edema and erythema
Grade 2A	Superficial ulcers, bleeding and exudates
Grade 2B	Deep focal or circumferential ulcers
Grade 3A	Focal necrosis (brown, black or gray discoloration)
Grade 3B	Extensive necrosis
Grade 4	Perforation

Source: Zargar SA, Kochhar R, Mehta S, et al. The role of fiberoptic endoscopy in the management of corrosive ingestion and modified endoscopic classification of burns. Gastrointest Endosc. 1991;37:165-9.

- *Grade 1 and 2A:* No stricture formation. Oral liquid diet can be started after 1–2 days.
- *Grades 2B/3A:* Most of the patients develop stricture.
- *Grade 3B:* 65% early mortality rate.

Management

- Immediate
  - *Intensive care unit (ICU):* Patient is kept in ICU.
  - *Wash and irrigation*
    - *Mouth:* Wash out the mouth with large volume of cold water.
    - *Eye:* Irrigate affected eye with large amount of saline or water. Fluorescein staining will determine corneal ulcerations.

> - Never induce emesis because it can worsen the complications.
> - Never neutralize with acid or base because the generated heat would destroy more tissue. Charcoal also is not useful. Use simple water.

  - *Examination:* Examine oropharyngeal injury and airway compromise and watch for perforation.
  - *Tracheostomy or intubation:* For relieving airway obstruction.
  - *Intravenous fluids and electrolytes:* For treating shock and acid-base imbalance.
  - *Maintenance of intake/output chart:* Monitoring of urine output for renal failure.
  - *Analgesic:* For relieving pain.
  - *Antibiotics and steroids:* Parenteral antibiotics for 3–6 weeks and steroids for 4–6 weeks (to prevent stricture) though given often, are not found useful.
  - *Feeding (depending upon the grade of injury):* Oral liquids can be started after 48 hours if patient can swallow without pain or vomiting. Some patients need nasogastric tube for feeding and maintenance of esophageal lumen.

- *Delayed*
  - *Esophagogram and EGD* are done every 2 weeks to monitor healing and development of stricture. Patients of corrosive injuries need lifelong follow-up.
  - *Management of stricture:*
    - Esophagoscopy and prograde dilatation
    - Gastrostomy and retrograde dilatation
    - Esophageal reconstruction and bypass.

> - **Caustic ingestion:** Oral burns may not correlate with severity of esophageal lesions. Alkaline agents penetrate deeper tissue layers. Watch for sign of airway obstruction because airway control must be the prime concern. Watch for features of mediastinitis (such as tachycardia, chest pain, fever, sepsis) and peritonitis.
> - **EGD:** It is controversial. It may lead to further injury. Early EGD may help in diagnosis and placements of feeding tube. It is terminated if a significant burn is seen. It is contraindicated after 12 hours.
> - **Strictures:** Caustic strictures are longer and tighter and usually refractory and have higher rate of complications during dilation.

FOREIGN BODIES

An ingested FB may be lodged in tonsil, base of tongue, vallecula, pyriform fossa or esophagus. A sharp fish bone and needle may go into the tonsillar crypts, base of tongue or vallecula. They can be easily removed as an office procedure.

Fish bone, chicken bone, needle and denture get lodged in the pyriform fossa. They may be removed under local anesthesia or general anesthesia.

> **Foreign body throat:** The most common site of impaction of 'fishbone' is palatine tonsil.

Common Foreign Bodies in Esophagus

Coin, piece of meat, chicken bone, denture, safety pin and marble piece.

> **Disc batteries:** Leaks of sodium and potassium hydroxides and mercury damage esophagus. They should be removed at the earliest as they lead to injury to mucosa (1 hour) and muscular layer (2–4 hours) and perforation (8–12 hours) if remains in esophagus. So their complications include stricture, perforation, tracheoesophageal fistula, mediastinitis and even death. Battery of 1.5 cm size should not remain for > 48 hours in the stomach of a child of < 6 years of age.

Risk Factors

- *Children:* Tendency to put the things in mouth.
- *Upper denture:* Lack of tactile sensation while chewing.

- ***Narrowed esophageal lumen:*** Patients with stricture and carcinoma can present with sudden obstruction after ingestion of piece of meat, fruit and vegetable.
- ***Psychotics.***
- ***Causes of loss of consciousness:*** Epileptic seizures, deep sleep and alcoholic intoxication.

Common Sites

- ***Cricopharyngeal sphincter:*** Most common site
- ***Bronchoaortic constriction***
- ***Cardiac end***

Sharp and pointed objects can lodge anywhere.

Most common site of esophageal foreign body in children: It is the upper esophageal sphincter.

Clinical Features

- ***Choking or gagging*** at the time of ingestion.
- ***Discomfort or pain*** usually increases on swallowing. Foreign body cervical esophagus usually presents with pain and tenderness in the lower part of neck. Constant substernal or epigastric pain indicates esophageal spasm or incipient perforation.
- ***Dysphagia:*** Obstruction may be total. Partial obstruction can become total due to edema.
- ***Drooling of saliva:*** It indicates total obstruction. Saliva may be aspirated and cause aspiration pneumonitis.
- ***Respiratory distress:*** Upper esophagus FB may compress posterior wall of trachea in children. Laryngeal edema can also occur.
- ***Indirect laryngoscopy:*** Pooling of secretions in the pyriform fossa. Foreign body may be seen protruding from postcricoid region.

Investigations

- ***X-rays soft tissue neck and chest posteroanterior and lateral views:*** Show location of a radiopaque FB (Figs 41.1 to 41.3). In children, multiple FBs from nasopharynx to the rectum are not uncommon and should be ruled out.
- ***Barium swallow for radiolucent foreign bodies:*** Patient swallows cotton soaked in barium or barium filled capsule. The esophagus shows filling defect (Figs 41.3A to C).

Management

- ***Esophagoscopy*** and removal of FB under general anesthesia. It is the most preferred and commonly employed modality of treatment.
- ***Hypopharyngeal speculum:*** This is good for the FBs lodged near the cricopharynx.
- ***Rigid esophagoscopy:*** It is done under general anesthesia. Any type of FB can be removed and taken

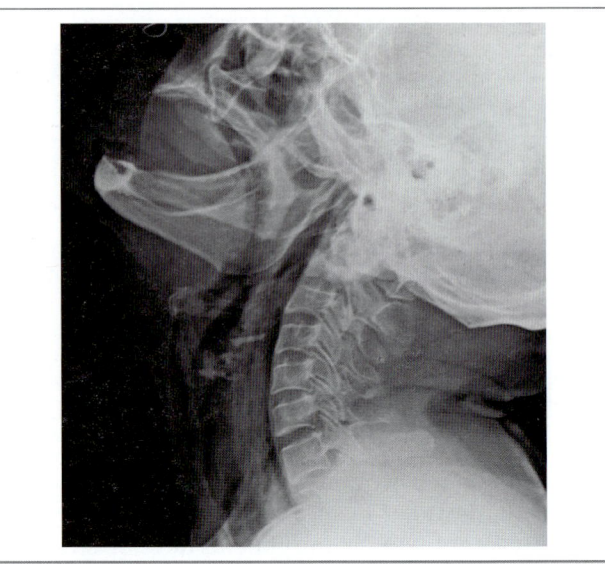

Fig. 41.1: X-ray soft tissue neck lateral view showing radiopaque foreign body (fishbone) in the laryngopharynx at the level of C4

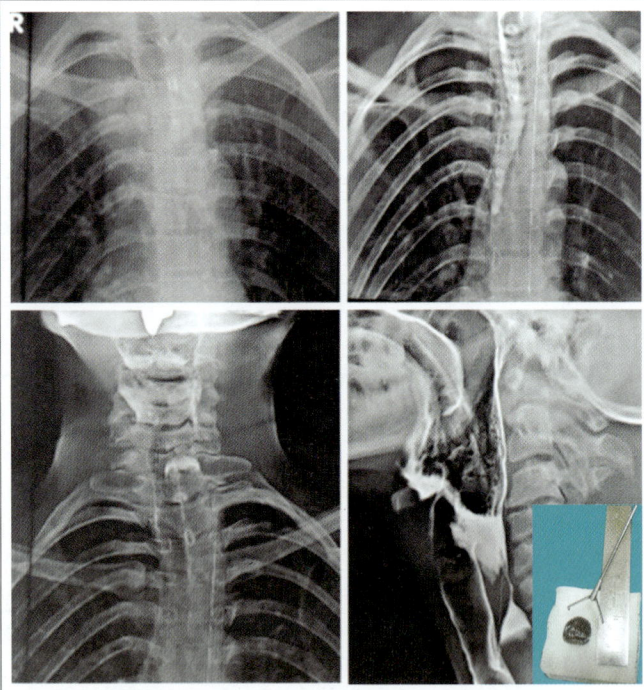

Fig. 41.2: Foreign body Sopari (inset) upper esophagus. X-ray (plain and Barium swallow) neck and chest PA and lateral views.
Courtesy: Dr Prashant B Desai (junior) and Bhavin H Patel, Surat, Gujarat

into the lumen of the scope. OT, anesthesia and indoor requirements increase the total cost to the patient.

- ***EGD:*** This economical and OPD procedure is done under local anesthesia and is good for the removal of small, soft and blunt FBs such as meat pieces and vegetable matters. It can be done even if the patient has jaw and spine problems. Even stomach and duodenum can

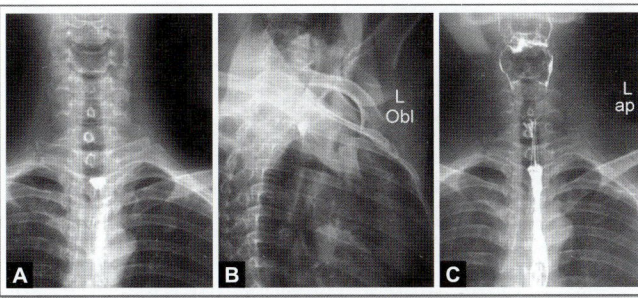

Figs 41.3A to C: Radio-opaque foreign body upper esophagus. (A) X-ray neck chest posteroanterior view; (B) X-ray neck chest Lateral view; (C) Barium swallow

be examined if needed in the same sitting. The main disadvantage is that big, pointed and impacted FBs cannot be removed and FBs cannot be taken into the lumen of scope as with rigid esophagoscope.

- *Cervical esophagotomy:* For impacted FBs or sharp hooks (partial dentures) above thoracic inlet.
- *Transthoracic esophagotomy:* For impacted FBs in thoracic esophagus.
- *Foreign body passed into stomach:* They usually pass with the stools, which should be examined every day. Purgatives should not be used. Indications for operative interference include:
  - Pain and tenderness in abdomen.
  - No progress of FB on serial X-rays taken at a few days interval.
  - Children (< 2 years): FB > 5 cm long usually does not pass through the turns of the duodenum.
  - Pyloric stenosis.

> **Cautions**
> - Never try to push FBs in the stomach.
> - Do not try to remove with Foley's or balloon catheters as there are chances of aspiration.
> - Glucagon will not relax esophageal strictures and rings.
> - Do not use papain (meat tenderizer) as it can digest esophagus itself.

Complications

- *Respiratory obstruction in infants and children:* Due to tracheal compression by the FB in upper esophagus and laryngeal edema.
- *Periesophageal cellulitis and abscess.*
- *Perforation of esophagus:* It can result in:
  - Mediastinitis
  - Pericarditis
  - Empyema or
  - Fatal bleeding from aorta.
- *Ulceration and stricture,* and
- *Tracheoesophageal fistula.*

GASTROESOPHAGEAL REFLUX DISEASE (GERD)

GERD refers to the damage of esophageal mucosa due to abnormal reflux of gastric content.

Etiology

Inappropriate function of lower esophageal sphincters (LES) permits reflux of gastric contents into esophagus. The conditions, which decrease LES tone, are following:
- Fatty foods, chocolate and peppermints.
- Tobacco smoking and alcohol.
- *Smooth muscle relaxants:* Anticholinergic, beta-adrenergic and calcium channel blockers.
- *Pregnancy:* High levels of progesterone.
- Sliding hiatus hernia.

Clinical Features

- *Typical:* Heartburn (burning sensation in the epigastric or substernal region) and acid regurgitation usually occur after meal when patient is recumbent.
  - Angina—like chest pain (worsens after sublingual nitroglycerin), while lying in bed at night.
  - Dysphagia (peptic stricture in esophagus), odynophagia (esophagitis) and belching.

Noncardiac chest pain: GERD accounts for 70% of noncardiac chest pain.

- *Atypical GERD symptoms or extraesophageal GERD:* They include nonproductive cough, hoarseness of voice, asthma like symptoms and dental erosions. The diagnosis is confirmed when symptoms respond to GERD therapy. The current GERD therapy consists of initial aggressive BID proton pump inhibitors (PPIs) followed by tapering to once daily in responders.

Nonproductive cough: GERD is among the most common causes of chronic cough. Other causes include postnasal drip, asthma and tuberculosis.

  - *Dental erosions:* Repeated long time exposure to acid can lead to loss of enamel and tooth structure.
- *Reflux laryngitis or laryngoesophageal reflux (LPR):*
  - Symptoms include hoarseness of voice, throat clearing, dysphagia, increased phlegm and globus sensation. LPR can cause laryngeal erythema, edema, vocal cord nodules, polyps, granulations, leukoplakia, cancer and pharyngeal ulcerations.

- Other signs include interarytenoid bar, arytenoids medial wall erythema and posterior pharyngeal wall cobblestoning.
- **Asthma-like symptoms:** About 70–80% asthma patients have GERD and treated with PPI. GERD-induced asthma is suspected in following cases.
  - Adult onset of asthma.
  - No family history of asthma or atopy.
  - Heartburn precedes onset of asthma.
  - Wheezing exacerbated with meals, exercise and supine position.
  - Nocturnal wheezing.

> *Reflux laryngitis or laryngopharyngeal reflux (LPR):* In cases of chronic hoarseness and cough or globus, first rule out neoplasm and then consider reflux laryngitis.

Diagnosis

- **Clinical:** History and response to therapy confirm the diagnosis.
- **Esophagogastroduodenoscopy (EGD):** Erosions and ulcerations at squamous-columnar junction (SCJ) in reflux esophagitis and findings of Barrett's esophagus.
- **Ambulatory 24-hour pH monitoring:** This gold standard test is done in refractory cases.
- **Bernstein test:** Infusion of 0.1 M HCl in esophagus reproduces chest pain.

Subgroups

The subgroups of GERD include:
- **Nonerosive reflux disease:** Nonerosive reflux disease patients have typical GERD symptoms, but do not show endoscopic findings.
- **Reflux esophagitis:** Biopsy shows mucosal changes.
- **Barrett's esophagus:** This predisposes to development of adenocarcinoma. Normal stratified squamous epithelium of distal esophagus is replaced by intestinal columnar metaplasia.

Treatment

The aims of the treatment are decreasing reflux, improving esophageal clearance and protecting esophageal mucosa.
- **Lifestyle modifications:** Patient's instructions include:
  - Weight loss.
  - Small and frequent meals.
  - Avoid fats, sweets, chocolate, tomatoes, onions, alcohol and caffeine at bedtime.
  - Finish dinner 3 hours before going to bed.
  - Elevation of head end of the bed during sleep.
- **Medical treatment:** It includes:
  - **Antacids.**
  - **H_2 receptor antagonists:** They (ranitidine) heal 50% cases of reflux esophagitis.
  - **Proton pump inhibitors:** PPI (such as omeprazole) heals 80% cases.
  - **Prokinetic drugs:** Prokinetic drugs (such as metoclopramide), which though do not heal esophagitis, improve esophageal clearance and gastric emptying and raise LES pressure. They should be taken 30 minutes before meal.
- **Antireflux surgery:** In Nissen's fundoplication, fundus of stomach is wrapped around LES.
  - **Indication:** Patients who do not respond to medical treatment and have normal esophageal peristalsis (confirmed by motility study) otherwise postoperative achalasia can occur.
- **Recent developments:**
  - Endoscopic suturing.
  - Injection of biopolymers in LES.
  - Radiofrequency delivery to gastroesophageal junction (GEJ).

Complications

- Esophagitis
- Ulcers in esophagus
- Hemorrhage
- Peptic stricture in esophagus
- Aspiration
- Barrett's esophagus.

BENIGN STRICTURES

The esophageal strictures occur when its muscular layer is damaged.

Causes

- **Intrinsic**
  - **Congenital:** Common in the lower third.
  - **Burns:** Corrosives or hot fluids.
  - **Trauma:** Impacted FBs and external injuries.
  - **Iatrogenic:** Pill-induced, nasogastric tube, sclerotherapy, radiation, and surgical anastomosis.
  - **Ulcers:** Reflux esophagitis, diphtheria and typhoid.
- **Extrinsic pressure causing narrowing**
  - Anomalous vessels and aneurysms.

Clinical Features

- Dysphagia first with solid and then with liquids.
- Regurgitation and coughing.
- Malnourishment.

Diagnosis

- *Barium swallow:* Shows number, extent and severity of strictures.
- *Esophagoscopy:* Diagnostic and therapeutic.

Treatment

- *Esophagoscopy and prograde dilatation with bougies under direct vision:* Patients need repeated dilatation.
- *Other types of dilators:*
  - **For uncomplicated short and straight strictures:** Mercury-filled rubber Maloney dilators
  - **For long, tight and tortuous strictures:**
    - Wire-guided rigid Savary-Gilliard dilators
    - Balloon dilators: Through-the-scope or wire-guided.
- *Gastrostomy:* It provides feeding to the patient and offers rest to the inflamed mucosa above the strictures. Prograde dilatation may be restored once inflammation subsides and lumen becomes visible. Patient is instructed to swallow a thread, which comes into the stomach, and then prograde or retrograde bouginage can be done.
- *Excision and reconstruction:* Strictured segment is excised and plastic reconstruction is done with stomach, colon or jejunum.

HIATUS HERNIA

It refers to displacement of stomach into the thorax. It is common in patients above 40 years of age.

Types

1. *Sliding hiatus hernia:* Raised intra-abdominal pressure can push the stomach into the thorax in the line of esophagus.
   Clinical features: Features of reflux esophagitis. It can cause ulceration, stenosis and hematemesis.
2. *Paraesophageal hiatus hernia or rolling hiatus hernia:* A part of the stomach and its peritoneal covering enters into the thorax by the side of esophagus. There is no reflux esophagitis because gastroesophageal junction (GEJ) remains below diaphragm and angle between the esophagus and stomach is maintained.
   Clinical features: The most common symptom is exertional dyspnea, which is caused due to the position of stomach in the thorax. Bleeding occurs in some patients.

Diagnosis

Barium swallow: Shows extent and type of hiatus hernia.

Treatment

- Conservative measures to reduce reflux esophagitis:
  - Head and chest raised during sleeping.
  - Avoid smoking.
  - Drugs for acidity and reflux esophagitis.
  - Control of obesity: Diet control and exercise.
  - Treat causes of raised intra-abdominal pressure.
- Surgical method is reduction of hernia and repair of diaphragmatic opening.

SCHATZKI'S RING

It is a web-like mucosal ring, which is seen at the SCJ or proximal to LES.

- *Clinical features:* Asymptomatic in 10% patients.
  - Young patient presents with episodic dysphagia to solids and sometimes liquids.
- *Diagnosis:* Barium swallow will confirm the diagnosis.
- *Treatment:* Pneumatic dilation.

PLUMMER-VINSON (PATTERSON BROWN-KELLY) SYNDROME

Plummer-Vinson (PV) syndrome predominantly affects middle aged females. It consists of atrophy of the mucous membrane of the alimentary tract, subepithelial fibrosis in lower part of laryngopharynx and iron deficiency anemia.

Clinical Features

- Dysphagia immediately after trying to swallow food.
- Iron deficiency anemia.
- Glossitis.
- Angular stomatitis.
- Koilonychias (spooning of nails).
- Achlorhydria.

Potential of Malignant Conversion

The PV syndrome may be associated with carcinoma of the tongue, buccal mucosa, pharynx, esophagus or stomach. About 10% of the patients develop postcricoid carcinoma.

Diagnosis

Barium swallow and esophagoscopy: A hypopharyngeal web (subepithelial fibrosis) can be seen in the postcricoid region.

Treatment

- *Oral/parenteral iron:* For correcting anemia. Serum level of iron is more important than hemoglobin.

- **Vitamins B_{12} and B_6.**
- **Esophagoscopy** and **dilatation** of webbed area with bougies.

INFECTIOUS ESOPHAGITIS

The three most common causes of infectious esophagitis are—*Candida*, cytomegalovirus (CMV) and herpes simplex virus (HSV). Patients are immunocompromised due to HIV-AIDS, post-transplant treatment and chemotherapy.

Etiology
- ***Candida albicans:*** It is the most common form and usually associated with HIV.
- Herpes simplex virus.
- Cytomegalovirus.
- Varicella-zoster virus.
- Human immunodeficiency virus.

Clinical Features
- ***Most common symptom:*** Odynophagia
- ***Other:*** Heartburn, nausea, fever and bleeding.

Treatment
- Management of immunocompromised condition.
- *Antifungal*
  - ***Fluconazole:*** 100–200 mg/day for 10–14 days.
  - ***Clotrimazole*** and ***nystatin:*** Topical 4–5 times a day.
  - ***Amphotericin B:*** In cases of granulocytopenia to prevent disseminated disease.
- *Antiviral*
  - ***Acyclovir for HSV:*** Intravenous 5–10 mg/kg every 8 hours till patient tolerate oral therapy.
  - ***Gancyclovir and foscarnet for CMV:*** Two-week full dose regimen followed by maintenance therapy for several weeks.

CRICOPHARYNGEAL SPASM

There occurs incoordination between relaxation of the upper esophageal sphincter (UES) and simultaneous contraction of the pharynx. UES fails to relax properly.

Causes
- Cerebrovascular strokes
- Parkinson's disease
- Bulbar polio
- Multiple sclerosis
- Muscular dystrophies.

DIFFUSE ESOPHAGEAL SPASM (DES)

In this motility disorder of smooth muscle, there occur spontaneous strong nonperistaltic contractions of the body of esophagus. There occurs degeneration of nerve processes but sphincter relaxation is normal.

Clinical Features
- Sudden dysphagia and substernal chest pain simulating angina pectoris in adults.
- Symptom improves with sublingual nitroglycerin.

Diagnosis
- ***Barium swallow:*** It shows segmented esophageal spasms, which appear like a rosary bead or a corkscrew.
- ***Manometry:*** Normal relaxation of the sphincter on swallowing and strong nonperistaltic uncoordinated esophageal contractions.

Treatment
- ***Medical:*** Calcium channel blockers and nitrates usually give good response.
- ***Surgical:*** Dilatation of lower esophagus and myotomy of esophagus extending from the arch of aorta to lower sphincter is done in severe refractory cases.

NUTCRACKER ESOPHAGUS

- There occur strong and high amplitude peristaltic esophageal contractions, which can be seen in manometric studies.
- Present with dysphagia and substernal pain like DES.
- Treatment is also similar to DES.

CARDIAC ACHALASIA

The characteristic features of this smooth muscle motility disorder are absence of peristalsis in the body of esophagus and high resting pressure in LES, which does not relax during swallowing.

Clinical Features
- ***Most common symptoms***, which persist and do not progress for years, include:
  - Dysphagia for liquids and solids.
  - Regurgitation of swallowed food especially in night. Choking and coughing awake the patient.
  - Chest pain.
- ***History of compensatory measures:*** Lifting of neck and carbonated drinks.
- ***Weight loss:*** It is minimal.
- ***Physical examination:*** It is unremarkable.

Diagnosis
- ***Barium swallow with fluoroscopy:*** It shows esophageal dilatation and failure of lower esophageal

sphincter to relax. Characteristic smooth tapering of lower esophagus leading to closed LES resembling rattail or bird's beak.
- *Manometry:* Shows low pressure in the body of esophagus (absent or abnormal peristalsis) and high pressure at LES (increased tone) which fails to relax.
- *Flexible endoscopy:* Rule out pseudoachalasia due to GEJ tumor especially in elderly patient with short history and weight loss.

Treatment

- *Endoscopic pneumatic dilatation:* It tears LES muscle fibers and thus reduces LES pressure. Perforation occurs in 5% of patients.
- *Modified Heller's operation:* Myotomy (incision of circular muscle fibers) of narrowed lower portion of esophagus is the definitive treatment.
- *Botulinum toxin injection in LES:* It block's cholinergic nerves and needs to be repeated every 2 years.
- *Medical:* Calcium channel blockers and nitrates.

SCLERODERMA OR PROGRESSIVE SYSTEMIC SCLEROSIS

Scleroderma affects mid and distal esophagus. The atrophy and fibrosis of esophageal smooth muscle result in decrease or absence of peristalsis (similar to achalasia) and incompetent LES (opposite to achalasia).

Clinical Features

The patients usually develop reflux esophagitis and stricture in distal part of the esophagus and may have hiatus hernia. So the clinical features include:
- Progressive dysphagia to solids and liquids like malignancy.
- Features of GERD due to decreased LES tone.
- Cutaneous lesions.

Diagnosis

- *Barium swallow:* Dilation and absence of peristalsis in distal two-third of the esophagus.
- *Motility studies:* Decreased smooth muscle contraction.

Treatment

No effective treatment except antireflux therapy.

ZENKER DIVERTICULUM

This pharyngeal pouch is a pulsion hypopharyngeal diverticulum where hypopharyngeal mucosa herniates

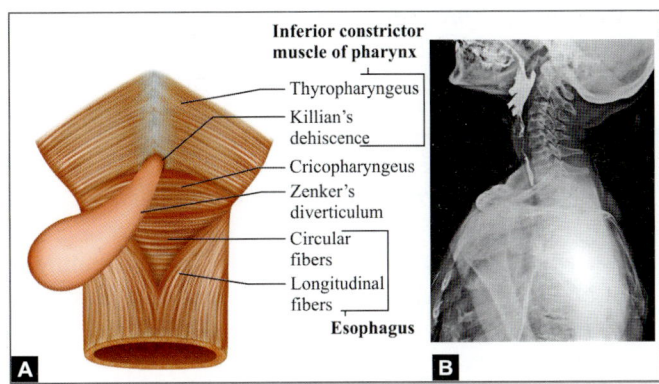

Figs 41.4A and B: (A) Zenker's diverticulum of hypopharynx; (B) Barium swallow. Carcinoma postcricoid and cervical esophagus. Note the prevertebral soft tissue widening

through the Killian's dehiscence which is a weak area between the thyropharyngeal and cricopharyngeal parts of the inferior constrictor muscle (Fig. 41.4A).

Etiology

The exact cause is not clear, but spasm of cricopharyngeal sphincter or its incoordinated contractions during the act of deglutition is considered to be an important predisposing factor. Patients are usually old adults.

Pathology

Herniation of pharyngeal mucosa, which extends behind the esophagus, begins in the midline and later on pouch extends and lie on the left. Mouth of the sac becomes wider than the opening of esophagus. Food usually enters into the sac.

Clinical Features

- *Most common symptoms* are halitosis, transfer dysphagia (difficulty initiating swallowing) and regurgitation of food days after ingestion.
  - *Dysphagia* may increase after a few swallows which fill the pouch with the food and then presses on the esophagus.
  - *Gurgling sound during swallowing.*
  - *Regurgitation of undigested food* at night (due to recumbent position) results in coughing and choking.
- *Loss of weight* and malnourishment.
- *Aspiration pneumonia.*

Diagnosis

- *Barium swallow* will show the site and size of diverticulum.
- *Esophagoscopy and nasogastric intubation are contraindicated* because of the risk of perforation of pouch.

Treatment

- *Diverticulectomy* (excision of pouch) or *cricopharyngeal myotomy* or both.

- **Dohlman's procedure:** Endoscopic diathermy of the partition wall between esophagus and pouch is preferred in poor risk debilitated patients.

GLOBUS HYSTERICUS PHARYNGEUS

- **Functional disorder** with no true dysphagia. Patient usually has fear of throat cancer.
- **Patient complains** of 'lump' in the throat. The feeling of lump is more marked between the meals when patient voluntarily and consciously swallows the saliva.
- **Clinical examination** is normal.
- **Management:** Rule out any organic cause and reassure the patient.

BENIGN NEOPLASMS

- Neoplasms of esophagus are rare and those found are usually malignant.

> Leiomyoma arises from the smooth muscle of esophagus wall. It accounts for two-third of all benign neoplasms.

- Other benign tumors include mucosal polyps, lipomas, fibromas and hemangiomas.
- They are usually pedunculated and seen in the esophageal lumen.
- **Treatment:** Endoscopic removal is not done because of the fear of perforation. They need surgical excision with external approach.

Leiomyoma

- **Clinical feature:** Tumor causes dysphagia when it exceeds the diameter of 5 cm.
- **Barium swallow:** Ovoid filling defect.

> **Endoscopy:** Submucosal swelling can be seen, but biopsy is not taken.

- **Treatment:** Enucleation of the tumor with thoracotomy.

CARCINOMA ESOPHAGUS

In India, esophagus is the fourth most common site of cancer in males and fifth in females. In Banglore registry it was found the third leading site of cancer for both males and females. (Source: ICMR, 2004). Incidence of esophageal malignancy is high in China, Japan, USSR and South Africa. It constitutes 3.6% (in affluent class) and 9.13% (in poor class) of all body cancers in India.

Risk Factors

- **Squamous cell carcinoma:** Usually occurs in proximal two-third of esophagus.
  - Black males
  - Smoking and alcohol consumption
  - Chewing of *paan*, *sopari* and tobacco
  - Diet rich in nitrates and pickled vegetables
  - Existing esophageal lesions:
    - Benign strictures
    - Cardiac achalasia
    - Diverticula
    - Corrosive injury
  - Premalignant conditions
    - Plummer-Vinson syndrome
    - Tylosis
    - Head and neck malignancy
    - Human papillomavirus.
- **Adenocarcinoma:** It occurs in distal one-third esophagus and GEJ.
  - White males
  - GERD and Barrett's esophagus
  - Hiatus hernia.

Pathology

Squamous cell carcinoma (SCC) is the most common type (93%) followed by adenocarcinoma (3%). Adenocarcinoma is seen in lower esophagus and may be an upward extension of the gastric carcinoma. The incidence of adenocarcinoma is on increase. Other types are very rare.

Spread

- **Direct:** Infiltrate esophageal wall and spread to trachea, left bronchus, aorta and pericardium. Recurrent laryngeal nerves involvement causes aspiration problems.
- **Lymphatic:** Depending on the part of esophagus cervical, mediastinal and celiac nodes may be enlarged. Cervical and thoracic lesions may involve supraclavicular nodes. Spread through submucosal lymphatics may lead to 'skip lesions'.
- **Blood borne:** Systemic distant metastases may occur in liver, lungs, bone and brain.

Clinical Features

- **Early symptoms** are substernal discomfort and preference for soft and liquid food.
- **Most common symptom** is gradually progressive dysphagia first to solids and then to liquids.
- Odynophagia and iron-deficiency anemia.
- Loss of weight and emaciation.
- Pain referred to the back indicates extension of tumor beyond esophageal walls.
- **Coughing, hoarseness of voice, pneumonia and mediastinitis:** They occur due to laryngeal paralysis and tracheoesophageal fistula formation.
- Hypercalcemia in some cases of SCC.

- **Squamous cell carcinoma of esophagus:** Prior head and neck cancer increases the risk of this cancer eightfold.
- **Dissemination:** There occurs rapid dissemination of mucosal cancer because esophagus does not have serosal layer.

Diagnosis

- **Barium swallow:** Narrowing and irregular esophageal lumen (uneven ulcerated edges apple core appearance) without proximal dilatation (Fig. 41.4B).
- **Esophagoscopy with biopsy** confirm the diagnosis.
- **Bronchoscopy:** For checking extension of tumor into the trachea and bronchi.
- **CT scan:** Accurately identify extent of tumor and metastatic disease.
- **Endoscopic ultrasound:** Assess depth of invasion.

Treatment

- T_1 *(involvement of lamina propria and submucosa)* or T_2 *(involvement of muscularis propria)* with N_0 (*no nodal metastasis*) surgery alone.
  - **Lower one-third esophagus:** The affected segment with proximal margin and fundus of stomach is excised with primary reconstruction of the food channel. Surgical mortality is 20%.
- T_3 *(involvement of adventia)* or N_1 *(nodal metastasis present):* Neoadjuvant chemotherapy/radiation before surgical resection.
  - **Upper two-third esophagus:** Radiotherapy is preferred as the great vessels and involvement of mediastinal nodes, which make the surgery difficult.
- **Late stages:** Palliative measures include:
  - Repeated dilation.
  - Esophageal intubation with Celestin or Mousseau-Barbin or a similar tube.
  - Gastrostomy or jejunostomy.
  - Laser Nd: YAG/photodynamic therapy ablation.
  - Chemotherapy.

Prognosis

- Usually esophageal carcinoma is diagnosed at a late stage and 5 year survival rate is poor (about 5–10%).

Self-evaluation Exercises

1. The features of mediastinitis include:
   a. Tachycardia
   b. Chest pain
   c. Fever
   d. All of the above

True (T)/False (F)

2. The most common site of impaction of 'fishbone' is palatine tonsil.
3. Oral burns of caustic ingestion always correlate with severity of esophageal lesions.
4. Alkaline burns do not penetrate deeper tissue layers.
5. Watch for sign of airway obstruction in corrosive poisoning because airway control must be the prime concern.
6. Esophagoscopy is controversial in corrosive poisoning as it may lead to further injury.
7. Early esophagoscopy in corrosive poisoning may help in diagnosis and placements of feeding tube, but is terminated if a significant burn is seen.
8. Esophagoscopy in corrosive poisoning is contraindicated after 12 hours.
9. Esophageal (Zenker's) diverticulum is treated by diverticulectomy and cricopharyngeal myotomy.

Fill in the blanks

10. In _____ syndrome, patient develops severe vomiting and chest pain after drinks and heavy dinner. X-ray of chest shows hydropneumothrorax.
11. In _____, the radiological findings include esophageal dilatation, rat-tail appearance, and failure of lower esophageal sphincter to relax.
12. _____ diverticulum occurs through Killian's dehiscence. It arises from posterior part of hypopharynx and causes regurgitation of undigested food.
13. _____ is the most common benign tumor of esophagus.
14. _____ carcinoma is the most common type of esophageal cancer.

Answers

1. d	2. T	3. F	4. F	5. T	6. T
7. T	8. T	9. T	10. Boerhaave's	11. Cardiac achalasia	
12. Esophageal (Zenker's)		13. Leiomyoma	14. Squamous cell		

Section 6: Larynx, Trachea and Bronchus

Chapter 42

Anatomy and Physiology of Larynx

⦿ Specific Learning Objectives
After going through the chapter, you should be able to answer the following questions:
- Describe the characteristic features of different laryngeal cartilages, ligaments and joints and their relations.
- Describe different parts of the larynx, their structures and the lymphatic drainage.
- Describe the various spaces of larynx and their importance in cases of cancer larynx.
- Enumerate laryngeal muscles, their nerve supply and functions.
- Describe the development of larynx. How is the larynx of infant and young children special from the adult larynx?
- What are the functions of larynx and their applied aspect?

ANATOMY OF LARYNX

The larynx lies in the middle and anterior part of neck opposite the third to sixth cervical vertebrae. During swallowing and phonation larynx moves in vertical as well as anteroposterior direction. The passive side to side movement of larynx produces a grating sensation called laryngeal crepitus.

CARTILAGES (FIGS 42.1 TO 42.4)

Larynx has 3 unpaired (thyroid, cricoid and epiglottis) and 3 paired cartilages (arytenoid, corniculate and cuneiform).
- **Hyaline:** Thyroid, cricoid and most part of the arytenoid cartilage (except its tip) are hyaline cartilages, which undergo ossification. The ossification, which begins first in thyroid at the age of 25 years and later in cricoid and arytenoids, is complete by 65 years.
- **Elastic:** The epiglottis, corniculate, cuneiform and tip of arytenoids are fibroelastic in nature. They do not ossify. Other example of elastic cartilage is auricular cartilage.
- **Thyroid:** This largest laryngeal cartilage has two alae, which meet anteriorly in midline and form an angle (Adam's apple) that is 90° in males and 120° in females. Vocal cords are attached in the middle of thyroid angle.
- **Cricoid:** This ring shaped cartilage has narrow anterior arch and expanded posterior lamina, over which articulate arytenoids.

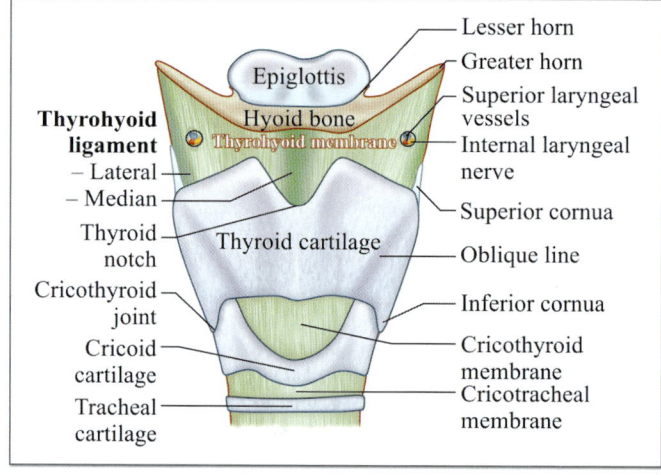

Fig. 42.1: Laryngeal framework—anterior view

- **Epiglottis:** This leaf-like, yellow, elastic cartilage forms anterior wall of laryngeal inlet. Petiole, a stalk-like process of epiglottis attaches it to the thyroid angle.
  - **Parts:** The anterior surface of epiglottis is attached to body of hyoid bone by hyoepiglottic ligament that divides epiglottis into two parts—suprahyoid and infrahyoid.
- **Arytenoid cartilages:** This pyramidal shape arytenoid cartilage has the following parts:
  - **Base:** It articulates with cricoid cartilage.
  - **Muscular process:** This lateral process provides attachment to intrinsic laryngeal muscles.

- **Vocal process:** This anterior process provides attachment to vocal ligament of vocal cord.
- **Apex:** Superiorly, it supports the corniculate cartilage in aryepiglottic fold.
- **Corniculate cartilage (of Santorini):** This articulates with the apex of arytenoids cartilage.
- **Cuneiform cartilage (of Wrisberg):** This rod shaped cartilage is situated in front of corniculate cartilage in the aryepiglottic fold.

JOINTS (FIGS 42.1 TO 42.4)

- **Cricoarytenoid joint:** This synovial joint is formed between the base of arytenoid and a facet on the upper border of cricoid lamina. Two types of movements are possible at this joint; rotatory and gliding. The rotatory movement occurs at a vertical axis and abducts and adducts the vocal cord. Arytenoids glide laterally and medially and help in closing and opening of the posterior part of glottis.
- **Cricothyroid joint:** This synovial joint is formed between the inferior cornua of thyroid cartilage and a facet on the cricoid cartilage.

MEMBRANES AND LIGAMENTS

Extrinsic (Figs 42.1 to 42.4)

- **Thyrohyoid membrane:** This membrane is pierced by neurovascular bundle of superior laryngeal vessels and internal laryngeal nerve. It connects thyroid cartilage to hyoid bone.
- **Hyoepiglottic ligament:** It connects the epiglottic cartilage to the body of hyoid bone.
- **Cricotracheal membrane:** It connects cricoid cartilage to the first tracheal ring.

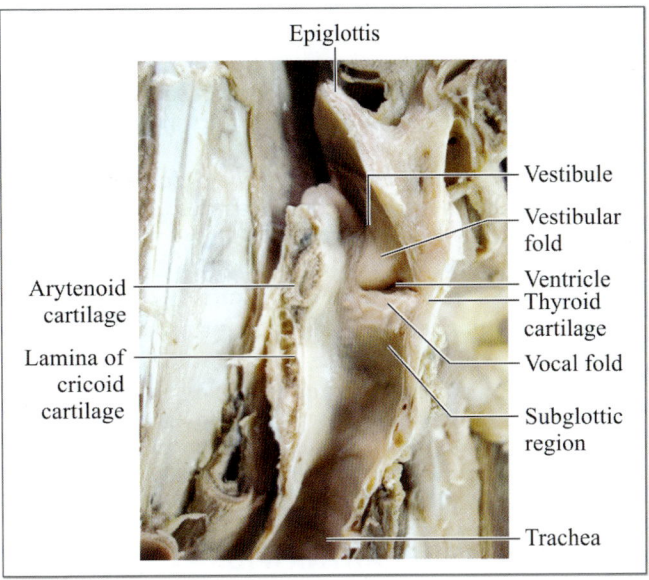

Fig. 42.3: Sagittal section of cadaveric larynx

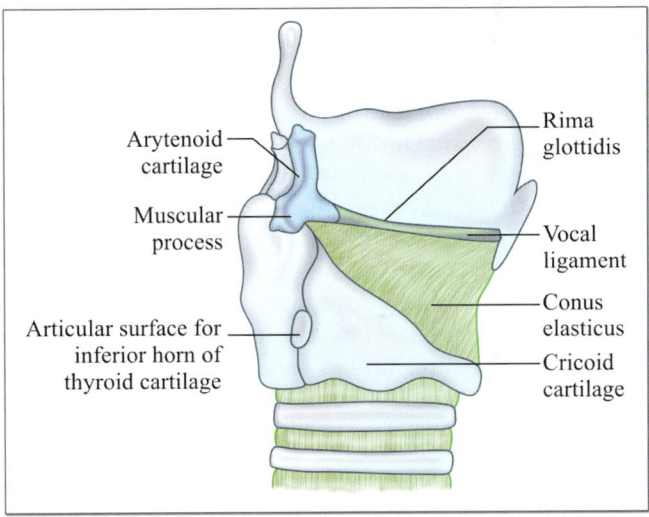

Fig. 42.4: Lateral view of larynx after removing right lamina of thyroid cartilages. See the laryngeal fibroelastic membrane and its attachment

Intrinsic (Figs 42.2 and 42.4)

- **Cricovocal membrane:** This triangular fibroelastic membrane has free upper border (vocal ligament), which stretches between middle of thyroid angle to the vocal process of arytenoids. The lower border is attached to the arch of cricoid cartilage.
  - **Conus elasticus:** The two sides of cricovocal membranes form conus elasticus. *Subglottic foreign bodies sometimes get impacted in the region of conus elasticus.*
  - **Cricothyroid membrane:** The anterior part of conus elasticus is thick and forms cricothyroid membrane, which connects thyroid cartilage to cricoid cartilage.

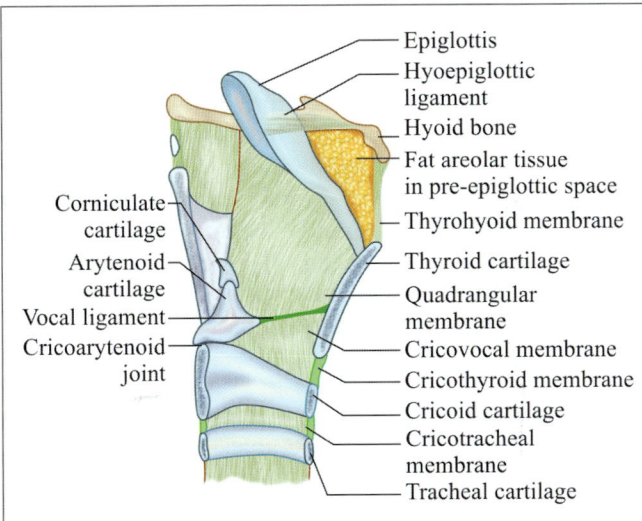

Fig. 42.2: Sagittal section of larynx

- **Cricothyrotomy:** Any airway obstruction above the vocal cord due to tumor and foreign body can be quickly, easily and effectively bypassed by piercing the cricothyroid membrane (cricothyrotomy).
- **Subglottic foreign bodies:** They sometimes get impacted in the region of conus elasticus.

- **Quadrangular membrane:** This is not well defined. It stretches between the epiglottis and arytenoids cartilages. Its free lower border forms the vestibular ligament, which lies in the vestibular fold (false cord). Its upper border lies in aryepiglottic fold.

Broyle's ligament: This is a small ligament which attaches the anterior commissure to the thyroid cartilage.

CAVITY OF THE LARYNX (FIGS 42.5 AND 42.6)

Superiorly laryngeal cavity communicates with laryngopharynx through the laryngeal inlet. Larynx ends at the lower border of cricoid cartilage (level of lower border of C_6) and becomes continuous with the trachea. The vestibular and vocal folds divide laryngeal cavity into three parts vestibule, ventricle and subglottic region.
- **Inlet of larynx:** During swallowing—the aryepiglottic folds, tubercle of epiglottis and arytenoids approximate and close the laryngeal inlet completely. This oblique entrance has following boundaries:
  - *Anterior:* Free margin of epiglottis.
  - *Lateral two sides:* Aryepiglottic folds.
  - *Posterior:* Interarytenoid fold.
- **Vestibule:** This region lies between the laryngeal inlet and vestibular folds. It has following boundaries:
  - *Anterior wall:* Posterior surface of epiglottis.

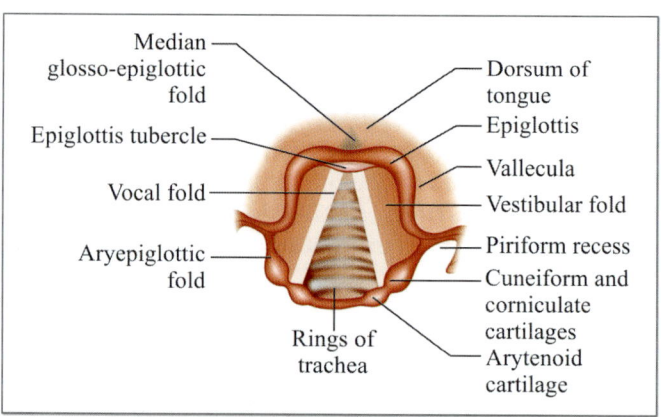
Fig. 42.6: Superior view of the inside of the larynx as seen during laryngoscopic examination during moderate respiration. Some of the subsites of oropharynx and laryngopharynx can also be noticed

  - *Lateral sides:* Aryepiglottic folds.
  - *Posterior wall:* Arytenoids.
- **Ventricle (sinus of larynx):** This deep elliptical space lies between vestibular and vocal folds and also called *ventricle of Morgagni*.
  - *Saccule:* This diverticulum of mucous membrane starts from the anterior part of ventricle and extends superiorly between vestibular folds and thyroid lamina. The secretions of mucous glands in the saccule provide lubrication for vocal cords.

- **Laryngocele:** This abnormally enlarged and distended saccule contains air.
- **Retention cyst:** The obstruction of duct of mucous gland in saccule can result in retention cyst.

- **Subglottic region (infraglottic larynx):** The subglottic region extends from below the vocal cords to lower border of cricoid cartilage.
- **Vestibular folds (false cords):** These folds of mucous membrane contain vestibular ligament (fibers of thyroarytenoid muscle) and mucous glands. They are situated anteroposteriorly across the laryngeal cavity.
- **Vocal folds (vocal cords):** These pearly white sharp bands extend between middle of thyroid angle and vocal processes of arytenoids. The vocal cord consists of a vocal ligament (upper edge of cricovocal membrane), which is covered with mucous membrane that has scanty subepithelial connective tissue.

Most common sites of laryngeal foreign bodies: They are seen in supraglottic region lying above the vocal cords.

- **Glottis (rima glottidis):** This area lies between vocal cords and arytenoids. Size and shape of glottis varies with the position of the vocal cords. Anterior two-third

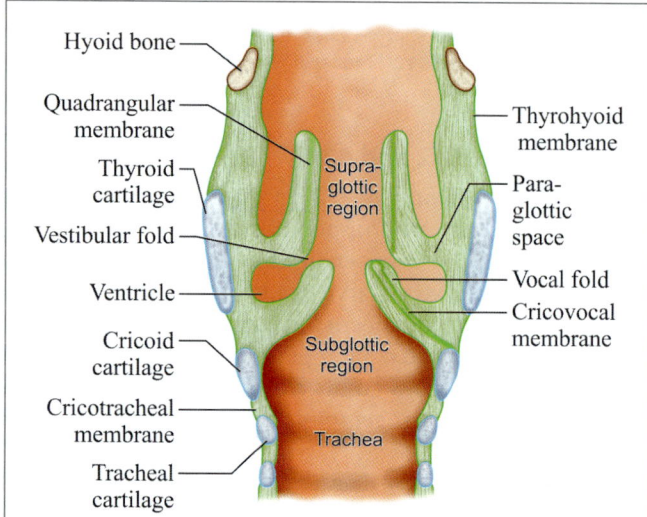
Fig. 42.5: Coronal section of larynx

of glottis is formed by membranous vocal cords while posterior one-third by vocal processes of arytenoids. Anteroposterior length of glottis is more in men (24 mm) than in women (16 mm).

The most narrow part of larynx: In adults, it is rima glottidis and in infants it is subglottic region.

MUCOUS MEMBRANE OF THE LARYNX

Epithelium of the mucous membrane is ciliated columnar except over the vocal cords and upper part of the epiglottis and aryepiglottic folds where it is stratified squamous. It lines the larynx loosely except over the posterior surface of epiglottis, true vocal cords and corniculate and cuneiform cartilages.

Mucous glands are abundant on the epiglottis, posterior part of the aryepiglottic folds and in the saccule. Vocal folds do not have mucous glands.

LYMPHATIC DRAINAGE

- *Supraglottic:* Lymphatics drain into upper deep cervical nodes through the thyrohyoid membrane.
- *Infraglottic:* Lymphatics drain into prelaryngeal (Delphian node) and pretracheal nodes (through cricothyroid membrane) and then to lower deep cervical and mediastinal nodes. Some lymphatics pierce cricotracheal membrane and directly drain into lower deep cervical nodes.
- *Glottic: Lymphatics in vocal cords are very scanty, hence glottic carcinoma rarely shows lymphatic metastases.*

SPACES OF THE LARYNX

- *Pre-epiglottic space of Boyer:* Anterior surface of infrahyoid epiglottis is separated from thyrohyoid membrane and thyroid cartilage by fat filled pre-epiglottic space. So it has following boundaries:
  - *Anterior:* Upper part of thyroid cartilage and thyrohyoid membrane.
  - *Superior:* Hyoepiglottic ligament.
  - *Posterior:* Infrahyoid epiglottis.
  - *Inferior:* Thyroepiglottic ligament.
  - *Communication:* Laterally it is continuous with paraglottic space.

Cancer of supraglottic larynx and base of tongue: They invade pre-epiglottic space.

- *Paraglottic space:* It communicates with pre-epiglottic space. This space is bounded by:
  - *Anterolateral:* Thyroid cartilage and cricothyroid membrane.
  - *Inferomedial:* Conus elasticus.
  - *Medial:* Ventricle and quadrangular membrane.
  - *Posterior:* Anterior part of pyriform fossa.

Spread of cancer larynx and laryngopharynx:
- Growths invading paraglottic space destroy cricothyroid membrane and present in the neck.
- Ventricle tumors invade paraglottic space and then spread transglottically.
- Vocal cord tumors involving thyroarytenoid muscle invade paraglottic space and then subglottic and extralaryngeal region.
- Lateral supraglottic tumors can travel to subglottic region through the paraglottic space along the inner surface of thyroid.
- Pyriform fossa tumor can come into endolarynx and fix vocal folds through the posterior part of paraglottic space.

- *Reinke's space:* This potential subepithelial space has scanty subepithelial connective tissue. It lies under the epithelium of vocal cords and superficial to its elastic layer. It is bounded by:
  - *Medial:* Epithelium of vocal cord
  - *Lateral:* Vocal ligament
  - *Above and below:* Arcuate lines
  - *Anterior:* Anterior commissure
  - *Posterior:* Vocal process of arytenoids.

Reinke's edema: Edema of Reinke's space results in fusiform swelling of the membranous vocal cords. Edema can also cause polypoidal degeneration of vocal cords.

MUSCLES OF LARYNX

There are two types of laryngeal muscles intrinsic (connecting laryngeal cartilages to each other) and extrinsic (connecting larynx to the surrounding structures).

Intrinsic Muscles

They are further divided into two—muscles acting on vocal cords and muscles acting on laryngeal inlet (Figs 42.7 to 42.9).
1. Vocal cords
   - *Abductors:* Posterior cricoarytenoid
   - *Adductors:*
     - Lateral cricoarytenoid
     - Interarytenoid (transverse and oblique arytenoids)
     - Thyroarytenoid (external part)
     - *Tensors:* Cricothyroid
     - *Relaxers*
       - Vocalis
       - Thyroarytenoid internal part

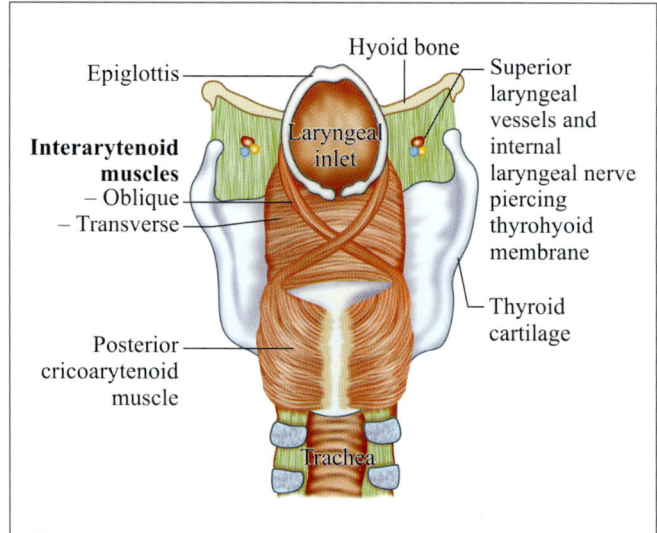

Fig. 42.7: Intrinsic muscles of larynx as seen on its posterior view

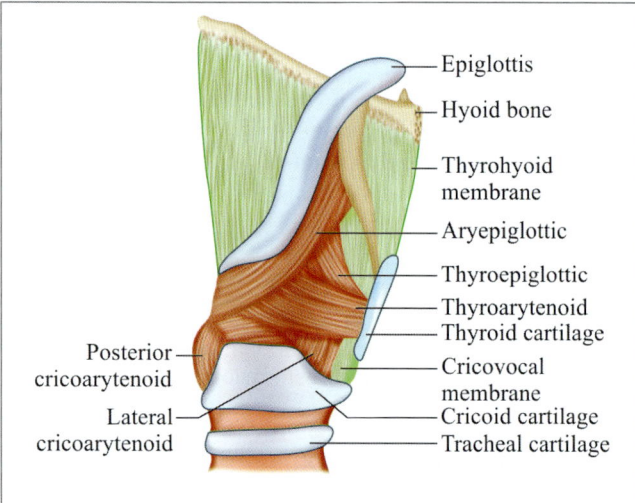

Fig. 42.8: Intrinsic muscles of larynx as seen on its lateral view

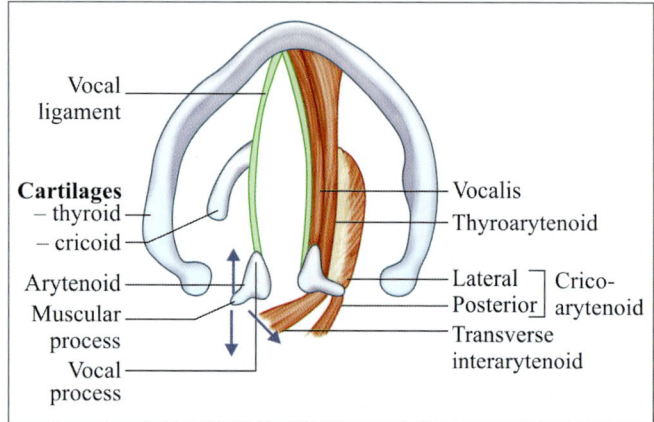

Fig. 42.9: Intrinsic muscles of larynx and their actions. Arrows indicate direction of movement of muscular process of arytenoid

2. Laryngeal inlet
   - **Openers:** Thyroepiglottic (part of thyroarytenoid)
   - **Closers:**
     - Interarytenoid (oblique part)
     - Aryepiglottic (posterior oblique part of interarytenoid)

Extrinsic Muscles

Elevators
1. *Primary elevators:* They are attached to the thyroid cartilage and include vertical pharyngeal muscles (stylopharyngeus, salpingopharyngeus and palatopharyngeus) and thyrohyoid.
2. *Secondary elevators:* They are attached to the hyoid bone and include suprahyoid muscles (mylohyoid, digastrics, stylohyoid and geniohyoid).

Depressors: They include infrahyoid strap muscles, which are sternohyoid, sternothyroid and omohyoid.

NERVE SUPPLY OF LARYNX (FIG. 42.10)

Larynx is innervated by vagus nerve. The motor neurons arise from the nucleus ambiguus of the medulla. The vagus nerve exits through the jugular foramen and then travels within the carotid sheath.

- *Motor supply:* All the intrinsic muscles of larynx are supplied by the recurrent laryngeal nerve except the cricothyroid muscle, which is supplied by the external laryngeal nerve, a branch of superior laryngeal nerve. Both recurrent and superior laryngeal nerves are the branches of vagus nerve (CN X), which carry the fibers of cranial part of accessory nerve (CN XI).
- *Sensory supply:* Larynx above the vocal cords is supplied by internal laryngeal nerve (branch of superior laryngeal). Larynx below the vocal cords is supplied by the internal branch of recurrent laryngeal nerve.
- *Recurrent laryngeal nerve:* The site of origin and course of right nerve is different from the left.
  - *Left recurrent laryngeal nerve:* It has intrathoracic course and arises from the vagus in the mediastinum at the level of arch of aorta. It loops around aortic arch and ascends into the tracheoesophageal gutter.
  - *Right recurrent laryngeal nerve:* It arises from the vagus at the level of subclavian artery and loops around subclavian artery and then ascends in the tracheoesophageal gutter. It does not have intrathoracic course.
- *Superior laryngeal nerve:* After arising from inferior ganglion of the vagus it descends behind the internal carotid artery. At the level of greater cornua of hyoid it divides into external and internal branches.
  - *External laryngeal nerve:* It travels in relation with superior thyroid artery and supplies cricothyroid.

Chapter 42 • Anatomy and Physiology of Larynx

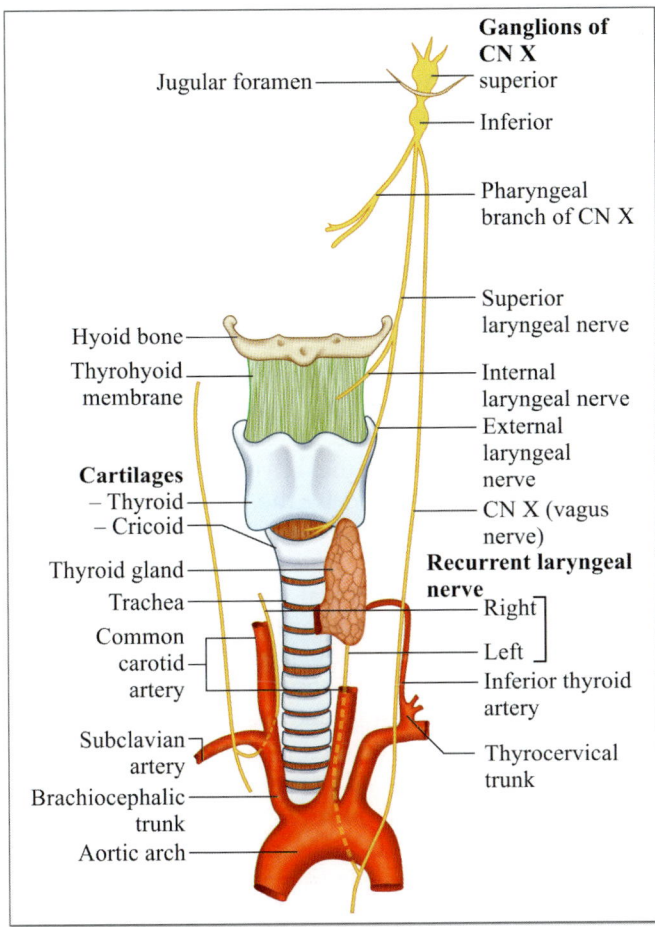

Fig. 42.10: Nerves supplying the larynx and their relations especially with arteries

- **Internal laryngeal nerve:** It pierces the thyrohyoid membrane along with the superior laryngeal vessels and supplies sensory innervation to the mucosa of supraglottic larynx and hypopharynx.

- **Galen's anastomosis:** It is the anastomosis between the branches of superior and recurrent laryngeal nerves.
- **Nonrecurrent recurrent laryngeal nerve (inferior laryngeal nerve):** It is often associated with anomalous retroesophageal right subclavian artery.
- **Glottic chink:** In cadaveric position of the vocal cords vocal chink is 14 mm. In full abduction it is about 19 mm. During the whisper, the position of vocal cord is paramedian.
- **Vocal cord palsy:** It is commonly caused by lesions of recurrent laryngeal nerve. Because of the intrathoracic course of left recurrent laryngeal nerve left vocal cord palsy is twice more common than right vocal cord palsy.

Cricothyroid and superior laryngeal nerve: The cricothyroid is the only intrinsic laryngeal muscle that is innervated by superior laryngeal nerve and not by the recurrent laryngeal nerve.

Table 42.1: Embryological development of larynx

Structure	Source
Laryngeal mucosa	Endoderm of cephalic part of foregut
Laryngeal cartilages	Mesenchyme
Epiglottis	Hypobranchial eminence
Upper part of thyroid cartilage	4th branchial arch
Lower part of thyroid cartilage, cricoid, corniculate, and cuneiform cartilages	6th branchial arch
Intrinsic muscles of larynx	6th branchial arch

DEVELOPMENT OF LARYNX

The hypobranchial eminence appears in the floor of primitive pharynx between the 2nd, 3rd and 4th branchial arches (Table 42.1). During the 3rd week of gestation, a median tracheobronchial groove appears in the floor of primitive foregut which deepens. The lateral septae (laryngotracheal septum) grow and fuse and separates the esophagus from trachea. The upper end of embryonic trachea forms the laryngeal inlet and lower end elongates and divides into two lateral lung buds. The hypobranchial eminence forms primitive epiglottis. Two swellings lateral to laryngeal fissure form arytenoids and aryepiglottic folds.

Infant Larynx

In comparison to the adult larynx, infant larynx has following significant differences:

- **Position:** Infant larynx is situated higher in the neck. Vocal cords lie at C3/C4 level and during swallowing go up to C1/C2 level. The epiglottis and soft palate forms a nasopharyngeal channel for breathing during suckling. Infant can simultaneously swallow and breathe. The milk passes over dorsum of tongue and sides of epiglottis while breathing occurs through nasopharyngeal channel formed by epiglottis and soft palate. In adults vocal cords lie at C5 level.
- **Cartilages:** Laryngeal cartilages in infants are soft and collapse easily.
    - **Epiglottis:** It is omega shaped.
    - **Arytenoids:** They are relatively large and cover significant posterior part of glottis.
    - **Thyroid:** It is flat.
    - **Cricoid:** The diameter is smaller than glottis.
- **Cricothyroid and thyrohyoid spaces:** They are very narrow. Hyoid bone overlaps thyroid and thyroid overlaps cricoid.

Tracheostomy in infants: The cricothyroid and thyrohyoid spaces are not appreciable landmarks during the tracheostomy in infants.

- *Size:* It is smaller and has a narrower lumen.
- *Shape:* It is conical and funnel-shaped.
- *Submucosal tissue:* It is thick and loose and becomes easily edematous in response to trauma or inflammation.

Subglottic edema in infants and young children: The subglottis has the complete cartilaginous ring (cricoid) and edema in this region occurs at the expense of lumen.

GROWTH OF LARYNX

Larynx has two phases of spurts in growth:
1. *First spurt:* It occurs at 3 years of life and larynx grows in width and length.

Congenital anomalies of larynx: First spurt of laryngeal growth in width and length at 3 years of life obviates the need for any airway surgery in certain congenital anomaly.

2. *Second spurt:* It occurs during adolescence.
   - *Thyroid angle:* It develops.
   - *Position:* Larynx gradually descends.
   - *Vocal cords:* They descend to C5 level and increase in length especially in males and lead to voice changes (Table 42.2).

FUNCTIONS OF LARYNX

The four main functions of larynx are—(1) respiration, (2) protection of lower respiratory tract, (3) phonation and (4) fixation of the chest.

Protection of Lower Airways

Larynx protects the lower respiratory tract:
- *Sphincteric closure of laryngeal opening:* During swallowing and vomiting, food entry into air passage is prevented by the closure of following three successive sphincters:
  - Laryngeal inlet
  - False cords
  - True cords

Table 42.2: Length of vocal cords in male and female children and adults

	Females		Males	
	Children	Adults	Children	Adults
Length of vocal cords in mm	6	15–19	8	17–23

- *Cessation of respiration:* When food comes in contact with the oropharynx, reflex generated by afferent fibers of ninth nerve ceases the respiration temporarily.
- *Cough reflex:* Coughing dislodges and expels any foreign particle that comes in contact with respiratory mucosa. Larynx acts as a watchdog of lungs and starts 'barking' at the entry of any foreign body.

Phonation and Speech

- *Aerodynamic myoelastic theory of voice production:* Like a wind instrument, larynx produces voice.
- *Speech:* Three phases in the production of speech:
  i. *Pulmonary phase:* It creates energy flow with inflation of lungs and expulsion of air. It provides a column of air to the larynx. The subglottic air pressure is generated by the exhaled air from the lungs with the help of contraction of thoracic and abdominal muscles.
  ii. *Laryngeal phase:* Vocal folds vibrate to create sound that is then modified in the next phase. The air pressure opens the adducted cords and small puffs of air are released. Vocal fold vibrations are not the result of laryngeal muscles. Vocal folds are adducted and pressure of moving air causes vibrations of the elastic vocal folds.
  iii. *Supraglottic/oral phase:* The laryngeal sound that is modified in the supraglottic/oral phase is considered a unique individual sound. Words of the sentences are formed by the muscles of pharynx, tongue and lips and teeth. The vibration of the vocal cords produces sound, which is amplified by mouth, pharynx, nose and chest. The modulator action of lips, tongue, palate, pharynx and teeth converts the sound into speech.

Frequency and intensity of sound: The air pressure produced by the lungs controls the intensity of sound. The frequency of vocal cord vibrations controls the pitch of sound. Different frequencies are produced with changes in length, breadth, elasticity and extension of vocal folds.

Respiration

The adduction of vocal cords during expiration and abduction of vocal cords during inspiration regulate the flow of air into the lungs.

Fixation of Chest

Closed larynx helps in the fixation of chest wall, which facilitates the action of various thoracic and abdominal muscles. This function plays an important role during digging, pulling and climbing, coughing, vomiting, defecation, micturition and childbirth.

Chapter 42 • Anatomy and Physiology of Larynx

Self-evaluation Exercises

1. Which of the following are not true for Reinke' space?
   a. Potential space with scanty subepithelial connective tissues
   b. Lies under the epithelium of vocal cords
   c. Lies superficial to elastic layer of vocal cords
   d. None of the above
2. Which of the following are true for the boundaries of Reinke' space?
   a. Above and below by the arcuate lines
   b. Anteriorly by anterior commissure
   c. Posteriorly by vocal process of arytenoids
   d. All of the above
3. The examples of elastic cartilages are:
   a. Auricular
   b. Epiglottis
   c. Corniculate and cuneiform
   d. Apices of the arytenoids
   e. All of the above
4. Hidden areas of the larynx are:
   a. Infrahyoid epiglottis
   b. Anterior commissure
   c. Subglottis
   d. Ventricle
   e. All of the above
5. The examples of elastic cartilages are:
   a. Thyroid
   b. Cricoid
   c. Greater part of arytenoids
   d. None of the above
6. Wrisberg's cartilage are:
   a. Cuneiform
   b. Fibroelastic
   c. Situated in aryepiglottic fold
   d. Does not undergo calcification
   e. All of the above

True (T)/False (F)

7. Hyaline cartilages do not undergo calcification.
8. Elastic cartilages undergo calcification.
9. Cricoid cartilage develops from VI branchial arch.
10. In male, thyroid angle is 120° while in female it is 90°.
11. Broyle's ligament is a small ligament which connects both vocal cords at the anterior commissure to the thyroid cartilage.
12. Epithelium of vocal cords is keratinizing stratified squamous.
13. Apex of pyriform fossa is not properly visible with indirect laryngoscopy examination.
14. The direct laryngoscopy examination is required to rule out malignancies of hidden areas of larynx and hypopharynx.
15. The pre-epiglottic and paraglottic spaces may be invaded by carcinoma arising in the laryngeal mucosa.
16. Edema of Reinke's space causes polypoid degeneration of vocal cords.
17. Edema of Reinke's space results in fusiform swelling of the membranous vocal cords.
18. The recurrent laryngeal nerve supplies all the intrinsic muscles of the larynx except the cricoarytenoid, which is innervated by inferior laryngeal nerve.
19. Vagus nerve supplies entire larynx except suproglottic part which is supplied by glossopharyngeal nerve.
20. Paralysis of recurrent laryngeal nerve does not affect cricoarytenoid.
21. The recurrent laryngeal nerve innervates laryngeal mucosa below the vocal fold whereas superior laryngeal nerve innervates laryngeal mucosa above the vocal fold.
22. Non recurrent-recurrent laryngeal nerve (Inferior laryngeal nerve) is often associated with anomalous retro-esophageal right subclavian artery.
23. In cadaveric position, vocal chink (Glottic chink) is 14 mm and in full abduction it is about 19 mm.
24. Anteroposterior depth of male glottis is 24 mm.
25. Ventricle of Morgagni is the laryngeal vestibule that is situated between the cords of larynx.

Contd…

Section 6 • Larynx, Trachea and Bronchus

Contd…

26. During the whisper, the position of vocal cord is median.
27. Vocal cord palsy is commonly caused by lesions of superior laryngeal nerve.
28. Because of the intrathoracic course of left recurrent laryngeal nerve left vocal cord palsy is twice more common than right vocal cord palsy.
29. Rate of topical absorption is poor in tracheobronchial tree and larynx.

Filling the blanks

30. The anastomosis between the branches of superior and recurrent laryngeal nerves (branches of vagus nerve) is called_____ .
31. Prelaryngeal lymph node in the region of the thyroid isthmus is called _____ .

Match the following

32. Adductors of vocal cord
33. Tensor of vocal cord
34. Abductor of vocal cord
35. Relaxer of vocal cord

A. Vocalis
B. Lateral cricoarytenoid
C. Cricothyroid
D. Posterior cricoarytenoid

Answers

1. d	2. d	3. e	4. e	5. d
6. e	7. F	8. F	9. T	10. F
11. T	12. F	13. T	14. T	15. T
16. T	17. T	18. F	19. F	20. F
21. T	22. T	23. T	24. T	25. F
26. F	27. F	28. T	29. F	30. Galen's anastomosis
31. Delphian node	32. B	33. C	34. D	35. A

Problem-oriented Cases (Spot Diagnosis)

1. A neonate female child presents with a unilateral parotid swelling with bluish overlying skin. The swelling increases when child is crying. There is no other abnormality.[1]
2. A HIV infected patient develops painless non tender parotid gland swelling. What is the most common cause?[2]
3. An adult male patient of 35 years age has been diagnosed as squamous cell carcinoma of left lateral border of anterior two-third tongue. The size of local ulceroinfiltrative lesion is 6 cm. The size of swelling of level 3 left cervical lymphadenopathy is 4 cm. General and systemic examination do not show any evidence of distant metastasis. Do TNM classification and staging of his cancer disease.[3]
4. A 50-year-old patient presents with 3 cm indurated infiltrative ulcerative lesion of right buccal mucosa. Cervical palpation reveals multiple nodes on the right side in the submandibular region. None of the node is more than 3 cm. Biopsy confirms the diagnosis of squamous cell carcinoma. Stage the disease and tell the best line of treatment.[4]
5. What will be the staging of a squamous cell carcinoma if the TNM classification has T_1, N_1 and M_0?[5]
6. A 40-year-old patient presents with frequent episodes of transient but severe unbearable throat pain that radiates to the ear and posterior part of tongue and is aggravated on swallowing. ENT head and neck examination does not show any positive findings.[6]
7. A 6-year-old child presents with sore-throat and fever of 2 days duration. Microbiology of throat swab reveals small, translucent beta-hemolytic colonies sensitive to *in vitro* bacitracin. Past history revealed severe allergic reaction to amoxicillin. Infection is not that serious and does not need parenteral antibiotic. Which antibiotic you think would be safe and effective.[7]
8. A child was scheduled for tonsillectomy. On the day of surgery he comes with URI (cough, cold, and fever). Will you proceed for surgery?[8]
9. A 10-year-old child after an episode of diphtheria develops hoarseness of voice. Laryngoscopy reveals right vocal cord palsy. In addition to the medical treatment what else would you like to do for the paralyzed vocal cord?[9]
10. A 5-year-old boy presents with recurrent upper respiratory tract infections, mouth breathing, and nasal obstruction. His parents observed that the child's hearing has deteriorated.[10]
11. A 15-year-old boy presents with right side nasal obstruction and episodes of profuse bleeding. On examination you see marked anemia and fullness of right cheek.[11]
12. A 45-year-old man presents with right side facial pain in temporoparietal and the lower jaw area. On examination you find right side conductive hearing loss and immobile soft palate.[12]

---

[1]Hemangioma, [2]Lymphoepithelial cysts, [3]Stage IV: $T_3N_2M_0$, [4]Stage III: $T_2N_1M_0$; Surgical excision of growth with supra-omohyoid neck dissection and post operative radiotherapy, [5]Stage III, [6]Glossopharyngeal neuralgia, [7]Azithromycin, [8]No. Wait for 3 weeks and treat the URI if needed with antibiotics, [9]Wait and watch for the spontaneous recovery, [10]Adenoid hypertrophy and otitis media with effusion, [11]Juvenile nasopharyngeal angiofibroma, [12]Trotter's syndrome

Chapter 43

Laryngeal Symptoms and Examination

> **Specific Learning Objectives**
> After going through the chapter, you should be able to answer the following questions:
> - What are the common symptoms of laryngeal and laryngopharyngeal disorders and their causes?
> - Describe the different methods of examination of larynx and laryngopharynx.
> - Name the findings which you will seek during the examination of larynx and laryngopaharynx and their causes?
> - What are the different causes of hoarseness of voice and how will you evaluate such patients?
> - What are the different types of stridors and their causes?
> - How will you examine and manage a child with stridor?

SYMPTOMS

The common laryngeal and laryngopharyngeal symptoms and their causes are mentioned in Box 43.1.

CLINICAL EXAMINATION

Clinical examination of larynx includes external examination of larynx, indirect laryngoscopy, fiber optic endoscopy (flexible and rigid), assessment of voice and cervical lymph nodes (Box 43.2). To elicit the post laryngeal crepitus (characteristic grating sound), cricoid is moved from side to side.

External Examination

It includes inspection (Fig. 43.1) and palpation (Box 43.2) of area of hyoid bone, thyroid cartilage, thyroid notch, cricoid cartilage and the tracheal rings for redness of skin, bulging or swelling, widening of larynx, surgical emphysema, change in contour or displacement of larynx, movements of larynx with deglutition and breathing and post laryngeal crepitus.

Indirect Laryngoscopy with Laryngeal Mirror

- **Laryngeal mirror:** It is used for the indirect examination of oropharynx, laryngopharynx and larynx. It is available in various sizes from 6 mm to 30 mm diameter.

> **Box 43.1: Larynx and laryngopharynx symptoms and their causes**
> - **Symptoms of voice:** Hoarseness, aphonia, puberphonia, easy fatigability of voice, rough, breathy, bitonal, dysphonic, whispered and feeble.
> - **Difficulty in respiration (respiratory distress/stridor):** Tumors, infection (acute laryngotracheobronchitis, diphtheria and epiglottitis in children), foreign bodies.
> - **Repeated clearing of throat:** Chronic laryngitis, benign and malignant tumors and laryngopharyngeal reflux (LPR)/gastroesophageal reflux disease (GERD).
> - **Pain in throat:** Ulcers (benign and malignant), perichondritis and arthritis.
> - **Difficulty in swallowing (dysphagia):** Epiglottitis, laryngeal paralysis and tumors of laryngopharynx.
> - **Coughing:** Aspiration of secretions due to laryngeal paralysis, infection, tumor, foreign bodies and LPR.
> - **Mass in the neck:** Cervical nodes, direct extension of growth and perichondritis laryngocele.

> *Laryngeal vs posterior rhinoscopy mirror (Fig. 43.2):* The posterior rhinoscopy mirror is smaller and its shaft is bayonet shaped, while the shaft of the laryngeal mirror is straight.

- **Method:** For indirect laryngoscopy (Figs 43.3A and B), patient sits erect with the head and chest leaning slightly towards the examiner. Patient protrudes out the tongue,

Box 43.2: Examination of larynx and laryngopharynx: Findings and their causes

External Examination
- **Inspection and palpation** (area of hyoid bone, thyroid cartilage, thyroid notch, cricoid cartilage and the tracheal rings). Note the following:
  - **Redness of skin:** Abscess, perichondritis, cancer
  - **Bulging or swelling:** Extension of cancer, metastatic and inflammatory lymph nodes
  - **Widening of larynx:** Growth of pyriform fossa
  - **Surgical emphysema:** Accidental and tracheostomy
  - **Change in contour or displacement of larynx:** Trauma and neoplasm
- **Movements of larynx** with deglutition and breathing:
  - **Present:** Normal
  - **Fixity:** Inflammation and malignant infiltration
- **Post laryngeal crepitus:**
  - **Present:** Normal
  - **Absent:** Postcricoid carcinoma, retropharyngeal abscess

Techniques of laryngoscopy (Table 43.1)
- Indirect laryngoscopy
- Rigid endoscopy
- Flexible endoscopy

Structures seen during laryngoscopy
- **Oropharynx:** Base of tongue, lingual tonsils, valleculae, glossoepiglottic folds and pharyngoepiglottic folds.
- **Larynx:** Epiglottis, aryepiglottic folds, arytenoids, ventricular bands, ventricles, true cords, anterior commissure, posterior commissure, subglottis and rings of trachea.
- **Laryngopharynx:** Pyriform fossa, postcricoid region, posterior wall of laryngopharynx.

Cervical lymph nodes

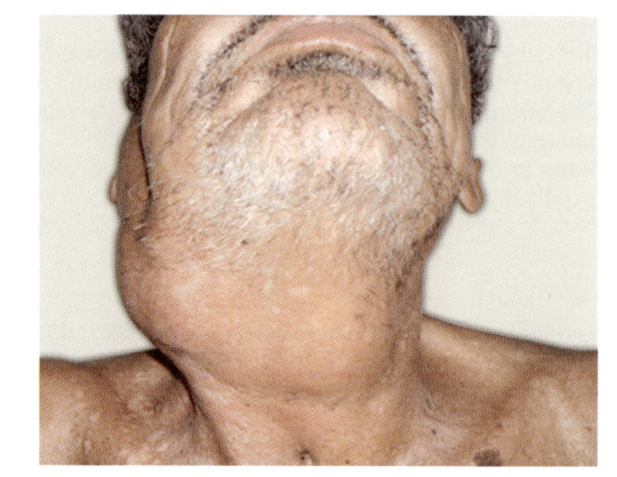

Fig. 43.1: Secondary metastatic neck nodes on right side involving levels Ib to V. Primary lesion was carcinoma of supraglottic larynx. Note the healed tracheostomy opening and widening of thyroid cartilage

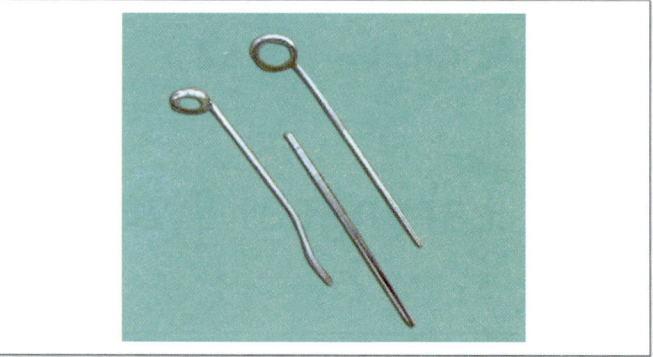

Fig. 43.2: Laryngoscopy and rhinoscopy mirrors with handle

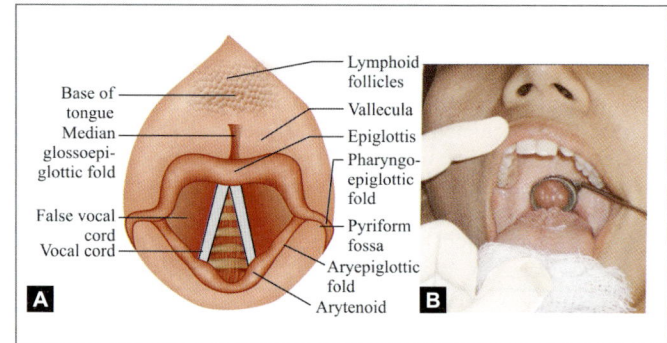

Figs 43.3A and B: Indirect laryngoscopy. (A) Structures seen; (B) Method

Table 43.1: Comparison of different techniques of indirect laryngoscopic examinations

Features	Laryngeal mirror	Rigid telescope	Flexible endoscope
Availability	Widely	Uncommon	Very uncommon
Cost	Most economical	Expensive	Most expensive
Color of image	Best and natural	Good	Moderate
Patient tolerance	Good	Moderate	Good
Photography quality	Not possible	Excellent	Good
Magnification	Absent	Maximum	Moderate
Stroboscopy quality	Not possible	Excellent	Good
Speech and singing observation	Difficult	Very difficult	Excellent
Vocal mechanics evaluation	Difficult	Not possible	Excellent
Biofeedback voice breathing therapy	Not possible	Possible	Excellent

which is wrapped in a piece of gauze cloth and then held by the examiner between the thumb and middle finger. Index finger of the examiner retracts out the patient's upper lip and moustache. To prevent fogging, a laryngeal mirror is always warmed over a spirit lamp or in hot water (some prefer savlon). It is advisable to test mirror's warmness on the back of hand before inserting into the mouth, because hot mirror can damage the mucosa. The warmed laryngeal mirror is introduced into the mouth and held firmly against the uvula and soft palate while the light is focused on the laryngeal mirror. Patient is asked to breathe quietly. Then the systematic examination begins of the oropharynx, laryngopharynx and larynx. Movements of both the cords are observed when patient takes deep inspiration (abduction of cords) and say "Aa" (adduction of cords) and "Eee" (for adduction and tension).

- **Failed mirror examination:** Topical anesthesia with 4% lignocaine facilitates laryngeal mirror examination. In some of the patients, laryngeal mirror examination cannot be performed due to anatomical abnormalities such as overhanging of epiglottis. It is also difficult in uncooperative and anxious patient and too much sensitive pharynx. In such cases, endoscopic examination is advised.

Endoscopy

The continuous light of endoscope helps in studying gross structure and function of larynx, while strobe light assesses mucosal health and vibration pattern. The comparison and an overview of different techniques of indirect laryngoscopic examination are given in Table 43.1. Both rigid and flexible laryngoscopes have fiberoptic lights and used under topical anesthesia in OPD. Rigid is introduced through mouth whereas flexible is passed through nose.

Stroboscopy

Stroboscope determines speed of cyclic motion, which appears slowed (strobe or running phase) or stopped (locked phase). Strobe light illuminates vocal folds at different points of different vibration cycles and creates illusion of slow motion. Strobe illumination helps in understanding mucosal scarring and distinguishing cysts from nodules.

Indications

Stroboscopy is valuable in following vocal fold conditions and may obviate the need for microlaryngoscopy:
- Stiffness
- Scar
- Submucosal injury
- Small vocal fold lesions
- Invasion depth of early cancer lesion
- Asymmetric mass or tension
- Follow-up after phonosurgery.

HOARSENESS OF VOICE

Any change in voice quality from harsh, rough or raspy voice to weak voice is usually referred as hoarseness. It is caused by laryngeal dysfunction. In cases of limited lungs or tracheobronchial tree diseases, voice becomes weak and damp.

Etiology

Hoarseness is a symptom and not a disease. The various causes of hoarseness are shown in Table 43.2. The conditions that interfere with the functions and structure of vocal cords include following:
- **Inappropriate approximation:** Vocal cord paralysis, fixation, tumors of vocal cords.

Table 43.2: Causes of hoarseness of voice (laryngeal disorders)

Infections	Acute and chronic laryngitis: • Influenza • Exanthematous fever • Laryngotracheobronchitis • Diphtheria, tuberculosis, syphilis, scleroma and atrophic laryngitis
Neoplasms	• Papilloma (solitary and multiple), hemangioma, chondroma, angiofibroma, fibroma and leukoplakia • Vocal nodule • Vocal polyp, amyloid tumor and contact ulcers • Cancer
Trauma	• Submucosal hemorrhage, laryngeal trauma (blunt and sharp) and foreign bodies • Intubation
Paralysis	Paralysis of vagus nerve and its branches recurrent and superior laryngeal
Fixation of cords	Arthritis and fixation of cricoarytenoid joints
Congenital	Cysts and web
Miscellaneous	• Dysphonia plica ventricularis • Myxedema and gout • Hysterical aphonia

- *Abnormal size:* Edema, tumor of vocal cord, partial surgical excision, fibrosis.
- *Abnormal stiffness:* It is decreased in paralysis and increased in spastic dysphonia and fibrosis.
- *Improper vibrations:* Congestion, submucosal hemorrhages, nodule and polyp.

History, Examination and Investigations

- *History:* Patient's occupation and habits, mode of onset and duration, and associated complaints should be noted.

> **Persistent hoarseness in elderly:** In cases of smokers and elderly people with hoarseness of more than 3 weeks, carcinoma vocal cord should be ruled out.

- *Examination:* Indirect laryngoscopy with mirror and endoscopy (rigid and flexible) for structural and functional assessment of the cords and cricoarytenoid joints.
  - Examination of neck, cardiovascular system and cranial nerves.
- *Investigations:*
  - Laboratory investigations to know infections and hypothyroidism.
  - Radiological examination such as X-ray chest, barium swallow.
  - Microlaryngoscopy and biopsy of the lesions.
  - Bronchoscopy in case of pulmonary causes.
  - Esophagoscopy in case of carcinoma esophagus and GERD.

STRIDOR

Stridor is a hallmark of laryngeal obstruction. It is an abnormal (stridulent or harsh) noise that is caused by a turbulent airflow in the impaired airway.

Types

Stridor may be heard during inspiration, expiration or both.
- *Inspiratory stridor:* It is because of obstruction from larynx and pharynx.
- *Expiratory stridor:* Expiratory stridor and prolonged expiratory phase are because of bronchial and low tracheal obstruction.
- *Biphasic stridor:* It is because of obstruction at the level of cervical trachea.

> **Stertor** is a snoring type of noise, which is made by nasopharyngeal and oropharyngeal obstruction.

Causes of Stridor

Various causes of stridor in infants and young children and adults are enumerated in Box 43.3.

> - **Acute stridor in children:** It is mostly caused by laryngotracheobronchitis, bacterial tracheitis, acute epiglottitis and laryngeal foreign bodies.
> - **Most common cause of stridor in adults:** It is carcinoma of larynx.

Box 43.3: Causes of stridor

Infants and Children
- *Nose:* Congenital choanal atresia, pyriform aperture stenosis and mid nasal stenosis.
- *Tongue:* Cretinism, hemangioma, lymphangioma, dermoid and lingual thyroid.
- *Mandible:* Micrognathia and Pierre-Robin syndrome.
- *Pharynx:* Congenital dermoid, adenotonsillar hypertrophy and retropharyngeal abscess.
- *Larynx:*
  - *Congenital:* Laryngeal web, laryngomalacia, cysts, vocal cord paralysis and subglottic stenosis.
  - *Inflammatory:* Epiglottitis, laryngotracheobronchitis (LTB) and diphtheria.
  - *Neoplastic:* Hemangioma and juvenile multiple papillomatosis.
  - *Traumatic:* Physical/chemical/thermal injury, external laryngeal trauma, foreign bodies and iatrogenic (bronchoscopy and prolonged intubation).
  - *Neurogenic:* Laryngeal paralysis.
  - *Miscellaneous:* Tetanus and tetany.
- *Trachea and bronchi:*
  - *Congenital:* Atresia, stenosis, tracheomalacia and tracheobronchial malacia.
  - *Inflammatory:* LTB and bacterial tracheitis.
  - *Neoplastic:* Tumors.
  - *Traumatic:* Foreign body and iatrogenic tracheal stenosis (prolonged intubation and tracheostomy).
- *Secondary external compression:*
  - *Congenital:* Vascular rings, esophageal atresia, tracheoesophageal fistula, congenital goiter and cystic hygroma.
  - *Inflammatory:* Retropharyngeal, parapharyngeal and retroesophageal abscess.
  - *Foreign body:* Esophagus.
  - *Tumors:* Thyroid.

Adults (in addition to the above causes)
- *Infections:* Ludwig's angina, peritonsillar abscess and tongue swelling.
- *Trauma:* Injury of larynx and trachea.
  - Fractures of mandible and maxillofacial injuries.
  - Caustic agent ingestion.
  - Radiation.
- *Neoplasms:* Malignancy of larynx, pharynx, upper trachea, tongue and thyroid.
- *Allergy:* Angioneurotic and drug sensitivity.
- *Obstructive sleep apnea.*

Assessment of Patient with Stridor

If the situation is not acute and does not require immediate intervention, diagnostic assessment must proceed further. Assessment of stridulous child includes focused history and examination and selected investigations involving endoscopy and imaging.

The clinical manifestations of impaired airway may include dyspnea and stridor, voice change (hoarseness), cough, local pain, restlessness, indrawing of intercostals, suprasternal, and supraclavicular spaces, and drooling. Bleeding and subcutaneous emphysema occur in cases of trauma.

- *Severity:* Severity of subcostal, intercostals and suprasternal recession is an indicator of the severity of airway impairment.
- *Cyanosis:* It is a late feature.
- *Nasal patency:* It can be assessed with a mirror, cotton wisp or bell of stethoscope.
- *Jaw and tongue:* Assess the jaw and tongue size.

> **Acute epiglottitis in a child:** Avoid examining a child's throat when epiglottitis is suspected.

Characteristic Features

Impairment in airway affects the feeding particularly in infants. Airway impaired babies typically "come up for air" during the breastfeeding. Bottle fed babies need small hole bottle and thickened feeds. Poor feeding may result in failure to thrive and poor weight gain. The following characteristic features indicate the cause of airway obstruction.

- *Stridor at birth:* Congenital laryngeal web, subglottic stenosis, tracheal narrowing and vocal cord palsy. Dynamic stridor evident in first few weeks of life indicates laryngomalacia.
- *Effect of position:*
  - *Prone position:* Stridor of laryngomalacia, micrognathia, macroglossia and innominate artery compression disappears when baby lies in prone position.
  - *Supine position:* Stridor in supine position occurs with a pedunculated laryngeal mass and micrognathia (results in tongue base occlusion).
- *Effect of crying:*
  - *Improvement:* Airway improvement during crying occurs in gross nasal obstruction, such as bilateral choanal atresia.
  - *Worsening:* In laryngomalacia, stridor is less at rest and during sleep and becomes worse by crying and feeding.
- *Progress:*
  - *A gradual increase in severity of stridor* implies subglottic hemangioma, mediastinal mass and cancer of upper airway.
  - *Rapid progression of airway impairment* with drooling is hallmark of acute epiglottitis, whereas bacterial tracheitis and laryngotracheobronchitis have relatively prolonged course.
- *Fever:* It indicates infective conditions such as laryngitis, epiglottitis, laryngotracheobronchitis or diphtheria.
- *Cough:* It is present in cases of tracheoesophageal fistula and tracheomalacia.
- *Hoarseness:* It suggests laryngeal papillomatosis and vocal cord palsy.
- *Dying spells:* Spells of apneas with cyanosis are common in severe tracheobronchomalacia.
- *Sequential auscultation:* Sequential auscultation with stethoscope over the nose, open mouth, neck and the chest helps in localizing the site of obstruction.
- *Birthmarks:* They are associated with subglottic hemangioma.
- *Sound of stridor:*
  - *Musical quality:* Laryngomalacia
  - *Breathy quality:* Vocal cord palsy
  - *Barking cough:* Tracheomalacia.

> - **Aspirations** occur in cases of vocal cord palsy, tracheoesophageal fistula and cleft larynx.
> - **Micrognathia and Pierre-Robin syndrome:** Stridor is due to falling back of tongue.
> - **Congenital vascular rings:** They cause both stridor and dysphagia.

Investigations

- Oxygen saturation monitoring is required.
  - Arterial blood gases estimation.
- *Endoscopy* and *intubation* in operation theater in cases of suspected epiglottitis.
- *X-ray chest PA view:* Ground glass appearance in bronchopulmonary dysplasia and mediastinal shift in cases of obstructive emphysema due to foreign body.
- *X-ray neck lateral view:* Demonstrate subglottis, oropharynx and nasopharynx.
  - Expiratory and inspiratory films (in older children): Diaphragmatic immobility is seen on the side of foreign body obstruction.
- *Videofluoroscopy* (in young children) for diaphragmatic screening and tracheomalacia.
- *Bronchography* with safer nonionic contrast media—demonstrates tracheobronchial stenosis and malacia.
- *MRI and helical CT:* For tracheal lesions, extrinsic compression and abnormal vasculature.

- **pH probe study:** For pH in upper esophagus and pharynx in cases of gastroesophageal reflux disease.
- **Ultrasound** of vocal cords for vocal cord palsy.

Endoscopy

A careful history, examination and selected needful investigations usually suggest a diagnosis, which needs to be confirmed by endoscopy. *See* Chapter 'Endoscopies'.

- **Flexible nasopharyngolaryngoscopy:** Ultrathin < 2 mm diameter endoscopes allow examination of even neonates without anesthesia. Vocal cord palsy and laryngomalacia can be seen.
- **Laryngotracheobronchoscopy:** This is gold standard in stridulous child assessment.
- **Microlaryngoscopy:** *See* Chapter 'Endoscopies'.
- **Bronchoscopy:** After bronchoscopy, child is intubated and detailed examination of the larynx and esophagus can be done. Larynx is examined again for active movements of vocal cords when the child is coming out of anesthesia and the tube has been removed.

Treatment

In acute cases of airway impairment, following things proceed simultaneously:

- **History taking:** Such as duration and foreign body.
- **Examination:** Such as severity of airway obstruction and oxygen saturation.
- **Active resuscitation:** Such as setting up humidified oxygen and preparation for intubation/tracheostomy. In cases of inadequate ventilation, airway must be secured through either medical or surgical means (Box 43.4). Oral airway helps in managing cases of nasal obstruction due to choanal atresia. Mini tracheostomy handles bronchopulmonary secretions.

> **Box 43.4: Technique and devices to secure an airway**
> - Oral airway
> - Orotracheal intubation
> - Nasotracheal intubation
> - Fiberoptic intubation
> - Laryngeal mask airway
> - Continuous positive airway pressure (CPAP)
> - Ventilating bronchoscope
> - Tracheotomy
> - Mini tracheostomy
> - Cricothyrotomy (laryngotomy)
> - Needle cricothyrotomy
> - Transtracheal needle ventilation
> - Percutaneous dilational tracheostomy
> - Surgical procedures in children to avoid tracheostomy
>   - Cricoid split
>   - Single stage laryngeal reconstruction

Self-evaluation Exercises

1. Aspiration occurs in cases of:
   a. Vocal cord palsy
   b. Tracheoesophageal fistula
   c. Cleft larynx
   d. All of the above
2. Acute stridor in children is mostly caused by:
   a. Laryngotracheobronchitis
   b. Bacterial tracheitis
   c. Acute epiglottitis
   d. Laryngeal foreign bodies
   e. All of the above

True (T)/False (F)

3. Avoid examining a child's throat when epiglottitis is suspected.
4. In micrognathia and Pierre-Robin syndrome, stridor is due to falling back of tongue.
5. Congenital vascular rings will cause stridor and not dysphagia.
6. The most common cause of stridor in adults is laryngitis.
7. If hoarseness persists for more than 3 weeks in an elderly smoker vocal cord nodules should be ruled out.

Answers

1. d
2. e
3. T
4. T
5. F
6. F
7. F

Chapter 44

Infections of Larynx

⊙ Specific Learning Objectives

After going through the chapter, you should be able to answer the following questions:
- How will you differentiate between the acute laryngotracheobronchitis and acute pediatric epiglottitis and manage them?
- What are the differences between adult and pediatric epiglottitis? What do you know about bacterial tracheitis?
- What are the differential diagnoses of edema larynx?

INTRODUCTION

Acute infections (such as croup and epiglottitis) of larynx are mainly seen in children and develop in hours to days. They present with respiratory distress and fever. The chronic infections (such as tuberculosis, leprosy and syphilis) of larynx are mainly seen in adults and exist for weeks to months. They usually present with hoarseness and pain and must be distinguished from malignancy. The list of infections of the larynx is given in Table 44.1.

Etiology/Risk Factors

Following are some etiologic and risk factors of larynx infections:
- Viral infections.
- Bacterial invasion takes place with *Streptococcus pneumoniae*, *Haemophilus influenzae*, *Hemolytic streptococci* and *Staphylococcus aureus*.
- Exanthematous fevers such as measles, mumps, and chickenpox.
- Vocal abuse
- Allergy
- Thermal and chemical burns of larynx due to inhalation and ingestion of hot and corrosive substances.
- Laryngeal trauma due to endotracheal intubation, endoscopy and laryngeal surgery.
- Foreign body
- Cricoarytenoid arthritis due to rheumatoid arthritis, systemic lupus erythematosus and Reiter's syndrome.
- Angioneurotic edema.
- Radiation-induced supraglottitis.

Table 44.1: Infections and manifestations of systemic disease of larynx

Acute infections	Chronic infections	Systemic diseases
Laryngotracheobronchitis	Tuberculosis	Rheumatoid arthritis
Bacterial tracheitis	Syphilis	Systemic lupus erythematosus
Pediatric epiglottitis	Leprosy (Hansen's)	Relapsing polychondritis
Diphtheria	Candidiasis	Sarcoidosis
Adult supraglottitis	Histoplasmosis	Wegener's granulomatosis
Whooping cough		Amyloidosis
Mumps, measles, chickenpox	Cryptococcosis	
	Actinomycosis	

ACUTE LARYNGOTRACHEOBRONCHITIS (LTB) CROUP OR LARYNGOTRACHEITIS

LTB is the most common cause of infectious respiratory obstruction in children.

Etiology/Risk Factors

- Croup is a viral infection (Parainfluenza type I and II and influenza A) and affect usually boys between 3 months and 5 years of age.
- Other uncommon viruses are adenovirus, respiratory syncytial, influenza, and measles viruses.
- Gram-positive cocci infection supervenes soon.
- Family members usually have cold and cough.

Pathology

The swelling of loose areolar tissue in the subglottic region causes airway obstruction and stridor. Thick tenacious secretions and crusts obstruct the airway.

Clinical Features

- The disease begins with symptoms of upper respiratory infection (URI) such as low grade fever, cold and cough.
- After several days of URI symptoms child develops hoarseness and brassy, barking and croupy cough.
- Intermittent inspiratory stridor becomes continuous.
- **Signs of upper airway obstruction:** Nasal flaring, suprasternal, infrasternal and intercostals recession.
- Stridor and dyspnea can lead to hypoxia, hypercapnia, tachycardia, hypoventilation and eventually death.

Diagnosis

X-ray of nasopharynx and neck may show tapered narrowing of the subglottis (steeple sign).

Differential Diagnosis

- **Bacterial tracheitis:** It is the complication of LTB and present with thick purulent respiratory secretions.
- **Epiglottitis:** The characteristic features include abrupt onset of high grade fever, dysphagia, dyspnea, hoarseness and toxic appearance without preceding and family history of flu-like symptoms (Table 44.2).

Treatment

- Following measures prevent laryngeal spasms:
  - Humidification (either hot or cold) softens crusts and tenacious secretions
  - Steam either from a vaporizer or shower
  - Cold steam from a nebulizer.
- **Hospitalization** is needed in cases of airway obstruction, cyanosis, restlessness, depressed sensorium, or toxic appearance.
- **Antibiotics:** Ampicillin (50 mg/kg/day in divided doses) for Gram-positive cocci and *H. influenzae*.
- **Intravenous fluids** for managing dehydration.
- **Steroids:** They reduce edema due to their anti-inflammatory effect, vasoconstriction and reduced vascular permeability.
  - Hydrocortisone 100 mg intravenous
  - Dexamethasone (0.6 mg/kg) intramuscular or oral
  - Nebulized budesonide.
- **Racemic adrenaline** (a mixture of D and L isomer) via nebulizer or respirator helps in reducing edema due to its vasoconstriction action. The child should be monitored for 3 hours (rebound effect) and then allowed to go home. It relieves dyspnea and may avert tracheostomy. Racemic epinephrine has fewer cardiovascular side effects.

Table 44.2: Differences between acute pediatric epiglottitis and laryngotracheobronchitis (LTB)

	Acute epiglottitis	Acute laryngotracheobronchitis
Pathogen	*H. influenzae* type B	Parainfluenza virus type I and II
Common age group	2–7 years	3 months to 5 years
Site of obstruction	Supraglottic larynx	Subglottic larynx
Prodromal flu symptoms	Absent	Present
Onset	Abrupt within hours	Gradual within days
Temperature	High grade	Low grade
Child's appearance	Toxic	Non-toxic
Cough	Usually absent	Barking seal-like
Dysphagia	Severe	Usually absent
Drooling of saliva	Present	Absent
Progression	Rapid	Slow
Family history of URI	Absent	Usually present
X-ray soft tissue neck	Thumb print sign on lateral view	Steeple sign on anteroposterior view

- **Intubation/tracheostomy:** In cases of airway obstruction. Tracheostomy is preferred when intubation is expected longer than 72 hours. Assisted ventilation may be needed. The endotracheal tube should be one size smaller.

PEDIATRIC EPIGLOTTITIS

In this life-threatening condition of children, there is marked edema of epiglottis which obstructs the airway.

Etiology/Risk Factors

- *H. influenzae* type B is the most common causative organism.
- Affects children of 2–7 years of age.
- Immunization against *H. influenzae* type B decreases the prevalence of this disease.

Clinical Features

- Abrupt onset of high grade fever, dysphagia, odynophagia, drooling of saliva, hoarseness of voice and respiratory distress.
- Child may sit upright (tripod position) with hyper-extended neck (Fig. 44.1).
- Inspiratory stridor, nasal flaring and retractions of suprasternal notch, supraclavicular and intercostals' spaces.
- Air hunger can rapidly progress to cyanosis, coma and death.
- Septicemia.

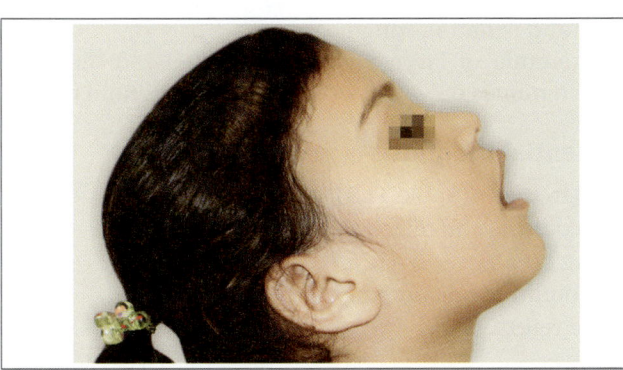

Fig. 44.1: Pediatric epiglottitis. Typical positioning (neck is flexed and head extended) of a child with partial upper airway obstruction

Diagnosis

- Red and swollen (fiery cherry-red) epiglottis and edema and congestion of other supraglottic structures.

Tongue depressor and indirect laryngoscopy examination can cause reflex laryngospasm and cardiorespiratory arrest and are not done in these cases. Laryngoscopic examination is done in OT, where facilities for intubation/tracheostomy are ready.

- ***X-ray soft tissue neck lateral view:*** Shows swollen epiglottis (thumb print sign).
- ***Throat swab and blood culture:*** *H. influenzae* type B can be seen in blood and epiglottis swab.

Differential Diagnosis

Acute LTB: Family members and child usually have preceding history of URI (*see* Table 44.2).

Treatment

- ***Intubation or tracheostomy*** under general anesthesia regardless of severity of respiratory distress is the first and top most priority and required for 1–3 days.
- ***Antibiotics:*** Ampicillin + sulbactam or third generation cephalosporin (cefataxime or ceftriaxone) intravenously is started immediately. They are effective against beta-lactamase positive *H. influenzae*.
- ***Intravenous fluids:*** For adequate hydration.
- ***Steroids:*** Hydrocortisone or dexamethasone IM or IV.
- ***Humidification*** and ***oxygen:*** Mist tent or croupette needed.

ADULT SUPRAGLOTTITIS

In this acute inflammatory condition, there is marked edema of supraglottic structures—epiglottis, aryepiglottic folds and arytenoids.

Etiology

Most common pathogens are *H. influenzae* and beta-hemolytic *streptococcus*.

Clinical Features

- Less acute and less toxic than pediatric epiglottitis.
- Sore throat and dysphagia are most common symptoms.
- Pale, boggy and edematous epiglottis and other supraglottic structures.
- Some patients have stridor, tachycardia or rapid progression and develop epiglottic abscess on lingual surface.
- Some patients develop epiglottic abscess on its lingual surface.

Diagnosis

- ***CBC:*** Leukocytosis
- ***Blood and pharynx culture:*** Usually negative (positive in cases of *H. influenzae*).

DIPHTHERIA

- Children below 10 years of age.
- Usually larynx is involved secondary to faucial diphtheria (*see* Chapter 'Pharyngitis and Adenotonsillar Diseases').

Clinical Features

- ***General:*** Gradual onset, low grade fever, sore throat, malaise, toxic look, tachycardia and thready pulse.
- ***Laryngeal:*** Hoarseness, croupy cough, inspiratory stridor, and increasing dyspnea.
- ***Diphtheritic membrane:*** Gray-white membrane on tonsil, pharynx, soft palate, larynx and trachea. On removal, it leaves a raw bleeding surface. The gray white pseudomembrane in larynx and trachea obstructs airway.
- ***Cervical lymphadenopathy:*** 'Bull-neck' appearance.

Diagnosis

Usually a clinical diagnosis but throat swab smear and culture confirm the diagnosis.

Treatment

- ***Diphtheria antitoxin:*** 100,000 units IV as saline infusion after sensitivity test.
- ***Antibiotics:*** Benzyl penicillin, 500,000 units IM every 6 hours for 6 days. Erythromycin to those who are allergic to penicillin.
- ***Maintenance of airway:***
  - Direct laryngoscopy removal of diphtheritic membrane and intubation to relieve obstruction.
  - Tracheostomy may be required.
- ***Complete bed rest*** for 2–4 weeks to guard against effect of myocarditis.

CHRONIC NONSPECIFIC LARYNGITIS

There are two types of chronic nonspecific laryngitis hyperemic and hypertrophic.

1. **Chronic hyperemic laryngitis:** It is a diffuse inflammatory condition, which symmetrically involves the true cords, ventricular bands, interarytenoid region and root of the epiglottis.
2. **Chronic hypertrophic (hyperplastic) laryngitis:** It may be either diffuse or localized. Localized varieties include dysphonia plica ventricularis; vocal nodules, vocal polyp, Reinke's edema, and contact ulcer.

The pseudostratified ciliated epithelium changes to squamous type. There may be hyperplasia and keratinization (leukoplakia) of squamous epithelium of the vocal cords (*see* Chapter 'Benign Tumors of Larynx').

Etiology/Risk Factors
- Infection in paranasal sinuses, teeth, tonsils and lungs.
- Occupational factors: Exposure to dust and fumes, such as in miners, gold, ironsmiths and chemical industries workers.
- Smoking and alcohol.
- Chronic coughing and clearing of throat.
- Vocal abuse.
- Gastroesophageal reflux disease (GERD).
- Inadequate hydration.

Clinical Features
- Hoarseness and easily tired voice.
- Constant hawking, dryness and intermittent tickling, and clearing the throat repeatedly.
- Discomfort in the throat.
- Dry and irritating cough.
- Hyperemia of larynx; vocal cords dull red; flecks of viscid mucus on vocal cords and interarytenoid region.

Differential Diagnosis
- Tuberculosis (Table 44.3) and leprosy.
- Sarcoidosis and relapsing polychondritis.
- Funguses.
- Autoimmune disorders.
- Acid reflux.
- Cancer.

Biopsy
Tissue should be sent for:
- Usual tissue stains
- Special fungal stains
- Acid-fast bacilli smears
- Fungal and acid-fast bacilli cultures.

> **Pachydermia laryngis:** The only symptom is hoarseness of voice. Diagnosis is made by biopsy, which shows acanthosis and hyperkeratosis. It is not premalignant.

Treatment
- Management of the infections of sinuses, tonsils, teeth and respiratory system (such as bronchitis, bronchiectasis and tuberculosis).
- Avoid smoking, alcohol, pollution, dust and fumes.
- Voice (speech) therapy.
- Steam inhalations.
- Expectorants.
- Management of GERD.

Table 44.3: Distinguishing features of tuberculosis, syphilis, malignancy and chronic nonspecific laryngitis

Features	Tuberculosis larynx	Syphilis larynx	Malignancy larynx	Chronic nonspecific laryngitis
Odynophagia	Severe	Absent	In advanced lesions	Absent
Weight loss	Present	Absent	In advanced lesions	Absent
Voice	Weak aphonic	Rough	Hoarse	Hoarse
Part of larynx affected	Usually arytenoid and interarytenoid region	Anterior one-third	Any part	Vocal cords
Lesion findings	Swelling (mamillated), superficial ragged ulcers, and granulations	Tertiary: Large nodules or deep ulcers; Secondary: diffuse laryngeal hyperemia	Ulcer with everted and irregular margins and induration	Congestion and edema
Sputum for AFB	Positive	Negative	Negative	Negative
VDRL test	Non reactive	Reactive	Non reactive	Non reactive
X-ray chest	Koch's chest	Normal	Cannon balls in advanced lesions (pulmonary metastasis)	Normal

Abbreviation: VDRL—venereal disease research laboratory

ATROPHIC LARYNGITIS (LARYNGITIS SICCA)

Atrophic laryngitis is associated with atrophic rhinitis (see Chapter 'Nasal Manifestation of Systemic Diseases'). There occurs atrophy of laryngeal mucosa and crust formation. It is rare.

Clinical Features
- Hoarseness of voice improves on coughing and removal of crust.
- Dry and irritating cough.
- Dyspnea occasionally due to laryngeal crusts.
- Atrophic mucosa covered with foul smelling crusts. Excoriating and bleeding mucosa on removal of crusts.

Treatment
- Humidification.
- Laryngeal sprays with glucose in glycerin or oil of pine.
- Expectorants containing ammonium chloride or iodides loosen the crusts.

TUBERCULOSIS

Tuberculosis of larynx is usually secondary to pulmonary tuberculosis and affects middle-aged males. The cases of primary tuberculosis of larynx are rare. Tubercle bacilli may reach the larynx by bronchogenic, lymphatic and hematogenous routes.

Pathology
- Tuberculosis involves posterior part of larynx. The common sites in order of decreasing frequency are interarytenoid region, ventricular bands, vocal cords and epiglottis.
- In bronchogenic spread, tubercle bacilli settle and penetrate the interarytenoid region.
- Laryngeal mucosa may become red and swollen due to cellular infiltration (pseudoedema). The submucosal tubercles caseate and ulcerate. Stages of perichondritis and cartilage necrosis are uncommon.

Clinical Features
- Weakness of voice followed by hoarseness is common.
- Severe pain radiating to ears, odynophagia, dysphagia, cough and weight loss.
- *Lesions:* Nonspecific inflammation to nodular, exophytic lesion and mucosal ulceration.
- *Vocal cords:* Hyperemia with impaired adduction (early sign) and mouse nibbled type ulcers.
- *Arytenoid and interarytenoid region:* Swelling (mamillated), superficial ragged ulcers and granulations overlying vocal process of arytenoids.
- *Epiglottis:* Pseudoedema causes 'turban epiglottis'.
- *Ventricular bands and aryepiglottic folds:* Swollen.
- *Mucosa:* Pale.

Turban epiglottis: It is due to the edema and tuberculous infiltration of the epiglottis.

Differential Diagnosis
Syphilis, malignancy and nonspecific chronic laryngitis (see Table 44.3). Biopsy will confirm the diagnosis.

Diagnosis
- *Mantoux test:* Purified protein derivative is usually positive even if there is no pulmonary involvement.
- *X-ray chest PA view:* Pulmonary tuberculosis.
- *Sputum examination:* For acid-fast bacilli and culture and sensitivity.
- *Biopsy:* To exclude carcinoma and distinguish from other condition.

Treatment
It consists of multidrug AKT therapy as per the culture and sensitivity report.

LUPUS

This indolent tubercle infection is usually associated with lupus of nose and pharynx and involves the anterior part of larynx.

Clinical Features
- Painless and usually asymptomatic condition.
- Findings: Lupus nose, involvement of epiglottis (may be completely destroyed), aryepiglottic folds and sometimes ventricular bands.
- Pulmonary tuberculosis: Absent.

Treatment
Antitubercular drugs offer good prognosis.

Lupus: It is a form of tuberculosis that eats away and destroys the epiglottis.

SYPHILIS

Laryngeal syphilis is rare.
- *Secondary syphilis:* Diffuse laryngeal hyperemia or coalescing maculopapular rash of supraglottic region.
- *Tertiary stage:* Diffuse, nodular, gummatous infiltrate. The nodules may ulcerate or coalesce and form larger nodules. The lesions may progress to chondritis, fibrosis and scarring. Laryngeal stenosis can occur.
- Biopsy and serological tests will confirm the diagnosis (see Chapter 'Sensorineural Hearing Loss').

LEPROSY (HANSEN'S DISEASE)

Laryngeal leprosy is a rare condition.

> The larynx is the second most common site of leprosy involvement in head and neck after the nose (ulceration and perforation).

- *Clinical features:*
  - Painless, erythematous or nodular edema of supraglottis extending to glottis.
  - Nodule may enlarge, ulcerate or heal by scar formation, which usually cause laryngeal stenosis.
- *Diagnosis:* Biopsy and nasal smear: Acid-fast staining shows *M. leprae* (Hansen's bacilli) in the foam cells.
- *Treatment:* Oral dapsone alone or with rifampicin are given for 5–10 years (For 1–2 years after the negative biopsy samples).

SCLEROMA

- *Etiology:* This chronic inflammatory disease is caused by *Klebsiella rhinoscleromatis (Frisch bacillus)*. Nose is the most common site of involvement (*see* Chapter 'Nasal Manifestation of Systemic Diseases').
- *Clinical features:*
  - Hoarseness, wheezing and dyspnea are the most common symptoms of laryngeal scleroma.
  - Smooth red swelling in subglottic region.
- *Diagnosis:* Biopsy
- *Treatment:*
  - *Antibiotics:* Streptomycin or tetracycline.
  - *Steroids:* To prevent fibrosis.
  - *Reconstructive surgery:* For subglottic stenosis.

EDEMA OF LARYNX

Edema glottidis refers to edema of the loose mucosa of supraglottic and subglottic regions. Vocal cords have sparse subepithelial connective tissue (*see* 'laryngeal causes of stridor and its treatment' in Chapter 'Laryngeal Symptoms and Examination').

Etiology

- *Infections:* Acute epiglottitis, LTB, laryngeal tuberculosis, syphilis of larynx, complications of parapharyngeal, peritonsillar and retropharyngeal abscesses and Ludwig's angina.
- *Trauma:* Laryngeal trauma, foreign body, thermal or caustic burns, inhalation of irritant gases and fumes.
- *Iatrogenic:* Surgery of tongue, floor of mouth, endoscopies and intubation.
- *Neoplasms:* Larynx and laryngopharynx malignancy.
- *Allergy:* Angioneurotic edema and anaphylaxis.
- *Radiation:* For larynx and pharynx malignancy.
- *Systemic diseases:* Nephritis, heart failure and myxedema.

Diagnosis

- Degree of airway obstruction and respiratory distress depend upon the cause and its severity.
- Inspiratory stridor.
- Indrawing of suprasternal, supraclavicular and intercostals spaces.
- Complete ear, nose and throat examination.
- *Indirect laryngoscopy:* Edema of supraglottic or subglottic region.
- *Direct laryngoscopy:* Needed in some pediatric patients.
- X-ray soft tissue neck.

Treatment

- *Management of the cause.*
- *Steroids:* In cases of epiglottitis, LTB or edema due to trauma, allergy or radiation.
- *Adrenaline* (1:1000) 0.3–0.5 ml IM repeated every 15 minutes if necessary for allergic or angioneurotic edema.
- *Intubation* of larynx or tracheostomy.

Self-evaluation Exercises

1. Which of the following are the facts about the pachydermia laryngis?
   a. Hoarseness of voice
   b. Diagnosis by biopsy, which shows acanthosis and hyperkeratosis
   c. Premalignant condition
   d. All of the above

True (T) or False (F)
2. Acute epiglottitis produces a typical 'Thumb sign' on X-ray soft tissue neck lateral view though it is not usually ordered.
3. Ceftriaxone (cephalosporin) is the first line of antibiotic in the management of acute epiglottitis.
4. In a child with suspected diagnosis of epiglottitis, securing an airway by intubation is the first line of treatment.
5. The child with acute laryngotracheobronchitis presents with stridor and respiratory distress.
6. Though avoided in acute laryngotracheobronchitis, X-ray soft tissue neck PA view shows typical 'steeple sign'.
7. Mouse nibbled appearance of vocal cords is the characteristic feature of laryngeal syphilis.
8. Turban epiglottis is due to the edema and tuberculous infiltration of the epiglottis.
9. Lupus, which is a form of tuberculosis, eats away and destroys the epiglottis.

Filling the blanks
10. Acute epiglottitis is common in children and is caused by _____ type B.
11. Acute laryngotracheobronchitis (croup) is the disease of children and is caused by _____ type 1, 2, and sometimes 3 and produces subglottic edema of larynx.

Answers
1. a, b
2. T
3. T
4. T
5. T
6. T
7. F
8. T
9. T
10. *Haemophilus influenzae*
11. Parainfluenza virus

Chapter 45

Benign Tumors of Larynx

⊙ Specific Learning Objectives

After going through the chapter you should be able to answer the following questions:
- What are the differences between vocal cord nodules and vocal cord polyp and how will you manage them?
- What are the differences between intubation and contact granulomas and how will you manage them?
- What are the differences Rinke's edema and leukplakia of vocal cords and how will you manage them?
- What are the differences between saccular cysts and laryngoceles and how will you manage them?
- What are the differences between solitary and multiple laryngeal papillomas and how will you manage them?

INTRODUCTION

Classification

Benign tumors of the larynx can be divided into three groups—non-neoplastic and neoplastic tumors, and saccular swellings (Table 45.1). The benign neoplastic tumors of the larynx are less common than malignant tumors. Laryngeal papillomas account for approximately 80% of all benign neoplasms of the larynx.

Risk Factors of Non-neoplastic Vocal Fold Mucosal Disorders

Non-neoplastic vocal fold mucosal tumor like masses occur as a result of infection, trauma, allergy, reflux, smoking and degeneration. They are seen more frequently than true benign neoplasms. Their risk factors are:
- ***An expressive and talkative persons:*** Most common
- ***Occupational:*** Extreme vocal demands, which may be related to family life, childcare, politics, religion, athletics, musical rehearsal and performance
- ***Tobacco smoking***
- ***Alcohol***
- ***Insufficient fluid intake***
- ***Infection***
- ***Allergy***
- ***Gastroesophageal reflux disease***
- ***Iatrogenic factors:*** Medicines (dry throat), endotracheal intubation and laryngeal instrumentations.

Table 45.1: Benign tumors of larynx

Non-neoplastic vocal fold mucosal disorders	Neoplastic	Saccular disorders
Vocal nodules	Recurrent respiratory papillomatosis	Ductal cysts
Vocal polyp	Juvenile type	Saccular cysts
Reinke's edema	Adult-onset type	Anterior
Contact ulcer	Chondroma	Lateral
Intubation granuloma	Hemangioma	Laryngopyocele
Leukoplakia	Granular cell tumor	Laryngocele
Amyloid tumors	Glandular tumors	Internal
	Rhabdomyoma	External
	Lipoma	Combined
	Fibroma	

VOCAL NODULES (SINGER'S NODULES)

Risk Factors

- Expressive and talkative persons, teachers, actors, vendors, singers, stock traders and school going children.
- Vocal trauma occurs when persons speak in unnatural low tones or high intensities.
- They are more common in school boys and in women.

Pathology

Vocal abuse or misuse leads to submucosal edema and hemorrhage, which undergo hyalinization and fibrosis. Hyperplasia of overlying epithelium appears as a nodule.

- **Site:** They are bilateral and occur at the area of maximum vibration of the cord. It is at the junction of anterior one-third and posterior two-thirds of the free edge of vocal cord (Fig. 45.1A).

Clinical Features

- *Hoarseness:* Chronic or repeated episodes.
- *Singers' complaints:* Vocal fatigue (reduced vocal endurance), difficulty in singing high notes softly, increased breathness (air escape), roughness, harshness and increased effort for singing.
- *Pain* in the neck on prolonged phonation.
- *Nodules:* Initially appear soft, reddish and edematous, but later on they look grayish or white in color.
- *Size:* Varies from pinhead to half a pea. One side may be bigger than other.

Diagnosis

The subtle nodules affect professional voice users and missed in laryngoscopy. They can be diagnosed with videostroboscopy.

Treatment

- *Medical:* Proper hydration and management of allergy and acid reflux.
- *Voice (speech) therapy:* Educating the patient in proper use of voice. Many early nodules disappear. Postoperative speech therapy prevents recurrence.
- *Surgery:* For chronic refractory or large nodules, precise removal with microdissection techniques is done under operating microscope (microlaryngoscopy). It avoids trauma to vocal ligament and mucosa. Patient is instructed not to speak for 4 days and gradual progression over 6 weeks to full voice.

VOCAL POLYP

Risk Factors

- Intermittent severe voice abuse, work in noisy environment and aspirin.
- Sudden shouting results in hemorrhage and submucosal edema.
- Unilateral hemorrhagic vocal cord polyp is more common in men (30–50 years age).

Clinical Features

- Sudden onset of hoarseness during extreme vocal abuse is the most common presentation.
- Chronic vocal huskiness or intermittent subtle aberrant sounds.
- Diplophonia (double voice) in some patients due to different vibratory frequencies of the two vocal cords.

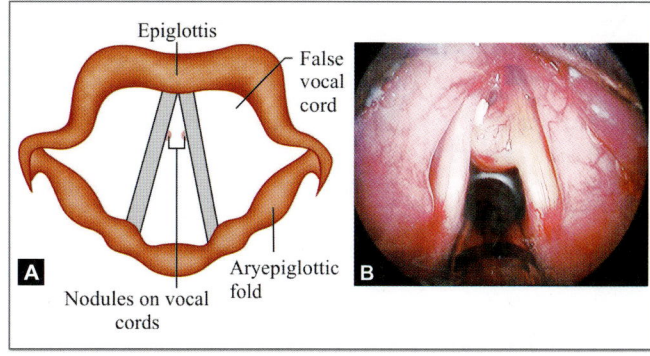

Figs 45.1A and B: (A) Bilateral vocal nodules; (B) Microlaryngoscopy right vocal chord polyp

Courtesy: Prof. Nitin M Nagarkar, AIIMS, Raipur

- Always unilateral at the junction of anterior one-third and posterior two-thirds of the free edge of vocal cord.
- Soft and smooth (dark and hemorrhagic in early stages) and polyp may become pedunculated. It flops up and down the glottis during respiration and phonation (Fig. 45.1B).

Treatment

- *Medical:* Stop anticoagulants and aspirin and manage acid reflux.
- *Voice therapy:* Early polyps may regress totally.
- *Surgery:* Microlaryngoscopic superficial surgical excision followed by speech therapy.

REINKE'S EDEMA (BILATERAL DIFFUSE POLYPOSIS)

Risk Factors

They include vocal abuse and long-term smoking. It is common in middle-aged women.

Pathology

Collection of fluid (edema) occurs in the subepithelial space of Reinke.

Clinical Features

- Female patients may complain of male voice.
- Hypermasculine voice with large polyps.
- Diffuse symmetrical swelling (pale watery bags of fluid) of superior surface and margins of both vocal cords.
- Rule out hypothyroidism.

Treatment

- *Lifestyle changes:* Cessation of smoking.
- *Voice therapy*
- *Microlaryngoscopy:* Polyp reduction with mucosal sparing facilitates epithelialization. Vocal cord stripping can lead to aphonia, high and husky voice. Some surgeons prefer to operate one side cord at a time.

CONTACT ULCER OR GRANULOMA

Risk Factors
- Faulty voice production, male lawyers, ministers, teachers and executives.
- Chronic coughing, throat clearing, psychological stress, conflict.
- Caffeine, alcohol, late-night eating habit and gastric reflux.

Pathology
Vocal processes of arytenoids hammer against each other and result in ulceration and granuloma formation.

Clinical Features
- *Most common symptom:* Unilateral mild pain over midthyroid cartilage. Pain can refer to ear.
- Hoarseness occurs when granuloma is large.
- Constant desire to clear the throat or coughing.
- Usually, unilateral ulcer with whitish exudates or bi-lobed granuloma (may become pedunculated) at the vocal process of arytenoids with congestion of arytenoids mucosa.

Treatment
- Antireflux regimen.
- Voice therapy.
- Injection of depot corticosteroids into lesion.
- Surgery should be the last resort because recurrence is predictable. Surgery consists of limited removal and leaving the base or pedicle undisturbed.

INTUBATION GRANULOMA

Risk Factors
They include rough endotracheal intubation, large tube, prolonged presence of tube between the arytenoids, rigid bronchoscopy and other direct laryngeal manipulation.

Pathology
Injury to vocal processes of arytenoids causes mucosal ulceration (perichondrial abrasions) and granuloma formation over the exposed cartilage. Granulomas usually mature and fall off.

Clinical Features
- Hoarseness is uncommon.
- Dyspnea occurs with large granulomas.
- Granuloma may be sessile to large and pedunculated attached to vocal process of arytenoid. Usually bilateral involving posterior thirds of true cords.
- Posterior glottic incompetence if severe tissue loss.
- Arytenoid fixation or interarytenoid synechium.

Treatment
- Wait and watch with antibiotics for several weeks.
- Speech therapy.
- *Surgery:* Only if conservative treatment fails, and granuloma (mature) persists. Endoscopic corticosteroid injection into the base of granuloma before removal is suggested. Stalk should be left behind. Topical application of mitomycin C may prevent recurrence.

LEUKOPLAKIA OR KERATOSIS
- *Risk factors:* Chronic laryngeal irritants.
- *Pathology:* The epithelial hyperplasia appears as a white plaque or warty growth and involves upper surface of either one or both vocal cords. It does not affect mobility of cord. In this precancerous condition, carcinoma in situ frequently supervenes.
- *Clinical features:*
  - Hoarseness
  - White plaque or warty growth on the upper surface of either one or both vocal cords.
- *Treatment:* Microlaryngoscopy stripping of vocal cords is needed. Histopathological examination of the tissues rules out any malignant change.

AMYLOID TUMORS
- Most patients are men in the age group of 50–70.
- Presents as a smooth plaque or a pedunculated mass.
- *Diagnosis:* Histopathology.
- *Treatment:* Microlaryngoscopic surgical excision.

> *Benign lesions of posterior larynx:* The conditions affecting posterior part of larynx include contact ulcer, pachydermia of larynx and intubation granuloma.

DUCTAL CYSTS
Blockage of ducts of seromucinous glands of laryngeal mucosa results in these retention cysts.

Common Sites
They include vallecula, aryepiglottic fold, false cords, ventricles and pyriform fossa.

Clinical Features
- Usually remain asymptomatic for long time and seen incidentally during examination.
- Hoarseness, cough, throat pain and dyspnea may occur in cases of very large cysts.
- An intracordal cyst presents with hoarseness similar to an epidermoid inclusion cyst.

Treatment

Marsupialization/removal in symptomatic patients.

SACCULAR CYSTS

Retention of secretion and distension of saccule occurs due to obstruction to the orifice of saccule and presents as a cyst in laryngeal ventricle.

Types

There are two types of saccular cysts—anterior and lateral.
- *Anterior saccular cyst* is small and present in the anterior part of ventricle and obscure anterior part of vocal cord.
- *Lateral saccular cyst* is large and may extend into the false cord, aryepiglottic fold and pyriform fossa and may appear in the neck through thyrohyoid membrane.
- *Laryngopyocele:* It is an infected lateral saccular cyst.

Clinical Features

- *Infants* with congenital lateral saccular cysts present with weak cry and stridor and cyanosis. Dysphagia may occur.
- *In adults* hoarseness is most common symptom.

Diagnosis

X-ray soft tissue neck lateral view and CT will confirm the diagnosis.

Treatment

- Endoscopic aspiration, marsupialization or CO_2 laser vaporization.
- *External approach for large lateral cysts:* Midline or lateral thyrotomy approach through thyrohyoid membrane.

LARYNGOCELE

Risk Factors

Trumpet players, glass-blowers and weight lifters.

Pathology

This air filled cystic swelling is dilatation of the saccule. It is said to arise from raised transglottic air pressure. There are three types of laryngocele; internal, external and combined or mixed (Fig. 45.2).
- *Internal:* It remains confined within larynx and presents as distension of false cord and aryepiglottic fold.
- *External:* Here distended saccule herniates through the thyrohyoid membrane and presents in neck. It produces a swelling in the neck on Valsalva and communicates with laryngeal ventricle. It can be seen on CT.
- *Combined or mixed:* Swellings can be seen both in the larynx, as well as outside in neck.

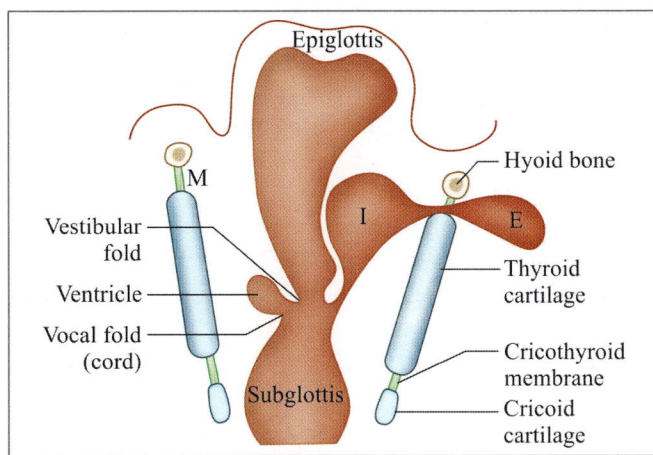

Fig. 45.2: Mixed type laryngocele showing internal (I) and external (E) components and their relations with thyrohyoid membrane (M)

Clinical Features

- Hoarseness and swelling in neck are common.
- Other symptoms in decreasing order of frequency include airway obstruction, dysphagia, sore throat, snoring and coughing.
- *External laryngocele:* Reducible swelling in the neck that increases in size on coughing and valsalva.

Diagnosis

X-ray soft tissue neck PA and lateral views with valsalva and CT scan show the presence and the extent of laryngocele.

Treatment

- Surgical excision through an external approach neck incision.
- Endoscopic marsupialization of an internal laryngocele.

- **Bryce's sign:** It is the gurgling sound produced on pressing the swelling of laryngocele.
- **Laryngocele in elderly persons:** Rule out saccule carcinoma because it can cause and present as laryngocele, which must be ruled out.

RECURRENT RESPIRATORY PAPILLOMATOSIS

Etiology

The disease is the response to mucosal infection by human papillomavirus (HPV) of the Papova class (subtype 6 and 11). They are of two types—juvenile and adult-onset. Juvenile variety is more common than adult-onset.

Juvenile Papillomas

- Patients are infants and young children.
- Papillomas are multiple and aggressive and involve wide area. They are rapidly recurrent.

- They are mostly seen on the true and false cords and the epiglottis. They can involve trachea and bronchi.
- They may spontaneously regress after puberty. They often recur and need multiple laryngoscopic removals.

Adult-Onset Papilloma

- Papilloma is usually smaller and limited to one site.
- They are usually less aggressive and do not recur.
- Most patients are males in the age group of 30–50 years.
- The most common sites are anterior half of vocal cord and anterior commissure.

Clinical Features

- Hoarseness and stridor (in juvenile type) are the most common presentations.
- Appear as glistening white irregular growths, which may be pedunculated or sessile.

Treatment

- Endoscopic removal under operative microscope can be done with
    - Cup forceps
    - Cryotherapy
    - Microelectrocautery
    - CO_2 laser offers precision and less bleeding
    - **Microdebrider:** It is helpful as the papillomas are friable and bleed while removing.

Other techniques, which are being tried and giving encouraging results include:
- Interferon therapy
- Indole-3-carbinol, derived from cabbage and broccoli
- Methotrexate
- Intralesional cidofovir
- 585 nm pulsed dye laser
- Photodynamic therapy
- Radiation
- Vaccines.

Multiple juvenile laryngeal papillomatosis:
- CO_2 laser is the best laser for multiple laryngeal papillomas.
- No modality of treatment can prevent recurrence.
- Malignant change is uncommon unless radiation has been used as a mode of treatment.

CHONDROMA

The clinical behaviors of chondroma and low-grade chondrosarcoma are similar.
- Mostly arise from cricoid cartilage and seen in subglottic region.
- Dyspnea common
- Dysphagia and sense of lump in throat when large tumor grows outward from the lamina of cricoid cartilage.
- Most patients are men in the age group of 40–60 years.

Laryngeal cartilaginous tumor: Cricoid cartilage is the most common site of laryngeal cartilaginous tumor.

HEMANGIOMA

There are two types: capillary and cavernous.

Infantile Hemangioma (Capillary)
- *Site:* Subglottic area.
- *Presentation:* Stridor in the first 6 months of life.
- *Associated findings:* Half of the children have hemangiomas on other parts of body particularly in head and neck region.
- *Prognosis:* Usually involutes spontaneously.
- *Treatment:* Steroids and tracheostomy in cases of respiratory obstruction. Vaporized with CO_2 laser.

Adult Hemangiomas (Cavernous)
- *Site:* Supraglottic larynx.
- *Treatment:* If asymptomatic no treatment. Steroid or radiation therapy may be employed. It cannot be treated with laser.

Self-evaluation Exercises

1. The most common site of vocal cord nodules is the:
    a. Junction of anterior and middle third
    b. Junction of posterior and middle third
    c. Middle part
    d. All of the above
2. Benign lesions affecting posterior part of larynx include:
    a. Contact ulcer
    b. Pachydermia of larynx
    c. Intubation granuloma
    d. All of the above

Contd...

Contd…

3. Which of the following are related with external laryngocele:
   a. Produces a swelling in the neck on Valsalva
   b. Communicates with laryngeal ventricle
   c. Seen on CT
   d. All of the above
4. The causes of vocal process ulcer include:
   a. Intubation injury
   b. Laryngopharyngeal acid reflux
   c. Adductor dysphonia
   d. All of the above
5. Multiple juvenile laryngeal papillomatosis is a pediatric benign tumor of larynx that is caused by:
   a. Herpes simplex
   b. Herpes zoster
   c. Human papillomavirus
   d. Epstein-Barr virus

True (T) or False (F)

6. The most common site of vocal cord nodules is the maximum vibratory area during speech.
7. Recurrence in multiple juvenile laryngeal papillomatosis is common and repeated excisions may be required and no modality of treatment can prevent recurrence.
8. Malignant change in multiple juvenile laryngeal papillomatosis is uncommon unless radiation has been used as a mode of treatment.
9. Bryce's sign is the gurgling sound produced on pressing the swelling of laryngocele.

Filling the blanks

10. _____ cartilage is the most common site of laryngeal cartilaginous tumor.
11. Laryngocele arises as a herniation of laryngeal mucosa from the saccule of the laryngeal ventricle through the _____ membrane.
12. _____ edema is usually associated with smoking and causes diffuse polypoid degeneration of vocal cords.
13. _____ laser is the best laser for the treatment of multiple laryngeal papillomas.

Answers

1. a	2. d	3. d	4. d	5. c	6. T
7. T	8. T	9. T	10. Cricoid	11. thyrohyoid	12. Reinke's
13. CO_2					

Chapter 46

Neurologic Disorders of Larynx

⊙ Specific Learning Objectives

After going through the chapter, you should be able to answer the following questions:
- What are the causes of different types of laryngeal palsies?
- How will you manage the unilateral and bilateral recurrent laryngeal nerve paralysis?
- How will you manage the unilateral and bilateral complete paralysis of larynx?
- How will you manage the unilateral and bilateral superior laryngeal nerve paralysis?
- What are the different phonosurgical procedures?

CLASSIFICATION OF LARYNGEAL PARALYSIS

Laryngeal paralysis may be divided into following categories:
- Congenital or acquired
- Unilateral or bilateral
- Complete or incomplete
- Abductor or adductor or both
- Sensory or motor or both

The nerve supply of larynx is discussed in detail in the Chapter 'Anatomy and Physiology of Larynx'.

POSITIONS OF VOCAL CORDS

Though not considered reliable indicator of lesion site, five positions of the vocal cords are traditionally described (Fig. 46.1).
- ***Median position:*** Vocal cord is in midline position such as in phonation. It may occur in recurrent laryngeal nerve (RLN) paralysis.
- ***Paramedian position:*** *Vocal cord is 1.5 mm away from midline such as in strong whisper.* It may occur in RLN paralysis.
- ***Intermediate (cadaveric) position:*** This is the neutral position of cricoarytenoid joint. Vocal cord is 3.5 mm away from the midline. Abduction and adduction take place from this position. This occurs when both recurrent and superior laryngeal nerves are paralyzed.
- ***Gentle abduction:*** Vocal cord is 7 mm away from midline such as during quiet respiration and paralysis of adductors.

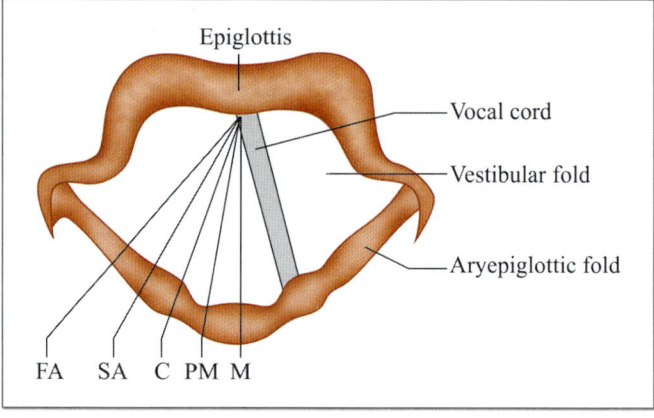

Fig. 46.1: Vocal cord positions

Keys: M, Median; PM, Paramedian; C, Cadaveric (Interme-diate); SA, Slight abduction; FA, Full abduction

- ***Full abduction:*** Vocal cord is 9.5 mm away from midline such as in deep inspiration.

Glottic Chink
- In cadaveric position of the vocal cords, vocal chink is 7 mm.
- In full abduction it is about 19 mm.

CAUSES OF LARYNGEAL PARALYSIS

In about 30% of cases no cause (idiopathic) can be ascertained even after thorough investigations. The causes of laryngeal paralysis are following:

- **Supranuclear (rare):** Strokes, tumor and trauma. Diffuse emboli in cerebral cortex may cause sustained abduction (aphonia) or inappropriate adduction (inspiratory stridor).
- **Nuclear (nucleus ambiguus in medulla):** Usually associated with paralysis of other cranial nerves.
  - Strokes
  - Tumors
  - Motor neuron disease
  - Polio
  - Syringobulbia
- **Vagus nerve**
  - **Intracranial**
    - Tumors of posterior fossa
    - Basal meningitis (tubercular)
  - **Jugular foramen (skull base)**
    - Fractures
    - Nasopharyngeal cancer
    - Glomus tumor
  - **Parapharyngeal space (neck)**
    - Penetrating injury
    - Parapharyngeal tumor
    - Metastatic nodes
    - Lymphoma
- **Recurrent laryngeal nerve (RLN) or low vagal trunk**
  - Neck trauma
  - Thyroid diseases and surgery
  - Cervical esophagus cancer
  - Cervical lymphadenopathy
  - Lung apex cancer
  - Cervical pleura tuberculosis
  - **Mediastinal lesions (left side only)**
    - Bronchogenic cancer
    - Thoracic esophagus cancer
    - Aortic aneurysm
    - Lymphadenopathy
    - Left atrial hypertrophy or dilatation
    - Intrathoracic surgery
- **Systemic causes**
  - Diabetes
  - Syphilis
  - Diphtheria
  - Typhoid
  - Streptococcal
  - Viral infections
  - Lead poisoning.

> **Vocal cord palsy**
> - Most common type of vocal cord palsy is recurrent laryngeal nerve palsy.
> - Because of the intrathoracic course of left recurrent laryngeal nerve left vocal cord palsy is twice more common than right vocal cord palsy.

UNILATERAL RECURRENT LARYNGEAL NERVE (RLN) PARALYSIS

- It leads to paralysis of all the intrinsic laryngeal muscles except the cricothyroid, which is supplied by the external branch of superior laryngeal nerve.
- The vocal cord may assume a median or paramedian position and does not move laterally (abduction) on deep inspiration.
- **Semon's law** states that in all progressive organic lesions, abductor fibers of the nerve, which are phylogenetically newer, are more susceptible than adductors that are phylogenetically older. So abductors are first to be paralyzed.
- **Wagner and Grossman hypothesis** states that cricothyroid muscle (supplied by external branch of superior laryngeal nerve), which has adduction function, keeps the cord in paramedian position.

Etiology

Bronchogenic carcinoma is a common cause. It is confirmed by X-ray chest, bronchoscopy and biopsy. It leads to left RLN paralysis. *See* also 'Etiology' Section.

> **Superior mediastinum tumor**
> - It impinges upon the arch of aorta and compresses left vagus nerve just before the origin of left RLN.
> - Hoarseness of voice is due to the left vocal cord palsy.

Clinical Features

- About one-third of the patients remain asymptomatic.
- Changes in voice gradually improve due to compensation. Healthy cord crosses the midline to meet the paralyzed cord.
- No problems of aspiration or airways obstruction occur.

> **Ortner's syndrome:** Paralysis of left RLN in cardiomegaly.

Treatment

Cases are asymptomatic and no treatment is required.

BILATERAL RECURRENT LARYNGEAL NERVE (ABDUCTOR) PARALYSIS

Etiology

Most common causes are neuritis and thyroid surgery.

Clinical Features

- The condition is often acute.
- Most common symptoms—dyspnea and stridor. They become worse on exertion and infection.
- Voice is good. There is no hoarseness.
- Vocal cords lie in median or paramedian position.

Treatment

For the treatment of dyspnea and stridor, these patients need surgery. Patient is treated with either permanent tracheostomy with a speaking valve or lateralization of the cord. Many patients need emergency tracheostomy when they suffer from upper respiratory tract infection.

- *Tracheostomy:* It relieves stridor and preserves voice, but tracheostomy needs regular care.
- *Lateralization of the cord:* In this surgery, vocal cord is moved and fixed in a lateral position. Though patient does not have tracheostomy, but it is at the expense of a good voice. The methods of lateralization of vocal cord are following:
  - *Arytenoidectomy (external approach or endoscopic):* Arytenoid cartilage is excised and the cord is fixed in a lateral position.
  - *Thyroplasty Type 2* (see 'Phonosurgery' Section).
  - *Endoscopic laser cordectomy (kashima operation):* This is usually accomplished with CO_2 laser.
  - *Nerve muscle implant:* Sternohyoid muscle with its nerve supply has been transplanted into the paralyzed posterior cricoarytenoid to bring some movement to the cord. The results are not encouraging.

UNILATERAL SUPERIOR LARYNGEAL NERVE (SLN) PARALYSIS

Isolated lesions of SLN are rare. They cause paralysis of cricothyroid and anesthesia of the supraglottic larynx.

Etiology

The involvement of external laryngeal nerve (branch of SLN) occurs in cases of thyroid surgery, tumors, neuritis or diphtheria. It causes cricothyroid paralysis.

Clinical Features

- *Weak and low pitch voice.*
- *Occasional aspiration:* Unilateral anesthesia of the larynx may pass unnoticed.
- *Askew position of glottis* (anterior commissure rotated to healthy side).
- *Shortening of vocal cord* with loss of tension (wavy appearance of paralyzed vocal cord).
- *Flapping of paralyzed vocal cord* (sags down during inspiration and bulges up during expiration).

BILATERAL SUPERIOR LARYNGEAL NERVE PARALYSIS

In this uncommon condition, both side cricothyroid get paralyzed along with anesthesia of supraglottis.

Etiology

- Surgical and accidental trauma.
- Neuritis (mostly diphtheria).
- Pressure by enlarged cervical nodes and neoplasms.

Clinical Features

- Episodes of coughing and choking during swallowing.
- Inhalation of food and pharyngeal secretions.
- Weak and husky voice.

Treatment

Neuritis cases may recover spontaneously. Chronic and repeated aspiration needs surgical management.

- Tracheostomy with a cuffed tube.
- Esophageal feeding tube.
- Epiglottopexy (a reversible procedure) closes laryngeal inlet and protects lungs from repeated aspiration.

UNILATERAL COMBINED (COMPLETE) PARALYSIS OF RECURRENT AND SUPERIOR LARYNGEAL NERVE

There occurs unilateral paralysis of all laryngeal muscles except the interarytenoid, which receives innervation from both the sides.

Etiology

- In thyroid surgery, both recurrent and external laryngeal nerves of one side may be damaged.
- Lesions of nucleus ambiguous lie in the medulla and posterior cranial fossa.
- Lesions of the vagus nerve proximal to the origin of superior laryngeal nerve in jugular foramen and parapharyngeal space.

The healthy cord is unable to approximate the paralyzed cord, which lies in cadaveric position, and results in hoarseness of voice and aspiration.

Clinical Features

- Hoarseness of voice.
- Aspiration of liquids through the glottis.
- Paralyzed vocal cord in cadaveric position.
- Glottic incompetence.
- Ineffective cough due to air waste.

Treatment

- *Speech therapy:* The healthy cord may compensate by moving across the midline and approximate paralyzed vocal cord.
- *Medialization of paralyzed vocal cord:*
  - *Injection* of teflon paste, collagen, autologous fat, or collagen derivative is injected lateral to the paralyzed cord endoscopically or transcervically.
  - *Thyroplasty type 1* (see 'Phonosurgery' Section).

- **Muscle or cartilage implant** is done through the laryngofissure approach. Bipedicled muscle graft or piece of cartilage is inserted between thyroid cartilage and vocal cord. The graft pushes the cord medially.
- **Arthrodesis of cricoarytenoid joint.** Through laryngofissure approach, arytenoid cartilage is rotated medially and fixed with a screw.

BILATERAL COMBINED (COMPLETE) PARALYSIS OF RECURRENT AND SUPERIOR LARYNGEAL NERVE

In this rare condition, there occurs total anesthesia of the larynx and all laryngeal muscles are paralyzed and both vocal cords lie in cadaveric position.

Clinical Features

- *Aphonia:* Vocal cords do not approximate.
- *Aspiration:* Because off incompetent glottis and laryngeal anesthesia.
- *Inability to cough:* It results in retention of secretions in the lungs.
- *Bronchopneumonia:* It occurs because of repeated aspirations and retention of secretions.

Patient will present with complete loss of speech, but there will be no difficulty in breathing because the vocal cords lie in cadaveric position.

Treatment

Surgical treatment is required to prevent aspiration.

Reversible surgeries

- *Tracheostomy:* Facilitates removal of pulmonary secretions and inhaled material.
- *Epiglottopexy:* Epiglottis is folded backwards and fixed to the arytenoids.
- *Vocal cord plication:* Through the laryngofissure approach, true and false cords are approximated with sutures after removing their mucosa.
- *Laryngotracheal separation*
- *Tracheoesophageal diversion*
- *Endolaryngeal stent*
- *Partial cricoidectomy*
- *Vertical laryngoplasty*

Irreversible surgeries

- *Total laryngectomy:* Indicated in cases of progressive and irreversible lesions and when speech is unserviceable.
- Subperichondrial cricoidectomy.
- Glottic closure.

Tracheal division and permanent tracheostome is the "Gold standard" surgical treatment for prevention of aspiration.

CONGENITAL VOCAL CORD PARALYSIS

Laryngomalacia is the most common cause of neonatal stridor. Vocal fold palsy is the second common cause of neonatal stridor.

Congenital unilateral paralysis is more common than bilateral. Bilateral palsy children have features of bilateral abductor such as respiratory distress and need tracheostomy.

Etiology

- Idiopathic
- Unilateral
    - Birth trauma: Intracerebral hemorrhage
    - Congenital anomaly of a great vessel or heart
- Bilateral paralysis
    - Hydrocephalus
    - Arnold-Chiari malformation
    - Meningitis
    - Cerebral or nucleus ambigus agenesis.

Clinical Features

- The high-pitched inspiratory and biphasic musical stridor.
- The cry is week.

Diagnosis

- *Awake flexible laryngoscopy* will confirm the diagnosis.
- *Magnetic resonance imaging (MRI) brain scan:* To rule out Arnold-Chiari malformations.

Treatment

About 70% noniatrogenic unilateral vocal fold palsies and 50% children of bilateral vocal cord palsies improves spontaneously.

- Tracheostomy is needed in 73% of the patients.
- Feeding can be done through slow flow nipple or nasogastric tube.
- For severe aspiration and dysphonia in unilateral palsy.
    - Injection of vocal fold with absorbable gelatin sponge (gelfoam) or polytetrafluoroethylene (teflon).
    - Medialization laryngoplasty (thyroplasty).
- For bilateral palsy
    - Endoscopic lateral cordotomy
    - *Arytenoidectomy:* Endoscopic or external approach.
    - *Arytenoidopexy:* External cervical approach.
    - Expand cricoid cartilage posteriorly with costal cartilage graft.

PHONOSURGERY

These surgical procedures improve the quality of voice.

Microlaryngeal Surgery

Excision of vocal cord lesions is done with microlaryngeal surgery or laser (*see* Chapter 'Endoscopies').

Local Injections

Injection of teflon paste, collagen, autologous fat, collagen derivative or gelfoam can be used to medialize and augment the vocal cord. Injections may be given percutaneous or transorally under the guidance of flexible laryngoscope or through microlaryngoscopy.

Laryngeal Framework Surgery (Thyroplasty)

Isshiki described four types of thyroplasty procedures, which produce functional alteration of vocal cords.

1. *Type I thyroplasty:* Medial displacement of vocal cord to improve voice quality.
2. *Type II thyroplasty:* Lateral displacement of vocal cord to improve the airway.
3. *Type III thyroplasty:* Shortening or relaxation of the vocal cord. Relaxed vocal cord lowers the pitch. The surgery is usually done in cases of mutational falsetto or gender transformation (female to male).
4. *Type IV thyroplasty:* Lengthening or tensioning of the vocal cord to elevate the pitch. Male character voice becomes female character. This procedure is done in cases of gender transformation, lax vocal cord, and vocal cord bowing due to aging or trauma.

Laryngeal Reinnervation Procedures

Through a window in thyroid cartilage, a segment of superior belly of omohyoid muscle along with its nerve (ansa hypoglossi) and vessels is implanted into the thyroarytenoid muscle. This procedure is supposed to innervate the paralyzed thyroarytenoid muscle.

Reconstructive and Rehabilitative Procedure

They are needed after tumor resection.

Self-evaluation Exercises

1. Which of the followings do not relate with superior mediastinum tumor?
    a. It impinges upon the arch of aorta
    b. Compresses left vagus nerve just before the origin of left recurrent laryngeal nerve
    c. Hoarseness of voice
    d. Left vocal cord palsy
    e. None of the above

True (T) or False (F)

2. In cadaveric position of the vocal cords, vocal chink is 7 mm and in full abduction it is about 19 mm.
3. During the whisper, the position of vocal cord is median.
4. Because of the intrathoracic course of recurrent laryngeal nerve left vocal cord palsy is twice more common than right vocal cord palsy.
5. Patient with combined paralysis of bilateral vocal cords will present with complete loss of speech, but there will be no difficulty in breathing because the vocal cords lie in cadaveric position.
6. Tracheal division and permanent tracheostome is the 'Gold standard' surgical treatment for prevention of aspiration.

Filling the blanks

7. Vocal cord palsy is commonly caused by lesions of _____ laryngeal nerve.
8. Paralysis of left recurrent laryngeal nerve in cases of cardiomegaly is called _____ syndrome.
9. Matching
    i. Thyroplasty Type I   a. Lateralization of vocal cord
    ii. Thyroplasty Type II   b. Lengthening (tightening) of vocal cord
    iii. Thyroplasty Type III c. Medialization of vocal cord
    iv. Thyroplasty Type IV   d. Shortening (relaxing) in length of vocal cord

Answers

1. e 2. T 3. F 4. T 5. T 6. T
7. Recurrent 8. Ortner's 9. i. c, ii. a, iii. d, iv. b

Chapter 47

Speech and Voice Disorders

> ### Specific Learning Objectives
> After going through the chapter, you should be able to answer the following questions:
> - What are the differences between ventricular dysphonia and puberphonia and how will you manage them?
> - What are the different types of spasmodic dysphonias and how would you manage them?
> - How will you manage a case of stuttering?
> - What do you know about: (1) Hysterical aphonia; (2) Phonasthenia; (3) Rhinolalia clausa; (4) Rhinolalia aperta?

Causes and evaluation of hoarseness of voice has been covered in Chapter 'Laryngeal Symptoms and Examination'.

DYSPHONIA PLICA VENTRICULARIS (VENTRICULAR DYSPHONIA)

In this condition ventricular folds (false cords) take over the function of true cords.

Etiology
- *Secondary:* In cases of impaired function of the true cord (paralysis, fixation, surgical excision and tumors), ventricular bands try to compensate phonatory function of true cords.
- *Functional:* Psychogenic.

Clinical Features
- *Voice*: Rough, low-pitched and unpleasant voice.
- *In functional cases:* In beginning voice is normal, but becomes rough later when false cords takes over the function of true cords.

Laryngoscopy
False cords approximate partially or completely on phonation and obscure the view of true cords.

Treatment
- *Secondary:* Ventricular dysphonia is difficult to treat.
- *Functional type:* Voice therapy and psychological counseling.

- *Broca's aphasia (motor or nonfluent aphasia):* The lesion lies near the primary motor cortex of dominant cerebral hemisphere. Patient's speech lacks rhythm and is reduced to the use of nouns and verbs in the wrong tense. Patient can hear and understand the speech. Patient can repeat single words, but not a full sentence. Patient's may have associated weaknesses in right lower face and right upper limb.
- *Wernicke aphasia (sensory or fluent aphasia):* Patient cannot comprehend the spoken word. Patient looks at the doctor as if s/he does not understand what the doctor is saying. So patient is mistaken as a case of hearing loss. Though patient's speech is intact, but usually it does not make any sense because of the misuse of words. Patient is not aware of his speech or comprehension problems.
- *Conductive aphasia:* Patient cannot repeat examiner's commands. The speech is fluent and comprehension remains intact. The lesion is in the arcuate fasciculus, which connects the Wernicke and Broca areas.

FUNCTIONAL (HYSTERICAL) APHONIA

- Usually seen in emotionally labile young females.
- This sudden onset aphonia is not associated with other laryngeal symptoms.
- Patient is usually able to whisper.
- *Laryngoscopy:* Vocal cords remain in abducted position and fail to adduct on phonation. The adduction of vocal cords occurs on coughing and sound of cough is good.
- *Treatment:* Reassurance and psychotherapy.

PUBERPHONIA (MUTATIONAL FALSETTO VOICE)

Failure in the change of childhood high-pitched voice to low-pitched male voice after puberty in boys is called **puberphonia**. However, the boy's physical and sexual developments are normal.

- **Pertinent anatomy:** After puberty, male larynx grows rapidly. Increase in length of vocal cords brings change in character of male voice. The female larynx changes a little.
- **Risk factors:** These boys are emotionally immature, feel insecure and show excessive fixation to their mother or sister. Psychologically, these boys try to avoid male responsibilities.

Treatment

- **Speech therapy and psychotherapy.**
- **Gutzman's pressure test:** The thyroid prominence is pressed in a backward and downward direction. It relaxes the overstretched cords and low tone voice is produced. In this way boy can learn to produce low tone voice and trains himself to produce syllables, words and sentences.
- **Prognosis** is usually good.

PHONASTHENIA

This is fatigue of phonatory muscles (thyroarytenoid and interarytenoid) and results in weakness of voice.

Risk Factors

Abuse or misuse of voice or after laryngitis.

Clinical Features

- Easy fatigability of voice.
- Indirect laryngoscopy findings on saying 'eeee':
  - **Thyroarytenoid weakness:** Elliptical space between the cords.
  - **Interarytenoid weakness:** Triangular gap near the posterior commissure.
  - **Weakness of both thyroarytenoid and interarytenoid:** Keyhole appearance of glottis due to combination of both elliptical space between the cords and triangular gap near the posterior commissure.

Treatment

- Voice rest and vocal hygiene.
- Periods of voice rest after excessive use of voice.

HYPONASALITY (RHINOLALIA CLAUSA)

Blockage of the nose or nasopharynx results in lack of nasal resonance in voice and is called **hyponasality**.

Etiology

- Rhinosinusitis
- Allergic and non-allergic rhinitis
- Nasal masses such as polyps and tumors
- Nasopharyngeal mass and adenoids
- Familial or habitual speech pattern.

HYPERNASALITY (RHINOLALIA APERTA)

The failure of the nasopharynx to cut off from oropharynx or undue passage between the oral and nasal cavities results in nasal resonance of all the words (even those words, which have little nasal resonance).

Etiology

- Velopharyngeal insufficiency:
  - Short soft palate: Submucous fibrosis
  - Cleft palate or submucous cleft palate
  - Paralysis of soft palate
  - Palatal perforation
  - After improper adenoidectomy
- Oronasal fistula
- Familial or habitual speech pattern.

SPASMODIC DYSPHONIA

Dystonia is action induced abnormal involuntary movements. Spasmodic dysphonia (focal dystonia of larynx) is an action induced laryngeal motion disorder.

Synonyms

Spastic dysphonia, spastic aphonia, phonic laryngeal spasm and coordinated laryngeal spasm.

Types

1. **Adductor:** Irregular hyperadduction of vocal folds.
2. **Abductor:** Intermittent abduction of vocal folds.
3. **Mixed type:** Combination of adductor and abductor.

Clinical Features

- The vocal cords are usually normal at rest but function abnormally with speaking.
- Reduced loudness of voice.
- Decreased speech intelligibility.
- Symptoms worsen is under stress or on telephone.
- **Factors improving symptom:**
  - Pinching of nose
  - Pressing the hand against the back of the head or into abdomen
  - Pulling on ear
  - Yawning, sneezing, singing, yelling, or humming.

Adductor Spasmodic Dysphonia

Abnormal involuntary co-contraction of the vocalis muscle results in inappropriate adduction of the vocal folds.

- Choked, strained, strangled and monotonal voice.
- Abrupt initiation and termination result in short breaks.
- Slow and harsh speech.
- Occasionally, compensatory pseudoabductor spasmodic dysphonia compensates for severe adductor laryngeal spasms by whispering.

Abductor Spasmodic Dysphonia

Abnormal co-contraction of the posterior cricoarytenoid results in inappropriate abduction of the vocal cords.
- Breathy and effortful voice.
- Abrupt termination results in aphonic whispered segments of speech.

Treatment

- Voice therapy.
- Alcohol, sedatives and tranquilizers provide transient improvement. Generally medical treatment is of little avail.
- Sectioning the recurrent laryngeal nerve.
- Selective denervation and reinnervation using the ansa cervicalis nerve.
- Thyroarytenoid myotomy.
- Injections of botox or collagen.

STUTTERING

Stuttering is a neurologic movement disorder in which abnormal, involuntary and inappropriate use of the speech muscles results in dysfluency. Stuttering is a result of increased muscle tension in the three subsystems of speech—respiratory, phonatory and articulatory. Muscles move too quickly and too far. Other cranial musculature (such as eyelids and muscles of facial expression) may also inappropriately contract.

Risk Factors

Too much attention or reprimands to childhood dysfluency between 2–4 years.

Prevention
Educate parents need not to overreact to child's dysfluency in early stages of speech development.

Clinical Features

- Characterized by hesitation to initiate, repetitions, prolongations or blocks in speech flow.
- Development of secondary mannerisms such as facial grimacing, eye blink or abnormal head movements.

Factors Relieving Stuttering

- Emotional arousal or sensory stimuli.
- Motor actions such as walking.
- Use of rhythmic patterns (metronome/monotone).
- Singing or speaking in a sing-song voice.
- Shouting.
- Foreign accent or slurred articulation.

Factors Aggravating Stuttering

The factors which may increase stuttering, include communicative pressures such as public speeches, personal interviews, counseling and meaningful negotiations.

Treatment

- Speech therapy and training
- Antidepressants though given are of no value.
- Small doses of injection botulinum toxin (1 unit or less, bilaterally) produce improvement in 50% cases.
- '**SpeechEasy**': Using both delayed and frequency altered auditory feedback in the ear devices (a frequency shift of +500 Hz with delayed auditory feedback of 60 m/sec) has shown significant improvement in fluency and normalcy of speech in both youth and adult subjects. It is marketed under the trademark 'SpeechEasy'.

Stuttering: It is the most common type of speech disorder.

Self-evaluation Exercises

1. Clinical features of phonasthenia include:
    a. Throat pain
    b. Easy fatigability of voice
    c. Triangular gap on phonation in the interarytenoid
    d. All of the above

2. Which is not related with Gutmann's pressure test?
    a. Pressure on the thyroid prominence in a backward and downward direction
    b. Improves the voice in cases of puberphonia
    c. Pressure relaxes the over stretched vocal cords
    d. Low-pitched voice can be produced
    e. All of the above

Filling the blanks

3. _____ is the most common type of speech disorder.
4. In dysphonia plica ventricularis, phonation is produced by the _____.
5. Functional aphonia always affects both vocal cords and they fail to _____.

Answers

1. d   2. e   3. Stuttering   4. False cords   5. Adduct

Chapter 48

Malignant Tumors of Larynx

⦿ Specific Learning Objectives

After going through the chapter, you should be able to answer the following questions:
- What are the etiological and predisposing factors and premalignant conditions of malignancy larynx?
- How would you evaluate the patients of cancer larynx? What are the anatomic divisions of larynx and how does cancer affect them?
- What are the various treatment options for cancer larynx and their indications?
- How will you manage a case of glottic cancer?
- How will you manage a case of supraglottic cancer?
- How will you rehabilitate the laryngectomy patients?

INTRODUCTION

National cancer registry (April 2005) reports that laryngeal cancer accounts for 2.63% of the whole body cancers (ICMR). Among the most common sites of cancer in males, larynx was found second in Delhi registry and third in Mumbai registry. Male-to-female ratio is 10:1. Indians are affected more than the people of Western countries. Patients are mostly in the age group of 40–70 years. Tumors of larynx can extend to hypopharynx and vice versa. Evaluation of persistent hoarseness is very important in smokers and elderly patients.

RISK FACTORS

Alcohol and smoking together increase the risk 50% greater than the additive risk of each.

- ***Smoking:*** It is a major (20 times riskier than nonsmokers) and the most common risk factor. Cigarette smoke contains carcinogenic benzopyrene and other hydrocarbons. Risk increases with increasing tobacco use. Filtered and light (air cured) tobacco has 50% lower risk than flue-cured or black tobacco. Passive smoking has also been implicated.
- ***Alcohol:*** Beer and hard liquor are riskier than wine.
- ***Radiation:*** Previous radiation to neck such as radiation for laryngeal papilloma can induce laryngeal carcinoma.
- ***Familial:*** Japanese and Russian have familial laryngeal malignancy that suggests genetic factors.
- ***Occupational and chemical:*** Exposure to asbestos, nickel compounds, certain mineral oils, mustard gas, petroleum products and glass-wool have been incriminated in the development of laryngeal cancer.
- ***Racial:*** Blacks are twice at risk than white Americans.
- ***Genetic:*** Either inactivation of tumor suppressive genes or activation of proto-oncogenes occurs.
- ***Human papillomavirus:*** About 40% laryngeal cancer specimens were found human papillomavirus (HPV)-positive. HPV (oncogenic Type 16) has been associated with head and neck cancer.
- ***Head and neck cancer:*** High incidence of second primary.
- ***Dietary:*** Phenols in drink and certain forms of tea such as mate (Latin America) and chimera (Brazil) have been recognized risk factors.
- ***Gastroesophageal reflux:*** Majority of cancer patients have associated reflux. Gastric acid reflux leads to chronic laryngeal irritation.
- ***Alkaline reflux:*** Achlorhydria and alkaline reflux (identified as laryngeal carcinogen) after gastric resection.
- ***Premalignant conditions:*** Leukoplakia, hyperkeratosis with atypia, and carcinoma *in situ* (CIS).

Premalignant Lesions

The five laryngeal squamous abnormalities, which run from benign to malignant, are as follows:

1. Hyperkeratosis
2. Hyperkeratosis with atypia
3. Carcinoma *in situ* (CIS)
4. Superficially invasive carcinoma
5. Invasive carcinoma.

Hyperkeratosis with atypia and CIS are managed satisfactorily by removing the strip of cord. Differentiation between severe hyperkeratosis with atypia and CIS is often difficult.

Preventive Measures

They include the following:
- Smoking cessation
- Reduced alcohol drinking
- Toxin free work environment
- Healthy diet and lifestyle.

EVALUATION

Clinical (Figs 48.1 and 48.2)

- Evaluate the hoarseness that persists for longer than 4 weeks. Large supraglottic and subglottic tumors can present with respiratory distress without any history of hoarseness of voice.
- Check for vocal cord mobility. Impairment or fixation occurs due to infiltration of thyroarytenoid muscle, cricoarytenoid joint or recurrent laryngeal nerve. It is an important finding for staging, management and prognosis of laryngeal cancer.
- Evaluate the extent of disease. Vallecula, base of tongue and pyriform fossa should be examined.
- A drawing showing the extent of disease must be made.
- Examine the neck for (Figs 48.1A and B).
  - Perichondritis and involvement of thyroid gland and strap muscles.
  - *Lymph node metastasis:* Note the size and number; whether mobile or fixed and unilateral, bilateral or contralateral.

- *Demarquay's sign:* Absence of elevation of the larynx during swallowing.
- *Supraglottic cancer:* It is the most aggressive of laryngeal cancers and has highest incidence of cervical nodal metastases.

Indirect Laryngoscopy

- *Mirror examination* offers best color and depth perception. Saliva and secretions should be swallowed. An intense gag reflex and difficult patient and anatomy may require supplemental examination.
- *Endoscopy:* Mirror examination is usually supplemented by fiber-optic rigid 70° or 90° telescope. The large channel of nasal flexible laryngoscopy even allows small biopsy without general anesthesia. If needed, the preparations for emergency tracheostomy should be kept ready. Any cartilage removed at tracheostomy should be submitted for histopathologic examination.
- *Photo or video documentation:* It allows dynamic study of laryngeal function.
- *Stroboscopy:* Normal mucosal wave indicates that lesion is superficial, and does not spread to the vocal ligament.

Imaging Study (Fig. 48.1B)

- *X-ray chest PA view:* Tuberculosis, pulmonary metastasis, mediastinal nodes or bronchogenic carcinoma.
- *CT and MRI:* Show the extent of tumor, invasion of pre-epiglottic or paraepiglottic space, destruction of cartilage, and lymph node involvement. Nodes greater than 1 cm or nodes with central necrosis are noted. Thyroid or cricoid cartilage destruction is better seen in CT. MRI T2W better highlights submucosal extension into the pre-epiglottic and paraglottic spaces.
  - *Whole-lung CT* is needed when X-ray chest shows any abnormality.

Imaging before biopsy: Imaging of the neck and airway before biopsy and endoscopy recognizes the need for emergent tracheostomy. A debulking biopsy with CO_2 laser or forceps may prevent the need for tracheostomy.

Detection of Recurrent/Residual Disease

Early recognition becomes difficult due to mucositis and edema of supraglottic laryngeal structures. Biopsy increases the chances of chondritis. The following imaging methods help:

- *Positron emission tomography (PET) Scan:* It is an accurate and effective means of showing recurrent and residual disease and distant metastasis.
- *CT scan:* It is more accurate than clinical examination.

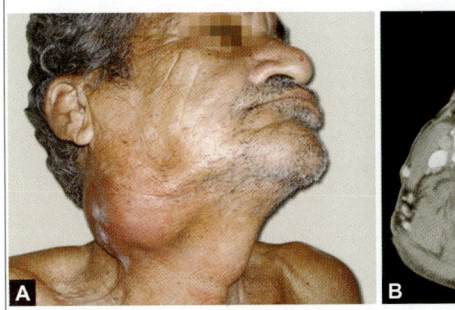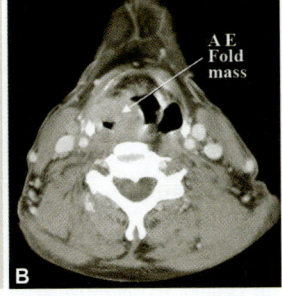

Figs 48.1A and B: (A) Carcinoma supraglottic larynx with secondary metastasis in neck involving levels I-B, II, III, IV and V. Note the healed tracheostomy opening; (B) CT scan neck. AE, aryepiglottic

- **Distant metastases:** The highest incidence of distant metastases in laryngeal cancer is seen in lungs.
- **Synchronous second primary:** In cases of carcinoma larynx the most common site of second primary (synchronous second primary) is bronchus.

Differential Diagnosis

The gross appearance of following conditions may be mistaken for malignancy. Biopsy will confirm the diagnosis.
- Fungal laryngitis
- Sarcoidosis
- Tuberculosis
- Wegener's granulomatosis

Direct Laryngoscopy Biopsy under General Anesthesia

It provides better view of the extent of disease and certain hidden areas, which are not seen during mirror examination such as infrahyoid epiglottis, anterior commissure, subglottis and ventricle. Telescopes may be passed through the scope for assessing subglottic and anterior commissure regions.
- *Microlaryngoscopy:* Small lesions of vocal cords are better visualized under operative microscope. It provides more accurate biopsy specimens without damaging the cord. Cord fixation is differentiated from arytenoid fixation by palpating the vocal process. The ventricular extension of growth is assessed with a laryngeal probe.

  The complete excisional biopsy of small suspected lesion with border of healthy tissue helps in determining the depth of invasion, which is difficult with small biopsy specimen of early lesions.
- *Supravital staining and biopsy:* Toluidine blue or Lugol's solution applied to the lesion is washed with saline. The dye is taken up in cases of CIS and superficial carcinomas. Leukoplakia does not take up dye. So, it helps in selecting the area for biopsy.
- *Autofluorescence laryngoscopy and lung imaging fluorescence endoscope (LIFE):* For evaluating laryngeal lesions.

Histopathology

Cordal carcinomas are mostly well differentiated whereas supraglottic lesions are anaplastic. Other variants of squamous cell carcinoma (SCC) include the following:
- Verrucous carcinoma
- Pseudosarcoma
- Basaloid squamous cell carcinoma.

Rare laryngeal malignancies are sarcomas, lymphoma, adenocarcinoma, neuroendocrine carcinoma and extramedullary plasmacytoma.

Laryngeal cancer: Squamous cell carcinoma accounts for 95% of all laryngeal malignancies.

STAGING (FIG. 48.2A AND TABLE 48.1)

For the purpose of staging American joint committee on cancer (AJCC) divides larynx into following three regions, which are further subdivided into several subsites.
1. *Supraglottis:* Suprahyoid epiglottis (both lingual and laryngeal surfaces), infrahyoid epiglottis, aryepiglottic folds (laryngeal aspect only), arytenoids, ventricular bands (or false cords) (Figs 48.2A).
2. *Glottis:* True vocal cords including anterior and posterior commissure (Figs 48.2A).
3. *Subglottis:* Below the glottis upto lower border of cricoid cartilage.

Transglottic tumors involve supraglottis and glottis across the ventricle, and usually cause fixation of the vocal cord. The clinical staging is supplemented with CT and MRI (Table 48.1). The staging and classification help to analyze outcomes of different modalities of treatment, and assists in predicting prognosis of disease.

MANAGEMENT

The treatment depends upon the site and extent of lesion, presence or absence of lymph node metastasis and distant metastases. The modalities of treatment include radiotherapy, surgery (conservation and total laryngectomy), chemotherapy and combined therapy.

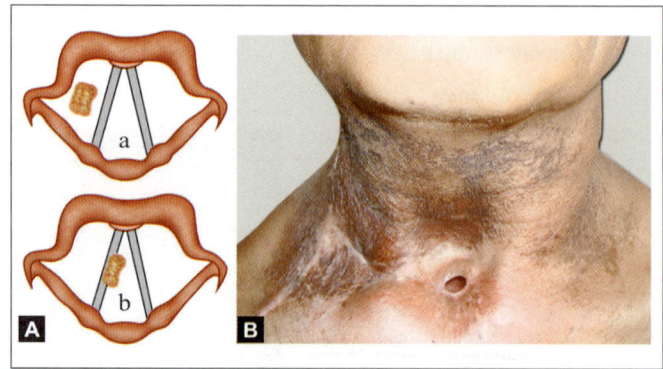

Figs 48.2A and B: (A) Carcinoma larynx. (a) Supraglottic; and (b) Glottic; (B) Narrowing of the tracheostome in an irradiated case of total laryngectomy with partial pharyngectomy and radical neck dissection of right side. Note the incision and skin changes after postoperative radiotherapy

Table 48.1: AJCC cancer staging (2002) and UICC TNM classification of carcinoma larynx and laryngopharynx

	Primary tumor (T-tumor)
T_X	Cannot be assessed
T_0	No tumor
T_{is}	Carcinoma *in situ* (CIS)
Supraglottis	
T_1	Tumor limited to only one subsite of supraglottis with normal vocal cord mobility
T_2	Tumor invades mucosa of more than one subsite of supraglottis or mucosa of any of the following structures without vocal cord fixation: glottis, medial wall of pyriform sinus, vallecula or base of tongue
T_3	Tumor limited to larynx with vocal cord fixation and/or involvement of any following structures: postcricoid area, preepiglottic or paraglottic space, or inner cortex of thyroid cartilage.
T_{4a}	Tumor invades thyroid-cricoid cartilage and any of the following extralaryngeal structures: esophagus, trachea, thyroid, infrahyoid strap muscles, or tongue muscles
T_{4b}	Tumor involves prevertebral space, mediastinum or encasing of carotid artery
Glottis	
T_1	Tumor involves only vocal cords, anterior or posterior commissure with normal vocal cord mobility
T_{1a}	Tumor involves only one vocal cord with normal vocal cord mobility
T_{1b}	Tumor involves both vocal cords with normal vocal cord mobility
T_2	Tumor spreads to supraglottis or subglottis with or without impaired vocal cord mobility
T_3, T_{4a} and T_{4b} similar to supraglottis	
Subglottis	
T_1	Tumor limited to subglottis with normal vocal cord mobility
T_2	Tumor spreads to glottis with or without impaired vocal cord mobility
T_3, T_{4a} and T_{4b} similar to supraglottis.	
Hypopharynx tumor size in greatest dimension	
T_1	Tumor ≤ 2 cm and limited to one subsite
T_2	Tumor > 2 cm, but ≤ 4 cm or invading > 1 subsite and without hemilarynx fixation
T_3	Tumor > 4 cm or with hemilarynx fixation.
T_{4a}	Tumor invades any of the following: thyroid-cricoid cartilage, hyoid bone, thyroid gland, esophagus, central compartment of soft tissue such as infrahyoid strap muscles and subcutaneous tissue.
T_{4b}	Tumor involves prevertebral fascia, mediastinum or encasing of carotid artery

Contd...

Contd...

Regional lymph nodes (N) size in greatest dimension
Similar to oral cancer. *See* Table 33.2 of Chapter 33 'Neoplasms of Oral Cavity'
Distant metastasis (M)
Similar to oral cancer. *See* Table 33.2 of Chapter 33 'Neoplasms of Oral Cavity'
Stage grouping for cancer of larynx and hypopharynx
Similar to oral cancer. *See* Table 33.2 of Chapter 33 'Neoplasms of Oral Cavity'

Radiotherapy

- Curative radiotherapy is given for early lesions $T_{1,2}$. The cords are mobile, and there is no involvement of cartilage and cervical nodes. The main advantage is preservation of voice.
- In cases of vocal cord cancer, radiotherapy gives 90% cure rate.
- In cases of superficial exophytic lesions of the tip of epiglottis and aryepiglottic folds, it gives 70–90% cure rate.
- The results are not good in cases of fixed cords, subglottic extension, cartilage invasion, and nodal metastases. These cases are candidates for surgery.

Carcinoma glottis: In comparison to supraglottis, nasopharynx and subglottic cancers, carcinoma glottis is the most radiosensitive tumor.

Surgery

To prove negative surgical margins, the specimen should be submitted for histopathological examination. Pathologist must be oriented by the surgeon.

- **Conservation surgery:** It preserves voice and avoids a permanent tracheal opening. Cases should be carefully selected:
  - *Cordectomy:* Excision of vocal cord via laryngofissure or endoscopy.
  - *Partial frontolateral laryngectomy:* Excision of vocal cord and anterior commissure.
  - *Partial horizontal laryngectomy:* Excision of supraglottis, which include epiglottis, aryepiglottic folds, false cords and ventricle.
- **Total laryngectomy:** The entire larynx is removed along with hyoid bone, pre-epiglottic space, strap muscles and one or more rings of trachea. Pharyngeal wall is closed primarily, and lower tracheal stump is sutured to the skin (Fig. 48.2B). The indications include T_{3-4} lesions and failure after radiotherapy or conservation surgery. It is combined with block dissection when nodal metastasis is present. It is not done in patients with distant metastasis.

- ***Hemithyroidectomy or subtotal thyroidectomy:*** The associated hemithyroidectomy or subtotal thyroidectomy is indicated in following conditions:
    - Palpable thyroid abnormality
    - Subglottic extension and tumors
    - T_4 glottic tumors
    - T_4 pyriform sinus tumors
    - Positive delphian nodes
    - Thyroid-cricoid cartilage destruction

Combined Therapy

Surgery may be combined with pre or postoperative radiation in a planned way to decrease the incidence of recurrence. Preoperative radiation may render fixed nodes resectable. Overall survival is better with postoperative radiotherapy, which is delivered within 5-7 weeks of surgery. Complications rate is higher with preoperative radiotherapy.

> ***Verrucous carcinoma of larynx:*** The treatment of choice is surgery.

Palliation Therapy

- Endoscopic significant debulking with laser or surgical forceps temporarily relieves the airway.
- Tracheostomy.
- Gastrostomy.

GLOTTIC CANCER

This is the most common laryngeal cancer. It has good prognosis because patients report early, and lymphatic spread is late. The most common sites are free edge and upper surface of vocal cord in its anterior and middle third.

Spread

- ***Local:*** Fixation of vocal cord is a bad prognostic sign and indicates involvement of thyroarytenoid muscle.
    - ***Anterior:*** Anterior commissure and then to the opposite cord
    - ***Posterior:*** Vocal process and arytenoid region
    - ***Upward:*** Ventricle and false cord
    - ***Downward:*** Subglottic region
- ***Lymphatic:*** There are not much lymphatic in vocal cords. Lymph node metastasis occurs when cordal lesions spread beyond the region of membranous cord.

Clinical Features

- ***Hoarseness of voice:*** An early and most common presentation, because of which glottic cancer is detected early. Cord cancer affects vibratory capacity.
- ***Airway obstruction:*** Large growth, accompanying edema or cord fixation may result in stridor.
- ***Lesion:***
    - Vocal cord thickening, raised nodule and ulcer.
    - Anterior commissure granulation tissue.

Treatment

- ***CIS:*** Endoscopic CO_2 laser application or stripping of vocal cord. If biopsy reveals invasive carcinoma, radiotherapy is given. Patient needs regular follow-up.
- ***Stage I:*** $T_1 N_0 M_0$
    - ***Middle third of vocal fold lesion:*** Radiotherapy (95% cure) or surgery (100% cure): endoscopic, CO_2 laser resection (cordotomy or cordectomy) or open cordectomy (laryngofissure). Surgery failures are given radiotherapy. But, radiotherapy failures may not be amenable to conservation surgery.
    - ***Extension to anterior commissure:*** Radiotherapy or frontolateral partial laryngectomy. In case of failure, total laryngectomy is indicated.
    - ***Extension to arytenoids:*** Surgery is preferred.
- ***Stage II ($T_2 N_0 M_0$):*** Normal cord mobility suggests growth limited to the surface whereas impaired mobility indicates invasion into intrinsic laryngeal muscles or paraglottic space. Invasion of paraglottic space or subglottic region may be associated with undetected invasion of laryngeal cartilages. With normal cord mobility, radiation gives 86% cure rate while it drops to 63% if cord mobility is impaired. In a case of postradiation edema, which persists for longer than 6 months, deep invasive recurrence must be ruled out.
    - Cord mobile and anterior commissure or arytenoids not involved: Radiotherapy gives good results (upper neck nodes are included in the radiation field). In cases of radiation failure, laryngectomy or partial vertical laryngectomy is indicated.
    - Anterior commissure and/or arytenoids involved or cord mobility impaired: Vertical hemi-laryngectomy or frontolateral laryngectomy. In cases of failure or recurrence, total laryngectomy is done.
- ***T_2 and early T_3:*** Supracricoid laryngectomy with cricohyoid-epiglottopexy.
- ***T_3 and T_4:*** Total laryngectomy combined with neck dissection (for palpable nodes).
- ***More advanced T_4:*** These lesions may be treated by combined therapy or palliative treatment.

SUPRAGLOTTIC CANCER

It is less common than glottic cancer. Prognosis is poor because patients report late, and lymphatic spread occurs early. Most common sites are epiglottis, false cords followed by aryepiglottic folds.

Spread
- **Local**
  - **Superior:** Vallecula and base of tongue.
  - **Lateral:** Pyriform fossa.
  - **Anterior:** Growths of infrahyoid epiglottis and anterior ventricular band extend into preepiglottic space, and penetrate the thyroid cartilage.
  - **Inferior:** Glottic region.
- **Lymphatic:** Lymph node metastasis occurs early. It usually involves upper and middle jugular nodes. Bilateral metastases may be seen in epiglottic lesion.

Clinical Features
Patients report late because supraglottic growths (Figs 48.1 and 48.2) remain silent for long time till they achieve enormous size and cause lymph node metastasis.
- **Most common symptoms:**
  - Throat pain
  - Dysphagia
  - Referred ear pain
  - Mass of lymph nodes in the neck
- **Late symptoms:**
  - Hoarseness of voice
  - Weight loss
  - Respiratory distress stridor
  - Halitosis
- **Lesion:** Either exophytic (suprahyoid epiglottis) or ulcerative (infrahyoid epiglottis).

Treatment
In addition to the factors of TNM staging, age of the patient and status of lung functions should be considered before planning the conservation surgery for supraglottic cancer.
- **Stage I:** T1 N0 M0: Radiation or excision with CO_2 laser.
  - **Suprahyoid epiglottic tumors:** Endoscopic excision with electrocautery or CO_2 laser.
  - **Infrahyoid epiglottic tumors:** Endoscopic laser partial laryngectomy.
- **Stage II:** $T_2 N_0 M_0$
  - **Good lung function:** Supraglottic laryngectomy with or without neck dissection. Vallecula and base of tongue upto the circumvallate papilla can be removed. Patient must be able to tolerate mild to moderate aspiration that may last for the rest of life. Other surgical procedures include subtotal laryngectomy with cricohyoidopexy and supracricoid partial laryngectomy.
  - **Poor lung function:** Radiotherapy.
- T_3 **and** T_4**:** Total laryngectomy with neck dissection and postoperative radiotherapy.

SUBGLOTTIC CANCER
Subglottic cancer is the least common laryngeal cancer.

Spread
- **Local:** One side growth of subglottis spreads around the anterior wall, and to the opposite side.
  - **Inferior:** Trachea.
  - **Upward:** Vocal cords are involved late so the hoarseness is a late symptom.
  - **Anterior:** Cricothyroid membrane, thyroid gland and infrahyoid ribbon muscles of neck.
- **Lymphatic:** Prelaryngeal (Delphian node), pretracheal, paratracheal and lower jugular nodes.

Clinical Features
These patients report late when the growth is significantly big and extensive.
- **Respiratory distress and stridor:** Most common feature.
- **Hoarseness of voice** due to infiltration of thyroarytenoid, recurrent laryngeal nerve or cricoarytenoid joint.
- **Lesion:** Raised submucosal nodule in anterior half.

Treatment
- T_1 **and** T_2**:** Radiotherapy.
- T_3 **and** T_4**:** Total laryngectomy and postoperative radiation, which include superior mediastinum.

ORGAN PRESERVATION THERAPY
The current trend in the management of cancer of larynx is developing towards chemotherapy+radiotherapy for preserving the larynx. Studies have shown that there is no difference in survival rate between the cases of total laryngectomy and combined chemotherapy+radiotherapy.

The patients who are candidates for total laryngectomy are given a course of chemotherapy. Those who have complete response (some include even partial response) are given complete radiotherapy. Those who have no response (some include even partial response) are treated with surgery, usually followed by radiotherapy. No difference in survival was found in these two groups.
- **Chemotherapy protocols:** They include:
  - Three-cycle regimen of cisplatinum (100 mg/m^2) and fluorouracil (5-FU) continuous infusion for 5 days at 15 or 21 days interval—most commonly used.
  - Three-cycle regimen of cisplatinum, bleomycin and 5-FU.

POST-LARYNGECTOMY REHABILITATION
Patient loses laryngeal speech after laryngectomy. Following methods may facilitate patient's communication. The current trend is for tracheoesophageal (TE) fistula speech. The artificial larynx is the least preferred ones. Good esophageal speech compares well with TE speech.

Esophageal Speech

Patient learns how to swallow air, and hold it in the upper esophagus. Then patient slowly ejects the air from upper esophagus, and speaks 6–10 words which are even though rough, are loud and understandable. Some patients learn to store air in stomach, which greatly improves duration of speech.

Artificial Larynx

It is useful when patients fail to learn esophageal speech. They are least socially acceptable because they draw unwanted attention to the speaker. Monotone sound production is its another limitation.

- *Electrolarynx:* This is transistorized, battery operated, portable device. It produces low-pitched sound which is further modulated into speech by the tongue, lips, teeth and palate. The vibrating disc is held against the soft tissues of the neck or oral cavity.
- *Transoral pneumatic device:* The expired air from the tracheostome vibrates the diaphragm of this device. The rubber diaphragm vibrations are carried by a plastic tube into the back of the oral cavity where modulators convert the sound into speech. It is rarely used.

Tracheoesophageal Fistula (TEF) Speech

The air is carried from trachea to esophagus/hypopharynx through a TEF. The vibrating column of air in the pharynx is modulated into speech. The lungs are used as bellows and produce greater air pressure across pharyngoesophageal (PE) segment that facilitates esophageal speech. The main disadvantage is aspiration into the trachea. The current prosthesis shunts the air from trachea to esophagus, and their inbuilt one-way valves prevent problems of aspiration.

TEF may be created either at the time of laryngectomy or 2–4 weeks after surgery or postoperative radiotherapy.

Prosthesis: There are two types of prostheses:
1. *Non-indwelling devices:* This is inserted in about 1–2 weeks after the TEF. Patients remove them daily for cleaning and maintenance.
   - Panje Voice Button (Hood Laboratories, USA)
   - Blom-Singer Duckhill Prosthesis (InHealth Technologies, USA)
2. *Indwelling prosthesis:* They are placed at the time of TEF, and remain in TEF. In case of problems they are replaced by the therapist or surgeon. They include:
   - Groningen Voice Button (Hood Laboratories, USA)
   - Provox and Provox 2 (Atos Medical AB, Horby, Sweden)
   - Blom-Singer Indwelling Voice Prosthesis (InHealth Technologies, USA).

- *Ashai technique:* It is a method of vocal rehabilitation in patients with laryngectomy.
- *Esophageal speech:* The dynamic component of phonation in esophageal speech after laryngectomy lies at pharyngoesophageal segment.

Self-evaluation Exercises

1. The first line of treatment of carcinoma larynx in stage I (T_1, N_0, M_0) is:
   a. Surgery or radiotherapy
   b. Combined surgery and radiotherapy
   c. Chemotherapy
   d. Immunotherapy
2. The first line of treatment of carcinoma larynx in stage III is:
   a. Chemotherapy
   b. Total laryngectomy followed by postoperative radiotherapy
   c. Preoperative radiotherapy
   d. Postoperative chemotherapy
3. The treatment of choice in verrucous carcinoma of larynx is:
   a. Surgery
   b. Radiotherapy
   c. Immunotherapy
   d. Chemotherapy
4. Which of the following are not the risk factors of carcinoma larynx?
   a. Genetic susceptibility
   b. Smoking, alcohol and previous ionizing radiation
   c. Gastroesophageal reflux disease (GERD)
   d. Exposure to wood dust, asbestos and volatile chemicals, nitrogen mustard
   e. None from the above

Contd…

Contd...

5. The dynamic component of phonation in esophageal speech in a case of laryngectomy lies at:
   a. Tracheostomy
   b. Mouth
   c. Pharyngoesophageal segment
   d. Gastroesophageal junction
6. Which is the most radiosensitive tumor among the following:
   a. Supraglottis
   b. Nasopharynx
   c. Carcinoma glottis
   d. Subglottic cancers

True (T)/False (F)

7. The most common and earliest symptom of carcinoma glottis is hoarseness of voice.
8. Supraglottic cancer is the most aggressive of laryngeal cancers and has the highest incidence of cervical nodal metastases.
9. The most common site in supraglottic region is aryepiglottic fold.
10. Ashai technique is a method of vocal rehabilitation in patients with laryngectomy.
11. In laryngectomy patients, Blom-Singer prosthesis diverts tracheal air into esophagus for voice production.

Filling the blanks

12. The highest incidence of distant metastasis in laryngeal cancer is seen in _____.
13. In cases of carcinoma larynx the most common site of second primary (synchronous second primary) is _____.
14. Absence of elevation of the larynx during swallowing is called _____ sign.

Answers

1. a	2. b	3. a	4. e	5. c	6. c
7. T	8. T	9. F	10. T	11. T	12. Lungs
13. Bronchus	14. Demarquay's				

Chapter 49

Management of Impaired Airway

> **Specific Learning Objectives**
>
> After going through the chapter, you should be able to answer the following questions:
> - What are the functions and indications of tracheostomy?
> - What are the different types of tracheostomy?
> - What special care will you take during the tracheostomy operation in infants and young children?
> - How will you take the postoperative care of tracheostomy and what are its complications?
> - What do you know about: (1) Cricothyrotomy; (2) Percutaneous dilatational tracheostomy; (3) Laryngomalacia?
> - How will you manage a case of foreign body larynx?
> - How will you manage a case of foreign body bronchus?
> - How will you manage a case of laryngotracheal trauma?

INTRODUCTION

A patient with impaired airway demands prompt attention from doctors. Failure to achieve a patent airway in cases of impaired airway, inevitably results in hypoxic brain injury and death.

TRACHEOSTOMY/TRACHEOTOMY

In tracheostomy, an opening in the anterior wall of trachea is created and converted into a stoma on the skin surface. The terms tracheostomy and tracheotomy have been used interchangeably. The tracheotomy means opening the trachea, which is a step of tracheostomy operation.

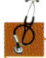

Tracheostomy facilitates breathing, suctioning, feeding, mobility, and early return of speech.

FUNCTIONS

- **Bypass the obstruction** in the upper airway (pharynx and larynx).
- **Ventilation:** Improves alveolar ventilation in cases of respiratory insufficiency in the following ways:
  - **Dead space:** Decrease the dead space by 30–50% (normal dead space is 150 ml).
  - **Resistance:** Reduces the resistance to airflow.
- **Protection:** Cuffed tracheostomy tube protects the tracheobronchial tree against aspiration of secretions and blood.
  - **Secretions:** Pharyngeal secretions in cases of bulbar paralysis and coma.
  - **Blood:** Bleeding from injuries of pharynx, larynx and maxillofacial region.
  - **Packing:** Allows packing of pharynx and larynx to control bleeding.
- **Suction:** Suction clearance of tracheobronchial secretions avoids the need for repeated bronchoscopy or intubation.
- **Intermittent positive pressure respiration (IPPR).**
- **Anesthesia:** Administration of anesthesia in cases of marked trismus due to oral submucous fibrosis.

If IPPR is expected to prolong beyond 72 hours, tracheostomy is preferred over endotracheal intubation.

INDICATIONS

The indications can be categorized in three groups—upper respiratory obstruction, retained secretions, and respiratory insufficiency. Prolonged intubation with mechanical ventilation is now the most common indication for tracheostomy; formerly, it was upper respiratory obstruction. Other indications include easier management of secretions and an adjuvant procedure during chest surgery, and major head and neck operations.

- **Upper respiratory tract obstruction:** *See* the causes of stridor in Chapter 'Laryngeal Symptoms and Examination'.
- Retained secretions
  - *Inability to cough:* Coma due to head injuries, cerebrovascular strokes, accidents, narcotic poisoning.
  - *Paralysis of respiratory muscles:* Due to spinal injuries, polio, Guillain-Barre syndrome and myasthenia gravis.
  - *Spasm of respiratory muscles:* Due to tetanus, eclampsia, strychnine poisoning.
  - *Painful cough:* Chest injuries, multiple rib fractures, pneumonia.
  - *Aspiration of secretions:* Bulbar polio, polyneuritis, bilateral laryngeal paralysis.
- **Respiratory insufficiency:** Emphysema, chronic bronchitis, bronchiectasis and atelectasis.

TIMINGS AND TYPES OF TRACHEOSTOMY

- **Emergent tracheostomy (slash trach):** It is required when intubation and laryngotomy (cricothyrotomy) are not feasible, and sudden airway distress is accompanied with impending death. The complication rate of emergency tracheostomy is as high as 21%. This emergent situation is an ideal indication for cricothyrotomy.

  The technique is more or less similar to elective tracheostomy. After the midline vertical cervical skin incision, a transverse incision is made along the lower border of cricoid cartilage in pretracheal fascia. The thyroid isthmus is dissected down (even cut with knife or diathermy) to expose upper three tracheal rings. Vertical tracheal incision involves second and third rings. Trachea is opened with a hemostat, and the tube inserted.
- **Urgent (awake) tracheostomy:** This is done in the operation theater under local anesthesia with minimal sedation. The patient has respiratory distress, and needs immediate surgical intervention.
- **Elective tracheostomy:** This tranquil, orderly and routine tracheostomy is a planned surgery. It is performed where all operative surgical facilities such as endotracheal intubation, local and general anesthesia, are available.
  - *Therapeutic:* It relieves not only the respiratory obstruction, but also allows removing tracheobronchial, secretions, and provides assisted ventilation.
  - *Prophylactic:* It is performed to prevent anticipated respiratory obstruction and aspiration of blood and secretions. The indications include extensive surgery of tongue, floor of mouth, mandibular resection or laryngofissure.
- **Temporary tracheostomy:** Elective tracheostomy is usually temporary, and is closed when causative disease is cured.
- **Permanent tracheostomy:** It is indicated in cases of bilateral abductor paralysis and laryngeal stenosis. In cases of laryngectomy and laryngopharyngectomy, a tracheostome is created where lower tracheal stump is stitched to the surface skin.

> **Tracheotomy:** It is the general opinion that the best time of doing tracheostomy is when you first think that patient needs tracheotomy. No one would like to end up in doing a 'slash' tracheotomy later!

LEVEL AND SITE OF TRACHEOSTOMY

On the bases of the site, tracheostomy has been divided into three groups—high, mid and low.

1. **High tracheostomy:** It is done at the level of first tracheal ring above the level of thyroid isthmus, which lies at the level of third and fourth tracheal rings. The high tracheostomy is generally avoided because of the postoperative risk of perichondritis of the cricoid cartilage and subglottic stenosis. In cases of carcinoma larynx with stridor when total laryngectomy would be done, high tracheostomy is indicated.
2. **Mid tracheostomy:** It is done through the second and third tracheal rings, and needs either division of the thyroid isthmus or its retraction upwards.
3. **Low tracheostomy:** It is done below the level of isthmus where trachea becomes deep, and lies close to large vessels. The tracheostomy tubes tend to impinge on suprasternal notch.

ANESTHESIA

General anesthesia with endotracheal intubation is preferred. It is particularly important in infants and children. No anesthesia is needed in unconscious patients and dire emergency conditions. In cases of malignancy larynx, it is usually done under local anesthesia (1–2% lignocaine with epinephrine infiltration).

POSITION

Patient lies in supine position. The neck is extended with a pillow under the shoulders to bring the trachea anteriorly.

STEPS OF OPERATION (FIGS 49.1 AND 49.2A AND B)

- *Skin incision:* A vertical midline cervical incision that extends from cricoid cartilage to just above the sternal notch is the most frequently used skin incision. A transverse incision—5 cm above the sternal notch—has the advantage of a cosmetically better scar.
- *Strap muscles:* Strap muscles are first separated in the midline and then retracted laterally. Pretracheal fascia is incised and elevated.
- *Thyroid isthmus:* The thyroid isthmus is either displaced upwards or divided between the clamps.
- *Trachea:* After injecting few drops of 4% lignocaine into the trachea (suppresses the cough), it is incised with a vertical incision in the region anywhere between second to fourth tracheal rings. The incision is then converted into a circular opening. Trachea may be fixed with a hook before the incision. The first tracheal ring is never damaged as it may result in perichondritis of cricoid cartilage and stenosis.
- *Tracheal hook (blunt and sharp):* Blunt tracheal hook retracts the thyroid isthmus, and exposes the trachea. It may also be used for retracting the strap muscles. When making incision in the tracheal wall, sharp tracheal hook is applied to the lower border of cricoid cartilage to stabilize the trachea.
- *Tracheal dilator:* It keeps the cut tracheal-edges open so that tracheostomy tube can be easily introduced. Its tip is blunt (*see* Chapter 'Instruments'). The blades spread out on approximating its rings. A curved artery forceps can also serve the purpose.
- *Tracheostomy tube:* An appropriate size of tracheostomy tube is inserted and secured by tapes (Fig. 49.3). *See* Chapter 'Instruments' for different types and sizes of tracheostomy tubes. To avoid surgical emphysema skin incision is not sutured. Gauge dressing is placed between the wound and tracheostomy tube.

TRACHEOSTOMY IN INFANTS AND CHILDREN

Great care is needed to prevent avoidable complications, which are not uncommon while doing tracheostomy in infants and young children. The following facts and precautions must be kept in mind:
- Stay strictly in midline. Position the child without neck or head deviation. Fix the larynx by putting a finger on either side of larynx. Put a vertical incision through skin, and down to the trachea.
- Trachea is soft and compressible in infants and children. The surgeon tends to displace trachea, and go deep or lateral to it; possibly injuring recurrent laryngeal nerve and common carotid artery. A bronchoscope or

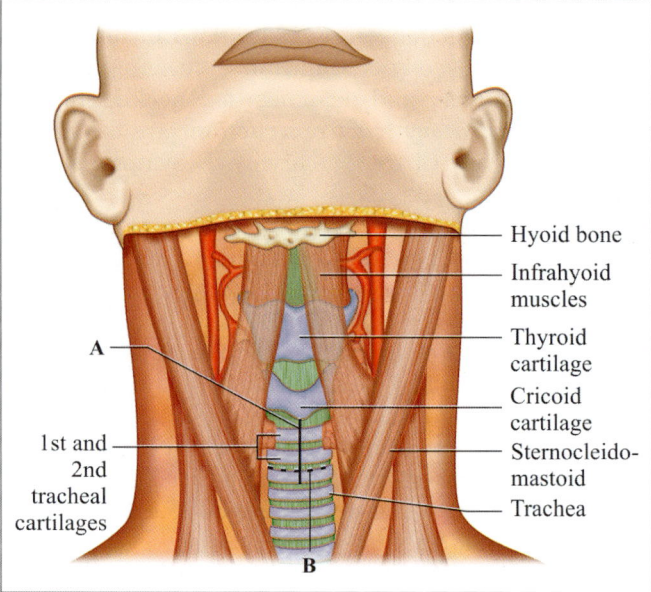

Fig. 49.1: Incisions for tracheostomy
Key: (A) Surface landmarks for the midline skin vertical incision for tracheostomy; (B) Horizontal skin incision for cricothyrotomy

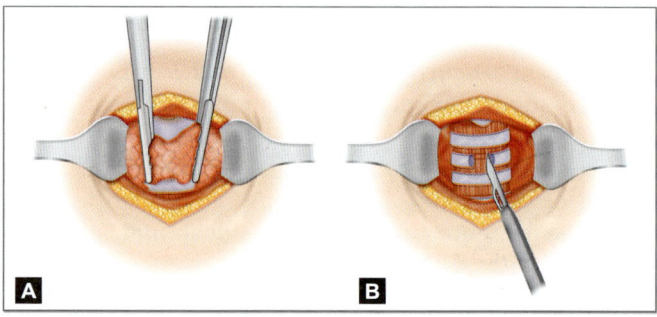

Figs 49.2A and B: Thyroid isthmus and tracheostomy. (A) Thyroid isthmus may be retracted superiorly or inferiorly, or transected and suture ligated; (B) Anterior section of a tracheal ring can be removed or a round window spanning two tracheal rings can be created

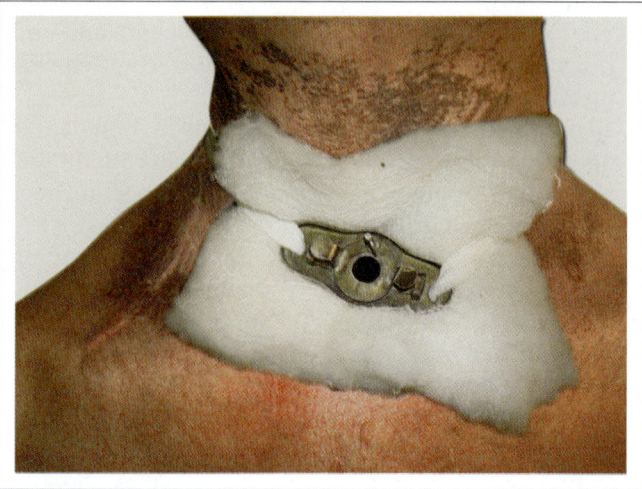

Fig. 49.3: Tracheostomy tube inserted and secured by tapes

an endotracheal intubation facilitates identification of trachea. Therefore, tracheostomy in infants and children is done under general anesthesia with endotracheal intubation.
- Too much extension of neck pulls thoracic structures into the neck. The vulnerable structures are pleura, innominate artery and thymus. The risk of making tracheostomy opening near suprasternal notch is high.
- The silk sutures, placed in the trachea on either side of midline, helps in proper incision of trachea. Trachea is only incised. The excision of a circular piece of anterior tracheal wall is never done.
- Tracheal lumen is narrow, and too much insertion of knife in trachea can easily injure posterior tracheal wall and esophagus causing tracheoesophageal fistula.
- Infolding of anterior tracheal wall while inserting the tracheostomy tube is avoided.
- Tracheostomy tube should be of proper diameter, length and curvature. A long tube can impinge on the carina, or go into right bronchus. Lower end of high curvature tube impinges on anterior tracheal wall, and its upper part compresses the tracheal rings or cricoid. Soft silastic and portex tubes are preferred over metallic tubes which cause more traumas. If a proper tracheostomy tube is not available, a pediatric endotracheal tube can be used.
- Postoperative X-ray chest and neck ascertains the position of tracheostomy tube.

POSTOPERATIVE CARE

- *Monitoring:* Watch for bleeding and displacement, and blocking of tube.
- *Paper pad and a pencil* for patient's communication as these patients cannot speak.
- *Suction of secretions:* Regular suction (hourly or half-hourly) depending on the amount of secretion for their removal.
  Use sterile catheters with a Y-connector that breaks suction force and avoids suction injuries to tracheal mucosa. Apply suction only when the catheter is taken out.
- *Proper humidification* that prevents crusting is achieved by using humidifier, steam tent, ultrasonic nebulizer, or keeping a boiling kettle in the room.
- *Crusting:* Few drops of normal or hypotonic saline or Ringer's lactate are instilled into the trachea every 2-3 hours to loosen crusts. Instillation of acetylcysteine (mucolytic agent) solution liquefies tenacious secretions, and loosens the crusts.
- *Tracheostomy tube care:* Inner cannula is removed, and cleaned regularly for the first 3 days to prevent respiratory distress. Outer tube is changed daily after 3-4 days of tracheostomy when a track is formed that facilitates easy tube placement.
  Periodical deflation of cuffed tube prevents pressure necrosis and dilatation of trachea.

DECANNULATION

Prolonged use of tracheostomy tube can cause tracheobronchial infections, tracheal ulceration, granulations, stenosis and unsightly scars. Therefore, decannulation (removal of tube) should be considered once the causative condition is under control.

Method: The tracheostomy tube is occluded, and the patient closely watched for respiratory distress. If there is no distress for 24 hours, the tube is removed, and the wound is taped. Wound healing usually takes place within a week. Rarely a secondary closure is required.

In children, decannulation is done using progressively smaller size tubes.

Decannulation in Infant and Young Child

As the decannulation in infant and young child carries more risk, the following cares should be observed:
- Decannulate the child in the operation theater where services of reintubation, anesthetist, headlight, laryngoscope, proper sized endotracheal tubes, and a tracheostomy tray are kept ready.
- After decannulation, the child is watched for several hours for respiratory distress, tachycardia and cyanosis. Blood gas determinations may be required.

Causes of Failed Decannulation

When decannulation fails in spite of all the measures, the following causes must be looked for. The patient requires endoscopic examination of the larynx, trachea and bronchi using telescopes or a flexible endoscope.
- Persistence of the cause for which tracheostomy was required.
- Granulations around the stoma and in trachea, where tip of the tracheostomy tube impinge.
- Tracheal edema.
- Subglottic stenosis.
- Incurving of tracheal wall at the site of tracheostome.
- Tracheomalacia.
- Psychological dependence on tracheostomy.
- Inability to tolerate the resistance of the upper airways (physiological dependence).

COMPLICATIONS

Complications of tracheostomy (Box 49.1) are traditionally categorized into three groups—immediate

> **Box 49.1: Complications of tracheostomy**
>
> - **Immediate**
>   - Hemorrhage
>   - Apnea
>   - Pneumothorax
>   - Vocal cord palsy
>   - Tracheoesophageal fistula
>   - Aspiration of blood
>   - False passage
> - **Intermediate**
>   - **Bleeding:** Reactionary and secondary
>   - Displacement of tube
>   - Obstruction of tube
>   - Subcutaneous emphysema
>   - Pneumomediastinum and pneumothorax
>   - Crusting in trachea
>   - Tracheitis and stomal cellulitis
>   - Tracheobronchitis
>   - **Severe infections:** mediastinitis, clavicular osteomyelitis, and necrotizing fasciitis
>   - Atelectasis and lung abscess
>   - Local wound infection and granulations
> - **Late (with prolonged use of tube):**
>   - Hemorrhage due to granulation tissue and innominate artery blowout
>   - Laryngeal stenosis
>   - Tracheal stenosis
>   - Tracheoesophageal fistula
>   - Difficult decannulation
>   - Persistent tracheocutaneous fistula
>   - Keloid or unsightly scar
>   - Corrosion of tracheostomy tube

(intraoperative), intermediate (few hours to days), and late (weeks and months).

> Pediatric, head injury, obese, burn and debilitated patients are more prone to complications.
> Hemorrhage and tube displacement are the major causes of tracheostomy deaths. The most common complications include hemorrhage (3.7%), tube obstruction (2.7%), and tube displacement (1.5%).

The common sites of *hemorrhage* are anterior jugular veins and thyroid isthmus. *Apnea* due to sudden washing out of CO_2, which was acting as a respiratory stimulus, may occur in a patient who had prolonged respiratory obstruction. Treatment includes administration of 5% CO_2 in oxygen (carbogen) or assisted ventilation.

Pneumothorax occurs due to injury to apical pleura. *Vocal cord palsy* occurs due to injury to recurrent laryngeal nerves. *Tracheoesophageal fistula* is the result of injury to posterior wall of trachea and esophagus.

Obstruction of tube can occur due to blood clot, partial displacement and impingement on posterior tracheal wall.

Innominate artery blows out due to erosion of its posterior walls. It carries 90% mortality rate. Direct digital pressure on the anterior wall of stoma tract is found effective. *Laryngeal stenosis* occurs due to cricoid cartilage perichondritis. *Tracheal stenosis* is the result of tracheal ulceration and infection. Tracheoesophageal fistula may occur due to cuffed tube and tip of tracheostomy tube. Problems of decannulation are more in infants and children.

CRICOTHYROTOMY (LARYNGOTOMY OR CONIOTOMY)

In this emergent procedure, an opening is made for airway through the cricothyroid membrane.

Indications

They include severe bleeding (maxillofacial injuries) foreign bodies, emeses, clenched teeth, repeated failed intubation, cervical spine injuries, burns and smoke inhalation.

Contraindications

They include infants and children, and inflammation and malignancy of larynx and surrounding area.

Technique

The neck is extended. Vertical midline cervical incision is made between the lower border of thyroid cartilage and upper border of the cricoid ring. Then, cricothyroid membrane is cut with a transverse incision, and subglottic larynx is entered. A small tracheostomy tube or any hollow tube like thing can be inserted to maintain airway. It is followed by tracheostomy, which is done at the earliest to avoid complications of cricothyrotomy such as perichondritis, subglottic edema and laryngeal stenosis.

PERCUTANEOUS DILATIONAL TRACHEOSTOMY

In percutaneous dilational tracheostomy (PDT), tracheostomy tube is introduced through the pretracheal skin and soft tissue without direct surgical visualization of trachea (Fig. 49.4).

Preoperative Criteria

- This minimally invasive, bedside procedure is performed only on intubated adult patients with long neck, which are admitted in the intensive care unit.
- Ability of the patient to hyperextend the neck.
- Easy reintubation in case of accidental extubation.

Contraindications

- **Absolute**
  - Need for emergency airway access

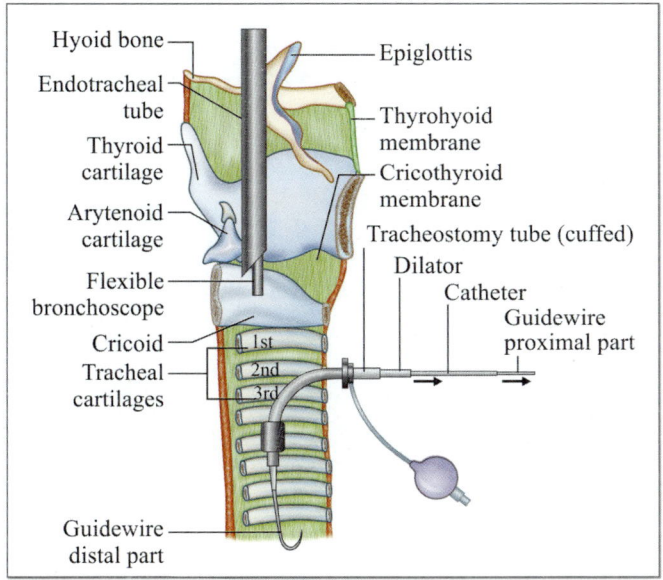

Fig. 49.4: Percutaneous dilational tracheostomy. After making skin incision and clearing pretracheal tissue, a guidewire along its sheath is introduced below the second tracheal ring. Guidewire, guide catheter, and dilator are advanced together after removing the guidewire sheath. Tracheostomy tube is loaded and advanced onto the dilator into the trachea. The procedure is done under bronchoscopic vision under general anesthesia

- *Relative*
  - Children younger than 12 years
  - History of difficult intubation
  - Anatomical
    - Cervical spine lesions causing limited extension of neck
    - Abnormality of trachea and larynx
    - Short and thick neck
  - Local tracheostomy site problems
    - Visible pulsating vessels
    - Active infection
    - Goiter
  - Hematological
    - Platelet count: less than 40,000/mm^3
    - Bleeding time: greater than 10 minutes
    - Prothrombin time or partial thromboplastin time: greater than 1.5 times of control
  - Positive end expiratory pressure: greater than 15 cm H_2O

Advantages

- Relatively easy to learn.
- The time required is considerably shorter.
- No need of operation theater and anesthesiologists team.
- Saves fees of operation theater and anesthesiologists team.
- No need to shift the patient from ICU.

Disadvantages

The PDT system set is expensive.

Technique

There are different systems and approaches to perform a percutaneous tracheostomy; the details of which are beyond the scope of this book.

IMMEDIATE AIRWAY MANAGEMENT

About 30% surgical anesthesia deaths are caused by impaired airway, which is usually due to inadequate ventilation, unrecognized esophageal intubation, and unanticipated difficult tracheal intubation. The methods to maintain airway during general anesthesia include jaw thrust, Guedel or laryngeal mask airway or an endotracheal tube.

Endotracheal Intubation

Endotracheal intubation is a quick method of establishing airway. The larynx is visualized with a laryngoscope and an endotracheal tube or a bronchoscope is inserted into the trachea. There is no need of anesthesia in emergency cases. Later on an orderly tracheostomy can be performed if needed. This avoids complications of an emergency tracheostomy, which are relatively frequent. Endotracheal tubes and their size selection are described in Chapter of 'Instruments'.

- **Difficult intubation:** In cases of difficult intubation, first pass a stylet and then rail road the endotracheal tube or take the help of flexible bronchoscope.
- **Dental wiring and jaws shutting:** In these cases nasal endotracheal intubation is done.

Other Procedures for Immediate Airway Management

- *Jaw thrust (Fig. 49.5):* In unconscious patients, extension of neck and lifting of mandible anteriorly displaces the tongue base anteriorly away from the posterior pharyngeal wall and widens and straightens the airway. Neck extension is not indicated in cases of cervical spinal injuries. The ventilation can be provided with face mask or Ambu bag.
- *Nasopharyngeal airway (trumpet) (Fig. 49.6A):* It is inserted into the hypopharynx through the nose and provide better patent airway from nose to laryngopharynx. In conscious patients it is better tolerated than oropharyngeal airway.
- *Oropharyngeal airway (Figs 49.6B to D):* This may be plastic or metallic. It brings the base tongue forward and widens the oropharynx. The ventilation can be provided with face mask or Ambu bag.

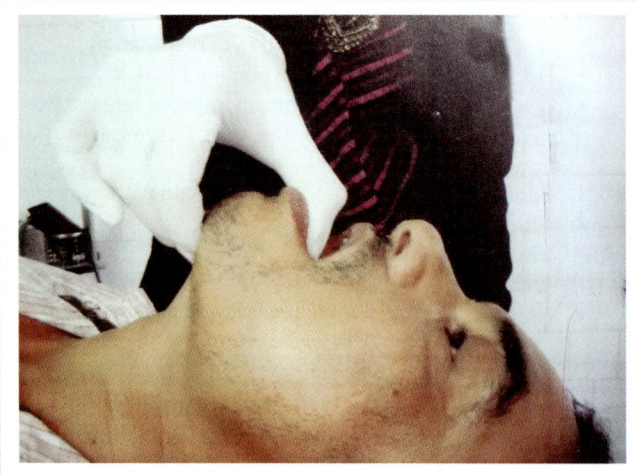

Fig. 49.5: Jaw thrust

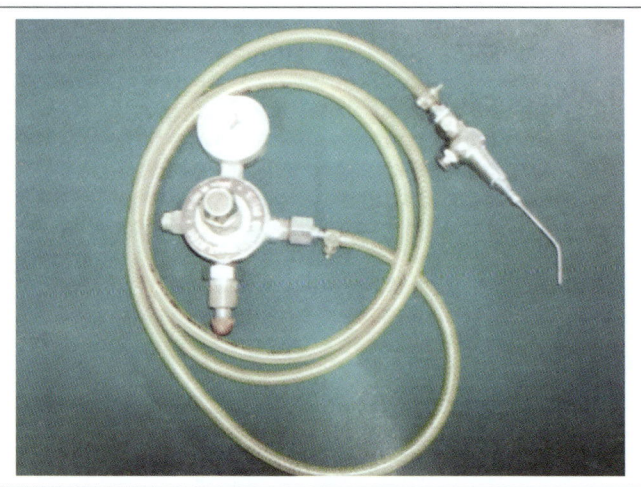

Fig. 49.7: Jet ventilation

- *Laryngeal mask airway (LMA) (Fig. 49.6E):* LMA consists of a tube and a distal end triangular laryngeal mask which fits over the laryngeal inlet in supraglottic region. The weight of patient decides the size of mask.
  - *Uses:* It is very useful in cases of unsuccessful intubation when standard mask ventilation is inadequate.
  - *Method:* The deflated cuff of mask is positioned over the larynx and than inflated. It is useful when face mask is ineffective and intubation is difficult.
  - *Disadvantages:* LMA does not prevent aspiration of gastric secretions. It cannot be used in patients with trismus.
  - *Contraindication:* It is contraindicated in cases of laryngeal obstruction.
- *Transtracheal jet ventilation (Fig. 49.7):* In this invasive method an intravenous catheter (12 or 14 gauge) is inserted into the subglottic region through the cricothyroid membrane. The direction of the catheter is kept towards the trachea and intraluminal position is confirmed by the aspiration with a syringe. After withdrawing the needle jet ventilation can be started through the catheter.
  - *Caution:* Expiration of air must be insured to avoid pulmonary barotrauma with pneumothorax, pneumomediastinum, and surgical emphysema.

Advantages of tracheostomy: Tracheostomy facilitates suctioning, feeding, mobility, early return of speech and decrease work of breathing.

CONGENITAL LESIONS OF LARYNX

Although the congenital laryngeal anomalies present with stridor, they can also cause dysphagia, aspiration, failure to thrive and dysphonia. Laryngoscopy (direct or flexible) usually diagnoses the problem while laryngotracheobronchial endoscopy will detect other synchronous airway lesions.

Congenital problems of aspiration and hoarseness of voice: Aspiration is more common with tracheoesophageal fistula, whereas hoarseness is more common with vocal cord palsy.

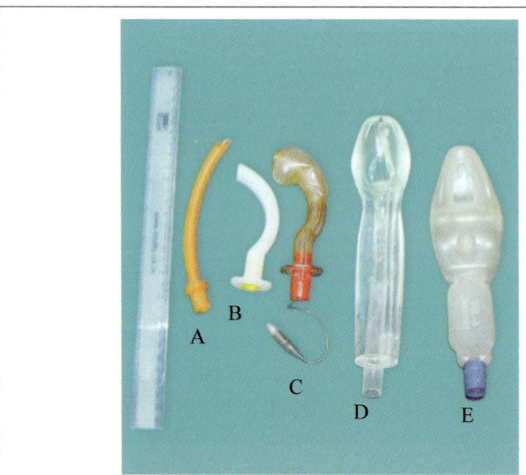

Fig. 49.6: Airway devices. (A) Nasopharyngeal airway; (B) Guedel oropharyngeal airway; (C) Cuffed oropharyngeal airway; (D) Sanjivani airway management oropharyngeal airway; (E) Laryngeal mask airway
Source: Dr AS Solanki, Consultant Anesthesiologist, Anand, Gujarat

LARYNGOMALACIA

This most common congenital laryngeal abnormality is characterized by excessive flaccidity of supraglottic larynx, which gets sucked in during inspiration.

Clinical Features

The newborn develops intermittent, low-pitched inspiratory stridor within the first 2 weeks of life. The severity of stridor increases on crying, but reduces in prone position. The stridor usually starts resolving after 9 months, and disappears by 2 years of age.

The cry is normal. Feeding difficulty, failure to thrive, and cyanosis occur infrequently. Children with laryngomalacia have high prevalence of gastroesophageal reflux disease (50–100%) and second synchronous airway lesions (17%).

Awake flexible laryngoscopy:
- Anterior prolapse of arytenoids mucosa.
- Short aryepiglottic folds.
- Posterior collapse of epiglottis.
- Elongated epiglottis is curled upon itself (omega-shaped). Aryepiglottic folds are floppy, and arytenoids are prominent.

Treatment

About 10% children need surgical intervention, which includes supraglottoplasty (aryepiglottoplasty). Tracheostomy may be needed.

> **Laryngomalacia:** It is the most common cause of stridor in childhood and usually occurs within the first 2 weeks of life.
> **Pathology:** It has multiple anatomic abnormalities, which include exaggerated omega-shaped epiglottis and short and inward collapse of aryepiglottic folds. Gastroesophageal reflux is probably secondary to increased negative intrathoracic pressure.

CONGENITAL VOCAL CORD PARALYSIS

Vocal fold (cord) palsy is the second most common cause of neonatal stridor after laryngomalacia. *See* Chapter 'Neurological Disorders of Larynx'.

CONGENITAL SUBGLOTTIC STENOSIS

It consists of abnormal thickening of cricoid cartilage or fibrous tissue below the level of the vocal cords. The subglottic diameter becomes less than 3.5 mm in full-term neonate (normal 4.5–5.5 mm) and 3 mm in premature neonate (normal 3.5 mm).

Clinical Feature

They depend upon the grade of stenosis. Upper respiratory infection (URI) causes increase in dyspnea and stridor. Cry is normal.

Direct Laryngoscopy and Bronchoscopy

The stenosis is confirmed and then grading is done.
- *Grade I:* Less than 50% obstruction
- *Grade II:* 51–70% obstruction
- *Grade III:* 71–99% obstruction
- *Grade IV:* No detectable lumen

> *Bronchoscopy in congenital subglottic stenosis:*
> - In case of premature neonate with subglottic stenosis, tip of 3 mm diameter bronchoscope cannot be passed through subglottis.
> - In a full term newborn with subglottic stenosis tip of 4 mm diameter bronchoscope cannot be passed.

Treatment

Many children, even though need observation, improve as the larynx grows. Grade-II or Grade-III/IV patients need tracheostomy. Decannulation may be tried when cricoid grows to sufficient size. Some children may need laryngotracheal reconstruction to expand cricoid ring.

LARYNGEAL WEB/ATRESIA

Laryngeal webs are rare. They can be of two types—anterior and posterior. Most severe type of laryngeal web is total atresia of larynx. The incomplete recanalization of larynx results in the web which is seen between the vocal cords, and has a concave posterior margin.

Clinical Features

The child presents with congenital airway obstruction, weak cry or aphonia. All patients need genetic screening and cardiovascular evaluation especially of aortic arch.

Treatment

- *Tracheostomy:* It is often required.
- Thin web needs cutting either with a knife or CO_2 laser.
- Thick web needs excision via laryngofissure, silicon keel placement and subsequent dilatations.

SUBGLOTTIC HEMANGIOMAS

Subglottic hemangiomas are benign vascular malformations and consist of endothelial hyperplasia.

Clinical Features

The infant remains asymptomatic for 3–6 months after birth. When hemangioma increases in size, the child presents with inspiratory or biphasic stridor which progressively increases in severity. Crying increases airway obstruction due to venous filling. The child has a normal cry. Some infants present with nonresolving croup. About 50% of

affected children have associated cutaneous hemangioma. Some children have associated mediastinal hemangioma.
- **Direct laryngoscopy with telescope or microscope:** Reddish-blue mass below the vocal cords can be seen. Biopsy may be associated with hemorrhage.
- **CT or MRI:** Assist in diagnosis.

Treatment
- **Tracheostomy and observation:** Many hemangioma regresses spontaneously.
- **Steroid:**
  - Dexamethasome 1 mg/kg/day for 1 week and then prednisolone 3 mg/kg in divided doses for one year.
  - Intralesional steroids and short-term intubation.
- **CO_2 and KTP lasers:** For small lesions.
- **Laryngofissure:** Surgical resection of circumferential or bilateral subglottic hemangiomas.

> *Congenital vascular lesions:* They grow a bit but then usually start regressing and do not need any treatment. Complete involution may take many years.

LARYNGOESOPHAGEAL CLEFT

The failure of the fusion of cricoid lamina results in laryngoesophageal cleft.

Clinical features: Coughing, choking and cyanosis occur during feeding. The child gets repeated aspiration pneumonia.

> *Causes of congenital stridor with a hoarse cry:* Laryngeal web, laryngeal paralysis and congenital laryngeal cyst.

FOREIGN BODIES OF AIR PASSAGES

Depending on the size and nature, a foreign body (FB) may lodge in the larynx, trachea, or bronchi. A large FB, which cannot pass through glottis, gets lodged in the supraglottic region. A small FB easily passes down into the trachea or bronchi. Sharp pointed foreign bodies (such as pins, needles, or fish bones) may stick in either larynx or tracheobronchial tree.

PREDISPOSING FACTORS

- **Age:** Children less than 5 years of age constitute more than 50% of the patients. They have a tendency to put the things in their mouth, which can go in either the food or the air passages.
- **Unconsciousness:** Unconscious adults (coma, deep sleep, alcoholic intoxication, or anesthesia) can inhale food, saliva, liquids, denture, and blood.
- **Disturbed swallowing:** Coughing, laughing, talking, crying, or tapping on back during swallowing can result in inhalation of food into air passages.
- **CN IX and CN X lesions:** Paralysis of pharynx and larynx can lead to aspiration problems.

NATURE OF FOREIGN BODIES

- **Nonirritating:** Plastic, glass or metallic items may remain symptomless for a long time.
- **Irritating:** Vegetables (peanuts, beans, seeds, areca nut) can cause diffuse reactive congestion and edema of the tracheobronchial mucosa (vegetable bronchitis). They may swell up, and cause airway obstruction and pulmonary suppuration.

CLINICAL FEATURES

Children may either hide or forget the incidence of foreign body (FB) inhalation. It is the suspicion of clinician that helps in diagnosis. The patients having air passage FB can pass through three stages:

1. **Inhalation:** This is the initial period of choking, gagging and wheezing that lasts for a short time. Small FB may be coughed out. If it is large, patient may get cyanosis and die.
2. **Latent:** During this symptom-free interval mucosa adapts to the presence of FB. It varies with the size and nature of the FB. Non-vegetable FB may go unnoticed for a long period of time.
3. **Manifestation:** Depending on the site, size, shape and nature of the FB, the obstruction, inflammation and trauma to the airway can give rise to following features:
   - **Laryngeal foreign body:** A large FB can kill the person. A relatively small FB can present with throat discomfort, hoarseness of voice, croupy cough, aphonia, inspiratory stridor, dyspnea, and hemoptysis.
   - **Tracheal foreign body:** A sharp FB produces coughing and hemoptysis. A small seed may move up and down the trachea, and produce audible slap, tracheal flutter, and palpatory thud. Biphasic stridor or asthmatoid wheeze is best heard when child's mouth is open.
   - **Bronchial foreign body:** Right bronchus is the most common site for FBs because it is wider and more in line with the tracheal lumen. A FB may either totally obstruct a lobar/segmental bronchus (atelectasis), or produce a check valve obstruction (obstructive emphysema) which allows only ingress of air (Fig. 49.8).
     - *Atelectasis:* Complete stop valve obstruction results in atelectasis of lung or its segment. Poor air entry is found on auscultation of the lower lobe on the back of the thorax.

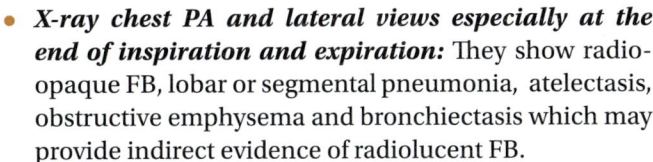

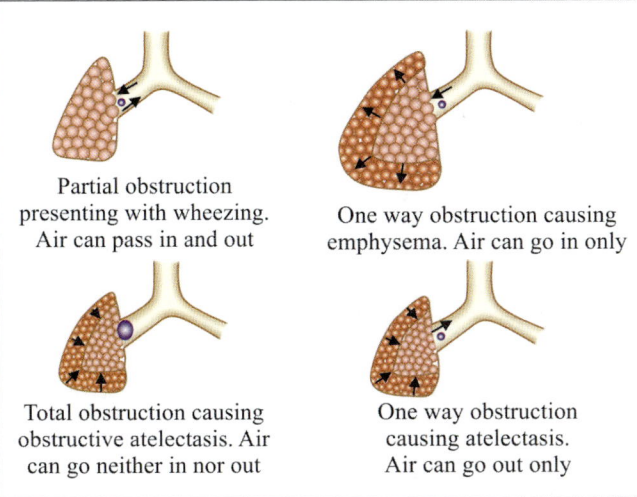

Fig. 49.8: Foreign body bronchus resulting in four types of bronchial obstruction

- **Obstructive emphysema:** Bronchial edema proximal to the FB and bronchial dilatation during inspiration produce a sort of check valve obstruction that allows entry of air with only inspiration.
- **Shifting foreign body:** Small FB may move from one bronchus to other bronchus or to trachea, and produce poor air entry in any lung.
- **Acute laryngotracheobronchitis:** Infection and chemical reaction of vegetable FB can produce the picture of acute laryngotracheobronchitis.
- **Spontaneous pneumothorax:** Emphysematous bulla may rupture.
- **Pulmonary infections:** A retained FB can give rise to pneumonitis, bronchiectasis or lung abscess.

Chronic and recurrent cough and pulmonary infection: In cases of chronic cough and recurrent pulmonary lesions (such as pneumonia, atelectasis, emphysema, pneumothorax, lung abscess and bronchiectasis) of the same side and region FB must be ruled out.

DIFFERENTIAL DIAGNOSES

Laryngotracheobronchitis (*see* Chapter 'Infections of Larynx').

Diagnosis

The detailed history, physical examination, and radiographs confirm the diagnosis.
- **X-ray soft tissue neck postero-anterior (PA) and lateral views in extended position:** Radio-opaque and sometimes, radiolucent foreign bodies can be seen in the larynx and trachea.
- **X-ray chest PA and lateral views especially at the end of inspiration and expiration:** They show radio-opaque FB, lobar or segmental pneumonia, atelectasis, obstructive emphysema and bronchiectasis which may provide indirect evidence of radiolucent FB.
- **Fluoroscopy/videofluoroscopy during inspiration and expiration.**
- **Bronchograms:** It delineates radiolucent foreign bodies and bronchiectasis.
- **CT scan:** HRCT/virtual bronchoscopy.
- **Laryngoscopy and bronchoscopy:** They are both diagnostic as well as therapeutic.

Jackson's dictum: In suspected cases of FB of air passages, bronchoscopy must be done as failure to do bronchoscopy is more disastrous than the complications of bronchoscopy.

MANAGEMENT

- **Medical:** Antibiotics, steroids and oxygen are administered immediately, and continued after the bronchoscopy.
- **Laryngeal foreign body**
    - **Cricothyrotomy or emergency tracheostomy:** These are done when Heimlich's maneuver fails.
    - **Direct laryngoscopy or laryngofissure:** FB is removed by direct laryngoscopy or by laryngofissure.
    - Heimlich's maneuver (Fig. 49.9):
        - *Indication:* A large bolus of food completely obstructing the larynx with total aphonia, and patient dying of asphyxia (impending death).

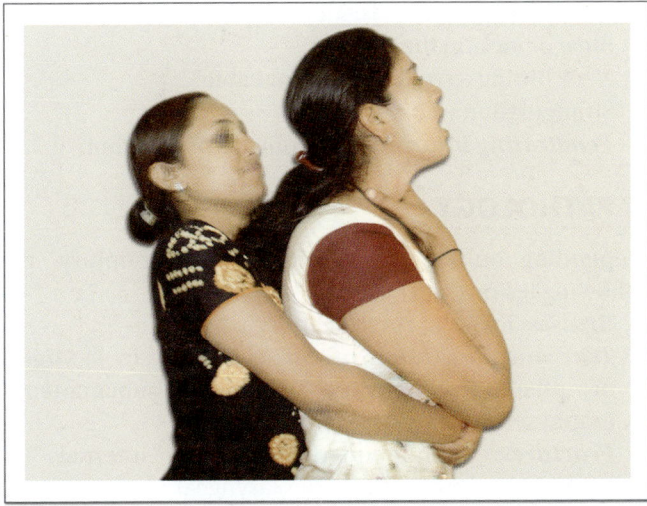

Fig. 49.9: Heimlich's maneuver. Standing behind the standing patient, sudden upward and backward thrusts just below the epigastric region squeeze the lungs' air, and may dislodge laryngeal foreign body

- **Contraindication:** Partially obstructing FB because maneuver can cause total obstruction.
- **Method:** First pounds on the back, and turns the patient upside down. Then, follows Heimlich maneuver. Standing behind the patient, and placing arms around patient's lower chest give four abdominal thrusts. The residual pulmonary air can dislodge the laryngeal FB.

- **Tracheal and bronchial foreign bodies**
  - **Bronchoscopy under general anesthesia:** Rigid bronchoscopy is the standard procedure for FB removal. Emergency removal is indicated only when the airway obstruction is present or FB is vegetable. The following methods are used for the removal of tracheobronchial FB:
    - Rigid bronchoscopy with or without a telescope.
    - Bronchoscopy with C-arm fluoroscopy.
    - Snares and basket or Fogarty's catheter balloon for rounded FB.
    - Bronchoscopy through the tracheostome.
    - Flexible fiberoptic bronchoscopy in selected cases.
    - Thoracotomy and bronchotomy for peripheral foreign bodies.
    - Lobectomy or pneumonectomy may be needed in cases of old unnoticed FBs.

> **Respiratory distress:** If a child with respiratory distress is becoming quiet, it indicates that the child is about to have respiratory collapse.

LARYNGOTRACHEAL TRAUMA

MODES OF INJURIES

- **Automobile accidents:** Most common.
- Blow or kick on the neck.
- Neck hitting a stretched wire or cable.
- Strangulation.
- **Penetrating injuries:** Sharp objects or gun shot.

PATHOLOGY

Depending on the mode and severity of injury, the following lesions can occur:
- **Bruises:** External cervical bruises.
- **Tear and laceration of mucosa:** Tears in laryngeal or pharyngeal mucosa results in subcutaneous emphysema.
- **Fractures:** Compound (external or internal) or comminuted fractures of the laryngeal framework are common after 40 years of age because of calcification of the laryngeal framework. Children laryngeal cartilages are more resilient, and usually escape injury.
  - Hyoid bone
  - Thyroid cartilage (vertical or transverse): Fracture of upper part of thyroid cartilage may cause avulsion of epiglottis and false cords. Fractures of lower part of thyroid cartilage can disrupt true vocal cords.
  - Cricoid cartilage
  - Upper tracheal cartilages
- **Hematoma and edema** of supraglottic or subglottic region.
- **Dislocation of joints**
  - **Cricoarytenoid joints:** The arytenoid cartilage can be displaced anteriorly, dislocated or avulsed.
  - **Cricothyroid joint:** Dislocation of cricothyroid joint can cause paralysis of recurrent laryngeal nerve which lies just behind the joint.
- **Laryngotracheal separation:** Trachea may get separated from the cricoid cartilage, and go into upper mediastinum injuring the recurrent laryngeal nerve.

CLINICAL FEATURES

Clinical features depend on the type and severity of the injury. They are following:
- Stridor.
- Hoarseness of voice or aphonia.
- Pain and difficulty in swallowing.
- Aspiration of food, blood and secretions.
- Local laryngeal pain more on speaking and swallowing.
- Hemoptysis due to mucosal tears.
- Cervical bruises or abrasions.
- Tenderness in the laryngeal area.
- **Subcutaneous emphysema:** It may increase on coughing and is due to mucosal tears of larynx and trachea.
- Flattening of thyroid prominence and anterior cervical contour.
- Gap and crepitus between fractured fragments of thyroid and cricoid cartilages or hyoid bone.
- Cricoid cartilage may get separated from larynx or trachea.

DIAGNOSIS

- **Laryngoscopy:** When the patient's condition allows indirect laryngoscopy examination can reveal edema, hematoma, mucosal lacerations, displacement of epiglottis, fragments of cartilage, asymmetry of larynx. Fiberoptic laryngoscopy (rigid or flexible) provides easier and better visualization. Direct laryngoscopy is relatively contraindicated as it may precipitate respiratory distress.
- **X-ray soft tissue neck lateral view:** It may show subcutaneous emphysema, mucosal swelling, fracture/displacement of epiglottis, thyroid and cricoid cartilages, hyoid bone, or change in the air column.

- **CT scan:** It reveals injuries of laryngeal cartilages in a better way. Three-dimensional reconstructions are very useful.

ASSOCIATED INJURIES

Rule out injury to head, cervical spine, chest, abdomen and extremities. X-ray chest may show pneumothorax. Gastrografin swallow will reveal esophageal tears.

COMPLICATIONS

- Laryngeal stenosis: Supraglottic, glottic or subglottic
- Perichondritis
- Laryngeal abscess
- Vocal cord paralysis

The chief danger of laryngeal trauma is respiratory distress (stridor).

TREATMENT

- Watch out for respiratory distress.
- Voice rest.
- Humidification of inspired air.
- **Steroids:** Steroids resolve edema and hematoma, and prevent scarring and stenosis.
- **Antibiotics:** They prevent perichondritis and cartilage necrosis.
- **Management of impaired airway:** In cases of laryngeal trauma, tracheostomy is preferred over endotracheal intubation which may be difficult and risky.
- **Open reduction:** It should be done in 3–5 days after injury, and definitely before 10 days.
  - **Wire and titanium miniplate:** For fractures of hyoid bone, thyroid or cricoid cartilage.
  - **Absorbable sutures:** Mucosal lacerations are repaired with vicryl.
  - Removal of loose fragments of cartilage and avulsed epiglottis and arytenoids.
  - **Anchoring:** Arytenoid and epiglottis are repositioned in their normal position.
  - **End to end anastomosis:** In cases of laryngotracheal separation.
  - **Internal splint of laryngeal structures:** A laryngeal stent or silicone tube may have to be left for 2–6 weeks. A silastic keel prevents webbing of anterior commissure.

Self-evaluation Exercises

1. The features foreign body bronchus include:
   a. History of coughing, choking and gagging.
   b. Foreign body lodges more often in the right bronchus and can be expelled spontaneously with coughing.
   c. X-ray chest may show either hyperinflated (emphysema) lung on one side or unilateral atelectasis (collapse) of lung.
   d. Best management for inhaled foreign body is bronchoscopy removal.
   e. All of the above.
2. Which of the following are related with the laryngomalacia:
   a. Stridor is relieved when child is put in prone position.
   b. Stridor disappears spontaneously as the child grows.
   c. Epiglottis appears omega-shaped.
   d. All of the above.
3. The causes of congenital stridor with a hoarse cry include:
   a. Laryngeal web
   b. Laryngeal paralysis
   c. Congenital laryngeal cyst
   d. All of the above

True (T)/False (F)

4. Respiratory dead space is approximately 150 ml and tracheostomy cuts down the dead space by 30–50%.
5. Flexible fiberoptic laryngoscopy is the best way to diagnose laryngomalacia.
6. In case of premature neonate with subglottic stenosis, tip of 3 mm diameter bronchoscope cannot be passed through subglottis.
7. In a full term newborn with subglottic stenosis tip of 4 mm diameter bronchoscope cannot be passed.

Filling the blanks

8. _____ is the most common cause of 'inspiratory stridor' 2–3 weeks after the birth.
9. _____ is the most common congenital anomaly of the larynx.
10. _____ is the most common site of congenital laryngeal web.
11. The chief danger of laryngeal trauma is _____.

Answers

1. e 2. d 3. d 4. T 5. T 6. T
7. T 8. Laryngomalacia 9. Laryngomalacia 10. Glottis
11. respiratory distress (stridor)

Section 7: Neck

Chapter 50

Anatomy of Neck

Specific Learning Objectives

After going through the chapter, you should be able to answer the following questions:
- Describe the different levels of cervical lymph nodes and their importance.
- Describe different types of neck dissection for the metastatic neck nodes and the structures removed and saved in them.
- Describe the arteries which supply to the thyroid gland and the landmarks of the laryngeal nerves which run along with them.

LYMPH NODES OF HEAD AND NECK

For the broad classification and the drainage of different groups of lymph nodes (Table 50.1).

- **Submental nodes:** Two to eight in number and lie on the mylohyoid muscle. The submental triangle is situated between right and left anterior bellies of digastric muscles and the hyoid bone.
- **Submandibular nodes:** They lie in relation with submandibular gland and facial artery. The submandibular (digastric) triangle is situated between anterior and posterior bellies of digastric muscle and bounded superiorly by the lower border of mandible and an imaginary line drawn between the angle of mandible and mastoid.
- **Parotid nodes:** They are in close relation with parotid salivary gland and are extraglandular (preauricular and infraauricular) and intraglandular.
- **Post auricular nodes (mastoid nodes):** They lie behind the auricle.
- **Occipital nodes:** They are at the apex of the posterior triangle and situated both superficial and deep into splenius capitus muscle.
- **Facial nodes:** They are situated along facial vessels and are named according to their location. Malar nodes lie near outer canthus.
- **Superficial lateral cervical nodes:** They lie along external jugular vein.
- **Deep lateral cervical nodes:** They lie deep to sternocleidomastoid muscle and in the posterior triangle. This group consists of three chains—internal jugular, spinal accessory and transverse.
- **Internal jugular chain:** It is further divided into upper (jugulodigastric node), middle and lower groups. They lie anterior, lateral and posterior to internal jugular vein and extends from digastric muscle to subclavian vein.
- **Spinal accessory chain:** It lies near the spinal accessory nerve in the posterior triangle. Upper nodes of this chain merge with upper jugular nodes.
- **Transverse cervical chain (supraclavicular nodes):** They are present in the lower part of the posterior triangle and lie horizontally along the transverse cervical vessels. The posterior cervical triangle lies between posterior border of sternocleidomastoid, anterior border of trapezius and the clavicle below.
  - **Scalene nodes:** These are medial group of supraclavicular nodes.
- **Anterior cervical nodes:** They are present between the two carotids and below the level of hyoid bone. They consist of two chains—anterior jugular chain and juxtavisceral chain.
  - **Anterior jugular chain:** It is situated along anterior jugular vein.
  - **Juxtavisceral chain:** It has three groups.
    i. **Prelaryngeal node (Delphian node)** lies on cricothyroid membrane.
    ii. **Pretracheal nodes** lie in front of the trachea, deep to pretracheal fascia.
    iii. **Paratracheal nodes (recurrent nerve chain)** lie along recurrent laryngeal nerve.
- **Lymph nodes not palpable clinically:**
  - **Retropharyngeal nodes**, behind the pharynx.
    - **Lateral group** lies close to base of skull at the level of atlas. **Rouviere** is most superior node.

Chapter 50 • Anatomy of Neck

Table 50.1: Classification of lymph nodes of head and neck

- **Nodes of upper horizontal chain**
  - *Submental nodes:* Afferents from chin, lower lip (only middle part), lower anterior gums, anterior floor of mouth and tip of tongue. Efferents to submandibular nodes and internal jugular chain.
  - *Submandibular nodes:* Afferents from lower lip (only lateral part), upper lip, cheek, nasal vestibule and anterior part of nasal cavity, gums and teeth (except lower anterior gums and teeth), medial canthus, soft palate, anterior pillar, anterior part of tongue, submandibular and sublingual salivary glands and floor of mouth (except central anterior part). Efferents to internal jugular chain.
  - *Parotid nodes:* Afferents from scalp (anterior to pinna), pinna, external auditory canal, face, buccal mucosa. Efferents to internal jugular and external jugular chain.
  - *Postauricular nodes (mastoid nodes):* Afferents—from scalp (posterior to pinna), posterior surface of pinna and skin of mastoid. Efferents to infra-auricular nodes and into internal jugular chain.
  - *Occipital nodes:* Afferents from scalp, skin of upper neck. Efferents to upper accessory chain of nodes.
  - *Facial nodes (midmandibular, buccinator, infraorbital and malar):* Afferents from upper and lower lids, nose, lips and cheek. Efferents to submandibular nodes.
- **Lateral cervical nodes (superficial and deep):** The **superficial external jugular group** drains into following deep internal jugular and transverse cervical nodes.
  - *Internal jugular chain*
    - *Upper deep cervical group (jugulodigastric node):* Afferents from oral cavity, oropharynx, nasopharynx, hypopharynx, larynx and parotid.
    - *Middle deep cervical group:* Afferents from oral cavity, oropharynx, hypopharynx, larynx, and thyroid.
    - *Lower deep cervical group:* Afferents from larynx, thyroid and cervical esophagus.
  - *Spinal accessory chain:* Afferents from scalp, skin of the neck, nasopharynx, occipital and postauricular nodes. *Efferents* to transverse cervical chain.
  - *Transverse cervical chain (supraclavicular nodes):* Afferents from accessory chain.
    - *Medial supraclavicular (scalene nodes):* Afferents from breast, lung, stomach, colon, ovary and testis.
- **Anterior cervical nodes**
  - *Anterior jugular chain:* Afferents from skin of anterior neck.
  - *Juxtavisceral chain*
    - *Prelaryngeal node (Delphian node):* Afferents from subglottic larynx and pyriform sinuses.
    - *Pretracheal nodes:* Afferents from thyroid gland the trachea. Efferents to paratracheal, lower internal jugular and anterior mediastinal nodes.
    - *Paratracheal nodes (recurrent laryngeal nerve chain):* Afferents from thyroid lobes, subglottic larynx, trachea and cervical esophagus.
- **Lymph nodes not clinically palpable**
  - *Retropharyngeal nodes: Lateral (Rouviere) and medial groups*—Afferent from nasal cavity, paranasal sinuses, hard and soft palate, nasopharynx, and posterior wall of pharynx. Efferents to upper internal jugular group.
  - *Sublingual nodes:* Afferents from anterior part of the floor of mouth and ventral surface of tongue. Efferents to submandibular and upper jugular nodes.

- *Medial group* lies near midline at lower level.
- *Sublingual nodes* lie deep along the lingual vessels.

The deep jugular groups receive in addition to their direct areas of drainage all the efferents from pericraniocervical ring, superficial cervical nodes and other paravisceral deep nodes (such as retropharyngeal, infrahyoid, prelaryngeal, pretracheal, paratracheal and subclavian). All the lymph from the head and neck finally drains into lower deep cervical group (terminal group). Efferents from the latter converge and form (right and left) jugular lymph trunks that descends on its vein to its termination at the jugulosubclavian venous junction (thoracic duct on left side).

Levels of Cervical Lymph Nodes (Figs 50.1 and 50.2)

The cervical lymph nodes are divided into different levels (Table 50.2), which is very important in cases of head and neck malignancies. On the bases of these levels various types of neck dissections are described (Table 50.3).

- **Anterior compartment nodes** lie between the medial borders of SCM muscles (or carotid sheaths), hyoid bone above and suprasternal notch below.
- **Ho's triangle in supraclavicular zone or fossa** lies between the medial and lateral ends of upper border of clavicle at the point where neck meets the shoulder. Metastasis in these nodes, which include lower part of levels IV and V, indicates an advanced stage of carcinoma nasopharynx.

NECK DISSECTION

This operation is used in the surgical management of cancer of the aerodigestive tract. It removes metastatic cervical lymph nodes and their surrounding fibrofatty tissues. See Table 50.3 for different types of neck dissection, their meanings and indications.

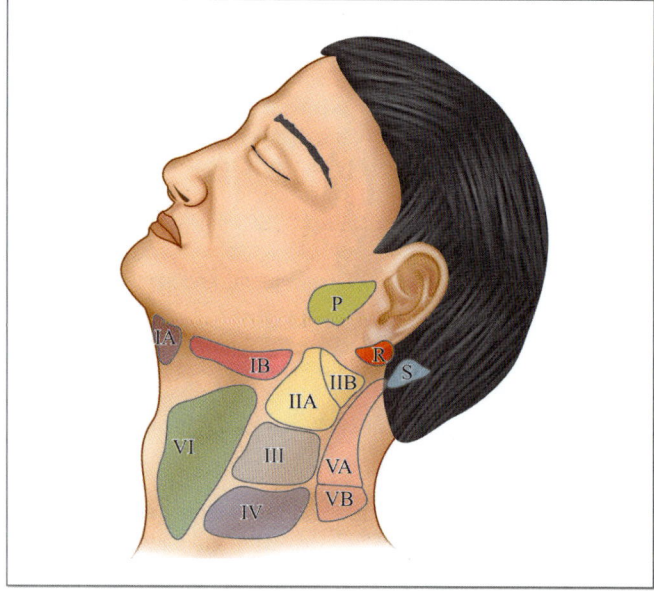

Fig. 50.1: Neck nodes regions
Key: P—parotid preauricular; R—retroauricular; S—suboccipital regions

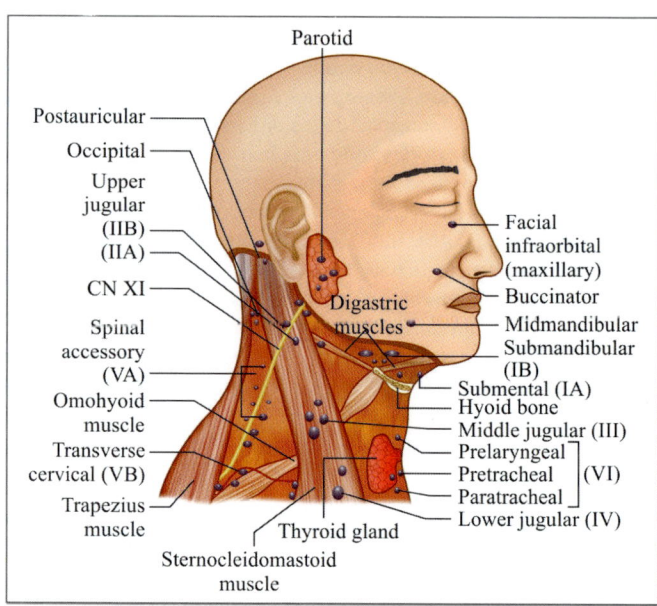

Fig. 50.2: Lymph nodes of head and neck. Neck nodes levels are mentioned in (parenthesis)

Table 50.2: Levels of cervical lymph nodes

- **Level I:** Submental nodes and submandibular nodes.
  - **Level IA:** Submental nodes.
  - **Level IB:** Submandibular nodes.
- **Level II:** Upper jugular (between skull base and hyoid bone).
  - **Level IIA:** Inferomedial to accessory nerve.
  - **Level IIB:** Superolateral to accessory nerve.
- **Level III:** Middle jugular (between hyoid bone and upper border of cricoid cartilage).
- **Level IV:** Lower jugular (between upper border of cricoid cartilage and clavicle).
- **Level V:** Posterior triangle group—subdivided into upper, middle and lower, corresponding to planes of levels II, III and IV.
  - **Level VA:** Spinal accessory nodes above the level of cricoid cartilage.
  - **Level VB:** Transverse cervical chains and supraclavicular nodes below the level of cricoid cartilage.
- **Level VI:** Anterior compartment nodes—prelaryngeal (precricoid or Delphian), perithyroidal, pretracheal, paratracheal.
- **Level VII:** Superior mediastinum nodes.
- **Lymph nodes not included:**
  - P: Parotid-preauricular
  - R: Retroauricular (mastoid)
  - S: Suboccipital
  - Others: Retropharyngeal and facial

Radical Neck Dissection (RND)

- **Structures removed:** All lymph nodes (level of I to V) and structures closely related to them that are present in the area between mandible and mastoid above, clavicle below, hyoid bone and contralateral anterior belly of digastric medially, and trapezius posteriorly.

Table 50.3: Classification of neck dissection

- **Radical neck dissection (RND):** Removes I, II, III, IV and V level of lymph nodes, submandibular salivary gland, tail of the parotid, omohyoid muscle, spinal accessory nerve, internal jugular vein and sternocleidomastoid muscle.
- **Modified radical neck dissection**
  - **Type I:** Preserves accessory cranial nerve (CN XI).
  - **Type II:** Preserves CN XI and internal jugular vein (IJV).
  - **Type III:** Preserves CN XI, IJV and sternocleidomastoid muscle (SCM).
- **Selective neck dissection:** Preserves CN XI, IJV and SCM.
  - **Supra omohyoid (or anterolateral):** Removes level I, II and III lymph nodes (cancer of oral cavity).
  - **Lateral:** Removes level II, III and IV lymph nodes (cancer of oropharynx, hypopharynx and larynx).
  - **Posterolateral:** Removes level II, III, IV, V and suboccipital lymph nodes (cancer or melanoma of posterior scalp or posterior upper neck).
  - **Anterior compartment:** Removes level VI lymph nodes (cancer of thyroid, subglottic, cervical trachea, hypopharynx).
- **Extended neck dissection:** Extended RND may include additional lymph node groups (retropharyngeal, parotid or level VI nodes) and nonlymphatic structures (external carotid artery, hypoglossal nerve, parotid gland, mastoid tip).

- **Lymph nodes:** Level of I to V lymph nodes present in submental, submandibular, and posterior triangle and internal jugular chain.
- **Salivary glands:** Submandibular and tail of parotid.
- **Muscles:** Sternocleidomastoid and omohyoid.
- **Internal jugular vein (IJV).**
- **Spinal accessory nerve.**

- ***Structures not removed:*** In RND, the lymph nodes, which are not removed are—postauricular, suboccipital, parotid (except those in the tail), facial, retropharyngeal and paratracheal. Following important structures are saved. because their injury can lead to morbidity and even mortality:
    - ***Arteries:*** Common carotid artery (CCA), internal carotid artery (ICA) and external carotid artery (ECA).
    - ***Nerves:*** Brachial plexus, phrenic nerve, vagus nerve, cervical sympathetic chain, marginal mandibular branch of facial, lingual and hypoglossal nerves.
- ***Incisions:*** Though RND alone can be performed, usually it is combined with the removal of primary tumor. Any one of the following incisions may be employed:
    - Schobinger
    - McAfee
    - Hockey-stick
    - Extensions from Gluck-Sorenson's incision, used for laryngectomy with neck dissection.
- ***Contraindications:*** They include:
    - Untreatable primary cancer
    - Distant metastases
    - Neck nodes fixed to deeper important structures.
    - Major systemic illnesses.

Modified Neck Dissection (Table 50.3)

It is similar to radical neck dissection but with certain modifications, which include preservation of one or more of the following structures:
- Spinal accessory nerve (CN XI)
- Internal jugular vein (IJV)
- Sternocleidomastoid muscle (SCM).

Selective Neck Dissection (Table 50.3)

In selective neck dissection, in addition to the three non-lymphatic structures (CN XI, SCM and IJV) certain levels of lymph nodes are not removed. There are different types of selective neck dissections.

Extended Neck Dissection (Table 50.3)

In addition to the structures removed in RND, extended neck dissection includes other lymph node groups (retropharyngeal, parotid or level VI nodes) and non-lymphatic structures (external carotid artery, hypoglossal nerve, parotid gland, mastoid tip).

> ***Elective neck dissection:***
> - It is the RND that is performed when there are no metastatic cervical lymph nodes.
> - In medullary carcinoma of thyroid, elective neck dissection is appropriate.

THYROID GLAND (FIG. 50.3)

It is made up of two lateral lobes and central isthmus. Lobes extend from thyroid cartilage to sixth tracheal ring. Isthmus overlies second to fourth tracheal rings. Sometimes a pyramidal lobe projects up from the isthmus on left side. Pretracheal layer of deep cervical fascia envelops the thyroid gland and trachea. Anterior relations include strap muscles, anterior jugular veins and SCM. Posterior relations are laryngopharynx, larynx, trachea and esophagus. The carotid sheath, which contains CCA, IJV and vagus nerve, lies lateral to the thyroid lobe. Cervical sympathetic trunk and thyrocervical trunk giving inferior thyroid artery lie posterior to carotid sheath.

Blood Supply and Related Laryngeal Nerves

- ***Superior thyroid artery and external laryngeal nerve (ELN):*** The ELN, a branch of superior laryngeal nerve supplying the cricothyroid muscle lies deep to the upper pole in ***sternothyrolaryngeal (Joll's) triangle***. The superior thyroid vessels running down the upper pole are very close to ELN, which can be damaged if superior thyroid vessels are ligated too high. ELN injury will limit the patient's vocal range (particularly in singers).
    - ***Joll's triangle:*** Boundaries of Joll's triangle include:
        - ***Lateral:*** Upper pole of thyroid gland and superior thyroid vessels.
        - ***Superior:*** Insertion of sternothyroid muscle.
        - ***Medial:*** Cervical midline.
        - ***Floor:*** Cricothyroid muscle.
        - ***Roof:*** Strap muscles.
- ***Inferior thyroid artery and recurrent laryngeal nerve (RLN):*** The RLN can be identified in the lower part of

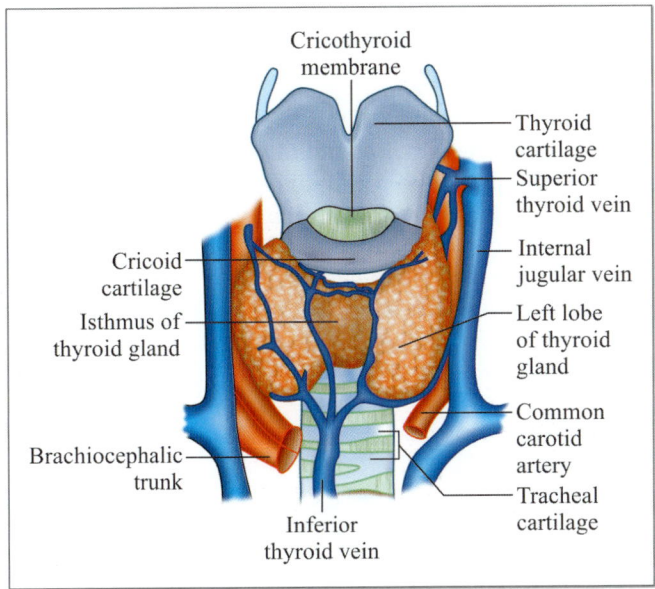

Fig. 50.3: Anterior surface of thyroid gland and its relations with carotid arteries and internal jugular vein

tracheoesophageal groove where it forms a boundary of the **Beahr's triangle**. RLN can be anterior, posterior or pass through the branches of inferior thyroid artery, which is traditionally ligated away from the thyroid lobe. The injury to RLN results in vocal cord palsy and hoarseness of voice. At the level of second or third tracheal ring in the region of Berry's ligament, RLN is intimately close to or pierce posterior surface of thyroid lobe. **Berry's ligament** is posterior condensation of pretracheal fascia where thyroid gland is tethered to trachea. The inferior thyroid artery arises from the thyrocervical trunk and pierces the prevertebral fascia medial to carotid sheath and enters into the posterior part of thyroid lobe.

- **Beahr's triangle:** The boundaries of Beahr's triangle include:
  - *Medial:* RLN in the lower part of tracheoesophageal groove. Occasionally RLN lie lateral to tracheoesophageal groove.
  - *Lateral:* Common carotid artery
  - *Superior:* Inferior thyroid artery
- **Thyroidea ima artery:** When present it may arise from aortic arch or innominate artery.

> **RLN triangle of Lore:** RLN traverses this from lateral to medial on right side and in tracheoesophageal gutter on left side. This triangle is bounded by trachea and esophagus (medially), retracted strap muscles (laterally) and inferior pole of thyroid (superiorly). The apex of the triangle faces thoracic inlet (inferiorly).

Venous Drainage

- **Superior and middle thyroid veins:** They drain into internal jugular vein.
- **Inferior thyroid veins:** They are multiple and drain into brachiocephalic vein.

Lymphatic Drainage

The lymphatic drainage of thyroid gland can be grouped into two categories—major and minor:
- *Major:* Major lymphatic drainage goes to;
  - Middle deep cervical (jugular) node level III.
  - Lower deep cervical (jugular) node level IV.
  - Posterior triangle nodes level V.
- *Minor:* Some of the lymphatics drain into:
  - Pre and paratracheal nodes level VI.
  - Superior mediastinal nodes level VII.

Lingual Thyroid

- **Incidence:** Very rare.
- **Pathology:** Ectopic thyroid situated in the posterior one-third of tongue. May be extra or only thyroid.
- **Clinical features:** Difficulty in respiration and swallowing if the mass on base of tongue is large.
- **Differential diagnoses:** Swellings of the base of tongue such as lingual tonsils, carcinoma, thyroglossal cyst, lymphoma and minor salivary gland tumor.
- **Treatment:** Surgical removal by suprahyoid transpharyngeal approach.

PARATHYROID GLANDS (FIG. 50.4)

- **Superior parathyroids:** They lie near the junction of medial and posterior surfaces of upper third of thyroid lobe at the level of cricoid cartilage superior to inferior thyroid artery. They are situated in or near the thyroid capsule. Their position is more consistent than the inferior parathyroids.
- **Inferior parathyroids:** They are posteriorly placed on the lower poles inferior to inferior thyroid artery.

> - **Thyroglossal cyst or fistula:** They occur in midline of neck when parts of thyroglossal duct persist. The cyst is generally seen near the hyoid bone but may also be found at the base of tongue (lingual cyst).
> - **Ectopic thyroid:** This tissue may be found in the midline of neck along the course of thyroglossal duct.

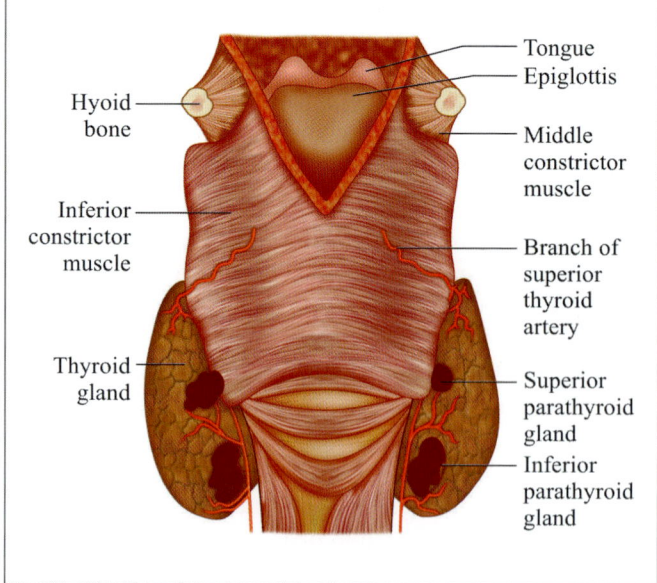

Fig. 50.4: Posterior surface of thyroid and parathyroid glands and laryngopharynx and cervical esophagus

Self-evaluation Exercises

1. Nerves which are not preserved in radical neck dissection include:
   a. Vagus
   b. Hypoglossal
   c. Phrenic
   d. None of the above

True (T)/False (F)

2. In selective neck dissection, only selective groups/levels of cervical lymph nodes are removed.
3. In medullary carcinoma of thyroid, elective neck dissection is inappropriate.

Answers

1. d   2. T   3. F

Chapter 51

Cervical Symptoms and Examination

> **Specific Learning Objectives**
>
> After going through the chapter, you should be able to answer the following questions:
> - What are the components of neck examination?
> - How will you perform the examination of neck lymph nodes?
> - How will you take the history and perform examination of thyroid patients?
> - How will you investigate a case of thyroid swelling?

NECK

HISTORY

The age of the patient (child, young adult or older adult) and location of the neck mass (midline neck, anterior triangle and posterior triangle) are particularly important in differentiation of congenital/developmental, inflammatory and neoplastic neck masses. Although the congenital/developmental swellings occur in children (< 15 years of age) and young adults (16–40 years of age), they are less common than inflammatory masses in these age groups. In contrast, neoplasia should be considered first in older adults (> 40 years of age). The specific history aspects and physical findings limit the number of diagnostic tests and can avoid unnecessary investigations.

> **Age specific swellings**
> - **Since birth:** Branchial fistula
> - **Newborn:** Sternomastoid tumor (torticollis or wryneck)
> - **Young children:** Branchial cyst and cystic hygroma
> - **Adults:** Inflammatory swellings
> - **Elderly people:** Secondary metastatic neck nodes

PHYSICAL EXAMINATION

Thorough physical examination gives an idea about the derivation of mass—inflammatory, congenital or neoplastic; vascular, salivary, thyroid or nodal. The key features of physical examination include:

- Site of the swelling according to anatomic lymphatic drainage and developmental areas.
- Size and extent of the mass and number of nodes.
- Relationship (fixation and displacement) to surrounding structures.
- Consistency of the mass.
- Presence of pulsation, thrills and bruits.
- Distinct odor of wet keratin and necrotic tumor.
- Transillumination.
- Radiotherapy effects.
- Depth of the swelling: Cutaneous, subcutaneous, deep or superficial to muscle.
- Complete head and neck evaluation including palpation and indirect laryngoscopy or flexible nasopharyngolaryngoscopy for upper aerodigestive tract especially for the primary sites of lymphatic drainage to the location of neck mass.

> - **Thyroglossal cyst:** This midline neck mass is recognized by its movement with swallowing. An ultrasound neck will evaluate for ectopic thyroid tissue.
> - **Carotid triangle swellings:** The most common causes of swellings in this region are paragangliomas, schwannomas, meningiomas and nodal metastases.

Examination of Lymph Nodes of Neck

Examination of neck nodes (Figs 51.1 and 51.2) needs a systematic approach. It is an important part of otorhinolaryngology, head and neck evaluation.

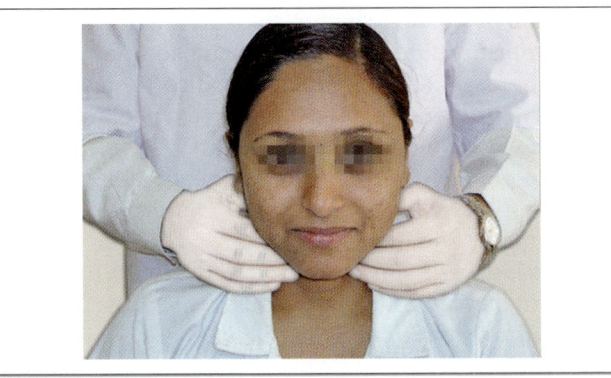

Fig. 51.1: Palpation of cervical lymph nodes

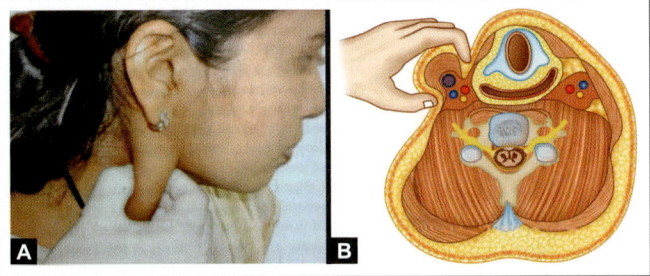

Figs 51.2A and B: Method of palpating deep cervical lymph nodes. The thumb and index finger grasping the sternocleidomastoid muscle palpate the deep jugular lymph nodes of region II, III, and IV

- *Method:* Palpation of cervical lymph nodes is carried out while standing behind the seated patient. Examiner uses both hands simultaneously with fingers semiflexed and adducted and thumbs in partial opposition. Slight flexion of neck achieves relaxation of muscles. Internal jugular chain (upper, middle and lower) groups lie deep to sternocleidomastoid muscle, which needs to be retracted. The nodes are explored systematically—the submental triangle, the submandibular glands and triangles (thumbs over buccinators); the retromandibular depressions (thumbs probing over parotids), the upper attachment of sternocleidomastoid, and the occipital attachment of trapezius. Palpation then continues along the vertical chains of cervical nodes which have superficial (associated with the external jugular and anterior jugular veins, the superficial cervical and anterior cervical groups) and deep nodes (upper, middle and lower deep cervical jugular nodes, alongside and embedded in areolar tissue near the carotid sheath but particularly those aspects surrounding the internal jugular vein) and then the juxtavisceral chain (prelaryngeal, pretracheal and paratracheal).
- *Findings:* During the inspection and palpation of these nodes, one must note their location, number, discrete/matted, size, consistency, tenderness and fixity. Inflammatory nodes are tender. Fixity can be either to overlying skin or deeper structures. Mobility of nodes is checked in both vertical and horizontal planes. Metastatic nodes are usually hard but metastatic melanoma and lymphoma nodes are soft.

THYROID GLAND

HISTORY

- *Age and sex:* Thyroid swellings (goiter) are more common in females. Hashimoto's disease is a disease of middle-aged women. Physiological goiter occurs frequently at puberty in girls. Deficiency of iodine in water and food is the cause of endemic goiter. Thyroid adenoma of middle-aged patients is usually toxic. Papillary carcinoma is common in young girls whereas follicular carcinoma occurs in middle-aged women. The anaplastic carcinoma occurs in old age. The patients of primary toxic goiter are usually young.
- *Onset, duration and progress:* Inflammatory diseases have short history. Thyrotoxicosis may appear in women having stress and strain. Sudden increase in the size of previous goiter is an ominous sign. Simple goiters grow very slowly, and may remain of the same size for years. Multinodular goiter and solitary nodules grow extremely slow. The papillary and follicular carcinomas also grow slowly for years before metastasizing. Anaplastic carcinoma grows fast.
- *Primary thyrotoxicosis:* These patients may or may not have goiter, and the brunt of attack falls on nervous system. The symptoms include loss of weight, staring or protruding eyes, preference for cold, excessive sweating, excitability, irritability, insomnia, tremors and muscle weakness. Enquire the patient regarding palpitation and exhaustion on strain.
- *Secondary thyrotoxicosis:* In this condition, long standing thyroid nodule, simple or multinodular goiter develops toxic features. In this disease, the brunt of attack falls on cardiovascular systems, and patients do not have protruding eyes and tremors. The cardiovascular symptoms include palpitation, ectopic beats, chest pain and dyspnea on exertion. Other features are cardiac arrhythmias, congestive cardiac failure and swelling of ankles.
- *Myxedema (hypothyroidism):* The symptoms include weight gain, intolerance to cold weather, dry skin, puffiness of face, dull expression, loss of hair and two-third of eyebrows, muscle fatigue, lethargy and mild hoarseness of voice.
- *Pressure effects:* Enquire about dyspnea (pressure on trachea), dysphagia (pressure on esophagus) and hoarseness of voice (pressure on recurrent laryngeal nerve).

- **Drugs:** Enquire about the medicines taken before the goiter or for the goiter.
- **Personal history:** Cabbage, kale and rape are goitrogens. Sea fish has low iodine contents.

EXAMINATION

General Examination

Look for the features of hyperthyroidism such as exophthalmos (staring), excitability, trembling, nervousness, sweating and wasting. Sleeping pulse rate must be recorded. Hypothyroidism causes weight gain, bradycardia, dry and rough skin and depression.
- *Abdominal examination:* In women with Hashimoto's disease, liver and spleen should be examined for cirrhosis.

Local Examination

Inspection and palpation of goiter are similar to examination of the swelling and neck, and include site, shape, size, extent, surface, pulsation, overlying skin, consistency, mobility and relation with neighboring structures. The thyroid swellings are palpated both from the front and behind (Fig. 51.3A). Thyroid swellings move on swallowing.
- *Uniform enlargement:* Gives shape of thyroid gland.
- *Nodule:* It may be single or multiple, and may occur either in isthmus or lobe.
- *Mobility:* Movements with deglutition are greatly limited in cases of chronic thyroiditis and malignancy. Extent of mobility should be checked in both horizontal and vertical dimensions.
- *Retrosternal extension (Fig. 51.3B):* It puts pressure on the great veins at the thoracic inlet and results in dilatation of subcutaneous veins over the upper part of chest. In these cases, it is not possible to get the lower limit of goiter on deglutition. Raising of both arms and touching both the ears result into facial congestion, cyanosis and distress.
- *Consistency:* Note whether the consistency is variable or uniform. Clinically, it is difficult to know whether the nodule is solid or cystic because the cystic fluid may be under great tension. The cellular swelling may have no tension, and feels soft. Ultrasonography neck examination easily differentiates between solid and cystic swellings. Stony hard consistency suggests malignancy and Riedel's thyroiditis.
- *Pulsation, bruit and murmurs (Fig. 51.4A):* It is usually present in toxic goiter, and is due to high vascularity.
- *Surrounding structures*
    - *Trachea:* It can be displaced and compressed from both the sides (scabbard trachea).
        - *Kocher's test:* Slight pressure on lobes produces stridor in cases of scabbard trachea.
    - *Esophagus:* Displacement or compression of esophagus will cause dysphagia.
    - *Recurrent laryngeal nerve:* Its involvement leads to vocal cord palsy and hoarseness of voice, and suggests malignancy.
    - *Carotid artery:* Benign large goiter just pushes the carotid sheath, and pulsation can be felt. Malignant goiter can encase the carotid artery and then carotid pulsations are not detected.
    - *Cervical sympathetic trunk:* Its involvement gives rise to Horner's syndrome and suggests malignancy.
        - *Horner's syndrome:* It consists of partial ptosis, enophthalmos, constricted pupil and anhidrosis of face.
- *Measurement of neck circumference:* Measurement at the most prominent part of goiter helps in determining the progress and results of treatment.
- *Metastasis:* In addition to the draining neck lymph nodes, surgeon should look for distant metastases in skull and pathological fractures of long bones.

Toxic Manifestations

The cardinal signs of primary toxic goiter include exophthalmos, enlargement of thyroid gland, tachycardia and tremors. In the secondary toxic goiter, exophthalmos

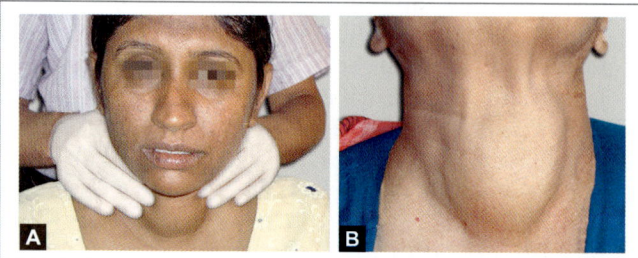

Figs 51.3A and B: (A) Thyroid palpation from behind. Fingers palpate lobes of the gland, and thumbs are placed on occipital region to keep the neck flexed; (B) Goiter; swelling is more on left side. Note the obliteration of suprasternal space that raises suspicion of retrosternal extension

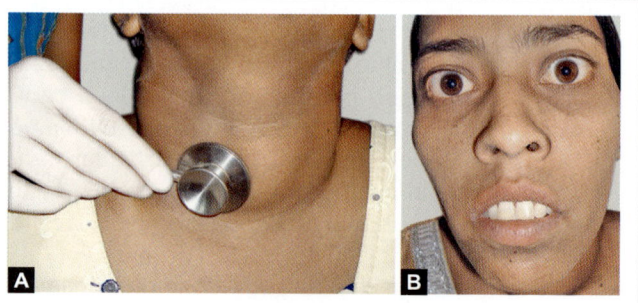

Figs 51.4A and B: (A) Auscultation of thyroid; (B) Exophthalmus in case of toxic goiter

and tremors are usually absent. The brunt of disease falls on cardiovascular system. Pulse becomes irregular in rate and rhythm. Atrial fibrillation and heart failure may supervene later on.

- **Exophthalmos:** It refers to protrusion of eyeball (Fig. 51.4B). The following signs should be looked for:
  - *Von Graefe's sign:* The upper eyelid lags behind when patient looks downward.
  - *Stellwag's sign:* It consists of upper eyelid retraction and infrequent winking.
  - *Joffroy's sign:* There is no forehead wrinkling when patient looks towards ceiling keeping the head downward. In cases of facial palsy, it is unilateral.
  - *Moebius sign of convergence:* Convergence of eyes becomes difficult.
  - *Dalrymple's sign:* The upper sclera becomes visible when patient has exophthalmos.
  - *Advanced features:* They include chemosis and ophthalmoplegia.
- **Tachycardia:** The sleeping pulse rate rises, and may vary from 90 to 180. Pulse becomes water hammer type.
- **Tremors:** Fine tremors of stretched fingers of stretched out arms are seen (Fig. 51.5A). In protruding tongue, fibrillar twitching can be seen (Fig. 51.5B). In advanced cases, whole body may shake and tremble.
- **Thyroid bruit:** It is present in Grave's primary thyrotoxicosis, and indicates increased vascularity. It is better present on the upper pole.

INVESTIGATIONS

There is a long list of thyroid function tests but the essential tests done routinely are mentioned here.

- **T_3, T_4 and TSH:** The levels of triiodothyronine (T_3), L-thyroxine (T_4) and TSH are reliable indicators of the functioning of thyroid gland (Table 51.1). If the TSH levels are normal, T_3 and T_4 estimations are usually not required.
  - *Free T_3 and T_4:* T_3 and T_4 are bound to serum proteins. The small amount biologically active hormones remain unbound and free, and have

Table 51.1: Levels of T_3, T_4 and thyroid-stimulating hormone (TSH) in thyroid disorders

Thyroid functions	Free T_3 (3.5–7.5 µmol l-1)	Free T_4 (10–30 nmol l-1)	TSH (0.3–3.3 mU l-1)
Euthyroid	Normal	Normal	Normal
Thyrotoxicosis	High	High	Low/undetectable
Myxedema	Low	Low	High
Developing hypothyroidism	Lower normal range	Lower normal range	High
T_3 toxicity	High	Normal	Low/undetectable

metabolic activity. T_3 is quick acting (few hours), and is a more important physiological hormone. T_4 acts more slowly (4–14 days). The free T_3 and T_4 are preferred, and the assay of total T_3 and T_4 are now becoming obsolete.

- *Pituitary-thyroid axis:* The secretion of TSH from pituitary depends upon the levels of T_3 and T_4, and is modified in a negative feedback mechanism. Thyrotropin-releasing hormone from hypothalamus also regulates the TSH secretion from pituitary gland.
- **Thyroid autoantibodies:** The levels of antibodies against thyroid peroxidase (thyroid microsomal antigen) and thyroglobulin are significantly high in many cases of autoimmune thyroiditis. In the follow-up cases of thyroid carcinomas, surgeon should not forget that anti-thyroglobulin antibody affects the levels of thyroglobulin.
- **X-ray chest and thoracic inlet:** It shows the retrosternal extension of goiter, tracheal deviation and compression and pulmonary metastasis.
- **Ultrasound neck:** It easily differentiates cystic nodules from the solid tumors. Ultrasound guided FNAC offer better results. Incidental thyroid swellings are frequently noticed during USG neck, and may not be clinically relevant.
- **CT, MRI and PET:** They are not suggested in routine study of thyroid swelling. Their indications include malignancy, retrosternal extension and recurrent thyroid swellings.
- **Isotope scanning:** It is indicated only in thyrotoxicosis to localize the area of overactivity in thyroid gland (single nodule or multinodular goiter) that has important implications for therapy. Whole-body scanning is indicated in operated patients of thyroid carcinoma to demonstrate metastases. Technetium (^{99m}Tc) is cheaper than radiolabelled iodine (^{123}I).

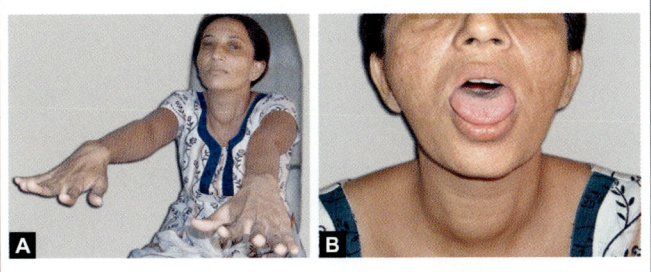

Figs 51.5A and B: (A) Fine tremors of stretched fingers of stretched out arms; (B) See for fibrillar twitching of the tongue

- *Fine-needle aspiration cytology (FNAC):* This simple, quick, economical and OPD procedure is the investigation of choice for discrete thyroid nodules. US-guided FNAC achieve more accurate sample material. The FNAC results may be nondiagnostic, non-neoplastic, follicular, suspicious of malignancy or malignant.
- *Serum calcitonin and carcinoembryonic antigen:* They are screening tests for medullary carcinoma.

Essential thyroid function tests done in routine: They are T_3, T_4 and TSH, thyroid antibodies, USG neck and FNAC.

Self-evaluation Exercises

1. Which of the following are not related with thyroglossal cyst?
    a. Midline neck mass
    b. Recognized by its movement with swallowing
    c. An ultrasound neck will evaluate for ectopic thyroid tissue
    d. None from the above
2. The most common causes of carotid triangle swellings are:
    a. Paragangliomas
    b. Schwannomas
    c. Meningiomas
    d. Nodal metastases
    e. All of the above
3. The essential thyroid function tests, which are done in routine, are:
    a. T_3, T_4 and TSH
    b. Thyroid antibodies
    c. USG neck
    d. FNAC
    e. All of the above

Answers

1. d   2. e   3. e

Pearls and Nuggets (Refresh your knowledge)

- *Dalrymple's sign:* This is the retraction of upper eyelid showing sclera above the cornea and is present in Grave's disease hyperthyroidism.
- *Thyroglossal duct:* The pyramidal lobe of the thyroid gland, which may be seen in an infant as a small lump on the anterior aspect of thyroid cartilage near the midline, is a remnant of thyroglossal duct. The thyroid gland develops from thyroglossal duct, which descends in the midline from the apex (foramen cecum) of the sulcus terminalis in the tongue.
- *Carotid triangle:* The most common causes of swellings in this region are paragangliomas, schwannomas, meningiomas, and nodal metastases.
- *Silent primary sites and metastatic neck nodes:* In patients with metastatic neck nodes when the primary lesion is not found upon physical examination including flexible/rigid endoscopy, biopsies from four silent primary sites should be taken. These four silent sites are nasopharynx, tongue base valleculae, pyriform sinus and tonsils (tonsillectomy).
- *Paragangliomas:* These vascular tumors are strongly enhancing on CT. They contain small regions of single void on most MRI pulse sequences.

Chapter 52

Neck Masses

Specific Learning Objectives

After going through the chapter, you should be able to answer the following questions:
- Differential diagnosis of neck swellings in children and young adults.
- What do you know about: (1) Carotid body tumors; (2) Parapharyngeal tumors; (3) Branchial cyst, sinus and fistula; (4) Thyroglossal cyst; (5) Cystic hygroma; (6) Scrofula; (7) Sternomastoid tumor; (8) Cervical rib?

The diagnostic tests employed in routine for neck masses are ultrasonography (USG), CT and MRI imaging, fine-needle aspiration cytology (FNAC) and biopsy.

LYMPHOMA

It is the third in male and sixth in female most common malignancy in India (ICMR, 2004).

Lymphoma, Hodgkin's disease and lymphosarcomas occur in all age groups, but are common in children and young adults. They account for up to 55% of all pediatric cancers.

- **Clinical features:** They include fever and hypertrophy of spleen, liver and Waldeyer's ring.
  - Eighty percent children with Hodgkin's disease have at least one neck mass whereas in lymphosarcomas, 40% children have this feature.
  - Lymph nodes are usually discrete, rubbery and nontender, and have progressive enlargement. Usually, there are no other ENT symptoms.
- **FNAC:** Needle biopsy is taken from a suspicious mass (single, dominant, supraclavicular, asymmetric), and studied by flow cytometry.
- **Open biopsy:** It provides complete histocytopathologic examination. Indications include uncooperative children, and when FNAC and flow cytometry results are equivocal or negative.
  - Biopsy from the site of abnormality of Waldeyer's ring, if any, is necessary for staging.

Extranodal lymphomas: Evaluation of gastrointestinal and central nervous system is required as *extranodal lymphoma* is common manifestation of non-Hodgkin's lymphoma.

CAROTID BODY TUMORS AND GLOMUS TUMORS

- **Clinical features:** They are:
  - **Site:** Around carotid bifurcation in carotid triangle.
  - **Nature:** Glomus tumors (chemodectoma) are pulsatile, compressible, and often rapidly refill on release of pressure.
    - Both bruit and thrill are present.
  - **Mobility:** Carotid body tumor can be moved from side-to-side, but not up or down.
  - **Tonsil:** In glomus vagus tumor, the tonsil may pulsate and be pushed medially.
- **Contrast CT, Gd-MRI and angiography:** They are diagnostic as the FNAC and biopsy are contraindicated. These tumors are highly vascular. Lyre's sign (splaying of internal and external carotid arteries) and extent of tumor can be seen.
- **Treatment:** Small tumor in a young patient is resected.
  - Arterial embolization aids in clearance of large tumors with less blood loss.
  - Radiotherapy is preferred in elderly patients or extensive tumors in high-risk patients.

- For more details of such tumor *see* 'glomus tumors of middle ear' in Chapter 'Tumors of Ear and Cerebellopontine Angle'.

SCHWANNOMAS OR NEURILEMMOMAS (PARAPHARYNGEAL TUMORS)

- *Clinical features:* These neurogenic tumors are solid.
  - They occur in parapharyngeal space, and displace the tonsil medially. Minor salivary gland tumors and metastatic nodes are also common in parapharyngeal space.
  - Vagus nerve tumor can cause hoarseness of voice.
  - Sympathetic chain tumors may present with Horner's syndrome.
- *Management:* Surgical exploration and excision are done after a thorough search for an unknown primary tumor.

> - **Carotid body tumor:** Embryologically it is believed to originate from neural-crest cell.
> - **Lyre sign:** Splaying apart of internal and external carotid arteries by carotid body tumor. It is seen on carotid angiography.

BRANCHIAL CYSTS

They are seen in late childhood and early adulthood.
- *Clinical features:* Initially, they appear as painful tender swelling with fever after an episode of upper respiratory tract infection (URI). They usually persist as soft, doughy, variably-sized masses even after the course of antibiotics.
- *Location:* Anterior triangle of neck
  - *Second branchial cleft cyst (common):* Deep to and along the anterior border of sternocleidomastoid muscle. Their remnant tract may course between carotid branches anterior to glossopharyngeal and hypoglossal nerves, and enter into oropharynx.
  - *First branchial cleft cyst (rare):* Along the inferior border of mandible, at the angle of mandible or just below the ear lobule. Their remnant tract may course towards the external auditory canal.
- *Ultrasonography:* It reveals cystic lesion.
- *FNAC:* Milky, mucoid or brownish fluid, which usually show cholesterol crystals.
- *Treatment:* Surgical excision of the cyst along with its tract after controlling the local infection with a course of antibiotics.

BRANCHIAL SINUS OR FISTULA

The tract ascends just beneath the deep cervical fascia along the carotid artery.

- *Course of tracts:* They are:
  - *Second branchial cleft sinus (common):* The tract passes between the second arch structures (external carotid artery, stylohyoid muscle and posterior belly of digastric) and third arch structures (internal carotid artery). This tract remains superficial to hypoglossal nerve. It perforates pharyngeal wall, and ends in tonsillar fossa.
  - *Third branchial cleft sinus (rare):* The tract passes deeper to both external and internal carotid arteries, but superficial to vagus and hypoglossal nerves. Its internal opening lies in piriform fossa.
- *Clinical features:* Both sinuses present with an external opening along the anterior border of sternocleidomastoid muscle.
- *Treatment:* Complete excision of the tract.

THYROGLOSSAL CYST

- *Clinical features:* Initially, it appears as painful tender swelling with fever after an episode of URI. It persists as soft, doughy, variably sized mass after a course of antibiotic.
  - *Location:* Midline of anterior neck (Fig. 52.1A).
  - *Pathognomonic sign:* Vertical movement with swallowing and on protrusion of tongue.
- *USG:* It differentiates the cyst from lymph node, dermoid cyst and thyroid tissue.
- *Radionuclide scan:* It is indicated if the cyst is present in the base of tongue to differentiate from undescended lingual thyroid.
- *Treatment:* Surgical excision of the cyst along with its tract and midportion of the hyoid (Sistrunk operation). The specimen should be sent for histopathological examination to rule out though rare concomitant cancer and thyroid tissue.

CERVICAL LYMPHANGIOMA (CYSTIC HYGROMA)

This cavernous lymphangioma is said to be the result of incomplete development and obstruction of normal

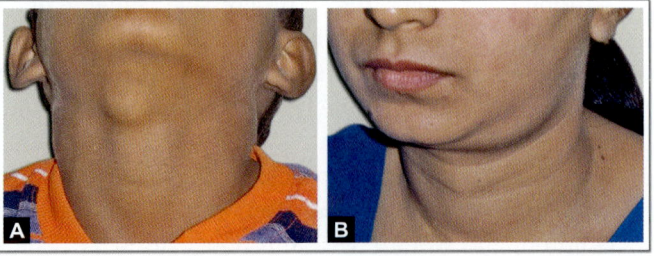

Figs 52.1A and B: (A) Thyroglossal cyst. Soft and doughy swelling in the midline of anterior neck in a child; (B) Tuberculous cervical lymphadenitis. Unilateral, painless, firm swelling in left submandibular region of a young adult female mimicking submandibular gland swelling. Excisional biopsy showed evidence of tuberculosis

lymphatic system (obstruction or sequestration of jugular lymph sac). Majority of them are present at birth, and becomes evident within the 1st year of life. Large swelling in neonates cause difficulty in labor. The extent is usually much more than what is apparent.
- *Most common site:* Posterior triangle.
- *Nature:* The swelling is fluctuant, diffuse, soft, spongy, and has indiscrete margins.
- *Diagnostic feature:* Transillumination.
- *Treatment:* The easily accessible mass is excised if it is affecting vital functions. Mutilating procedures are not performed.
  - *Sclerotherapy:* Due to the high-risk of recurrence and complications, it may be tried in extensive lesions.

DERMOID CYST

This slow-growing painless cystic swelling is most commonly seen in children and young adults.
- *Most common sites:* Midline submental swelling.
- *Differential diagnosis:* Epidermal or sebaceous cyst lies superficially in the skin whereas dermoid cyst lies deep in cervical fascia, and skin moves freely over it.
- *Treatment:* Complete surgical excision.

TUBERCULOUS CERVICAL LYMPHADENITIS (SCROFULA)

Tuberculosis (TB) is a common cause of cervical lymphadenopathy (Fig. 52.1B). It is the most common presentation of extrapulmonary TB.
- *Organisms:* Both bovine and human bacilli.
- *Route of entry:* Tonsil.
- *Clinical features:* Patients who are often children and young adults are usually asymptomatic and have no evidence of active TB. They present with:
  - *Lymphadenitis:* Unilateral, painless, firm, erythematous swelling in the posterior triangle. Matting together of a substantial number of lymph nodes is common. The tuberculous process is usually limited to one group of lymph nodes.
  - *Cold abscess:* The caseated node can liquefy and breakdown, and result in the formation of cold abscess (Figs 52.2A and B).
  - *Collar stud abscess:* The pus can erode the deep cervical fascia, and flows into the space beneath the superficial fascia.
  - *Discharging sinus:* The overlying skin may become reddened, and lead to discharging sinus.
- *Tuberculin skin test:* It is almost always positive (> 10 mm induration).
- *X-ray chest posteroanterior view:* Children and immunosuppressed adults usually have concurrent pulmonary TB.

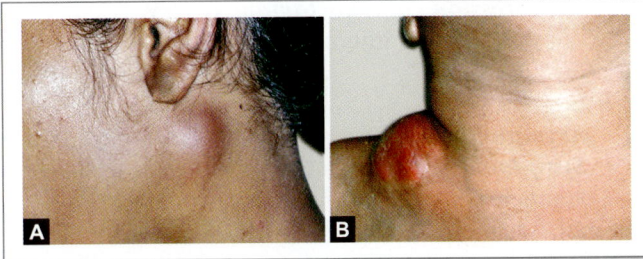

Figs 52.2A and B: (A) Tuberculous cervical lymphadenitis with cold abscess. Unilateral, painless, soft and erythematous swelling behind the left angle of mandible in a young adult female. Pus was aspirated; (B) Tuberculous cervical lymphadenitis with cold abscess. Right supraclavicular painless, soft and erythematous swelling in a 3 year child

- *FNAC:* It generally shows granulomata but acid-fast bacilli are seen in immunosuppressed patients.
- *Culture:* It differentiates tuberculous lymphadenitis from that caused by other mycobacteria or fungi.
- *Treatment:* Multi-drugs AKT (depending on the culture and sensitivity report) and complete excision without drains to avoid fistulization.
  - *Unresolving abscess:* It needs excision along with its surrounding fibrous capsule and nodes.
  - *Active pulmonary TB:* In these cases tubercular cervical lymph nodes are not removed.

STERNOMASTOID TUMOR

Birth trauma results in fibrosis and later shortening of sternocleidomastoid muscle in newborns.
- *Clinical features*
  - *Torticollis:* Face is turned to opposite side and head is laterally flexed on ipsilateral shoulder.
  - *Neck mass:* Palpation of mass in sternocleidomastoid.
- *Treatment*
  - *Conservative:* Active and passive neck movements and positions in early stages.
  - *Surgery:* Division of sternocleidomastoid muscle is done in persistent cases.

CERVICAL RIB

An extra rib occasionally arises from the seventh cervical vertebra, and attaches to first rib. It results in compression of subclavian artery and brachial plexus, which pass between anterior and middle scalene muscles over the first rib. Arterial compression may result in aneurysm and mural thrombus formation, and emboli can go to the distal arterial system of upper limb.
- *Clinical features*
  - *Neck mass:* Bony hard lump in supraclavicular region.
  - *Compression of lower part of brachial plexus:* Tingling and numbness along the upper side of forearm and hand.

- **Compression of subclavian artery:** Cold and numb hand and intermittent claudication of upper limb.
- **Treatment**
  - **Asymptomatic cases:** No treatment is required.
  - **Symptomatic cases:** The cervical rib is excised by supraclavicular or transaxillary approach.

THYMIC CYST

- **Origin:** Very rare tumor that arises from thymic remnant (derived from third pharyngeal pouch).
- **Site:** Anywhere from angle of mandible to the midline of neck (thymus descends through neck to mediastinum).
- **Clinical features:** Cystic or solid swelling in children or adults anterior and deep to middle third of sternocleidomastoid muscle.
- **Treatment:** Surgical excision.

PLUNGING RANULA

It has been discussed in Chapter 'Neoplasms of Oral Cavity'.

Self-evaluation Exercises

1. Biopsy is contraindicated in:
   a. Carotid body tumor
   b. Glomus tumors of middle ear
   c. Nasopharyngeal angiofibroma
   d. All of the above
2. Which of the followings are not congenital lesions:
   a. Branchial sinus
   b. Thyroglossal cyst
   c. Cystic hygroma
   d. Branchial cyst
   e. None from above

True (T)/False (F)

3. Eighty percent children with Hodgkin's disease have at least one neck mass.
4. Embryologically carotid body tumor is believed to originate from neural-crest cell.
5. The external opening of second arch branchial fistula lies along the anterior border of sternocleidomastoid muscle. The fistulous tract passes deep to digastric muscle between the internal and external carotid arteries.
6. Extranodal lymphoma is a common manifestation of non-Hodgkin's lymphoma.
7. Thyroglossal cyst arises from remnants of thyroglossal duct.

Filling the blanks

8. _____ sign (splaying of internal and external carotid arteries) is the feature of carotid body tumor.
9. _____ is the most common pediatric cancer.

Answers

1. d	2. e	3. T	4. T	5. T	6. T
7. T	8. Lyre's	9. Lymphoma			

Chapter 53

Neoplasms of Thyroid

> **Specific Learning Objectives**
>
> After going through the chapter, you should be able to answer the following questions:
> - What are the etiological, predisposing and risk factors of thyroid neoplasms?
> - What are the differential diagnoses of thyroid nodule and adenoma and their management?
> - How will you evaluate a case of suspicious/high risk thyroid swelling? What are the different types of MEN?
> - What are the differential diagnoses of malignant tumors of thyroid gland and how will you manage them? What is Hurthle cell carcinoma?
> - What are the different types of thyroid surgeries and their indications and complications?

INTRODUCTION

Colloid and adenomatous nodular goiters are most common. Carcinoma of thyroid gland is uncommon. Adenoma is the most common benign thyroid neoplasm. In the endemic areas of goiter, mortality rate from thyroid cancer is about 10 times more. Although there is no age bar, majority of follicular, medullary and anaplastic carcinoma patients are elderly. In adolescent and young adults, thyroid carcinoma is mainly of papillary type.

PREDISPOSING (RISK) FACTORS

- *Iodine deficiency and elevated thyroid-stimulating hormone (TSH) levels:* Relationship between iodine deficiency, endemic goiter and thyroid cancer (especially follicular type) is well-known. Dietary deficiency of iodine affects T_3 and T_4 production. Prolonged TSH stimulation causes abnormal thyroid gland to under go malignant change.
    - *Prevention:* Dietary iodine supplementation reduces the incidence of thyroid cancer.
- *Solitary thyroid nodule:* The incidence of malignant change in solitary nodule is 10–20%.
- *Ionizing radiation:* It causes papillary carcinomas.
- *Genetic predisposition:* Hyperthyroidism, goiter and thyroid cancer run in families. Genetic-based medullary carcinoma is found in several variants of multiple endocrine neoplasia (MEN) syndromes.
- *Autoimmunity:* Thyroid lymphoma frequently occurs in cases of autoimmune lymphocytic thyroiditis (Hashimoto's disease).

- *Cowden syndrome:* It includes skin tags, multiple hamartomas and tumors of breast and thyroid (follicular and papillary carcinoma).
- *Gardners syndrome:* Patient has familial colonic polyposis and thyroid cancer.

THYROID NODULE

Box 53.1 shows the classification of thyroid neoplasms. The nodules are demarcated but not encapsulated. Many have gelatinous consistency with areas of degeneration or calcification.

- *Risk factors:* The malignancy risk factors of a solitary nodule (Fig. 53.1A) include the following:
    - *Age:* Patients under 14 or over 65 years of age
    - *Sex:* Male
    - *Enlarging* in spite of suppressive doses of thyroxine
    - *Past history of:*
        - Ionizing radiation
        - Thyroid cancer
    - Family history of thyroid cancer.

TYPES OF THYROID NODULES

Colloid (Adenomatous) Nodule

- *Pathology:* Benign hyperplasia of follicular cells which become more sensitive to TSH. The follicles are filled with colloid.
- *Treatment:* Suppressive therapy with thyroid hormone which decrease the secretion of TSH.

Box 53.1: Classification of thyroid neoplasms

Benign—adenoma (most common)
- Follicular
- Microfollicular
- Hurthle cell
- Embryonal

Malignant
- Primary
  - Follicular epithelium
    - Papillary adenocarcinoma (60–80%)
    - Follicular adenocarcinoma (10–20%)
    - Anaplastic carcinoma (5–10%)
  - Parafollicular cells
    - Medullary carcinoma (5%)
  - Lymphoid cells
    - Lymphoma
- Secondary
  - Metastatic from—kidney, lung, colon and breast
  - Direct spread local infiltration from—carcinoma of larynx and postcricoid region.

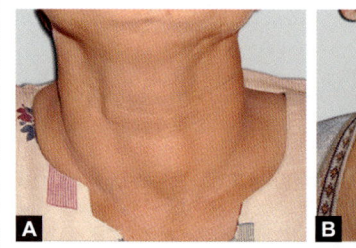 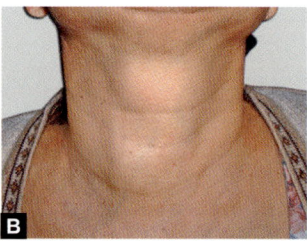

Figs 53.1A and B: (A) Left lobe thyroid nodule in euthyroid patient; (B) Hashimoto thyroiditis. Right-side painful thyroid swelling of 5 days duration in 45-year-old lady

Follicular Adenoma

- ***Pathology:*** Encapsulated well defined benign neoplasm of follicular cells. *It is the most common tumor of thyroid.*
- ***Sequele:*** Cystic degeneration, hemorrhage, fibrosis, calcification.
- ***FNAC:*** It does not differentiate benign from malignant. In malignancy biopsy shows capsular/vascular invasion so the removed adenoma must be submitted for histopathology.

Hurthle Cell Adenoma

- Hurthle cells are oncocytes which have plenty of mitochondria.
- Rest of the features are similar to follicular adenoma.

Thyroid Cyst

- About 25% of thyroid nodules have cystic component.
- ***Causes:***
  - Simple thyroid, parathyroid and thyroglossal cysts.
  - Cystic degeneration or hemorrhage in follicular adenoma and colloid nodule.
  - Cystic change in papillary carcinoma.
- ***USG:*** It will differentiate cyst from solid swellings.
- ***FNAC:***
  - ***Clear and colorless fluid:*** Parathyroid cyst (fluid tested for parathoromone).
  - ***Brown fluid:*** Cystic degeneration or Hemorrhage in colloid nodule or adenoma or simple thyroid cyst.
  - ***Red or bloody fluid:*** Papillary carcinoma.
  - ***Columnar cells:*** Thyroglossal cyst.
  - ***USG guided FNAC from solid component of cyst:*** To know the exact nature of lesion.
- ***Treatment:***
  - ***Less than 4 cm size:*** Aspiration and suppression therapy with thyroid hormone. Surgical excision in case of recurrence.
  - ***More than 4 cm size:*** Surgical excision.

Regenerative Nodule

In some cases of Hashimoto's disease when patient is somewhat hypothyroid TSH may stimulate certain follicular cells to form a localized swelling.

Malignant Nodule

Patients with thyroid cancers can present as thyroid nodule.

Dominant Nodule

In many cases of multinodular goiter only one nodule is clinically visible and rest of the nodules may either be palpable during surgery or seen on USG. This dominant nodule can be malignant.

Autonomous (Toxic) Nodule

- ***Pathology:*** Single hot nodule that hyperfunctions independent of the TSH.
- ***Etiology:*** Mutation in TSH receptors of follicular cells and multiplication of follicular cells
- ***Thyroid scan:*** Higher uptake by the nodule than rest of the thyroid.
- ***T_3, T_4, TSH:*** Mild thyrotoxicosis (high T_3 and T_4) with low TSH.
- ***Treatment:***
  - ***Surgery:*** Total lobectomy with isthmusectomy.
  - ***Radioactive iodine thyroid ablation.***
  - ***Intranodular injection of ethanol:*** May be repeated but risk of recurrent laryngeal nerve injury.

EVALUATION OF THE THYROID NODULE

The history, examination and investigations are discussed in detail in Chapter 'Cervical Symptoms and Examination'. Investigations for malignant thyroid nodules are discussed in other section of this Chapter.

Chapter 53 • Neoplasms of Thyroid

- **Thyroid adenoma:** Adenoma is the most common benign thyroid neoplasm. In contrast to nodule, it is encapsulated. They are not premalignant, and rarely become toxic. Capsular or vascular invasion indicates malignancy.
- **Clinical features:** It usually presents as a solitary nodule or a dominant nodule in multinodular goiter in middle-aged females.

FNAC MANAGEMENT OF THYROID NODULE

Treatment will depend on the report of FNAC (93% sensitivity and 96% specificity). It can have following reports.
- **Malignant:** Evaluate the patient for surgery.
- **Suspicious for malignancy:** Evaluate the patient for surgery.
- **Nondiagnostic or insufficient material:** FNAC must be repeated and if still inconclusive.
  - **No risk factors:** Follow up
  - **Risk factors present:** Evaluate the patient for surgery
- **Benign:**
  - **Cystic:** Aspiration
    - **No recurrence:** Follow up
    - **Recurrence:** Repeated aspirations
      1. **No recurrence:** Follow up
      2. **Recurrence:** Evaluate the patient for surgery
  - **Solid:** Advised thyroid scan
    - **Hot**
      1. **Toxic:** Evaluate the patient for surgery or radioactive iodine ablation
      2. **Nontoxic**
         a. **Small:** Follow up
         b. **Large:** Evaluate the patient for surgery
    - **Not hot:** T_4 suppression
      1. **No regression:** Evaluate the patient for surgery
      2. **Regression:** Continue with thyroid suppression therapy.

Consistency of different types of thyroid nodules:
- **Cysts:** Cystic if filled with fluid
- **Colloid nodules:** Doughy
- **Papillary and medullary cancers:** Hard rubber
- **Anaplastic cancer:** Hard, fixed and craggy
- **Lymphomas:** Diffuse swelling.

Thyroid nodules: Six to seven percent of adult females and 1–2% of adult males will show a thyroid nodule on thorough clinical examination.

THYROID CARCINOMA

The clinical features of thyroid cancer include:
- Solitary nodule
- Rapidly enlarging pre-existing goiter of long duration
- Hard and fixed thyroid
- Enlarged neck nodes
- Neck pain and referred otalgia
- Distant metastases
- Pressure features
  - **Trachea:** Stridor
  - **Esophagus:** Dysphagia
  - **Recurrent laryngeal nerve:** Hoarseness of voice and vocal cord palsy.

TYPES OF THYROID CARCINOMA

Papillary Adenocarcinoma

It accounts for 60–80% of all thyroid malignancies. Unlike follicular carcinoma it occurs in areas which do not have iodine deficiency.
- **Pathology:** Fibrovascular stalk with malignant cells form a papilla (papillary carcinoma). Prominent nucleoli give typical 'Orphan Annie eye' appearance. Cystic changes can occur. Laminated calcium bodies (psammoma bodies) are also seen. Lymphatic metastasis is more common than distant metastatic.
- **Age:** It is most common in fifth decade of life. It is the only thyroid cancer of children.
- **Clinical features:** It presents as firm non-capsulated thyroid nodule. It is usually (80%) multicentric, and involves both thyroid lobes.
- **Lymphatic metastases:** There is high incidence of enlarged level III–VII neck nodes. Primary tumor may remain impalpable (occult primary).
- **Distant metastases:** Pulmonary metastasis is more common than bony metastasis.
- **Classification:** On the bases of size and extension, they are categorized into the following groups:
  - **Minimal (microcarcinoma) less than 1.0 cm:** They are often seen as incidental findings at USG neck. Their incidence far exceeds that of papillary carcinoma. Conservative approach is justified in management.
  - **Intrathyroidal greater than 1.0 cm.**
  - **Extrathyroidal:** Extend outside thyroid capsule or with lymph node metastases.
- **Prognosis:** Ten year survival from intrathyroid cancer is over 90% whereas from extrathyroidal, it falls to 60%. In

older age group, it is more aggressive, and may invade larynx and trachea.

If God ask you to choose a cancer to suffer from, which one would you like to have?[1]

Follicular Adenocarcinoma

It accounts for only 10–20% of all thyroid malignancies. Hematogenic distant metastasis is more common than lymphatic spread.
- *Age:* It is most common in the sixth decade of life and seldom seen under 30 years of age.
- *Clinical features:* It usually presents as a new solitary thyroid nodule. It may present as malignant change in a thyroid swelling of many years duration. Some patients may present with features of secondary metastases.
- *Metastases:* In contrast to papillary carcinoma, bony and pulmonary metastases are more common than lymphatic metastasis.
- *Classification:* In contrast to papillary carcinoma, it has well defined capsule. Depending upon the breach of capsule, patients are divided into two groups.
- *FNAC:* It will not be able to differentiate between follicular adenoma and carcinoma. Lobectomy is required to know whether a follicular neoplasm is benign or malignant.

Medullary Thyroid Carcinoma

It accounts for only 5% of all thyroid malignancies. It arises from parafollicular C cells which secrete calcitonin and carcinoembyogenic antigen. Calcitonin levels have diagnostic and surveillance importance.
- *Clinical features:* As a part of multiple endocrine neoplasia (MEN) syndrome it is familial and frequently multifocal and bilateral and presents at a younger age. Sporadic cases are often unifocal. Middle and upper part of thyroid lobe swelling with cervical nodes in elderly people. Later on pain, dyspnea, dysphagia and hoarseness of voice appear.
- *MEN syndrome (Box 53.2):* MEN IIA is an autosomal dominant condition. Medullary thyroid carcinoma occurs in association with pheochromocytoma and hyperparathyroidism. *If affected family member has genetic mutation on the RET proto-oncogene, prophylactic total thyroidectomy should be considered after excluding pheochromocytoma.*
- *Tumor marker:* The levels of serum calcitonin are valuable.
- *Metastasis:* Fifty percent patients have distant metastasis in mediastinum, lung or bone at the time of presentation.

> **Box 53.2: Types of Medullary thyroid carcinoma and Multiple endocrine neoplasia (MEN) syndrome**
>
> **Sporadic (80%):** Unifocal
> - **Familial (20%):** Multifocal bilateral and in young patients
>   - **MEN type II A (Sipple syndrome):** Consists of medullary thyroid carcinoma, hyperparathyroidism (30%), pheochromocytoma (50%) and Hirschsprung disease.
>   - **MEN type II B (rare):** Consists of medullary thyroid carcinoma, pheochromocytoma, mucosal and intestinal neuromas and Marfanoid habitus.
>   - **Non MEN familial (rare).**

Lymphoma and Anaplastic Carcinoma

They are uncommon tumors. They present as rapidly increasing swelling of neck in elderly women.
- *Lymphoma (B-cell non-Hodgkins type):* It usually occurs in females who have Hashimoto's autoimmune lymphocytic thyroiditis (Fig. 53.1B).
- *Anaplastic cancers:* It can appear in long-standing goiter patients as a rapidly growing tumor associated with referred otalgia and hoarseness of voice. This aggressive tumor is highly metastatic and invades larynx, pharynx and esophagus.
  - *Prognosis:* Treatment is not effective. Patient usually dies within 1 year of presentation. It has very poor prognosis.
- *Investigations:*
  - *Thyroid function tests:* T_3, T_4 and TSH.
  - *Thyroid antibodies.*
  - *FNAC and open biopsy (or tru-cut):* Appropriate immunocytochemistry is essential to distinguish these two tumors because the treatment and prognosis of these cancers are different.
- *CT scan:* Neck and chest for anaplastic, and whole body for lymphoma.
- *Lactate dehydrogenase, ESR, bone marrow and trephine:* For thyroid lymphoma.

> **Biopsy:** Thyroid lymphoma and anaplastic carcinoma need open biopsy before the beginning of therapy.

Hurtle Cell Carcinoma (Oncocytic Carcinoma)

- *Clinical:* It presents as thyroid nodule but lesions are multifocal and bilateral.
- *Spread:* Both distant and lymphatic metastasis occur. Prognosis is poor as it is more aggressive than papillary and follicular carcinoma. It does not take up I^{131}.
- *FNAC:* Show only Hurthle cells. Malignancy is decided on histopathology.
- *Treatment:* Hurthle cell adenoma needs lobectomy and isthmusectomy. Completion thyroidectomy with

---
[1] Papillary adenocarcinoma of thyroid

clearance of paratracheal nodes is done on the biopsy report of capsular/vascular invasion. Palpable lateral nodes need neck dissection.

INVESTIGATIONS OF THYROID CARCINOMA

- **T_3, T_4 and TSH:** Their abnormal levels indicate non-neoplastic lesions and medical treatment (hyper and hypothyroidism) (Fig. 53.2).
- **Thyroid antibodies:** They are not mandatory but help in interpretation of serum thyroglobulin levels after surgery.
- **FNAC:** This safe, quick, cheap and effective OPD procedure is mandatory. It requires experienced cytopathologist.
- **X-ray chest:** It can show tracheal deviation, mediastinal extension, lymph nodes enlargement and pulmonary metastasis.
- **X-ray neck and thoracic inlet:** In addition to tracheal deviation and compression, other findings are:
  - *Benign lesion:* Rim or eggshell calcification
  - *Multinodular goiter:* Heavy irregular calcification
  - *Papillary carcinoma:* Finely stippled area due to calcification in Psammoma bodies.
  - *Medullary carcinoma:* Bilateral calcification at the upper lateral portion of gland.
- **Ultrasound:** This easy, quick and cheap method of assessment helps in the following ways:
  - Measure tumor size
  - Diagnose multinodular goiter
  - Exclude contralateral lesion
  - Distinguish purely cystic (up to 1 mm diameter) nodules from complex cysts with solid (up to 3 mm diameter) component.
  - Demonstration of Psammoma bodies.

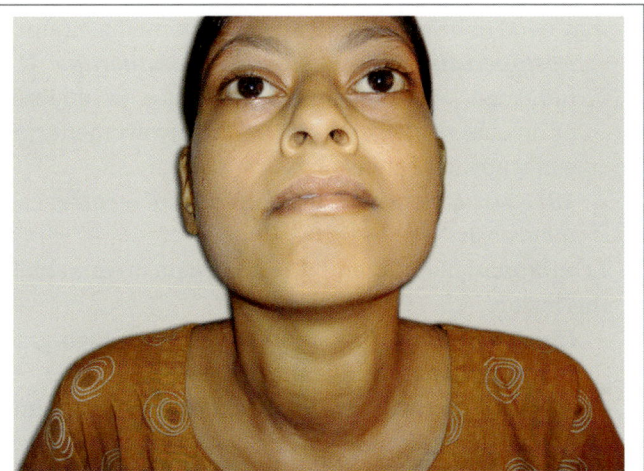

Fig. 53.2: Toxic goiter

- Disadvantage: It cannot reliably distinguish benign from malignant lesions.
- **Scintigraphy:** It differentiates between cold (non-functional) and hot (functioning) nodule of more than 5 mm diameter.
  - *Technetium-99m:*
    - *Solitary cold nodule:* It may be adenoma, carcinoma, cyst or dominant nodule in non-palpable multinodular goiter. The chances of malignancy of cold nodule are 20%.
    - *Hot nodules:* They are unlikely to be malignant.
  - *Metaiodobenzylguanidine:* It is useful in suspected cases of MEN as it is taken up by pheochromocytoma and medullary thyroid carcinoma.
  - *^{67}Ga citrate (gallium scanning):* It is useful in detecting lymphoma in long-standing cases of Hashimoto's disease.
  - *^{131}I:* It is used after surgery to ablate residual thyroid tissue. It also searches and treats metastases.
- **Computed tomography:**
  - *Neck and thorax:* It shows involvement of larynx, trachea, pharynx, esophagus, major vessels and retrosternal extent, and pulmonary metastasis and nodal deposits in neck and mediastinum.
  - *Abdominal:* It is done for lymphoma staging, and in suspected cases of pheochromocytoma.
- **Magnetic resonance imaging:** It has good soft tissue contrast. MR angiography assesses vessel involvement.
- **Serum calcium and calcitonin:** They are indicated in medullary carcinoma.
- **Excision biopsy:** Small-lateral tumors need lobectomy with removal of isthmus and a small portion of opposite lobe. The small isthmus nodule needs removal of central portion of gland with 1 cm safe margin.

Thyroglobulin and calcitonin: These serum markers are used to track thyroid carcinoma after its treatment.

TNM CLASSIFICATION AND STAGING OF THYROID CARCINOMA

Table 53.1 shows TNM classification and staging of thyroid carcinoma. Patients with differentiated papillary and follicular carcinoma under 45 years of age do not have stage III and IV, whereas histological diagnosis of anaplastic carcinoma puts the patient directly in stage IV.

TREATMENT OF THYROID CARCINOMA

Treatment of thyroid carcinoma requires multidisciplinary approach and includes:
- **Surgery** for the primary tumor and lymphatic metastasis (neck dissection). Thyroid surgeries include:

Contd...

Contd...

- **Lobectomy or hemithyroidectomy:** Complete removal of one thyroid lobe and isthmus.
- **Subtotal thyroidectomy:** Bilateral removal of more than one half of thyroid gland plus isthmus.
- **Near-total thyroidectomy:** Complete removal of one lobe, isthmus and removal of greater than 90% of opposite lobe.
- **Total thyroidectomy:** Removal of both sides lobes, and central isthmus.
- **Completion thyroidectomy:** Conversion of lesser operation into a near-total or total thyroidectomy.

- **Radioactive Iodine** for ablating residual thyroid tissue and metastases.
- **External beam radiotherapy** after surgery, and in cases of lymphoma.
- **Thyroxin therapy** to suppress the TSH levels.
- **Chemotherapy** in high-grade and more-advanced lymphoma.

Table 53.1: TNM classification and staging of thyroid carcinoma

Primary tumor (T)	
T_x	Unable to assess primary tumor
T_0	No evidence of primary tumor
T_1	Intrathyroid tumor up to 2 cm greatest dimension
T_2	Intrathyroid tumor more than 2 cm, and less than 4 cm in greatest dimension
T_3	Intrathyroid tumor more than 4 cm and limited to sternothyroid muscle
T_4	Tumor involving subcutaneous tissue and neighboring organs like larynx, trachea, esophagus, RLN; very advanced involve carotid artery and prevertebral fascia or mediastinal vessels
Regional lymphadenopathy (N) (cervical and upper mediastinal nodes)	
N_x	Unable to assess regional lymph nodes
N_0	No evidence of regional metastasis
N_{1a}	Metastasis to level VI nodes
N_{1b}	Metastasis to any level from I to V or VII nodes
Distant metastases (M)	
M_x	Unable to assess for distant metastases
M_0	No distant metastases
M_1	Distant metastases
TNM staging (under 45 years) for papillary and follicular carcinoma	
Stage I	Any T, any N, and M_0
Stage II	Any T, any N, and M_1
TNM staging for papillary and follicular (over 45 years) and medullary carcinoma (any age)	
Stage I	$T_1 \, N_0 \, M_0$
Stage II	$T_{2-3} \, N_0 \, M_0$
Stage III	$T_4 \, N_0 \, M_0$; $T_{1-4} \, N_1 \, M_0$
Stage IV	$T_{1-4} \, N_{0-1} \, M_1$
TNM staging for anaplastic carcinoma	
Stage IV	Any T, any N and any M

Source: AJCC Cancer Staging Manual. 7th ed. (2010)

- **Papillary and follicular adenocarcinoma:** In contrast to squamous cell carcinoma of head and neck region, distant metastasis in this differentiated thyroid carcinoma is not a death sentence. About 50% patients receiving radioiodine for pulmonary metastasis live for 10–15 years. Bony metastasis has poor prognosis. Hematogenous spread is more common with follicular than papillary carcinoma.
    - $T_{1-2} \, N_0 \, M_0$ **in females under 45 years:** Tumor in lobe—lobectomy/isthmusectomy with 1 cm margin; TSH suppression with thyroxin and thyroglobulin surveillance.
    - $T_2 \, N_0 \, M_0$ **in males or greater than 45 years:** Total thyroidectomy, immediate postoperative radioiodine ablation of residual normal thyroid tissue, TSH suppression with thyroxine (usually 200 mcg daily), and thyroglobulin surveillance for life.
    - T_3 **or** $T_{1-4} \, N_1 \, M_{0-1}$**:** Total thyroidectomy, selective neck dissection (nodal surgery depending upon the extent of lymphatic involvement), immediate postoperative radioiodine ablation of residual normal thyroid tissue, TSH suppression with thyroxine, and thyroglobulin surveillance for life.
        - *Clinically N_0 neck:* Level VI should be always dissected, and levels II–V and VII must be palpated during surgery.
        - *Clinically N_1 neck (levels II–V):* Selective neck dissection involving these levels; modified radical, radical or extended radical neck dissection depending on the size and extent of disease.
    - **Postoperative external beam radiotherapy:** It is indicated when operative clearance is doubtful, or in cases of extensive nodal involvement.
- **Medullary carcinoma:** It needs total thyroidectomy with modified radical or radical neck dissection, which may need to be extended into superior mediastinum.
    - **Postoperative external beam radiotherapy:** It is indicated when operative clearance is doubtful, or in cases of extensive nodal involvement with extracapsular extension.
    - **131I-MIBG:** It may be used in cases of recurrence or metastasis.
- **Lymphoma:** Radiotherapy is the main treatment for this lesion.
    - **Chemotherapy:** It is indicated in high-grade histology and more advanced disease.
- **Anaplastic carcinoma:** Unfortunately, no treatment is effective in this thyroid cancer. Radiotherapy achieves regression but early recurrence usually occurs. Patient with stridor needs isthmus split tracheostomy.

Prognostic factors of thyroid carcinoma are the following:
- **Age:** Patients under 45 years of age do better.
- **Sex:** Females do better.
- **TNM staging:** Higher the stage, poorer is the prognosis.
- **Histology:** Tall cell variant of papillary carcinoma and marked invasion of follicular carcinoma have poorer prognosis. Anaplastic carcinoma has very poor prognosis.
- **Treatment:** Delay treatment, extensive surgeries and inadequate facilities offer poorer prognosis.
- **Surgeon:** Experienced surgeon can offer best treatment.
- **AGES or AMES criteria:** **A**ge (>45), **G**rade histologic, **M**etastasis, **E**xtracapsular spread, **S**ize (>4 cm).

THYROID SURGERY

Indications (3Cs: Cancer, Compression and Cosmetic)

- Large thyroid swelling
- Hyperthyroidism
  - Toxic nodule
  - Grave's disease
- Malignant tumors of thyroid
- Suspicion of cancer on FNAC and risk factors
- Pressure symptoms:
  - *Dyspnea:* Pressure on trachea
  - *Dysphagia:* Pressure on esophagus
  - *Hoarseness of voice:* Erosion of recurrent laryngeal nerve.
  - *Thoracic inlet syndrome:* Retrosternal extension causing *Pemberton's sign (respiratory distress, engorgement of veins and suffusion of face on raising the arms above the head).*

Preoperative Evaluation

See the Chapter 'Cervical Symptoms and Examination' for the evaluation that consists of the history, examination and investigations.

Anesthesia and Position

General anesthesia with endotracheal intubation and patient kept in supine position with extended neck.

Types of Thyroid Surgeries

They are described in the treatment section of thyroid carcinoma in this chapter.

Operative Steps

- *Skin incision:* A horizontal skin incision in a crease just above the suprasternal space extending between the anterior margins of two sternocleidomastoid muscles cutting skin and subcutaneous tissue.
- *Flaps:* After cutting the platysma, subplatysmal superior (up to thyroid notch) and inferior (up to suprasternal space and clavicle) flaps are raised.
- *Strap muscles:* Midline cervical fascia incision separates the two sternohyoid muscles which are retracted laterally exposing the thyroid and sternothyroid muscle. The later is separated from thyroid and retracted laterally along with the sternohyoid muscles. This will fully expose the thyroid lobes and isthmus which must be palpated. If the thyroid is very big then many surgeons cut the strap muscles and even the sternocleidomastoid.
- *Middle thyroid vein:* It is identified and ligated. It drains into internal jugular vein.
- *Inferior thyroid veins:* They form a venous plexus on the anterior surface of trachea and are ligated and cut.
- *Thyroid ima artery:* It may be seen in some cases and must be ligated.
- *Inferior thyroid artery:* Recurrent laryngeal nerve (RLN) may run anterior, posterior or through the branches of inferior thyroid artery so is at great risk while ligating this vessel. They have intimate relations near ligament of Berry so be dealt very carefully there. *See* Chapter 'Anatomy of Neck' for the detail relations of thyroid, parathyroid, their vessels and related nerves.
- *Superior thyroid artery and vein:* External branch of superior laryngeal nerve runs posterior and medial to superior thyroid vessels and must not be injured while ligating these vessels. The upper pole of thyroid is retracted laterally and anteriorly.
- *Parathyroid glands:* Parathyroid glands and their blood supply must be preserved. If accidently removed they are sliced and implanted back into the sternocleidomastoid muscle.
- *Isthmus:* In cases of hemithyroidectomy or lobectomy, after incising pretracheal fascia thyroid isthmus is separated from trachea and cut between two clamps. The normal side of isthmus is ligated with 3/0 vicryl. In cases of subtotal, near total and total thyroidectomy, isthmus is not cut and the above steps are repeated on the opposite side. The steps of ligation of vessels vary from surgeon to surgeon and case to case.
- *Drainage:* Complete hemostasis is achieved and wound is irrigated with normal saline and betadine and suction drainage is kept in position and sutured properly.
- *Closure:* Strap muscles are sutured together with 3/0 vicryl and wound is closed in two layers.

Complications

They include iatrogenic trauma during surgery, anesthesia complications and postoperative complications of surgery.

- **Injury to laryngeal nerves:** Injury to external and recurrent laryngeal nerve will cause voice problem. Trauma to trachea, esophagus and great vessels is rare.
- **Parathyroid glands:** Their accidental removal will lead to hypocalcemia and tetany (numbness and tingling of lips, hands and feet) one to four days after surgery. So the calcium levels are checked regularly and patients are given calcium and vitamin D.
- **Injury to cervical pleura:** It will cause pneumothorax.
- **Hematoma and airway impairment:** If large hematoma can put pressure on trachea and cause respiratory distress and would need immediate evacuation.
- **Hypothyroidism:** Subtotal, near total and total thyroidectomy patients will develop hypothyroidism after 4 to 6 week and need lifelong thyroid hormone therapy.

Self-evaluation Exercises

1. Which of the following are true for papillary and follicular carcinoma of thyroid:
    a. Low-risk patients are females under 45 years and high-risk patients are all males, and over 45 years females.
    b. Low-risk tumors include less than 1 cm size papillary and minimally invasive follicular carcinoma.
    c. High-risk tumors include more than 2 cm size papillary and follicular carcinomas.
    d. All of the above.

True (T)/False (F)

2. Thyroid lymphoma and anaplastic carcinoma need open biopsy before the beginning of therapy.

Answers
1. d   2. T

Pearls and Nuggets (Refresh your knowledge)

- **Thyroid nodules:** Six to seven percent of adult females and one to two percent of adult males will show a thyroid nodule on thorough clinical examination.
- **Parafollicular cells of thyroid:** These cells are **neural crest cells** that migrate into 4th pharyngeal pouch and present adjacent to thyroid follicles.

Chapter 54

Deep Neck Infections

⊙ Specific Learning Objectives

After going through the chapter, you should be able to answer the following questions:
- Describe the applied anatomy of various deep neck spaces. What are the sources of infection and microorganisms causing deep neck infections?
- How will you differentiate peritonsillar abscess from parapharyngeal abscess and then manage them? Mention their complications.
- How will you differentiate between prevertebral and retropharyngeal abscesses and manage them?
- What do you know about Ludwig's angina?
- What are the differential diagnoses of trismus?

INTRODUCTION

Deep space neck infections are potentially lethal infections and need immediate appropriate treatment. These spaces are situated between the three layers of deep cervical fascia. On the basis of hyoid bone, deep neck spaces can be divided into several groups (Box 54.1 and Fig. 54.1).

Box 54.1: Classification of deep neck spaces

Suprahyoid
- Face
  - Buccal
  - Canine
  - Space of body of mandible
  - Masticator
    - Masseteric
    - Temporal
    - Pterygoid
  - Temporal
  - Parotid
- Neck
  - Peritonsillar
  - Parapharyngeal
  - Submandibular
    - Sublingual space (superior)
    - Submaxillary space (inferior)

Infrahyoid
- Visceral

Entire length of neck
- Vascular: Carotid sheath
- Prevertebral
- Danger space or alar space
- Retropharyngeal

PERTINENT ANATOMY

Peritonsillar Space

It is situated between the capsule of tonsil and the superior constrictor muscle. Medial wall of the parapharyngeal space is the lateral wall of the peritonsillar space and is formed by the superior constrictor muscle and buccopharyngeal fascia.

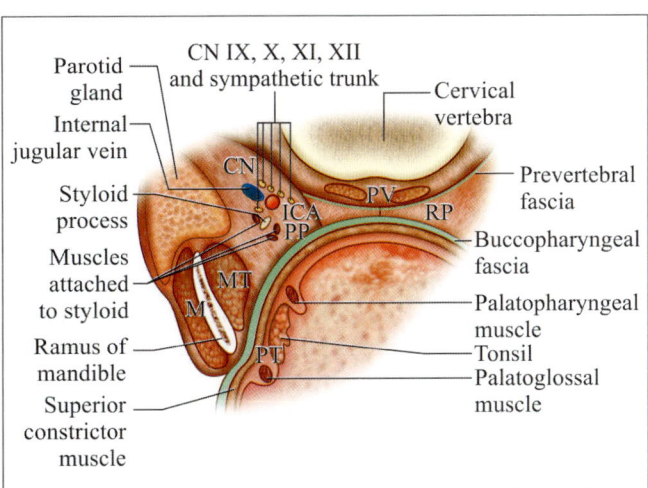

Fig. 54.1: Deep neck abscesses

Abbreviations: ICA, Internal carotid artery; M, Masseter muscle; MT, Medial pterygoid muscle; PP, Parapharyngeal space; PT, Peritonsillar space; PV, Prevertebral space; RP, Retropharyngeal space

Parapharyngeal Space or Pharyngomaxillary Space or Lateral Pharyngeal Space

This pyramid-shaped space has its base towards the skull base while its apex is towards the hyoid bone.

- *Boundaries:*
  - *Medial:* Buccopharyngeal fascia, which covers the superior constrictor muscles. It forms lateral wall of the peritonsillar space.
  - *Posterior:* Prevertebral fascia, which covers prevertebral muscles and transverse processes of the cervical vertebrae.
  - *Lateral:* Medial pterygoid muscle and mandible in anterior part, and the deep lobe of the parotid gland in the posterior part.
- *Compartments:* Styloid process and the structures attached to it divide the parapharyngeal space into anterior and posterior compartments.
  - *Anterior compartment:* It is medially related to the tonsillar fossa, and laterally to the medial pterygoid muscle.
  - *Posterior compartment:* It is related medially to the posterior part of lateral pharyngeal wall, and laterally to the parotid gland. The contents of this compartment are the following structures:
    - Internal carotid artery
    - Internal jugular vein
    - Cranial nerves 9th, 10th, 11th and 12th
    - Cervical sympathetic trunk
    - Upper deep cervical nodes.
- *Communications:* Parapharyngeal space communicates with the following spaces:
  - Retropharyngeal
  - Submandibular
  - Parotid
  - Carotid
  - Visceral.

Retropharyngeal Space

- *Boundaries and extent:*
  - The retropharyngeal space lies between the buccopharyngeal fascia covering the pharyngeal constrictor muscles, and the prevertebral fascia covering the vertebrae and prevertebral muscles.
  - It extends from the skull base to the bifurcation of trachea in mediastinum.
- *Compartments:*
  - A midline fibrous raphe divides this space into two compartments (spaces of Gillette) one on each side.
  - An abscess of retropharyngeal space causes unilateral bulge.
- *Contents:* The space contains retropharyngeal nodes.
- *Communications:*
  - It communicates with the parapharyngeal space.
  - Retropharyngeal space infection can pass down into the mediastinum behind the esophagus.

Danger Space

It lies just posterior to retropharyngeal space in between the alar fascia (anteriorly) and prevertebral fascia (posteriorly). These are the two layers of preverterbral layer of deep cervical fascia. It contains only loose connective tissue and extends from skull base to mediastinum. So the *infection of this space can cause mediastinitis*. During the surgical drainage, both the dangerous and retropharyngeal spaces are treated as one unit. A dissecting finger is used to disrupt the partition between these two spaces.

Prevertebral Space

- It lies between the vertebral bodies and the prevertebral fascia and extends from the skull base to coccyx.
- Infection usually comes from the caries spine.
- An abscess of this space produces a midline bulge.

Submandibular Space (Fig. 54.2)

- *Boundaries:*
  - The submandibular space lies between the mucous membranes of floor of the mouth and tongue, and the superficial layer of deep cervical fascia.
  - It extends between the hyoid bone and mandible.
- *Compartments:* Mylohyoid muscle divides this space into two compartments. These compartments communicate with each other around the posterior border of the mylohyoid muscle.
  - *Sublingual compartment:* Lies above mylohyoid.
  - *Submaxillary and submental compartment:* It lies below the mylohyoid.

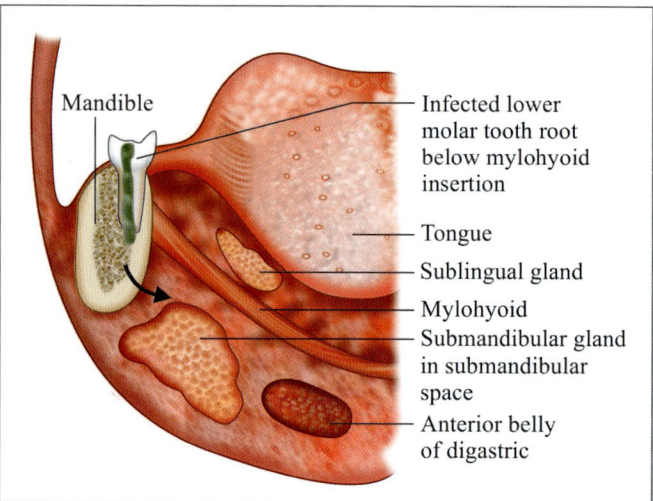

Fig. 54.2: Submandibular space. Coronal section showing pathway for pus

Masticator Space

- **Boundaries and extent**
  - *Superior:* Base of skull
  - *Inferior:* Lower border of mandible
  - *Lateral:* Superficial lamina of investing layer of deep cervical fascia making parotid capsule.
  - *Medial:* Muscles of mastication (masseter, medial and lateral pterygoids, and insertion of temporalis) and mandible.

> *CT with contrast enhancement:* It is the most valuable investigation in deep neck infections.

PERITONSILLAR ABSCESS (QUINSY)

Quinsy is a collection of pus in the peritonsillar space.

Source of Infection

Tonsillitis is the source of infection. The crypta magna gets infected and sealed off. An intratonsillar abscess develops which subsequently bursts through the tonsillar capsule into the peritonsillar space. The peritonsillitis sets up, and results in an abscess. It is a mixed infection of *Streptococcus pyogenes*, *Staphylococcus aureus* and anaerobic organisms.

Clinical Features

- *Age:* Most patients are adults. Children are rarely affected. Acute tonsillitis is more common in children.
- *Side:* Usually unilateral.
- *Local features:* They are–
  - *Pain:* Unilateral severe throat pain.
  - *Referred otalgia:* CN IX supplies tonsil and ear.
  - *Odynophagia* can lead to drooling of saliva from the angle of mouth and dehydration.
  - *Hot potato voice:* Muffled and thick speech.
  - *Halitosis:* Foul breath due to oral sepsis and poor hygiene.
  - *Trismus:* Due to spasm of pterygoid muscles.
- *General:* Following features of septicemia are usually present in all deep space neck infections.
  - Fever (up to 104°F) with chills and rigors
  - General malaise, body pain and headache
  - Nausea and constipation.
- *Physical findings (Fig. 54.3):* They show:
  - *Anterior pillar and soft palate:* Congestion and swelling anterior and superior to the tonsil.
  - *Tonsil:* Enlarged but gets buried in and hidden behind the edematous anterior pillar and soft palate. Tonsillar exudate may be seen.
  - *Uvula:* Swollen, edematous and pushed to the opposite side.

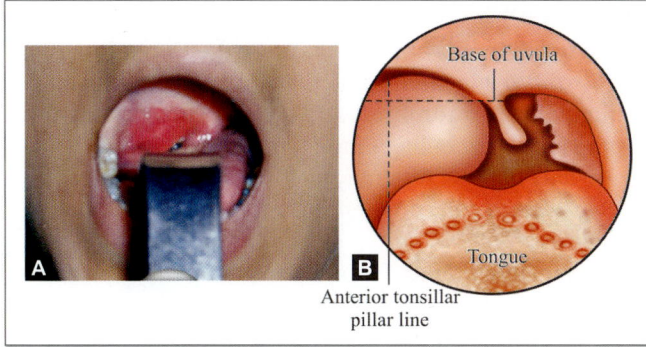

Figs 54.3A and B: (A) Peritonsillar abscess right side; (B) Site of incision and drainage lies just lateral to the junction of vertical anterior faucial pillar line and horizontal base of uvula line

  - *Cervical lymphadenopathy* of jugulodigastric lymph nodes. Swelling is tender and painful.
  - *Torticollis:* Neck is tilted towards side of abscess.

Treatment

- *Medical:* The conservative measures are taken in cases of all the deep-space neck infections. They may possibly cure the patient and include:
  - Hospitalization.
  - Intravenous fluids to combat dehydration.
  - Suitable antibiotics covering both aerobic and anaerobic organisms.
  - *Analgesics and antipyretics (paracetamol):* Aspirin can increase the chances of bleeding.
  - *Oral hygiene:* It is maintained by hydrogen peroxide or saline mouthwashes.
- *Surgical (incision and drainage of abscess)*
  - *Indications:* Frank abscess formation.
  - *Method:* With the help of a guarded knife, a small stab incision is made at the point of maximum bulge above the upper pole of tonsil, or the junction of anterior pillar and base of uvula (Fig. 54.3B). The site is touched by phenol (carbolic acid) prior to incision. A sinus- or artery-forcep is inserted to open and drain the abscess. It may need to be repeated the following day to drain any reaccumulation. Peritonsillar abscess forceps can also be used for drainage of peritonsillar abscess. *See* Chapter 'Instruments'.
  - *Interval tonsillectomy:* Tonsillectomy is done 4–6 weeks after an attack of quinsy.
  - *Abscess or hot tonsillectomy:* It cuts down the cost remarkably. It avoids risk and morbidity of second anesthesia and surgery as abscess is drained simultaneously. The risk of rupture of abscess during anesthesia and operative bleeding should be kept in mind.

Complications

Though rare in this era of antibiotics, they include:
- *Parapharyngeal abscess* may result in edema of larynx, jugular vein thrombosis and spontaneous carotid artery and jugular vein bleeding.
- *Airway obstruction* may need tracheostomy.
- *Septicemia* can cause endocarditis, nephritis and brain abscess.
- *Aspiration of pus* (spontaneous rupture of abscess) will cause pneumonitis and lung abscess.

PARAPHARYNGEAL SPACE ABSCESS

Syn: Pharyngomaxillary and lateral pharyngeal space abscesses

Sources of Infections

- *Oropharynx:* Bursting of peritonsillar abscess, pharyngitis, tonsillitis and adenoiditis.
- *Dental:* Infections of usually lower last molars.
- *Suppurative otitis media:* Bezold's abscess and petrositis.
- *Extensions:* Infections of parotid, retropharyngeal and submaxillary spaces.
- *Injuries:* Penetrating injuries of neck.
- *Iatrogenic:* Injection local anesthetic for tonsillectomy and mandibular nerve block.

Clinical Features

- *Common features:* The patients with parapharyngeal abscess usually present with:
  - Fever
  - Odynophagia
  - Sore throat
  - Torticollis (due to spasm of prevertebral muscles)
  - Toxemia.

Other features depend upon the compartment involved.
- *Anterior compartment:*
  - Prolapse of tonsil and tonsillar fossa
  - Trismus due to spasm of medial pterygoid muscle
  - Cervical swelling behind the angle of jaw
  - Odynophagia.
- *Posterior compartment:*
  - Pharyngeal bulging behind the posterior pillar.
  - Cranial nerve palsies: CN 9, 10, 11 and 12 palsies will cause dysphagia, hoarseness, nasal regurgitation and palsies of palate, larynx and tongue.
  - Horner's syndrome: Involve sympathetic chain.
    - Anhidrosis
    - Partial ptosis
    - Enophthalmos
    - Constricted pupil
  - Swelling in parotid region.

Complications

- Airway obstruction due to edema of larynx.
- Thrombophlebitis of jugular vein.
- Retropharyngeal abscess.
- Infection of mediastinum and carotid sheath.
- Carotid artery bleeding.

Treatment

- *Medical:* Intravenous antibiotics to combat infection.
- *Surgical drainage under general anesthesia:* Preoperative tracheostomy is required in cases of marked trismus and airway obstruction. A horizontal incision is made 2–3 cm below the angle of mandible. Abscess is approached and drained with blunt dissection along the inner surface of medial pterygoid muscle towards styloid process. A drain is usually inserted. Transoral drainage has the danger of injuring great vessels, and is avoided.

ACUTE RETROPHARYNGEAL ABSCESS

Most patients are children below 3 years of age.

Sources of Infection

Suppuration of retropharyngeal lymph nodes occur secondary to:
- Infection in the adenoids, nasopharynx, posterior nasal sinuses and nasal cavity.
- Penetrating injury of posterior pharyngeal wall and cervical esophagus.
- Petrositis due to acute mastoiditis.

Clinical Features

- Dysphagia and respiratory distress (stridor) are prominent symptoms because abscess obstructs the air and food passages.
- Croupy cough may be present.
- Torticollis: Stiff neck and extended head.
- Unilateral bulging in posterior pharyngeal wall on one side of the midline.

Diagnosis

- *X-ray soft tissue neck lateral view:* Shows widening of prevertebral space and presence of gas.
- *CT scan:* Shows retropharyngeal abscess (Fig. 54.4A).

Treatment

- *Medical:* Systemic intravenous antibiotics.
- *Incision and drainage of abscess:* Rupture of abscess may occur during intubation. Child is kept in supine and head-low position. A vertical incision is made in the most fluctuant area of the abscess on the lateral part

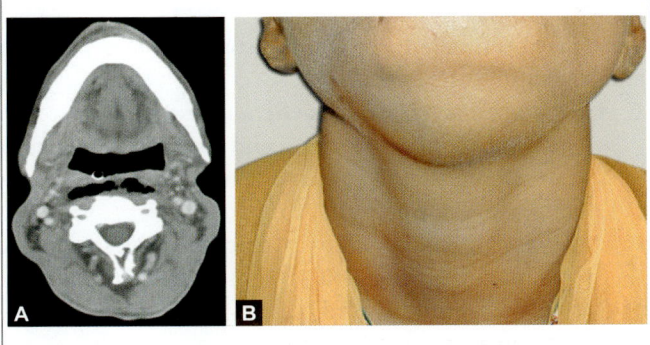

Figs 54.4A and B: (A) CT scan neck axial section. Retropharyngeal abscess (Prof Swati Shah, GCR MC, Ahmedabad); (B) Ludwig's angina. Submental and submandibular tender swelling in a 20-year old lady

of the posterior pharyngeal wall. Suction must be ready and handy to prevent aspiration of pus.
- *Tracheostomy:* In cases of a large abscess causing respiratory distress and laryngeal edema.

CHRONIC RETROPHARYNGEAL ABSCESS OR PREVERTEBRAL SPACE ABSCESS

It is common in adults and rare in children.

Sources of Infection

- *Tuberculosis of cervical spine (Pot's spine):* It presents swelling in the midline of posterior pharyngeal wall because infection is behind prevertebral fascia.
- *Tuberculosis of retropharyngeal lymph nodes:* It presents swelling on the side of the midline as the infection is in the retropharyngeal space.

Clinical Features

- Mild discomfort in throat and dysphagia.
- Posterior pharyngeal wall: Fluctuant swelling centrally or on one side of midline.
- Cervical tuberculous lymph nodes.

Diagnosis

X-ray and CT cervical spines: Shows caries of the cervical spine and abscess.

Treatment

- *Medical:* Full course of multi-drugs antitubercular therapy is started and continued after the surgery.
- *Incision and drainage of abscess:* A vertical incision is made along the anterior border (for low abscess) or posterior border (for high abscess) of sternocleidomastoid muscle.

LUDWIG'S ANGINA

It is the infection of the submandibular space.

Bacteriology

- Infections involve both aerobes and anaerobes.
- *Most common causative microorganisms:* α *Hemolytic streptococci, staphylococci* and *bacteroides.*
- Rarely *Haemophilus influenzae, Escherichia coli* and *Pseudomonas* are noted.

Sources of Infection

- *Dental infections (80%):* Lower premolars roots remain above the mylohyoid line and will cause sublingual space abscess. The lower molar roots go below the attachment of mylohyoid muscle and cause submaxillary space abscess (Fig. 54.2).
- *Others:* Submandibular sialadenitis, injuries of oral mucosa and fractures of the mandible.

Clinical Features

- Presenting complaints are marked difficulty in swallowing, odynophagia and trismus.
- There occurs swelling in the floor of mouth. The tongue is pushed up and back if the infection happens to be involving the sublingual space.
- Once the infection spreads to the submaxillary and submental spaces, the submandibular regions become swollen and tender (Fig. 54.4B), and feel woody hard. There is marked cellulitis of these areas. The frank abscess is uncommon
- In advanced cases, airway is threatened. Tongue is progressively pushed upwards and backwards. Laryngeal edema may ensue.

Treatment

- *Systemic antibiotics and incision and drainage* are the main element of management. Drainage material must be submitted for culture and sensitivity.
- *Incision and drainage:*
  - Intraoral approach for abscess of sublingual space.
  - External approach for submaxillary space abscess.
    - *Method:* A transverse incision extending between angles of mandible is made. A vertical blunt dissection in midline leads to drainage of serous fluid (not frank pus) and provides significant relief.
- *Tracheostomy* in cases of respiratory distress.

Complications

- *Spread of infection:* Parapharyngeal and retropharyngeal spaces and mediastinum.
- *Impairment of airway:* Edema of larynx and tongue.
- *Septicemia and aspiration* pneumonia.

ABSCESS OF SPACE OF BODY OF MANDIBLE

- **Sources of infection:** Periapical abscess of bicuspids and first and second molars of lower jaw.
- **Clinical features:** Patient presents with a painful tender swelling on the facial or/and lingual surface of the lower part of the body of mandible. Redness of surrounding gingiva may be seen in some patients. The affected tooth feels long and becomes tender. Tenderness can be elicited in buccal or/and lingual sulcus.
- **Treatment:** Antibiotics and surgical drainage.

MASTICATOR SPACE ABSCESS

In comparison to parapharyngeal abscess patient is not acutely ill.

Sources of Infections

- Pericoronitis or impacted third molars.
- Posterior spread of infection of body of mandible space.

Clinical Features

- **Severe painful swelling:** It extends over ramus of mandible and obliterates subangular depression.
    - Fluctuation is usually absent.
- **Marked trismus:** It results from irritation of masseter and medical pterygoid muscle.
- **Dysphagia.**
- **Induration of posterior sublingual tissue** making the tongue depression difficult.

Treatment

Parenteral antibiotics for 1 week and incision and drainage.

TRISMUS

(L. fr. G. trismos, a creaking, rasping; Synonym: Lockjaw) Persistent contraction of masseter muscle leads to inability to open the mouth. In the past, tetanus was a common cause but in India now, the most common cause is oral submucous fibrosis.

Causes

They can be divided into three groups—acute painless, acute painful, and chronic.

1. **Acute painless trismus (medical causes)**
    - **Tetanus:** Spasms of neck and abdominal muscles and convulsions occur due to the painful tonic muscular contractions.
    - **Tetany:** It occurs due to calcium deficiency and hypoparathyroidism. It is characterized by muscle twitches, cramps and carpopedal spasm, severe laryngospasm and seizures.
    - **Strychnine poisoning:** It stimulates all parts of the central nervous system. The muscles are relaxed in between the convulsions.
2. **Acute painful trismus (ENT causes)**
    - **Peritonsillar abscess**
    - **Parapharyngeal abscess of anterior compartment**
    - **Ludwig's angina**
    - **Alveolar infection** especially of last molar region.
    - **Acute parotitis:** Mumps and bacterial parotitis.
    - **Acute temporomandibular arthritis**
    - **Condylar fracture of mandible:** History of trauma and painful swelling. OPG will confirm the diagnosis.
    - **Acute otitis externa** especially furuncle.
3. **Chronic trismus (ENT causes)**
    - **Oral submucous fibrosis**
    - **Ankylosis of temporomandibular joint**
    - **Malignancy** of buccal mucosa, tonsil, retromolar trigone, pterygopalatine fossa, maxillary sinus, and parotid.

Sequela

- Poor oral hygiene.
- Difficulty in enjoying sumptuous meals.
- Difficult mouth and throat examination and surgical interventions.
- **Endotracheal intubation:** In cases of emergency and anesthesia, endotracheal intubation becomes troublesome, and patient may need tracheostomy.

Self-evaluation Exercises

1. Patient of parapharyngeal abscess develops:
    a. Trismus
    b. Fever
    c. Swelling that pushes the tonsil medially
    d. Spreads laterally posterior to sternocleidomastoid
    e. All of the above
2. The spaces involved in Ludwig's angina are:
    a. Sublingual
    b. Submental
    c. Submandibular
    d. All of the above

Contd...

Contd…

True (T)/False (F)
3. CT with contrast enhancement is the most valuable investigation in deep neck infections.
4. Parapharyngeal abscess occurs due to caries/extraction of molar tooth.

Filling the blanks
5. In peritonsillar abscess (Quinsy), there occurs collection of pus in the peritonsillar space that lies _____ to superior constrictor muscle of pharynx.
6. Trismus in peritonsillar abscess (Quinsy) is due to spasm of _____ pterygoid muscle.
7. The parapharyngeal abscess lies _____ to medial pterygoid muscle.
8. The otogenic parapharyngeal abscess is caused by _____.

Answers
1. e 2. d 3. T 4. T 5. Medial
6. Medial 7. Medial 8. Petrositis

Problem-oriented Cases (Spot Diagnosis)

1. A 20-year-old boy presents with throat pain and easy fatigable voice. During indirect laryngoscopy both vocal cords approximate well but leave a triangular gap in the interarytenoid region.[1]
2. A middle aged chronic smoker male patient has been suffering from hoarseness of voice for 2 years. On indirect laryngoscopy, reddish areas of mucosal irregularity are seen on both vocal cords. What will be your line of management?[2]
3. A 3-year-old boy presents with hoarse voice and slight respiratory distress. The child is having multiple laryngeal papillomas, which also involve glottis. Which is the best line of treatment?[3]
4. A patient of carcinoma larynx involving anterior commissure and vocal cord has perichondritis of thyroid cartilage. What will be your line of treatment?[4]
5. An adult patient who is a chronic smoker has squamous cell carcinoma of larynx. The local laryngeal lesion is involving unilateral vocal and false cords. Vocal cords are mobile. There are no neck nodes. Do the TNM classification and staging according to American joint committee on cancer classification.[5]
6. A 4-year-old child presents in emergency with mild respiratory distress. Laryngoscopy reveals multiple juvenile papillomatosis of the larynx. What will be your first line of treatment when the immediate facility for microlaryngoscopy surgery is not available?[6]
7. A 30-year-old patient comes back to hospital with gradually increasing respiratory distress in 4 days. The patient was on mechanical ventilation and had orotracheal intubation for 2 weeks. Patient was ok after removing the endotracheal tube and was discharged. It seems that the patient has developed tracheal stenosis. What would be your next line of treatment?[7]
8. A tracheostomy patient with Portex tracheostomy tube in position develops severe respiratory distress due to the blockage of the tube. What immediate action will you take? (*Hint:* Portex tracheostomy tube does not have separate inner cannula).[8]
9. A five-year-old child is afebrile but weak and exhausted from a week of paroxysmal coughing with inspiratory whoops, frequently associated with vomiting. The parents admit that childhood vaccinations were not given. Blood samples reveals lymphocytosis of 44000/mm^3. What is your most likely diagnosis?[9]
10. A 35-year-old patient develops trismus, fever, and swelling that is pushing the tonsils medially and spreading laterally posterior to sternocleidomastoid. He had extraction of third molar caries tooth few days back.[10]
11. A 50-year-old man who is smoker and alcoholic develops gradually progressive lymphadenopathy in the upper cervical region. On thorough ENT examination, no primary site of cancer was seen. What will be your next diagnostic step?[11]
12. During microlaryngoscopy CO$_2$ laser surgery an ignition of the endotracheal tube is seen. What will be your immediate step?[12]

[1]Phonasthenia, [2]Microlaryngoscopy and biopsy, [3]Microlaryngoscopy and excision, [4]Laryngectomy and postoperative radiotherapy, [5]Stage II: $T_2N_0M_0$, [6]Tracheostomy, [7]Intravenous steroids, [8]Immediate removal of Portex tracheostomy tube, [9]Whooping cough (pertussis), [10]Parapharyngeal abscess, [11]Fine needle aspiration cytology (FNAC), [12]Remove endotracheal tube and reestablish the airway

Section 8: Operative Procedures and Instruments

Chapter 55

Middle Ear and Mastoid Surgeries

Specific Learning Objectives

After going through the chapter, you should be able to answer the following questions:
- What are the indications and complications of myringotomy and grommet insertion?
- Describe the different approaches of mastoid operations and their indications.
- Describe the indications, steps and complications of simple mastoidectomy
- Describe different types of mastoidectomy and their indications.
- What surgical treatments are used for conductive hearing loss? Describe different types of tympanoplasty and the grafts used in them.

MYRINGOTOMY AND TYMPANOSTOMY TUBES (GROMMET)

Myringotomy refers to an incision of the tympanic membrane (TM) to drain middle ear fluid, which may be suppurative or nonsuppurative (Fig. 55.1).

Ventilation tube (grommet) (Fig. 55.2) is inserted through myringotomy incision for draining middle ear fluid as well as for providing aeration in case of malfunctioning Eustachian tube (ET).

Intratympanic glomus tumor: Myringotomy/grommet insertion are contraindicated in suspected cases of intratympanic glomus tumor because they can cause profuse bleeding in such patients.

Indications for Myringotomy
- *Indications in acute otitis media (AOM)*
  - *Bulging eardrum*
  - *Acute excruciating pain*
  - *Unresponsive to antibiotics:* Incomplete resolution with opaque drum and persistent conductive hearing loss.
  - *Complications:* Facial paralysis, labyrinthitis and meningitis with bulging tympanic membrane.

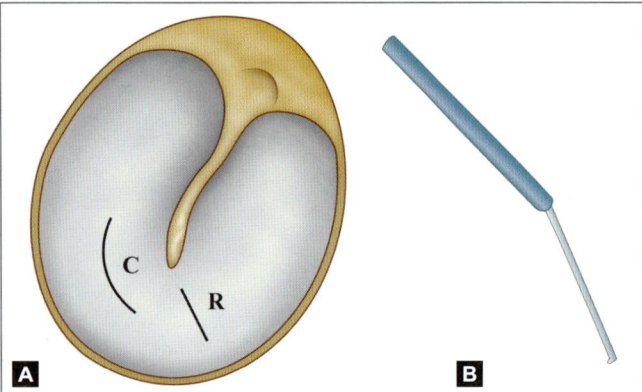

Figs 55.1A and B: Myringotomy. (A) Incisions: C, Circumferential for acute suppurative otitis media (ASOM) and R, radial for otitis media with effusion (OME); (B) Myringotome

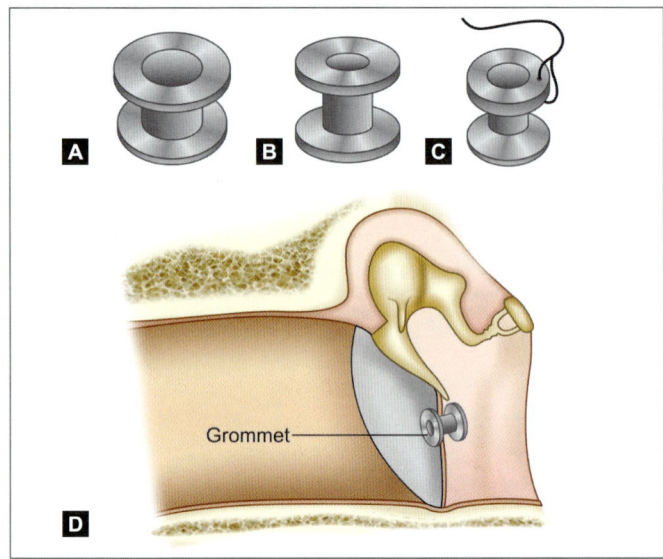

Figs 55.2A to D: Ventilation tubes. (A) Tuebingen ventilation tube; (B) Sheehy teflon ventilation tube; (C) Shepard teflon ventilation tube with wire; and (D) Grommet in position

- *Otitis media with effusion (OME).*
- *Aero-otitis media* to drain middle ear fluid and unlock the Eustachian tube.

  - *Tympanostomy tubes (grommet):* They provide longer lasting drainage of middle ear effusion than myringotomy and indicated in OME.
  - *Atelectatic ear:* Grommet for long term aeration.

Anesthesia
- *General anesthesia*
  - In children and uncooperative adults.
  - Acutely inflamed tympanic membrane.
- *Local anesthesia:* In cooperative adults.

Technique
- *Requirement:* The procedure is always done under operating microscope. Clean wax and debris from external auditory canal (EAC).
- *Site, size and shape of incision:* Perform myringotomy in anterior portion preferably anteroinferior quadrant of TM using a sharp myringotome (Fig. 55.1B). Myringotomy may be done by a fine micro-knife. Either radial or circumferential incision is employed.
  - *Acute otitis media (AOM):* A circumferential incision in the posteroinferior quadrant of pars tensa avoids injury to incudostapedial joint.
  - *Otitis media with effusion (OME):* A small radial incision may be used in the posteroinferior or anteroinferior quadrant of pars tensa.
  - *Grommet:* The size of incision should be just enough to admit the grommet.
- *Cautions:* Following precautions should be taken:
  - *Thick tympanic membrane (TM):* A deep incision that cuts through TM is required.
  - *AOM:* In cases of acute inflammation distinction between the TM and posterior meatal wall is lost. Avoid putting incision in the posterior meatal wall.

Operative microscope: The objective piece of microscope commonly used for ear microsurgery is 200–300 mm.

Postoperative Care
- *Topical antibiotic ear drops* in presence of mucoid effusion reduce otorrhea.
- *Swimming:* Surprisingly, studies found no difference in rates of otorrhea in patients who swam or not with or without earplugs.
- *Hearing tests.*
- *Follow-up:* Twice a year otoscopy/microscopy to assess:
  - Status of tympanostomy tube
  - Tympanic membrane (TM) for perforation, retraction pocket, atelectasis and cholesteatoma.

Complications
Complications are uncommon in experienced hands.
- *Otorrhea:* Most common complication.
- *Myringosclerosis:* It is of little functional importance.
- *Trauma:* External auditory canal lacerations and injury to ossicles such as incudostapedial joint and stapes.
  - If jugular bulb is high and floor of the middle ear dehiscent, injury to jugular bulb can cause profuse bleeding.
- *Tympanic membrane:*
  - Perforation
  - Atrophy
  - Retraction
  - Atelectasis
  - Cholesteatoma.
- *Grommet:*
  - Migration or loss of tube into middle ear
  - Early extrusion
  - Plugging of tube.
- *Anesthetic complications.*

MASTOIDECTOMY (BOX 55.1)

Mastoidectomy is an operation in which mastoid antrum is opened and air cells are removed. This operation can be done either alone or in association with tympanoplasty. Tympanoplasty consists of eradication of middle ear disease and reconstruction of the hearing mechanism.

Surgical Approaches (Figs 55.3 and 55.4)
Depending upon the experience of surgeon and nature and extent of the lesion, middle ear and mastoid operations can be done with endaural and postaural approach.
- *Postaural (or Wilde's) incision (Fig. 55.4A):* This postaural incision begins at the highest attachment

Box 55.1: Types of mastoidectomies

- *Simple mastoidectomy* (cortical mastoidectomy or Schwartz operation)
- *Canal wall-up procedures* (intact posterior meatal wall or closed procedures)
  - With facial recess approach
  - Without facial recess approach
- *Canal wall-down procedures* (open procedures)
  - Radical mastoidectomy
  - Modified radical mastoidectomy
  - Bondy procedure
- *Tympanoplasty* (reconstructive surgery)
  - During the primary surgery
  - Second stage

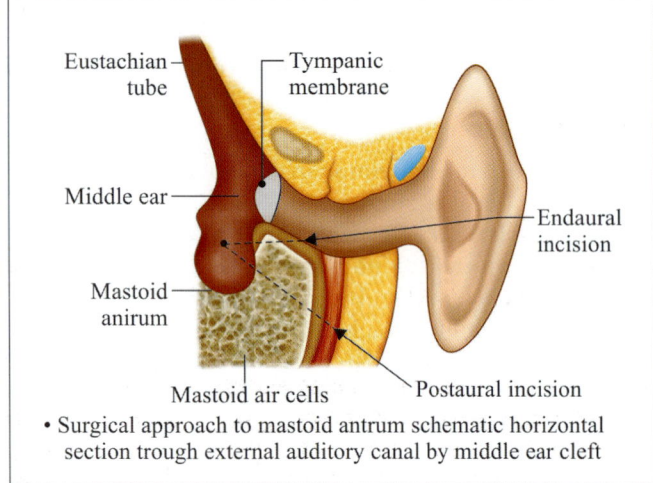

Fig. 55.3: Postaural and endaural approaches to mastoid antrum

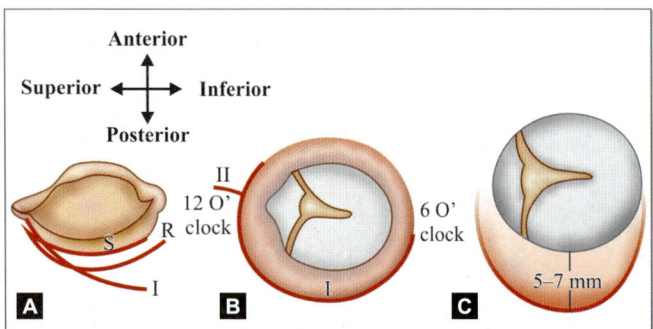

Figs 55.4A to C: Surgical approaches. (A) Postaural incisions (S, Sulcus (Retroauricular); R, Retrosulcus; and I, Infants incision); (B) Endaural incision (I, Lempert I posterior meatal wall semicircular incision and II, Lempert II upward curvilinear 12 o'clock incision); and (C) Endomeatal incision (Rosen)

of the pinna and ends at the mastoid tip. The incision may lie either 1 cm behind or in the retroauricular groove. In children upto 2 years of age, the postaural incision must be slanting posteriorly to avoid lower part of the mastoid. In these children, mastoid process is not developed and stylomastoid foramen from where facial nerve emerges is located more superficially. The slanting incision avoids cutting facial nerve which is superficial.

- ■ *Indications:* They include:
  - ◆ Cortical mastoidectomy
  - ◆ Radical and modified radical mastoidectomy
  - ◆ Tympanoplasty
  - ◆ Decompression of facial nerve
  - ◆ Endolymphatic sac operation.
- **Endaural approach (Fig. 55.4B):** Lempert's incision employed for the endaural approach has two parts:
  1. *Lempert I:* This semicircular horizontal incision is made at the bony cartilaginous junction in the posterior meatal wall. The incision extends from 12 o'clock to 6 o'clock position.
  2. *Lempert II:* This curvilinear vertical incision begins from the 1st incision at 12 o'clock and passes upwards between tragus and the crus of helix (incisura terminalis) without cutting the aural cartilage.
  - ■ *Indications:* Both mastoid and external canal surgeries can be done.
    - ◆ *Osteoma and exostosis of EAC*
    - ◆ *Tympanoplasty*
    - ◆ *Atticoantrotomy:* Atticoantral cholesteatoma
    - ◆ *Modified radical mastoidectomy:* Cholesteatoma of attic, antrum and mastoid.
- **Endomeatal or transcanal approach (Fig. 55.4C):** Rosen's stapedectomy incision is an example of endomeatal incision. A posterior tympanomeatal flap is raised to enter into the middle ear. Posterior meatal wall skin is raised and annulus dislocated from the sulcus. Rosen's incision consists of two parts:
  1. *I incision:* A small vertical incision begins at 12 o'clock position near the annulus.
  2. *II incision:* A curvilinear incision 5–7 mm away from the annulus begins at 6 o'clock position and meets the 1st incision in the posterosuperior region of deep bony canals.
  - ■ *Indications:* It offers nice view of the middle ear:
    - ◆ Exploratory tympanotomy
    - ◆ Stapedectomy
    - ◆ Inlay myringoplasty
    - ◆ Ossicular reconstruction.

Anesthesia

Under general anesthesia or local anesthesia.

Position of Patient

Patient lies in supine position with head turned to the side so that operation ear is on upper side.

CORTICAL MASTOIDECTOMY

Syn: Simple or complete mastoidectomy or Schwartz operation

Cortical mastoidectomy refers to complete exenteration of all accessible mastoid air cells without removing the posterior meatal wall.

Indications

- Acute coalescent mastoiditis with or without subperiosteal abscess.
- Acute otitis media with reservoir sign (not resolving with medical treatment).

- Masked mastoiditis.
- Primary step to perform:
  - Cochlear implantation.
  - Endolymphatic sac surgery.
  - Decompression of facial nerve.
  - Labyrinthectomy.
  - Cerebrospinal fluid (CSF) otorrhea.
  - Access to cerebellopontine angle (acoustic neuroma), skull base, and petrous apex (translabyrinthine or retrolabyrinthine procedures).

Steps of Operation

- *Incision:* A postaural incision cuts through soft tissues and reaches upto the periosteum without cutting the temporalis muscle. Mastoid retractors (Jansen's or Mollison's) retract soft tissues after the postaural incision and elevation of flaps. The pressure on the edges of the incision provides hemostasis. Lempert's endaural retractor is used in cases of endaural approach. Lempert's endaural speculum can be used to spread open the meatus when giving local injection or making an endaural incision.
- *Exposure of mastoid:* Periosteum is cut in the line of postaural incision. A horizontal incision is made along the lower border of temporalis muscle. A branch of superficial temporal artery is usually encountered and may need ligation or cauterization. Periosteum is elevated from the lateral surface of mastoid and posterosuperior region of bony meatus. Farabeuf's periosteal elevator is used for elevation of periosteum from the mastoid cortex. Tendinous fibers of sternocleidomastoid muscle need sharp cutting near the mastoid tip.
- *Identification of mastoid antrum:* Mastoid cortex is drilled out to enter into the mastoid antrum. In adults mastoid antrum lies 12–15 mm deep to the suprameatal triangle (Macewen's triangle). Mastoid gouges may be used to remove mastoid bone. Horizontal semicircular canal, aditus ad antrum and short process of incus are identified. Mastoid suction tips helps in aspirating blood, discharge, irrigation water and bone dust and pieces.
- *Removal of mastoid air cells:* Lempert's mastoid curette (scoop) removes bony septa and granulations in mastoid antrum and air cells. The electrical drill and burs are replacing the use of gouges and curettes. All the accessible mastoid air cells are removed. Zygomatic cells in the root of zygoma and retrosinus cells behind the sinus between sinus plate and cortex are also removed. The bony plate of tegmen tympani above, sinus plate behind and posterior meatal wall in front though exposed are not removed (Figs 55.5 and 55.6). Try to identify following structures in the newly created mastoid cavity:

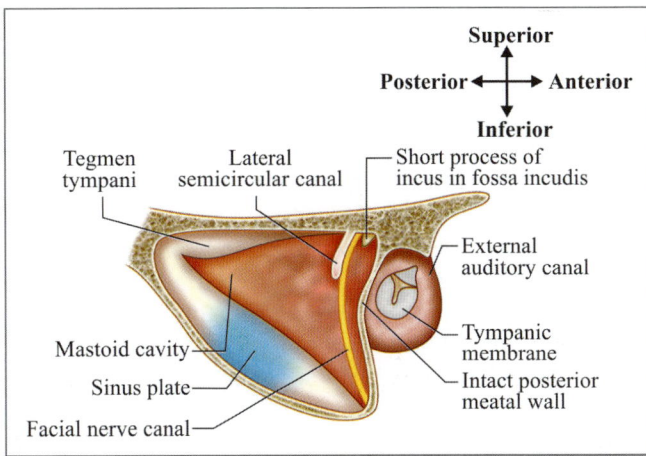

Fig. 55.5: Simple cortical mastoidectomy with intact posterior meatal wall

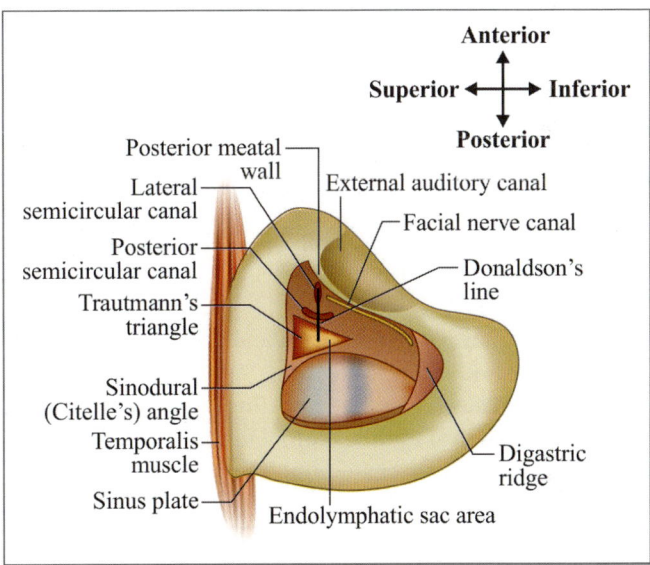

Fig. 55.6: Cortical mastoidectomy cavity—landmarks and structures seen

- **Sinodural (Citelle) angle:** It lies between the tegmen antri (middle cranial fossa) and the sigmoid sinus.
- **Solid angle:** This solid bone angle, which lies medial to antrum, is formed by the three semicircular canals.
- **Trautmann's triangle:** This bony plate of posterior surface of petrous bone lies behind the mastoid antrum. It is bounded by following structures:
  - Sigmoid sinus
  - Bony labyrinth
  - Superior petrosal sinus.
- **Donaldson's line:** This line passes through the lateral semicircular canal bisecting the posterior semicircular canal. The endolymphatic sac that appears as thickening of the posterior cranial fossa dura (double layered) is situated inferior to Donaldson's line.

- ***Removal of mastoid tip:*** Removal of the lateral wall of mastoid tip will expose muscle fibers of posterior belly of digastric. Edges of the mastoid cavity should be beveled (saucerization of edges) so that soft tissue sits in and obliterates the cavity.
- ***Closure of wound:*** After cleaning the bone dust from the wound and mastoid cavity (thorough irrigation with saline), the wound is closed in two layers. If there is infection or excessive bleeding, a drain may be kept at the lower end of incision for 1 to 2 days. The EAC is packed with ribbon gauze impregnated in antimicrobial agent. It avoids stenosis of ear canal. Mastoid bandage is applied.

Postoperative Care

- ***Antibiotics:*** They are started before the surgery and continued postoperatively for at least 1 week. Perioperative swab for culture from the mastoid helps in identifying the microorganisms and selecting the antibiotic.
- ***Mastoid drain:*** It is usually removed in 1–2 days.
- ***Removal of stitches:*** They are removed usually on the 6th day.

Complications

- Perioperative injuries to:
  - Facial nerve
  - Horizontal semicircular canal: Patient develops vertigo and jerky nystagmus
  - Sigmoid sinus (profuse bleeding)
  - Dura mater of middle cranial fossa-CSF leak
  - Dislocation of incus-conductive hearing loss
- ***Postoperative:*** Wound infection and wound breakdown.

RADICAL MASTOIDECTOMY (FIG. 55.7)

Radical mastoidectomy eradicates disease from the middle ear and mastoid and exteriorizes mastoid, middle ear, attic and antrum into the external ear by removing the posterior meatal wall. The structures removed are—cholesteatoma, granulations, remnants of TM, malleus, incus (not the stapes), chorda tympani and mucoperiosteal lining. The opening of ET is closed with a piece of muscle or cartilage.

There is no reconstruction of hearing system. As the posterior meatal wall is removed, the entire area of middle ear, attic, antrum and mastoid is converted into a single cavity. The basic aim is to exteriorize the diseased area for inspection and cleaning. This radical surgery is now not done frequently.

Closure of Eustachian tube (ET): It prevents infection of middle ear from the nasopharynx.

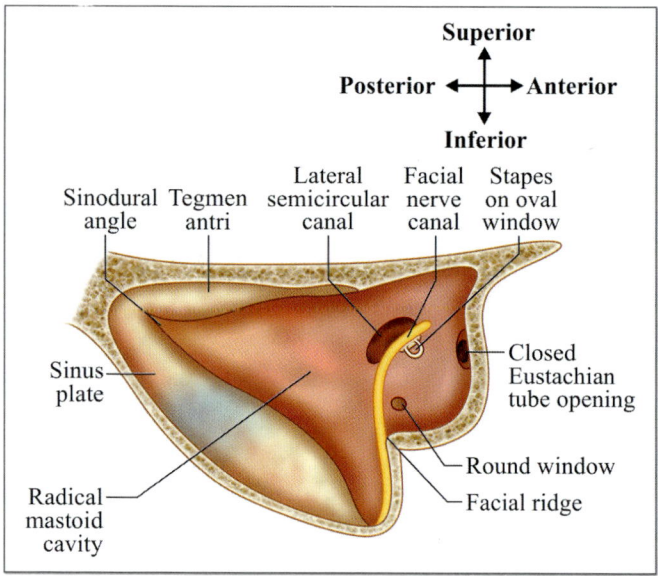

Fig. 55.7: Radical mastoidectomy cavity

Indications

- CSOM with intracranial complications.
- Cholesteatoma invading Eustachian tube, round window niche, perilabyrinthine or hypotympanic cells.
- Revision surgery to eradicate chronic inflammatory disease and remnant cholesteatoma.
- Disease in petrous apex.
- Glomus tumor.
- Carcinoma middle ear: If en bloc removal of temporal bone is not feasible then radical mastoidectomy followed by radiotherapy may be considered.

Steps of Operation

(*See* Cortical Mastoidectomy)
- ***Incision:*** Postaural or endaural.
- ***Exposure of mastoid area:*** The periosteum from the lateral mastoid surface is elevated. This extends from the root of zygoma to the area behind the suprameatal triangle and from suprameatal crest (continuation of inferior temporal line) to the lower part of mastoid tip. The wound is retracted.
- ***Exposure of attic and antrum:*** The cortical mastoid bone is drilled out from the suprameatal triangle, spine of Henle, root of zygoma and upper part of superior meatal wall till the exposure of attic and antrum. The tegmen antri and lateral semicircular canal are identified.
- ***Removal of 'bridge' and facial buttresses:*** Deeper part of superior bony meatal wall bridging over the notch of Rivinus is taken off carefully without damaging the deeper middle ear structures. The removal of anterior buttress (anterior spine of the notch) and posterior

buttress (posterior spine of the notch), which form the lateral attic wall, will expose the regions of attic, aditus ad antrum, facial canal and ossicles. The diseased incus and the malleus are removed.

- *Lowering of facial ridge:* The deeper part of posterior meatal wall lying over the vertical part of facial nerve called **facial ridge** is removed as much as possible within the safety of facial nerve. It makes mastoid cavity easily inspected and cleaned during the postoperative care.
- *Debridement of middle ear:* Remnants of TM, annulus, sulcus tympanicus, middle ear mucoperiosteum, cholesteatoma, polyp, granulation tissue, malleus and incus are removed step by step. Stapes is left intact. ET mucosa is curetted and plugged with tensor tympani muscle or piece of cartilage.
- *Cavity inspection and irrigation:* Ensure complete exteriorization of the mastoid antrum and cavity and middle ear including attic into the EAC. Bony overhangs are removed and cavity is smoothened with polishing burr. Saucerization of the cortical edges of mastoid must be done. Irrigate the cavity and wound with saline or ringer to remove blood and bone dust.
- *Meatoplasty:* A concha based flap from posterior and superior meatal wall is raised and turned into the mastoid cavity. It covers the area of the facial ridge and facilitates epithelialization of the mastoid cavity. A crescent of conchal cartilage is excised to widen the meatus. It facilitates access to cavity for inspection and cleaning during the postoperative care.

> Meatoplasty is also done as an isolated procedure in cases of sagging auricle, which is seen in older people. The obstruction of the ear canal causes hearing loss and retention of wax.

- *Mastoid obliteration:* If the ultimate mastoid cavity becomes very large, it may be obliterated with temporalis muscle or other musculofascial tissues. Due care must be taken to remove any remnant cholesteatoma, which must not be buried underneath.
- *Closure of wound:* The mastoid cavity is packed with betadine ribbon gauze. The wound is closed in two layers. Mastoid bandage is applied.

> **Mastoid surgery:**
> - Aim of mastoid surgery in unsafe CSOM is rendering the ear safe.
> - Techniques, which are used to control bleeding from bone during mastoid surgery, include bone wax, bipolar cautery over the bleeding area and diamond drill.
> - Cutting drill over the bleeding area will not control bleeding.

Postoperative Care

- *Antibiotic:* It is given for 7–14 days.
- *The bandage and packing:* They are removed as per the liking of the surgeon from 1–7 days. Skin stitches are removed on 6th or 7th day. Some prefer changing of the pack at weekly intervals and others leave the cavity unpacked with regular suction and cleaning till the epithelialization of the cavity.
    - Look for any signs of perichondritis or infection.
- *Cavity care:* The epithelialization of cavity takes 2–3 months. The cavity is checked every 4–6 months in the first year and then annually. The debris is removed. Granulation tissue which delays the healing is either removed or chemically cauterized.

Complications

- *Perioperative injury to:*
    - Facial nerve resulting in facial paralysis.
    - Dura or sigmoid sinus.
    - Stapes dislocation can result in labyrinthitis sensorineural hearing loss (SNHL) and vertigo.
    - Severe conductive hearing loss due to removal of the ossicles and tympanic membrane.
- *Perichondritis*
- *Cavity problems:*
    - Nonhealing of cavity.
    - Regular after care.

MODIFIED RADICAL MASTOIDECTOMY

In this modification of radical mastoidectomy, hearing mechanism and middle ear cleft structures are preserved as far as possible. Only irreversibly damaged tissues are removed. Preservation and conservation of middle ear structures help in reconstruction of the hearing mechanism.

Modified radical mastoidectomy eradicates disease from the attic and mastoid and exteriorizes both into the EAC by removal of the posterior meatal and lateral attic walls (Fig. 55.8). The remnant of TM, functioning ossicles and the reversible mucosa and function of the ET, are preserved.

Indications

- Atticoantral cholesteatoma.
- Chronic otitis media with limited disease.

Operation

The operative steps, postoperative care and complications are similar to radical mastoidectomy and the differences are following:

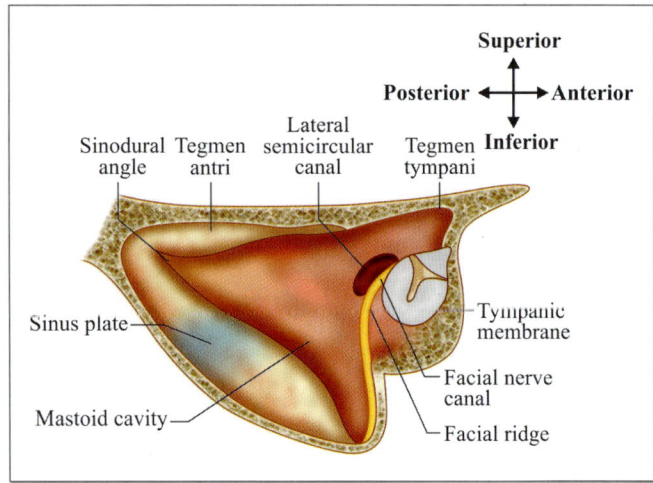

Fig. 55.8: Modified radical mastoidectomy cavity

Table 55.1: Types of tympanoplasty (Wullstein) (TM, tympanic membrane)

Types	Defect	Position or contact of graft
Type I (myringoplasty)	TM perforation	TM or malleus
Type II	TM perforation with erosion of malleus	Incus or remnant of malleus
Type III Myringostapediopexy or columella tympanoplasty	Malleus and incus absent	Stapes superstructure
Type IV	Stapes superstructure absent	Stapes footplate
Type V Fenestration operation	Stapes footplate fixed	Fenestra in horizontal semicircular canal

- **Removal of disease and preservation of healthy tissue:** Cholesteatoma, granulations and unhealthy mucosa are removed. Incus and head of malleus are preserved. They are removed only if cholesteatoma engulfs them or extends medial to them. Healthy pars tensa and middle ear structures are left undisturbed.
- **Tympanoplasty:** Reconstruction of TM and ossicular chain can be done (mastoidectomy with tympanoplasty operation) at the same sitting or in second stage.

TYMPANOPLASTY

These surgeries are done under operating microscope with the help of microsurgical instruments.
- **Tympanoplasty:** The tympanoplasty operation consists of both eradication of middle ear disease and reconstruction of hearing mechanism including tympanic membrane and ossicles. It may be done with or without mastoidectomy.
- **Myringoplasty:** The limited repair of tympanic membrane is called *myringoplasty*.
- **Ossiculoplasty:** The limited reconstruction of ossicular chain is called *ossiculoplasty*.

Indications
Conductive hearing loss due to the following causes:
- CSOM tubotympanic and atticoantral cholesteatoma (mastoidectomy with tympanoplasty).
- Trauma to tympanic membrane and ossicles.
- Tympanosclerosis.
- Deep retraction pockets.
- Congenital middle ear defects such as fixity of malleus head and congenital cholesteatoma.

Types of Tympanoplasty (Wullstein)
Wullstein described five types of tympanoplasty (Table 55.1). Several modifications in the Wullstein classification have been reported in the literature, which mainly pertain to the types of ossicular reconstruction (Fig. 55.9).
- **Cavum minor and tympanoplasty IV:** In type IV tympanoplasty graft is placed between the oval and round windows to create an air pocket around the round window. This narrow middle ear space, which is called *cavum minor* is a mucosa lined space that extends from the Eustachian tube to the round window. Sound

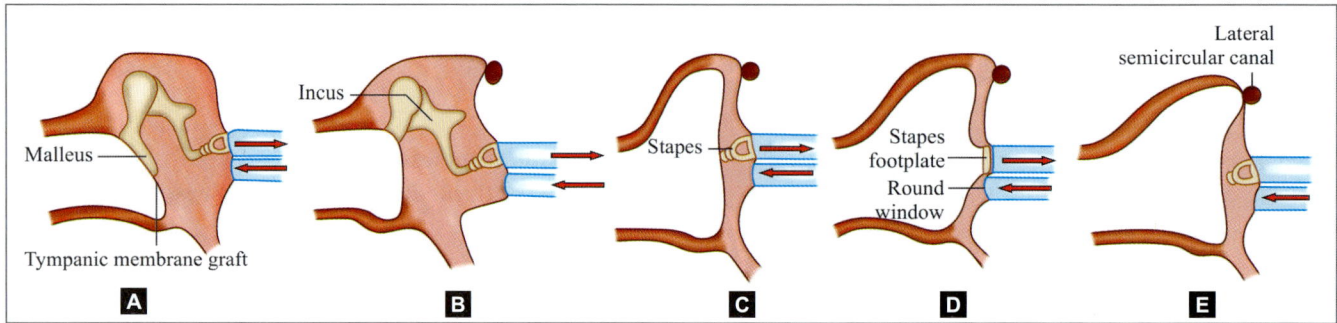

Figs 55.9A to E: Types of tympanoplasty. Tympanic membrane graft touches (A) Malleus (Type I); (B) Incus or ramnant of malleus (Type II); (C) Stapes superstructure (Type III); (D) Mobile stapes footplate (Type IV); and (E) Lateral semicircular canal (Type V)

Chapter 55 • Middle Ear and Mastoid Surgeries

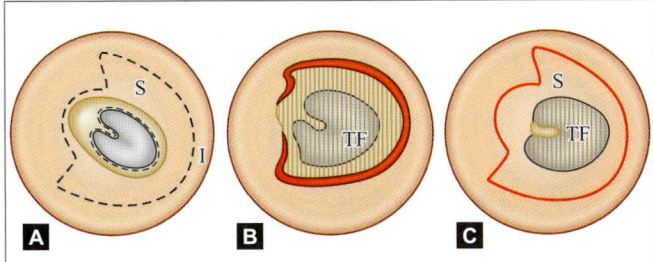

Figs 55.10A to C: Overlay myringoplasty. (A) Incision (I) to raise the meatal skin (S) and epithelium of tympanic membrane (TM); (B) Placement of temporalis fascia graft; and (C) Replacement of meatal skin and epithelium of TM

waves in this Type IV tympanoplasty directly hit on the footplate while the round window has been shielded by the cavum minor.
- **Tympanoplasty V:** In Type V tympanoplasty a window is created (fenestration) on horizontal semicircular canal and covered with a graft.

Myringoplasty

The simple closure of TM perforation is called myringoplasty.
- **Graft materials:** The most commonly used graft materials are temporalis fascia and tragal perichondrium. The other graft material includes fascia lata, cartilage and homograft (dura, vein, cadaver TM).
- **Techniques:** There are following three techniques—
  - **Underlay technique:** In this technique, graft is placed medial to the tympanic annulus. It requires opening of the middle ear (tympanotomy), which provides an opportunity to examine the ossicles and other middle ear structures.
  - **Overlay technique (Fig. 55.10):** Graft is placed lateral to fibrous layer of the TM. It requires careful removal of squamous epithelium from the lateral surface of remnant TM.
  - **Midlay technique:** Graft is placed in between the fibrous and mucosal layers of TM.

Ossiculoplasty

- **Indications:** Ossicular reconstruction is required in cases of destruction of ossicular chain mostly caused by chronic suppurative otitis media (CSOM).
  - **Destruction of ossicles**
    - *Necrosis of long process of incus:* Most common.
    - *Loss of stapes superstructure:* It leaves behind a mobile footplate and malleus.
    - *Destruction of malleus, incus and the stapes superstructure:* They leave behind only the mobile footplate. It is common in cholesteatoma.
  - **Fixation of ossicles**
    - *Ankylosis of stapes footplate (otosclerosis and tympanosclerosis):* The correction of ankylosis of stapes consists of removal of the superstructures stapes and its replacement by prosthesis.
    - *Fixation of the head of malleus in the attic (tympanosclerosis and congenital):* It needs removal of the head of malleus and entire incus. Then a contact is established between handle of malleus and the stapes.
- **Graft materials:** They are:
  - **Autografts (Fig. 55.11):** The most commonly used are autograft ossicles (incus transposition and sculptured ossicles) and tragal cartilage.
  - **Homograft:** Ossicles and membrane.
  - **Prosthetic implants:** They are made of ceramic (hydroxy appetite), teflon, gold and titanium.
    - *Total ossicular replacement prosthesis (TORP):* It bridges the gap between TM and stapes footplate.
    - *Partial ossicular replacement prosthesis (PORP):* It provides a direct contact between TM and stapes head.

> **Grafts**
> - Autograft temporalis fascia acts as a scaffold in tympanoplasty.
> - Denatured homograft TM has no antigenic property.

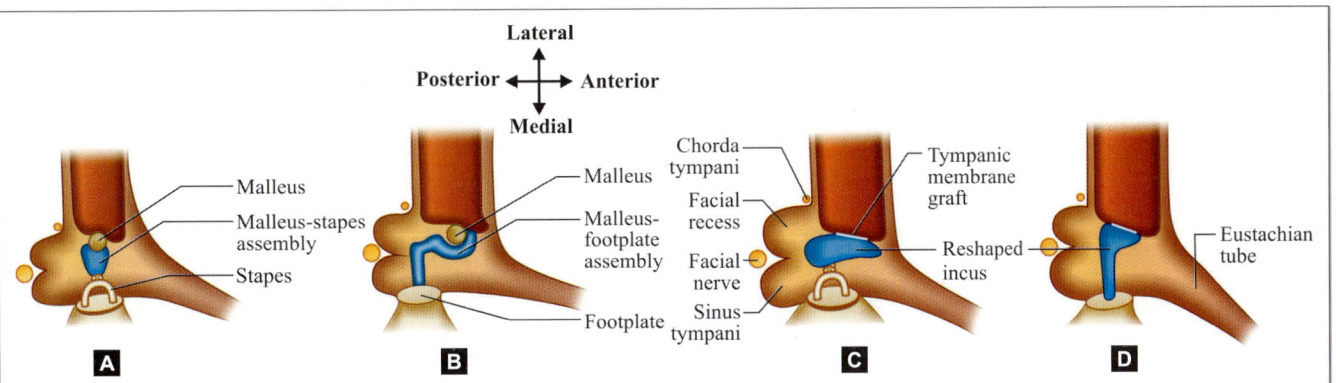

Figs 55.11A to D: Ossicular reconstruction. (A) Malleus-stapes assembly; (B) Malleus-footplate assembly; (C) Reshaped incus between stapes head and tympanic membrane graft; and (D) Reshaped incus between stapes footplate and tympanic membrane graft

Self-evaluation Exercises

1. The objective piece of operative microscope commonly used for ear microsurgery is:
   a. 100
   b. 200–300
   c. 400
   d. All of the above
2. The techniques, which are used to control bleeding from bone during mastoid surgery, include:
   a. Bone wax
   b. Bipolar cautery
   c. Diamond drill
   d. All of the above

True (T)/False (F)

3. The aim of mastoid surgery in unsafe chronic suppurative otitis media (CSOM) is good hearing.
4. Cutting drill over the bleeding area will not control bleeding in mastoid surgery.
5. Eustachian tube is not obliterated surgically in radical mastoidectomy.
6. Closure of Eustachian tube in radical mastoidectomy prevents infection of middle ear from the nasopharynx.
7. Autograft temporalis fascia acts as a scaffold in tympanoplasty.
8. Denatured homograft tympanic membrane has antigenic property.

Answers

1. b	2. d	3. F	4. T	5. F
6. T	7. T	8. F		

Chapter 56

Operations of Nose and Paranasal Sinuses

Specific Learning Objectives

After going through the chapter, you should be able to answer the following questions:
- What are the different steps of diagnostic nasal endoscopy and mention the structures you would be examining?
- What are the indications, contraindications and complications of endoscopic sinus surgery?
- What do you know about: (1) Antrum puncture; (2) Inferior meatus antrostomy; (3) Caldwell-Luc operation
- What are the indications and different techniques of nasal septal surgery?

SINUS OPERATIONS

The current trend for treating the sinonasal diseases is functional endoscopic sinus surgery (FESS), which will be dealt in detail but it is important to have knowledge of external approaches, which used to be the mainstay of treatment in recent past. FESS is considered for patients with refractory rhinosinusitis or its complications. The success rate of FESS is good in patients with chronic or recurrent rhinosinusitis while it is low in cases with recurrent polyps, severe allergies, past external procedures and immunocompromised state.

DIAGNOSTIC NASAL ENDOSCOPY (SINUSCOPY) (FIG. 56.1)

The brighter illumination, magnification, and angled view of endoscopes (sinuscopes) facilitate examination of all the cleft and crevices of nose and nasopharynx.

Indications

Sinuscopy facilitates in diagnosing the following:
- Nose, paranasal sinuses (PNS) and nasopharynx diseases.
- Locate the site of nose bleed.
- Biopsy from nose, PNS and nasopharynx lesions.
- Assess the response to treatment of nose, PNS and nasopharynx diseases.

Instruments

- 4 mm 0° and 30° sinuscopes.
- 2.7 mm 0° and 30° sinuscopes in cases of children and narrow nasal cavity.
- Freer's elevator.
- Suction cannula.
- Biopsy forceps.
- Antifog solution/savlon to avoid fogging.

Techniques

- **Anesthesia:** Mix 4% xylocaine in equal quantity of oxymetazoline hydrochloride. Instill these drops into the nose and then pack nasal cavity with packing impregnated with this solution.
- **Position of patient:** Patient is kept in either sitting or supine position (Fig. 56.1).
- **Method:** For thorough and complete examination, the scope is passed through the standard three paths. The examination is conducted while inserting and withdrawing the scope.

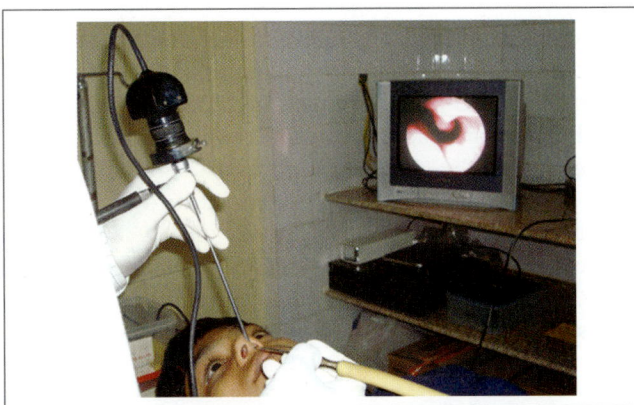

Fig. 56.1: Sinuscopy examination with CCTV attachment. Right hand holds the suction cannula

- **First pass (0° sinuscope):** It examines the nasal vestibule, nasal cavity in general, septum, inferior meatus and nasopharynx.
    - The scope is passed up to the nasopharynx through the inferior meatus. Slight pressure over the lacrimal sac may show the opening of nasolacrimal duct in the inferior meatus.
    - Note the septal deviation or spur, nature of nasal discharge, and color of mucous membrane, opening of the eustachian tube, walls of nasopharynx, and upper surface of soft palate.
- **Second pass (0° sinuscope):** It examines the posterior part of middle turbinate, sphenoethmoidal recess, superior meatus, superior turbinate and openings of the sphenoid sinus (in the posterior wall of sphenoethmoidal recess between the nasal septum and superior turbinate) and posterior ethmoid sinuses (in the superior meatus).
    - The scope is passed medial to the posterior part of middle turbinate and progresses up to the sphenoethmoidal recess between the nasal septum and superior turbinate.
- **Third pass (30° sinuscope):** It examines the structures of osteomeatal complex in the middle meatus such as uncinate process, bulla ethmoidalis, hiatus semilunaris, sinus of turbinate (space lateral to middle turbinate), basal lamina and the frontal recess.
    - The sinuscope is passed into the middle meatus usually from the anterior aspect but in some cases it is entered from behind where it is wider and the structures are examined from behind forward. If needed middle turbinate can be gently retracted medially with the help of Freer elevator.
- **Complication:** Bleeding can occur due to improper manipulation of instruments and is usually controlled by the application of vasoconstrictor pledgets.

ENDOSCOPIC SINUS SURGERY (ESS)

The endoscope has revolutionized the diagnosis and treatment of diseases of nose and paranasal sinuses. Now the first line of surgical treatment of rhinosinusitis is FESS. FESS has demonstrated success rates of 76–98%.

The philosophy of FESS is minimal (functional) surgery with mucosal preservation to achieve physiological drainage and ventilation of sinuses and healing. FESS targets the diseased sinuses and normal sinuses are left alone. Aggressive removal of mucosa is avoided as it leads to postoperative healing problems.

Indications

- *Recurrent and chronic rhinosinusitis,* which do not respond to medical therapy.
- *Nasal polyps* both ethmoidal and antrochoanal.
- *Foreign body.*
- *Septoplasty*
- *Dacryocystorhinostomy (DCR)*
- *Epistaxis* especially uncontrolled posterior bleeding and ligation of sphenopalatine artery.
- *Headache and facial pains:* Due to nasal septal deviation and concha bullosa.
- *Complications of rhinosinusitis* such as orbital abscess.
- *Cerebrospinal fluid (CSF) rhinorrhea:* Traumatic and iatrogenic. Patch material includes mucosal grafts, fascia grafts and synthetic products.
- *Fungal mycetoma:* CT shows heterogeneous lesion and microcalcifications.
- *Juvenile nasopharyngeal angiofibroma.*
- *Tumors of nose and paranasal sinuses* such as inverted papillomas.
- *Failed previous surgeries* such as external maxillary, ethmoidal and frontal procedures.
- *Mucoceles* (frontoethmoid and sphenoid)-marsupialization.
- *Encephalocele*
- *Pituitary tumors*
- *Optic nerve decompression*
- *Orbital decompression* in Graves' disease.
- *Choanal atresia*

Maxillary sinusitis: Most common predisposing factor linked to maxillary sinusitis is mucosal swelling in ethmoid infundibulum.

Contraindications

The contraindications include following conditions, which are better tackled by the external approaches:
- Intracranial complications.
- Orbital cellulitis with visual field defects.
- Osteomyelitis.
- Aggressive fungal infections such as mucormycosis.

Anesthesia

- *Local anesthesia with sedation:* ESS in adults is usually done under local anesthesia and sedation. It improves safety, as manipulations of orbital periosteum and dura are painful. The standby anesthesiologist monitors the vital parameters such as blood pressure, pulse, respiration, temperature and oxygen saturation.
- *General anesthesia:* It is preferred in pediatric patients, anxious adults, in anticipated long cases and computer-assisted navigation systems.

Preparations

Topical decongestants and anesthetics are administered in nose before the patient comes to operation theater (OT).

Local injection 1% lignocaine with 1:100,000 epinephrine is infiltrated in the middle turbinates and area just anterior to them. Depending on the site and extent of surgery other areas can also be infiltrated. A small Foley catheter no. 8 or expandable sponges in nasopharynx prevents blood pooling in oropharynx.

Position of Patient

Patient is placed in supine position. A slight reverse Trendelenburg position with patient rotation towards surgeon helps in reducing blood loss and makes surgeon comfortable.

Techniques

The endoscopes and microsurgical instruments provide better precision in the removal of tissue and avoid unnecessary stripping of mucosa. There are two techniques of ESS—Messerklinger (anterior to posterior) and Wigand (posterior to anterior).

1. *Messerklinger technique:* It consists of anterior to posterior approach. It includes following steps:
   - *Removal of uncinate process and exposure of infundibulum:* Uncinectomy and infundibulotomy are done with the help of either back-biting forceps or sickle knife and Blakesley forceps.
   - *Identification and widening of maxillary sinus ostium:* Maxillary ostium is situated in the posterior part of infundibulum and becomes visible after uncinectomy. It is enlarged anteriorly and posteriorly.
   - *Anterior ethmoidectomy:* Removal of ethmoidal bulla (bullectomy) is performed with curette or Blakesley forceps.
   - *Frontal sinusotomy:* Exposure and cleaning of frontal sinus ostium is done in the event of frontal sinus disease. Many do this step in last. The position of frontal sinus opening varies depending on the insertion of uncinate process. It is situated lateral to anterior attachment of middle turbinate, medial to lamina papyracea, anterior to anterior ethmoidal artery and posterior to agger nasi cells.
   - *Identification of roof of ethmoid:* Remove the remaining anterior ethmoidal cells and identify the middle turbinate basal lamella.
   - *Posterior ethmoidectomy (removal of posterior ethmoidal cells):* The thin basal lamella separates the anterior ethmoidal cells from the posterior ethmoid cells. It is penetrated in the lower and medial part and the diseased posterior ethmoid cells are removed.
   The presence of posterior ethmoid Onodi cells, which extends into sphenoid bone lateral and superior to sphenoid sinus, places the optic nerve at risk.
   - *Sphenoid sinusotomy:* Opening of the anterior wall of the diseased sphenoid sinus is done in last. The inspissated secretions and pus is aspirated. The sinus can be entered either by directly enlarging the opening of the sphenoid sinus or through the created anterior and inferior ethmoid cavity.
   - *Packing:* Small Merocel packing in middle meatus keeps the middle turbinate medial and prevents adhesions.
2. *Wigand technique:* It involves posterior to anterior approach and include following steps:
   - Partial resection of middle turbinate.
   - Opening of posterior ethmoidal cells.
   - Removal of anterior wall of sphenoid sinus.
   - Identification of skull base within sphenoid sinus.
   - Removal of anterior ethmoids.
- *Advanced techniques:*
   - *Powered instruments:* Powered instrument such as soft tissue shaver (microdebrider) helps in removing polyps and soft tissue masses. Bone cutting drills are used during the surgery of frontal sinus and lacrimal sac.
   - *Image-guided navigation:* The computer-aided ESS is of great assistance in revision surgeries and when operating near the optic nerve and base of skull. When anatomical landmarks are disturbed by the pathology. Anatomy can be distorted due to previous surgery, mucocele and extensive polyposis and intracranial and orbital extensions.

Postoperative Care

- *Watch for swelling:* Elevation of head and local ice to nose reduce swelling.
- *Monitoring* of visual and mental status.
- *Watch for subcutaneous emphysema:* Small fracture of lamina papyracea can cause subcutaneous emphysema, which can increase due to positive pressure ventilation, coughing, vomiting and blowing of nose.
- *Antibiotics:* Intraoperative as well as postoperative for 7–10 days.
- *Steroids:* Reduces mucosal edema and manage allergy.
- *Analgesics* relieve the pain.
- *Other agents:* Allergy management, antifungal agents, and leukotriene inhibitors; and irrigations are administrated as per the need of the case.
- *Removal of nasal packing:* It is removed at the time of discharge that is usually 24 hours after the surgery.
- *Topical saline and decongestants:* Saline nasal spray and a short course of nasal decongestant after the removal of nasal packing.
   - Nasal saline irrigations remove blood clots, crusts and secretions.
- *Removal of stenting:* Plan for the stent removal if that is used.

Section 8 • Operative Procedures and Instruments

Table 56.1: Minor and major complications of endoscopic sinus surgery

Minor	Major	
	Orbital	Intracranial
Minor bleeding	Lamina papyracea injury	CSF rhinorrhea, stroke
Hyposmia	Orbital hematoma	Fracture of skull base
Synechia	Extraocular muscle injury:	Intracranial bleeding
Headache	Diplopia	Meningitis, brain injury
Periorbital ecchymosis	Injury optic nerve: Blindness	Carotid injury, death
Periorbital emphysema	Decreased visual acuity	Pneumoencephalus
Dental pain	Nasolacrimal duct or sac injury	**Others:** Anosmia, bleeding
Facial pain		

- **Avoid strenuous activity and nose blowing** and medicines that increase risk of bleeding.
- **First postoperative visit:** It varies from patient to patient and is usually after 3–6 days. Some patients need frequent cleaning while others may need none. Debridement of old blood and crusts promotes healing and restores mucociliary function. Fixed clots and crusts are not removed as they cause damage to mucosa and bleeding. Middle turbinate should not get lateralized.

Complications (Table 56.1)

They are divided into two categories: Minor and major.

> The most common minor complication of FESS is the adhesions and major complications are bleeding, blindness and intracranial injury.

- **Subcutaneous emphysema:** See postoperative care.
- **Bleeding:** The common arteries injured are posterior septal artery below sphenoid sinus and arteries from the internal maxillary artery into middle turbinate. Injury to carotid artery needs immediate angiography for balloon occlusion.
- **Orbital hematoma:** Rapidly expanding orbital hematoma occurs due to the injury to anterior or posterior ethmoidal artery.
  - *Clinical features:* It leads to elevated intraorbital pressure and blindness.
  - *Treatment:* It needs immediate removal of the nasal pack, administration of steroids, control of bleeding (cautery or clipping), reduction of intraorbital pressure (orbital decompression or lateral canthotomy and cantholysis) and ophthalmologist consultation.
- **CSF leak:** The overlay and the underlay graft materials used in cases of CSF leak include nasal mucosa, fascia (temporalis), fat, muscle, acellular dermal graft, and bone or cartilage. Fibrin glue adds support and assists healing.

> *Anterior ethmoidal artery*: It is located at frontoethmoidal suture line. It lies 24 mm posterior to the anterior lacrimal crest.

ANTRAL PUNCTURE OR PROOF PUNCTURE

In antral puncture (AP), medial wall of maxillary sinus is punctured in the region of inferior meatus for antral irrigation (lavage).

Indications

- **Diagnostic:** For collecting the specimen of the antral contents for cytological (early malignancy) and identification of microorganisms (staining, culture and sensitivity).
  - Thin amber-colored fluid with cholesterol crystals indicates antral cyst.
  - Blobs of mucopus indicate hyperplastic sinusitis.
  - In cases of suppuration, foul smelling pus mixes with irrigating saline.
- **Therapeutic:** For washing out the pus in chronic and subacute maxillary sinusitis.

Contraindications

- **Acute maxillary sinusitis:** In this condition AP can lead to osteomyelitis.
- **Underdeveloped maxilla** with thick bony wall.
- **Fracture maxilla.**
- **Children** (<3 years).

Anesthesia and Position

- **Local anesthesia and sitting position in adults:** A pack of 4% lignocaine with adrenaline in inferior meatus is kept for 10–15 minutes. Middle meatus is decongested, which help in opening the maxillary ostium and easy return of fluid.
- **General anesthesia and tonsillectomy position:** They are used in children and anxious uncooperative adults.

Instruments

Lichtwitz trocar cannula and Hagginson's syringe (*see* Chapter 'Instruments') are used for proof puncture (antral lavage). It perforates the lateral wall of inferior meatus. This area is easily accessible and safe.

Technique

The medial wall of maxillary antrum is punctured through the lateral wall of inferior meatus with Lichtwitz trocar

Chapter 56 • Operations of Nose and Paranasal Sinuses

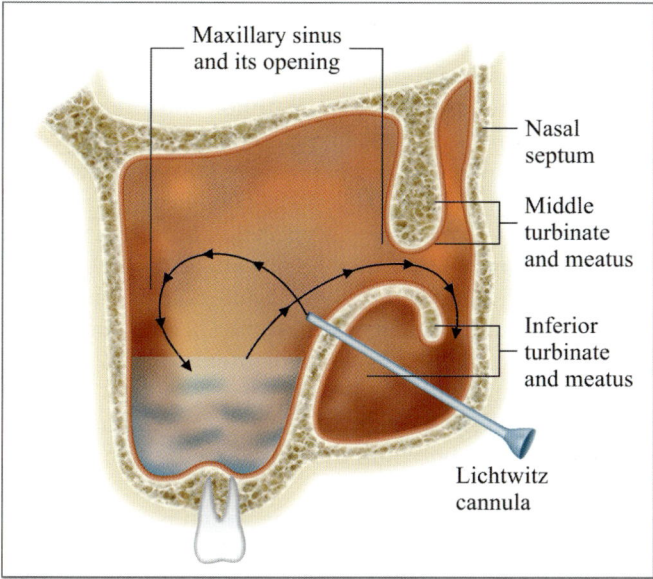

Fig. 56.2: Antrum puncture. The medial wall of maxillary antrum is punctured with Lichwitz trocar and cannula

and cannula (Fig. 56.2). A point 1.5–2.0 cm posterior to anterior end of inferior turbinate and near the attachment of concha in inferior meatus is selected for puncture because the bone is very thin here and is easily pierced. The direction of the trocar and cannula is towards the ear. After piercing the nasoantral wall, trocar is removed. The cannula is advanced gradually till it reaches the posterior antral wall and then is withdrawn a little. The antrum is then irrigated with 37°C 20 ml normal saline (Fig. 56.3A) or Hagginson's syringe (Fig. 53.3B) till the return is clear. The cannula is removed and a pack is kept in the inferior meatus if bleeding is present.

Complications

- *Swelling of cheek:* It can occur if cannula goes into soft tissues over the anterolateral wall of the maxilla. Puncture of the posterior antral wall will result in the swelling of posterior part of cheek.
- *Orbital injury and cellulitis:* They occur when trocar and cannula perforates the floor of orbit.
- *Bleeding:* It may be brisk in some cases.

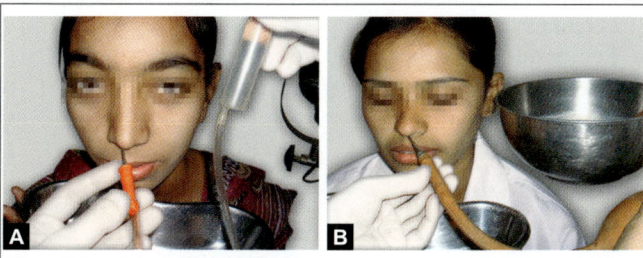

Figs 56.3A and B: (A) Proof puncture (antral lavage). Antrum is irrigated with 20 ml syringe; (B) Antrum irrigation with Hagginson's syringe

- *Air embolism:* Though rare it may prove fatal. Avoid air insufflation into the antrum after irrigation.

INFERIOR MEATAL ANTROSTOMY

In this procedure, an opening is made in the medial wall of maxillary antrum in the inferior meatus.

- *Indication:* Refractory cases of chronic purulent maxillary sinusitis.
- *Contraindications:* Polypoidal hypertrophy, osteitis and suspected malignancy.
- *Anesthesia and position:* It can be done under local or general anesthesia.
- *Technique:* After fracturing the inferior turbinate medially and superiorly with a large periosteal elevator, the lateral wall of inferior meatus is perforated with a curved hemostat. This perforation is further enlarged to 1.5–2 cm diameter close to the floor of nose with Kerrison's bone forceps, Luc's or side-biting ring forceps. The sinus content pus/debris is aspirated by suction. *See* Chapter 'Instruments'.
- *Complications:* They are occasional and include bleeding and injury to nasolacrimal duct. Packing into the sinus and nose is done in cases of severe bleeding.

CALDWELL-LUC OPERATION

Caldwell-Luc operation, which was described by George Caldwell in 1893 and Henry Luc in 1897, consists of two antrostomies: canine fossa (through sublabial approach) and inferior meatus (intranasally). It allows for both dependent drainage and irrigation. It has a long history in the treatment of paranasal sinus diseases.

This operation has held on its own for 100 years. Until the last quarter of the 20th century, this operation was the mainstay of treatment for chronic sinusitis. The postoperative factors coupled with advances in CT scan and endoscopes, culminated in the development of FESS. Though some infrequent indications still remain, FESS has now replaced the Caldwell-Luc operation as the treatment of choice in sinusitis.

Indications

The main indication is chronic maxillary sinusitis.
- Complications of acute maxillary sinusitis.
- Removal of foreign bodies or root of tooth.
- Dental cyst.
- Oroantral fistula.
- Biopsy in suspected cases of neoplasm.
- Recurrent antrochoanal polyp.
- Fracture of maxilla or blow out fractures of the orbit.
- Horgan's transantral ethmoidectomy.
- Pterygopalatine fossa surgery such as ligation of maxillary artery and vidian neurectomy.

- In combination with endoscopic approach—orbital decompression and removal of inverting papillomas.

Contraindication

It is contraindicated in children below 17 years of age.

Anesthesia

General anesthesia with cuffed endotracheal intubation is preferred but can even be done under local anesthesia.

Position

Patient is placed in supine position and face is turned slightly to the opposite side. Head end of the table is raised.

Instruments

See the Chapter on 'Instruments'.

Techniques (Figs 56.4A and B)

- *Preparation:* Nose is packed with cotton pledgets soaked in topical decongestant and 4% xylocaine. Local 1% or 2% lignocaine with epinephrine (1:100000) is infiltrated in gingivobuccal and gingivo labial sulcus.
- *Incision:* Lip retractor retracts the upper lip. Cheek retractor can also be used for making a horizontal incision with its ends upward in the gingivolabial sulcus below the canine fossa. The incision cuts through mucous membrane and periosteum. In children this incision is made above the level of secondary dentition, which can be seen in plain radiograph.
- *Mucoperisoteal flap:* Periosteum elevator is used for elevating the periosteum and soft tissues. The mucoperiosteal flap is raised superiorly up to the level infraorbital nerve, which should not be stretched and damaged.
- *Canine fossa antrostomy:* Using 4 mm osteotome and hammer or a drill, a window is made in the antrum through the canine fossa. Killian's nasal gouge (bayonet-shaped) can be used for opening the maxillary antrum.

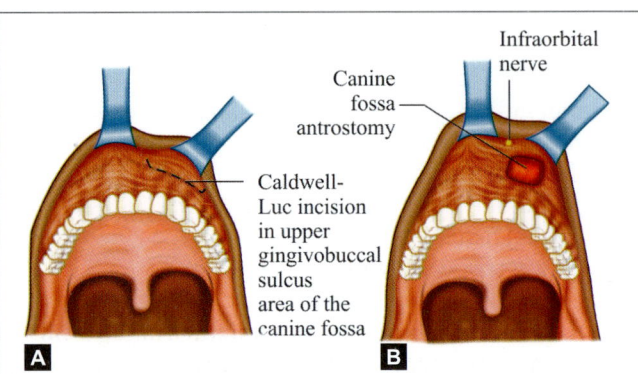

Figs 56.4A and B: Caldwell-Luc operation. (A) Incision; (B) Canine fossa antrostomy

The window is enlarged as necessary using Kerrison's punch or Citelli sphenoid punch.

- *Removal of disease:* The maxillary sinus pathology and diseased mucosa (cyst, benign tumor, and foreign body) can be removed with elevators, curettes and forceps. Luc's forceps can be used to remove polyps, growth and bone pieces.
- *Intranasal antrostomy:* A curved hemostat is pushed into the antrum below the inferior turbinate at least 1 cm behind the anterior end of middle turbinate (to avoid damage to nasolacrimal duct). This opening is widened to about 1.5 cm in diameter with Kerrison's and side biting forceps.
- *Endoscopic examination:* The maxillary sinus can be examined through both the antrostomies with the help of endoscopes.
- *Packing:* Ribbon gauze packing which is impregnated with liquid paraffin or Furacin (0.2% w/w nitrofurazone) ointment is prepared. One end of the packing is brought out from the nasoantral window into the nose and the rest is packed in maxillary antrum. Packing is also done in the nose. Dressing forceps (Tilley's, Wilde's or Hartmann's) is used for packing. The packing takes care of bleeding.
- *Closure:* Sublabial incision is closed with absorbable suture.

Postoperative Care

- *Local ice packs:* They prevent edema, hematoma and discomfort.
- *Pack removal:* Sinus and nose packing is usually removed in 24–48 hours.
- *Antibiotic:* Postoperative antibiotic is given for 1 week.
- *Instruction to patient:* Avoid blowing of nose for 2 weeks because it can cause surgical emphysema.

Complications

- Bleeding is controlled with packing.
- Anesthesia of the cheek may last for few weeks or months and occurs due to stretching or injury to infraorbital nerve. Gentle sublabial retraction prevents this complication.
- Anesthesia of teeth (devitalized teeth).
- Facial asymmetry.
- Recurrent sinusitis and polyposis.
- Dacryocystitis due to injury to nasolacrimal duct.
- Sublabial oroantral fistula.
- Osteomyelitis of maxilla.

SURGERY OF NASAL SEPTUM

If needed the trimming of enlarged turbinates, nasal valves repair and correction of external nose deformity are done together with the correction of deviated nasal septum

(DNS). The two surgeries commonly performed on nasal septum are submucosal resection (SMR) and septoplasty. Both the operations are done now with sinuscope. The indications, contraindications, anesthesia, position and postoperative care and complications are more or less similar. The main difference is in the technique of operation.

Indications

- *DNS* causing nasal obstruction, recurrent headaches, rhinosinusitis, obstructive sleep apnea and otitis media.
- *Recurrent epistaxis* from spur and convex side of DNS.
- *Septorhinoplasty* for external nasal deformities.
- *Hypophysectomy:* Trans-septal trans-sphenoidal approach.
- *Vidian neurectomy:* Trans-septal approach.
- *Septal cartilage graft:* It is obtained for rhinoplasty and repair of CSF leak.
- *Endoscopic sinus surgery:* If DNS is obstructing access to middle meatus, frontal recess and nasolacrimal sac.

Contraindications

- *Children:* A conservative surgery (septoplasty) should be considered in children.
- *Acute URI*
- *Medical:* Bleeding diathesis and uncontrolled diabetes and hypertension.

Anesthesia

- *Local anesthesia with sedation:* It is preferred in adults. Topical and local xylocaine with epinephrine provides both analgesia and decongestion. Infiltration of nasal septum with 1% xylocaine and 1:100,000 epinephrine in subperichondrial and subperiosteal planes is done with 27-guage needle. The injection begins at caudal end of septum and then goes posteriorly and includes both sides of septum and floor around maxillary crest.
  - In cardiac patients, oxymetazoline is preferred over epinephrine. Maximum dose of xylocaine is 4–7 mg/kg.
- *General anesthesia with endotracheal intubation* is used for children and too much anxious adults.
- *Position:* Patient is placed in reclining position and head end of the table is raised.

Techniques

Septoplasty is replacing SMR. ESS provides better visualization and facilitates mucoperichondrial elevation. The CO_2 laser can be used in some cases of septal spurs.

SUBMUCOUS RESECTION OF NASAL SEPTUM (SMR)

- *Incision:* A curvilinear incision cutting only mucoperichondrium is made above the caudal end of septal cartilage at the mucocutaneous junction. The incision can be made on any one side of the nose depending upon the surgeons' preference.
- *Mucoperichondrial and periosteal flap:* It is elevated in the plane beneath the perichondrium and periosteum. Long bladed nasal speculums (Killian's or St Clair Thomson's) keep mucoperiosteal flaps away.
- *Incision of the cartilage:* Cartilage is incised posterior to the first incision without cutting the opposite side of mucoperichondrium. An elevator is passed through the cartilage incision and mucoperichondrial and periosteal flap is raised from the opposite side of nasal septum. Freer's double ended elevator can be used for the elevation of flaps.
- *Removal of cartilage and bone:* The cartilage and bone that lie between the two flaps are removed with the help of Ballenger swivel knife and Luc's forceps. Bony spur, ridge and maxillary crest are removed with the help of gouge (4 mm unguarded osteotome or Killian's bayonet-shaped nasal gouge) and hammer or double action bone nibbling forceps. Preservation of 1 cm strip of cartilage along the dorsal and caudal border of the septum (L-strut) prevents collapse of the dorsum of nose and retraction of columella (Fig. 56.5).
- *Closing:* After achieving hemostasis, one or two stitches may be applied in mucoperichondrial incision.
- *Packing:* Ribbon gauze, which is smeared with furacin ointment or liquid paraffin, is packed in each side of nose. Dressing forceps (Tilley's, Wilde's or Hartmann's) is used for nasal packing. It prevents collection of blood between the flaps.

SEPTOPLASTY

Septoplasty is a conservative septal surgery and retains maximum possible septal framework. Mucoperichondrial and mucoperiosteal flap is raised only on concave side.

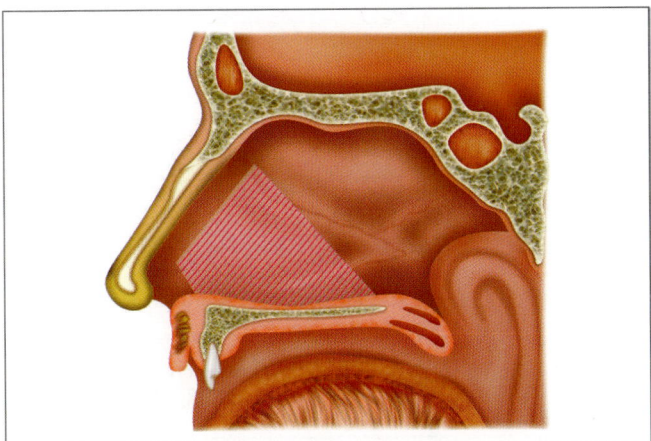

Fig. 56.5: Submucosal resection (SMR) of large central septal segment preserving L-strut (1 cm dorsal and 1 cm caudal septal segment)

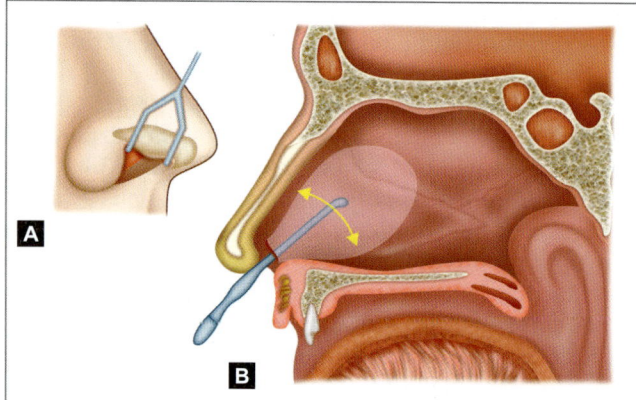

Figs 56.6A and B: Septoplasty. (A) Incision (Killian and hemitransfixion); (B) Plane of dissection (Cottle elevator creating subperichondrial pocket)

- **Incision**: A 2–3 mm curvilinear incision is made above the caudal end of septal cartilage on the concave side (Fig. 56.6). A transfixion or hemitransfixion incision is employed in cases of caudal dislocation.
- **Flaps and tunnels:** Mucoperichondrial flap is raised only on the concave side and superior tunnel is created. Mucoperiosteal flap is elevated on both the sides of maxillary crest and two inferior tunnels are created. The superior and inferior tunnels on concave side are joined after cutting the fibrous tissue with sharp knife.
- **Septal cartilage:** It is separated from the vomer and ethmoid plate (Fig. 56.7).
- **Maxillary crest:** If needed, it is fractured to realign the septal cartilage.
- **Bony septum:** It is corrected by removing deformed parts.

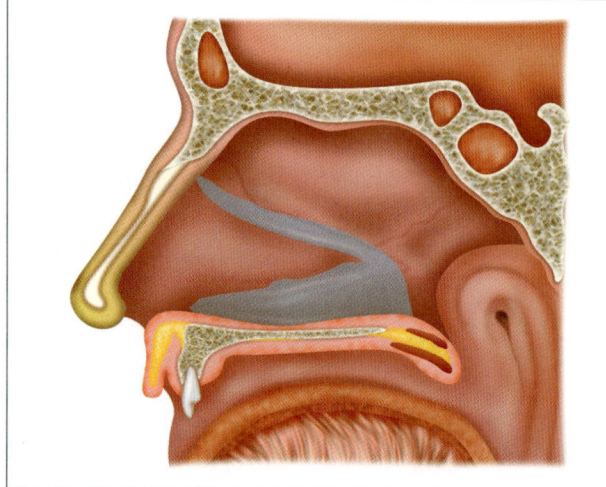

Fig. 56.7: Septoplasty. Separation of septum from the perpendicular plate of ethmoid and trimming of the inferior cartilaginous portion displaced from the maxillary crest

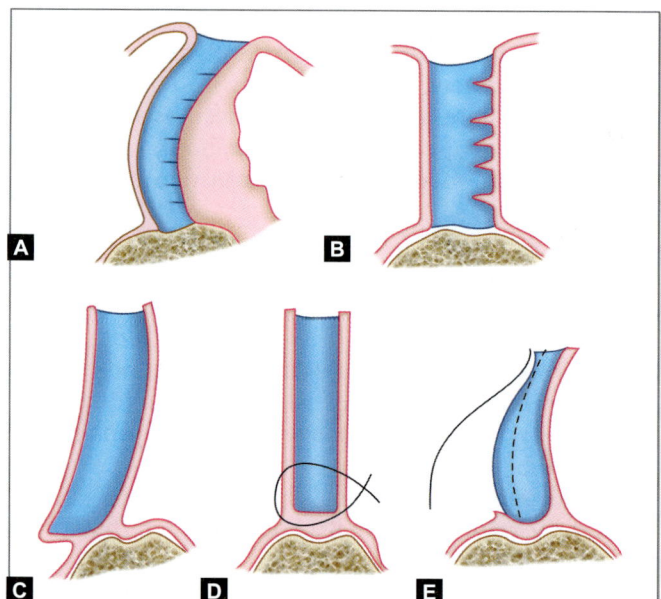

Figs 56.8A to E: Septoplasty techniques. (A and B) Scoring of the cartilage on concave side removes the interlocked cartilage stresses; (C and D) Excising the dislocated lower end of septal cartilage and replacing on the anterior nasal spine or in the groove of nasal crest of maxilla; (E) Shaving the convexity of septal cartilage

- **Deformed septal cartilage:** It can be corrected by scoring, cross hatching, morcelizing, shaving or wedge excision (Fig. 56.8).
- **Other options:**
  - **Septorhinoplasty:** Some cases need separation of septal cartilage from upper lateral cartilages, implantation of cartilage either in the columella or dorsum of nose.
  - **Endoscopic sinus surgery:** Sinuscope provides better visualization and facilitates 'flaps' elevation.
  - **Laser surgery:** The CO_2 laser can be used in selective septal spurs and 2–3 mm height mucoperichondrium and cartilaginous spur are completely excised. The opposite side mucoperichondrium is left intact.
- **Closure:** Trans-septal sutures keep the mucoperichondrial flaps together and prevent hematoma. Nose is packed.

POSTOPERATIVE CARE

- **Position:** Patient is kept in semi-sitting position that prevents oozing of blood and swelling.
- **Diet:** A soft diet in the first two days minimizes active mastication and prevent bleeding.
- **Analgesics** control pain.
- **Antibiotic** for 5–7 days.
- **Nasal packs:** They are removed usually after 24 hours. Subsequently regular regimen of saline water flushing, gentle suctioning and application of antibiotic ointment is started.

- **Decongestant** nasal drops and steam inhalations for 5 days.
- **Sutures** are removed on 5th or 6th day.
- **Instructions:** Patient is instructed to avoid strenuous exercise, trauma to the nose, blowing and frequent picking of nose for about 3 weeks.

COMPLICATIONS

In addition to the complications of anesthesia following complications can occur after septal surgery:
- **Hemorrhage:** Repacking of nose is required in severe reactionary bleeding. The other two types of hemorrhage include primary (during surgery) and secondary (5–7 days after surgery due to infection).
- **Septal hematoma:** It needs immediate evacuation followed by intranasal packing on both sides of septum with equal pressure.
- **Septal abscess:** It occurs due to infection of septal hematoma. It needs immediate incision and drainage.
- **Perforation:** It occurs when both sides of septal mucosa are perforated at the same level.
- **Saddle nose deformity and tip ptosis:** They occur when too much of septal cartilage is removed along the dorsal border.
- **Columella retraction:** It can occur when caudal strip of nasal cartilage is removed.
- **Failure:** Persistence of deviation is usually the result of inadequate surgery, which needs revision operation.
- **Flapping of nasal septum:** In this condition two mucoperichondrial flaps move with respiration to the right or left. It happens when too much septal framework is removed.
- **CSF leak:** Never manipulate perpendicular plate of ethmoid before incising it as it can damage cribriform plate and cause CSF leak.
- **Toxic shock syndrome:** This staphylococcal (sometimes streptococcal) infection is characterized by nausea, vomiting, purulent secretions, hypotension and rash.
    - **Treatment:** It consists of removal of packing (which may be the cause), proper hydration of patient, maintenance of blood pressure and administration of proper antibiotics.
- **Synechia:** Injuries to mucosal fold and turbinates at the same level can lead to formation of adhesions. Asymptomatic synechia do not need any treatment. They need excision if they cause nasal obstruction. The two raw surfaces are kept apart for 2 weeks with polyethylene or silastic sheet.

Self-evaluation Exercises

True (T)/False (F)
1. The anterior ethmoidal artery is located at frontoethmoidal suture line.
2. The anterior ethmoidal artery lies 12 mm posterior to the anterior lacrimal crest.
3. Most common predisposing factor linked to maxillary sinusitis is mucosal swelling in ethmoid infundibulum.
4. In Caldwell-Luc operation, entry into the maxillary sinus is made through the canine fossa (canine fossa antrostomy).
5. The complete removal of septal cartilage in the operation of submucosal resection of septum results in hump of cartilaginous nasal dorsum.

Answers
1. T 2. F 3. T 4. T 5. F

Chapter 57

Adenotonsillectomy

> ### ⊚ Specific Learning Objectives
> After going through the chapter, you should be able to answer the following questions:
> - What are the indications and contraindications of adenotonsillectomy?
> - Which are the different surgical techniques for adenotonsillectomy?
> - What is the difference between tonsillectomy and tonsillotomy?
> - What are the different operative steps of adenotonsillectomy and how will you take postoperative care?
> - What are the complications of adenotonsillectomy?
> - How will you manage postoperative bleeding and velopharyngeal insufficiency?

In addition to proper history and detailed clinical examination, following points need special consideraton to prevent operative and postoperative complications of adenotonsillectomy.

A unilateral tonsil enlargement in children can be due to lymphoma while in adults epidermoid carcinoma may be the cause. An excisional biopsy is indicated in these conditions.

INDICATIONS FOR TONSILLECTOMY

Recurrent infections and upper airway obstruction are the most common indications for tonsillectomy.

Absolute
- Chronic or recurrent tonsillitis:
  - More than six episodes in 1 year, or
  - Five episodes per year for 2 years, or
  - Three episodes per year for 3 years, or
  - Two weeks or more of lost school or work in a year.
- Peritonsillar abscess: In children after 4–6 weeks of abscess; in adults after second attack.
- Tonsillitis causing febrile convulsions.
- Cardiac valvular disease associated with recurrent streptococcal tonsillitis.
- Hypertrophy of tonsils causing:
  - Excessive snoring or sleep disturbances
  - Obstructive sleep apnea
  - Cor pulmonale
  - Dysphagia
  - Interfere with speech.
- Suspicion of malignancy-asymmetric tonsillar hypertrophy.

Relative
- Diphtheria carriers, who are not responding to antibiotics.
- Streptococcal carriers, who are infecting others.
- Chronic tonsillitis with bad taste or halitosis.
- Recurrent sore throats or upper respiratory infections (URI).
- Recurrent streptococcal tonsillitis in a patient with valvular heart disease.
- Tender cervical adenitis.
- Difficulty in eating.
- Tonsillolithiasis.
- Orofacial and dental abnormalities.
- Failure to thrive.
- Enuresis.
- Obstructive tonsils in infectious mononucleosis not responding to medical therapy.

Part of other Operations
- Palatopharyngoplasty for obstructive sleep apnea (OSA) syndrome.
- Glossopharyngeal neurectomy. CN IX is severed in the bed of tonsil.
- Removal of styloid process.

INDICATIONS FOR ADENOIDECTOMY

Adenoidectomy may be done alone or in combination with tonsillectomy. Adenoids are usually removed first and the nasopharynx is packed. Adenoidectomy prevents recurrence of dental abnormalities after orthodontic treatment.

- Adenoid hypertrophy causing
  - Excessive snoring
  - Mouth breathing
  - OSA syndrome or sleep disturbances
  - Cor pulmonale
  - Failure to thrive
  - Enuresis
  - Dysphagia
  - Speech abnormalities such as rhinolalia clausa
  - Craniofacial growth abnormalities
- Purulent adenoiditis
- Recurrent rhinosinusitis
- Middle ear infections
  - Chronic secretory otitis media
  - Recurrent acute otitis media
  - CSOM (safe type) with recurrent ear discharge
- Dental malocclusion

The common indications of adenoidectomy include nasal obstruction due to adenoidal hyperplasia, recurrent acute otitis media and otitis media with effusion in children.

CONTRAINDICATIONS

- Anemia: Hemoglobin less than 10 g%.
- Acute upper respiratory tract infection or acute tonsillitis. Children with acute URI (cough, cold, and fever) should wait for 3 weeks and get treatment.
- Overt or submucous cleft palate: Conservative adenoidectomy can be considered. Leaving the lower portion of adenoidal pad intact prevents velopharyngeal insufficiency.
- Bleeding disorders such as leukemia, purpura, aplastic anemia, hemophilia.
- Epidemic of polio.
- Uncontrolled systemic disease such as diabetes, cardiac disease, hypertension and asthma.
- During the period of menses in females.

Children under 3 years are at more surgical risks.

SURGICAL TECHNIQUES

- ***Guillotine method:*** It may be employed in mobile tonsil without any fibrosis. Fibrosis of the tonsillar bed occurs due to repeated infections. This technique has been abandoned.
- ***Dissection and snare method (with sharp instrumentation):*** More operative bleeding but less postoperative pain.
- ***Electrocautery (Bovie and bipolar):*** Less operative bleeding but more postoperative pain.
- ***Laser:*** CO_2 or KTP laser surgery.
- ***Cryosurgery:*** Tonsil is frozen with two applications of cryoprobe for 3–4 minutes each time and then allowed to thaw. Tonsils undergo necrosis and then fall off and leave a granulating surface. Bleeding is less because of the thrombosis of vessels.

NEWER TECHNOLOGIES

- ***Harmonic scalpel:*** Ultrasonic technology cuts and coagulates tissues. Tonsillectomies have been done but cannot be used for adenoidectomy. Each blade used for operation increases the cost.
- ***Coblation:*** This technology utilizes the radio-frequency bipolar electrical current. It claims effective dissection with less postoperative pain from thermal injury. It has been used for completion tonsillectomy, adenoidectomy (for small adenoid pads and not for large obstructive adenoids) and intracapsular tonsillectomy. Tonsillotomy leaves behind small amount of tonsil tissue covering the constrictor muscle.
- ***Powered instrumentation:*** Microdebrider shaver allows precise, rapid and safe removal of tissue. It can be used for adenoidectomy (endoscopic nasal surgery) and tonsillotomy (intracapsular tonsillectomy).

PREOPERATIVE MEASURES

- No solid food by mouth for 8 hours; clear liquids may be allowed for 3 hours before surgery.
- Sedation with midazolam hydrochloride (0.5–1 mg/kg) 30 minutes before surgery.
- Intravenous antibiotic such as ampicillin 20 mg/kg up to 1 g.
- Intraoperative dexamethasone (0.5 mg/kg) especially in OSA and children younger than 3 years.

ANESTHESIA

The operation is usually done under general anesthesia with endotracheal intubation. In cooperative adults, it may be done under local anesthesia.

Section 8 • Operative Procedures and Instruments

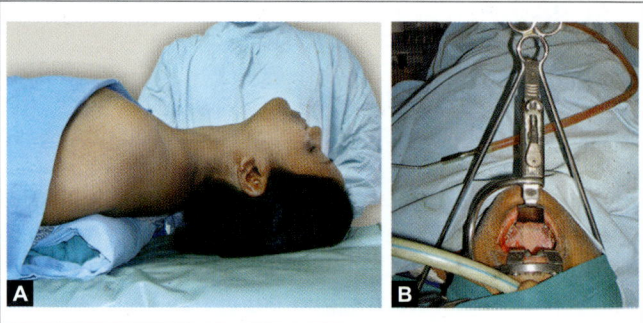

Figs 57.1A and B: Adenotonsillectomy. (A) Rose position. The patient lies supine. The head is extended by putting a sandbag beneath the shoulders; (B) Boyle-Davis gag in position

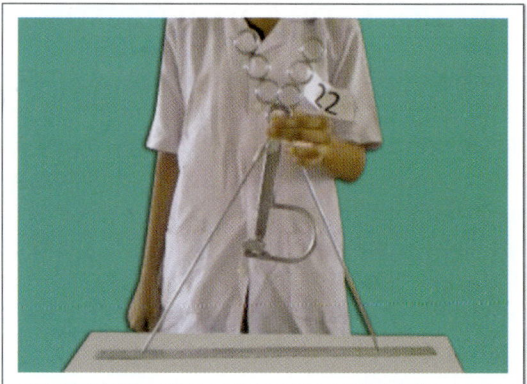

Fig. 57.2: Displaying the positions of Boyle-Davis mouth gag, Draffins bipods and Magauran plate

POSITION

Rose's position (Fig. 57.1A): Supine position with extended head (place a pillow under the shoulders). A rubber ring under the head stabilizes head and prevents its hyperextension.

SURGICAL INSTRUMENTS

See the Chapter 'Instruments'.

OPERATIVE STEPS

When both the tonsils and adenoids are removed in one sitting, adenoids are removed first. Depending upon the indication, either tonsils or adenoids may be removed alone.

Adenoidectomy

- *Opening of mouth:* Boyle-Davis mouth gag is used for opening the mouth and retracting the tongue anteriorly and inferiorly (Figs 57.1B and 57.2). The built in tongue depressor along with the closed mouth gag is inserted in the mouth after depressing the lower jaw. The mouth gag is opened gradually. It is suspended from Draffin's bipods that extends the neck and head. The two pods are assembled together as per the height at which the tongue blade of the Boyle-Davis mouth gag is suspended. The lower ends of the pods are placed in one of the several depressions of the Magauran's plate.
- *Laryngopharyngeal packing:* Put a throat pack, which prevents blood and secretions entering esophagus and aspiration of laryngeal clot and leakage of air, oxygen and anesthetic agent.
- *Examination:* Nasopharynx and adenoids are examined after retracting the soft palate with curved end of the tongue depressor. Tonsil dissector and anterior pillar retractor can also be used for retracting the soft palate and uvula.
- *Digital palpation:* It helps in the following:
  - Assesses adenoids size.
  - Pushes the lateral adenoid masses towards the midline.
  - Assesses evidence of submucous cleft palate and abnormal vessels.
- *Adenoid curette:* St. Clair Thomson's curette with guard shaves off the adenoid mass and holds it and prevents from slipping. Introduce a proper size of adenoid curette with guard into nasopharynx and feel the posterior border of nasal septum. Press the adenoid curette backward and engage the adenoids. The LaForce adenotome may also be used instead of adenoid curette. Shave the adenoids with gentle sweeping movement of adenoid curette.
  - *Caution:* Flexion of head at this stage will avoid injury to the odontoid process.
    - Remove the lateral adenoid masses with smaller curettes.
    - Remove the remaining small tags of adenoids with punch forceps, smaller plain adenoid curette, Luc's forceps or conchotome.
- *Hemostasis:* Achieve the hemostasis with packing. Persistent bleeders may be cauterized under direct vision. Very occasionally, postnasal pack is required for refractory cases of bleeding.

Adenoidectomy: It should be modified or avoided in cases of submucous cleft palate.

Tonsillectomy (Dissection and Snare Method)

- *Opening of mouth:* Boyle-Davis mouth gag is introduced and held in position with Draffin's bipods.
- *Laryngopharyngeal packing:* See 'Adenoidectomy' Section.
- *Tonsil holding:* Tonsil is grasped and pulled medially with tonsil holding forceps (Allis clamp, tenaculum, or

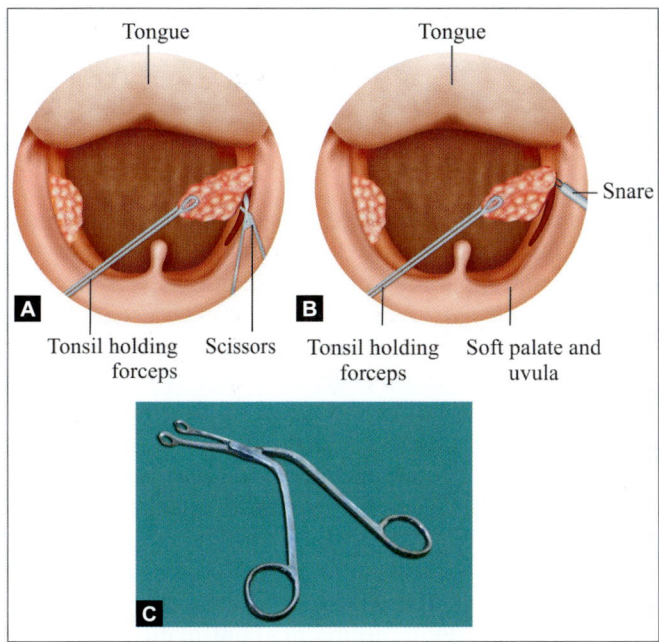

Figs 57.3A and B: Tonsillectomy. (A) A blunt curved scissor is dissecting tonsil from the peritonsillar tissue while tonsil is grasped with tonsil holding forceps and pulled medially; (B) Wire loop of tonsillar snare threaded over the tonsil onto its pedicle and cut; (C) Tonsil holding forceps

Denis Browne) (Fig. 57.3). Luc's forceps may also be used for this purpose.
- **Incision:** The mucous membrane where it reflects from the tonsil to anterior pillar is incised either with sharp instrument or electrocautery. Tonsil dissection forceps with teeth (Waugh's) can also be used for putting incision in the mucous membrane and dissection of tonsil. The incision is extended along the upper pole between the tonsil and posterior pillar. Electrocautery must not touch metal instruments such as mouth gag and Yankauer suction. Yankauer's suction tube is used for suction.
- **Dissection:** With the help of a blunt curved scissor or tonsil dissector (Thompson dissector or a Fischer knife), separate the tonsil capsule from the bed of tonsil. Begin the dissection from the upper pole. Tonsil dissector and anterior pillar retractor dissect the tonsil and retract the anterior pillar to inspect the fossa for any bleeding. Retraction of the upper pole medially and towards tongue facilitates the dissection. It is continued until lower pole is reached. Tonsil scissors can also be used for sharp dissection of the tonsils and cutting the ligatures.
    - **Caution:** Preserve the mucosa and muscle of the posterior pillar to prevent postoperative nasopharyngeal stenosis.
- **Snare:** Eve's tonsillar snare is threaded over the lower pole tonsil pedicle, which is amputated with snare and tonsil removed. When firmly closed, the snare crushes and cuts the pedicle and minimizes the bleeding.
- **Packing:** A gauze sponge placed in tonsillar fossa for few minutes obtains pressure hemostasis.
- **Other side:** Procedure is repeated on the other side.
- **Removal of packs:** Remove the packs from tonsillar fossa and nasopharynx.
- **Hemostasis:** Bleeding is usually controlled using electrocautery on a low wattage. Large bleeders may be clamped and ligated with the help of tonsillar artery forceps. Straight and curved tonsil artery forceps (such as Negus artery forceps) are used to catch the bleeding point and ligating the bleeder. Negus Knot tyer helps in tying the ligature knot up to the tip of curved artery forceps that holds the vessel. Tonsil needle is used for sewing the tonsillar pillars together for controlling the bleeding, when it is not controlled by ligation and cauterization of bleeding points. In these cases if gauze is kept in the tonsillar fossa that must be removed within 48 hours.
    - **Caution:** Suture ligatures with needle may inadvertently ligate external maxillary and lingual arteries or damage internal carotid artery.
- **Irrigation and cleaning:** Irrigate nasopharynx, oropharynx, oral and nasal cavity thoroughly and evacuate secretions and blood clots from laryngopharynx. Stomach may also be suctioned.

POSTOPERATIVE CARE

- **Immediate general care:** This includes:
    - **Position:** Patient is kept in tonsillar position till full recovery from anesthesia.
    - **Monitor vital signs** such as pulse, respiration and blood pressure.
    - **Watch for bleeding** from the nose and mouth, vomiting, swelling (surgical emphysema), pain, and respiratory distress.
    - **OSA and cor pulmonale:** In these cases pulse oximetry and planned mechanical ventilation is important for persistent hypercapnia until Pco_2 levels return to normal.
- **Diet:** Plenty of cold fluids such as cold milk or ice cream. Sucking of ice cubes helps in relieving pain. The child may take soft diet on the second day such as custard, jelly, boiled eggs, porridge or slice of bread soaked in milk. Solid foods subsequently are allowed as tolerated.
- **Oral hygiene:** Saline gargles 3–4 times a day. Mouth should be washed with plain water after every feed.
- **Analgesics:** Paracetamol with or without codeine.
- **Antibiotics:** For a week.
- **Instruction on discharge:** Patient is instructed to report immediately if there is any bright red colored bleeding from nose or mouth.

Post-tonsillectomy earache: This referred otalgia occurs through the glossopharyngeal nerve.

Atlantoaxial dislocation: It can occur in children during adenotonsillectomy and esophagoscopy and due to nasopharyngeal infection.

COMPLICATIONS

The complications are mainly related to pain, bleeding (0.3% to 5%), respiratory obstruction and pulmonary edema and may even result in death. Complications are divided here into three groups: immediate, delayed and rare.

Immediate

- *Primary hemorrhage:* Bleeding during the operation is usually controlled by pressure, ligation or electrocoagulation. Certain analgesic such as ketorolac should be avoided. Application of tannic acid, bismuth subgallate or hemostatic agents may be helpful. Coagulopathy must be ruled out. Residual remnants of adenoid tissue should be completely removed.
- *Reactionary hemorrhage:* Bleeding after the recovery from anesthesia on the day of surgery is usually controlled by removing the clot, applying pressure or vasoconstrictor. Clot may prevent the clipping action of the superior constrictor muscle on the vessels. Immediate postoperative bleeding from nose and mouth or vomiting of dark colored blood and rising pulse rate indicate bleeding from the operative site. Topical decongestant nasal drops may help in controlling nasopharyngeal bleeding. In cases of refractory bleeding, patient is taken back to operation room and ligation or electrocoagulation of the bleeding vessels is done under general anesthesia. Postnasal pack may be needed in children with adenoidectomy.
- *Injury:* Oral cavity and oropharyngeal structures such as tonsillar pillars, uvula, soft palate, tongue, superior constrictor muscle and teeth can be injured during tonsillectomy. Eustachian tube, pharyngeal musculature and vertebrae injuries during adenoidectomy can be prevented by avoiding hyperextension of neck and undue pressure of curette.
- *Aspiration and foreign bodies:* Such as blood, tissue of tonsil or adenoids and tooth.
- *Pulmonary edema:* It can occur in cases of OSA and cor pulmonale.
- *Edema of tongue, nasopharynx and palate:* Need replacement of nasal trumpet and intravenous steroids.
- *Edema:* Face or eyelids.
- *Surgical emphysema:* Due to superior constrictor muscle injury.

Delayed

- *Secondary hemorrhage:* Bleeding seen between 5th–10th postoperative days is the result of sepsis and premature separation of the membrane.
  - *Clinical features:* The common presentation is blood-stained sputum but bleeding may be profuse.
  - *Management:* If bleeding is not controlled after removal of clot and topical application of dilute adrenaline, hydrogen peroxide and with pressure, then patient is taken to operation room. Under general anesthesia, bleeding vessel is electrocoagulated or ligated. Approximation of pillars with mattress sutures or external carotid ligation may be required in rare cases. Transfusion of blood or plasma may be needed. Systemic antibiotics control the infection.
- *Infection:* It may cause parapharyngeal abscess and otitis media.
- *Pulmonary complications:* Aspiration of blood, mucus or tissue fragments may lead to atelectasis or lung abscess.
- *Scarring:* Soft palate and pillars.
- *Tonsillar remnants:* The remaining tonsil tags or tissue may cause repeated infection.
- *Hypertrophy of lingual tonsil:* It is compensatory to the loss of palatine tonsils.
- *Velopharyngeal insufficiency:* Hypernasality is a complication of adenoidectomy. It is usually managed by speech pathologist. But refractory cases may need reconstructive surgery (pharyngeal flap, sphincteroplasty or posterior pharyngeal wall augmentation).
- *Nasopharyngeal stenosis:* It occurs due to scarring after excessive damage to nasopharyngeal mucosa (roof, posterior and lateral walls) and resection of posterior tonsillar pillar. These children are difficult to manage.
- *Recurrence:* Remaining adenoids and tonsil tissue may grow again. If plica triangularis near the lower pole of tonsil is not removed along with tonsil, it may get hypertrophied.
- *Atlantoaxial subluxation (Grisel's syndrome):* It leads to stiff neck and spasm of sternocleidomastoid and deep cervical muscles. Treatment includes intravenous antibiotics and cervical traction.

Self-evaluation Exercises

1. The common indications of adenoidectomy in children include:
    a. Nasal obstruction due to adenoidal hyperplasia
    b. Recurrent otitis media
    c. Otitis media with effusion
    d. All of the above
2. Atlantoaxial dislocation can occur in children due to:
    a. Adenotonsillectomy
    b. Nasopharyngeal infection
    c. Esophagoscopy
    d. All of the above

True (T)/False (F)

3. Children for tonsillectomy coming with acute upper respiratory infections should wait for 3 weeks and get treatment for URI.

Filling the blanks

4. Post-tonsillectomy referred earache occurs through the _____ nerve.

Answers

1. d   2. d   3. T   4. glossopharyngeal

Chapter 58

Endoscopies

> ### Specific Learning Objectives
> After going through the chapter, you should be able to answer the following questions:
> - What are the indications and contraindications of direct laryngoscopy and microlaryngoscopy?
> - What are the advantages and disadvantages of flexible laryngoscopy and direct laryngoscopy?
> - What are the differences between flexible and rigid bronchoscopy and esophagoscopy?
> - What are the indications and contraindications of bronchoscopy?
> - What are the indications and contraindications of esophagoscopy?
> - What are the complications of laryngoscopy, bronchoscopy and esophagoscopy?

DIRECT LARYNGOSCOPY/ MICROLARYNGOSCOPY

Laryngoscope used for direct laryngoscopy (DLS) may have either single or twin light carrier which is connected to a cold light source through a flexible cable. The size of laryngoscope is selected as per the age of the patient. The oropharynx, hypopharynx and larynx are visualized directly with the help of laryngoscope.

- Laryngoscope of microlaryngoscopy (MLS) is self-retaining laryngoscope. It can be fixed on the chest by a chest piece so that hands of the surgeon remain free for the surgery. MLS is performed under the magnification of an operating microscope (Fig. 58.1). Microlaryngeal surgery needs special laryngoscopes, forceps, and scissors. (Figs 58.2A to G). Other types of laryngoscopy have been described in Chapter 'Laryngeal Symptoms and Examination'.

INDICATIONS

Direct laryngoscopy/microlaryngoscopy can be performed for both diagnostic as well as therapeutic purposes.
- **Diagnostic**
  - *Infants and young children*.
  - *Difficult anatomy and patient:* Strong gag reflex and overhanging epiglottis.
  - *Symptoms:* Hoarseness, dyspnea, stridor and dysphagia.

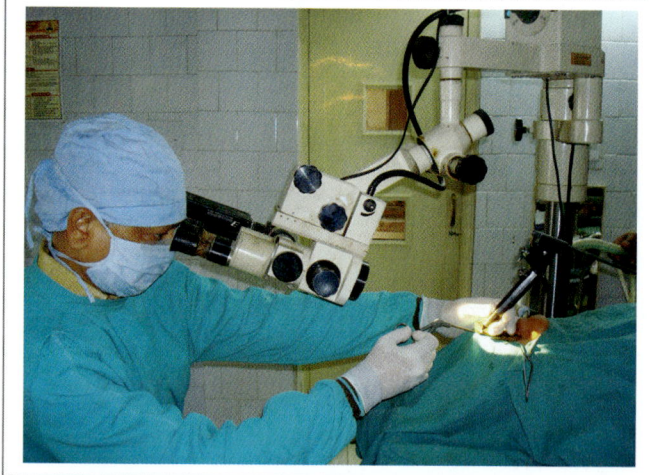

Fig. 58.1: Microlaryngoscopy procedure

  - ***Examination of hidden areas:*** Following areas cannot be adequately seen during mirror laryngoscopy:
    - *Oropharynx:* Base of tongue and valleculae.
    - *Hypopharynx:* Lower part of pyriform fossa.
    - *Larynx:* Infrahyoid epiglottis, anterior commissure, ventricles and subglottic region.
  - ***Biopsy:*** Tumors of base of tongue, vallecula, laryngopharynx and larynx.
- **Therapeutic**
  - ***Benign swellings:*** Removal of papilloma, fibroma, vocal nodule, polyp and cyst.

Chapter 58 • Endoscopies

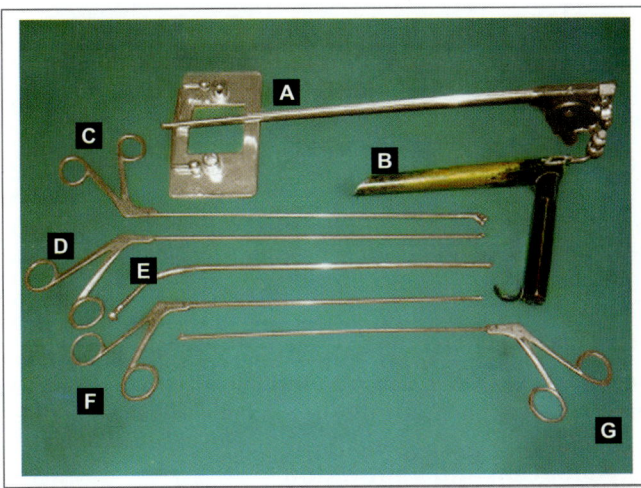

Figs 58.2A to G: Microlaryngoscopy instruments. (A) Laryngoscope holder and chest support; (B) Anterior commissure operating laryngoscope; (C) Laryngeal forceps, upward-angled large size cupped jaws; (D) Laryngeal forceps, side-angled medium size cupped jaws; (E) Suction tube; (F) Laryngeal forceps, upward-angled fine cupped jaws; and (G) Laryngeal forceps, up-cutting angled scissor

- *Malignant lesions:* Early carcinoma of larynx and laryngopharynx.
- *Foreign bodies:* Oropharynx, hypopharynx and larynx.
- *Strictures:* Dilatation of laryngeal strictures.

CONTRAINDICATIONS

- Lesions of cervical spines.
- Stridor (usually need prior tracheostomy).
- Recent coronary occlusion.
- Cardiac decompensation.

ANESTHESIA

- Usually done under general anesthesia.
- Infants and young children do not need any anesthesia for diagnostic DLS.

POSITION

Patient lies in supine position. Head is elevated 10–15 cm by placing a pillow under the occipital region or by raising head flap of operation table. Neck is flexed and the head is extended (barking dog position).

Objective piece of operative microscope: 400 mm focal length of objective piece of operative microscope is used for microlaryngoscopy.

PROCEDURES

- *Protection of teeth and lips:* Examine the patient for neck stability, loose teeth and dentures. Eyes are protected with a shield and the patient is draped. A gauze piece protects the upper teeth against trauma.
- *Lubrication:* Lubricate laryngoscope with liquid paraffin or xylocaine jelly.
- *Holding of scope:* Left hand holds the handle of laryngoscope. Right hand retracts the lips and guides the introduction of laryngoscope and handle suction and forceps.
- *Introduction of scope:* Laryngoscope is introduced on right side of the tongue and is then moved to the midline. That brings the epiglottis in view.
- *Lifting of epiglottis:* The lifting of epiglottis forward (without levering laryngoscope on the upper teeth or jaw) provides view of the interior larynx.
- *Interior of larynx:* The tip of anterior commissure laryngoscope is advanced further between the vestibular folds (to examine the ventricles and anterior commissure) and the vocal cords (to examine the subglottic region).
- *Structures examined:* The structures, which are examined serially, include tongue base, valleculae, epiglottis, pyriform sinuses, aryepiglottic folds, arytenoids, postcricoid region, false cords, ventricles, vocal cords, anterior and posterior commissure, subglottic region and mobility of vocal cords and arytenoids.
- *Telescope:* Angled (90°) telescopes facilitate examination of the undersurface of vocal cords and subglottic region.

Practical tips for DLS/MLS
- Protects the lips and teeth. Lips are easily pinched between the laryngoscope and teeth or gingiva. Upper teeth are easily broken by levering the laryngoscope on them.
- Position the head. Extend the neck. Head rests on the occiput (sniffing position). This position provides the best access to anterior areas.
- Exclude contraindications for extending the neck: Fusion, instability, Down syndrome.

Do not biopsy both sides of the vocal folds (such as nodules) close to the anterior commissure to prevent formation of web.

POSTOPERATIVE CARE

- *Position:* Patient is kept in coma position, which prevents aspiration of blood and secretions.
- *Observation:* Watch for any spitting of blood, respiratory distress and cyanosis. They can be due to laryngeal spasm, laryngeal edema, or aspiration of blood.

COMPLICATIONS

- Injury to lips, tongue and teeth
- Bleeding
- Laryngeal spasm and edema.

FLEXIBLE NASOPHARYNGOLARYNGOSCOPY

See Chapter 'Laryngeal Symptoms and Examination.'

- **Flexible laryngoscopy:** If you have difficulty in seeing into nasopharynx and oropharynx request the patient to breath through nose that will clear the soft tissue obstruction.
- **Valsalva maneuver:** By requesting the patient to perform this maneuver we can better visualize the pyriform sinuses because it will distend them.

BRONCHOSCOPY

Bronchoscopy is of two types—rigid bronchoscopy and flexible bronchoscopy.

INDICATIONS FOR BRONCHOSCOPY

- *Diagnostic*
    - *Symptoms*
        - Dyspnea or stridor
        - Hemoptysis
        - Unexplained chronic cough
        - Hoarseness of voice
        - Fever or chest pain suggestive of pulmonary infections
    - *X-ray chest findings*
        - Atelectasis: Segment, lobe or lung
        - Opacity: Segment or lobe
        - Obstructive emphysema
        - Hilar or mediastinal shadows
        - Pleural effusions
    - *Vocal cord paralysis*
    - *Collection of bronchial secretions:* For culture and sensitivity, acid-fast bacilli, fungus, and malignant cells.
- *Therapeutic*
    - Foreign body removal.
    - Suction clearance of secretions, blood clots or inspissated mucus plugs: Head injuries, chest trauma, thoracic and abdominal surgery and coma.
    - Assessment or placement of endotracheal tubes or double lumen tubes.
    - Guided percutaneous tracheostomy.
    - Thermal ablation and removal of tumors.
    - Debridement of benign stenosis.
    - Balloon dilation.
    - Placement of airway stent.

RIGID BRONCHOSCOPY

For instruments *see* Chapter 'Instruments'.

Advantages

Large instruments can be passed through the larger lumen of rigid bronchoscope. It is advantageous in the following conditions:
- Removal of foreign bodies.
- Suctioning in profuse hemoptysis.
- Placements of noncompressible silastic airway stent.
- Coring out tumors.
- Tamponading to a bleeding source.

Anesthesia

Usually done under general anesthesia but can be done with topical surface anesthesia and conscious sedation.

Oxygenation and Ventilation

- Intermittent apneic to spontaneous/assisted.
- Tidal volume through closed system or open system of side port Venturi jet ventilation.

Position

Patient lies in supine position. Neck is flexed on thorax and head is extended on atlanto-occipital joint.

Techniques

- *Lubrication of scope:* Lubricate proper size bronchoscope with liquid paraffin or xylocaine jelly.
- *Protection of teeth and lips:* Examine the patient for neck stability, loose teeth and dentures. Eyes are protected with a shield and the patient is draped. A gauze piece or teeth guard protects the upper teeth against injury.
- *Holding of scope:* The shaft of bronchoscope is held in right hand like a pen. Left hand thumb retracts the upper lip and teeth while index finger lifts lower teeth and guides the introduction of bronchoscope with bevel up.
- *Introduction of scope:* Bronchoscope is directed perpendicularly until the uvula is passed. It is introduced usually on the right side of the tongue and is then moved to the midline. It brings the epiglottis in view.
- *Larynx:* Tip of epiglottis is identified while lifting the base of the tongue. Glottis is exposed when epiglottis is lifted forward. Bronchoscope is introduced either directly or after exposing the glottis with the help of a spatular type laryngoscope especially in infants, young children and short neck or thick tongue patients.
    - Rotate the bronchoscope 90° clockwise to bring its beveled tip in the axis of glottis and enter into the trachea. Rotate back the scope into its original position.
- *Tracheobronchial tree:* Gradually advance the scope and examine the entire tracheobronchial tree. Head and neck are flexed to the left while examining the right bronchial tree and to the right for left side bronchial

tree. In this way, axis of bronchoscope corresponds with trachea and bronchi. Examine openings of all the segmental bronchi.
- ***Telescope:*** Straight and angled telescopes provide magnification and facilitate detailed examination.
- ***Biopsy:*** Take biopsy of the lesion.
- ***Collection of secretions:*** Collect secretions for exfoliative cytology and culture and sensitivity of microorganisms.

> ***Precautions for rigid bronchoscopy***
> - Select proper size of bronchoscope as per the patient's age.
> - No force is applied against closed glottis.
> - Avoid repeated removal and introduction of bronchoscope as far as possible. Prolonged procedure (> 20 minutes) may cause postoperative subglottic edema in infants and children.
> - Maintain intravenous line and administer injections of antibiotic and steroid especially in infants and children.

Postoperative Care
- ***Position:*** Patient is kept in coma position, which prevents aspiration of blood or secretions.
  - Patient is kept in humid atmosphere.
- ***Observation:*** Watch for any spitting of blood, respiratory distress (inspiratory stridor, suprasternal retraction) and cyanosis. They can be due to laryngeal spasm, laryngeal edema, or aspiration of blood. These patients may need tracheostomy.

Complications
- Injury to teeth and lips.
- Transient fever especially after bronchoalveolar lavage.
- Bleeding and hemoptysis in cases of inflamed or malignant tissue.
- Hypoxia and cardiac arrest.
- Laryngeal spasm and edema.

FLEXIBLE FIBEROPTIC BRONCHOSCOPY

Flexible fiberoptic bronchoscope (FOB) is replacing rigid bronchoscope but its utility is limited in children because of the problems of ventilation (Table 58.1).

> ***Tracheobronchial tree and larynx:*** Rate of topical absorption is highest.

Advantages
- Magnification and better illumination.
- Better documentation with facility of video recording.
- Smaller size allows examination of subsegmental bronchi.
- Easy to do even under topical anesthesia.

Table 58.1: Comparative advantages and disadvantages of flexible and rigid bronchoscopy and esophagoscopy

Feature	Flexible	Rigid
Need of admission	Out-door procedure	Needs admission and preanesthetic check up
Anesthesia	Usually topical	Usually general
Examination	Better due to bright illumination and magnification	Relatively poor
Facility of OT and anesthetist	Not required	Required
Jaws, cervical spines lesion, ICU patients, trismus	Can be done	Very difficult and risky
Biopsy	Small pieces	Large pieces
Foreign bodies (FB)	Only small FBs; FBs cannot be retracted in to endoscope	Any FB; FBs can be retracted in to endoscope
Hemorrhage control	Not possible	Possible
Airway and ventilation (bronchoscopy)	Not possible	Possible
Video recording	Excellent	Very difficult
Postoperative care and complications	Minimal	Relatively more
Relatives and assistants	See on TV monitor	Not possible
Cost	Economical	Expensive

Abbreviation: OT—Operation theater

- It can be performed in cases of neck or jaw abnormalities or critical illness (bedside examination).
- The suction/biopsy channel helps in removing secretions, inspissated mucous plugs or small foreign bodies.
- Flexible bronchoscope can be passed through endotracheal tube.

> ***Bronchoscopy biopsy of the right upper lobe carina/spur:*** It is the most dangerous site for biopsy because of the risk of injury to underlying right pulmonary artery.

- ***Flexible bronchoscopy:*** It offers visions of segmental bronchi and the upper lobe bronchi, which are beyond the reach of rigid bronchoscopes.
- ***Rigid bronchoscopy:*** It is superior in taking biopsy and culture specimens, removing foreign bodies and in surgical intervention such as dilatation.

ESOPHAGOSCOPY

Esophagoscopy is of two types—rigid esophagoscopy and flexible esophagoscopy.

INDICATIONS

- *Diagnostic*
    - **Symptoms:** Dysphagia, odynophagia, aphagia, sensation of a lump or "sticking" in throat, retrosternal burning, hematemesis and persistent regurgitation.
    - **Signs:** Vocal cord palsy.
    - **Investigation findings**
        - Radiological evidence of extrinsic or intrinsic esophageal disorders.
        - Abnormal esophageal manometry.
        - Abnormal esophageal pH recording.
    - **Diseases:** Malignancy esophagus, cardiac achalasia, strictures, infectious esophagitis, diverticulum, reflux esophagitis, hiatus hernia, esophageal varices, caustic ingestion, secondary neck node with unknown primary, surveillance for second primary, penetrating trauma to thorax to rule out esophageal injury.
- *Therapeutic*
    - Foreign body
    - Impacted food
    - Dilatation of esophageal strictures, stenosis and cardiac achalasia.
    - Removal of benign neoplasms such as fibroma, papilloma, and cysts.
    - Insertion of Soutar's or Mousseau-Barbin tube in palliative treatment of esophageal carcinoma.
    - Tracheoesophageal puncture after total laryngectomy.
    - Treatment of diverticulum and varices.

CONTRAINDICATIONS OF ESOPHAGOSCOPY

- *Absolute:*
    - Coagulopathy.
    - Perforation of esophagus: Spontaneous, traumatic or iatrogenic.
- *Relative contraindications:* Advanced heart, liver or kidney disease.
- *Contraindications of rigid esophagoscopy:* In most of the following conditions, new generations of flexible gastroscopes can be used successfully (*see* Table 58.1).
    - **Severe trismus:** It does not allow passage for esophagoscope. Small size flexible gastroscopes can be passed through nose.
    - **Cervical spine lesions:** Cervical trauma, spondylosis, Pott's spine, osteophytes, or kyphosis.
    - **Receding mandible.**
    - **Aneurysm of aorta:** May rupture and cause fatal hemorrhage.

RIGID ESOPHAGOSCOPY

For instruments *see* Chapter 'Instruments'. The size of the esophagoscope is selected as per the age of the patient. Handle at the proximal end of esophagoscope indicates the direction of the bevel at the distal end.

A rigid bronchoscope may be used for performing esophagoscopy but the rigid esophagoscope cannot be used for bronchoscopy.

Advantages

- More amenable to therapeutic indications especially removal of foreign bodies.
- Better visualization of proximal one-third of esophagus.

Disadvantages

- General anesthesia.
- More cost and morbidity to patient.
- More complications such as dental trauma and esophageal perforation.
- Concomitant examination of stomach and intestine not possible.
- Not amenable to cases of trismus or cervical spine degenerative diseases.

Anesthesia

It is usually done under general anesthesia with endotracheal intubation.

Position

- Patient is placed in supine position. Head is elevated by 10–15 cm. Neck is flexed on chest. Head is extended at atlanto-occipital joint. This position brings the axes of mouth, pharynx and esophagus in a straight line and facilitates passage of esophagoscope. Shoulders are at the edge of operation table and head rests on a special headrest or hold by an assistant.
- A right-handed surgeon sits on the left of the long axis of the patient.
- The assistant, instrument table, light source and suction are on right side of surgeon.

Techniques (Fig. 58.3)

- *Protection of teeth and lips:* Examine the patient for neck stability and loose teeth or dentures. Eyes are protected with a shield and the patient is draped. A gauze piece or teeth guard protects the upper teeth against injury. Left hand thumb retracts the upper lip and teeth while index finger lifts lower teeth.

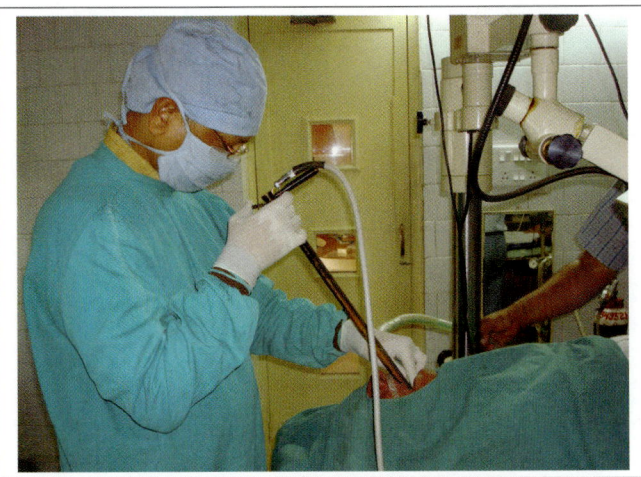

Fig. 58.3: Procedure of esophagoscopy

- **Lubrication of scope:** Lubricate proper size esophagoscope with liquid paraffin or xylocaine jelly.
- **Holding of scope:** Esophagoscope is held by its proximal end in right hand and introduced into right side of mouth lateral to the tongue and advanced towards the middle of base of tongue.
- **Laryngopharynx:** Esophagoscope is further advanced gently by the left thumb and index finger. Identify epiglottis, endotracheal tube and arytenoids.
- **Cricopharyngeal sphincter:** Keep the tip of esophagoscope in midline and behind the larynx. Lift the scope with the help of left thumb and open the hypopharynx. Slow, gentle and sustained pressure of the scope tip on the cricopharyngeal sphincter opens it. Then the tip of scope is guided into the esophagus. A fine bougie or an additional dose of muscle relaxant may be used if needed. Advance the scope constantly seeing the esophageal lumen.

Caution: Application of too much force on cricopharyngeal sphincter is the most common cause of cervical esophageal perforation.

- **Aortic arch and left bronchus:** Indentations of aortic arch (aortic pulsation seen and felt) and left bronchus lie about 25 cm from the incisors. During this time, head of the patient is slightly lowered, which brings the esophageal lumen in the line of the scope.
- **Cardiac end:** Head and shoulders are kept below the level of the table. The head, which is slightly higher than the shoulders, is moved slightly to the right. The esophagoscope now points to the left anterior superior iliac spine. Cardia has redder and more velvety (rugose) mucosa.
- **Withdrawing:** Inspect the esophageal wall again while withdrawing the esophagoscope.

Postoperative Care

- **Features of esophageal perforation:** Watch for the pain in interscapular region, surgical emphysema of neck and chest, and abrupt rise of temperature.
- **Diet:** Sips of plain water may be given if there is no evidence of esophageal perforation.

Complications

- **Injury** to lips, teeth, and pharynx.
- **Perforation of esophagus:** This is the most dreaded complication and usually occurs near cricopharyngeal sphincter (Killian's dehiscence). Surgical emphysema develops within an hour. It may be complicated with an abscess in retropharyngeal space or mediastinum. The features of thoracic esophageal perforation include–
  - Pain in the interscapular region
  - Surgical emphysema
  - Abrupt rise of temperature.
- **Compression of trachea:** It occurs especially in children when esophagoscope is pressed on posterior tracheal wall. It causes obstruction to respiration and cyanosis and needs immediate withdrawal of esophagoscope.

Esophageal perforation:
- **Features:** Fever after esophagoscopy.
- **Diagnosis:** Swallow study confirms diagnosis.
- **Treatment:** Early intervention to repair is most desirable. Drain the perforation to prevent complications.

FLEXIBLE ESOPHAGOSCOPY

Advantages

- An outdoor procedure.
- No general anesthesia. It is done under local anesthesia with or without intravenous sedation.
- Less morbidity.
- It can be done in abnormalities of spine or jaw.
- Gastroscope allows examination of stomach and duodenum.
- Good illumination and magnification.
- Accurate diagnosis of the mucosal diseases.

Disadvantages

- Narrow channel limits the size of instruments and removal of certain foreign bodies.
- Foreign body cannot be retracted into the endoscope (like rigid esophagoscope) so more chances of injuring esophagus.
- Laryngopharynx and proximal one-third esophagus (less distensible with insufflations) may not be examined adequately.

Common Indications
- Precision biopsies.
- Removal of small foreign bodies or benign tumors.
- Dilatation of webs or strictures.
- Injection of sclerosing agents in bleeding varices.

Endoscope and Instruments
Esophagoscope is available in wide range of diameter smallest being 5.0 mm. There are separate channels for optics, suctioning (secretions), insufflations, and instruments (for biopsy, foreign bodies, sclerotherapy and laser ablation). Set up also includes light source, camera and video processing unit.

Techniques
- The patient is usually in left lateral position or in supine and gentle extension of neck with a shoulder roll.
- Lubricated scope (with xylocaine jelly) is introduced into the mouth through a plastic mouth block and advanced into the pharynx, postcricoid region and esophagus (Fig. 58.4).
- The esophagoscope can be deflected in any direction and secretions can be aspirated.
- Air or water insufflation opens the lumen of esophagus and the endoscope is advanced further.

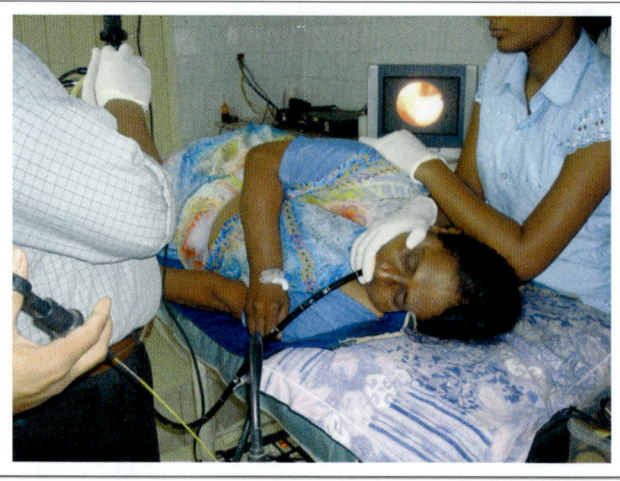

Fig. 58.4: Flexible esophagoscopy. Note the biopsy forceps in the hand of assistant

Self-evaluation Exercises

1. Features of esophageal perforation include:
   a. Fever after esophagoscopy
   b. Swallow study confirms diagnosis
   c. Early intervention to repair is most desirable
   d. Drain the perforation to prevent complications
   e. All of the above
2. Which focal length of objective piece of operative microscope is usually used for microlaryngoscopy?
   a. 100 mm
   b. 200 mm
   c. 300 mm
   d. 400 mm
   e. Any mm
3. Rigid bronchoscopy is superior to flexible bronchoscopy in:
   a. Taking biopsy and culture specimens
   b. Removing foreign bodies
   c. Surgical intervention such as dilatation
   d. All of the above

True (T)/False (F)

4. Application of too much force on cricopharyngeal sphincter is the most common cause of cervical esophageal perforation during esophagoscopy.
5. Flexible bronchoscopy offers visions of segmental bronchi and the upper lobe bronchi which are beyond the reach of rigid bronchoscopes.
6. Rate of topical absorption is highest in tracheobronchial tree and larynx.

Answers

1. e 2. d 3. d 4. T 5. T 6. T

Chapter 59

Instruments

⊙ Specific Learning Objectives
After going through the chapter, you should be able to identify and tell the uses of the described instruments.

INTRODUCTION

There is vast number of ENT instruments used for diagnostic, therapeutic and surgical purposes. The figures show quite good number of instruments but the description covers only frequently asked instruments. For the further details regarding the method of use and indications, the reader should refer to the related Chapters such as 'Symptoms and Examination' and Section of 'Operations'.

OPD INSTRUMENTS

Figures 59.1 to 59.5 show OPD instruments. For the related details, *see* Chapters of 'Symptoms and Examination' of respective Sections.

- **Dressing forceps (Figs 59.1A, I and J):** Tilley's dressing forceps has a box joint. Its bayonet-shaped or bent at an obtuse angle prevents the hand of the surgeon from obstructing the line of vision. Hartmann's dressing forceps is similar to Tilley's forceps and has a screw joint and the serrated and grooved jaws. Wilde's dressing forceps acts on spring action.
  - *Uses:* They are used for nasal packing, ear dressing and removal of foreign bodies.
- **Ear speculum (Figs 59.1B to D):** This cone-shaped speculum has tapered end that is inserted into the cartilaginous portion of the external auditory canal (EAC) after retracting the pinna. The black or dull finished speculums are used in operations as they prevent reflection of light. Various sizes and shapes of the ear speculums are available. The use of the largest ear speculum that can easily enter the canal is safe and provides better view.
  - *Use:* It is used for examination and operations of the EAC, tympanic membrane (TM) and middle ear.
- **Otoscope (Fig. 59.1E):** It has its own illumination. The source of light is housed in its handle. It also provides magnification. Some of the otoscopes have Siegel's speculum (pneumatic otoscope).
  - *Use:* It helps in examining the EAC and tympanic membrane (TM). It is especially useful in examining the ears and nose of infants and bedridden patients.
- **Tuning fork (Fig. 59.1F):** See Chapter 'Hearing Evaluation'.
  - *Use:* They are used for Rinne, Weber and other tuning fork hearing tests.
- **Barany noise box (Fig. 59.1H):**
  - *Use:* Used for masking purposes during the tuning fork hearing tests (*see* Chapter 'Hearing Evaluation').

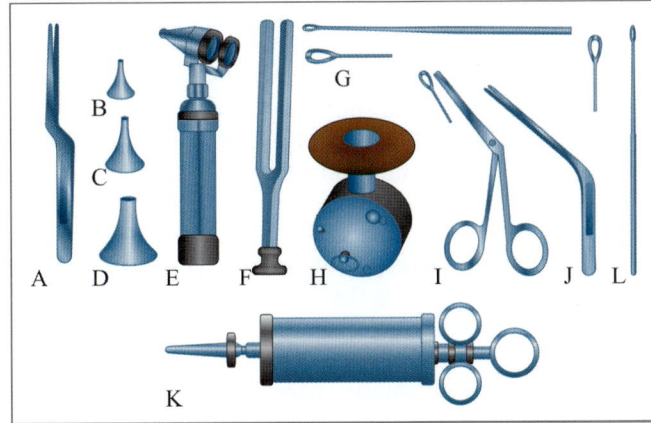

Figs 59.1A to L: OPD ear instruments. (A) Jansen dressing forceps bayonet shaped; (B) Plastic ear speculum; (C) Hartmann ear speculum; (D) Boucheron ear speculum; (E) Heine Otoscope with plastic ear specula; (F) Tuning fork; (G) Billeau ear loop; (H) Barany noise box with soft rubber; (I) Lucae ear dressing forceps; (J) Troeltsch dressing forceps angular; (K) Ear syringe; (L) Weber-Loch ear curette
Source: Karl Storz, Germany

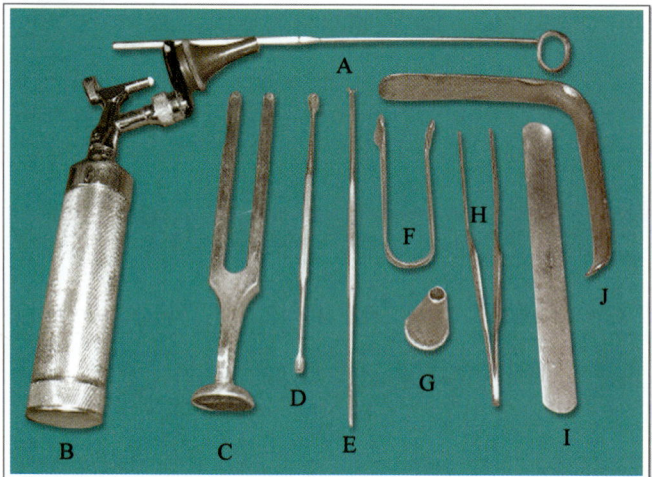

Figs 59.2A to J: OPD instruments. (A) Laryngeal mirror; (B) Otoscope; (C) Tuning fork; (D) Ear vectis and curette; (E) Jobson-Horne probe with round serrated end applicator and curette end; (F) Thudicum nasal speculum; (G) Ear speculum; (H) Bayonet-shaped ear dressing forceps; (I) Straight tongue depressor; (J) L-shaped tongue depressor

- **Aural syringe (Fig. 59.1K):** This metal syringe consists of a cylinder with a well-fitting piston and a nozzle. *See* Chapter 'Diseases of External Ear'.
  - **Use:** It is used for ear syringing to remove EAC wax and foreign bodies.
- **Blunt probe:**
  - **Use:** It is used for palpation of polyp, growths and swellings in the ear and nose.
- **Laryngeal mirror (Fig. 59.2A):** The shaft of the laryngeal mirror is straight (mirror sizes 6–30 mm diameter). *See* Chapter 'Laryngeal Symptoms and Examination'.
  - **Use:** For indirect laryngoscopy examination of oropharynx, laryngopharynx and larynx.
- **Thudicum nasal speculum (Fig. 59.2F):** It consists of U-shaped metal spring with two blades at its ends. The size is chosen according to the age of patient and size of the nose. The nasal speculum is held in the left hand and it assists in widening the vestibule. *See* Chapter 'Nasal Symptoms and Examination'.
  - **Uses:** They are used for nasal examination and during surgery of the nose.
- **Lack's L-shaped tongue depressor (Fig. 59.2J):** One blade is slightly bent at the end. The bent end is used for holding and it supports the little finger of the examiner. The other blade depresses the tongue and is used like a lever to depress anterior two-third of the tongue with the fulcrum over the lower teeth.
  - **Caution:** Touching of the posterior one-third of the tongue usually leads to the gag reflex and not tolerated by the patient.
  - **Uses:** It is used for examining the oral cavity and the pharynx. In addition to the depressing of tongue, it can also be used for:
    - Squeezing the tonsil
    - Retraction of cheek
    - Test for gag reflex
    - To check nasal air blast
    - Spatula test for suspected case of tetanus
    - Posterior rhinoscopy examination
    - Checking out for loose teeth
    - Intraoral surgical procedure
    - Checking postnasal bleeding.
- **Postnasal mirror:** Mirror is smaller than laryngeal mirror and the shaft is bayonet-shaped.
  - **Use:** It is used for examining the nasopharynx and posterior part of nasal cavity. *See* Chapter 'Nasal Symptoms and Examination'.

> The posterior rhinoscopy mirror is smaller and its shaft is bayonet-shaped, while the shaft of the laryngeal mirror is straight.

- **Jobson-Horne probe with ring curette (Figs 59.2E and 59.3):** It has two ends: round serrated end applicator and curette end.
  - **Use:** One end of the Jobson-Horne's probe is used for applying cotton to clean ear discharge. The other end (ring curette) is used to remove the ear wax and foreign body.
- **Siegel's pneumatic speculum (Fig. 59.4):** It is fitted with a convex lens and is attached to a rubber bulb through plastic tubing. The rubber bulb assists in alternately increasing and decreasing pressure in the EAC. Its convex lens provides magnification.
  - **Uses:**
    - *Mobility of tympanic membrane (TM):*
    - *Fistula test: See* Chapter 'Evaluation of Vertigo'.

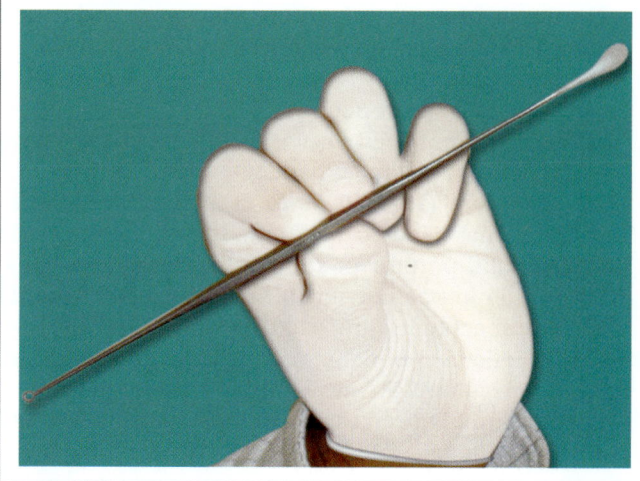

Fig. 59.3: Jobson-Horne's probe. Applying cotton to clean the ear

Chapter 59 • Instruments

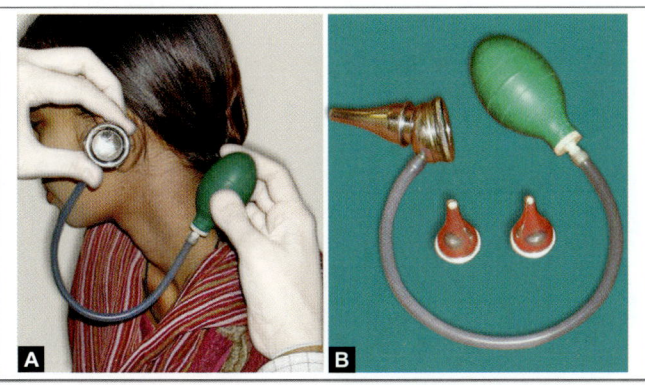

Figs 59.4A and B: Siegel's examination. (A) Method; (B) Siegel's pneumatic speculum

- *Aural toilet:* Suction of ear secretions in acute and chronic suppurative otitis media.
- *Topical ear medicines:* Pushing of medicines through the central perforation of TM.
- **Eustachian catheter and Politzer's bag (Fig. 59.5):** Eustachian catheter is a 12–15 cm metal cannula. It has a ring at its base that indicates the direction of its curved tip. It looks similar to the antral washing cannula, in which opening is not at the tip but a little proximal to it. An olive-shaped tip of the Politzer's bag is introduced into the nose.
  - *Uses (see Chapter 'Disorders of Eustachian Tube'):*
    - Politzer test and Eustachian tube catheterization for testing the functioning of Eustachian tube.
    - To inflate the middle ear.
    - To instill medicines into middle ear.
    - To remove foreign body from the nose.
    - For suctioning the secretions and discharge.

MASTOID AND EAR MICROSURGERY

Figure 59.6 shows speculum, retractors and suction cannula. Figure 59.7 shows bone cutting instruments. Figure 59.8 show elevators and suction cannula. See Chapter 'Middle Ear and Mastoid Surgeries'.

- **Endaural speculum (Fig. 59.6A):** There are many types of endaural speculum like Lempert's. This curved speculum is similar to Vienna model.
  - *Use:* It spreads open the meatus and is used when giving local injection or making an endaural incision.
- **Myringotome (Fig. 59.6F):**
  - *Use:* For puncturing TM and placing grommets.
- **Mastoid self-retaining retractors (Figs 59.6B to D):** There are many other types of mastoid retractors like Mollison's and Jansen's. The catch prevents its closure and the blades hold apart the edges of the incision.
  - *Uses:*
    - *Mastoidectomy:* They retract soft tissues after incision and elevation of flaps. The pressure on the edges of the incision provides hemostasis.
    - *Other operations:* This self retaining retractor may be used in other surgeries, such as laryngofissure, craniotomy, burr-holing and external ethmoidectomy.
- **Lempert's endaural retractor (Fig. 59.6G):** It has three blades. The two lateral blades retract the flaps. The third central blade with holes retracts the temporalis muscle superiorly. The central blade with its hole is fixed to the body of the retractor.
  - *Use:* In the endaural approach mastoidectomy.
- **Mastoid suction tips (Figs 59.6E and 59.8C to F):** This bent cannula has an obtuse angle and a hole that can be used to regulate the force of suction. The hole can be

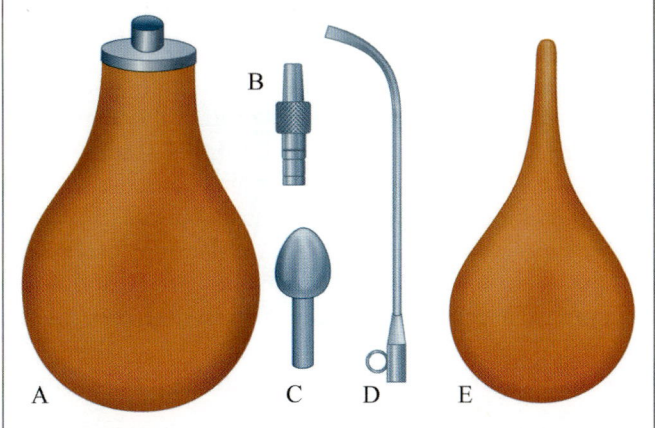

Figs 59.5A to E: Eustachian tube instruments. (A) Politzer air bag 8 ounce capacity; (B) Metal connector Eustachian catheter to Politzer air bag; (C) Nasal tip for use with Politzer air bag; (D) Hartmann Eustachian catheter; (E) Soft rubber air bag (2.5 ounce capacity)
Source: Karl Storz, Germany

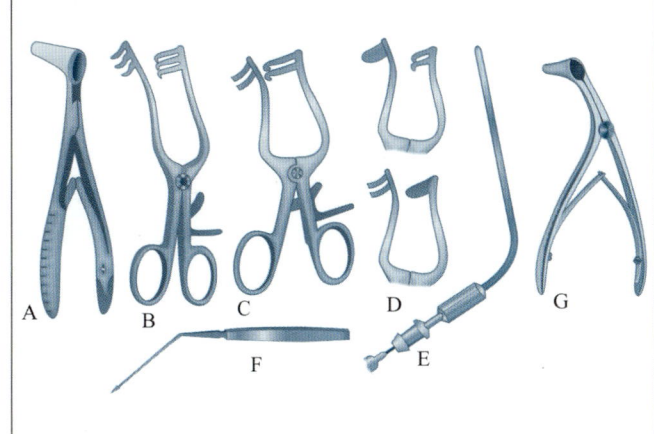

Figs 59.6A to E: Ear surgery instruments retractors. (A) Hartmann speculum; (B) Wullstein retractor; (C) Plester retractor 2 x 2 prongs; (D) Plester retractors with biprong blade and solid blade for left and right side; (E) Ferguson suction tube with finger cut-off and stylet; (F) Myringotome; (G) Lempert's endaural retractor
Source: Karl Storz, Germany

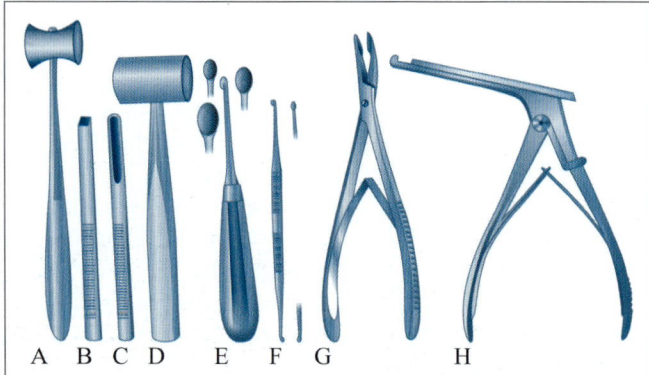

Figs 59.7A to H: Ear surgery bone cutting instruments. (A) Cottle mallet; (B) Trautmann mastoid chisel; (C) Trautmann mastoid gauge; (D) Lucae mallet; (E) Spratt mastoid curette; (F) House curette; (G) Beyer-Rongeur light curved jaws; (H) Kerrison Rongeur
Source: Karl Storz, Germany

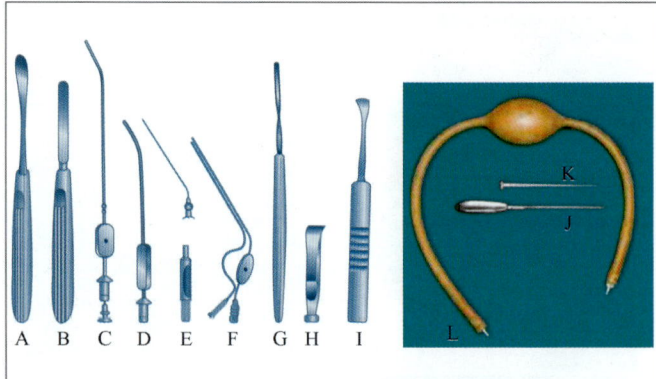

Figs 59.8A to I: Ear surgery instruments, elevators and suctions. (A) Jansen elevator; (B) Plester elevator; (C) Plester suction tube with finger cut-off and stylet; (D) Zoellner suction tube with finger cut-off; (E) Fisch adaptor for suction cannula with finger cut-off luer cone; (F) Fisch suction irrigator; (G) Lempert elevator; (H) Farabeuf's elevator; (I) Fisch elevator. Antrum puncture instruments. (J) Lichtwitz trocar; (K) Cannula; (L) Higginson's syringe
Source: Karl Storz, Germany

closed by placing a finger tip on it. Fine suction tips are used for microsurgery.
  ▪ *Use:* Suction of blood, secretions, irrigation water and bone dust.
● *Mastoid gouges (Fig. 59.7C):* They are of various sizes and have a concave edge and rounded margins. The electrical drill and burrs are replacing the use of gouges.
  ▪ *Uses:*
    ♦ *Mastoidectomy:* Remove bone in mastoid surgery.
    ♦ *Caldwell-Luc operation:* Used for canine fossa antrostomy for opening the maxillary antrum.
    ♦ *Exostosis:* Excision of exostosis EAC.
● *Mastoid curette (scoop) (Figs 59.7E and F):* There are many other types of mastoid curette like Lempert's.
  ▪ *Use:* It removes bony septa and granulations in mastoid surgery.
● *Farabeuf's periosteal elevator* (Fig. 59.8H)
  ▪ *Use:* It is used for elevation of periosteum from the mastoid cortex in mastoidectomy.

OPERATIONS OF NOSE AND PARANASAL SINUSES

See Chapter 'Operations of Nose and Paranasal Sinuses'.

ANTRUM PUNCTURE (FIG. 59.8J to L)

● *Lichtwitz trocar and cannula:* It perforates the lateral wall of inferior meatus. This area is easily accessible and safe region. After piercing the nasoantral wall, trocar is removed (*see* Chapter 'Operations of Nose and Paranasal Sinuses').
  ▪ *Use:* It is used for proof puncture (antral lavage).
● *Higginson's syringe:*
  ▪ *Use:* Irrigating maxillary antrum with normal saline.

INFERIOR MEATAL ANTROSTOMY

● *Tilley's harpoon*
  ▪ *Use:* Intranasal antrostomy in the inferior meatus.
  ▪ *Advantage:* Removes bony chips when it is withdrawn. So they do not remain in maxillary sinus.
● *Tilley's antral burr*
  ▪ *Use:* It enlarges and smoothens the hole made by harpoon in intranasal inferior meatal antrostomy.
● *Rose's sinus douching cannula:* The hook outside indicates the direction of the tip.
  ▪ *Use:* It is used for the irrigation of maxillary sinus through the inferior meatus window after intranasal antrostomy or Caldwell-Luc operation.

NASAL FRACTURE REDUCTION FORCEPS

● *Walsham's forceps (Fig. 59.9A):* Rubber tubing may be used to cover one blade to protect the skin of the external nose (*see* Chapter 'Maxillofacial Trauma').
  ▪ *Use:* They are used for the disimpaction and reduction of the fractures of nasal bones.
● *Asch's septum forceps (Fig. 59.9B):* The forceps are bent at an obtuse angle. When they are closed, there remains a gap between the blades that prevent the crushing of the nasal septum.
  ▪ *Use:* Lifting and reducing fractures of nasal septum.

NASAL SEPTAL AND SINUS SURGERY

Figure 59.10 shows instruments of endoscopic sinus surgery. Figures 59.11 and 59.12 show instruments of nasal and septal surgeries.

Chapter 59 • Instruments

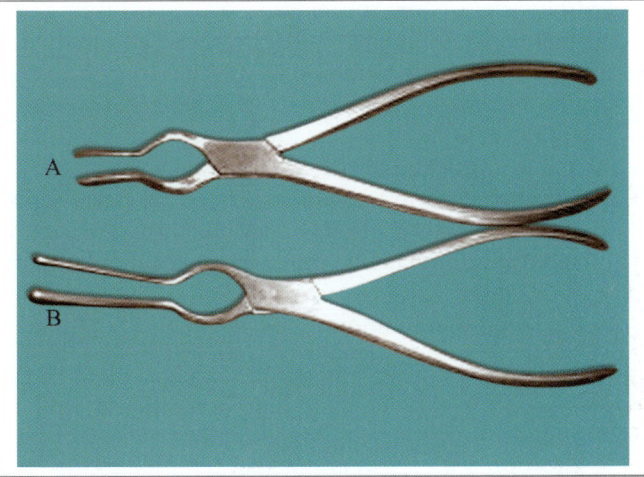

Figs 59.9A and B: (A) Walsham forceps; (B) Asche's forceps

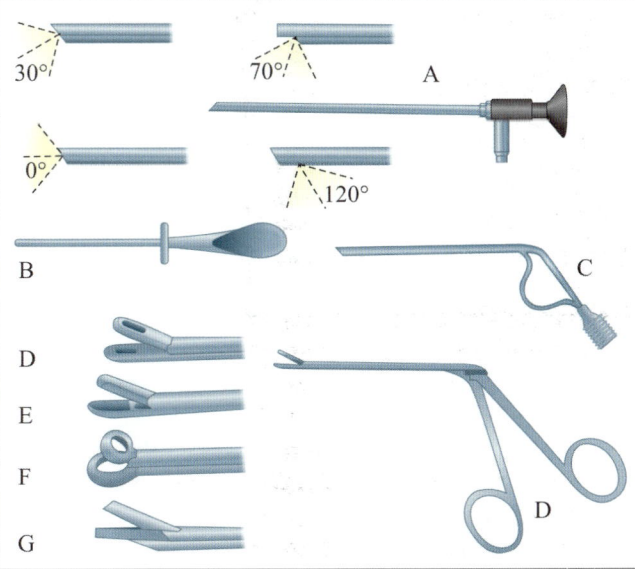

Figs 59.10A to G: Instruments of endoscopic sinus surgery. (A) Hopkins telescopes 4 mm with fiber optic light transmission (0°, 30°, 70° and 120° Sinuscopes); (B) Trocar and cannula for sinuscopy; (C) Suction irrigation tube with channel for inflow and outflow; (D) Blakesley ethmoid forceps; (E) Takahashi ethmoid forceps; (F) Hartmann nasal cutting forceps; (G) Struycken narrow blade nasal cutting forceps for removal of turbinates
Source: Karl Storz, Germany

- **Bone forceps (Fig. 59.11):** Double action bone nibbling forceps are bent at an obtuse angle and have four joints with double lever systems that allow the blades to close and open to a limited extent in a narrow deep cavity. They have strong grasp.
  - *Use:* They are used for removing the bony part such as deviated nasal septum.
- **Chisels (Figs 59.11D, E and J):** In comparison to an elevator they have head.
  - *Uses:* Various nasal and paranasal sinus surgeries.

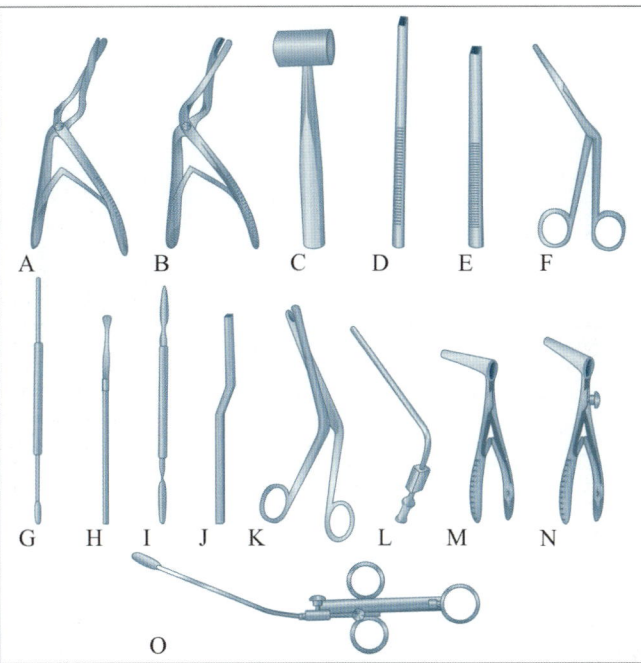

Figs 59.11A to O: Instruments for nasal surgery. (A) Jansen Middleton septum bone forceps with through cutting blades; (B) Jansen septum bone forceps; (C) Cottle mallet; (D) Cottle chisel with depth markings; (E) Masing chisel double guarded; (F) Heymann nasal scissors medium size; (G) Freer elevator double ended; (H) Freer septum chisel straight end; (I) Killian elevator double ended; (J) Killian claus septum chisel with V-shaped cutting edge; (K) Luc septum bone forceps; (L) Ferguson suction tube with finger cut-off and stylet; (M) Killian-Struycken nasal speculum; (N) Cottle nasal speculum with set screw; (O) Krause nasal snare
Source: Karl Storz, Germany

- **Heymann turbinectomy scissors (Fig 59.11F):** It has a bend in the center that offers better field of vision. Its narrow stout blades have blunt tips.
  - *Use:* Removal of inferior turbinate.
- **Elevators (Figs 59.11G, I and 12E):** There are various shapes and sizes of periosteum elevators. In comparison to a chisel, it does not have a head. A rest is provided for a finger and the edge is blunt. Freer, Cottle and Killian have two dissecting faces (ends).
  - *Septal surgery:* They are used for the elevation of mucoperichondrium/mucoperiosteum in nasal septum operation. The sharper spade like end begins the dissection in submucoperichondrial plane. Its flat and dull end elevates the flap in an atraumatic way especially in nasal septal surgery.
  - *Endoscopic sinus surgery:* For manipulating uncinate process, middle meatus and bulla ethmoidalis.
  - *Caldwell-Luc operation and mastoidectomy:* For elevating the periosteum and soft tissues.
  - *Tympanoplasty:* For separating temporalis fascia from temporalis muscle.
- **Nasal speculum (Figs 59.11M, N and 59.12 and J):** There are many other types of nasal speculum like

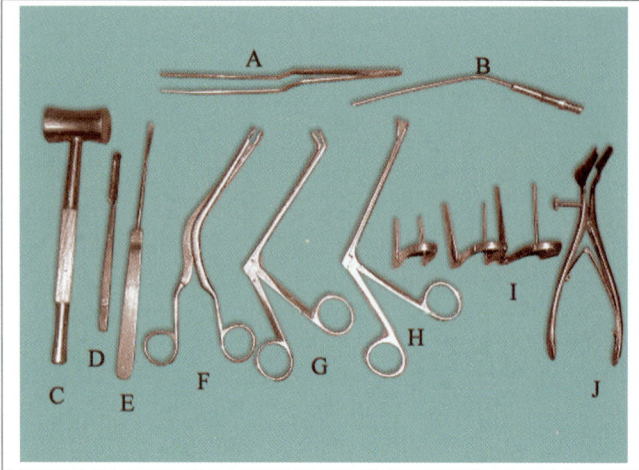

Figs 59.12A to J: Instruments for septal surgery. (A) Nasal dressing forceps bayonet-shaped; (B) Suction cannula; (C) Mallet with both sides plain faces; (D) Septum gouge, straight, round cutting edge, without notch; (E) Periosteum elevator; (F) Luc's forceps with fenestrated jaws; (G) Takahashi ethmoidal forceps upward curved with oval cup-shaped; (H) Takahashi ethmoidal forceps straight oval cup-shaped; (I) Three sizes of nasal speculum; (J) Septum speculum with joint and set screw

St. Clair Thomson's and Killian's. Its long blades are concave from inside. They keep mucoperiosteal flaps away.
- **Uses:** It is used in septal surgery such as submucosal resection (SMR) and septoplasty.
- *Mallet or hammer (Figs 59.11C and 59.12C):* It consists of handle, shaft and a head.
  - **Uses:** To give gentle blows on the gouge for removing spur and doing osteotomy in rhinoplasty.
- *Nasal gouges (Fig. 59.12D):* There are many types of nasal gouges. Killian's bayonet-shaped gouge has rounded and concave, or "V" shaped edge for a better grip on the septal bone.
  - **Uses:**
    * *Nasal septum surgery:* It is used for removal of septal spurs, bony crests, ridges and maxillary crest.
    * *Caldwell-Luc operation:* For canine fossa antrostomy and opening the maxillary antrum.
- *Luc's forceps (Fig. 59.12F):* These have a screw joint. The blades are fenestrated and cup-shaped with sharp edges. The tissue caught by the blades may bulge out through the fenestra for a better grip.
  - **Uses:**
    * *Nasal surgery:* To remove polyps (to grasp and avulse), growth and bone/cartilage during Caldwell-Luc operation and septal surgery.
    * *Punch biopsy:* From nose, oral cavity and pharynx.
    * *Tonsillectomy:* For holding the tonsils.
    * *Adenoidectomy:* For removing the tags of adenoids after the use of adenoid curette.

- *Ballenger's swivel knife:* The blade of this knife (available in different sizes) revolves automatically and changes direction while cutting the cartilage anteroposteriorly, downwards and posteroanteriorly. The blade is fitted by swivel joints to the handle so that the blade can rotate through 360° in the joints.
  - **Method:** It is introduced in a cut of the nasal septal cartilage and is pushed backwards, then downwards and finally forwards to remove a quadrangular piece of the septal cartilage.
  - **Use:** In SMR operation.

MOUTH GAGS AND RETRACTORS

- *Jennings mouth gag (Figs 59.13A and 59.14A):*
  - **Method:** It is placed in the centre of the mouth. The blades of this mouth gag fit over the alveolar margins and not over the teeth.
  - **Advantages:** Unlike Doyen's gag, it can be fitted to edentulous patients and does not damage the teeth.
- *Doyen's mouth gag (Figs 59.13B and 59.14C):* It keeps the mouth open for intraoral tongue surgery.
  - **Method:** It is applied on one side of the mouth on molar teeth. Its curved blades fit over the teeth. The lower jaw is depressed by the surgeon and the closed mouth gag is introduced in between the jaws and is gradually opened. It remains open by a ratchet.
  - **Uses:**
    * Operations of the oral cavity, such as tongue-tie release and excision of early tongue cancer.
    * Oral toilet in an unconscious patient for keeping the airway free.
    * Improving the movements of the temporomandibular joint ankylosis with trismus.
    * Prevent tongue bite in epileptics.
  - **Disadvantages:**
    * Chances of teeth damage.
    * Not used in edentulous patients.

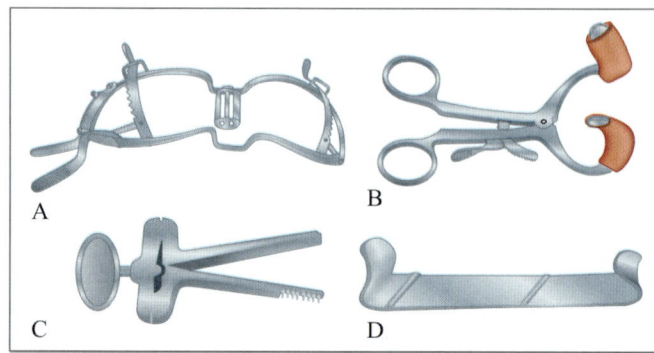

Figs 59.13A to D: Mouth gags. (A) Whitehead mouth gag with tongue depressor; (B) Doyen-Jansen mouth gag; (C) Heister mouth gag; (D) Roux cheek retractor
Source: Aesculap®, Germany

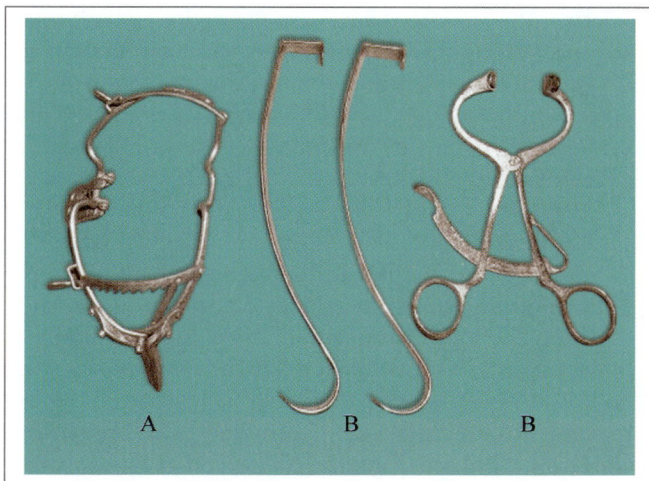

Figs 59.14A to C: Different types of mouth retractors. (A) Whitehead mouth gag with tongue depressor; (B) Hajek's retractors; (C) Doyen's pattern mouth gag

- **Cheek retractor (Fig. 59.13D):** It has a handle and a blade which is molded to fit snugly into the angle of the mouth. It retracts the cheek and exposes the teeth, gums and jaws.
  - *Uses:* It is used for making an incision for Caldwell-Luc operation and for interdental wiring for fractures of the maxilla and mandible.
- **Hajek' lip (cheek) retractor (Fig. 59.14B):** This is S-shaped retractor has two different types of ends. One end is bent at right angle and is used for retracting the upper lip. The other end is bent in a curved manner and is used by the assistant or the surgeon for supporting his thumb against the head of the patient. This end can be used for cheek retraction.
  - *Uses:* It retracts the upper lip during Caldwell-Luc operation and maxillectomy operations.

ADENOTONSILLECTOMY

See Chapter 'Adenotonsillectomy' and Figures 59.15 to 59.17.
- **Boyle-Davis mouth gag (Figs 59.15A to D and 59.16B):** This mouth gag remains open because of the ratchet. Tongue blades of various sizes are available. It opens the mouth and retracts the tongue anteriorly and inferiorly.
  - *Uses:* It is used for the surgeries of the oral cavity, oropharynx and nasopharynx such as
    - Tonsillectomy
    - Adenoidectomy
    - Snoring surgeries like uvulopalatopharyngoplasty
    - Palatal surgeries
    - Repair of cleft palate
    - Excision of angiofibroma
    - Removal of antrochoanal polyp
    - Craniovertebral anomalies

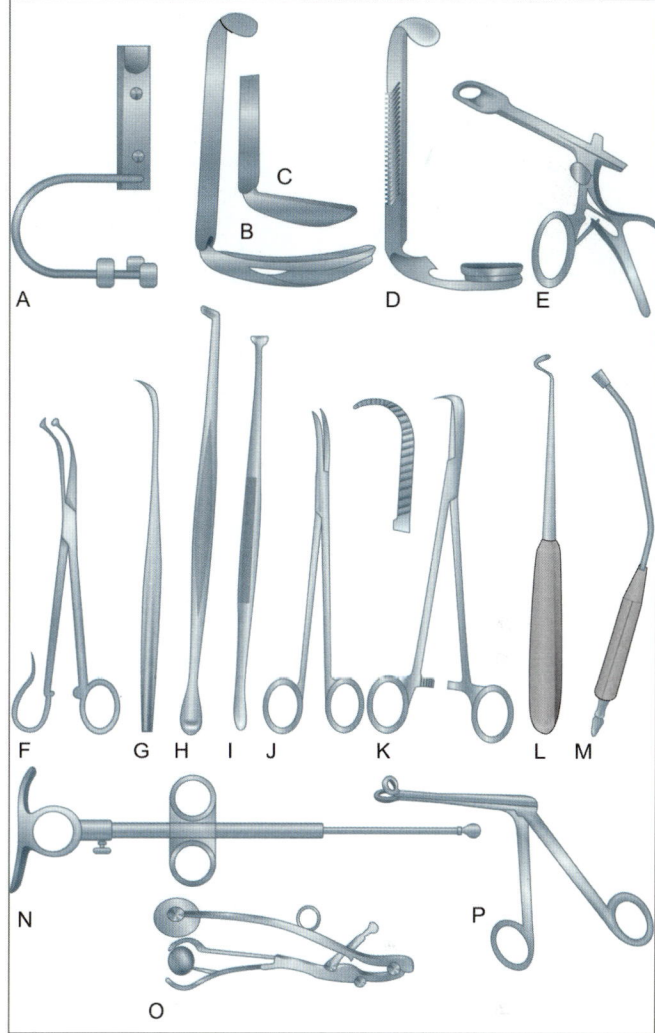

Figs 59.15A to P: Instruments of adenotonsillectomy. (A) Frame of Boyle Davis gag with interchangeable inserts suitable for many tongue depressors; (B) Russel Davis tongue blade with a groove for holding endotracheal tube, and protecting it from moving, kinking, or closure by teeth; (C) McIvor tongue blade; (D) Gast tongue blade with groove for endotracheal tube and lateral slot; (E) Sluder-Ballenger tonsillotome with blade and handle; (F) White tonsil holding forceps; (G) Abraham tonsil knife; (H) Henke Tonsil dissector; (I) Hurd tonsil dissector and pillar retractor; (J) Tonsil scissor; (K) Negus tonsil artery forceps; (L) Hurd ligature needle; (M) Yankauer suction tube; (N) Eves tonsil snare; (O) Corwin tonsil hemostats with spring clamp and sliding collar for holding gauze pad in position; (P) Hartmann tonsil punch forceps
Source: Aesculap, Germany

- **Method:** The built in tongue depressor along with the closed mouth gag is inserted in the mouth after depressing the lower jaw. The mouth gag is opened gradually. It is suspended from Draffin's bipods.
- **Draffin's bipod (Fig. 59.16A):** There are two pods and each has four rings in a row. The two pods are assembled together as per the height at which the tongue blade of the Boyle-Davis mouth gag is suspended. The lower ends of the pods are placed

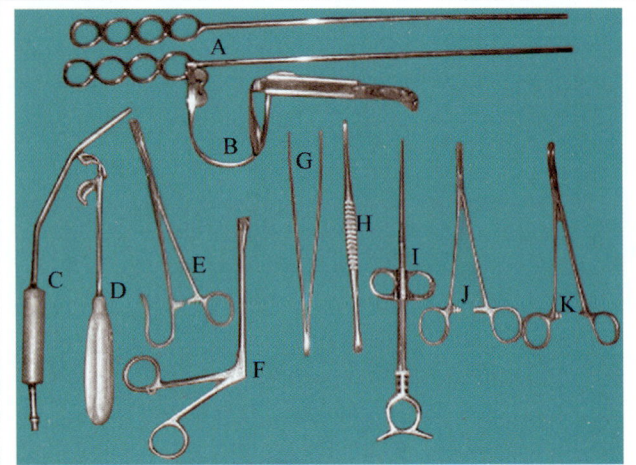

Figs 59.16A to K: Instruments of adenotonsillectomy. (A) Draffin suspension apparatus (two bipods); (B) Boyle Davis mouth gag with tongue depressor; (C) Yankauer's tonsil suction tube; (D) St. Clair Thomson's adenoid curette with guard; (E) Peacock Vulsellum tonsil holding forceps; (F) Tonsil holding forceps; (G) Waugh's tenaculum tonsil dissection forceps with teeth; (H) Tonsil dissector and retractor; (I) Eves tonsil snare; (J) Straight tonsil artery forceps; (K) Curved tonsil artery forceps

in one of the several depressions of the Magauran's plate.
- *Use:* They are used along with Boyle-Davis mouth gag.
- **Tonsil holding forceps (Denis Browne's):** They resemble Luc forceps, but their fenestrated jaws are not sharp. The upper jaw sits within the larger lower jaw. There are many other types of tonsil holding forceps (Figs 59.15F and 59.16E and F).
  - *Use:* These are meant for holding the tonsil during tonsillar dissection. Luc forceps may also be used.
- **Tonsil knife (Fig. 59.15G):** This is sickle-shaped knife.
  - *Use:* It is used for making the first mucosal incision of tonsillectomy at the upper pole of tonsil.
- **Tonsil dissector and anterior pillar retractor (Fig. 59.15I):**
  - *Uses:*
    * *Tonsillectomy:* Its blunt end is used to dissect the tonsil. Its C-shaped bent end is used to retract the anterior tonsillar pillar and helps in inspecting the fossa for any bleeding. The retraction of anterior pillar also provides better visualization of tonsil especially fibrosed tonsil before surgery so that tonsil holding forceps can be applied properly.
    * *Nasopharynx:* It can be used in retracting the soft palate and uvula during adenoidectomy and for examining the nasopharynx.
- **Tonsil scissors (Fig. 59.15J):** These are long scissors with slightly bent blunt tips.
  - *Use:* They are used for sharp dissection of the tonsils and cutting the ligatures. They can also be used for tongue tie release and uvulectomy for long uvula.
- **Tonsil needle (Fig. 59.15L):** It consists of needle and handle. The sharp curved needle is at a right angle to the long handle.
  - *Use:* It is used for sewing the tonsillar pillars together for controlling the bleeding, which is not controlled by ligation and cauterization of bleeding points.
- **Yankauer's suction tube (Figs 59.15M and 59.16C):** This long suction cannula consists of large handle and covered tip that prevents damage to mucosa.
  - *Uses:* It is used for suction in tonsillectomy and other oral, oropharyngeal and nasopharyngeal operations.
- **Eve's tonsil snare (Figs 59.15N and 59.16I):**
  - *Use:* When firmly closed, it crushes and cuts the pedicle and minimizes the bleeding.
  - *Method of application:* The index and the middle fingers are passed into the two rings on the outer tube of the snare, and the thumb is introduced in the ring of the central movable slide. The loop of the fully opened snare wire is threaded on the tonsil holding forceps. The snare wire loop is pushed down up to the lower pole of the tonsil. On closing by pushing the slide into the tube with the thumb, the snare wire loop is withdrawn into the tube of the snare and the tonsil is removed.
- **Conchotome (Fig. 59.15P):** This punch biopsy forceps open like the jaws of a crocodile and is bent at an obtuse angle. The upper smaller ring sits inside the larger lower ring.
  - *Uses:* It is used for punching out pieces of the turbinates. It is also used for removing the tags of adenoids and taking punch biopsy.
- **Draffin's bipod (Fig. 59.16A):** There are two pods and each has four rings in a row. The two pods are assembled together as per the height at which the tongue blade of the Boyle-Davis mouth gag is suspended. The lower ends of the pods are placed in one of the several depressions of the Magauran's plate.
  - *Use:* They are used along with Boyle-Davis mouth gag.
- **St. Clair Thomson's adenoid curette (Figs 59.16D and 59.17B):** There are two varieties: (1) with cage (guard); and (2) plane without cage (guard). The curette shaves off the adenoid mass while the guard holds the adenoid tissue and prevents from slipping. The sharp transverse blade cuts adenoids and holds them in a cage with the help of the fangs in the cage. Remaining tags of adenoids are removed by a smaller plain adenoid curette, Luc forceps or conchotome.
  - *Use:* For adenoidectomy it is held in dagger holding fashion. The plane curette is used to remove adenoid tissue around the Eustachian tube.

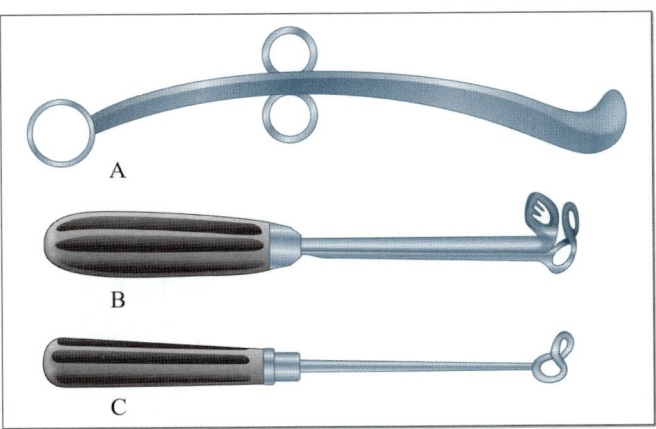

Figs 59.17A to C: Instruments of adenoidectomy. (A) LaForce adenotome; (B) St. Clair-Thompson adenoid curette with catcher; (C) Beckmann adenoid curette

- **Caution:** The neck flexion avoids subluxation of atlanto-occipital joint. Bring the adenoid tissue from lateral wall to midline by right index finger. Keep the curette with cage in midline.
- **Tonsil dissection forceps with teeth (Waugh's) (Fig. 59.16G)**
    - **Use:** It is used for putting incision in the mucous membrane and dissection of tonsil.
- **Tonsil artery forceps (straight and curved) (Figs 59.16J and K):** The tip of Negus artery forceps (Fig. 59.15K) is sharply curved and is used as replacement forceps to ligate the bleeding point.
    - **Use:** The straight forceps is used to catch the bleeding point and is replaced by curved forceps before tying a ligature.
- **Negus knot tyer:** It has a blunt forked end and slips the ligature knot beyond the curved tip of the artery forceps.
    - Use: It helps in tying the ligature knot up to the tip of curved artery forceps that holds the vessel.

INCISION AND DRAINAGE OF QUINSY

- **Peritonsillar (Quinsy) abscess forceps (Fig. 59.18):** These bayonet-shaped quinsy forceps have a sharp trocar point with a shoulder that prevents deep entry. See Chapter 'Deep Neck Infections' for other related details.
    - **Use:** It is used for drainage of peritonsillar abscess.
    - **Method:** The sharp trocar tip of closed forceps is inserted into the abscess and then forceps are opened like a sinus forceps to drain the pus.

ENDOSCOPES

There are two types of illumination in the rigid hollow tube scopes, Jackson and Negus. The illumination is distal in Jackson type and proximal in Negus type (Table 59.1).

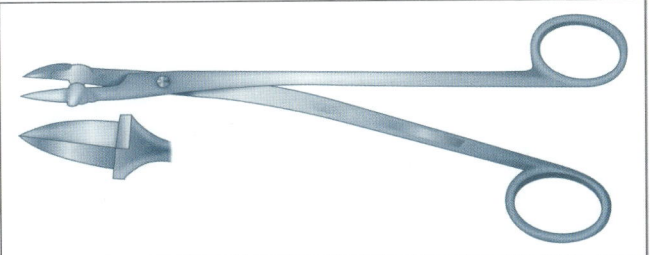

Fig. 59.18: Peritonsillar abscess forceps

Table 59.1: Comparison between two types of illumination (Jackson and Negus) in traditional hollow tube rigid scopes

Characteristics	Jackson pattern	Negus pattern
Location of illumination	Distal	Proximal
Brightness	Less bright	More bright
Number of illuminants	One	Two
Visibility of forceps tip	Good	Poor
Chances of secretions covering illuminant	Frequent	Occasional
Width of scope	Narrow	Broader
Vision	Relatively poor	Better
Introduction	Easy	Relatively difficult

Figures 59.19 and 59.20 show the instruments used for laryngoscopy and bronchoscopy and esophagoscopy respectively. For further related details, see Chapter 'Endoscopies'.

Laryngoscopes

Laryngoscope used for direct laryngoscopy has light carrier which is connected to a cold light source through a flexible cable. There are several models of laryngoscopes (Figs 59.19A to K). The size of laryngoscope is selected as per the age of the patient. The larynx and hypopharynx are visualized directly with the help of laryngoscope.

- **Direct laryngoscope (Jackson) (Fig. 59.19A):** This U-shaped laryngoscope consists of a metal tube with illumination at the distal end (through which laryngoscopy is performed) and a right-angled handle.
    - **Uses:** They are used for direct laryngoscopy. Some laryngoscopes have a detachable posterior blade for inserting bronchoscope and esophagoscope.

Bronchoscope

Bronchoscope (Fig. 59.20A) consists of a hollow metal tube. Jackson type has distal illumination. There are openings (vents) at the distal part of the tube for the aeration of the side bronchi. The size of bronchoscope should be selected as per the age of the patient (Table 59.2).

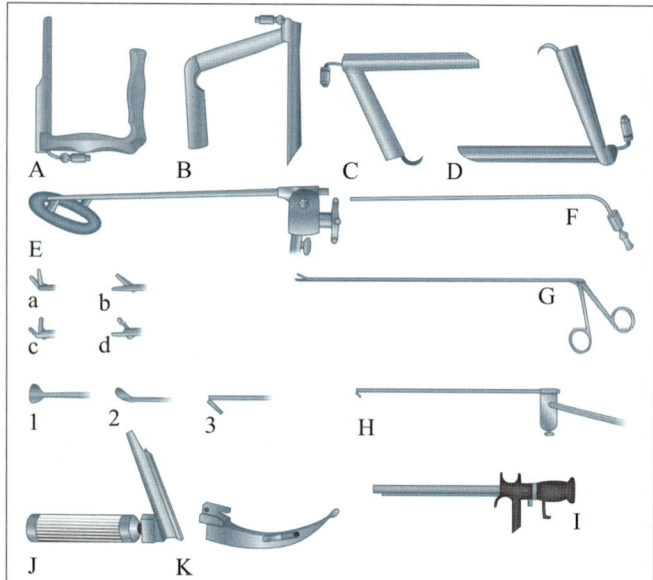

Figs 59.19A to K: Laryngoscopic instruments. (A) Jackson laryngoscope; (B) Holinger anterior commissure laryngoscope; (C) Kleinsasser operating laryngoscope; (D) Stange hour glass operating laryngoscope; (E) Ricker Kleinsasser laryngoscope holder and chest support for adult and children; (F) Suction tube; (G) Kleinsasser laryngeal forceps: (a) angled scissor, (b) straight alligator, (c) angled cupped jaws, (d) straight cupped jaws; (H) Handle for use with Kleinsasser laryngeal instruments: (1) straight knife, (2) curved knife, (3) blunt laryngeal hook; (I) Hopkins lateral Telelaryngopharyngoscope 90°; (J) Magill folding laryngoscope; (K) McIntosh folding laryngoscope
Source: Karl Storz, Germany

Esophagoscope

Esophagoscope (Fig. 59.20K) appears similar to the bronchoscope but does not have vents. It is used for diagnostic and therapeutic esophagoscopy. The size of the esophagoscope is selected as per the age of the patient. Handle at the proximal end of esophagoscope indicates the direction of the bevel at the distal end.

A bronchoscope may be used for performing esophagoscopy but the esophagoscope cannot be used for bronchoscopy.

TRACHEOSTOMY

- **Tracheal dilator (Fig. 59.21 TD):** The blades spread out on approximating its rings. Its tip is blunt. A curved artery forceps can also serve its purpose.
  - *Use:* It keeps the cut tracheal edges open so that tracheostomy tube can be easily introduced.
- **Tracheal hook (blunt and sharp)**
  - **Blunt:** It retracts the thyroid isthmus and exposes the trachea. It may also be used for retracting the strap muscles.

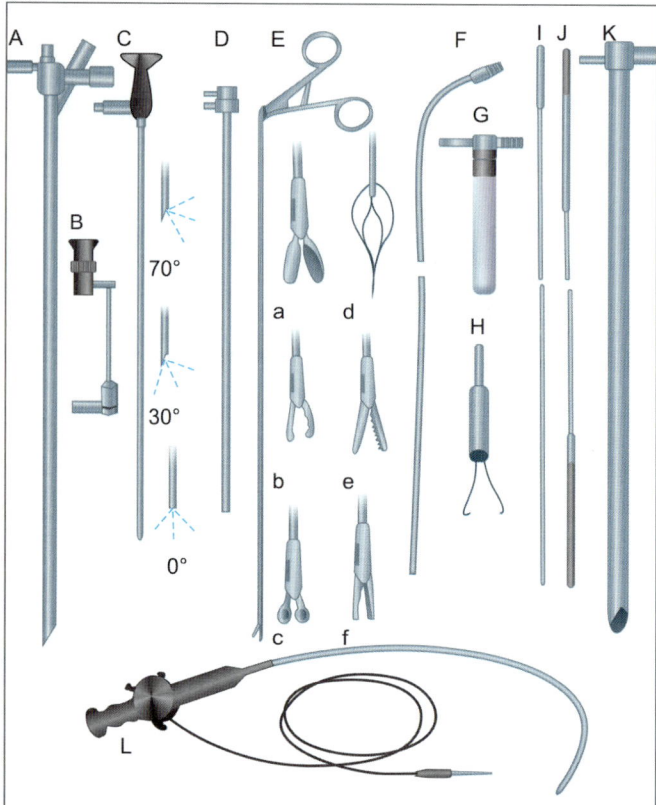

Figs 59.20A to K: Bronchoesophagoscopy instruments. (A) Bronchoscope tube; (B) Adjustable magnifier; (C) Hopkins telescope: 0°, 30°, and 70°; (D) Rubber telescope guide; (E) Forceps: peanut grasping (a), universal biopsy and grasping (b), circular cup biopsy (c), foreign body basket (d), alligator grasping (e), and rotating sharp pointed (f); (F) Rigid suction tube; (G) Specimen collector may be attached directly to suction tubes; (H) Sponge holder for sterile smear cytology; (I) Cotton carrier; (J) Bougie; (K) Oval esophagoscope tube; (L) Broncho fiberscope with instrument channel
Source: Karl Storz, Germany

Table 59.2: Size of bronchoscope and the age of patient

Age group	Size of bronchoscope lumen (mm)
Preterm neonates	2.5–3.0
1–2 years	3.5–4
3–9 years	4.5–5
9–14 years	6

- **Sharp:** It retracts the lower border of cricoid cartilage and thus stabilizes the trachea when making incision in the anterior wall of trachea.

Types of Tracheostomy Tubes (Figs 59.21 and 59.22)

There are various types of tubes. *See* Box 59.1 for the classification of tracheostomy tubes.

They can be grouped on the bases of cuff, fenestra, length, number of lumen and the material. Some of the commonly used tubes are described here.

Chapter 59 • Instruments

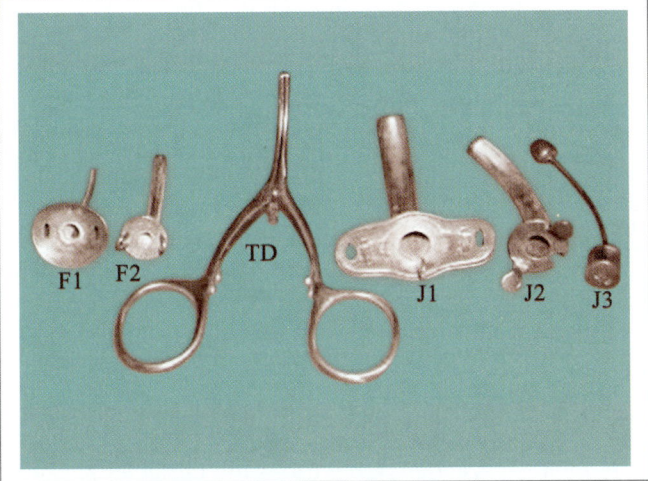

Fig. 59.21: Metallic tracheostomy tubes and tracheal dilator (TD). Fuller's bivalved tracheostomy tube has two tubes outer two blades (bivalve) tube (F1) and inner fenestrated tube (F2). Jackson's tracheostomy tube has three parts: outer tube (J1), inner tube (J2) and an obturator (J3)

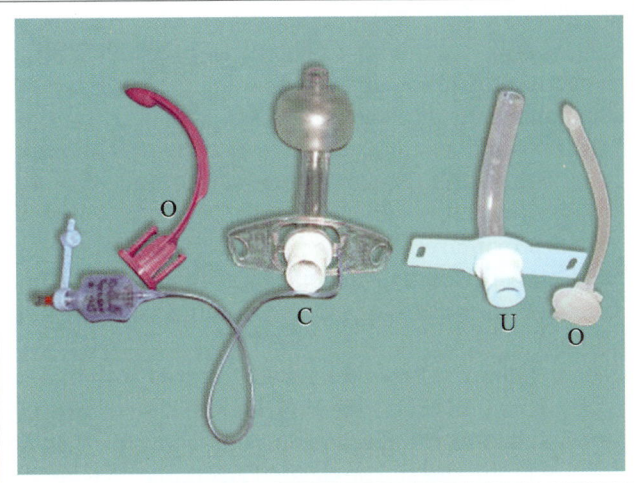

Fig. 59.22: Nonmetallic tracheostomy tubes. Cuffed (C) and Uncuffed (U) tubes with their obturator (O)

- ***Fenestra at the upper curvature of the tube:*** It helps in speech production or in weaning from tracheostomy.
- ***Extra length tracheostomy tubes:*** They are used in cases of thick or swollen pretracheal tissue, a growth and stenosis in trachea and postcricoid growth pressing trachea.
- ***Adjustable flange long tube:*** The flange can be adjusted.
- ***Single lumen (cannula) tube:*** It has only one cannula.
- ***Double lumen (cannula) tube:*** It has inner cannula and outer cannula.
- ***Metallic tubes:*** They are formed from the alloy of silver, copper and phosphorus.
- ***Polyvinyl chloride (PVC) tubes:*** They are disposable (single use) and thermolabile. They adjust to tracheal lumen.
- ***Silicone tubes:*** The advantages include less crusting and no adherence of bacteria and secretions.
- ***Siliconized PVC tubes:*** They offer advantages of both PVC and silicon tubes.
- ***Silastic tubes:*** They are soft and non-irritating and minimize the crusting.
- ***Rubber tubes:*** They are most economical.
- ***Armored tubes:*** The plastic tubes are reinforced by a spiral or rings of stainless steel. They do not get kinked.

Fuller's Bivalved Tracheostomy Tube

It has two tubes outer and inner (Figs 59.21, F1 and F2). The inner tube is slightly longer than outer tube. The two blades (bivalve) of the outer tube when pressed together can be easily inserted into the tracheostomy opening. There is no need of a pilot and a tracheal dilator. The central hole in the inner tube provides a chance to breathe when tube is blocked by a finger, cork or secretions. The tip of the compressed outer tube is not so blunt and may cause injury.

Box 59.1: Classification of tracheostomy tubes

- **On the basis of cuff**
  - Uncuffed
  - Cuffed tubes
    - Single cuff tube
    - Double cuff tube
    - Low pressure cuff tube
- **On the basis of fenestra at the upper curvature of tube**
  - Tubes without fenestra
  - Single fenestrated tube
  - Multiple fenestrated tube
- **On the basis of length of the tube**
  - Standard length
  - Extra length tracheostomy tube
    - Adjustable flange long tube
- **On the basis of number of lumens (cannula)**
  - Single lumen (cannula) tube – Nonmetallic
  - Double lumen (cannula) tube – Jackson and Fuller
  - Suction-aided tracheostomy tubes – Metallic
- **On the basis of the material**
  - Metallic
    - Jackson
    - Fuller
  - Nonmetallic
    - Polyvinyl chloride (PVC)
    - Silicone
    - Siliconized PVC
    - Silastic
    - Rubber tube
  - Mixed
    - Armored tubes

Chevalier Jackson's Tracheostomy Tube

Traditionally, it is made of silver or German silver which is nonirritating. It has three parts—outer tube, inner tube and an obturator (Figs 59.21, J1 to J3).

1. **Outer tube:** Outer tube fits into the tracheostomy opening. When the inner tube is removed, the outer tube continues to serve the function. Shield is attached to the proximal end of outer tube and is fixed to the neck by a tape threaded through the holes of the shield. Lock fitted on the shield fixes the inner tube inside the outer tube.
2. **Inner tube:** The inner tube is slightly longer than outer tube. It can be fixed to the shield of the outer tube by a lock. The longer inner tube does not allow the blocking of outer tube and can be cleaned and replaced regularly.
3. **Obturator (pilot):** The obturator is passed in the outer tube and helps in the introduction of tube into the trachea. Its blunt rounded end is inserted into the outer tube after removing the inner tube. It is used for inserting the tracheostomy tube into the trachea. When tube is inserted in its position, pilot is withdrawn and inner tube is inserted back into the outer tube.

Metallic tubes cannot be used during radiotherapy and MRI. Metal tubes become radioactive by irradiation. Patient cannot speak with patent tube in position. The speaking valve can be used with metallic tubes.

Nonmetallic Tracheostomy Tubes (Fig. 59.22)

These tubes are usually larger than the metallic tubes and are available with or without pressure cuff. These tubes are useful for patients undergoing radiation therapy (metal tubes become radioactive by irradiation) and MRI.

- **Cuffed tracheostomy tube:** The external bulb in cuffed tubes tells the status of inside cuff.
  - **Indications:** Cuff tracheostomy tubes are required when patients need anesthesia or intermittent positive pressure respiration. It is used in unconscious patient or when patient is on a respirator.
  - **Advantages:** The inflated cuff prevents not only aspiration of secretions into the trachea, but also prevents air leak and keeps the position in tube.
  - **Precautions:** Cuff should be deflated every 2 hours for 5 minutes to prevent pressure damage to the trachea. In the current two cuffs tube, inflation of the cuff can be alternated. The current low pressure cuff tubes may not damage the trachea and avoids tracheal stenosis.
- **Cuffed suction aid tracheostomy tube:** The inbuilt suction channel reaches above the cuff and helps in sucking out pharyngeal secretion collected above the cuff.

Cuffed tracheostomy tube: Suction is done before deflating the cuff. It avoids the aspiration of accumulated pharyngeal secretions into the trachea.

Nonmetallic tracheostomy tubes are useful for patients undergoing radiation therapy and MRI. They are less traumatic to trachea.

Size of Tracheostomy Tube

Tracheostomy tubes are of different sizes or numbers. Larger the number, greater is the inner diameter. In adults, tubes of inner diameter varying between 6 mm and 9 mm or 10 mm are used. Sometimes, size of tube (Jackson's or Negus) is expressed in French gauge (FG), which is about three times the size of internal diameter. It means 8 mm internal diameter will have approximately 24 FG.

FG = outer diameter x π (π = 3.14 or approx 3)

- **Children:** An appropriate size of tracheostomy tube should be selected as per the age of the patient (Table 59.3).

AIRWAY DEVICES

See Chapter 'Management of Impaired Airway' for laryngeal mask airway, oropharyngeal airway and nasopharyngeal airways, etc.

Table 59.3: Size of tracheostomy tube and the age of patient

Age group	Tracheostomy tube size lumen (mm)
Preterm neonates	2.5–3.0
1–2 years	3.5–4
3–6 years	4.5–5
6–12 years	5.5–6
12–14 years	7
Adults	8–9

Section 9: Related Disciplines

Chapter 60

Diagnostic Imaging

⦿ Specific Learning Objectives
After going through the chapter, you should be able to identify the normal structures and the abnormalities seen in the routinely performed conventional X-rays and CT and MRI scans of head and neck region.

The increased availability of new imaging modalities are making the accurate diagnostic process easier and replacing the conventional radiology. It is the key to good otolaryngology practice. ENT surgeon must be able to recognize the most appropriate test to fit the clinical context. Though the simple and least expensive imaging [conventional X-rays and ultrasound (US)] should be preferred, but in complex problems, more expensive scans [Computerized tomography/Magnetic resonance imaging (CT/MRI)] are more cost-effective as they lead to early and confident diagnosis and management. If frequent imaging studies are expected, then nonradiation-dependent modalities (MRI and US) must be preferred as they avoid the adverse effects of the radiation (especially in children and young) such as cancer and genetic defects.

CONVENTIONAL RADIOLOGY

X-rays are absorbed differently by soft tissue, bone, gas and fat. X-ray of chest is requested commonly for preanesthetic assessment to exclude tuberculosis, pulmonary metastasis and bronchogenic carcinoma.

Temporal Bone (Fig. 60.1)

- ***Areas of translucency (semitransparent):*** Their causes are cholesteatoma, mastoidectomy, malignancy, eosinophil granuloma, tuberculosis of mastoid, multiple myeloma, glomus and large antral and periantral mastoid air cells.
- ***Law's view (lateral view of mastoid):*** Sagittal plane of the skull is parallel to the film; X-ray beam is projected 15° cephalocaudal. Key areas of the mastoid (attic, aditus and antrum) are not seen well.
  - ***Structures seen:*** External auditory canal (EAC) superimposed on internal auditory canal (IAC), mastoid air cells, tegmen, lateral sinus plate and temporomandibular joint.
- ***Schullar's view:*** This frequently used view is similar to Law's view, but X-ray beam is projected 30° cephalocaudal and prevents superimposition of two sides of mastoid bones.
  - ***Structures seen:*** EAC superimposed on IAC, mastoid air cells, tegmen, lateral sinus plate, condyle of mandible, sinodural angle and atticoantral region (key areas for cholesteatoma and its erosion).
  - ***Clinical applications:*** Extent of pneumatization, sclerotic mastoid, destruction of intercellular septa (mastoiditis), location of sinus plate (position of sigmoid sinus) and tegmen (roof of middle ear and floor of middle cranial fossa), cholesteatoma and longitudinal fracture of petrous pyramid.

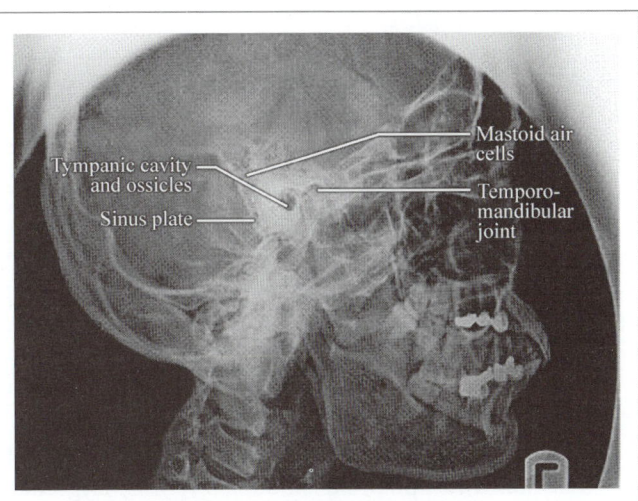

Fig. 60.1: X-ray mastoid left–normal
Source: Dr Jayesh Patel, Consultant Radiologist, Anand, Gujarat

- **Stenver's view:** Long axis of the petrous bone lies parallel to the film.
  - *Structures seen:* Entire petrous pyramid, arcuate eminence, internal auditory meatus, labyrinth with its vestibule, cochlea and mastoid antrum.
- **Towne's view:** This is an anteroposterior view of skull with 30° tilt from above and in front. It shows both petrous pyramids, which can be compared.
  - *Structures seen:* Both side temporal bones, arcuate eminence, superior semicircular canal, mastoid antrum, IAC, tympanic cavity, cochlea and EAC.
  - *Clinical applications:* Acoustic neuroma and apical petrositis.
- **Transorbital view:** This is an anteroposterior view of skull. Orbitomeatal line is at right angles to the film. X-ray beam passes through the orbit.
  - *Structures seen:* IAC, cochlea, labyrinth and both petrous pyramids projected through the orbits.
  - *Clinical applications:* Acoustic neuroma and petrous pyramid.
- **Submentovertical view:** Vertex remains near the film and X-ray beam is projected from the submental area.
  - *Structures seen:* EAC, mastoid cells, middle ear, eustachian tube, IAC, foramen ovale and spinosum, carotid canal, and sphenoid, posterior ethmoid and maxillary sinuses (seen best in that order), zygoma, zygomatic arches, mandible along with coronoid and condyle processes.

Nose and Paranasal Sinuses

The most common view taken for paranasal sinus is Water's view and second one is Caldwell view.

- **Common radiological findings:**
  - Slight haziness in sinuses due to mucosal thickening.
  - Presence of cyst (missing tooth in dentigerous cyst).
  - An opacity with horizontal level due to fluid in chronic sinusitis.
  - Opacity due to sinusitis, antrochoanal polyp (maxillary sinus) and malignancy (opacity beyond the sinus limit due to erosion).
  - Dense opacity with regular outline (osteoma).
  - Multilocular swelling expanding the bone (osteoclastoma).
- **Water's view (occipitomental view):** Nose and chin touch the film and X-ray beam is projected from occipital side. Open mouth view shows sphenoid sinus. Petrous bones are projected below the maxillary sinuses. Fractures of right and left nasal bones and their lateral displacement can be seen.
  - *Structures seen (Fig. 60.2):* Maxillary (seen best), frontal and sphenoid sinuses, zygoma, zygomatic arch, nasal bones, frontal process of maxilla, superior orbital fissure and infratemporal fossa.

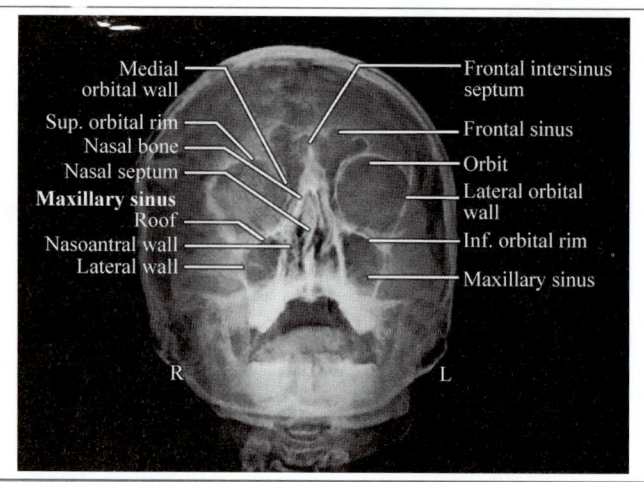

Fig. 60.2: X-ray PNS Water's view–normal
Source: Dr Jayesh Patel, Consultant Radiologist, Anand, Gujarat

- **Caldwell view (occipitofrontal view):** Nose and forehead touch the film and X-ray beam is projected 15–20° caudally. Frontal and ethmoidal sinuses are seen well in this view.
  - *Structures seen:* Frontal, ethmoid and maxillary sinuses, frontal process of zygoma, zygomatic process of frontal bone, superior margins of orbits, lamina papyracea, superior orbital fissures and foramen rotundum.
- **Lateral view**
  - *Structures seen (Fig. 60.3):* Anterior and posterior extents of sphenoid, frontal and maxillary sinuses, sella turcica, ethmoid sinuses, alveolar process, condyle and neck of mandible.
  - *Right and left oblique views:* For seeing the posterior ethmoid sinuses and the optic foramen.

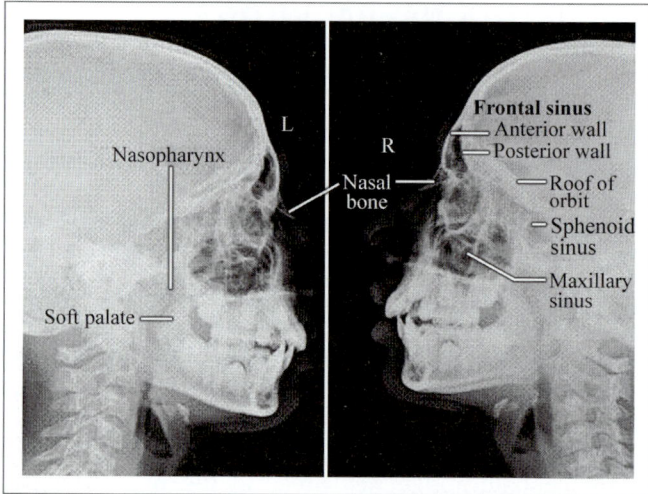

Fig. 60.3: X-ray nasal bones lateral view left and right showing fracture of septal cartilage
Source: Dr Jayesh Patel, Consultant Radiologist, Anand, Gujarat

- *Lateral views of nasal bones:* To see fracture line, depression or elevation of the fractures segment. Lower part of nasal bones, which is thin, fracture more frequently. Groove for ethmoidal nerve and vessels may look like fracture line.
- *Occlusal view of nasal bone:* Film is held between the teeth and X-ray beam is projected perpendicular to the film. It shows fracture line and lateral displacement of the nasal pyramid clearly.

Neck, Larynx and Pharynx

- *Lateral view of neck (Fig. 60.4)*
  - *Structure seen:* Outline of base of tongue, vallecula, hyoid bone, epiglottis and aryepiglottic folds, arytenoids, false and true cords with ventricle in between them, thyroid and cricoid cartilages, subglottic space and trachea, prevertebral soft tissues, cervical spines and pretracheal soft tissues and thyroid.
  - *Clinical applications:*
    - *Radio-opaque foreign bodies* of larynx, pharynx and upper esophagus.
    - *Acute epiglottitis*
    - *Retropharyngeal abscess:* Retropharyngeal widening with fluid level and straightening of cervical spines, and/or tuberculosis of cervical vertebrae.
    - *Position of tracheostomy tube*, T-tube and laryngeal stent.
    - *Laryngeal stenosis*.
    - *Fractures of larynx and hyoid bone* and their displacement.
    - *Compression of trachea* by thyroid or retropharyngeal masses.
    - *Osteophytes in cervical vertebrae* and injuries of spine.
- *Posteroanterior view of neck:* It helps in differentiating between a foreign body of larynx and esophagus (lateral view is also needed). It shows compression or displacement of trachea by lateral neck masses such as thyroid swellings.
- *Soft tissue lateral view nasopharynx:* For soft tissue masses in the nasopharynx, soft palate, roof and posterior wall of nasopharynx.
  - *Clinical applications:*
    - *Adenoids*
    - *Angiofibroma:* Soft tissue density arising from posterosuperior wall of nasopharynx and interrupting the airway.
    - *Antrochoanal polyp:* Soft tissue density with a column of air between the mass and posterior wall of nasopharynx.
    - *Foreign body nose and tumor.*
    - *Choanal atresia:* Interruption of air column from nose to nasopharynx.
- *Submandibular salivary gland:* Radio-opaque calculus can be seen.

Barium Swallow

For further detail, *see* 'Barium Esophagography' in Chapter 'Pharyngeal Symptoms and Examination'.

Foreign bodies (FBs) of airway and esophagus: Figures 60.5 to 60.9 shows various FBs of respiratory passage, cricopharynx and esophagus. For more Figures *see* FBs Esophagus in Chapter 'Disorders of Esophagus'.

ORTHOPANTOMOGRAM

A pantomograph is a panoramic radiograph machine. It permits visualization of entire maxillary and mandibular dentition, alveolar arches and contiguous structures on a single extraoral film.

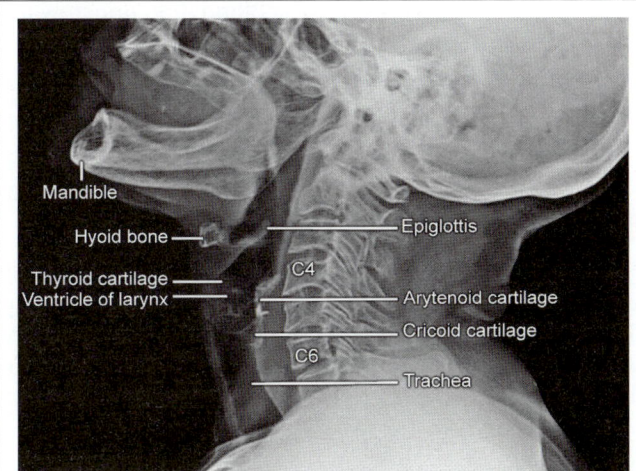

Fig. 60.4: X-ray soft tissue neck and nasopharynx lateral view
Source: Dr Jayesh Patel, Consultant Radiologist, Anand, Gujarat

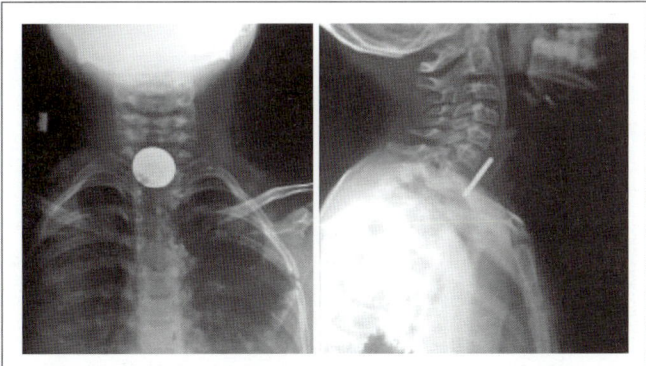

Fig. 60.5: FB (coin) in cricopharynx. X-ray neck and chest PA and lateral views

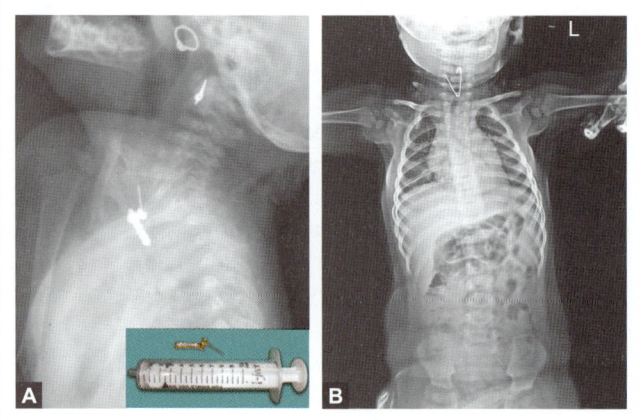

Fig. 60.6: FBs Esophagus. (A) X-ray neck and chest lateral view showing radio-opaque FB in upper esophagus (Earring shown inset); (B) X-ray chest and neck PA view showing FB (open safety pin) in cricopharynx
Courtesy: Dr. Alpesh Fefar, Surendranagar, Gujarat

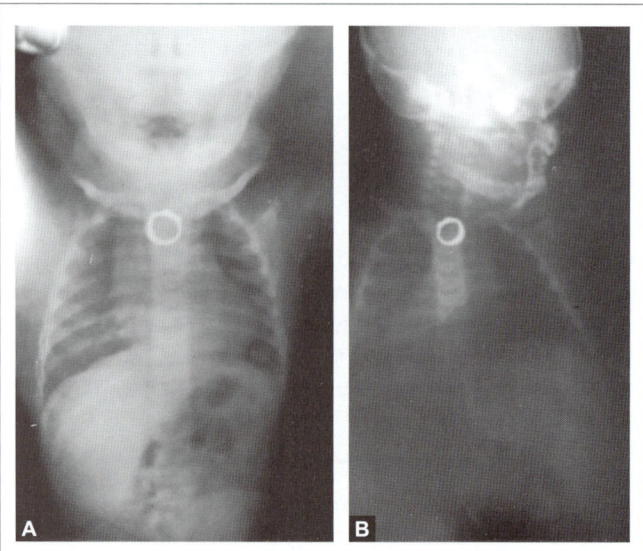

Figs 60.7A and B: FB (ring) upper esophagus. (A) X-ray neck and chest PA; (B) Lateral view
Courtesy: Dr. Alpesh Fefar, Surendranagar, Gujarat

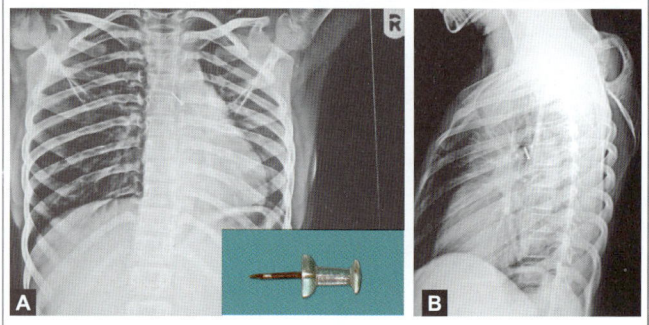

Figs 60.8A and B: FB (Notice board pin) bronchus. (A) X-ray chest PA view; (B) X-ray chest Lateral view; FB shown in inset
Courtesy: Dr. Alpesh Fefar, Surendranagar, Gujarat

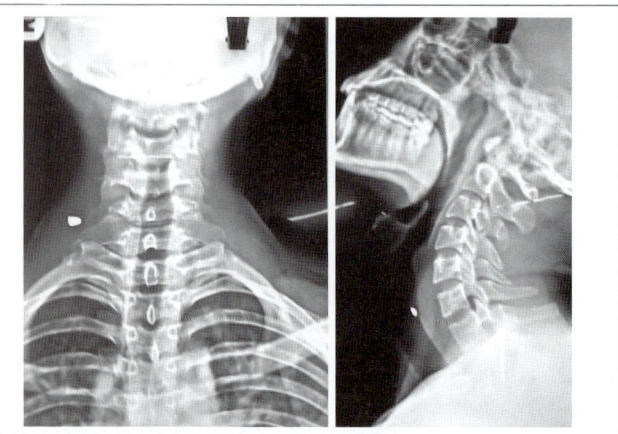

Fig. 60.9: Penetrating metallic FB in lower part of sternocleidomastoid muscle. X-ray neck PA and lateral view. Note the Lateral view is giving the illusion of FB trachea.
Courtesy: Dr. Alpesh Fefar, Surendranagar, Gujarat

Box 60.1: Echogenicity of various tissues

- *Fat:* Moderate degree of internal echoes.
- *Skeletal muscle:* Less echogenic than fat.
- *Solid mass:* Well-defined margins with variable echogenicity, but less echogenic than fat.
- *Cyst:* Few internal echoes, but strong echogenic back wall.
- *Calcium and bone:* Strongly echogenic.

ULTRASOUND

Ultrasound (US) requires an experienced operator. It is inexpensive, quick, reliable, noninvasive and effective investigation.

US allows differentiation between solid and cystic masses and assessment of margins and texture of neck swellings (Box 60.1).

- *Doppler ultrasound:* It measures blood flow of vessels.
- *Color doppler:* Flowing blood appears either red or blue, which depends upon the blood direction, towards or away from the transducer.
- *Power doppler:* It can demonstrate tissue perfusion.

Ultrasound: It is better than CT in differentiating solid from cystic lesions.

COMPUTERIZED TOMOGRAPHY

Computerized tomography (CT) is now becoming readily available and fast replacing the need of plain X-rays (Fig. 60.10). CT is quite commonly used to diagnose refractory cases of rhinosinusitis and for staging head and neck malignancies.

Due to the high degree of over-lap between the densities (gray tones), it is difficult to differentiate between lymph nodes, muscles and vessels.

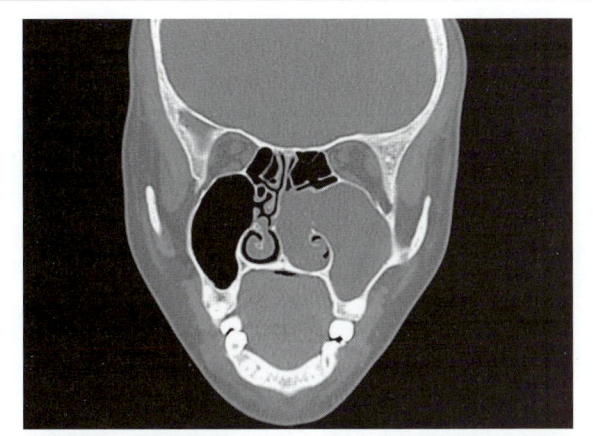

Fig. 60.10: CT scan plain coronal section nose and paranasal sinuses showing antrochoanal polyp
Source: Dr Amit Goyal, AIIMS, Jodhpur

- ***Spiral CT:*** Helical or spiral CT scans a volume of tissue and provides better quality images than the conventional CT.
- ***Contrast CT:*** Intravenous contrast agents allow identification of rim enhancement in pathological lymph nodes and increase the definition of primary tumors.
- ***CT angiography:*** The facilities enhance characteristics of tissues in both arterial and venous phases of imaging.
- ***Processing of volumetric data:*** The volumetric data can be processed to produce—
  - *Multiplanar images:* Sagittal and coronal
  - *Three-dimensional (3D) images*
  - *Virtual endoscopy:* Such as laryngoscopy, bronchoscopy and sinuscopy.

MAGNETIC RESONANCE IMAGING

High contrast resolution and multiplanar imaging capability make MRI ideal for intracranial, spinal and musculoskeletal imaging.

Machines

Clinical MRI machines operate at magnetic field strengths of between 0.5 and 2.0 tesla (T). Higher the field strength of the magnet, higher the signal-to-noise ratio and higher is the quality of MRI. The open access magnets allow interventional procedures.

Imaging Protocols

- ***T1W:*** Because of high soft tissue discrimination, T1W images show exquisite anatomical details (Fig. 60.11A).
- ***T2W:*** The pathological lesions increase T2 de-phase times, which produce higher signal than surrounding normal tissue in T2W images (Fig. 60.11B).

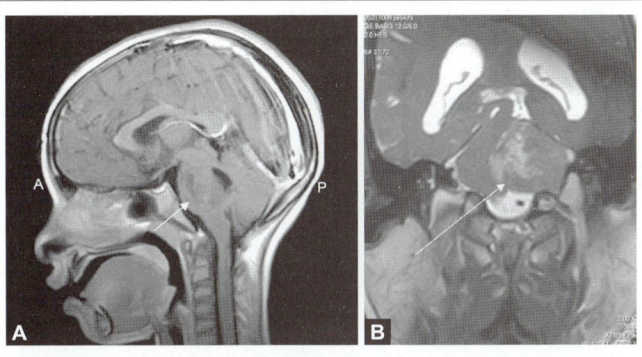

Figs 60.11A and B: (A) MRI head sagittal section T1-weighted; (B) MRI head axial section T2-weighted
Source: Dr Ritesh Prajapati, Consultant Radiologist, Anand, Gujarat

The combination of T1W and T2W images is good for characterizing fluid containing structures, solid components and hemorrhage.

- ***Gadolinium-enhanced T1W:*** Intravenous gadolinium reduces T1 relaxation time and enhances lesions, which appear as high signal intensity areas (improved delineation of tumor margins relative to the lower signal of muscle, bone, vessel and globe).
- ***Magnetic resonance angiography:*** It uses specific sequences and demonstrates flowing blood.

- **MRI, Doppler and ultrasound:** These imaging technologies do not use ionizing radiation.
- **MRI contraindication:** It should not be used in the third trimester of pregnancy.
- **Acoustic neuroma:** MRI is superior to CT in diagnosis of acoustic neuroma.

INTERVENTIONAL RADIOLOGY

Ultrasound and CT guidance can be employed to choose shortest route from skin to the lesion. US, which is quick and flexible, allows needle path in real time without radiation hazard. Some of the indications are:
- Percutaneous biopsy
- Drainage of abscess and fluid collection
- Percutaneous gastrostomy
- High local dose of chemotherapy to feeding vessels of tumor.
- Angioplasty and vascular stenting.
- Therapeutic embolization.

COMPUTED TOMOGRAPHY (CT) ANATOMY OF EAR, NOSE, THROAT, HEAD AND NECK

- Ear and temporal bone (Figs 60.12 to 60.15)
- Nose and paranasal sinuses (Figs 60.16 to 60.23)

Section 9 • Related Disciplines

- Oral cavity and oropharynx (Figs 60.24 and 60.25)
- Laryngopharynx and neck (Figs 60.26 and 60.27)
- Larynx and neck (Fig. 60.28)

High resolution CT scan: This is best to assess temporal bone lesions including fractures.

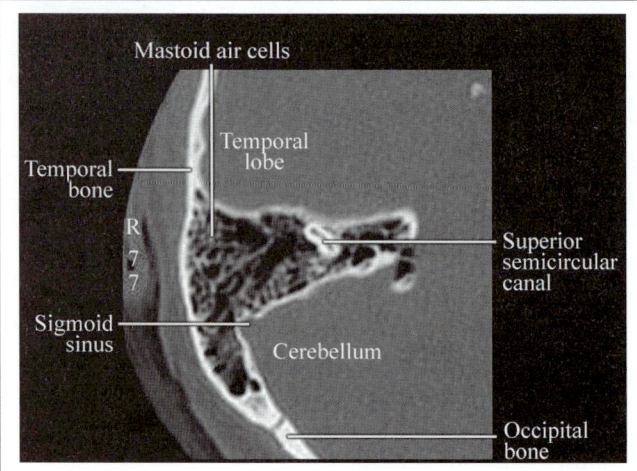

Fig. 60.12: CT scan axial section. Pneumatization of temporal bone

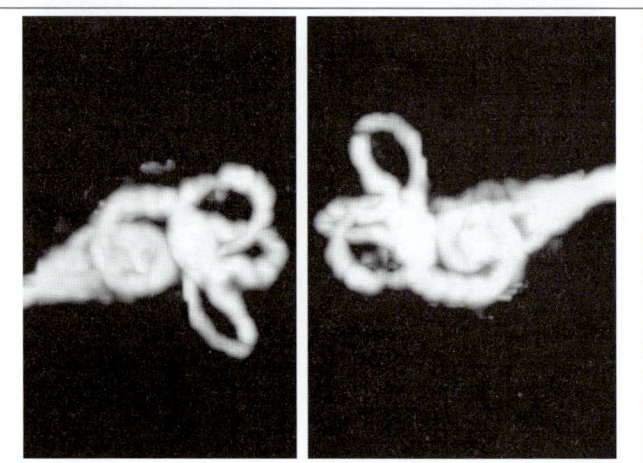

Fig. 60.15: MRI temporal bone showing membranous labyrinths of both the sides
Source: Dr Amit Goyal, AIIMS, Jodhpur

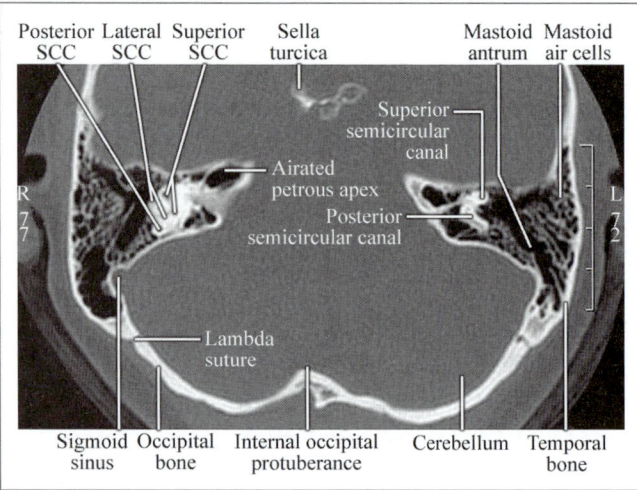

Fig. 60.13: HRCT temporal bone axial section showing vestibular anatomy

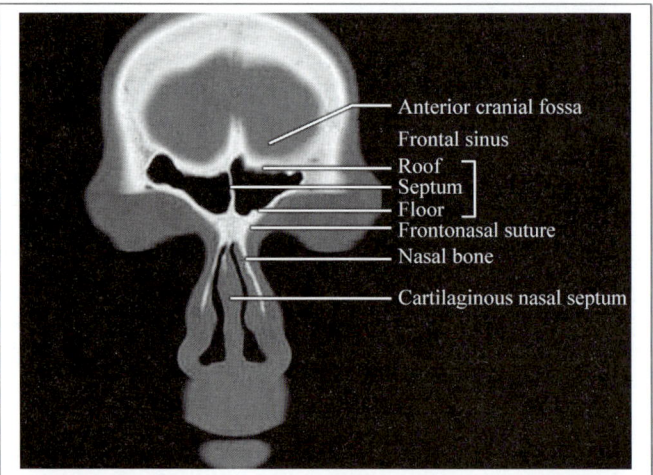

Fig. 60.16: CT PNS coronal section showing frontal sinuses

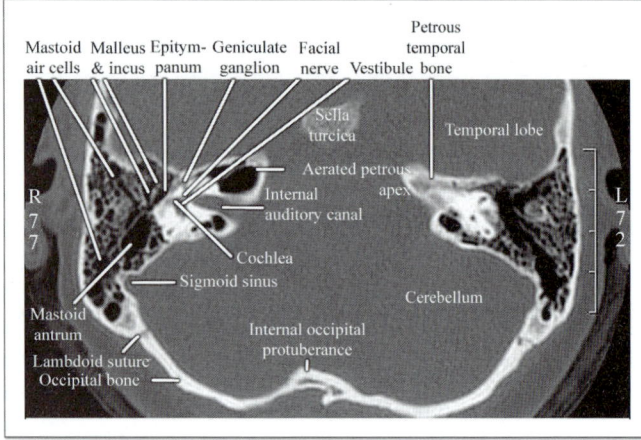

Fig. 60.14: HRCT temporal bone axial section showing internal auditory canal

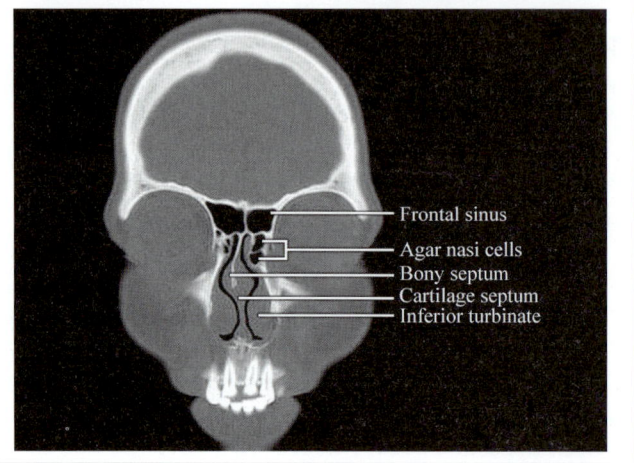

Fig. 60.17: CT PNS coronal section showing agger nasi cells

Chapter 60 • Diagnostic Imaging   481

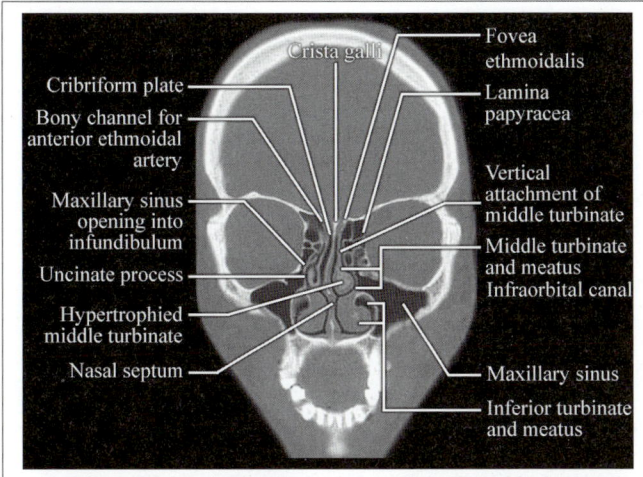

Fig. 60.18: CT PNS coronal section showing ethmoidal and maxillary sinuses

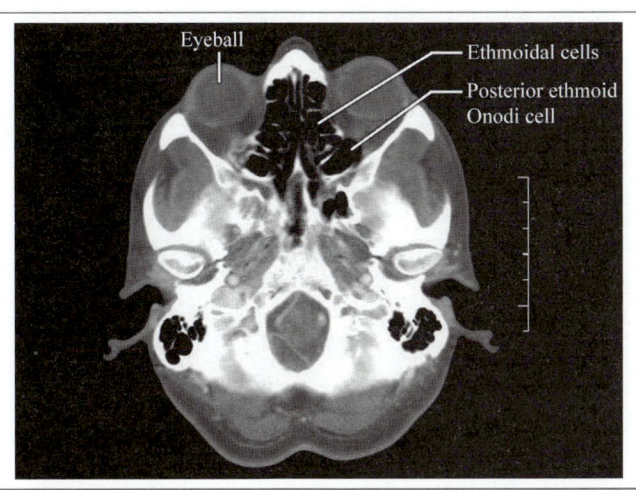

Fig. 60.21: CT scan head axial sections showing nose and paranasal sinuses

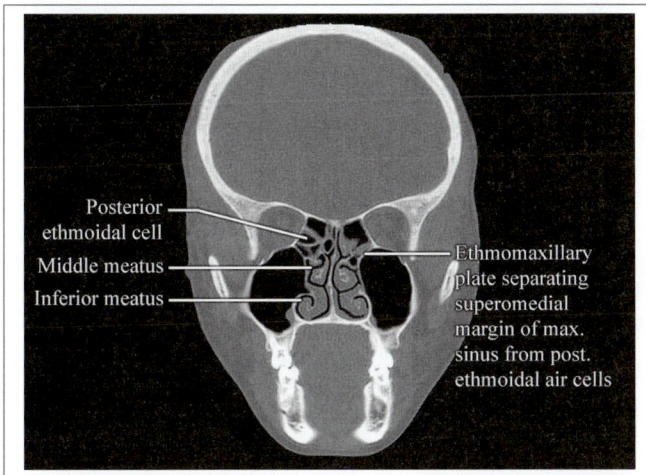

Fig. 60.19: CT scan nose and paranasal sinuses coronal section

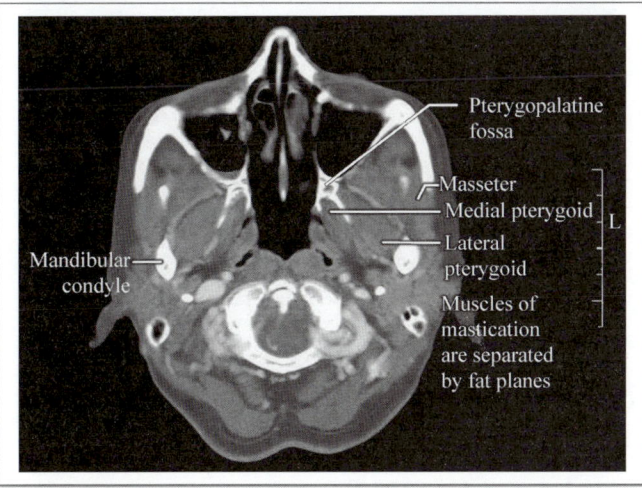

Fig. 60.22: CT scan head axial sections showing nose and paranasal sinuses

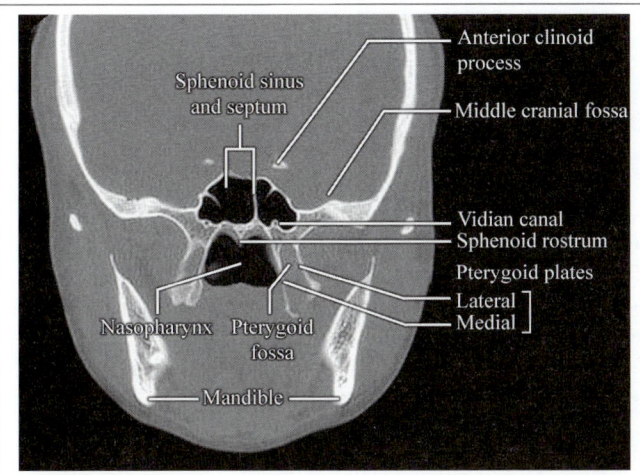

Fig. 60.20: CT PNS coronal section showing sphenoidal sinuses

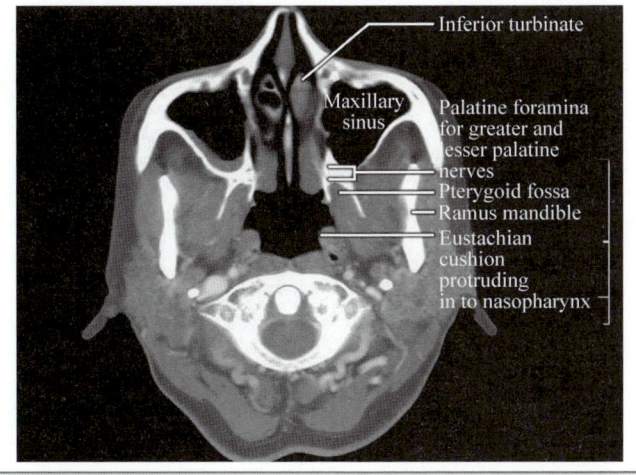

Fig. 60.23: CT scan head axial sections showing nose and paranasal sinuses

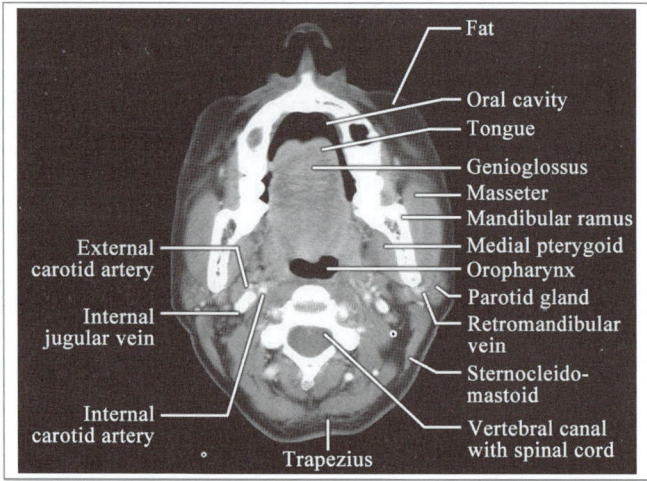

Fig. 60.24: CT scan oral cavity and oropharynx

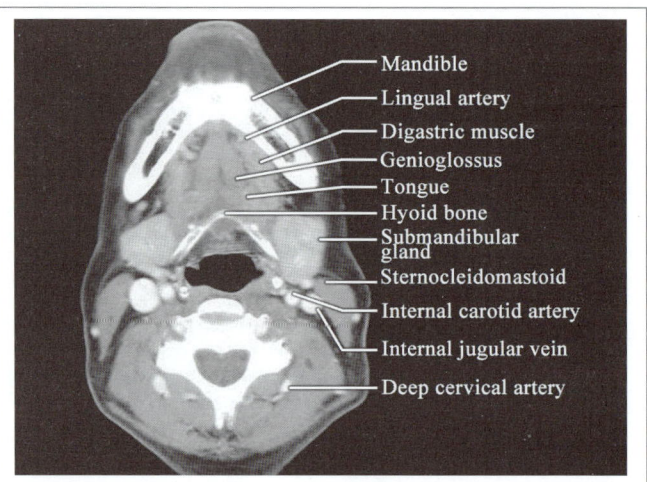

Fig. 60.26: CT scan laryngopharynx

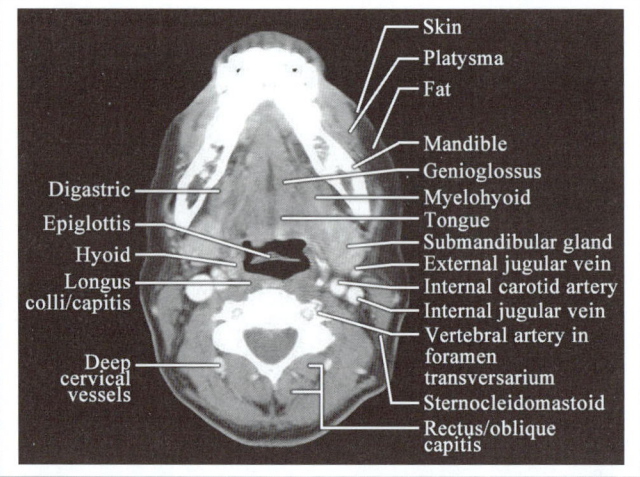

Fig. 60.25: CT scan oropharynx

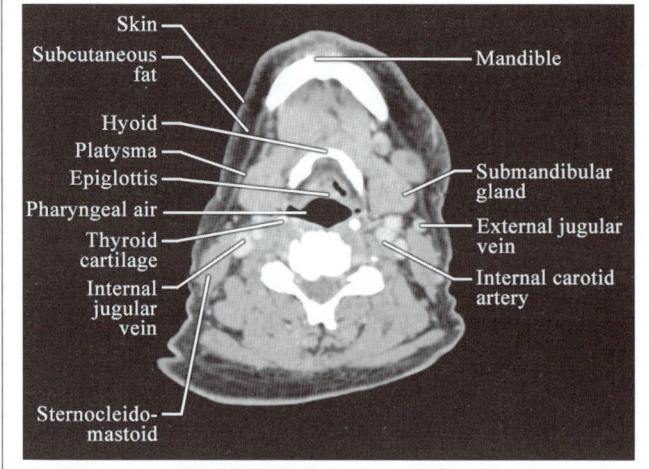

Fig. 60.27: Axial CT scan at hyoid bone level show necrotic nodes at level IA on left side

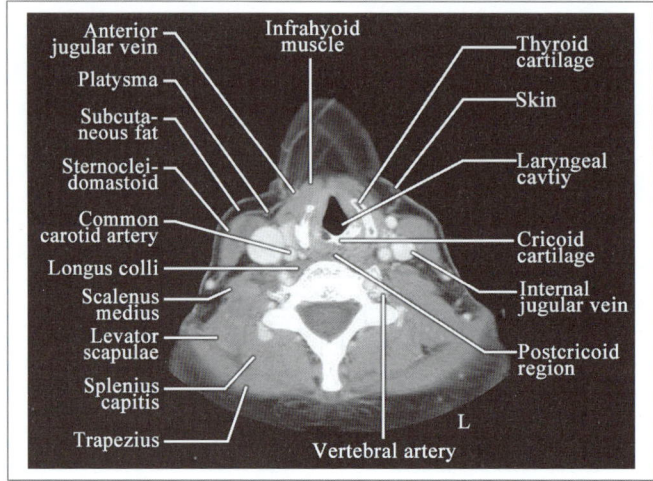

Fig. 60.28: CT neck with contrast showing larynx and other cervical structures

Self-evaluation Exercises

1. The imaging technologies, which do not use ionizing radiation, are:
   a. MRI
   b. Doppler
   c. Ultrasound
   d. All of the above

True (T)/False (F)

2. High resolution CT scan is best imaging technique to assess temporal bone fractures.
3. Ultrasound is better than CT in differentiating solid from cystic lesions.
4. MRI should not be used in the third trimester of pregnancy.
5. MRI is superior to CT in diagnosis of acoustic neuroma.

Answers

1. d   2. T   3. T   4. T   5. T

Chapter 61

Radiotherapy and Chemotherapy

⊙ Specific Learning Objectives
After going through the chapter, you should be able to answer the following questions:
- What are the different sources and modes of radiotherapy?
- What are the advantages and disadvantages of preoperative and postoperative radiotherapy?
- What are the complications of radiotherapy and how will you take care of the patients during and after radiotherapy?
- What are the advantages and disadvantages of adjuvant and neoadjuvant chemotherapy?
- What do you know about organ preservation therapy?

RADIOTHERAPY

Radiation oncology has emerged as a separate medical specialty. Radiotherapy forms an integral part in the management of head and neck malignancies. It may be used either alone or in combination with surgery and/or chemotherapy. It is used alone (curative radiotherapy) in early cancers (such as glottic cancer) to preserve the function of the organ. As an adjuvant to surgery or chemotherapy, it can increase the survival rate in more advanced lesions. Palliative radiotherapy in advanced lesions, when total control of disease is not expected, helps in controlling local symptoms of pain, bleeding and obstruction to air and food channels. It has also been found useful in the treatment of benign vascular lesions (angiofibroma and glomus tumor) and to control excessive scar formation in cases of keloids.

BASIC PHYSICS

There are various types of waves. Wave is a periodic disturbance in a medium or space. The chief characteristics of a wave are: speed of propagation, frequency, wavelength and amplitude.

Electromagnetic Radiations

The energy of electromagnetic radiations (a stream of photons) can be regarded as waves propagated through space (need no supporting medium). They travel in a vacuum with the speed of light. Photon travels at speed of light. It is a particle with zero rest mass consisting of a quantum (minimum amount by which energy or angular momentum of a system can change) of electromagnetic radiation. Electromagnetic spectrum is the range of wavelengths over which electromagnetic radiation extends. The longest waves are radio waves (Table 61.1) while the shortest are cosmic rays. Gamma rays produced from a ^{60}Co correspond to a wavelength of 10^{-12} m and 1.3 million electron volts (MeV). Energies of 3–5 electron volts (eV) (correspond to less than 10^{-6} m) are required to break chemical bonds.

Ionizing Radiations (Box 61.1)

The sufficiently high energy of ionizing radiations result in ionization in the medium through which they pass. In biological tissue, their effect can be very serious, as a consequence of the ejection of an electron from a water molecule and the oxidizing or reducing effects of the resulting highly reactive species.

Table 61.1: Range of wavelength (in meters) in electromagnetic spectrum

Radio waves	10^5–10^{-3} m
Infrared waves	10^{-3}–10^{-6} m
Visible light (VIBGYOR 400–700 nm)	4–7×10^{-7} m
Ultraviolet	10^{-7}–10^{-9} m
X-rays	10^{-9}–10^{-11} m
Gamma rays	10^{-11}–10^{-14} m
Cosmic rays	Less than 10^{-14} m

Box 61.1: Ionizing radiations

- Stream of high energy particles
  - Electrons
  - Protons
  - α-particles
- Short wavelength electromagnetic radiations (photon beams)
  - Ultraviolet rays
  - X-rays
  - Gamma rays

- **Photon beams:** X-rays and gamma rays are the most common radiations. X-rays are produced when high-energy electrons bombard a metallic target. Gamma rays are emitted by radioactive material cobalt-60.
- **Electron beam:** It is a type of particle radiation. It is the second most common forms of radiotherapy, which have rapid dose build up and sharp dose fall off with very little scatter. Electron beams are produced by linear accelerator, betatron and microtron. They boost up the radiation dose to the target area and avoid radiation to adjoining spinal cord.
- **Particle radiations:** Fast neutrons, α-particles, protons and pions are under trial. Neutron radiations are used in cancer of salivary glands.

Radiation Units

They are expressed in terms of energy that is deposited in a unit of material.
- **Rad (radiation absorbed dose):** One rad is equivalent to 100 ergs deposited per gram of material.
- **Gray (Gy):** One Gy is equivalent to 1 joule deposited per kilogram of material.
- **Rad and Gy:** 100 rads = 1 Gy = 100 centigrays (cGy), so 1 rad = 1 cGy.

Sources of Radiation

High energy of radiations penetrate deeper. Old X-ray machines, which were used for superficial skin and lip tumors, produced less energy [only in kilovolts (kV)]. Newer machines produce radiations of high energy in million volts (MV) and penetrate deeper and are used for deep seated tumors. They do not affect skin and bone. The common sources for radiotherapy are:

- **Kilovoltage machines:** They are becoming obsolete and consist of superficial (50–150 kV) and ortho (200–400 kV) voltage X-ray machines that produce X-rays of 50–400 kV.
- **Cobalt-60 machine:** This is the most commonly used source for radiotherapy. It uses radioactive cobalt-60 that produces gamma rays of 1.17 and 1.33 MeV. The radioactive cobalt-60 has its natural decay time. It needs replacement every 5 years.
- **Linear accelerator:** These megavoltage machines can produce photon and electron beams of 4–25 MV depending on whether an intervening metallic target is used in machine or not. They work on electricity. Other examples are betatron and microtron.
- **Radioactive material:** Radium-226 used in the form of needles has been replaced by safer radionuclides, which include Cesium-137 pellets, Iridium-192 wire, Gold-198 seeds and Iodine-125.

THERAPEUTIC WINDOW

There are some intrinsic differences in the properties of tumor and normal cells. A therapeutic dose of radiation in a radiosensitive tumor has wide "therapeutic window," which results in 95% chances of tumor control and 5% chances of normal tissue complications. In contrast radioresistant tumors have narrow "therapeutic window," which means a therapeutic dose of radiation has 95% chances of tumor control with very high chances of normal tissue damage. The following techniques exploit this therapeutic window concept:

- Three-dimensional treatment planning and delivery
- Brachytherapy
- Intraoperative radiotherapy
- Use of high-LET (linear energy transfer) and charged particle radiations
- Altered fractionation schedule
- Use of radiosensitization and radioprotective schedule.

MODES OF RADIOTHERAPY

- **External beam therapy (teletherapy):** It uses photon and electron beams. They project to the target area through the skin from a distance. The main advantages of megavoltage radiotherapy are its better precision, skin sparing, diminished bone absorption and increased dose to deep tumor.
- **Brachytherapy:** It uses radioactive material, which are placed in close contact with the tumor.
  - **Interstitial implants:** Needles (^{226}Ra and ^{137}Cs), wires, ribbons and seeds are inserted into the tumor.
    - **Shorter half-life:** ^{198}Au and ^{125}I have shorter half-life and are permanently left in the tissues.
  - **Intracavitary implants:** The radioactive material is placed in a hollow cavity next to the tumor for either minutes, hours or days. Examples include nasopharynx and maxillary antrum.
  - **Recent developments:** The following recent developments is again making brachytherapy popular, which was abandoned due to the hazards of radiation to the physician, nurses and other personnel:
    - After-loading techniques (^{192}Ir)
    - Safer radionuclides
    - Computerized dosimetry

Currently, high-dose rate remote after-loading devices are available, which push ^{192}Ir via a set of interstitial catheters. Computers control dwelling time throughout the implant.

- **Unsealed radionuclide therapy:** Radioactive isotopes are given either orally or intravenously. They are concentrated by metabolic pathways in malignant tissue, which receive large radiation doses. The normal tissues are relatively spared. The best example is the radioactive iodine treatment of differentiated thyroid carcinoma of follicular cell origin.

Radioactive iodine: It cannot be used in the ablation of medullary carcinoma of the thyroid.

COMBINED MODALITY TREATMENT

- **Curative radiotherapy** for small cancerous lesions not only cures the cancer but also has the advantage of preserving the function of the organ. The curative dose ranges from 65–75 Gy (6,500–7,500 rads/cGy).
- **Palliative radiotherapy** is given in advanced inoperable tumors, distant metastases and poor nutrition and diseases of heart, lung, liver and kidney.
- **Combination therapy** combines radiotherapy with surgery and chemotherapy. Radiotherapy can be given before, after and even during the surgery to achieve better control of disease. Each modality has its own advantages and disadvantages; however postoperative radiotherapy is the most common and well established.

Preoperative Radiation

- *Advantages*
  - **Reduce size of tumor:** It reduces the tumor bulk and can convert inoperable tumor into operable one.
  - **Better response:** Response to radiation is better because of the better oxygenation of tissues, which is affected in operated cases.
  - **Blocks lymphatics:** Radiation blocks the lymphatics and the chances of dissemination of tumor cells during surgery are less.
  - **Decrease spread:** It decreases the chances of microscopic spread beyond palpable tumor mass and occult metastasis to lymph nodes.
- *Disadvantages*
  - **Central core of tumor:** The central part of large tumor responds poorly to radiation because of poor oxygenation.
  - **Postoperative complications:** Radiation induced reduction in the vitality of tissues increases the chances of postoperative complications such as delayed healing, flap necrosis, fistulae formation and carotid blowouts.

Postoperative Radiation

- *Advantages*
  - **Limited disease:** It is more effective as the remaining tumor mass after the radical surgery is limited.
  - **Better planning:** As the extent of disease is well defined after the surgery, radiotherapy can be better planned for the suspected areas of residual disease.
  - **Operation:** Surgical resection is easier and postoperative complications are lesser in comparison to the cases of preoperative radiotherapy.
- **Disadvantages:** Blood supply of the tissues is affected, which results in relative hypoxic cells that respond poorly to radiation.
- *Indications:*
  - When the margins of growth are reported positive or very close.
  - In the presence of invasion of bone or cartilage.
  - Extracapsular invasion of lymph nodes.
  - Neck nodes are multiple or the size of a node is greater than 3 cm.

Radiotherapy and Chemotherapy

Chemotherapy can be used before, during and after radiotherapy.

- **Induction chemotherapy** (before radiotherapy) reduces the bulk of tumor and may help in organ preservation. The vascularity of the lesion is maintained and enhanced.
- **Concomitant chemotherapy** acts as a radiosensitizer and improves the effect of radiation on the tumor cells. Methotrexate and bleomycin are good radiosensitizers.
- **Adjuvant chemotherapy** is used after radiation. It helps in controlling distant metastases.

PLANNING OF RADIOTHERAPY

Shells are prepared for accurate treatment of tumor and sparing adjacent normal and critical structures. The treatment simulator consists of diagnostic X-ray machine with image intensification facilities. It allows distance adjustment to make rectangles of any size. The introduction of blocks shapes the radiation beam to shield normal critical structures.

The histology nature, site, size and extent of tumor and its draining lymph nodes must be known. The primary tumor and its draining lymph nodes are included in the radiation field. Extent of tumor can be found by clinical examination (palpation under anesthesia) and imaging (CT/MRI) studies.

Factors Affecting Response to Radiotherapy

- Smaller the tumor, better is the response.
- Tumors of lymphoid tissues are very radiosensitive.

- Anaplastic tumors and embryonal tumors are also radiosensitive.
- The differentiated squamous cell carcinomas do not respond well.
- Adenocarcinomas, sarcomas and bone tumors have low sensitivity.

Effect of smoking on the radiotherapy response: Patients who smoke while on radiation therapy appear to have lower response rates and shorter survival durations than those who do not; therefore, patients should be advised stop smoking before beginning radiation therapy.

Intensity Modulated Radiation Therapy (IMRT)

The aim of any radiotherapy is to deliver entire dose to the tumor and none to normal tissue. The IMRT is current step in that direction. In the past, customized cerrobend and multileaf collimators used to shape the beam. They allowed the field to be shaped to cover area of interest. In three-dimensional conformal radiotherapy, isodose curves conform closely to tumor shape but close normal tissues are not spared.

IMRT delivers the dose as a gradient across the area of interest. The main advantage of IMRT is sharper gradient between tumor tissue and normal tissue.

Techniques: There are three techniques of IMRT:
1. **Dynamic IMRT:** It is similar to tomotherapy unit, which circle around patient.
2. **Stepwise delivery:** It is similar to three-dimensional conformal radiotherapy.
3. **Step and soot IMRT:** It is the hybrid of former two where multiple beam arrangements are used but leaves are changed in real time.

Cyberknife stereotactic surgery: In this robotic arm technique, radiation is delivered by 6-MV linear accelerator under image guidance. It precisely hits the target area sparing the adjacent normal tissue. The indications include acoustic neuroma and recurrence of cancer after curative radiotherapy.

COMPLICATIONS OF RADIOTHERAPY

Complications depend on the site of lesion, dose delivered and its daily fractions. They can be early and late. Higher the total dose and larger the daily fraction, more are the complications. Acute radiation side effects are caused by changes in tissues, which are composed of rapidly proliferating cells. The delayed effects are caused by changes in tissues, which have slow proliferating cells.

Early Complications

The acute side effects manifest by the second to third week of radiotherapy and resolve within 4-6 weeks after completion.
- Radiation sickness (anorexia and nausea)
- Mucositis (ulcers in mouth and pharynx): Acute radiation mucositis generally persists for 8–12 weeks after radiation.
- Xerostomia: Dryness of oral cavity mucosa leads to difficulty in chewing, swallowing and speaking.
- Skin reactions are erythema, pruritus dry and wet desquamation of skin (Fig. 61.1)
- Pharyngeal edema: Dysphagia, odynophagia
- Laryngeal edema: Hoarseness of voice, respiratory distress (stridor)
- Fungal infections: Irradiated patients are prone to develop candida infection in oral cavity and pharynx.
- Hematopoietic suppression.

Late Complications

- Permanent xerostomia (dryness of mouth) if major salivary glands are included within the treatment field.
- Atrophy of skin and subcutaneous fibrosis: Facial alopecia in treated regions, pigmentation, telangiectasias and submental edema.
- Teeth decay: Radiation to alveolar process and salivary glands. Xerostomia facilitates caries of teeth.
- Osteoradionecrosis especially of mandible
- Trismus due to fibrosis of temporomandibular joint and muscles of mastication
- Transverse myelitis
- Eye: Radiation to retina and lens leads to retinopathy and cataract
- Endocrinal deficit: Radiation to thyroid and pituitary
- Malignancy: Thyroid cancer and orbital osteosarcoma.

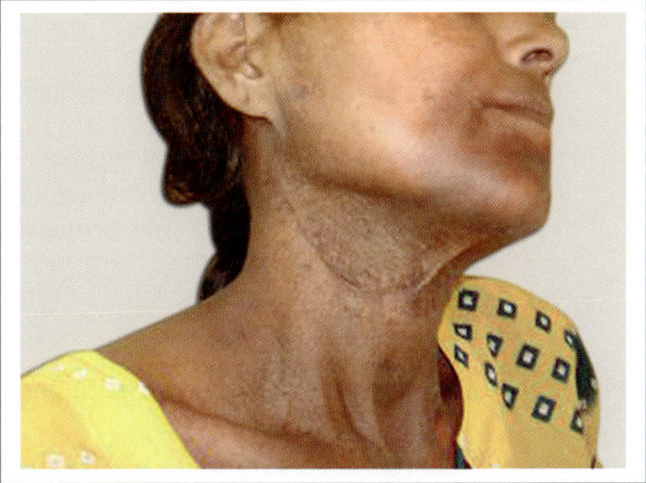

Fig. 61.1: Skin reactions after postoperative radiotherapy

- Ear: Otitis media with effusion and internal ear damage causing hearing loss and vertigo.
- Brain necrosis: Somnolence syndrome.

Lhermitte's sign: This rare sign is seen after radiation of cervical spines. On flexing the neck, patient develops electric current like sensation in arms, dorsal spine and both legs.

Patient Care during Radiotherapy

- *Nutrition:* Diet should be rich in protein, vitamins and iron. Nasogastric tube feeding is started if needed. Blood transfusion is given if patient has severe anemia.
- *Teeth care:* Prior dental evaluation and extraction if needed are of paramount importance and prevent osteoradionecrosis of mandible. Wound of extraction must heal before the beginning of radiotherapy.
- *Skin care:* Skin reactions were common with old superficial and orthovoltage X-ray machines. The current megavoltage therapy does not much affect the skin. Electron beam therapy to skin can also result in skin reactions. Following cares are taken:
  - Keep the skin dry and avoid soap, water and wet shaving.
  - Avoid sunlight.
  - Avoid abrasive dressing and clothing and adhesive plaster for dressings, which peels off the desquamated skin.
  - Skin should be covered with soft cloth, which can provide free aeration to the skin.
  - Moisturizers minimize and soothe the skin symptoms. For moist desquamated skin, use antibiotic ointment. Topical steroid creams relieve itching and pain.
- *Mouth care:* Dryness of mouth (xerostomia) and ulcerations (mucositis) are common and interfere with feeding. Following cares are taken:
  - Avoid alcohol, tobacco, spicy food and irritating mouthwashes containing alcohol.
  - For xerostomia, pilocarpine (100-200 mg po tid) is given from the beginning and continued for months after completion. Patients with permanent xerostomia will need frequent intake of plenty of liquids between and during meals. Artificial saliva preparations are also helpful.
  - Milk of magnesia neutralizes the acid pH and prevents caries of teeth and soothes and protects inflamed mucosa.
  - Xylocaine viscous relieves pain and discomfort of mucositis and facilitates food taking. Patients with severe oral or pharyngeal symptoms may require gastric tube feeding.
  - Oral candida is usually treated by topical application of nystatin and clotrimazole. Systemic antifungal therapy is needed for the fungus, which lie beneath organic debris.

Amifostine: It decreases the xerostomia but is expensive and side effects may be severe.

CHEMOTHERAPY

Chemotherapy can be used either alone or in combination with surgery and radiotherapy. The drugs, which are found effective in head and neck squamous cell cancers are, methotrexate, cisplatin, bleomycin and 5-fluorouracil. Adriamycin has been used for adenoid cystic carcinoma and dacabazine for melanomas. Lymphomas (both Hodgkin and non-Hodgkin types) have multifocal origin and are managed with chemotherapy.

WORK-UP BEFORE CHEMOTHERAPY

- *History and clinical examination:* Exclude kidney, heart and lung diseases.
- *CBC:* Hemoglobin, total and differential WBC count and platelet count. Many drugs are myelosuppressive.
- *Urine examination.*
- *Biochemistry:* Blood urea nitrogen and creatinine and liver function tests. Methotrexate and cisplatin are nephrotoxic.
- *Radiology:* X-ray chest, CT scan/MRI (to know extent of disease) and ultrasound abdomen for liver/spleen.
- *Pulmonary function tests:* Bleomycin causes interstitial pulmonary fibrosis.
- *ECG:* Adriamycin has cardiotoxicity.
- *Audiogram:* Cisplatin causes high frequency hearing loss.
- *Nutritional status.*

TOXICITY OF ANTICANCER DRUGS

Anticancer drugs act not only on rapidly dividing cancer cells but also normally dividing cells of hair follicles, gastrointestinal mucosa and bone marrow. They can cause alopecia, stomatitis, nausea, vomiting, diarrhea, anemia, leukopenia and thrombocytopenia (Table 61.2). Some drugs have selective action on certain systems, such as kidney (methotrexate and cisplatin), nerves (vincristine and cisplatin), heart (adriamycin) and bladder (cyclophosphamide).

Table 61.2: Chemotherapeutic agents for head and neck malignancies

Drugs, Doses, Indications and Response rate (RR)	Acute toxicity	Delayed toxicity
• **Alkylating agents**		
Cisplatin [squamous cell carcinoma (SCC)] 50–100 mg/m^2 IV 3 weekly (RR 28%)	Severe nausea and vomiting	Nephrotoxicity, ototoxicity, neuropathy
Carboplatin (RR 22%) 360 mg/m^2 IV, 4 weekly	Severe nausea and vomiting	Myelosuppression, prolonged anemia
Cyclophosphamide 100–400 mg/m^2/d; 1–1.5 g/m^2 IV every 3–4 weeks (SCC, neuroblastoma, leukemia, lymphomas, multiple myeloma)	Nausea and vomiting with higher doses	Neutropenia, alopecia, hemorrhagic cystitis
Ifosfamide (RR 26%) 1.5–2.5 g/m^2 twice weekly		Myelosuppression, alopecia, confusion; mesna prevents cystitis
• **Antimetabolites**		
Methotrexate (SCC, acute leukemia, lymphomas) 2.5–5 mg/d orally; 20–25 mg IM twice weekly; 500–1,000 mg/m^2 IV every 2–3 weeks (RR 31%)	None Citrovorum factor (leucovorin) rescue for doses over 100 mg/m^2	Mucositis (oral and GIT ulcers), myelosuppression, acute renal failure, rash, hepatotoxic
5-Fluorouracil (SCC; RR 15%) 15 mg/kg/d IV for 3–5 days every 3 weeks	None	Nausea, mucositis, diarrhea, myelosuppression and dacryocystitis
• **Antibiotics**		
Bleomycin (SCC, lymphoma, RR 21%) Up to 15 units/m^2 IM/IV/SC twice weekly	Allergic reactions, fever and hypotension	Fever, pulmonary fibrosis, dermatitis (skin rash), mucositis
Adriamycin (lymphoma, sarcoma, salivary gland cancer, esthesioneuroblastoma) 60–90 mg/m^2 IV monthly	Vesicant, nausea, vomiting, diarrhea	Cardiotoxicity, mucositis, myelosuppression, alopecia
Mitomycin 10–20 mg/m^2, 6–8 weekly	Severe vesicant; nausea	Bone marrow depression, hemolytic-uremic syndrome
• **Vinca Alkaloids**		
Vincristine (SCC, lymphoma, rhabdomyosarcoma) 1.5 mg/m^2/week (max 2 mg)	Severe vesicant	Areflexia, neurotoxicity, alopecia, myelosuppression, paralytic ileus, syndrome of inappropriate antidiuretic hormone secretion and constipation
Vinblastin 0.1–0.2 mg/kg (6 mg/m^2) IV	Mild nausea and vomiting; severe vesicant	
• **Taxanes**		
Paclitaxel (Taxol) (RR 38%) 135 mg/m^2 IV infusion 24 hours every 3 weeks [squamous cell carcinoma (SCC)] *Docetaxel (Taxotere) (RR 38%)* 60–100 mg/m^2 IV 3 weekly	Mild nausea vomiting; hypersensitivity reaction (premedicate with diphenhydramine and dexamethasone)	Myelosuppression, neuropathy Edema (fluid retention), neutropenia, neuropathy
• **Supporting Agents**		
Leucovorin 10 mg/m^2, 6 hourly IV/oral	None	Enhances toxic effects of fluorouracil
Mesna 20% of ifosfamide dosage	Nausea, vomiting, diarrhea	None

New agents under investigation: Topoisomerase-I inhibitors, gemcitabine (pyrimidine antimetabolite), vinorelbine (semisynthetic vinca alkaloid), trimetrexate, edatrexate, and piritrexim.

> **Indications for chemotherapy include:**
> - To make radiotherapy more effective for the tumor.
> - Combined with radiotherapy for organ-preservation therapy especially of laryngeal cancers.
> - Induction or neoadjuvant therapy facilitates less extensive local surgery.
> - To control symptoms in metastatic disease.

PALLIATIVE CHEMOTHERAPY

Palliative chemotherapy includes use of cytotoxic drugs either singly or in combination in advanced, recurrent or metastatic disease just to relieve the symptoms. It is not well proved that they prolong life. The response duration to commonly used single agents tends to be 2–4 months. The complete response was observed in less than 5%. Some of the combination chemotherapy regimens, which have been used and improve the response rates, are the following:
- Cisplatin and 5-fluorouracil
- Cisplatin and methotrexate
- Carboplatin and 5-fluorouracil
- Cisplatin and bleomycin
- Cisplatin, methotrexate and bleomycin
- Cisplatin, vinblastine and bleomycin
- Cisplatin, methotrexate, vinblastine and bleomycin.

> ***Bleomycin:*** This antineoplastic drug causes pulmonary toxicity.

COMBINED MODALITY THERAPY

The chemotherapy may be used either before, during or after other modalities of treatment, such as surgery and radiotherapy. The three general approaches, which have been undertaken for the sake of improving primary treatment program by using combined modality therapy, are—induction, chemoradiation and adjuvant therapy.

Induction or Anterior Chemotherapy (Neoadjuvant Chemotherapy)

When chemotherapy is used before surgery or radiation, it is called induction or anterior chemotherapy. It helps in reducing tumor burden and micrometastases, which can occur during surgery or before radiation. This neoadjuvant chemotherapy has better compliance and tolerance in downstaging patients. It eliminates problems of poor vascularity (after surgery and radiotherapy) and helps in preservation of organ function. The combination of cisplatin and 5-fluorouracil is the most commonly used neoadjuvant chemotherapy.

Chemoradiation

In cases of unresectable tumors, concurrent radiotherapy and chemotherapy may result in additive or synergistic enhancement and is used to improve local and regional control.

Adjuvant or Posterior Chemotherapy

Chemotherapy used after surgery or radiation is aimed to cure micrometastases and decrease distant metastases.
- ***Advantages:*** The potential advantages are:
    - Surgery is not delayed.
    - No blurring of tumor margins as it occurs in neoadjuvant chemotherapy.

> **Organ Preservation**
>
> The radical surgery of stage III and IV tumors results in loss of speech, loss of swallowing function, or disfigurement. The neoadjuvant chemotherapy followed by radiotherapy has been used to preserve functions for tumors of hypopharynx, larynx and oropharynx. The patients who achieve either partial or complete response with neoadjuvant chemotherapy go for radiotherapy, while nonresponders go for radical surgery. No significant survival difference is reported in either group (*see* Chapter 'Malignant Tumors of Larynx').

PREVENTION OF CANCER

LIFESTYLE MODIFICATIONS

The lifestyle factors, which accounts for a majority of avoidable cancer, include:
- Chewing of *paan, sopari* and tobacco.
- Smoking and alcohol.
- Occupational risks.
- Obesity, parity and length of lactation (breast cancer).
- High intake of fat and specific fatty acids (breast, colon, prostate and lung cancer).
- Exposure to ultraviolet light (use of sunscreens protects skin from sunlight).
- Exercise, folate and calcium supplementation, fruit and vegetable intake and dietary fiber (colorectal cancer and adenomas).

CHEMOPREVENTION

It is an important area of research. It consists of administration of drugs, which inhibit carcinogenesis or reverse a premalignant condition.
- ***Indications:*** Following high-risk patients have been identified for chemoprevention:
    - Past history of cancer (for preventing second cancer).
    - Premalignant lesions, such as leukoplakia.
    - Risks due to family history, lifestyle and occupation.
- ***Pharmacological agents:*** The following agents have been tried in different designs (induction, maintenance and adjuvant) in head and necks malignancies:

Chapter 61 • Radiotherapy and Chemotherapy

- **Retinoids (synthetic and natural analogs of vitamin A):** Retinoids have both acute toxicities (dryness of conjunctiva and oral mucous membrane, cheilitis, skin desquamation, hypertriglyceridemia, bone tenderness, arthralgia and myalgia) as well as chronic toxicities (teratogenic, hepatotoxic and bone remodeling).
  - Vitamin A (retinol)
  - β-all-transretinoic acid (retinoid)
  - 13-cis retinoic acid (isotretinoin)
  - Etretinate (aromatic ethyl ester derivative).
- **Carotenoids:** β-carotene is a major source of vitamin A in diet. Carotenoids results in yellowing of skin.
- **α-tocopherol** (vitamin E)
- **Calcium and selenium**
- **N-acetyl cysteine:** It is relatively nontoxic.
- **Epidermal growth factor receptor.**
- **Farnesyl transferase**
- **Aspirin and cyclooxygenase-2 inhibitors.**
- **Other diet and pharmacological agents, which are under investigations include:** Soy isoflavones, folic acid, dietary fat and fish oils, raloxifene, sulindac and polyphenols in green tea.

- **Further information about ongoing trials:** It can be obtained from USA's Chemoprevention Branch of National Cancer Institute. www.cancer.gov/cancer_information.

Self-evaluation Exercises

True (T)/False (F)
1. Sensitivity to radiation is more on the well oxygenated peripheral cells of carcinoma than the hypoxic central cells of carcinoma.

Filling the Blanks
2. _____ sign is seen after radiation of cervical spine. On flexing the neck, patient develops electric current like sensation in arms, dorsal spine and both legs.
3. Radioactive iodine cannot be used in the ablation of _____ carcinoma of the thyroid.
4. The chemotherapy used after surgery or radiotherapy for cancer is called as _____ chemotherapy.
5. The antineoplastic drug, _____ causes pulmonary toxicity.

Answers
1. T
2. Lhermitte's
3. medullary
4. adjuvant
5. bleomycin

Chapter 62

Laser Surgery and Cryosurgery

⊙ Specific Learning Objectives
After going through the chapter, you should be able to answer the following questions:
- What do you know about LASER and cryosurgery?
- What are the indications, advantages and disadvantages of commonly used lasers in ENT?
- What is the role of cryosurgery in ENT?
- What do you know about photodynamic therapy and radiofrequency surgery?

LASER

LASER is an acronym for **L**ight **A**mplification by **S**timulated **E**mission of **R**adiation. Laser light is the brightest monochromatic (one wavelength) light. In addition to diagnostic medicine and surgery, the laser is used in research laboratories, communications, surveying, manufacturing, lecture pointers, printers, CD players and engraving. Bar code scanners are used in supermarkets and shops.

RELATED PHYSICS

- ***Spontaneous emission of radiation:*** In a stable atom, there are equal number of protons and electrons. Electrons revolve around the nucleus in one or several discrete orbits. The orbits closure to nucleus, have lower energy levels than the larger shells, which are away from nucleus. The interaction of electron with photon (called absorption), which is a quantum of light, makes the atom excited. During excitation, an electron of low energy level can go into higher energy orbit. But within a very short time (10^{-8} sec) the electron spontaneously drops back to its lower level and gives up energy difference. During this process, atom emits extra energy as photon of light, which is called as spontaneous emission of radiation.
- ***Stimulated emission of radiation:*** If a photon of correct energy hits an excited atom, it results in emission of two identical photons, which have same frequency and energy and travel in same direction. This stimulated emission of radiation, which was described by Einstein, is the basic fundamental principle of laser science.
- ***Radiant laser energy:*** The stimulated radiation is amplified with the help of two mirrors in an optical resonating chamber, which is filled with an active medium, such as Ar, Nd:YAG or CO_2. An electric current excites this active medium, which can consist of molecules, atoms, ions semiconductors or even free electrons in an accelerator. Mirrors reflect the photons back and forth. One of the two mirrors is partially transmissive, which emits some of the radiant energy as laser.

Properties of Radiant Laser Energy
The radiant laser energy is a type of electromagnetic radiations. It has following qualities that distinguish it from disorganized light of a bulb:
- ***Monochromatic***, i.e. same wavelength (single color)
- ***Collimated*** (unidirectional)
- ***Coherent:*** Both temporally (waves of light oscillating in a phase) and spatially (photons are equal and parallel)
- ***Extremely intense.***

CONTROL OF LASER

The variables of lasers, which can be controlled, are power (watts), spot size (millimeters) and exposure time (seconds).
- ***Irradiance (W/cm^2):*** It considers surface area of focal spot. It is more useful measure than power, which may be kept constant. Irradiance varies directly with power

and inversely with spot size. The laser lens setting (focal length) and working distance combinations decide the size of focal spot. Larger the focal spot (unfocussed, away from focal plane), lower the irradiance. Smallest the focal spot (focused in focal plane), highest the irradiance, which results in precise cutting and vaporization.

- **Depth of focus:** The beam waist presents over a range of distances called depth of focus.
- **Fluence (J/cm^2):** It is a measure of the total amount of laser energy per unit area. It varies directly with exposure time (seconds). Working in pulsed mode or in continuous mode can change fluence.

Transverse Electromagnetic Mode (TEM)

TEM determines the shape of laser spot. It refers to the distribution of radiant energy of laser beam across the focal spot. The different modes of TEM are:

- **TEM_{00}:** Laser spot is circular on cross-section. The power density is greatest at the center and progressively diminishes peripherally (Gaussian distribution).
- **TEM_{01} and TEM_{11}:** Beams cannot be focused to a small spot and have complex distribution of energy. It results in predictable tissue vaporization.

TISSUE EFFECT

The tissue deals with incident laser energy in four ways:
1. **Reflects:** No effect on the tissue
2. **Absorbs:** Results in interaction with tissue and varies with laser's wavelength
3. **Transmits:** No effect on the tissue
4. **Scatters:** Spreads the energy and limits the penetration depth. Shorter the wavelength, more is the scattering.
   - **Levels of heating and tissue changes:** The primary form of interaction of absorbed laser with tissue is heating, the level of which decides the following changes:
     - **60–65°C:** Protein denaturation and blanching of tissue.
     - **100°C:** Vaporization of intracellular water, vacuole formation, craters and tissue shrinkage.
     - **Several 100°C:** Carbonization, disintegration, smoke, destruction and gas generation.

Zones of tissue damage:
- **Central area of tissue vaporization:** In the center of the wound is an area of tissue vaporization that makes a crater and carbon flakes.
- **Middle area of thermal necrosis:** Central crater is surrounded by an area of necrosis. Small vessels, nerves and lymphatics are sealed.
- **Outer area of thermal conductivity and repair:** This is the outermost area that heals with passage of time.

The short laser pulse minimizes the lateral thermal damage.

Uses of LASER energies:
- **Photothermal:** To cut, coagulate and vaporize
- **Photoacoustic:** To break stones (lithotripsy)
- **Photochemical:** Photodynamic therapy for destroying cancer tissue
- **Photodissociation (LASIK Lasers):** To reshape cornea in cases of refractive errors.

LASER IN OTOLARYNGOLOGY

The laser can be ultraviolet, which result in heating and photodissociation of chemical bonds, but most commonly used lasers emit either visible [Argon (Ar) and Potassium-titanyl-phosphate-532 (KTP-532) lasers] or infrared light [carbon dioxide (CO_2) laser]. Properties of commonly used lasers and their ENT applications are given in Table 62.1.

- **Most commonly used:** CO_2, neodymium:yttrium-aluminium-garnet (Nd:YAG), KTP-532 and Ar.
- **Other:** Ar tunable dye laser and flash lamp pumped dye laser.
- **Under investigations:** Erbium:YAG (Er:YAG) and holmium:YAG (Ho:YAG) lasers.

> - **Visible lasers:** Ar and KTP-532
> - **Invisible lasers:** CO_2, Nd:YAG, Excimer, Ho:YAG and Er:YAG
> - **Lasers need optical fibers:** Ar, KTP-532, Diode, Nd:YAG, Ho:YAG and Er:YAG
> - **Lasers for ear surgery:** CO_2, Ar, KTP-532 and Er:YAG

Carbon Dioxide (CO_2) Laser

CO_2 laser requires aiming beam of helium neon laser. It is the most commonly used laser in ENT surgery. It is transmitted through an articulating arm and can be used free-hand for microscopic surgery, attached to microscope and adapted to rigid bronchoscope. Its main limitation is that it cannot pass through the flexible endoscopes.

It is effective not only in vaporizing tissues, but it also provides bloodless field. Surgery can be performed in cases of hypertension, bleeding dyscrasias and coagulopathies. The other advantages are precision surgery and less postoperative edema and pain.

- **Advantages:**
  - Negligible scattering and reflection
  - Absorption independent of color
  - Minimal thermal effect on adjacent tissue
- **Indications:**
  - **Nose:** Papillomas, rhinophyma, telangiectasis, nasal polyps, choanal atresia and turbinate hypertrophy.
  - **Oral cavity:** Leukoplakia, erythroplakia, small superficial cancers and debulking of large, recurrent or inoperable tumors.

Table 62.1: Properties of commonly used lasers and their ENT applications

	Ar laser	Nd:YAG laser	CO_2 laser
Electromagnetic range	Visible	Invisible infrared	Invisible infrared
Color	Blue-green	Colorless	Red light of helium-neon
Wavelength	0.488 and 0.514 µm	1.064 µm	10.6 µm
Extinction length*	80 m	40 m	0.03 mm
Transmitted through	Clear aqueous tissue	Clear liquids	
Absorption by	Hemoglobin, pigmented tissue	Darkly pigmented tissue, charred debris	Water, tissue with high water content
Scattering	Less	More	Negligible
Clinical applications	Portwine stains, hemangiomas, telangiectasis, stapedotomy	Obstructive lesions of trachea, bronchus, esophagus; vascular, lymphatic lesions	Extremely versatile, used in ear, nose and throat lesions
Precision	Good	Less	Good

Abbreviations: Ar, Argon; Nd:YAG, Neodymium:Yttrium-Aluminium-Garnet; CO_2, Carbon Dioxide
*Extinction length: The thickness of water necessary to absorb 90% of the incident laser energy

- **Oropharynx:** Recurrent tonsillitis and hypertrophy, tonsillar and pharyngeal tumors, tongue T_1 and limited T_2 cancer.
- **Larynx:** Papilloma, web, stenosis (glottic, subglottic, and posterior), capillary hemangiomas, vocal nodule, Reinke's edema, leukoplakia of cord, polypoid degeneration of cord, arytenoidectomy, T_1 midcordal carcinoma without anterior commissure involvement, suprahyoid supraglottic T_1 cancer, laryngocele, cysts and granulomas.
- **Trachea and bronchi:** Recurrent papillomatosis, tracheal stenosis, granulation tissue and bronchial adenoma, debulking of obstructive malignant lesions of trachea and bronchi.
- **Plastic surgery:** Benign and malignant tumors of skin, vaporization of nevi and tattoos
- **Ear:** Stapedotomy and acoustic neuroma.

Argon Laser

Argon laser passes through clear fluid and is absorbed by hemoglobin and pigmented tissues.
- *Indications:*
  - **Vascular lesions:** Photocoagulation of portwine stain, hemangioma and telangiectasia.
  - **Retinal lesions:** It passes through the clear aqueous tissues (cornea, lens and vitreous).
  - **Ear microsurgery:** Its uses in ear microsurgery are lysis of middle ear adhesions, spot welding or tympanoplasty grafts.
    - **Stapedotomy:** A drop of blood is kept on stapes footplate before its use in stapedotomy.

Potassium-Titanyl-Phosphate-532 Laser (KTP-532)

KTP laser has wavelength of 532 nm (blue-green) and comparable with Ar laser. It falls in visible spectrum and is selectively absorbed by pigment and more strongly by hemoglobin. Hand-held probe facilitates its use in endoscopic sinus surgery and microlaryngeal surgery. The optical fiber delivery can be manipulated through rigid bronchoscope.
- *Indications:* It is first choice in the following conditions:
  - **Ear:** Stapedotomy.
  - **Nose:** Polyps, concha bullosa, epistaxis, turbinate hypertrophy and telangiectasia.
  - **Oral cavity:** Verrucous and T_1 carcinoma, leukoplakia, erythroplakia, early tongue cancer T_1, lymphangioma.
  - **Oropharynx:** Recurrent tonsillitis and hypertrophy, uvulopalatopharyngoplasty in obstructive sleep apnea, T_1 and T_2 carcinoma.
  - **Larynx:** Laryngocele, cyst, granulomas, stenosis (glottic, posterior and subglottic), bilateral vocal cord paralysis, recurrent respiratory papillomas, suprahyoid supraglottic T_1 carcinoma and obstructing carcinoma.
  - **Skin:** Pigmented dermal lesions.

Neodymium:Yttrium-Aluminium-Garnet Laser (Nd:YAG)

Nd:YAG laser can be transmitted by flexible endoscopes and has effective coagulative properties. It controls the bleeding well. The flexible fiberoptic delivery system allows its use with flexible endoscope.

It is excellent for tissue coagulation, but the precision is poor as the tissue damage is widespread and depth of tissue penetration is less predictable. It can be used in combination with CO_2 laser.
- *Indications:* It is advantageously used for following lesions as control of bleeding (dangerous in bronchoscopy) is more secure.

- **Obstructive malignant tumor** of trachea, bronchus and esophagus.
- **Vascular lesions:** Hereditary hemorrhagic telangiectasia of nose.
- **Lymphatic disorders:** Lymphangioma.

Advantages of LASER:
- High precision
- Easy and rapid tissue ablation
- Less postoperative pain and edema.

Disadvantages
- High cost of machine and maintenance
- Special training of healthcare personnels
- Special precautions and safety measures to prevent hazards of laser.

Complications and Safety

The laser is a potentially dangerous instrument. The utmost caution is required to prevent accidents, which can injure not only patient but also health care personnel present in operation room.

- **Education of staff:** The operating surgeon and anesthesiologist must have proper experience and training. Nursing and operation theater personnel should be conversant with safety measures before operating laser.
- **Protection of eye:** Protective eyeglasses with side protectors, which are specific for the wavelength of each laser (blue-green glasses with optical density of 6 for Nd:YAG laser; orange yellow glasses for Ar, KTP or dye lasers), must be worn by the patient, surgeon, anesthetist, assistants, nurses and all other personnel present in operating room. They prevent accidental burns to cornea, retina and lens. Patient's eyes are protected by a double layer of saline moistened eye pads.
- **Protection of skin:** All exposed parts of the patient such as skin, mucous membranes and teeth are protected by saline soaked towels, pads or sponges that are moistened periodically.
- **Evacuation of smoke:** Two separate suctions, one for the blood and mucous and the other for smoke and steam (laser vaporization of tissues) are used.
- **Anesthetic gases and equipment:** The endotracheal tube fire is the dreaded complication. Only non-inflammable gases (such as halothane and enflurane) are used. During the CO_2 laser, red rubber tube is wrapped by reflective metallic foil. Cuff of endotracheal tube is inflated with saline water, which may be colored by methylene blue that helps in warning about the leak of cuff. Tubes are further protected with saline soaked cotton. The colorless or white polyvinyl or silicone tube that does not have any black or dark marking or a lead lined marking along the side, is safest with the use of Nd:YAG laser.

Management of laser induced endotracheal tube fire:
- Stop ventilation
- Saline irrigation
- Immediately withdraw the burnt tube and introduce new tube
- Intravenous steroids
- Bronchoscopy: To assess the damage to tracheobronchial tree. Patient may need repeated bronchoscopies after operation.

PHOTODYNAMIC THERAPY (PDT)

PRINCIPLE

Photosensitizing agent is taken up preferentially by the malignant cells, which are then exposed to specific wavelength of laser (such as Ar tunable dye laser with a wavelength of 630 nm). Laser activates the photosensitizing agent and destroys the cancer cells. The photosensitizer photofrin (dihematoporphyrin ether or DHE) is given intravenously.

Light activation of photoconcentrated DHE results in mitochondrial damage and apoptosis in malignant cells. Erythrocyte leakage and endothelial damage of vessels cause ischemic necrosis of tumor tissue.

INDICATIONS

- Cancer of skin, larynx, nasopharynx, aerodigestive tract and endobronchial region.
- Recurrences after radiation and surgery.
- Superficial cancers of larynx have been treated with PDT. It has got US FDA approval for treating obstructing esophageal and endobronchial tumors and minimally invasive endobronchial non-small cell carcinoma.

SIDE EFFECTS

The main side effect of PDT is generalized skin photosensitization. Patient should use sun-protective clothing and avoid exposure to sunlight.

RADIOFREQUENCY SURGERY

Radiofrequency (RF) surgery reduces the volume of tissues. This minimally invasive surgery can be done as an OPD procedure.

INDICATIONS

Radiofrequency cuts and coagulates tissues with minimal lateral tissue damage. It can be used in the following disorders:
- **Nasal obstruction:**
  - Reduction of hypertrophied inferior turbinates.

- **Snoring and obstructive sleep apnea (OSA):**
  - Reduction of redundant soft palate and uvulopalatoplasty
  - Reduction of fullness in base of tongue.
- **Lingual thyroid**
- **Tonsillotomy**
- **Microlaryngeal surgery** to remove granuloma, papilloma and cyst
- **Myringotomy**
- **Rhinophyma**
- **Cosmetic:** Removal of skin lesions.

MATERIAL AND METHOD

The machine generates electromagnetic waves of very high frequency (350 kHz to 4 MHz). Usually 460 kHz RF is delivered through the probe, which is inserted into the tissue and causes ionic agitation. Heating of the tissue causes protein coagulation and tissue necrosis. There is no charring. The scar formation occurs in 3 weeks. RF reduces the size of tissue. The parameters, which can be controlled are:

- Power in watts
- Temperature in degrees of celsius
- Resistance in ohms
- Treatment time in seconds
- Energy in joules (watts × seconds).

CRYOSURGERY

PRINCIPLE

At –30°C and below, rapid freezing of tissues and slow thawing results in the destruction of tissue. This principle is used in cryosurgery, which has been used to treat benign, premalignant and malignant lesions.

The freezing agents are used either by an open method (liquid nitrogen spray or CO_2 snow) or through a closed system cryoprobe, which is based on Joule-Thomson effect (rapid expansion of compressed gas through a small hole produces cooling). The freezing agents employed in closed systems probes are—liquid nitrogen, nitrous oxide and CO_2. The probes are available in different sizes and designs and produce a tip temperature of –70°C. The thermocouples of probes can be inserted into the tissue to monitor the temperature.

Tissue Effect

The cell death occurs through following mechanisms:
- **Dehydration** occurs due to crystallization of intracellular and extracellular water that increases electrolytes concentration. The pH changes and urea and dissolved gases increase to reach toxic concentrations, which cause cell death.
- **Denaturation** of cell membrane lipoproteins makes cell membrane permeable to cations. Thawing of cells, which become full of cations, results in lysis of cells.
- **Thermal shock** arrests the cellular respiration.
- **Vascular stasis** of both arterial and venous blood results in ischemic infarction. Cryosurgery is useful in the treatment of vascular lesions (hemangioma, angiofibroma and glomus tumors) because thrombosis of capillaries results in less bleeding.
- **Autoantibodies** specific to the frozen tumor tissues may provide tissue specific immunity to subsequent recurrence.

Technique

- **Anesthesia:** Cryosurgery can be done under local anesthesia, mild sedation and even without anesthesia because tissue freezing itself causes numbness.
- **Freezing:** The cryoprobe is applied into or upon the tissues for 3–8 minutes. It results in rapid freezing.
- **Thawing:** Frozen tissue is allowed to thaw slowly.
- **Repetitions:** The procedure may be repeated as required to achieve the best result.
- **Thermocouple:** It ensures freezing at an adequate depth.
- **Healing:** The wound heals by secondary intention. The slough usually falls in 3–6 weeks.

INDICATIONS

The increasing availability and popularity of laser is fast declining the indications of cryosurgery. Its lower cost still makes it an option in developing countries.

- **Benign vascular tumors:** Hemangiomas (skin, oral cavity, oropharynx) angiofibroma and glomus tumor.
- **Premalignant lesions:** Leukoplakia of oral cavity and solar keratosis (precancerous condition of skin). The scarring is less and quality of regenerated epithelium is better than diathermy.
- **Malignant lesions:** Intraepithelial carcinoma (Bowen's disease) and basal cell carcinoma of skin. Palliation of advanced, recurrent and residual tumors. Debulking of tumor facilitates deglutition and respiration. It reduces bleeding and relieves pain. Cryotherapy does not cause necrosis of bone and cartilage, which underlie the lesion. Recurrent tumors and ill-defined lesions are not good cases for cryotherapy.
- **Nose:** Reduction of turbinates improves the airway. In allergic rhinitis, it controls sneezing and rhinorrhea.
- **Tonsils:** Cryodestruction in high risk patients.

ADVANTAGES

- **Anesthesia:** No need of general anesthesia. Therefore, good for high risk patients.

Chapter 62 • Laser Surgery and Cryosurgery

- **Bleeding:** The patients with bleeding disorders or coagulopathies can be managed.
- **Palliation** in multiple and recurrent cancers where second course of radiotherapy cannot be used.
- **Minimal after effects**, such as discomfort and pain.
- **Minimal scarring:** Good for sites known for keloid development.
- **OPD:** Cryosurgery can be done as an OPD procedure.
- **Lower cost** in comparison to laser.

DISADVANTAGES

- **Excisional biopsy** and histopathological assessment of tumor margins are not possible.
- **Depth** of freezing is unpredictable.
- **Side effects:** Causes skin depigmentation and loss of hair (destruction of hair follicles).

> **Cryosurgery**
> - In cryosurgery, liquid nitrogen is applied at –30°C.
> - The cryoprobe is kept for 3–8 minutes so that area is frozen rapidly reaching a temperature of about –70°C.

HYPERBARIC OXYGEN THERAPY (HBOT)

Hyperbaric oxygen therapy is breathing pure oxygen in a pressurized room or tube. It is a treatment for decompression sickness, serious infections, arterial gas embolism and wounds that won't heal due to diabetes and radiation injury.

In a hyperbaric oxygen therapy chamber, the air pressure is increased to three times higher than normal air pressure. Lungs can gather more oxygen. Blood carries this oxygen throughout the body. This helps fight bacteria and stimulate the release of growth factors and stem cells, which promote healing.

INDICATIONS

- Sudden idiopathic sensorineural hearing loss and tinnitus: The results are better if therapy is started earlier. In various studies, improvements have been reported in 30–80% of the patients.
- Acoustic trauma
- Noise-induced hearing loss
- Malignant otitis externa
- Mucormycosis of paranasal sinuses
- Skin flaps with compromised blood supply
- Radiation tissue damage
- Healing problems in diabetes
- Crush injuries
- Osteomyelitis
- Bell's palsy.

COMPLICATIONS

It is generally a safe procedure but treatment does carry following potential risks: Temporary myopia, Tympanic membrane rupture, Lung collapse, Seizures and Fire of the treatment chamber.

Self-evaluation Exercises

1. Which of the following are visible lasers:
    a. CO_2
    b. Argon
    c. Nd:YAG
    d. KTP-532
2. Which of the following laser does not need optical fiber:
    a. CO_2
    b. Argon
    c. Nd:YAG
    d. KTP-532
3. Management of laser induced endotracheal tube fire include:
    a. Stop ventilation
    b. Saline irrigation and immediate withdrawal of the burnt tube
    c. Intravenous steroids
    d. Bronchoscopy to assess damage
    e. All the above

True (T)/False (F)

4. Argon laser is useful for middle ear surgery.
5. To cause cell death in cryosurgery, temperature should at least reach –30°C.
6. In cryosurgery, liquid nitrogen is applied at –30°C.
7. The cryoprobe is kept for 3–8 minutes so that area is frozen rapidly reaching a temperature of about –70°C.

Answers

1. b, d
2. a
3. e
4. T
5. T
6. T
7. T

Chapter 63

Human Immunodeficiency Virus Infection

Specific Learning Objectives
After going through the chapter, you should be able to answer the following questions:
- What are the mode of transmission and classifications of HIV infection?
- How the immunity is affected in HIV infection and decides the course of disease?
- How will you evaluate the HIV/AID patients and manage them?
- Describe the ear, nose, throat, head and neck manifestations in the HIV/AID patients.

HIV/AIDS

In 1986, the first case of acquired immunodeficiency syndrome (AIDS) was seen in India and surveillance of human immunodeficiency virus (HIV) infection/AIDS was started. National AIDS Control Organization (NACO) reports that Manipur, Maharashtra, Nagaland, Punjab and Daman & Diu (descending order) have high seropositivity rates per thousand persons screened for HIV. Among the cases of AIDS reported to NACO, maximum number of AIDS cases (in descending order) were in Tamil Nadu, followed by Maharashtra, Gujarat and Andhra Pradesh. About 85% were due to sexual relationship while nearly 3% were due to blood and blood products and about 2.5% due to perinatal transmission.

Transmission
The primary modes of HIV infection transmission and high-risk groups are:
- ***Sexual contact:*** Homosexual (especially receptive anal intercourse), heterosexual (promiscuous individuals, prostitutes and truck drivers) and bisexual.
- ***Skin piercing devices:*** Non-sterile needles, syringes and other skin piercing devices, and needle sharing in intravenous drug abuse.
- ***Transfusion of blood and its products:*** Common in hemophiliac, thalassemic and dialysis patients.
- ***Mother to child:*** Prenatal (transplacental), perinatal (during birth) and postnatal. The chances of vertical HIV transmission from an infected mother to her infant depend on the stage of maternal disease, type of delivery, birth order and concurrent sexually transmitted disease (STD) such as syphilis. They are approximately 25%.
- ***Health care workers:*** Contact with blood and body fluids such as amniotic, pleural, peritoneal or pericardial fluids carries high risk. Risk from specimens of urine, stool, saliva, sputum, tears, sweat and vomitus is negligible.

Human Immunodeficiency Virus (HIV)

HIV is composed of nucleocapsid core, structural proteins and a membrane envelope. It is a retrovirus of the Lentivirus subfamily. The nucleocapsid core contains two identical genomic RNA strands of about 10,000 nucleotides. HIV infection has a long incubation time and slow progression of disease.
- ***Types:*** HIV infection of human beings are of two types:
  1. ***HIV Type1:*** Most common and very pathogenic.
  2. ***HIV Type2:*** Less common and less pathogenic.

Human immunodeficiency virus (HIV): Reverse transcriptase of this virus produces DNA from viral RNA.

Immunology
- ***CD4 count:*** HIV infects CD4 T-lymphocytes and macrophages, which have CD4 surface marker and are associated with helper inducer function of the immune system. Once CD4 lymphocytes count falls below 500 cells/mm^3 (normal 600–1500 cell/mm^3), the myriad of AIDS defining pathological conditions start appearing. Death usually occurs within 2–3 years, once CD4 cell count falls below 200 cell/mm^3.

- **Immunity:** The slow but progressive impairment of both humoral and cell-mediated immunities makes the patient susceptible to opportunistic infections and neoplasms, culminating in AIDS. The impairment of macrophage function results in impaired chemotaxis and phagocytosis with increased susceptibility to candidiasis and toxoplasmosis. Decreased immunoglobulin production due to lack of T-cell stimulation of B cells makes the person vulnerable to encapsulated microorganisms such as *Streptococcus pneumoniae*.

> - **Immunity:** HIV mainly affects the cell mediated immunity.
> - **CD4 count:** Opportunistic infections and malignancies arise when CD4 count falls below 200/mm^3.

Classification and Course of Disease

The HIV infection runs through the following stages:

I. **Initial viremia:** HIV infection begins with initial viremia, which produces mild fever, headache, body aches, macular skin rash and lymph nodes enlargement. This clinical picture, which resembles infectious mononucleosis, subsides in 1–2 weeks. The HIV is then taken up by lymphatic system (lymph nodes, tonsils and adenoids). This initial viremia lasts for a few weeks and then no virus is detected in plasma. Antibody test becomes positive in 2–4 months of infection.

II. **Latent period:** This asymptomatic period lasts for a long period of about 10 years, HIV is replicating in the lymphoid tissue. CD4 T-helper cell count and function slowly deteriorate.

III. **Advanced disease:** AIDS features start appearing after several years, when CD4 T-cell count falls significantly and patient becomes susceptible to opportunistic infections. Death usually occurs within 2 years of the appearance of clinical signs and symptoms of AIDS.

- **CD4 Count:** The disease can be categorized further as per the CD4 counts:
  - 500 or more
  - 200 to 499
  - Less than 200

Diagnosis

Anti-HIV antibodies, detected by ELISA and Western blot, occur within 3 months of HIV infection. CD4 count and HIV viral load accurately ascertain the HIV infection and patient's immune status. The important tests, which are done to diagnose and treat HIV infection and its progression, are:

- **ELISA test:** Screening test (sensitivity > 99.9%).
- **Western blot test:** Confirmation test.
- **CD4 cell count (Normal 600–1500/mm^3):** CD4 lymphocyte percentage is more reliable than CD4 count. Falling counts indicate progression of disease. Count <200/mm^3 and <20% indicates high risk of AIDS progression.
- **PCR:** Quantitative test to measure viral load, which correlates with progression of disease.

Other tests which may also be carried out, include:

- **Complete blood count:** Anemia, leukopenia especially lymphopenia and thrombocytopenia.
- **Beta 2-Microglobulin level:** It is a prognostic test, which indicates macrophage monocyte stimulation. The levels rise at seroconversion and continue to rise with progression of disease.
- **P-24 antigen:** The presence of P-24 core protein of HIV indicates active HIV replication. This is an earliest test, which becomes positive even before the seroconversion.

Treatment

It consists of four elements: Treatment for opportunistic infections and malignancies, antiretroviral treatment (Table 63.1), hematopoietic stimulating factors and prevention of opportunistic infections.

- **Treatment for opportunistic infections and malignancies:** Patients who have good response to antiretroviral treatment, do not need maintenance treatment of opportunistic infections such as—
  - **M. avium:** Clarithromycin with ethambutol.
  - **Lymphoma:** Chemotherapy, radiation and dexamethasone for CNS lesions.
  - **Cytomegalovirus:** Valacyclovir, ganciclovir and foscarnet.
  - **Candidiasis** (esophageal or recurrent vaginal): Fluconazole.
  - **Herpes simplex and zoster:** Acyclovir, famciclovir, valacyclovir and foscarnet.
  - **Kaposi sarcoma:** Limited cutaneous lesions (observation, intralesional vinblastin); Extensive cutaneous lesions (chemotherapy, radiation); and visceral lesion (combination chemotherapy).
- **Antiretroviral treatment (Table 63.1):** Highly active antiretroviral therapy (HAART) has been reported to threefold decrease in mortality and a sixfold decrease in opportunistic infections. It consists of nucleoside reverse transcriptase inhibitors (NRTI), non-nucleoside reverse transcriptase inhibitors (NNRTI) and protease inhibitors (PI). Nucleoside analogues includes zidovudine (AZT), didanosine (ddI), zalcitabine (ddC) and stavudine (d4T). Reverse transcriptase inhibitor is lamivudine (3TC). Protease inhibitors are saquinovir, ritonavir and indinavir.
  - **Indications:** CD4 cell count<350 cells/mcL (< 200 cells/mcL in cases of higher risk for toxicity); Symptomatic HIV disease; Very high viral loads > 100,000/mcL.

Table 63.1: Antiretrovirals

Nucleoside reverse transcriptase inhibitors (NRTI)	Zidovudine, lamivudine, tenofovir, emtricitabine, stavudine, didanosine, abacavir, apricitabine, elvucitabine, racivir
Non-nucleoside reverse transcriptase inhibitors (NNRTI)	Nevirapine, efavirenz, etravirine, rilpivirine
Protease inhibitors (PI)	Ritonavir, atazanavir, lopinavir, darunavir, indinavir, saquinavir, nelfinavir, amprenavir, fos-amprenavir, tipranvavir
Fusion inhibitors	Enfuvirtide

- *Goal:* Viral load < 50–75 copies/mcL.
- *Monitoring:* Watch for toxicity and adverse reactions; CD4 cell count and viral load; drug resistance.

- *Side effects of indinavir (protease inhibitor):* They include breast hypertrophy, central adiposity, hyperlipidemia, insulin resistance and nephrolithiasis.
- *Ritonavir:* It inhibits HIV protease.
- *Highly active antiretroviral therapy (HAART):* HAART in HIV infection is associated with following:
  - Reduced incidence of opportunistic infections.
  - Decrease in viral mRNA copies/mL of blood.
  - Increase in CD4 count.
  - Decrease in rate of emergence of drug resistance.

- *Hematopoietic Stimulating Factors:*
  - *Epoetin alfa (erythropoietin):* In cases of anemia it avoids blood transfusions.
  - *Human G-CSF (filgrastim) and granulocyte-macrophage colony-stimulating factor GM-CSF (sargramostim):* They increase neutrophil count.
- *Prevention of opportunistic infections:* The decision to begin prophylactic therapy of opportunistic infections depends on following factors:
  - CD4 count.
  - Evidence of severe immune suppression such as oral candidiasis.
  - Past history of infection.

EAR, NOSE, THROAT, HEAD AND NECK MANIFESTATIONS OF HIV / AIDS

CERVICAL ADENOPATHY

Baseline palpable adenopathy is common in HIV infection.
- *Indications for biopsy:* FNAC can avoid open biopsy. The indications of biopsy include:
  - Single big node
  - Progressive enlargement of adenopathy
  - Marked constitutional symptoms
  - Cytopenia and raised ESR.
- *Causes:* Cervical lymphadenopathy can be due to:
  - *Infection:* Typical and atypical tuberculosis, histoplasmosis, toxoplasmosis and cat-scratch disease.
  - *Malignancy:* Lymphoma, carcinoma and Kaposi sarcoma.

NEOPLASMS

Four cancers are currently included in CDC classification of AIDS—Kaposi sarcoma, non-Hodgkin lymphoma, primary lymphoma of brain and invasive cervical carcinoma.
- *Most common neoplasms:* They are—
  - Kaposi's sarcoma
  - Non-Hodgkin's lymphoma
  - Lymphoepithelial cysts of parotid gland
- *Uncommon neoplasms:* They include—
  - Hodgkin's lymphoma
  - Cutaneous neoplasms: Squamous cell carcinoma.

Kaposi's Sarcoma

It is the most common malignant lesion of AIDS. It can occur at any stage of HIV infection.
- *Clinical features:* This multicentric non-invasive neoplasm respects the fascial planes and involves skin, mucosa and viscera.
  - *Lesions:* They appear as non-blanching, purplish (in light skinned people) or brownish (in dark skinned people) papules or nodules. These slightly raised lesions may vary in size (millimeters to centimeters).
  - *Site:* In oral cavity the most common site is palate. The exophytic lesions of tongue and gingivae may also be seen. The lesions can involve posterior pharyngeal wall and other sites such as eyelids, conjunctiva, pinna, face and neck.
- *Differential diagnoses:* It should be differentiated from angioma or pyogenic granuloma.
- *Diagnosis:* Biopsy shows excessive proliferation of spindle cells of vascular origin, endothelial cells, extravasation of red blood cells and hemosidrin laden macrophages.
- *Treatment:*
  - *Systemic chemotherapy:* Rapidly progressive dermatologic or visceral disease needs liposomally encapsulated doxorubicin intravenously every 3 weeks.
  - *Local:* Milder forms do not need any specific treatment and usually respond to antiretroviral therapy. Other forms of local management include:
    - Localized radiation
    - Intralesional vinblastin
    - Cryotherapy
- *Prognosis:* The ultimate survival is usually determined by infections and not by Kaposi's sarcoma.

Non-Hodgkin's Lymphoma (NHL)

It is the second most common AIDS-associated malignancy. NHL is an aggressive late stage disease and occurs in 10–30% of AIDS patients.

1. **Types:** Both nodal, extranodal (about 90%) and CNS lymphomas (about 40%) may be seen when CD4 counts fall below 200/mm^3.
2. **Clinical features:** Fever, night sweat, weight loss and non-tender rapidly enlarging neck mass.
3. **Treatment:** Chemotherapy and radiotherapy show poor control.

Lymphoepithelial Cysts of Parotid Gland

Lymphoepithelial cysts are bilateral and multiloculated and contained within parotid fascia. They usually involve the tail of parotid. Other parotid lesions include Kaposi's sarcoma, non-Hodgkin's lymphoma and parotitis.

- **Clinical features:** Asymptomatic bilateral parotid swellings are not uncommon in HIV infections. Reactive lymphocytes infiltrate parotid tissue. The salivary flow and amylase are normal.
- **Treatment:** Parotidectomy is advocated if needle aspiration fails. Intralesional tetracycline sclerosis and low dose of radiation have also been tried.
- **Prognosis:** In children, it indicates strong anti-HIV response and longer survival.

NOSE AND SINUSES

Acute and chronic sinus problems are common.
- Both aerobic and anaerobic infections are common.
  - Uncommon pathogens: *Legionella, Alternaria, Cryptococcus, Candida* and *Acanthamoeba*.
  - Fungal sinusitis (*Aspergillus* and *Mucormycosis*): It is rapidly invasive and extends intracranially.
- **Treatment:** In persistent and recurrent cases of sinusitis, in addition to antibiotics, long course of guaifenesin and topical steroids help in resolving the disease.
  - Surgical treatment is considered in invasive fungal infections.

> *Indications of antral puncture sinus lavage:* It should be done if patient does not respond to medications and when local and systemic complications arise.

NASOPHARYNX

Kaposi's sarcoma and NHL can involve nasopharynx.

EAR

- **External ear:** Kaposi's sarcoma of pinna and seborrheic dermatitis, which may get secondarily infected, are common.
  - Aural polyps due to *Pneumocystis carinii*.
- **Middle ear:** Serous and acute otitis media occur due to adenoid hypertrophy.
  - Most common pathogens (decreasing frequency): *Streptococcus pneumoniae, Haemophilus influenzae* and *Morexella catarrhalis. Staphylococcus, Pseudomonas* and *Pneumocystis carinii* are rare.
- **Sensorineural hearing loss:** Usually due to cytomegalovirus (CMV) affecting inner ear or CN VIII.
- **Ramsay Hunt syndrome or Herpes zoster oticus:** It has been reported in up to 16% of AIDS patients. Reactivation of latent varicella zoster virus can occur.

ORAL CAVITY

Oral candidiasis or hairy leukoplakia is highly suggestive of HIV infection in patients who have no other obvious cause of immunodeficiency. Kaposi's sarcoma lesions may ulcerate and become secondarily infected. Aphthous ulcers and xerostomia can also occur.

- **Candidiasis:** Oral candidiasis is the most common oral manifestation of AIDS. HIV candidiasis patients have high rate of progression to AIDS. It presents with tender, white and pseudomembranous lesions. Candida infection of esophagus causes severe odynophagia.
  - **Types:** (1) The pseudomembranous lesions are removable white plaques. (2) Erythematous lesions are red friable plaques.
  - **Treatment:** Patients who do not respond to clotrimazole (10 mg troche 4 or 5 times a day) can be treated with fluconazole (50–100 mg orally once a day for 3–7 days).
    - *Angular cheilitis:* Fissures at the sides of the mouth are usually due to Candida. They are treated topically with ketoconazole cream (2%) twice a day.
    - *Candidal esophagitis:* Fluconazole 200 mg OD for 10–14 days. The patients, who do not respond, should be evaluated for other causes of esophagitis such as herpes simplex and CMV.
- **Hairy leukoplakia:** This oral cavity lesion is seen almost exclusively in HIV patients. About half of the HIV infected patients with hairy leukoplakia develops AIDS in 16 months (Fig. 63.1).
  - **Pathogens:** Epstein-Barr virus and papillomavirus.
  - **Clinical feature:** It manifests as white vertically corrugated patches on the lateral border of tongue. The lesion may be flat or slightly raised. It is not usually troubling to patients and sometimes regresses spontaneously. The vertical parallel lines have fine or thick hairy projections.
- **Herpes simplex stomatitis:** Vesicular and extremely painful lesions may coalesce and form large ulcers of several centimeters. They are quite common.
  - Angular cheilitis can also be seen.

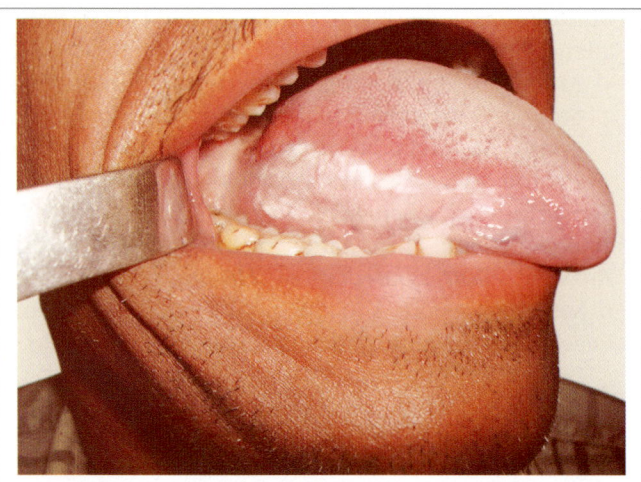

Fig. 63.1: Hairy leukoplakia lateral margin of anterior two-third tongue. Note the slightly raised lesion with hairy projections

- *Gingivitis and periodontitis:* They presents as tender bleeding gums and erythema at the gum-line.
  - *Treatment:* It usually responds to professional dental cleaning and chlorhexidine rinses.
- *Acute necrotizing ulcerative gingivitis (ANUG) and necrotizing stomatitis:* They indicate severe AIDS and present as red and swollen gingival lesions that undergo necrosis and destruction of periodontal soft tissue.
  - *Treatment:* Metronidazole 400 mg TDS for 5 days and referral to oral surgeons.
- *Aphthous ulcers:* The treatment of these painful ulcers include:
  - Fluocinonide topical application six times a day.
  - Dexamethasone swishes (0.5 mg in 5 mL elixir TDS).
  - Lidocaine 10% spray.
  - Thalidomide 50 mg orally daily and increasing to 100–200 mg daily. This teratogenic analgesic should be prescribed only to refractory patients who are at zero risk of procreation. The most common side effects include sedation and peripheral neuropathy.

OCCUPATIONAL EXPOSURE

Health care providers such as doctors (especially surgeons), nurses and laboratory staff while handling the blood, body fluids and other secretions may contract the disease. Each and every sample handled should be considered as potentially infected. The risk is usually due to:

Needle-stick injury: Hollow injection needle is more dangerous than solid suture needle. The risk of contracting HIV infection is 1:250.

- Cuts with contaminated knife or other sharp instruments.
- Exposure of open wound including area of dermatitis or even normal skin to infected blood or body fluid. Gloves and gown/coat are protective.
- Large mucous membrane exposure by splatter of blood.

Management of Needle Stick Injury

- Immediately wash the area thoroughly with water without soap and apply an antiseptic.
- Though the seroconversion takes time, ELISA test is done at the earliest to establish negative baseline for worker's compensation. The test is repeated at 6 weeks, 3 months and 6 months.
- Zidovudine therapy, 200 mg every 4 hours for 6 weeks, at the earliest has shown to decrease the rate of seroconversion after needle stick injury. The side effects of drug should be kept in mind.

Prevention

- Wear gloves. Wash hands before and after the contact.
- Handle the blood, body fluid and laboratory specimens as potentially infectious.
- Immediately place used syringes in impermeable container; never recap or manipulate needle.
- Wear gowns, protective glasses and mask when splatter with blood or body fluids is expected, such as bronchoscopy, tracheostomy and oral surgery.
- Linen soiled with blood and body fluid and secretions must be handled as potentially infectious.
- Wear mask for the opportunistic respiratory infections such as tuberculosis.

Care of Endoscopes

After the use, endoscopes should be wiped with alcohol and then immersed in 2% glutaraldehyde for 10 minutes. The flexible scopes then must be rinsed in water and air-dried.

Chapter 63 • Human Immunodeficiency Virus Infection

Self-evaluation Exercises

1. Highly active antiretroviral therapy (HAART) in HIV infection is associated with following:
    a. Reduced incidence of opportunistic infections
    b. Decrease in viral mRNA copies/mL of blood
    c. Increase in CD4 count
    d. Decrease in rate of emergence of drug resistance
    e. All of the above
2. Which of the following are not the side effects of indinavir (protease inhibitor)?
    a. Breast hypertrophy and central adiposity
    b. Hyperlipidemia
    c. Insulin resistance
    d. Nephrolithiasis
    e. None from above
3. Oral manifestations of HIV include:
    a. Oral candidiasis
    b. Hairy leukoplakia
    c. Recurrent aphthous ulcers
    d. All of the above

True (T)/False (F)

4. A single hollow bore needle prick has 1:500 chances of HIV seroconversion.
5. Reverse transcriptase of the HIV produces RNA from viral DNA.
6. HIV mainly affects the cell mediated immunity.
7. Opportunistic infections and malignancies arise in HIV infection when CD4 count falls below 500/mm^3.
8. Kaposi's sarcoma is the least common malignancy seen in AIDS patients.
9. Ritonavir inhibits HIV protease.

Answers

| 1. e | 2. e | 3. d | 4. F | 5. F |
| 6. T | 7. F | 8. F | 9. T | |

Pearls and Nuggets (Refresh your knowledge)

- **Esophageal perforation:** Fever after esophagoscopy heralds perforation. Swallow study confirms diagnosis. Early surgical repair is important. Draining the perforation may prevent complications. Antibiotics can mask the clinical features.
- **Caustic ingestion:** Oral burns may not correlate with severity of esophageal lesions. Alkaline agents penetrate deeper tissue layers.
- **Management caustic ingestion:** Watch for sign of airway obstruction because airway control must be the prime concern. Watch also for the features of mediastinitis (such as tachycardia, chest pain, fever, sepsis) and peritonitis.
- **Symptoms of laryngopharyngeal reflux:** They include in descending order of frequency hoarseness, cough, globus pharyngeus, throat clearing and difficulty in swallowing. Gastrointestinal symptoms are absent in more than 50% of patients with gastroesophageal reflux diseases (GERD).
- **Laryngoscopy in laryngopharyngeal reflux:** It shows posterior laryngitis, pachydermia, Reinke's edema, and granulomas.
- **Complications of laryngopharyngeal reflux:** GERD may be a risk factor for subglottic stenosis and laryngeal cancer.
- **Squamous cell carcinoma of esophagus:** Prior head and neck cancer increases the risk of this cancer eight-fold.
- **Airway:** Before aggressive ventilation, always confirm the placement of an endotracheal or tracheotomy tube by observing:
    - Humidification in the tube upon expiration
    - Affirm CO_2 return
    - Auscultation for bilateral breath sounds to rule out main-stem bronchi placement.
- **Bronchoscopy biopsy of the right upper lobe carina/spur:** It is the most dangerous site for biopsy because of the underlying right pulmonary artery.
- **Apical lung tumor:** It can manifest into **Horner syndrome** because of the compression of the structures that pass through the scalene interval and cross the first rib. Preganglionic sympathetic axons leave the spinal cord in the T_1 ventral ramus and synapse in the superior cervical ganglion and innervate the face, scalp, and orbit.
- **Brook's tumor:** It is of basal cell origin.
- **Hereditary lipid proteinosis:** It most commonly involves larynx.
- **Montogomery tube:** This silicon T-tube is used in ENT procedure.

Index

Page numbers followed by *b* refer to box, *f* refer to figure, *fc* refer to flow chart and *t* refer to table, respectively.

A

Abbe-Estlander flap 284
Abductor paralysis 375
Abductor spasmodic
    dysphonia 381
Abscess 120, 185, 188, 339, 427
    cerebellar 124, 125, 127
    cerebral 124
    cervical 305
    chronic retropharyngeal 429
    cold 415
    collar stud 415
    epidural 122
    extradural 118, 122, 208, 209
    forceps, peritonsillar 471, 471*f*
    incision and drainage of 427-429
    intratonsillar 307
    laryngeal 401
    lingual tonsillar 307
    lung 394
    mastoid 118
    meatal 118, 121
    parapharyngeal 118, 121, 305, 428, 430
    parotid 273
    perisinus 122, 126
    peritonsillar 305, 427, 427*f*, 430
    postauricular 118, 120
    pyemic 127
    retropharyngeal 118, 121, 429*f*, 477
    rupture of 125
    septal 197, 232, 449
    subdural 123, 209
    subperiosteal 208
Absorption 16
Accidents
    cerebrovascular 313
    motor vehicle 235
Achalasia, cardiac 300, 342, 344
Achlorhydria 341
Acids 336
    reflux 364
Acinic cell carcinoma 276
Acoustic neuroma 36, 137, 157, 165, 165*f*, 166, 435, 479

Acoustic reflex 47
    measurement 40
    neural pathways 47
    pathways 47*f*
Acoustic therapies 37, 37*b*
Acoustic trauma 63, 497
Acquired immune deficiency
    syndrome (AIDS) 154, 261, 287, 498
Actinomycosis 273, 361
Adamantinoma 248
Adducter spasmodic
    dysphonia 380
Adenocarcinoma 162, 252, 277
    follicular 418, 420, 422
    papillary 418, 419, 422
Adenohypophysis 296
Adenoidectomy 105, 107, 451, 452, 468, 469
    instruments of 471*f*
Adenoiditis, purulent 451
Adenoids 99, 289-291, 477
    palatine 291*t*
Adenolymphoma 276
Adenoma, pleomorphic 247, 275, 280, 317, 329
Adenopathy, cervical 500
Adenotonsillar disease 303
Adenotonsillar hypertrophy, chronic 307
Adenotonsillectomy 450, 452*f*, 469
    instruments of 469*f*, 470*f*
Adiadochokinesia 134
Aditus ad antrum 9
Adjustable flange long tube 473
Adriamycin 489
Aero-otitis media 107, 433
Aflatoxin 249
Agger nasi 174
    cells 174, 177, 480*f*
Agoraphobia 144, 146
Agranulocytosis 269, 305
Air bone gap 43, 44, 55
Air conduction 40, 41
    hearing aid 77
Air embolism 445
Air pressure 94
Airway
    breathing and circulation 236
    devices 396*f*, 474

    impairment of 429
    maintenance of 363
    nasopharyngeal 304, 395, 396*f*
    obstruction 308, 386, 428
    protection of 180
    resistance syndrome,
        upper 311
Alae nasi movements 187
Alkaline nasal irrigation 215
Alkaline reflux 382
Alkalis 336
Allergen, elimination of 140
Allergic rhinitis, classification of 226*f*
Allergy 2, 106, 114, 308, 358
    management of 105
    testing 97
Alopecia, facial 487
Alport's syndrome 70
Alveolar ridge
    lower 256
    upper 256
Alveolus
    lower 256
    upper 185, 256
Ameloblastoma 248, 280, 281
American Academy of
    Otolaryngology-Head and
    Neck Surgery 139*b*
American Joint Committee on
    Cancer 251*t*, 326
American sign language 74
Amifostine 488
Ammonia 181, 187
Amoxicillin 106
Amphotericin B 342
Amyloidosis 361
Analgesic 61, 86, 104, 337, 427, 443, 453
Analog hearing aids 78
Anemia 127
    iron deficiency 341
Anesthesia 56, 390, 391, 423, 446, 451, 457, 458, 496
    general 384, 442, 444, 447
Aneurysm 167
Angina 313
Angioedema 223
Angiofibroma 210, 246, 477
    excision of 469

Angiography
    carotid 318
    vertebral 167
Angiotensin converting
    enzyme 227
Angular cheilitis 501
Angular stomatitis 341
Animal bites 235
Ankyloglossia 263, 270
Annulus tympanicus 7
Anomalies
    congenital 150
    craniofacial 261
    craniovertebral 469
Anosmia 173, 187, 231
    causes of 188
Anoxia 70
Antibiotics 87, 88, 104, 105, 118, 124, 192, 203, 217, 245, 307, 337, 362, 363, 401, 436, 443, 453
    aminoglycoside 61, 62
    antipseudomonal 93
    first line of 203
    intravenous 204
    second line of 203
    systemic 86, 115, 232, 429
    therapy 106, 122, 123, 127
Antibody, antinuclear 71
Anticancer drugs, toxicity of 488
Anticholinergics 206
Antidiphtheric serum 306
Antigen, carcinoembryonic 412
Antihistamines 106, 201, 225
Anti-IgE antibody therapy 225
Antireflux surgery 340
Antral sign 318
Antrochoanal polyp 210, 211, 477, 479
    removal of 469
Antrostomy, intranasal 446
Antrum puncture 204, 445f, 466
Aorta, aneurysm of 460
Aortic arch 296, 461
Apex syndrome, orbital 207, 208
Aphasia
    conductive 379
    fluent 379
    nominal 125
    nonfluent 379
Aphonia 377
Aphthous stomatitis, recurrent 268
Aphthous ulcer 269f
Apicitis, petrous 121
Aplasia, alexander 69
Apnea 394
    hypopnea index 311, 315
Aponeurosis, pharyngeal 289
Appetite 6, 181
Aquino's sign 163
Arch
    palatoglossal 291

    palatopharyngeal 291
    second branchial 19
    zygomatic 239
Argon laser 494
Arnold's nerve 5
Arnold-Chiari malformation 58, 131
Arousal index 311
Arousal test 73
Arrhythmias, cardiac 313
Arterial dissection 36
Arterial embolization 193
Arterial ligation 194
Arteries 405
    caroticotympanic 29
    carotid 410
    cerebellar 150
    cochlear 19
    ethmoidal 194
    facial 174
    infraorbital 174
    maxillary 13, 174, 194
    ophthalmic 174
    petrosal 150
    sphenopalatine 174
    subclavian 302
    supplying middle ear 13t
    vestibulocochlear 19
Arthritis, rheumatoid 71, 361
Artificial larynx 388
Aryepiglottic folds 365
Arytenoidectomy 376, 377
Asch's septum forceps 238, 466, 467f
Ashai technique 388
Aspergillus niger 90
Asphyxia, cyclic 233
Aspiration 231, 340, 359, 377
    pneumonia 343, 429
Aspirin triad syndrome 205
Asthma 231, 340
Ataxic gait 29
Atelectasis 107, 394, 398, 433
Atherosclerosis 36
Atlantoaxial dislocation 454
Atlantoaxial subluxation 454
Atresia 87
    choanal 233, 442, 477
    correction of 234
Atresioplasty, endoscopic 234
Atrophic rhinitis, secondary 215
Atrophy 433
Attacks
    acute 138, 140
    drop 139
Atticoantrotomy 434
Atticotomy 113
Audible systolic bruit 162
Audiogram 35, 43, 65, 79, 130, 139
    otosclerosis 55f

Audiometric tests 40
Audiometry 31, 55, 60, 106, 166
    impedance 40, 46
Auditory canal
    external 4, 5, 12, 19, 24-26, 30, 35, 52, 72, 78, 85, 98, 102, 103, 106, 141, 160, 164f
    internal 165
Auricle 4, 19, 33
    disorders of 85
    keloid of 161
    melanoma of 161
    squamous cell
        carcinoma of 161
Auricular artery, branches of 150
Auricular nerve, posterior 150
Autoantibodies 496
Autofluorescence
    laryngoscopy 384
Autoimmune disease 154, 268
Autoimmune disorders 364
Autoimmunity 155, 417
Autonomic nervous system 175
Autosomal dominant,
    congenital 70
Autosomal recessive,
    congenital 70
Awake flexible laryngoscopy 377, 397

B

Bacillus proteus 102, 126
Bacteria, anaerobic 272
Bacterial endocarditis, subacute 305
Bacterial rhinosinusitis, acute 200, 201, 221
Bacteroides fragilis 110, 125
Ballenger's swivel knife 468
Barany noise box 463
Barium swallow 300, 300f, 302, 332, 333, 338, 341-343, 343f, 345, 477
Barotrauma 102, 143
Barrett's esophagus 340
Basal cell
    carcinoma 161, 186f, 198
    hyperpalsia theory 112
Basaloid squamous cell
    carcinoma 384
Basilar membrane 15
Basilar migraine 144
Beahr's triangle 406
Beam radiotherapy, external 422
Beam therapy, external 485
Beckmann adenoid curette 471f
Behçet's disease 66
Behçet's syndrome 269
Bell's palsy 154, 155, 497
Bell's phenomenon 155, 155f
Bernstein test 340

Berry's ligament 406
Bezold's abscess 118, 121, 121*f*
Bilevel positive airway pressure 314
Bill's island 12
Binaural tests 41
Bing test 40, 43
Biopsy 214, 217, 218, 219, 250, 260, 265, 326, 327, 334, 345, 364, 365, 420, 456, 459, 500
Birth injuries 70
Bleomycin 489, 490
Blepharoplasty 221
Blepharospasm 157
Blink reflex 166
Blood
    aspiration of 394
    borne infection 102, 142
    culture 127
    disorders 269
    loss 192, 221
    oxygen saturation 313
    sugar 218
    transfusion of 498
    vessels 191
Body equilibrium, maintenance of 28
Body mass index 313
Body tumor, carotid 413, 414
Boerhaave's syndrome 336
Bondy procedure 114
Bone 171
    anchored hearing aid 66, 76, 79
    conduction 40, 41
        absolute 31, 40, 52
        hearing aid 73, 77
    destruction of 112
    erosion 118
    forceps 467
    fractures, bilateral temporal 154
    hyoid 400
    lacrimal 171
    palatine 171
Bony cochlea, cross section of 15*f*
Bony labyrinth 14, 20, 53
    ossification of 53
Bony septum 448
Bony skeleton, enlargement of 185
Boucheron ear speculum 463*f*
Boyle-Davis mouth gag 452*f*, 469
Brachial plexus 415
Brachytherapy 322, 485
Brain abscess 118, 124, 209
    otogenic 124
    rupture 125*f*
Brainstem 166
    evoked response audiometry 40, 48, 48*f*, 48*t*, 68, 71, 72, 166
    implant, auditory 84
    infarct 36
Branhamella catarrhalis 102

Brisk jerky nystagmus 142
Broca's aphasia 379
Brompheniramine 225
Bronchi 358, 494
Bronchial obstruction, types of 399*f*
Bronchial tree 224
Bronchitis, asthmatic 221
Bronchoaortic constriction 338
Bronchoesophagoscopy
    instruments 472*f*
Bronchography 359
Bronchopneumonia 377
Bronchoscope tube 472*f*
Bronchoscopy 345, 360, 397, 399, 400, 458, 459, 503
    flexible 459
Brook's tumor 503
Brown's sign 162
Brudzinski's sign 124
Bruises 400
Bruit 410
Bryce's sign 371
Buccal mucosa, leukoplakia of 264*f*
Bulbar polio 342
Bull's eye lamp 3
Bulla ethmoidalis 173
Bullous lichen planus 266
Burns 235
    corrosive 336
Bursa, nasopharyngeal 290
Bursitis, pharyngeal 322

C

Caldwell-Luc approach 211
Caldwell-Luc operation 242, 445, 446*f*, 466-468
Caloric tests 133, 133*f*, 142
Canal
    atresia of 19
    auditory 4
    paresis 133
    semicircular 14, 15, 27
    wall-down procedure 114, 433
    wall-up procedure 113, 433
Canalithiasis 132, 136
Cancer 364
    anaplastic 419, 420
    glottic 386
    head and neck 382
    hypopharyngeal 331*f*
    laryngeal 384
    papillary 419
    phobia 298
    prevention of 490
    subglottic 387
    supraglottic 383, 386
Candida albicans 90, 266, 342

Candidiasis 266, 361, 499, 501
    chronic hypertrophic 266
Canine fossa antrostomy 446, 446*f*
Carbogen, inhalation of 65
Carbon dioxide laser 493
Carboplatin 489
Carcinoma 35, 141, 162, 164*f*, 280, 335
    anaplastic 418, 420, 422
    buccal mucosa 285, 286*f*
    esophagus 344
    follicular 422
    gingiva 284
    glottis 385
    hard palate 286
    in situ 383
    invasive 383
    larynx 384*f*
    lips 283
    lymphoepithelial 277, 325
    maxillary sinus 249
    medullary 412, 418, 421, 422
    mucoepidermoid 276
    nasal cavity 251*t*
    nasopharyngeal 291, 320
    oncocytic 420
    oral tongue 284
    papillary 421
    posterior pharyngeal wall 328, 333
    pyriform sinus 331
    retromolar trigone 287
    soft palate 328
    supraglottic larynx 383*f*
    tongue 284*f*
    tonsil 327
    verrucous 286, 384
Carhart's notch 55
Carhart's tone decay test 45
Carotenoids 491
Carotid artery
    external 13, 194
    internal 13, 329, 425, 426
Carotid system
    external 174
    internal 174
Cartilage
    cricoid 400
    incision of 447
    septal 170, 173, 448
Cartilaginous tumor, laryngeal 372
Catecholamines 163
Caudal septal deviation 173, 230
Cells
    frontoethmoid 177
    lymphoid 418
    marginal 13
    papilloma, transitional 248
    parafollicular 418
    perilabyrinthine 13
    perisinus 13
    retrofacial 13

tumor, granular 280, 281
zygomatic 13
Cellulitis 90, 445
    orbital 208, 209t
    periesophageal 339
Cementoma 248
Central auditory tests 40
Central nervous system 21, 28, 29, 142, 145
Cephalometric radiogram, lateral 315
Cerebellar artery
    anteroinferior 145
    posteroinferior 145
    superior 145
Cerebellopontine angle 165
    boundaries of 165
    lesions 152
    tumors 35, 154, 165f
Cerebellum 118, 166
    degenerative lesion of 131
Cerebrospinal fluid 16
    otorrhea 118, 123, 435
    rhinorrhea 242, 442
Cerebrum 181
Ceruminoma 161
Cervical chain, transverse 402, 403
Cervical esophagus, perforation of 336
Cervical lymph nodes
    levels of 403
    palpation of 409f
Cervical lymphadenitis,
    tuberculous 414f, 415
Cervical nodes
    anterior 402, 403
    lateral 403
    superficial lateral 402
Cervical spine, tuberculosis of 429
Chandler classification 208t
Charge syndrome 58
Chemoradiation 490
Chemosis 127
Chemotherapy 252, 320, 328, 422, 484, 486, 488
    adjuvant 486
    concomitant 486
    induction 486
    palliative 490
    protocols 387
    systemic 322, 500
Chest pain, noncardiac 339
Chevalier Jackson's
    tracheostomy tube 474
Chevallet vertical fracture 229f
Chloroquin 62
Chlorpheniramine 225
Choanal atresia, unilateral 188
Cholesteatoma 99, 107, 109, 110, 112, 122, 124, 126, 141, 167, 433
    acquired 111, 111fc
    congenital 111, 113, 157

    primary acquired 111, 113
    spread of 112
    structure 10, 110f
    types of 111, 111t
Chondritis 86, 90
Chondroma 247, 372
Chondrosarcoma 162, 253
Chorda tympani 8, 150
    nerve 11, 56
Chordoma 317
Choristoma 317
Chraniopharyngioma 317
Ciliary dysfunction 105
Ciliary dyskinesia 101, 205
Cirrhosis 282
Cisplatin 489
Citelli's abscess 118, 121
Citelli's angle 12
Cleft cyst, second branchial 414
Cleft lip 230, 261
    congenital 171
Cleft palate 99, 101, 105, 230, 261
    repair of 469
    submucous 296, 309
Cleft sinus, second branchial 414
Clemastine 225
Clotrimazole 342
Coalescent mastoiditis, acute 118
Cochlea
    aqueduct of 15
    membranous 15
Cochleosacculotomy 141
Cogan's syndrome 66, 141
Cold air caloric test 134
Collet-Sicard syndrome 321
Colloid nodule 417, 419
Columella retraction 449
Columellar septum 172
Columnar cells 418
Combination therapy 328
Commando operation, external
    neck incision of 285f
Complete blood count 64, 71, 119, 192, 224, 499
Concha bullosa 173
Conductive hearing loss,
    causes of 52b, 53fc
Condyle, fractures of 241
Confrontation test 125
Congenital stridor, causes of 398
Coniotomy 394
Continuous positive airway
    pressure 314, 360
Cor pulmonale 308, 313, 450, 451
Cord, lateralization of 376
Cordectomy 385
Coronavirus 303
Corti
    organ of 16, 26

    tunnel of 17
Corticobulbar fibers, bilateral 75
Corticospinal tracts, bilateral 75
Corticosteroids 106, 225, 266
    short-course of 269
Costen's syndrome 58
Cottle test 187, 188, 189f
Cotton wool test 187
Cough 359, 377, 391
    nonproductive 339
    painful 391
    whooping 361
Cowden syndrome 417
Coxsackievirus infections 303
Cranial fossa
    anterior 242, 252
    middle 6, 118, 122, 242
    posterior 118, 122
Cranial nerves, examination of 298
Craniopharyngioma 291
Crepitus, post-laryngeal 333f
Crest
    maxillary 448
    vestibular 14
Cricoarytenoid joint, arthrodesis of 377
Cricoidectomy, partial 377
Cricothyrotomy 360, 394, 399
Crista ampullaris 16
Crocodile tears 154
Crohn's disease 335
Crouzon's syndrome 70
Crowe-beck test 127
Crush injuries 497
Cryosurgery 451, 496, 497
Crypta magna 292
Cryptococcosis 361
Crypts, secondary 292
Cupulolithiasis 136
Cutaneous horn 161
Cyanosis 2
Cyberknife stereotactic surgery 487
Cyclophosphamide 489
Cylindroma 276
Cystadenoma lymphomatosum,
    papillary 276
Cystic carcinoma, adenoid 252, 276, 317
Cysts 160, 185, 419, 478
    arachnoidal 167
    branchial 121, 414
    ductal 370
    mucous 329
    nasoalveolar 198
    nasolabial 185, 186f
    preauricular 19, 86
    retention 292
    saccular 371
    thymic 416
    thyroglossal 406, 408, 414, 414f
Cytomegalovirus 303, 499

D

Dacryocystitis 446
Dacryocystorhinostomy 442
Dalrymple's sign 411, 412
Danger space 426
Dead labyrinth 133
Deafness 249
Decompression 158
    orbital 442
Deep neck
    abscesses 425*f*
    infections 425
    spaces, classification of 425*b*
Deferoxamine 62
Deformity 185
    external 231
Dehydration 272, 496
Deiter's cells 17
Delphian node 386, 402, 403
Demarquay's sign 383
Dental caries 282
Dental cysts 185
Dental infections 429
Dental malocclusion 451
Dental wiring 395
Dermatitis, contact 89
Dermoid 185
    cyst 160, 185, 190, 198, 280, 282, 415
        simple 198
        submental 282
Desferioxamine 62
Diabetes mellitus 154
Dichotic test 41
Dietary deficiency 263
Diphenhydramine 225
Diphtheria 2, 305, 361, 363
    antitoxin 363
Diphtheroids 215
Diplopia 128, 249
Distortion evoked otoacoustic emission 49
Distraction techniques 73
Diverticula 344
Diverticulectomy 343
Diverticulum, hypopharyngeal 289, 301
Dix-Hallpike maneuver 132
Dix-Hallpike test 132*f*, 136
Dizziness 143, 163
    causes of 140*t*
    pathophysiology of 29
    types of 140
Dohlman's procedure 344
Doll's-eye test 132
Donaldson's line 12, 435
Dorello's canal 29
Double lumen tube 473
Double ring sign 243
Down's syndrome 70, 99, 101
Doyen's mouth gag 468

Drainage, lymphatic 13, 176, 179, 255-257, 290, 291, 293-295, 406
Drug therapy 225
Duct
    cochlear 15
    endolymphatic 16
    frontonasal 237
    incision of 274
    nasolacrimal 446
    semicircular 16
    thyroglossal 412
Dysgeusia 134, 258
Dysmetria 29
Dysphagia 299, 300, 304, 309, 338, 341, 343, 355, 423, 430, 450, 451
    causes of 301*b*
    lusoria 302*f*
Dysphonia
    plica ventricularis 379
    spasmodic 380
    ventricular 379
Dysplasia
    benign 265
    fibrous 247*f*
    minimal 265
Dyspnea 423

E

Eagle's syndrome 33, 329
Ear
    anatomy of 4
    development of 19*t*
    discharge 112, 114, 116, 119
        recurrent 451
    drops 88, 104
    external 36, 501
    fluids, inner 16
    inner 19
    lymphatic drainage of 13*t*
    microsurgery 494
    middle 19, 26, 33, 35, 36, 52, 105
    polyp 35, 113, 116
    speculum 463
    surgery 35, 142
    trauma 89
    wax 91
Earache 32, 163, 304
    post-tonsillectomy 454
Ecchymosis, periorbital 238
Ectoderm 19
Edema 400, 454
    mucosal 105
    peripheral 313
    pulmonary 454
Electrocochleography 40, 48, 61, 140
Electrolarynx 388
Electromyogram 313
Electron beam 485

Electroneurography 152
Electronystagmography 134, 140
Emphysema
    obstructive 399
    subcutaneous 394, 400, 443, 444
    surgical 356, 454
Empyema 204
    mastoid 119
    subdural 118
Encephalitis 209
Encephalocele 442
    extranasal 198
Endaural speculum 465
Endoderm 19
Endolymph 16
    flow of 28
    overaccumulation of 138
Endophlebitis 126
Endoscope 97, 471
    care of 502
Endoscopic sinus surgery, instruments of 467*f*
Endoscopy 112, 114, 250, 298, 333, 334, 344, 357, 359, 360, 383, 456
    flexible 343
Endotracheal intubation 234, 395, 430, 447
Endotracheal tube 469*f*
Enuresis 309, 450, 451
Enzyme-linked immunosorbent assay (ELISA) 224, 305
    test 499
Eosinophilia 226
Epidermosis 110
Epiglottic tumors, infrahyoid 387
Epiglottitis 362
    acute 359, 362, 477
    pediatric 361, 362, 363*f*
Epiglottopexy 377
Epiphora 155, 238, 249
Epistaxis 190, 229, 231, 308, 442
    anterior 191
    balloon 194*f*
    causes of 190, 190*b*
    posterior 191, 193
    recurrent 447
    sites of 191
Epithelial carcinoma, WHO classification of 320*t*
Epithelioma 198, 199
Epithelium 289
    olfactory 174
Epitympanum 8
Epstein-Barr virus 60, 304, 320
Epulis granulomatosa 281
Epulis gravidarum 281
Epworth sleepiness scale 313, 314*t*
Erythema multiforme 269
Erythrocyte sedimentation rate 64
Erythroleukoplakia 265
Erythromycin 62

Erythroplakia 265
    tongue 265f
Escherichia coli 88, 110, 125, 126, 215, 429
Esophageal injury, corrosive 337t
Esophageal rupture, cervical 336
Esophageal sphincter
    lower 295, 335
    upper 295, 335, 342
Esophagitis 340
    candidal 501
    infectious 342
    monilial 335
Esophagogastroduodenoscopy 340
Esophagoscopy 300, 302, 338, 341-343, 345, 459
    flexible 461, 462f
    procedure of 461f
Esophagotomy
    cervical 339
    transthoracic 339
Esophagus 33, 288, 294, 294f, 410, 419
    abdominal 295
    cervical 295
    disorders of 335
    evaluation of 300
    lower 300f
    nutcracker 342
    perforation of 336, 339, 461
    squamous cell carcinoma of 345, 503
    thoracic 295
    upper 300f
Esthesioneuroblastoma 489
Estradiol nasal spray 215
Ethmoid 171
    anterior 187
    posterior 179
    roof of 443
    sinus, malignancy of 252
Ethmoidal artery, anterior 444
Ethmoidectomy
    anterior 443
    external 206, 211
    intranasal 206
    posterior 443
Eustachian catheter 98, 98f
Eustachian tube 9, 10f, 32, 35, 47, 55, 96, 96f, 96t, 97, 99, 101, 102, 114
    anatomy 95, 95f
    catheterization 98
    closure of 436
    disorders of 95
    dysfunction 101
    endoscopy 97
    examination of 31, 97
    function 97, 97t
    instruments 465f
    mucosa of 96
    obstruction 99
    pharyngeal opening of 290
    physiology of 96

Eve's tonsil snare 470
Ewald's law 131
Excision biopsy 421
Exophthalmos 188, 207, 411
Exostoses 160, 466
Extension 289, 428
External auditory canal
    disorders of 87
    examination of 31
    furuncle of 120, 120t
    nerve supply of 6f
External ear
    diseases of 85t
    malignant tumors of 161
Extracorporeal shock wave lithotripsy 275
Eyeball
    displacement of 238
    fixation of 127
Eyelids, inflammatory edema of 207
Eyes 224, 249
    movements 313

F

Facial nerve
    branches of 149, 149f
    course of 148
    decompression of 435
    examination of 31
    hyperkinetic disorders of 157
    motor nucleus of 148
    palsy causes of 154, 154b
        complications of 154
    topographical lesions of 153f
Facial pain, atypical 33
Farabeuf's periosteal elevator 466
Fascia
    buccopharyngeal 289
    pharyngobasilar 289
Fenestra cochlea 9, 15
Fenestra vestibuli 9
Fever 119, 126, 304, 359
    exanthematous 102
    pharyngoconjunctival 303
    rheumatic 305
    scarlet 305
Fiberoptic bronchoscopy, flexible 459
Fibers
    gustatory 148
    sympathetic 11
Fibroma
    irritation 280, 281
    ossifying 248
Fibrosarcoma 162
Fibrosis 115
    cystic 101, 205, 209
    subcutaneous 487
Fibrous dysplasia, monostotic 247
Fick and Cody tack procedures 141

Fine needle aspiration
    cytology 260, 412, 321
Finger friction test 40, 41
Fissure, palpebral 238
Fistula 31, 414
    collaural 87
    large 242
    oroantral 242
    perilymphatic 57, 118, 131, 142, 143
    postauricular 116
    sign 141
    test 31, 131, 141, 464
        false negative 131
        false positive 131
    thyroglossal 406
Fits, epileptic 125
Fitzgerald-Hallpike bithermal
    caloric test 133
Flaps 423, 448
Fluconazole 342
Fluids
    intravenous 337, 362, 363
    nasal regurgitation of 299
Fluoroscopy 342, 399
Foley's catheter 193, 193f
Follicular tonsillitis and
    diphtheria, acute 306t
Fordyce's spots 266
Fowler's alternate binaural loudness
    balance test 44
Fractures 400
    blowout 239
    bone 157t
    condylar 221, 242
    Le Fort classification of 240f
    mandibular 221, 242
    maxilla 444
    maxillofacial 235
    orbital 235
    pure blowout 239
Frenzel glass 132
Frenzel maneuver 98
Frey's syndrome 11, 154, 278
Frisch bacillus 366
Frog-face deformity 318
Frost bite 4, 86
Fuller's bivalved
    tracheostomy tube 473, 473f
Functional endoscopic
    sinus surgery 173, 177, 204
Fundoscopy 124
Fungal rhinosinusitis, allergic 219
Fungal sinusitis
    allergic 209
    chronic invasive 219
Fungi, causative 219
Furuncle 185, 196
Furunculosis 90, 119
Fusiform bacilli 305
Fusion inhibitors 500

G

Galvanic test 134
Gamma knife surgery 167
Gancyclovir 342
Gardners syndrome 417
Gastric junction, esophageal 300f
Gastroesophageal reflux 295, 382
　　disease 205, 300, 335, 339, 364, 368
Gastrostomy 341
Gelle's test 40, 43
Geniculate body, medial 27
Gentamicin, intratympanic
　　injections of 141
Geographical tongue 270, 270f
Gingivitis 502
Gingivostomatitis, herpetic 267, 267f
Glasgow coma scale/score 221
Glioma 247
　　extranasal 198, 247
Globus hystericus pharyngeus 344
Glomerulonephritis, acute 305
Glomus jugulare 162
　　tumors 141
Glomus tumor 35, 36, 157, 162, 413
　　intratympanic 432
Glomus tympanicum 162
Glossectomy, partial midline 315
Glossitis 341
　　migratory 270
Glottis 376, 384
Glycerol test 139
Goiter, multinodular 421
Granulation 115, 116
　　tissue 113
Granuloma 370
　　cholesterol 99, 107, 113, 167
　　nonhealing midline 214
　　pyogenic 280, 281
Granulomatous disorders 262
Graves' disease 442
Greater palatine artery 174
Greater superficial petrosal nerve 149
Grisel's syndrome 454
Grunwald, lateral sinus of 174
Guedel oropharyngeal airway 396f
Guillain-Barre syndrome 154
Guillotine method 451
Gums 259
Gutzman's pressure test 380

H

Habenula perforata 56
Haemophilus influenzae 92, 102, 124, 201,
　　272, 361, 429, 501
Hagginson's syringe 445f
Hair cells 17, 138
　　functions of 26
　　outer 17t
　　vestibular 28f
　　inner 17, 17t, 26
Hair follicles 5
Hairy leukoplakia 259, 501, 502f
Hairy tongue 259, 270
Hajek lip retractor 469
Halitosis 299, 427
Haller cells 177
Hallucination, auditory 35
Hamartoma 317
Hamman's sign 336
Hand, foot and mouth disease 268
Handicap, degree of 44
Hansen's disease 366
Hard palate 256, 259
　　hemangioma 259f
Hartmann ear speculum 463f, 465f
Hartmann eustachian catheter 465f
Hashimoto thyroiditis 418f
Hay fever 223
Head and neck, lymph nodes of 404f
Head thrust test 132
Headache 33, 127, 128, 205, 231, 442
Hearing loss 40, 44, 51, 52, 55, 61, 66, 91, 99,
　　114, 116, 139, 143, 162, 166
　　causes of 40
　　classification of 51
　　conductive 39, 41, 42, 44, 45, 51, 52,
　　　52t, 55, 57, 59, 93, 99, 102, 111, 119
　　degree of 44, 66
　　noise-induced 26, 63, 497
　　non-organic 67
　　normal and conductive 43
　　sensorineural 35, 40-45, 51, 52, 52t, 59,
　　　60fc, 71fc, 75, 94, 107, 152
　　severity of 40, 44
　　sudden sensorineural 64
　　types of 39, 40, 44
Hearing tests 72, 115, 433
　　types of 40b
Hearing, physiology of 24, 24f
Heart failure, congestive 313
Heartburn 295, 300
Heerfordt's syndrome 154
Heimlich's maneuver 399f
Heine otoscope 463f
Heller's operation, modified 343
Hemangioma 160, 198, 248, 276, 280, 281,
　　329, 372
　　adult 372
　　capillary 160, 248
　　cavernous 160, 248
　　infantile 372
　　subglottic 397
　　tongue 281f
Hemangiopericytoma 248, 317
Hematoma 87, 400, 424
　　auricular 86f
orbital 238, 444
　　septal 188, 197, 229, 231, 234, 238, 449
Hemisphere, cerebellar 134
Hemithyroidectomy 386, 422
Hemorrhage 340, 394, 449
　　cerebellar 144, 145
　　primary 454
　　secondary 454
Hemostasis 452, 453
Hennebert's sign 61, 131, 138
Hereditary hemorrhagic telangiectasia 194
Hereditary lipid proteinosis 503
Herpangina 268, 303
Herpes labialis 267, 267f
Herpes lesions 156f
Herpes simplex 71, 499
　　infection
　　　primary 267
　　　recurrent 267
　　　secondary 267
　　stomatitis 501
　　virus 267, 304
Herpes zoster oticus 92, 156, 501
Herpetiform aphthous stomatitis 268
Heymann turbinectomy scissors 467
Hiatus hernia 301, 335, 341
　　paraesophageal 341
Hiatus semilunaris 174
Higginson's syringe 466
His, hillocks of 19
Histeliberger's sign 166
Histoplasmosis 361
Hitzelberger's sign 6
Hodgkin's disease 413
Holinger anterior
　　commissure laryngoscope 472f
Holman-Miller sign 318
Homonymous hemianopia,
　　contralateral 125
Hopkins telescope 472f
Hormones 140
Horner's syndrome 147, 321, 410, 503
Hot fomentation 204
Hot nodules 421
Hot tonsillectomy 427
House-Brackmann system 150, 151t
Human immunodeficiency
　　virus (HIV) 261, 498
　　infection 282, 498
Human papillomavirus 248, 282, 325,
　　382, 344
Hump nose 197
Hurthle cell
　　adenoma 418
　　carcinoma 420
Hutchinson's teeth 61, 218
Hutchinson's triad 61
Hydration, inadequate 364
Hydrops, endolymphatic 59, 138
Hydroxyzine 225

Hygroma, cystic 414
Hyperkeratosis 383
Hypermotility 301
    disorder 335
Hypernasality 380
Hyperplasia 105
    adenoid 105
Hypertension 36, 313
    pulmonary 308
Hypertrophy, adenoid 451
Hyperventilation 134, 144, 146
Hypomotility 301
Hyponasality 380
Hypopharynx 293, 295, 456
    cancer of 385
    structures of 293f
    subsites 294, 331
    tumors of 331, 385
    Zenker's diverticulum of 343f
Hypophysectomy 447
Hypopnea 311
Hyposmia 187, 231
Hypotension, orthostatic 134
Hypothyroidism 75, 154, 227, 424
Hypotympanum 8
Hyrtl's fissure 118

I

Ifosfamide 489
Immotile cilia syndrome 181
Immunity 499
Immunoglobulins 180
Immunosuppressant therapy 141, 214
Immunotherapy 220, 225
Implant, cochlear 66, 74, 76, 81, 435
In vitro tests 224
Incision, postaural 433
Infarction, cerebellar 144, 145
Infections 59, 70, 196, 242, 454
    acute 191
    fungal 205
    pulmonary 399
    routes of 102, 124, 142
    sources of 115, 427, 428, 430
    spread of 92, 429
    viral 106, 154
Inflammation
    meningeal 142
    mucosal 301
Injuries 454, 461
    corrosive 344
    modes of 241, 400
    orbital 445
    penetrating 242, 336, 400

Intermittent positive pressure respiration 390
Intranasal provocation test 224
Intraoral devices 314
Intrathecal fluorescein 243
Intubation 221, 337, 362, 363, 366
    granuloma 368, 370
    orotracheal 360
Invagination theory 111
Invasion, stages of 125
Invasive fungal sinusitis, acute 218
Ipratropium 206
    bromide nasal spray 201
Irritation, meningeal 123
Ischemia, vascular 155
Isthmus 6, 95, 423
    nasopharyngeal 290
    oropharyngeal 291
Itraconazole 219

J

Jackson's tracheostomy tube 473f
Jacobson, vomeronasal organ of 182
Jansen dressing forceps 463f
Jansen elevator 466f
Jansen middleton septum
    bone forceps 467f
Jarjavay fracture 229, 229f
Jaundice, neonatal 70
Jaw thrust 395, 396f
Jennings mouth gag 468
Jervell and Lange-Nielson syndrome 70
Jet ventilation 396f
Jobson-Horne's probe 464, 464f
Joffroy's sign 411
Joints
    cricoarytenoid 400
    cricothyroid 400
    dislocation of 400
Joll's triangle 405
Jugular bulb, thrombosis of 127
Jugular chain, internal 402, 403
Jugular foramen 375
    syndrome 163, 321
Jugular fossa, dehiscent roof of 8
Jugular lymph nodes 127
Jugular vein 127
    internal 404, 426
    ligation of 127
    thrombosis 121
Jugular wall 8
Jugulodigastric node 403
Juvenile nasopharyngeal
    angiofibroma 317, 319t, 442
Juvenile papillomas 371
Juxtavisceral chain 402, 403

K

Kallmann syndrome 188
Kaposi's sarcoma 280, 282, 287, 499-500
Kartagener's syndrome 181, 209
Kashima operation 376
Keloid 32f
Keratitis
    exposure 154
    interstitial 61
Keratoacanthoma 161
Keratoma 110
Keratosis 370
    obturans 35, 90
    pharyngitis 307
    seborrheic 198
Kernig's sign 124
Ketoconazole 219
Kidneys 214
    disease 191
    function tests 60
Kiesselbach's plexus 174, 190
Killian's dehiscence 289, 343
Killian's nasal gouge 446
Killian-Jamieson's space 295
Kissing tonsils 308f
Klebsiella ozaenae 215
Klebsiella pneumoniae 201
Klebsiella rhinoscleromatis 366
Kleinsasser operating
    laryngoscope 472f
Klippel-Feil syndrome 70
Kobrak test, modified 134
Kocher's test 410
Koilonychias 341
Koplik's spots 303
Korner's septum 13
Krause's nasal snare 211
Krause's nodes 321

L

Labyrinth 36
    blood supply of 18
    endolymphatic 53
    membranous 15, 53
Labyrinthectomy 141, 435
Labyrinthine
    artery 150
    fistula 118, 131, 141, 142
    segment 149
Labyrinthitis 60, 118, 122, 136
    bacterial 60
    hyperactive 142
    serous 118, 142
    suppurative 118, 142
    viral 60
Lacrimation, gustatory 154

Lamier Hackemann's space 295
Laryngeal nerve
    chain, recurrent 403
    external 405
    internal 294
    paralysis
        bilateral recurrent 375
        bilateral superior 376
        unilateral recurrent 375
        unilateral superior 376
    recurrent 375, 405, 410, 419
    superior 377
Laryngeal paralysis
    causes of 374
    classification of 374
Laryngectomy
    partial 332
        frontolateral 385
        horizontal 385
Laryngitis
    atrophic 365
    chronic
        hyperemic 364
        hypertrophic 364
        nonspecific 364, 364t
    fungal 384
    sicca 365
Laryngocele 371
    external 371
Laryngofissure 398, 399
Laryngomalacia 396, 397
Laryngopharyngeal reflux
    complications of 503
    symptoms of 503
Laryngopharynx 33, 293, 300, 312, 356, 461, 480
Laryngoplasty, vertical 377
Laryngoscopy 360, 379, 394, 399, 400, 503
    direct 384, 397, 398, 399, 456
    flexible 315, 458
    indirect 333, 338, 355, 356f, 366, 383
    techniques of 356
Laryngotracheitis 361
Laryngotracheobronchitis 361, 362, 362t, 399
Laryngotracheobronchoscopy 360
Larynx 33, 224, 295, 312, 356, 456, 458, 480, 494
    and hyoid bone, fractures of 477
    benign tumors of 368, 368t
    cancer of 385
    congenital lesions of 396
    edema of 366
    infections of 361
    interior of 457
    malignant tumors of 382
    movements of 356
    neurologic disorders of 374
    verrucous carcinoma of 386
    widening of 356

Laser 194, 451, 492, 495
    cordectomy, endoscopic 376
    surgery 448, 492
Lederman's classification 250, 250f
Leiomyoma 344
Lempert's endaural retractor 465
Leprosy 154, 217, 361, 366
Leucovorin 489
Leukemia 141, 269, 270, 305, 489
Leukocytosis 272
Leukoplakia 285, 368, 370
    candidal 266
    erosive 265
    homogenous 264
    nodular 265
    oral 264
Leukotriene modifier 206, 225
Levator palate 96
Levator veli palatini muscle 96
Lhermitte's sign 488
Lichen planus
    erosive 266
    erythematous 266
    oral 265
    reticular 265
Lichtwitz trocar and cannula 466
Ligation, endoscopic 194
Limen nasi 172
Linea temporalis 12
Lingual tonsils, diseases of 307
Lips 255, 256, 259
    reading 76
Little's area 174, 190, 191
Liver disease 191
Lobectomy 422
Loop diuretics 61, 62
Lubrication 301, 457
Luc's abscess 118, 121
Luc's forceps 468
Ludwig's angina 429, 429f, 430
Lumbar puncture 123, 124, 126, 127, 128
Lumen
    contents of 31
    obstruction 301
Lupus vulgaris 217
Luschka pouch 323
Lyme disease 154
Lymph nodes 305, 329, 402-404
    cervical 306, 356, 404t
    classification of 403f
    examination of 408
    metastases 284, 383
    post-facial 257
    regional 322t, 327t, 385
    submandibular 176
Lymphadenitis 415
Lymphadenopathy
    cervical 363, 427
    regional 283, 422

Lymphangioma 276, 280, 281, 495
    cervical 414
Lymphatic metastasis, regional 283
Lymphoid tissue, mucosa associated 289
Lymphoma 162, 280, 317, 325, 328, 413, 418-420, 422, 489
    extranodal 413
Lymphonodular pharyngitis, acute 303
Lyre's sign 413, 414

M

MacEwen's triangle 12f
    boundaries of 12
Macrotia 85
Macula 16, 18
    saccular 28
Maggots nose 245
Maggots, removal of 245
Malignancy, sign and symptoms of 275
Malignant tumor, obstructive 495
Malleus
    destruction of 439
    head of 55
Malnutrition 282
Mandible
    condylar fracture of 430
    fractures 235
        Dingman's
            classification of 241f
Mandibulofacial dysostosis syndrome 70
Manometry 302, 343
Mantoux test 365
Marcus-Gunn pupil 75
Margin, superior 173
Mask airway, laryngeal 360, 396
Mass 185, 205, 249
    parapharyngeal 329
    pediatric 210
Mast cell stabilizers 225
Mastoid
    abscesses, types of 120f
    air cells 12
        removal of 435
    antrum 6, 11-13, 434f, 435
    curette 466
    drain 436
    examination of 31
    exposure of 435
    lymph nodes,
        suppuration of 119
    nodes 402, 403
    obliteration 437
    self-retaining retractors 465
    suction tips 465
    surgery 437
        postauricular 161f
    tip, removal of 436
    types of 12, 12f

Mastoidectomy 105, 123, 127, 433, 434, 456, 466, 467
    cortical 119, 434, 435
    radical 114, 436, 436f
    simple 433
    types of 433b
Mastoiditis 116, 118, 120, 142, 435
    acute 6, 118, 120, 120t
    coalescent 119
Maxilla 171
    carcinoma of 242
    fractures of 242
    infections of 242
    osteomyelitis of 208, 446
Maxillary carcinoma,
    classifications of 250f
Maxillary sinus
    carcinoma of 248
    malignancy 249f
    ostium of 177
Maxillectomy, medial 319
Maximal stimulation test 152
McGovern's technique 234
Measles 303
Meatal segment 149
Meatoplasty 437
Meatus
    middle 171, 173
    size of 31
    superior 171
Median rhomboid glossitis 266
Mediastinitis 344, 394
Mediastinum tumor, superior 375
Medullary infarction, lateral 145
Melanoma 198, 280, 287, 317
    malignant 252
    nose 199
Melkersson's syndrome 156
Membrane, diphtheritic 363
Ménière's disease 16, 27, 36, 44, 130, 131, 133, 136, 138, 138f, 139b, 139f, 141, 145
Meniett device therapy 141
Meningeal artery
    branches of 150
    middle 13
Meningioma 248
    extracranial 248
    intracranial 248
Meningitis 73, 118, 123, 127, 209, 232
    meningogenic 142
    neonatal 70
Meningoencephalocele 198
    extranasal 247
    intranasal 246
Meningo-neurolabyrinthitis 61
Mesoderm 19
Messerklinger technique 443
Metaiodobenzylguanidine 421
Metastasis 167, 410
    lymphatic 161, 285, 286, 419

Metastatic cervical lymph nodes 199
Metastatic neck nodes, secondary 356f
Methotrexate 489
Methylene blue dye 98
Metronidazole 204
Michel aplasia 69
Microdebrider 372
Micrognathia 359
Microlaryngeal surgery 378, 496
Microlaryngoscopy 360, 384, 456
    instruments 457f
    laryngoscope of 456
    procedure 456f
Microscopy 106, 112, 114
Microtia 85, 86f, 87
Middle ear
    inflation of 106
    parts of 7f, 8
Midlay technique 439
Migraine 144, 146
Migration
    epithelial 6
    theory 111
Mikulicz's disease 277, 278
Mitomycin 489
Mobius syndrome 154
Moebius sign 411
Mold spores 225
Mondini aplasia 69
Moniliasis 266
Monoamine oxidase 2
Mononucleosis, infectious 154, 304, 305
Monotic test 41
Montogomery tube 503
Morexella catarrhalis 102, 201, 501
Morgagni, sinus of 290, 321
Moro's reflex 73
Motility disorders 301
Motion sickness 144, 146
Motor fibers, branchial 148
Motor neuron facial paralysis
    lower 152
    upper 152
Motor paralysis, contralateral 125
Mouth
    angle of 155
    care 488
    commissure of 255
    dryness of 487
    floor of 256, 259, 301
    gags 468
    opening of 452
    retractors 468
        types of 469f
    vestibule of 185
Mucocele 203, 207, 280, 282, 442
    frontoethmoidal 207
    maxillary 207
Mucormycosis 218
Mucosa 31, 294, 365

    buccal 256, 259
    tear and laceration of 400
Mucosal lesions, oral 262, 262b, 269
Muller's maneuver 313, 315
Multi-drugs antitubercular therapy 116
Multiorgan disease 214
Multiple endocrine neoplasia
    (MEN) syndrome 417, 420
Multiple juvenile laryngeal
    papillomatosis 372
Multiple sleep latency test 313
Mumps 2, 271
    measles, chickenpox 361
Murmurs 410
Muscles 96, 404
    extraocular 58
    intratympanic 11
    masseter 425
    palatal 296
    skeletal 478
    sternocleidomastoid 121f, 409f
Muscular coat 289
Muscular dystrophies 342
Mycetoma, fungal 442
Mycobacterial disease, tuberculous 273
Mycobacterium leprae 217
Mycobacterium tuberculosis 116
Mycoplasma pneumoniae 92
Myelitis, transverse 487
Myocardial infarction 313
Myoclonus 36
Myotomy
    cricopharyngeal 343
    hyoid 316
Myringitis 103
    bullosa 92, 103
    granular 93
Myringoplasty 438, 439
    inlay 434
    overlay 439f
Myringosclerosis 433
Myringotomy 105, 107, 119, 158, 432, 432f, 496

Myxedema 409

N

Nails, spooning of 341
Nares, atresia of 197
Nasal airflow 180f
Nasal alkaline wash 218
Nasal allergy 102
Nasal balloon 193
Nasal bones 171, 198f, 237, 477
    bilateral fracture of 237f
    fracture 238f
    unilateral fracture of 237f

Nasal cavity 185, 251
   decongestion of 176
   examination of 186
   lateral wall of 171
   nerve supply of 175
   patency of 187
   posterior 191
Nasal continuous positive
   airway pressure 314
Nasal crusts, removal of 218
Nasal decongestants 225
Nasal dermoid 198f, 247
Nasal discharge 205, 308
Nasal dorsum 197
   depression of 173
Nasal endoscopy 205, 441
   examination 202
Nasal fracture 237f
   reduction forceps 466
Nasal furuncle 186f
Nasal gouges 468
Nasal mastocytosis 209
Nasal mucosa and biopsy, scrapings of 217
Nasal musculature 170
Nasal myiasis 232, 245
Nasal obstruction 180, 187, 188, 205, 227, 231, 308, 495
   bilateral 188
   causes of 188, 189fc, 210
   unilateral 188
Nasal packing
   anterior 192
   posterior 193
Nasal polyps 209, 442
Nasal pruritus 223
Nasal reflexes 181
Nasal regurgitation 242
Nasal septal bleeding, persistent 194
Nasal septum 172, 230
   bleeding polyp of 248
   blood supply of 175f
   disorders 229
   flapping of 449
   fractures of 229, 229f
   perforation of 232
   structure of 172f
   submucous resection of 447
   surgery 448, 468
Nasal skin 170
Nasal smear 224
Nasal speculum 186f, 467
Nasal steroid spray 204
Nasal stuffiness, bilateral 223
Nasal surgery 316, 468
   instruments for 467f
Nasal synechia, prevention of 233
Nasal topical ipratropium bromide 225
Nasal valve 172, 188, 189f
   disorders 188

   external 188, 189f
   internal 188, 189f
Nasal vestibulitis 196, 198f
Nasogastric intubation 343
Nasopharyngeal carcinoma,
   malignant tumors 317
Nasopharyngolaryngoscopy,
   flexible 97, 298, 313, 360, 458
Nasopharynx 33, 185, 191, 289, 295, 297, 298, 454, 470, 501
   benign tumors of 317
   examination of 298b
   functions of 290
   malignant tumors of 317, 322t
Nasotracheal intubation 360
Natal trauma 230
Neck 312, 408, 421
   anatomy of 402
   circumference, measurement of 410
   dissection 403
      classification of 404t
      extended 404, 405
      modified 405
      radical 322, 404
   mass 413, 415
   nodes
      examination of 298
      regions 404f
   swelling 249, 326
Necrosis, thermal 493
Necrotizing otitis media, acute 105
Needle stick injury 502
   management of 502
Neoadjuvant chemotherapy 490
Neodymium:yttrium-aluminium-garnet laser 494
Neoplasms 154, 185, 190, 209, 358, 500
   benign 344
   vascular 36
Nerve 405
   accessory 29
   auriculotemporal 5, 6, 7
   chain, recurrent 402
   cochlear 165
   conduction velocity 153
   cranial 8, 33, 167, 249, 426
   cross-section of 151f
   disorders, facial 148
   excitability test 152, 155
   facial 5, 6, 9f, 33, 56, 92, 148, 165, 166, 176, 236
   glossopharyngeal 7, 29, 33
   graft 158
   injury, pathophysiology of 150
   intratympanic 11
   laryngeal 405, 424
   muscle implant 376
   nucleus, facial 149f
   olfactory 175, 181, 187

   palsy, facial 47, 116, 122, 150, 151, 158
   structure 151f
   vestibular 20
Neural pathways, auditory 20, 27
Neuralgia, glossopharyngeal 33, 58
Neurectomy, vestibular 141
Neurilemmomas 414
Neuritis, peripheral 187
Neuroblastoma, olfactory 253
Neurofibroma 161, 198, 247
Neuronitis, vestibular 137
Neutropenia, cyclical 269
Nicotine stomatitis 266
Nodal metastases, cervical 321
Nodes
   facial 402, 403
   postauricular 402, 403
   prelaryngeal 402, 403
   pretracheal 402, 403
   retropharyngeal 402, 403
   sublingual 403
   submandibular 402, 403
   submental 402, 403
   supraclavicular 402, 403
Nodule 289, 369
   autonomous 418
   malignant 418
Noise trauma 63, 70
Nonallergic rhinitis, types of 226
Nonerosive reflux disease 340
Non-Hodgkin's lymphoma 501
Non-nucleoside reverse
   transcriptase inhibitors 499, 500
Nonsquamous cell carcinoma 280
Non-treponemal tests 61
Nose 312, 493, 494, 496
   anatomy of 169
   and paranasal sinuses 33, 441, 476
      complaints of 184t
      malignant tumors of 246
      operations of 441, 466
      tumors of 246, 246t, 442
   blood supply of 174, 174b
   cellulitis of 196
   external 169, 185
   floor of 185
   osteocartilaginous framework of 169
   patency of 185
   physiology of 179
   structure, external 170f
   swelling, external 186f
   vestibule of 172
Nucleoside reverse transcriptase
   inhibitors 499, 500
Nucleus
   lower part of 148
   upper part of 148
Nutrition 488
Nutritional deficiency 331

Nystagmus 28, 94, 128, 139
   degree of 131
   irritative type of 142
   spontaneous 31, 130
Nystatin 342

O

Obesity 309
   morbid 315
Obstructive sleep apnea
   pathophysiology of 312
   symptoms of 312b
Oculomotor palsy 125
Oculo-oro-genital syndrome 269
Odynophagia 299, 300, 364, 427
Ohngren's classification 250, 250f
Ohngren's line 250f
Olfactory bulb 181, 187
Olfactory disorders, causes of 187
Olfactory nerves, injury of 175
Onchodystrophy 70
Oncocytoma 276
Onodi cells 178
Ophthalmoplegia, internuclear 58
Optic nerve decompression 442
Optimum discrimination score 45
Optokinetic test 132
Oral cancer, classification of 283t
Oral cavity 33, 214, 255, 258, 312, 480, 493, 494, 501
   anatomy of 255
   benign tumors of 280
   cancers of 285
   carcinoma of 282
   neoplasms of 280
   subsites of 283
   tumors of 280t
Oral communication, auditory 74
Oral lesions, drug induced 270
Oral submucous fibrosis,
   management of 264b
Orbit 185, 239, 249, 318
Orbital fissure syndrome,
   superior 207, 208, 250
Organ preservation therapy 387
Oroantral fistula, sublabial 446
Oropharyngeal airway 396
Oropharynx 33, 291, 295, 298, 305, 312, 356, 428, 456, 494
   functions of 292
Orthopantomogram 477
Ortner's syndrome 375
Osler-Weber-Rendu disease 194
Ossicles
   destruction of 439
   fixation of 439
Ossicular necrosis 99, 107, 113

Ossiculoplasty 438, 439
Osteitis 119, 208
Osteogenesis imperfecta 54
Osteoma 160, 247, 434
Osteomeatal complex 173, 173f
   cadaveric dissection of 172f
Osteomyelitis 208, 497
   clavicular 394
   frontal bone 208
Osteosarcoma 162
Ostium 177
   accessory 177
Ostmann's pad 95
Otalgia 32, 34b
   causes of 33b, 34fc, 103
   primary 32
   secondary 33
   severe 92
Otic capsule 19, 20, 53
Otic labyrinth 53
Otitic barotrauma 107
Otitic hydrocephalus 118, 127
Otitis externa 53, 85, 87, 88, 90, 103
   acute 89, 430
   allergic 89
   bullous 92
   chronic 89
   granular 89
   malignant 92, 497
Otitis media 9, 36, 53, 73, 101, 105, 117, 433
   acute 53, 56, 101, 106, 117, 122, 124, 126, 142, 305, 433
   chronic 110
   healed chronic 110
   intracranial complications of 33
   recurrent 105, 308, 451
   serous 55, 308
   suppurative 117, 123, 158, 428
   syphilitic 116
   unilateral 107
Otogenic suppurative
   thrombophlebitis 126
Otolaryngology 1
Otolith 18
   membrane 18
   organs 27
      macula of 18f
Otomycosis 90
Otorhinolaryngology 1
Otorhinorrhea 242, 243
Otorrhea 33-35, 92, 103, 163, 433
   causes of 103
   purulent 164
   recurrent 34
Otosclerosis 25, 36, 47f, 51, 52, 56, 439
   cochlear 54
Otosclerotic lesions, types of 54f
Otoscopy 7, 30, 35, 55, 93, 106, 112, 114, 162
Otospongiosis 54
Oxygen therapy, hyperbaric 65, 497

Oxyhemoglobin desaturation,
   degree of 313
Oxymetazoline 225

P

Pain 34, 119, 258, 338, 369, 427
   abdominal 304
   facial 442
   throat 304
Painful trismus, acute 430
Painless trismus, acute 430
Palate 301
Palpation 31, 185, 299, 328
Pancytopenia 269
Panendoscopy 261
Pansinusitis 203f
Papilledema 127, 128, 160, 198, 280, 328
Papilloma
   adult onset 372
   inverted 248
Papillomavirus 280
Paracusis willisii 52, 55
Paraganglioma 317, 412
Parainfluenza virus 303
Paralabyrinthitis 141
Paralysis
   facial 9, 94, 105, 118, 156f, 163
   palatal 105
Paranasal sinuses 169, 185b, 187, 203f, 210f, 318, 479f, 481f
   anatomy of 176
   development and growth of 179t
   development of 179
   examination of 185
   mucormycosis of 497
   mucous membrane of 178
   opening of 171f
   physiology of 182
Parathyroids
   glands 406, 423, 424
   inferior 406
   superior 406
Paratracheal nodes 402, 403
Parkinson's disease 342
Parosmia 188
Parotid duct, opening of 259
Parotid gland 6, 150, 236, 273f
   lymphoepithelial cysts of 501
   swelling of 273f, 275f
   tail of 275f
Parotid nodes 402, 403
Parotidectomy, superficial 277
Parotitis, acute 430
Paroxysmal positional vertigo,
   benign 57, 132, 136, 137f
Pars flaccida 7

Pars tensa 7
Passavant's ridge 290, 291
Patterson Brown-Kelly syndrome 331, 341
Pediatric epiglottitis, acute 362t
Pediculosis 2
Pemphigoid, cicatricial 267
Pemphigus vulgaris 267
Pendred's syndrome 70
Penicillin 218
Percutaneous dilational tracheostomy 360, 394, 395f
Perennial allergic rhinitis 223
Perez bacillus 215
Perichondritis 86, 87f, 90, 401, 437
Perilabyrinthitis 141
Perineurium 150
Periodontitis 502
Periosteum, inflammation of 119
Peripheral nerve injury, classification of 151f
Petrositis 118, 121, 122
Peutz-Jeghers syndrome 261
Pharyngeal wall 288, 288f
    posterior 289, 294, 299
Pharyngectomy, partial 332
Pharyngitis 303
    bacterial 261, 303
    irritative 303
    tonsillitis, membranous 305
    viral 303
Pharynx 224, 228, 288
    evaluation of 297
Phelps sign 163
Phenylephrine 225
Phlebectasias 281
Phonasthenia 380
Photodissociation 493
Photodynamic therapy 495
Photon beams 485
Pickwickian syndrome 311
Pierre-Robin syndrome 359
Piezoelectric actuator 79
Piezoelectric sensor 79
Pillar 299
    retractor, anterior 470
Pinna 24, 31
    avulsion of 86
    development of 19f
    nerve supply of 5f
    rewarming of 86
Pitch 38
Pituitary fossa 178f
Pituitary thyroid axis 411
Pituitary tumors 442
Placode, auditory 20
Plasmacytoma 248, 317
Plastic ear speculum 463f
Plastic surgery 494
    facial 221
Pleura, cervical 424

Plummer-Vinson syndrome 331, 333, 335, 341, 344
Pneumatic dilatation, endoscopic 343
Pneumatic otoscopy 58
Pneumocystis carinii 501
Pneumomediastinum 394
Pneumonia 344
Pneumothorax 394
    spontaneous 399
Politzer's bag 465
Politzer's test 98, 98f
Polyarteritis nodosa 154
Polychondritis 232, 234
    relapsing 87, 361
Polycyclic hydrocarbons 249
Polycythemia 314
Polymerase chain reaction 105
Polymorphic reticulosis 214
Polyps 113, 115, 188, 210, 224
    causes of 35b
    choanal 188
    ethmoidal 210
Polysomnography 309, 313
Polyvinyl chloride tubes 473
Postcricoid carcinoma 294
Postcricoid malignancy 333f
Posture test 186
Pot's spine 429
Potassium iodide 215
Potato tumor 198
Pott's puffy tumor 208
Pressure equalization tube 141
Probe test 242
Proliferative verrucous leukoplakia 265
Promontory 9, 15
Propantheline bromide 140
Prophylaxis 60, 64, 91, 157
    antimicrobial 105
    surgical 105
Proptosis 127, 188, 249
Prosthesis, indwelling 388
Proteus mirabilis 125
Proteus vulgaris 215
Proton pump inhibitors 340
Protympanum 8
Pruritus 34
Prussak's space 11
Psammoma bodies 261, 421
Pseudoephedrine 225
Pseudomembranous candidiasis, acute 266
Pseudomonas aeruginosa 88, 92, 110, 125
Pseudomonas pyocynea 126
Pseudosarcoma 384
Psoriasis 89
Pterygoid canal, arteries of 13
Pterygoid muscle, medial 425
Puberphonia 380

Puberty 227
Pulsation sign 162
Pulse oximetry 313
Punch biopsy 468
Pure tone 31, 38, 68
    audiogram 63, 68, 83
    audiometry 38, 43, 43f, 52, 60
Pus, aspiration of 428
Pyocele 207
Pyogenes 102
Pyramid 9, 150
Pyriform fossa
    cancer of 294, 332
    mass 332f
Pyrosis 295

Q

Queckenstedt's test 127
Quinine toxicity 62
Quinsy, incision and drainage of 471

R

Radial flow theory 16
Radiant laser energy 492
Radiation 69
    electromagnetic 484
    mucositis 269
    sources of 485
    spontaneous emission of 492
    stimulated emission of 492
    therapy 319
        intensity modulated 319, 487
    tissue damage 497
    units 485
Radical mastoidectomy, modified 114, 122, 434, 437, 438f
Radical neck dissection, modified 404
Radioactive iodine 422, 486
    thyroid ablation 418
Radioallergosorbent test 224
Radiotherapy
    complications of 487
    modes of 485
    palliative 486
Radkowski classification 319
Ramsay Hunt syndrome 6, 92, 156, 501
Ranula 280, 282
Rapid strep tests 305
Rathke's pouch 290, 317
Recess
    anterior 6
    cochlear 14
Red reflex 162
Reflux
    esophagitis 340

laryngitis 339, 340
laryngoesophageal 339, 340, 503
Rehabilitation
   auditory 73
   post-laryngectomy 387
Reinke's edema 368, 369
Reissner's membrane 15
Respiratory disturbance index 311, 313
Respiratory infections, upper 450
Respiratory mucosa 174
Respiratory muscles
   paralysis of 391
   spasm of 391
Respiratory obstruction 339
Respiratory papillomatosis, recurrent 371
Respiratory tract obstruction, upper 391
Retinoids 491
Retropharyngeal abscess, acute 428
Retropharyngeal lymph nodes,
   tuberculosis of 429
Retropharyngeal space 425, 426
   infection 305
Rhabdomyosarcoma 162, 164, 190, 253, 317
Rhinitis medicamentosa 227
Rhinitis
   allergic 222, 226, 226f
   atrophic 187, 211, 214, 231
   chronic 105
   diphtheritic 203
   drug induced 227
   emotional 227
   gustatory 227
   honeymoon 227
   hypertrophic 205
   influenzal 201
   irritative 203
   nonairflow 227
   nonallergic 222, 226
   recurrent 308
   sicca 216
   vasomotor 226, 227
Rhinolalia aperta 380
Rhinolalia clausa 308, 380
Rhinophyma 170, 185, 198, 496
Rhinoplasty 5, 172, 221, 238
Rhinorrhea 223
   excessive 227
Rhinoscopy
   anterior 185, 186, 186f, 189fc, 205, 297, 298
   posterior 31, 97, 185, 186, 297, 298
Rhinosinusitis 200, 209
   acute 200
   chronic 200, 202, 204, 205t, 231, 442
      hyperplastic 205, 221
   classification 200
   complications of 206, 207b, 442
   infectious 200
   pediatric 179
   recurrent 200, 231, 442, 451
   subacute 200
   viral 200
Rhinosporidiosis 218
Rhinosporidium seeberi 218
Rhinotomy, lateral 248
Rhinovirus 303
Rhytidectomy 221
Ricker Kleinsasser
   laryngoscope 472f
Rigid bronchoscopy 458, 459
Rigid esophagoscopy 338, 460
Rigid nasal endoscope 97, 298
Ring sign 126
Ringertz tumor 248
Rinne test 31, 40, 41, 42f, 52
Ritonavir 500
Rodent ulcer 185, 186f, 198
Romberg's test 134
Rose's sinus douching cannula 466
Rosenmuller, fossa of 96, 289, 290
Rosenthal's canal 15
Round window reflex 25
Rouviere's node 291

S

Sac
   decompression, endolymphatic 141
   endolymphatic 16, 138, 141
   surgery, endolymphatic 435
Saccular cyst
   anterior 371
   lateral 371
Saddle nose deformity 197, 213, 232, 449
Sade classification 93
Salicylates 62
Saliva
   dribbling of 155
   drooling of 338
Salivary gland 33, 153f, 404
   cancer 489
   disorders of 271
   malignancy of 261, 277
   neoplasms of 275
   submandibular 477
   tumors 275, 275t, 280, 287, 325
Samter's triad 205, 209
Sanjivani airway management
   oropharyngeal airway 396
Santorini, Fissures of 5
Saprophytic fungal infection 219
Sarcoidosis 154, 216, 278, 361, 384
Sarcoma 253, 280, 325, 489
   osteogenic 253
Sardana's approach 319
Scabies 2
Scala media 15
Scala tympani 15
Scala vestibuli 15
Scalene nodes 403
Scarpa's ganglion 20
Scars 31, 185
   atrophic 98
Schatzki's ring 335, 341
Schaumann's bodies 147
Scheibe aplasia 69
Schirmer's test 153, 153f, 166, 278
Schneiderian papilloma 248
Schwabach's test 31, 40, 43
Schwann cells 147
Schwannoma 167, 247, 414
   vestibular 165
Schwartz operation 434
Schwartz sign 55
Scleroderma 343
Scleroma 366
Sclerosis, multiple 36, 66, 137, 144, 145, 342
Sclerotherapy 415
Scope, lubrication of 458, 461
Scutum 10
Seasonal allergic rhinitis 223
Sebaceous adenoma 160
Sebaceous cyst 5, 160
Seborrhea 89
Semicircular canal
   lateral 10, 14
   posterior 15
Semon's law 375
Sensitivity index test 44
Sensory neuroepithelium 18
Sensory system, cochlear 24
Septal cartilage 448
   caudal dislocation of 229
   fractures of 476f
Septal surgery,
   instruments for 468f
Septicemia 127, 428, 429
Septodermoplasty 194
Septoplasty 231, 442, 447, 448f
   techniques 448f
Septorhinoplasty 238, 447, 448
Sequelae, symptoms of 112
Sessions's classification 319
Sexually transmitted disease 2, 498
Sheehy teflon
   ventilation tube 432f
Shepard teflon
   ventilation tube 432f
Shock, thermal 496
Shrapnell's membrane 7
Sialadenectomy 274
Sialadenitis, viral 261
Sialoendoscopy 275
Sialography 260, 273
Sialolithiasis 274
Siegel's examination 465f
Siegel's speculum 43, 131, 464, 465f
Sigmoid sinus thrombosis 126

Silastic tubes 473
Singer's nodules 368
Sinodural angle 435
Sinuscopy 205, 441
Sinuses 31, 185, 224
    branchial 414
    cavernous 178*f*, 208*f*
    empyema, maxillary 204
    ethmoid 206, 251
    ethmoidal 177, 186, 203*f*
    frontal 177, 178, 186, 187, 206, 237, 480*f*
    maxillary 173*f*, 176, 178, 186, 187, 203*f*, 206, 251, 481*f*
    mucus drainage of 178
    operations 441
    ostium, maxillary 443
    preauricular 19, 86, 86*f*
    pyriform 294
    surgery, endoscopic 179, 206, 207, 248, 442, 444, 447, 448, 467
    thrombosis, cavernous 127, 208, 209, 209*t*, 232
    tympani 9, 9*f*
Sinusitis 105, 200, 308
    fungal 211, 218
    maxillary 442
    recurrent 446
Sistrunk operation 414
Sjögren's syndrome 261, 277, 278
    primary 277
    secondary 277
Skeletal deficiency,
    mandibular 315
Skin 494
    atrophy of 487
    care 488
    glands 5
    incision 392, 423
    lesions 217, 269
        superficial 161
    nasomaxillary 186*f*
    protection of 495
    redness of 356
    tests 224
Sleep apnea 180, 231, 311
    central 311
    mixed 311
    obstructive 299, 308, 309, 311, 358, 450, 496
    syndrome, obstructive 311
Sleep sonography 309
Slowly progressive
    hearing loss 112
Sluder's neuralgia 33, 221
Smell
    disorders of 181
    loss of 187
    sense of 185, 187
Smooth muscle relaxants 339
Snare 211, 311, 453

Sodium fluoride 55
Soft palate 299, 427
Soft tissue injuries 235, 236
Solitary cold nodule 421
Solitary thyroid nodule 417
Sore throat 299
    recurrent 450
Sound, conduction of 24
Spatula test 187
Speech
    audiometry 40, 45, 73, 139
    discrimination score 45
    discrimination tests 83
    esophageal 388
    noise 39
    reading 76
    recognition score 45
    types of 38*t*
Sphenoethmoidal mucocele 207
Sphenoethmoidal recess 172
Sphenoid sinus 178, 204, 206
    malignancy of 252
    neoplasms of 203
    relations of 178*f*
    walls 178*f*
Sphenoid sinusotomy 443
Sphenopalatine artery,
    endoscopic ligation of 194
Sphenopalatine neuralgia 33
Sphincter
    cricopharyngeal 338, 461
    esophageal 295
Spinal accessory chain 402, 403
Spinal accessory nerve 404
Spine, cervical 34, 301, 429
Spondee words 45
Sports injuries 235
Spurs 230
Squamous cell 13
    carcinoma 162, 198, 199, 276, 280, 320, 325, 331, 335, 344, 384, 489
Squamous epithelium 115
Squamous metaplasia theory 112
Squamous papilloma 247, 317
S-shaped deformity 230
St. Clair Thomson's
    adenoid curette 470, 471*f*
Stange hour glass
    operating laryngoscope 472*f*
Stapedectomy 55, 56, 57*f*, 143, 434
    piston 57*f*
Stapedial otosclerosis 54
Stapedial reflex 47, 153
Stapedotomy 56, 494
Stapes fixation, congenital 55
Stapes footplate
    ankylosis of 439
    fixation of 54*f*
Stapes mobilization 55
Stapes superstructure, loss of 439

Staphylococcus aureus 88, 92, 102, 110, 196, 361, 427
Staphylococcus epidermidis 92
Steam inhalation 204
Stellwag's sign 411
Stenger test 67
Stenosis
    laryngeal 394, 401, 477
    nasopharyngeal 454
Stensen's duct 273*f*
Steroids 66, 155, 217, 220, 362, 363, 366, 398, 401, 443
    intratympanic 65
    nasal spray 225
    therapy 65
Strap muscles 392, 423
Streptococcal tonsillitis, recurrent 450
Streptococcus haemolyticus 125, 201
Streptococcus pneumoniae 102, 124, 125, 272, 361, 499, 501
Streptococcus pyogenes 272, 303, 305, 427
Streptococcus viridans 272
Stria vascularis 15, 16
Stridor 358, 359
    biphasic 358
    causes of 358, 358*b*
    expiratory 358
    inspiratory 358
    sound of 359
Stroboscopy 357, 383
Strokes, cerebrovascular 342
Stylalgia 329
Styloid process 150, 293, 296
Stylomastoid artery 150
Stylomastoid foramen 149*f*
Subclavian artery
    abnormal right 302*f*
    compression of 416
Subclavian steal syndrome 144
Subglottic stenosis, congenital 397
Sublingual tissue, posterior 430
Submandibular duct, opening of 259
Submocous fibrosis, oral 262, 263*f*, 264*f*, 430
Sudden sensorineural hearing loss,
    causes of 64*b*
Sunderland classification 151
Suppurative otitis media
    acute 31, 51, 103, 432*f*
    chronic 31, 32, 35, 51-53, 93, 107, 109, 110, 141, 169, 164, 308, 439
    complications of 117, 117*f*, 118*f*
Suppurative sialadenitis, acute 272
Supraglottitis, adult 361, 363
Supraorbital ridge 237
Supratonsillar fossa 292
Surgery 143, 220, 250
    septal 231, 232, 467
    types of 113
Sutures, absorbable 401
Sweat glands, tumors of 198

Swelling 31, 185, 356
    benign 328, 456
    carotid triangle 408
    classification of 198t
    facial 249
    over mastoid region 119
    submandibular 285
Synechia 449
Syphilis 61, 136, 217, 361, 364t, 365
    acquired 217
    congenital 61, 131, 141, 217
    secondary 61, 365
    tertiary 61
Systemic diseases 59, 118, 154, 205, 262
    nasal manifestation of 213
Systemic lupus
    erythematosus 66, 361

T

Tachycardia 411
Taste buds 257
Taste, sense of 258
Teeth 259
    anesthesia of 446
    care 488
Tegmen cells 13
Temporal bone 36, 123, 156, 475, 480
    air cells of 13f
    fractures of 94, 102
    pneumatization of 118
Temporal lobe
    abscess 125
    auditory cortex 27
    of cerebrum 118
Temporalis fascia graft,
    placement of 439f
Temporomandibular arthritis,
    acute 430
Temporomandibular joint 6, 33, 34
    ankylosis of 430
    disease 36
Tensor tympani 8, 11, 36
    muscle, canal of 9
Tensor veli palatini muscle 96
Teratoma 317
Thoracic esophagus,
    rupture of 336
Thorax 421
Thornwaldt's disease 322
Throat
    swab 363
    repeated clearing of 355
Thrombophlebitis, lateral sinus 118, 126
Thrombus, extension of 126
Thudicum nasal speculum 186, 464, 464f
Thyroid 33, 301
    adenoma 419
    antibodies 420, 421

artery
    inferior 405, 423
    superior 405, 423
auscultation of 410f
autoantibodies 411
bruit 411
carcinoma 419, 421, 422t
    investigations of 421
    medullary 420
    treatment of 421
    types of 419
cartilage 400
cyst 418
disorders 411t
function tests 412, 420
gland 405, 409
    anterior surface of 405f
isthmus 392, 392f
lingual 406, 496
neoplasms,
    classification of 418b
nodules 417, 419, 424
    evaluation of 418
    types of 417, 419
palpation 410f
parafollicular cells of 424
scan 418
stimulating hormone 60, 71, 411t, 417
surgeries 423
    types of 423
veins
    inferior 406, 423
    middle 423
Thyroidectomy
    completion 422
    subtotal 386, 422
Thyroplasty 376, 378
Thyrotoxicosis
    primary 409
    secondary 409
Thyroxin therapy 422
Tilley's antral burr 466
Tinnitus 35, 55, 58, 61, 65, 91, 139, 162, 166
    causes of 35f
    classification and causes of 36b
    management program 36
    pulsatile 163
Tip cells 13
Tip ptosis 188
Tissue, biopsy of 218
Titanium abutment 79
Titanium fixture 79
Tobey-Ayer test 127
Tone decay test 40
Tongue 256, 259, 261, 301, 304
    base of 291, 299
    carcinoma of 292
    depressor 259
    edema of 454
    lesions of 262, 270

    malignancy 284f
    tie 270
Tonsillar crypts 292
Tonsillar cyst 307
Tonsillar pillars 299
Tonsillar remnants 454
Tonsillar space, anterior 292
Tonsillectomy 293, 304, 307, 450, 452, 453f,
                    468-470
    interval 427
Tonsillitis 105
    chronic 305, 450
    recurrent 305
Tonsillolingual sulcus 293
Tonsillolithiasis 450
Tonsillotomy 496
Tonsils 299, 247, 496
    and adenoids, functions of 289
    artery forceps 471
    bed of 292, 292f
    crypts of 292f
    dissector 470
    holding forceps 470
    lingual 289, 291
    malignancy 305
    nasopharyngeal 289, 290
    palatine 289, 291t, 292
Tornwald's disease 291
Torticollis 427
Torus mandibularis 280
Torus palatinus 280
Torus tubarius 95, 290
Total laryngectomy 377, 385
Total ossicular replacement prosthesis 439
Total thyroidectomy 422
Toxic goiter 421f
Toxic shock syndrome 449
Toxoplasmosis, rubella,
    cytomegalovirus (TORCH) 71
Toynbee's maneuver 102
Toynbee's test 98
Trachea 358, 392, 410, 419, 494
    compression of 461, 477
Tracheal dilator 392, 472, 473f
Tracheal hook 392, 472
Tracheal stenosis 394
Tracheitis 394
    bacterial 361, 362
Tracheobronchial larynx 459
Tracheobronchial tree 458, 459
Tracheobronchitis 394
Tracheocutaneous fistula,
    persistent 394
Tracheoesophageal fistula 339, 388, 394
Tracheostomy 234, 304, 316, 337, 362, 363,
                376, 377, 390, 391, 392,
                392f, 396-398, 429, 472
    complications of 394b
    elective 391
    emergency 399

    low 391
    mid 391
    permanent 391
    tubes 390, 392, 393, 473, 474
        classification of 473b
        corrosion of 394
        metallic 473f
        nonmetallic 473f, 474
        position of 477
        size of 474, 474t
        types of 472
    types of 391
Tragal cartilage pointer 150
Transantral ethmoidectomy 211
Transient evoked otoacoustic
    emission 49, 72
Transient ischemic attack 145
Transillumination test 202
Transoral pneumatic device 388
Transtracheal jet ventilation 396
Transtracheal needle ventilation 360
Trauma 56, 59, 70, 433
    accidental 154, 230
    facial 221
    iatrogenic 56
    laryngeal 401
    laryngotracheal 400
    maxillofacial 235
    penetrating 87, 143
Trautmann's triangle 12, 435
Treacher-Collins syndrome 70
Treponemal tests 61
Trigeminal nerve 75, 175
    branches of 179
    ophthalmic division of 29, 179
Trigeminal neuralgia 33, 75
Trimethoprim-sulfamethoxazole 214
Trimethoprim-sulfisoxazole 106
Tripod fracture 239
Trismus 249, 258, 263, 427, 430, 460
Trotter's method 192
Trotter's syndrome 321
Tubal blockage, acute 99
Tubal occlusion, stages of 102
Tubal tonsil 289, 290
Tubercular otitis media 116
Tuberculin skin test 415
Tuberculosis 2, 217, 361, 364t, 365, 384
Tubotympanic recess,
    endoderm of 19
Tuebingen ventilation tube 432f
Tullio's phenomenon 61, 132, 141, 143
Tumors 59, 64, 85, 242, 301, 358
    amyloid 368, 370
    benign 189
    central core of 486
    intracanalicular 165f, 166
    intracranial 188
    intratympanic 162
    malignant 189, 325

    marker 420
    nodes 326
    parapharyngeal 329, 414
    primary 283, 422
    reduce size of 486
    sternomastoid 415
    types of 321
Tuning fork tests 31, 35, 41, 41t, 42
Turban epiglottis 365
Tylosis 344
Tympanic artery
    anterior 13
    superior 13
Tympanic membrane 6, 7f, 8f, 10, 19, 25f, 26, 32, 32f, 52, 56, 85, 93, 99, 162, 433, 439f
    atrophic 93, 107
    central perforation of 115f
    diseases of 85t
    disorders of 93
    examination of 5, 31
    hydraulic action of 25
    layers of 7f
    mobility of 464
    perforation of 93, 106, 110f, 116, 119
    traumatic rupture of 93
Tympanic plexus 8, 11
Tympanocentesis 104
Tympanograms 46, 47f
    types of 46t
Tympanomastoid surgery 158
Tympanomastoid suture 150
Tympanomeningeal hiatus 118
Tympanometry 5, 40, 46, 83, 105, 106, 114, 116, 433, 434, 438, 467
Tympanoplasty, types of 438, 438t
Tympanosclerosis 55, 93, 99, 107, 115, 439
Tympanostomy tube 105, 107, 432, 433
    status of 433
Tympanotomy
    exploratory 64, 434
    posterior 9f, 84
Tympanum
    dimensions of 8f
    six boundaries of 8f

U

Ulcer 31, 185, 263, 340
    aphthous 305, 502
    contact 368, 370
    traumatic 305
Union for International
    Cancer Control 326
Upper airway obstruction
    management of 304
    signs of 362
Uremia 154
Utricle 15, 28

Utricular macula 28
Uvula 299, 427
Uvulopalatopharyngoplasty 313, 314
Uvulopalatoplasty 316
    laser assisted 316

V

Vagus nerve 5-7, 33, 375
Valsalva maneuver 31, 32, 106, 131, 458
Valsalva test 98
Valvular heart disease 450
van Der Hoeve syndrome 54, 70
Varicella-zoster virus 92, 156
Vascular rings, congenital 359
Vasovagal reflex 6
Venous drainage 13, 19, 293, 406
Ventilation 97, 390
    tubes 432f
Vermis 134
Vertebrae, cervical 477
Vertigo 55, 56, 94, 163
    attacks 138
    central 133t, 147
    cervical 144, 146
    evaluation of 29, 130
    musculoskeletal 146
    pathophysiology of 29
    peripheral 133t, 147
    phobic postural 144, 146
    spells 145, 147
    spontaneous 142
Vesicle 263
    auditory 20
Vestibular aqueduct syndrome, large 14
Vestibular artery
    anterior 19
    posterior 19
Vestibular disorders
    central 29, 144
    peripheral 29, 136
Vestibular lesions
    central 132
    peripheral 132
Vestibular nerve
    inferior 21, 165
    superior 20, 165
Vestibular neuritis, acute 136, 137
Vestibular organs, hair cells of 18f
Vestibular system
    central 27
    peripheral 27
    physiology of 27
Vestibule 14, 185, 188
    aqueduct of 14
Vestibulo-ocular reflex 21, 132
Vestibulospinal tract 21
Videofluoroscopy 359, 399

Vidian nerve 176
Vidian neurectomy 176, 447
Vinca alkaloids 489
Vincent's angina 268, 305
Viral labyrinthitis, acute 137
Viral rhinosinusitis, attacks of 200
Vision
    blurring of 128
    loss of 249
Vocal cord 365
    mobility 333
    paralysis 401, 458
        congenital 377, 397
    plication 377
    positions 374, 374f
    shortening of 376
Vocal fold lesion,
    middle third of 386
Vocal nodules 368
    bilateral 369f
Vocal polyp 369
Voice
    hoarseness of 344, 357, 357t, 386, 387, 423
    symptoms of 355
    test 31, 40, 41
    therapy 369

Von Bekesy, traveling
    wave theory of 26
Von Graefe's sign 411
Von Recklinghausen disease 165
Von Troeltsch anterior pouch 11

W

Wagner and Grossman hypothesis 375
Waldeyer's ring 289, 289f, 413
Wallenberg's syndrome 144, 145
Walsham's forceps 238, 466, 467f
Wart 160
Warthin's tumor 276
Wax granuloma 91
Weber's test 31, 40, 42, 42f, 52
Weber-Ferguson's incision 251
Wegener's granulomatosis 66, 154, 206, 213, 213f, 214t, 361, 384
Wernicke aphasia 379
Western blot test 499
Wharton's duct
    calculus 274f
    opening, appearance of 274f
Whiplash vertigo 146

Wigand technique 443
Woodruff's plexus 190
Wound, closure of 436, 437
Wullstein retractor 465f

X

Xeroderma pigmentosa 282
Xerostomia 258, 277
    permanent 487
Xylometazoline 225

Y

Yankauer's suction tube 470
Young's operation 215
    modified 215
Young's syndrome 209

Z

Zenker's diverticulum 335, 343
Zona arcuata 15
Zona pectinata 15
Zygoma 239